美国骨科医师学会骨科知识更新
肩部与肘部

Orthopaedic Knowledge Update: Shoulder and Elbow

〔美〕格雷戈里·P.尼克尔森 (Gregory P. Nicholson)　主编

查晔军　主译

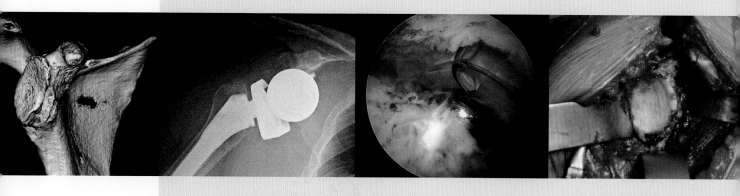

Wolters Kluwer ｜ AAOS AMERICAN ACADEMY OF ORTHOPAEDIC SURGEONS ｜ 北京科学技术出版社

著作权合同登记　图字：01-2023-3627

图书在版编目（CIP）数据

肩部与肘部 / (美) 格雷戈里·P.尼克尔森(Gregory P. Nicholson) 主编；查晔军主译. -- 北京：北京科学技术出版社，2024.4
（美国骨科医师学会骨科知识更新）
书名原文: Orthopaedic Knowledge Update: Shoulder and Elbow
ISBN 978-7-5714-3156-3

Ⅰ.①肩… Ⅱ.①格…②查… Ⅲ.①肩关节—外科学②肘关节—外科学 Ⅳ.①R687.4

中国国家版本馆CIP数据核字（2023）第134553号

策划编辑：何晓菲	电　　话：0086-10-66135495（总编室）
责任编辑：何晓菲	0086-10-66113227（发行部）
责任校对：贾　荣	网　　址：www.bkydw.cn
封面设计：申　彪	印　　刷：雅迪云印（天津）科技有限公司
图文制作：北京创世禧电脑图文设计有限公司	开　　本：889 mm×1194 mm　1/16
责任印制：吕　越	字　　数：1000 千字
出版人：曾庆宇	印　　张：42
出版发行：北京科学技术出版社	版　　次：2024年4月第1版
社　　址：北京西直门南大街16号	印　　次：2024年4月第1次印刷
邮政编码：100035	ISBN 978-7-5714-3156-3

定　　价：468.00元

主译简介

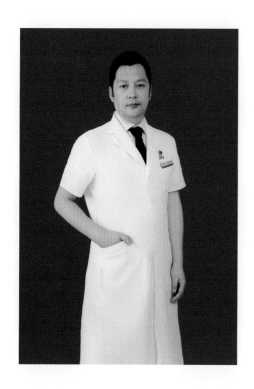

查晔军 主任医师，北京大学、首都医科大学副教授，硕士研究生导师。国家区域医疗中心北京积水潭医院郑州医院执行院长，北京积水潭医院创伤骨科主任助理、骨科冲击波诊疗中心副主任。

社会任职包括 AO Trauma 讲师，国际矫形与创伤外科学会（SICOT）中国部肩肘外科专业委员会委员，中华医学会骨科学分会创新与转化学组青年委员会委员，中国医师协会骨科医师分会青年委员会上肢创伤学组副组长、非公医疗学组委员兼秘书长，北京医学会创伤学分会委员、骨科学分会创伤骨科学组委员兼秘书，中国研究型医院学会关节外科专业委员会肘关节外科研究学组委员兼秘书，北京整合医学学会心理行为医学专业委员会副主任委员，《中华肩肘外科电子杂志》编委，《中国医刊》特邀编委，《中国骨与关节损伤杂志》青年编委，《中华创伤骨科杂志》特邀编委，《北京医学》通讯编委。

审译者名单

主译 查晔军

审阅 蒋协远 公茂琪

译者（按姓氏拼音顺序）

顾航宇

郭　祁

李国珅

刘　刚

米　萌

孙志坚

王　京

肖　丹

肖鸿鹄

查晔军

张玉富

周　力

周　源

前　言

肩肘外科持续快速发展，《美国骨科医师学会骨科知识更新：肩部与肘部》主要关注肩肘外科的最新进展。本书简明但深入地为临床骨科医师展示了肩肘外科的最新文献和各相关领域的研究进展，对肩肘外科专业的医师会有很大的帮助，住院医师和研究者也可从来自世界各地的编委和章节作者们所提供的丰富的专业知识中受益。

本版更新了"反肩关节置换术的运动学和生物力学"一章。几乎所有的上肢骨科专科医师都知道，疼痛综合征的发生率较高，但是其诊断和治疗很困难，"肩肘关节的复杂区域疼痛综合征"一章对其相关定义、流行病学、评估方法和治疗的内容进行了更新。本书还包括基础科学和关节镜的相关章节，并对肩锁关节损伤、肩胛上神经损伤和肩胛骨功能障碍等知识进行了更新。本书使用了较大篇幅介绍了与肩袖损伤相关的内容，涉及多个章节，讨论了肩袖损伤的治疗方法、肌腱愈合的最新研究以及加强肩袖愈合的方法等。

《美国骨科医师学会骨科知识更新：肩部与肘部》的编者都是各自领域的领军人物，他们与章节作者们组成了优秀的团队，在本书的准备、写作和编辑中付出了极大的努力并取得了出色的成果，美国骨科医师学会（AAOS）的成员也一直积极推动着本书的出版工作，笔者非常感谢他们对本书的贡献。笔者非常感谢能有机会成为本书主编，也非常荣幸被 AAOS 成员选举为本项目的负责人。再次感谢参与本书编写和出版的所有编者、章节作者、AAOS 成员及其他人员为本书做出的出色贡献。希望本书能够对所有肩肘外科医师有所帮助。

主编 Gregory P. Nicholson, MD

目录

第五部分　关节炎与关节成形术

第六部分　创伤与骨折

第一部分

基础科学

栏目编委：
Patrick J. McMahon, MD

第一章　肩关节的解剖与功能

Yoshimasa Fujimaki, MD, PhD; Daisuke Araki, MD, PhD; Richard E. Debski, PhD

引言

肩关节的活动范围较肌肉骨骼系统中的其他主要关节都大。这是因为周围的骨与软组织的结构为肩关节提供了灵活性及稳定性。当肌肉拉动手臂时，单纯的骨结构不能提供足够的稳定性，必须由肌肉和软组织来维持肩关节稳定。肩部运动涉及整个肩部复合体，包括肩胸关节，它是上肢运动的基础。

骨解剖学

肱骨头

肱骨近端是椭圆形的肱骨头，它是盂肱关节的一部分。肱骨头被透明关节软骨覆盖着，关节软骨至干骺端边缘的骨性过渡是肱骨解剖颈的标记。肱骨头后倾角的定义为关节面相对于矢状面的方位。该夹角最常以肘关节通髁轴与肱骨头关节软骨或干骺端边缘的前后轴之间的夹角作为参考（图 1-1）。[1-3]肱骨头的后倾角具有很大的个体差异性；在肩关节置换术中，肱骨解剖颈被用作截骨术的参考。[4-5]

None of the following authors nor any immediate family member has received anything of value from or owns stock in a commercial company or institution related directly or indirectly to the subject of this chapter: Dr. Fujimaki, Dr. Araki, and Dr. Debski.☆

☆各章的这一部分介绍的是本章编著者是否接受了商业公司资助，了解这些情况可使读者更客观地看待他们的研究成果。按原著版权方要求，简体中文版保留该部分英文内容。

一项纳入 24 个肱骨头表面形态数据的三维研究发现，关节表面的平均曲率半径为 23.9 mm（22.5~25.8 mm）。[2]球度偏差为 0.20 mm（0.15~0.26 mm），为曲率半径的 0.8%。肱骨头后倾角在肱骨头上缘和下缘中间平面的测量值为 18.6°（2.5°~40.0°），但角度大小因测量位置的不同而有所差异（图 1-2）。该研究的结论是，肱骨头的软骨 - 干骺端界面的前方中点可能是一个有价值的标记，经此点测量的肱骨头后倾角数值与使用关节表面的质心计算的后倾角相近。[2]

投掷运动员双侧盂肱关节的活动范围似乎不同。具体而言，与非优势肩相比，优势肩有更大的外旋角度和较小的内旋角度。[6]分别分析 25 名投掷运动员和 25 名非投掷运动员（对照）的优势肩和非优势肩，在运动范围、松弛程度、肱骨头后倾角以及肩胛盂后倾角四个方面进行比较，发现与非优势肩相比，投掷运动员优势肩的肱骨头后倾角和肩胛盂后倾角增加。外展 90° 和 45° 时，优势肩的外旋角度增加，而内旋 90° 时减少。非投掷运动员的双肩在这些方面没有任何数值上的显著差异。

这种运动角度改变的原因是，由于重复的微创伤，优势肩的生理适应导致前囊的选择性伸展和后囊的收紧。由于施加的应力，骨结构也可能发生适应。外科医师应该仔细检查高水平的顶级运动员，以确定他们在运动范围和骨骼特征方面的双侧差异。

结节间沟

肱骨沟已被用作骨折复位或肩关节置换术中假体对线的标志。[7-8]一项纳入 50 个肱

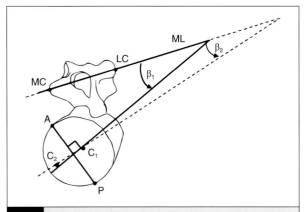

图 1-1 肱骨头后倾角示意图。肱骨头后倾角与通髁轴、矢状面上的软骨 - 干骺端界面和关节面的质心相关。AP= 轴面，β_1= 软骨 - 干骺端界面处的后倾角，β_2= 关节面质心的后倾角，C_1= 关节面的球心，C_2= 关节面的质心，LC= 外上髁，MC= 内上髁，ML= 通髁轴。经允许引自 Harrold F, Wigderowitz C：A three-dimensional analysis of humeral head retroversion. *J Shoulder Elbow Surg* 2012; 21(5): 612–617.

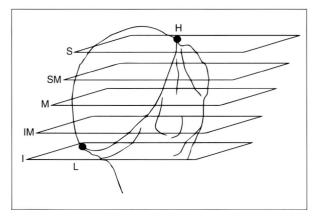

图 1-2 示意图显示肱骨头被垂直于骨干轴线的 5 个平行面划分为 6 个部分。H= 软骨 - 干骺端界面的最高点，I= 下平面，IM= 下中平面，L= 软骨 - 干骺端界面的最低点，M= 中平面，S= 上平面，SM= 上中平面。经允许引自 Harrold F, Wigderowitz C：A three-dimension alanalysis of humeral head retroversion. *J Shoulder Elbow Surg* 2012;21(5):612–617.

骨的形态计量学研究发现，结节间沟的平均长度为 8.1 cm（6.7~10.4 cm），相当于肱骨长度的 25.4%（16.3%~32.5%）；中点宽度为 10.1 mm（7.3~15.5 mm），相当于肱骨宽度的 49.7%~54.5%；深度为 4.0 mm，相当于肱骨深度的 18.8%。结节间沟壁形成的角度为 106°。这些参数之间没有相关性。[9]

肩胛盂

肩胛盂是梨形中间的凹陷，从肩胛体向外侧延伸，为盂肱关节的承窝。CT 检查常被用于评估肩胛骨冠状面和矢状面旋转对肩胛盂后倾角的影响。评估肩胛骨时可使用基于 3 个解剖学标记的坐标系进行测量：肩胛盂的中心、肩胛冈与肩胛骨内侧缘的交点以及肩胛下角的最远端点。[10] 在肩胛骨的静止位置单独测量解剖学肩胛盂后倾角，为 2.0°（±3.8°）。解剖学肩胛盂后倾角与临床肩胛骨后倾角的差异取决于原始轴位 CT 图像中肩胛骨的位置，二者平均相差 6.9°（0.1°~22.5°）。这些结果表明，肩胛骨在冠状面或矢状面就算仅有 1° 的错位，也将导致肩胛盂后倾角测量的不准确。当使用 CT 测量肩胛盂后倾角时，必须考虑具体

轴向重建平面。[10]

盂唇和关节囊的解剖学

盂唇

盂唇由一圈纤维组织及纤维软骨过渡区组成，该过渡区通过增加肩胛盂的深度起到被动稳定的作用。此外，它也是盂肱关节的关节囊和肱二头肌长头腱（LHBT）的主要附着部位。[11]

盂唇呈卵圆形，形状和下面的肩胛盂边缘一致，其与肩胛盂的后下部连接最牢固。[12] 盂唇对盂肱关节稳定性的作用已有论述。[13-14] 越来越多的学者认为肩关节上盂唇前后向（SLAP）损伤是肩部疼痛和不稳定的根源之一。盂唇损伤（如 SLAP 损伤）更常采用 MRI 或肩关节镜进行诊断，因此，准确理解盂唇的正常变异至关重要[15]（图 1-3）。

一些研究表明，盂唇的前上部解剖存在广泛的变异。一项纳入 546 例接受肩关节镜检查的患者的临床研究发现，73 例（13.4%）盂唇前上部有解剖变异：18 例（3.3%）仅有 1 个盂唇下孔；47 例（8.6%）有绳状盂肱中韧带；8 例（1.5%）

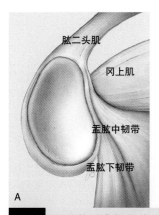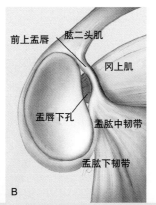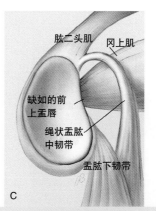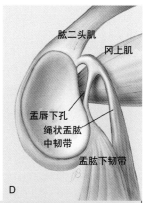

图 1-3　盂唇的正常解剖（A），孤立的盂唇下孔（B），盂唇下孔伴绳状盂肱中韧带（C），前上盂唇缺失伴绳状盂肱中韧带（D）。经允许转自 Moseley H 及 Overgaard B: The anterior capsular mechanism in recurrent anterior dislocation of the shoulder: Morphological and clinical studies with special reference to the glenoid labrum and glenohumeral ligaments. *J Bone Joint Surg Br* 1962;44(4):913–927.

盂唇前上部缺失，伴有绳状盂肱中韧带。[16]这些变异的存在与盂唇前上部磨损、异常的盂肱上韧带以及在 90° 外展时手臂被动内旋增加呈正相关（图 1-4）。

一项纳入 691 例患者的研究发现，98 例（14.2%）的盂唇前上部有 3 种不同的解剖变异，分别为下隐窝［17 例（2.46%）］、盂唇下孔［53 例（7.67%）］和盂唇前上部缺失伴绳状盂肱中韧带［28 例（4.05%）］。[17]其中两个变异（盂唇下孔和盂唇前上部缺失伴绳状盂肱中韧带）与 Ⅱ 型

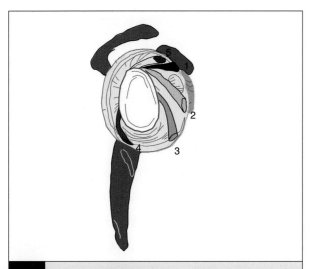

图 1-4　右肩关节囊韧带示意图。1= 盂肱上韧带，2= 盂肱中韧带，3= 盂肱下韧带前束，4= 盂肱下韧带后束，5= 肱二头肌长头腱

SLAP 损伤显著相关。尽管盂唇的变异似乎不会导致不稳定，但它们可能会增加内旋，并使肩部易发生盂肱上韧带和盂唇前上部损伤。

盂肱关节囊

盂肱关节囊包绕盂肱关节，维持滑膜环境，可以在关节处于活动范围的极限时提供稳定性。[18-19]目前的文献描述，盂肱上韧带、盂肱中韧带、盂肱下韧带由关节囊前部增厚形成，加强了关节囊的前下部，可使肱骨头紧贴肩胛盂（图 1-5）。

实验研究以及计算研究通常针对关节囊的上部区域，但最近的研究数据表明，盂肱关节的前方和后方关节囊之间具有显著的相互作用和多种功能。[20-22]其中一项研究在有或没有机械连接的情况下，对肱骨向前施加 25 N 的力，然后采用有限元模型确定牵引位置相邻及不相邻关节囊区域的最大主应变分布和形变。[22]结果表明，在肩胛骨和肱骨之间传递力时，关节囊之间具有显著的相互作用。关节囊局部区域不应该单独用于实验或计算分析盂肱关节囊的功能。反之，应该将盂肱关节囊作为一片连续的纤维组织进行评估。研究发现，盂肱关节囊的机械性质与平行或垂直于它的盂肱韧带相似。[21]这一发现进一步支持了关节囊是一片连续的纤维组织的观点。

一项解剖学研究对 27 例标本进行了组织学检

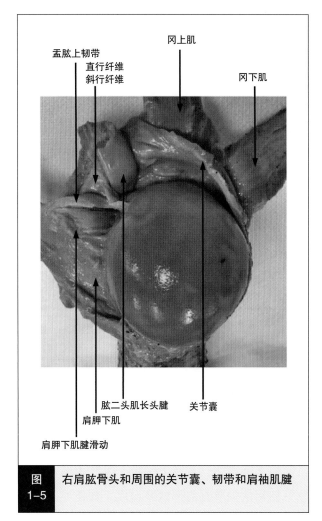

图 1-5　右肩肱骨头和周围的关节囊、韧带和肩袖肌腱

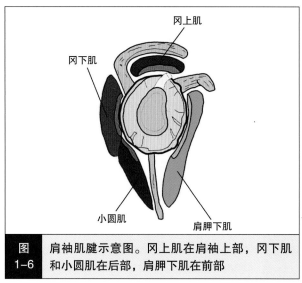

图 1-6　肩袖肌腱示意图。冈上肌在肩袖上部，冈下肌和小圆肌在后部，肩胛下肌在前部

查，得出的结论是：在显微镜下，盂肱上韧带是由直行纤维和斜行纤维组成的稳定结构。[23]该研究表明，盂肱上韧带不仅可以连接和稳定盂肱关节，还可以通过插入肱骨结节间沟，从而加固和稳定肱二头肌长头腱。

肌肉和肌腱解剖学

肩袖

肩袖由冈上肌、冈下肌、肩胛下肌和小圆肌的肌腱组成，这些肌腱可以为盂肱关节运动提供动力（图 1-6）。为盂肱关节提供稳定性是肩袖的主要功能之一。在手臂外展的过程中，肩袖将肱骨头拉入肩胛盂内，以允许三角肌抬高手臂。[24]这个运动模式为凹压效应。如果没有肩袖的作用，肱骨头就会向上移出关节窝，三角肌的效率就会降低。

关节窝在前后方向上最容易受到剪切力的干扰，因为关节窝前后向的深度比上下向的深度要小。[25]在正常肩关节中，肩胛下肌向前、冈下肌和小圆肌向后的拮抗合力将肱骨头压入肩胛盂。对尸体解剖分析发现，当模拟肩胛下肌、冈下肌和小圆肌的肌腱肩袖麻痹时，盂肱关节向上不稳定。[26]

冈上肌

冈上肌起自肩胛冈上方的冈上窝。公认的观点是，冈上肌和其他肌腱止于肱骨解剖颈外侧的大结节和小结节上。然而，这种模式最近受到了质疑。研究发现，冈上肌在肌肉的前半部分有一个长的腱状部分，它总是附着于大结节最深凹陷的最前面区域；在 21% 的标本中，它也附着于小结节的最上面区域。[27]冈上肌呈三角形，内侧至外侧的平均最大长度为 6.9 mm，平均最大厚度为 12.6 mm。冈下肌在肌肉的上半部分有一个长的腱状部分，它向前弯曲并延伸到大结节最深凹陷的前外侧区域。冈下肌呈梯形，内侧至外侧的平均最大长度为 10.2 mm，平均最大厚度为 32.7 mm。因此，该研究发现大结节上的冈上肌的大小比以前认为的要小得多；大结节的这个区域实际上被大量的冈下肌所占据。研究人员提出，以前认为只涉及冈上肌腱的肩袖撕裂可能也涉及大量的冈下肌腱成分。[27]

冈上肌收缩使肩部的盂肱关节外展。在开始外展的前 10°~15°，冈上肌是肩部外展的主要肌肉；外展超过 30° 后，三角肌成为主要的外展肌。冈上肌有助于抵抗由上肢重量引起的肩部向下的重力。[28]

冈下肌

冈下肌较厚，呈三角形，占据肩胛骨的冈下窝。肌肉由起源于冈下窝内侧 2/3 的粗纤维和来自其表面脊部的肌腱纤维形成；也起源于覆盖其上并将其与大圆肌和小圆肌分隔开的冈下筋膜。[29]纤维汇聚形成肌腱，走行于与肩胛骨相对的脊柱外侧边缘，穿过盂肱关节囊的后部，止于肱骨大结节的中间凹陷。

冈下肌的主要功能是使肩关节中的肱骨部分后伸和外旋。当手臂固定时，冈下肌外展肩胛骨的下角。冈下肌和小圆肌外旋肩关节并协助盂肱关节后伸。[29]最近的一项研究检查了在冠状面外展和矢状面前屈时，肱骨轴向旋转中穿过盂肱关节的几个肌肉区域的瞬时力臂。[30]研究发现，冈下肌和小圆肌是最重要的外旋肌。

肩胛下肌

肩胛下肌起源于肩胛骨的前表面，通过喙突和肩胛颈的外侧，在肩胛盂水平变成腱状。在其止点处，肩胛下肌的腱性部分与盂肱关节囊的纤维混合并附着于小结节。其余的止点由肌肉组成，位于小结节下方。最近的研究发现，肩胛下肌止点的形态近端宽，远端为锥形，呈逗号状。[31]止点由近端肌腱部分和远端肌肉部分组成。除近端裸露区域外，男性标本肩胛下肌止点处的大小明显大于女性标本的。

肩胛下肌是肩袖中最大和最强的肌肉。肩胛下肌向内旋转（内旋）肱骨头。当手臂抬起时，肩胛下肌将肱骨向前和向下拉。[32]肩胛下肌也可防止肱骨头前移脱位。研究发现，肩胛下肌是最重要的内旋肌。[30]肩胛下肌损伤的诊断有时很困难，关节镜和开放手术在评估某些撕裂方面的能力有限。研究者在一项肩胛下肌腱撕裂的 MRI 研究中发现，诊断成像对诊断和评估肩胛下肌损伤的程度很重要。临床医师必须了解几种不寻常的肩胛下肌腱撕裂类型。全层撕裂可能很难被发现，因为瘢痕组织附着于大结节，酷似正常肌腱纤维。由于喙肱韧带的稳定作用和正常的下部肩胛下肌的附着，即便是广泛的肩胛下肌腱撕裂也可能不表现出肌腱回缩。瘢痕组织可以防止磁共振关节造影剂的泄漏。

小圆肌

小圆肌的上 2/3 起自肩胛骨腋侧的后表面。其余的 1/3 起自两个腱膜薄层，其中一个将小圆肌与冈下肌分离，另一个将其与大圆肌分离。小圆肌的纤维斜行向上和向下进入大结节的最低部。在 31 个尸体标本中，接近一半的小圆肌周围有一个独立的筋膜鞘包绕，另一半有一个围绕冈下肌和小圆肌的联合筋膜鞘。[33]所有肩关节在肩胛盂颈部的下部均有一个粗壮的筋膜韧带。支配小圆肌的运动神经分支在急转弯后，总是走行于该悬韧带与小圆肌之间。这些发现可能对理解孤立性小圆肌萎缩有意义。

冈下肌和小圆肌除了在肩关节内收、后伸和水平外展中发挥作用外，还可与三角肌后部一起使肱骨外旋。

肱二头肌

肱二头肌长头腱起源于肩胛盂上唇和肩胛盂上结节，其关节内部分在结节间沟内，离开盂肱关节之前绕过肱骨头。[34]它起源于盂唇，并构成盂唇的一部分。肱二头肌短头腱起源于喙突，来自每个起点的肌腹汇聚形成肱二头肌。[35]

一项纳入 101 具尸体标本的肩部的研究发现，肱二头肌长头腱起源于肩胛盂上唇和肩胛盂上结节的类型不同。[36]该研究描述了 4 种起源类型：完全后方（28 例）、后方优势（56 例）、相等（17例）、和完全前方（0 例）。所有肩部的肱二头肌长头腱均起源于肩胛盂唇和肩胛盂上结节。这项研究的结果可以帮助临床医师评估肱二头肌长头腱的起源和治疗如 SLAP 损伤等疾病。

肱二头肌长头腱的关节内部分通常宽而平，关节外部分较小而圆。肌腱直径 5~6 mm，长度约 9 cm。[35] 旋肱前动脉提供肱二头肌长头腱关节部分的血供。肌腱的更远端部分无血管走行，有利于其在结节间沟鞘内的滑动运动。[37]

手臂从中立位开始前屈和内旋时，肱二头肌长头可在盂肱关节中最多滑动 18 mm。[38] 肱二头肌长头在肩关节屈曲、后伸、外展、内旋、外旋和前方稳定性中具有重要作用。

肩胸关节的功能

肩胛骨是肩关节运动的基础，肩袖在胸廓和手臂之间的运动链中起连接的作用。肩胸运动是由肩胸关节和盂肱关节产生的（图 1-7）。肩胛骨在胸部的运动对于上肢的正常功能是必不可少的。[39] 肩胸关节不是可动关节。然而，在手臂运动期间，肩胛骨和胸部之间会发生大量的运动。在肩关节外展中，每 3° 中有 2° 发生在盂肱关节，1° 发生在肩胸关节。[40] 手臂运动时肩胸的协调运动称为肩胛肱骨节律。

在一项使用电磁运动传感器和表面电极检测 20 名健康受试者的肌肉活动的研究中，研究者发现当受试者的手臂主动和被动地抬高时，肩胛骨在胸部上的方向和位置是不同的。[41] 被动抬高期间肌肉活动水平的降低，导致肩胛胸廓运动学发生了改变，包括肩胛骨上旋和外展角度的改变。最明显的区别是在手臂中等幅度抬高时观察到的。当手臂主动抬起时，肩胛骨的上旋角度明显更大。这一

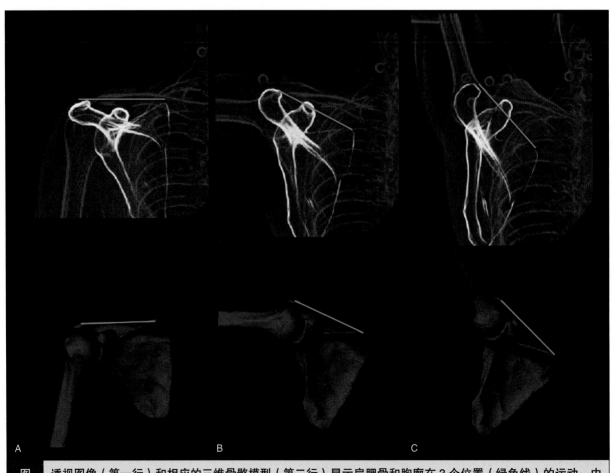

图 1-7 透视图像（第一行）和相应的三维骨骼模型（第二行）显示肩胛骨和胸廓在 3 个位置（绿色线）的运动：中立位（A）、外展 90° 位（B）和最大上举位（C）

发现提示斜方肌（特别是前锯肌）在肩胛骨上旋中的重要作用，特别是在手臂中等幅度抬高时。在体格检查时应该仔细评估这些肌肉和肩胛骨的上旋角度，特别是它们在手臂中等幅度抬高时的情况。

一项活体 MRI 研究评估了肩胛骨的三维运动，从外旋 90° 到内旋 90°，肱骨处于 90° 外展位。[42] 在整个运动过程中，肩胸关节的运动约占 12.5%。当上臂位置由外旋 90° 变为内旋 60° 时，大部分运动来自盂肱关节。当内旋超过 60° 时，肩胛骨开始明显向前倾斜。[42] 肩胸运动对于肩部正常功能是重要的，上述发现有力地支持了这一观点。

总结

肩关节由复杂的骨性结构和软组织结构组成，可提供大范围的运动并保持稳定。其复杂的解剖结构在个体之间有很大差异，必须正确建模才能了解其正常功能和病理状态。为了适当地恢复正常的解剖和关节功能，外科医师必须在诊断和手术过程中考虑患者的解剖变异。

参考文献

［1］ Crockett HC, Gross LB, Wilk KE, et al: Osse-ous adaptation and range of motion at the glenohumeral joint in professional baseball pitchers. *Am J Sports Med* 2002;30(1):20-26.

［2］ Harrold F, Wigderowitz C: A three-dimensional analysis of humeral head retroversion. *J Shoulder Elbow Surg* 2012;21(5):612-617.

Surface topography data for 24 cadaver humeral heads were collected using a handheld digitizer and a surface laser scanner to determine variability in retroversion of the cartilage-metaphysis interface in the axial plane. The results suggested that the cartilage-metaphyseal interface has a high degree of variability and is not a suitable landmark for osteotomy procedures.

［3］ Hill JA, Tkach L, Hendrix RW: A study of glenohumeral orientation in patients with anterior recurrent shoulder dislocations using computerized axial tomography. *Orthop Rev* 1989;18(1):84-91.

［4］ Robertson DD, Yuan J, Bigliani LU, Flatow EL, Yamaguchi K: Three-dimensional analysis of the proximal part of the humerus: Relevance to arthroplasty. *J Bone Joint Surg Am* 2000;82(11):1594-1602.

［5］ Pearl ML, Volk AG: Retroversion of the proximal humerus in relationship to prosthetic replacement arthroplasty. *J Shoulder Elbow Surg* 1995;4(4):286-289.

［6］ Kvitne RS, Jobe FW, Jobe CM: Shoulder instability in the overhand or throwing athlete. *Clin Sports Med* 1995;14(4):917-935.

［7］ Angibaud L, Zuckerman JD, Flurin PH, Roche C, Wright T: Reconstructing proximal humeral fractures using the bicipital groove as a landmark. *Clin Orthop Relat Res* 2007;458:168-174.

Three-dimensional geometry of the bicipital groove was quantified in 49 dried humeri. The anterior offset of the bicipital groove was found to be almost constant from proximal to distal relative to the intramedullary axis. The distal bicipital groove at the level of the surgical neck is a reasonable landmark for establishing humeral head retroversion.

［8］ Itamura J, Dietrick T, Roidis N, Shean C, Chen F, Tibone J: Analysis of the bicipital groove as a landmark for humeral head replacement. *J Shoulder Elbow Surg* 2002;11(4):322-326.

［9］ Wafae N, Atencio Santamaría LE, Vitor L, Pereira LA, Ruiz CR, Wafae GC: Morphometry of the human bicipital groove (sulcus intertubercularis). *J Shoulder Elbow Surg* 2010;19(1):65-68.

Morphometric study of the bicipital groove and humerus in 50 dry humeri confirmed the variability of length, thickness, width, and angle measurements of the bicipital groove.

［10］ Bryce CD, Davison AC, Lewis GS, Wang L, Flemming DJ, Armstrong AD: Two-dimensional glenoid version measurements vary with coronal and sagittal scapular rotation. *J Bone Joint Surg Am* 2010;92(3):692-699.

Three-dimensional CT scans of 36 cadaver scapulae were evaluated while being rotated in 1° increments in the coronal and sagittal planes to investigate the effect of scapular rotation on glenoid version. Misalignment of 1° or more in the coronal or the sagittal plane created inaccuracy in measurement.

［11］ Dunham KS, Bencardino JT, Rokito AS: Anatomic variants and pitfalls of the labrum, glenoid cartilage, and glenohumeral ligaments. *Magn Reson Imaging Clin N Am* 2012;20(2):213-228, x.

Normal glenoid labrum, articular cartilage, and gleno-humeral ligament anatomy and variants were evaluated. Pitfalls were described related to interpreting conventional and arthrographic MRI.

[12] Stoller D: *Magnetic Resonance Imaging in Orthopaedics and Sports Medicine.* Philadelphia, PA, Lippincott, Williams & Wilkins, 2007.

[13] Moseley H, Overgaard B: The anterior capsular mechanism in recurrent anterior dislocation of the shoulder: Morphological and clinical studies with special reference to the glenoid labrum and glenohumeral ligaments. *J Bone Joint Surg Br* 1962;44(4):913-927.

[14] Pagnani MJ, Deng XH, Warren RF, Torzilli PA, Altchek DW: Effect of lesions of the superior portion of the glenoid labrum on glenohumeral translation. *J Bone Joint Surg Am* 1995;77(7):1003-1010.

[15] Powell SN, Nord KD, Ryu RKN: The diagnosis, classification, and treatment of SLAP lesions. *Oper Tech Sports Med* 2012;20:46-56.

The clinical features of SLAP lesions were reviewed, with mechanism of injury, physical examination, classification, associated lesions, normal and pathologic anatomy, and a treatment algorithm.

[16] Rao AG, Kim TK, Chronopoulos E, McFarland EG: Anatomical variants in the anterosuperior aspect of the glenoid labrum: A statistical analysis of seventy-three cases. *J Bone Joint Surg Am* 2003;85(4):653-659.

[17] Kanatli U, Ozturk BY, Bolukbasi S: Anatomical variations of the anterosuperior labrum: Prevalence and association with type II superior labrum anteriorposterior (SLAP) lesions. *J Shoulder Elbow Surg* 2010; 19(8):1199-1203.

Retrospective evaluation of 713 consecutive shoulder arthroscopies for anterosuperior labral variations and coexisting labral pathologies found that some anatomic variants of the anterosuperior labrum were associated with the development of SLAP lesions.

[18] Burkart AC, Debski RE: Anatomy and function of the glenohumeral ligaments in anterior shoulder instability. *Clin Orthop Relat Res* 2002;400:32-39.

[19] Tischer T, Vogt S, Kreuz PC, Imhoff AB: Arthroscopicanatomy, variants, and pathologic findings in shoulderinstability. *Arthroscopy* 2011;27(10):1434-1443.

Information on shoulder anatomy and pathology related to shoulder stability was synthesized to improve clinical diagnoses and surgical treatment.

[20] Moore SM, Stehle JH, Rainis EJ, McMahon PJ, Debski RE: The current anatomical description of the inferior glenohumeral ligament does not correlate with its functional role in positions of external rotation. *J Orthop Res* 2008;26(12):1598-1604.

The strain distribution in the inferior glenohumeral ligament was observed in five cadaver shoulders at 0°, 30°, and 60° of external rotation while a 25-N anterior load was applied. The complex strain distributions suggested that the inferior glenohumeral capsule should be treated as a continuous sheet of fibrous tissue.

[21] Rainis EJ, Maas SA, Henninger HB, McMahon PJ, Weiss JA, Debski RE: Material properties of the axillary pouch of the glenohumeral capsule: Is isotropic material symmetry appropriate? *J Biomech Eng* 2009; 131(3):031007.

A combined experimental and computational protocol was used to characterize the mechanical properties of the axillary pouch of the glenohumeral capsule, which were found to be the same in the longitudinal and transverse directions.

[22] Moore SM, Ellis BJ, Weiss JA, McMahon PJ, Debski RE: The glenohumeral capsule should be evaluated as a sheet of fibrous tissue: A validated finite element model. *Ann Biomed Eng* 2010;38(1):66-76.

Finite element models were used to determine the distribution of maximum principal strain and deformed shape of the glenohumeral capsule at the apprehension position. The study concluded that discrete capsular regions should not be isolated for experimental or computational analysis of glenohumeral capsule function.

[23] Kask K, Põldoja E, Lont T, et al: Anatomy of the superior glenohumeral ligament. *J Shoulder Elbow Surg* 2010;19(6):908-916.

Twenty-seven cadaver shoulder specimens were examined to provide a detailed anatomic description of the superior glenohumeral ligament and its relationship to the rotator cuff interval. The superior glenohumeral ligament was found to be a constant macroscopic structure consisting of direct and oblique fibers.

[24] Harryman DT II, Sidles JA, Clark JM, McQuade KJ, Gibb TD, Matsen FA III: Translation of the humeral head on the glenoid with passive glenohumeral motion. *J Bone Joint Surg Am* 1990;72(9):1334-1343.

[25] Wuelker N, Korell M, Thren K: Dynamic glenohumeral joint stability. *J Shoulder Elbow Surg* 1998;7(1): 43-52.

[26] Thompson WO, Debski RE, Boardman ND III, et al: A biomechanical analysis of rotator cuff deficiency in a cadaveric model. *Am J Sports Med* 1996;24(3):286-292.

[27] Mochizuki T, Sugaya H, Uomizu M, et al: Humeral insertion of the supraspinatus and infraspinatus: New

anatomical findings regarding the footprint of the rotator cuff. *J Bone Joint Surg Am* 2008;90(5):962-969.

The humeral insertions of the rotator cuff were investigated in 113 cadaver shoulders. The supraspinatus was found to have a long tendinous portion in its anterior half, which always inserted into the anteriormost area of the highest impression on the greater tuberosity.

[28] Ackland DC, Pandy MG: Lines of action and stabilizing potential of the shoulder musculature. *J Anat* 2009;215(2):184-197.

The lines of action were determined for 18 major muscles and muscle subregions crossing the glenohumeral joint of the human shoulder. Computer simulations then predicted the contribution of these muscles to joint shear and compression forces during scapular plane abduction and sagittal plane flexion.

[29] Clemente C: *Gray's Anatomy of the Human Body*, ed 30. Philadelphia, PA, Lea & Febiger, 1985.

[30] Ackland DC, Pandy MG: Moment arms of the shoulder muscles during axial rotation. *J Orthop Res* 2011; 29(5):658-667.

The moment arms were determined for 18 major muscle subregions crossing the glenohumeral joint with axial rotation of the humerus during coronal plane abduction and sagittal plane flexion. The inferior infraspinatus and the teres minor were found to be the most important external rotators.

[31] Ide J, Tokiyoshi A, Hirose J, Mizuta H: An anatomic study of the subscapularis insertion to the humerus: The subscapularis footprint. *Arthroscopy* 2008;24(7): 749-753.

The morphology of the subscapularis insertion to the humerus was elucidated in 40 cadaver shoulders. The insertion site anatomy was broad proximally and tapered distally in a comma shape.

[32] Morag Y, Jamadar DA, Miller B, Dong Q, Jacobson JA: The subscapularis: Anatomy, injury, and imaging. *Skeletal Radiol* 2011;40(3):255-269.

Anatomy and MRI findings in injured subscapularis tendons were compared with normal anatomy.

[33] Chafik D, Galatz LM, Keener JD, Kim HM, Yamaguchi K: Teres minor muscle and related anatomy. *J Shoulder Elbow Surg* 2013;22(1):108-114.

The complex anatomy surrounding the teres minor muscle was evaluated.

[34] Ghalayini SR, Board TN, Srinivasan MS: Anatomic variations in the long head of biceps: Contribution to shoulder dysfunction. *Arthroscopy* 2007;23(9):1012-1018.

Current knowledge of anatomic variants and management of LHBT lesions was discussed, with a report of congenital absence of the LHBT in three patients. A classification system was proposed for symptomatic lesions and congenital absence of the LHBT.

[35] Elser F, Braun S, Dewing CB, Giphart JE, Millett PJ: Anatomy, function, injuries, and treatment of the long head of the biceps brachii tendon. *Arthroscopy* 2011; 27(4):581-592.

An update was provided on the anatomy and biomechanical properties of the LHBT, with an evidencebased approach to current treatment strategies for disorders of the LHBT.

[36] Tuoheti Y, Itoi E, Minagawa H, et al: Attachment types of the long head of the biceps tendon to the glenoid labrum and their relationships with the glenohumeral ligaments. *Arthroscopy* 2005;21(10):1242- 1249.

[37] Ahrens PM, Boileau P: The long head of biceps and associated tendinopathy. *J Bone Joint Surg Br* 2007; 89(8):1001-1009.

Current views on the pathology of LHBT lesions were described. The anterior circumflex humeral artery feeds the articular portion of the LHBT, but the distal portion of the tendon is avascular.

[38] Braun S, Millett PJ, Yongpravat C, et al: Biomechanical evaluation of shear force vectors leading to injury of the biceps reflection pulley: A biplane fluoroscopy study on cadaveric shoulders. *Am J Sports Med* 2010; 38(5):1015-1024.

The LHBT was evaluated in eight fresh-frozen cadaver shoulders to measure its course in common arm positions. Shear and compressive force vectors as well as the excursion of the tendon also were determined.

[39] Kibler WB, McMullen J: Scapular dyskinesis and its relation to shoulder pain. *J Am Acad Orthop Surg* 2003;11(2):142-151.

[40] Karduna AR, McClure PW, Michener LA: Scapular kinematics: Effects of altering the Euler angle sequence of rotations. *J Biomech* 2000;33(9):1063-1068.

[41] Ebaugh DD, McClure PW, Karduna AR: Three-dimensi-onal scapulothoracic motion during active and passive arm elevation. *Clin Biomech (Bristol, Avon)* 2005;20(7):700-709.

[42] Koishi H, Goto A, Tanaka M, et al: In vivo threedimensi-onal motion analysis of the shoulder joint during internal and external rotation. *Int Orthop* 2011; 35(10):1503-

1509.

Open MRI was used to examine the right shoulder of 10 healthy volunteers to assess the three-dimensional motion of the scapula from 90° of external rotation to 90° of internal rotation with the humerus in 90° of abduction. The scapulothoracic joint was found to contribute approximately 12.5% of the entire motion.

第二章　肩袖肌腱损伤与愈合的基础科学

Sarah Ilkhani-Pour, MSE; Andrew A. Dunkman, BA; Louis J. Soslowsky, PhD

引言

　　肩部是人体肌肉骨骼系统中非常复杂的区域之一。盂肱关节的球窝特征使其具有比其他关节更大的活动范围。盂肱关节的复杂性和灵活性是肩袖肌腱经常受伤的原因，导致患者出现疼痛、残疾和经济损失。肩部损伤和退变的频繁发生为临床医师和研究者研究其生物学、病理学和管理提供了动力。最近，对肩袖肌腱的研究集中在分子层面上，包括影响生物力学的因素、退变的原因以及生物结构和机械功能之间的相互作用。临床研究、动物模型研究和新的成像技术提供了深入认识肩袖肌腱愈合的手段，并可指导修复技术的选择、术后护理和康复。

肩袖的解剖、组成和结构

　　组成肩袖的 4 块主要的肌肉是冈上肌、冈下肌、小圆肌和肩胛下肌。这些肌肉赋予了盂肱关节稳定性，并参与手臂的运动。这些肌肉的肌腱都插入肱骨的近端。在这些肌腱中，冈上肌腱最常受伤，这是因为其位于喙肩弓下，易于受损，且血供较差。因此，大多数关于肩袖肌腱愈合的研究都聚焦于冈上肌腱。

　　Ⅰ型胶原被认为占肩袖肌腱干重的 85%，而冈上肌腱含有大量的Ⅲ型胶原，并且其糖胺聚糖含量相对较高。冈上肌腱受到显著压迫，并表达常见于软骨的细胞外基质蛋白。研究者已经开始量化特定蛋白聚糖在冈上肌腱中的分布。夹心酶联免疫吸附测定可用于检测生前健康的尸体肩部的冈上肌腱中饰胶蛋白聚糖、聚集蛋白聚糖和双糖链蛋白聚糖的浓度。饰胶蛋白聚糖通常与肩袖的张力和承重相关，在 6 个区域中的浓度恒定。聚集蛋白聚糖和双糖链蛋白聚糖分别与肌肉压缩和重塑的活跃性相关，在冈上肌腱的前部和后部中浓度较高。由于冈上肌腱前部是最容易受到损伤的区域，因此了解该部位的蛋白聚糖浓度特别有价值。[1]

　　大多数肩袖损伤发生在冈上肌腱 - 骨结合部。由于化学物质从肌腱过渡到骨时浓度骤然变化，因此该区域承受着显著的浓度巨变应力。从工程学的角度理解这些特性有助于改进治疗方案和外科技术。虽然插入位点分为 4 个不同的区域，但实际上，这 4 个区域间的转变是渐进的和连续的。第一区，即肌腱本身（类似肌腱中间物质的区域），主要含有排列良好的Ⅰ型胶原纤维。第二区，即纤维软骨区，主要含有Ⅱ型和Ⅲ型胶原，且蛋白聚糖浓度增高。随着矿化的继续，矿物质浓度显著增高，最后两个区域为矿化纤维软骨和骨。研究者最近使用拉曼光谱术进一步研究了这一过渡带。这种新的定量研究矿物质组成的方法揭示了插入位点中矿物质与胶原蛋白的比例和晶体组织呈线性增加的趋势[2]（图 2-1）。

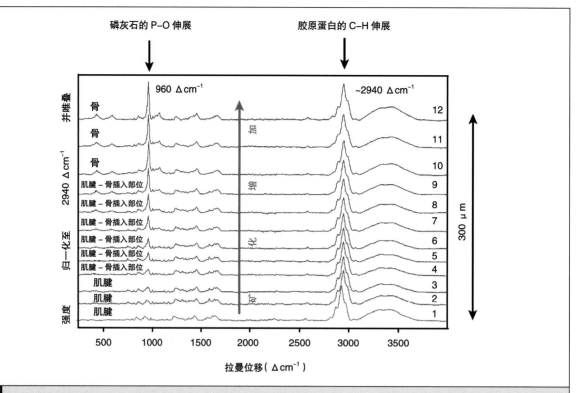

图 2-1 跨大鼠肩部肌腱－骨插入部位的矿物质组成的拉曼光谱量化图表。所有光谱都通过胶原蛋白的 C-H 伸展进行归一化，然后列于 y 轴，以便更好地进行比较。矿物质含量以 960△cm⁻¹ 磷灰石的 P-O 伸展来表示，可以看到沿着从肌腱到骨骼的方向逐渐增加。经允许引自 Wopenka B，Kent A，Pasteris JD，Yoon Y，Thomopoulos S：The tendon-to-bone transition of the rotator cuff: A preliminary Raman spectroscopic study documenting the gradual mineralization across the insertion in rat tissue samples.*Appl Spectrosc* 2008;62(12):1285-1294.

修复和术后愈合的失败使得这种浓度梯度无法重新创建和恢复，一定程度上导致了再撕裂的高发生率。

肩袖肌腱的生物力学

肩袖的主要功能是机械性的，包括稳定肩关节和使肩关节运动。肩袖肌腱具有黏弹性、非线性和非均匀的材料特性。了解肩袖肌腱的生物力学特性有助于深入了解肩袖撕裂的预防、修复和康复。最近的研究成果包括测量体内肩袖形变的技术、对未受伤肌腱的材料性质的量化、对撕裂进展的观察以及对系统性改变是如何影响肩袖肌腱力学的认识。

活体测量

无创成像技术有助于评估肩袖肌腱的愈合。在 X 线立体摄影测量分析中，使用静态 X 线片对

目标材料中的标记物进行了分析。以不锈钢丝缝合为标记，在绵羊肩袖肌腱准确测量到缝合线迁移了约 1 mm。[3] 这种技术可能适用于跟踪手术修复后间隙形成的情况。同样，低剂量 CT 被用来定位植入患者体内的标记物。[4] 低剂量 CT 的误差在 0.7 mm 以内，标记物间的距离受手臂位置和肩袖内标记物位置的影响。以上所述技术只能用于静态成像，不能用于评估组织的功能特性。为了突破这一限制，双平面 X 线分析通过高速射线图像跟踪植入的钽珠并测量肩袖组织的动态变形。在活体犬模型中，这项技术可区分修复成功的、修复失败的和健侧的冈下肌。[5] 修复成功的肌腱收缩约 19%，在修复后 28 周内僵硬度上升 70%。修复失败的肌腱尽管瘢痕组织变硬，但并没有收缩。该技术的误差在 0.1 mm 以内，并且有助于体内组织变形的功能分析。二维斑点跟踪超声技

术已被用于未受伤的、健康的冈上肌腱，以确定体内应变。[6]该技术可检测冈上肌腱浅侧（囊侧）和深侧（关节侧）之间的应变差异，以及肌腱对肌肉等张和等长收缩的不同反应。这些发现可能预示，一种不同的修复分层撕裂的技术即将诞生。

材料特性

有限元模型可帮助医师计算、分析肩袖的机械力学改变。冈上肌腱的三维有限元模型已被用于确定发生在肌腱前缘关节侧的最大拉伸应力，以说明该部位较高的撕裂频率。[7]这项分析首次使用了冈上肌的三维有限元模型，且受到其各向同性和均匀性假设的限制。在其他研究中，例如，对尸体标本的冈上肌腱组织的体外力学测试发现，冈上肌腱具有高度的不均匀性和非线性力学特点。[8-9]在整个测试过程中使用偏光设置可使胶原纤维排列量化。拉伸模量是应力－应变曲线线性区域中的应力与应变之比。拉伸加载期间，无论是纵向（平行于纤维方向）还是横向（垂直于纤维方向）的拉伸，拉伸模量和纤维排列都取决于所在

肌腱内的区域。在纵向加载中，取自冈上肌腱后部的标本的拉伸模量比取自前部肌腱或内侧肌腱的标本的更低，在囊侧和关节侧区域之间没有张力模量差异。类似地，纤维排列在后部样本中最混乱，在中间样本中有序（图 2-2）。肌腱材料特性也可用于区分正常和撕裂的肩袖肌腱。当使用动态剪切机械测试测量时，来自巨大肩袖撕裂患者的活检标本显示出明显低于正常肌腱的储能模量。[10]通过储能模量可以测量黏弹性材料中储存的弹性能。撕裂的肌腱在机械力学性能上较弱，储能模量可能是未来研究的有用参数。机械力学性能降低可能造成肌腱大量撕裂，从而导致修复失败。

肌腱之间的机械相互作用

肩袖撕裂，从小范围的、可处理的，进展到大范围的甚至修复失败的过程，是临床中的重要问题。使用羊冈下肌撕裂模型研究撕裂的大小和肌腱应变之间的直接关系，发现与较小的撕裂相比，较大的撕裂容易在较低的负荷下出现修复失败。[11]撕裂在进展开始时只有 1.7% 的应变，这表明即使是很小的撕裂也可能进展。在这项研究中，

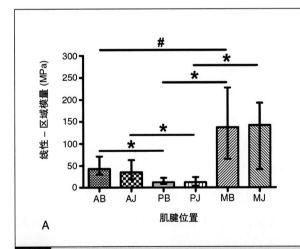
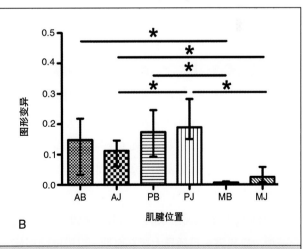

图 2-2　描述拉伸模量和胶原组织的区域变化的图表。两图都标明了中位数和四分位数之间的范围。冈上肌腱的弹性模量具有区域性差异。A. 后部样本的模量始终低于内侧和前部样本。B. 图形变异是衡量胶原纤维组织紊乱的指标，在冈上肌腱上是不均匀的。排列得越整齐的区域往往具有较高的模量，而排列较无序的区域（具有较高的循环方差）往往具有较低的模量值。#= 趋势性，*= 显著性，AB= 前方滑囊，AJ= 前关节，PB= 后方滑囊，PJ= 后关节，MB= 内侧滑囊，MJ= 内侧关节。经允许引自 Lake SP, Miller KS, Elliott DM, Soslowsky LJ: Effect of fiber distribution and realignment on the nonlinear and inhomogeneous mechanical properties of human supraspinatus tendon under longitudinal tensile loading. *J Orthop Res* 2009; 27（12）:1596–1602.

冈下肌腱被分离并与其他肩袖肌腱分开进行测试。然而，在体内，由于肩袖内各肌腱一起工作，稳定盂肱关节并使盂肱关节运动，因此多项研究分析了冈上肌腱和冈下肌腱之间的机械相互作用。解剖尸体肩部，保留完整的冈上肌腱和冈下肌腱，对冈上肌腱所受的负荷、肌腱撕裂大小、肩胛骨外展角度、关节旋转角以及冈上肌腱修复的存在与否进行了研究，以确定它们对冈上肌腱和冈下肌腱应变的影响。[12-14]使用这些数据建立多元回归模型发现，肩关节外展角度和冈上肌腱负荷是冈下肌腱和冈上肌腱应变的显著预测因子。[15]这些发现表明，在中立位旋转中，通过限制负荷并将手臂保持在30°外展位，可以减缓撕裂的进展，有助于修复后管理。

系统性改变

研究人员试图了解与肩袖肌腱病变和撕裂相关的危险因素。最近，系统性改变，如高胆固醇血症、糖尿病、年龄相关的骨丢失和吸烟等，已被证实与肩袖肌腱病变和撕裂相关。在一项临床研究中，肩袖撕裂患者的总胆固醇、甘油三酯和低密度脂蛋白水平明显高于有肩痛但无肩袖撕裂的患者（图2-3）。肌腱或细胞外基质上的胆固醇沉积（黄色瘤）可能改变肌腱的力学、增加其损伤易感性并影响其愈合。此外，高胆固醇血症患者的血流受限可能会进一步加重肩袖肌腱的不良血供。[16]这项研究证实了高胆固醇血症和肩袖撕裂之间的相关性，但没有确定这两者的因果关系。使用动物模型的研究表明，高胆固醇血症显著影响肌腱的弹性模量。[17]

早前的研究发现糖尿病患者骨量减少和骨折愈合减缓，故研究人员诱导大鼠高血糖，以模拟糖尿病对手术修复后肌腱－骨愈合的影响。正如预期的那样，高血糖大鼠的修复质量较差，胶原纤维组织和纤维软骨形成明显较少，肩袖修复在采用约为对照组动物中修复部位负荷的一半时即失效。因此，对于血糖水平控制不佳的患者，可能需要特殊考虑。[18]

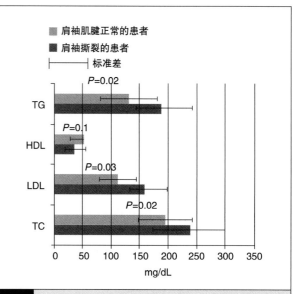

图 2-3　本图显示了一项临床研究结果，该研究比较了肩袖肌腱正常的患者和肩袖撕裂的患者的甘油三酯（TG）、高密度脂蛋白（HDL）、低密度脂蛋白（LDL）和总胆固醇（TC）水平。肩袖撕裂的患者高胆固醇血症的发生率比肩袖肌腱正常的患者更高。经允许引自 Abboud JA, Kim JS: The effect of hypercholesterolemia on rotator cuff disease. *Clin Orthop Relat Res* 2010;468（6）:1493–1497.

雌激素缺乏导致骨吸收增加，从而造成骨密度降低。双侧卵巢切除的大鼠的骨密度降低，但同时服用双膦酸盐的大鼠，其骨密度增高，失效应力明显增高。与对照组大鼠相比，所有雌激素缺乏的大鼠（无论是否服用双膦酸盐）纤维软骨和插入部位组织较差、刚度增加、拉伸模量增加。因此，增高患者的骨密度可能有助于防止肩袖修复失败。[19]最近的研究评估了尼古丁对大鼠模型中正常冈上肌腱机械力学性能的影响。摄入尼古丁的大鼠，其冈上肌腱的弹性模量明显高于对照组，因此研究人员推测，尼古丁可能与吸烟者的肩袖撕裂的风险增高相关。[20]

肌腱变性和撕裂

动物模型

大鼠肩关节是应用最广泛的肩袖动物模型。

大鼠肩部的骨骼解剖与人类相似，二者的冈上肌均穿过肩峰下方。大鼠肩部的功能也与人类肩部的功能接近。大鼠肩胛骨的位置意味着其肩部的前屈相当于人类的外展。急性肩袖肌腱剥脱可改变大鼠的步态，这一发现支持该观点。[21]在急性肩袖肌腱剥脱的早期和晚期两个时间点，大鼠步长的减少与冈上肌功能的降低是一致的；第二次肌腱剥脱会导致额外的有害影响。这种步态分析技术在后续研究中进行了改进，例如，添加了测量大鼠移动过程中地面反作用力的力板。[22]单侧冈上肌分离修复后，大鼠步态的改变是短暂的；早期的步长、峰值垂直力、峰值折断力和峰值侧向力都发生了变化，但所有参数在修复后 4 周内恢复到对照组水平。

家兔肩胛下肌也被建议作为肩袖动物模型。[23]虽然家兔肩峰不明显，但其肩胛下肌腱穿过另一由肩胛上结节、喙突、肩胛骨下结节和喙肱肌组成的骨性隧道有借鉴意义。

慢性撕裂

慢性肩袖撕裂与退行性改变和萎缩有关。与来自正常肩部的标本相比，来自冈上肌腱撕裂患者的肌腱活检样本的纤维结构丧失、肌腱细胞呈圆形、细胞密度增加、血供增加、胶原蛋白着色能力降低。[24]这些来自冈上肌腱中部的活检标本显示变性发生在整个肌腱，而不仅仅是在撕裂端。通过衰减全反射傅里叶变换红外光谱术可以区分不同大小的肩袖撕裂的肌腱活检标本的化学和结构特性。[25]撕裂的肌腱Ⅰ型、Ⅱ型和Ⅲ型胶原含量降低。小撕裂的变化主要涉及脂质和一些蛋白聚糖，而在大撕裂中，胶原蛋白的变化最大，由此可得出撕裂大小与变性加重之间存在关联。

肩袖撕裂患者的肌肉活检标本显示出明显的差异，这取决于肩袖撕裂的大小[26]。其中，脂肪浸润是最明显的差异，与对照组的肌肉活检标本相比，大块撕裂在肌纤维之间和Ⅰ型肌纤维的肌质内有显著的脂质聚集。虽然脂肪浸润这个术语通常用来描述肌肉组织的萎缩和伴随的脂肪沉积，

但这些脂肪细胞的起源尚未确定。大量撕裂导致肌原纤维数量减少、纤维间结缔组织增加、慢肌纤维的线粒体含量增加、冈上肌的血供增加。脂性萎缩更常见于肩部的较大撕裂或冈上肌腱前部撕裂。[27]回顾性分析显示，脂肪浸润的程度与患者的年龄、症状出现与确诊之间的时间长短以及累及的肌腱数量有关。[28]如果撕裂涉及 1 个以上的肌腱，则脂肪变性发生得更快，进展得更快。多元回归分析显示，肌腱回缩量、外展扭矩和血清维生素 D 水平是冈上肌脂肪变性的独立预测因素，血清维生素 D 水平低与脂肪变性增加有关。[29]肌肉收缩部分的两种成分（α- 骨骼肌肌动蛋白和肌球蛋白重链多肽 -1）的表达水平与冈上肌脂肪变性的增加相关。[30]这种肌肉基因表达的增加表明脂肪变化不是因肌肉纤维变性而发生的，而是因为肌肉再生失败。

动物模型已被用于研究与慢性肩袖撕裂相关的退行性改变。在过去，在大鼠模型中很难诱导脂肪浸润。对大鼠冈上肌腱急性横断的研究发现肌肉收缩、肌节缩短、肌肉萎缩和肌腱变性，但脂性萎缩很少见。[31-32]即使到了高龄，大鼠也没有出现明显的脂性萎缩。[33]肌肉的改变是短暂的，但肌腱变性随着时间的推移而进展。与人类不同，大鼠的瘢痕形成会将肌腱重新连接到肱骨，从而重建负荷。在大鼠单侧冈下肌 – 冈上肌腱脱离后观察到的受到损伤的冈上肌腱和冈下肌腱的变化与人类慢性撕裂活检结果一致，这些变化包括面积增加、松弛百分比（一种黏弹性的测量值，描述给定应变下负载随时间减少的量）增加、解体，以及细胞密度和细胞的圆整度增加。[34]肌腱复位的效果随着损伤程度的增加而减少，从而确保冈上肌的变化不是暂时的。

与先前的研究不同，这项研究没有发现肌肉的脂性萎缩。然而，切断肩胛上神经确实会导致脂肪变性（肌内和肌细胞内脂肪含量增加）以及冈下肌和冈上肌萎缩，并上调成脂转录因子和成肌转录因子[35]（图 2-4）。类似的脂肪变性在小鼠

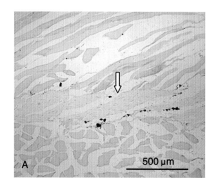
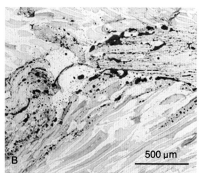
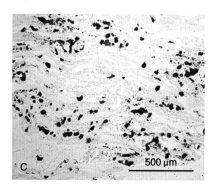
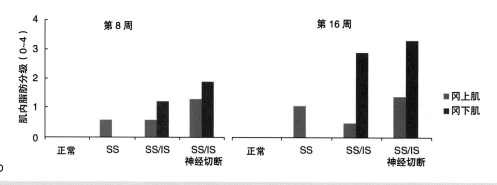

图
2-4

图 A~C 是来自大鼠模型研究的油红 O 染色的组织切片。A. 正常冈上肌（冠状面的纵切面，厚 10 μm）显示很少的肌内脂肪沉积和肌细胞内脂肪滴。在肌肉的中心可以看到冈上肌腱（箭头），在肌腱的上方和下方可以看到肌纤维。B. 切断冈上肌腱和冈下肌腱 16 周后的冈下肌。可见许多脂肪沉积（红色）。C. 切断肌腱和神经 16 周后的冈下肌显示高水平的肌内脂肪（红色）。D. 第 8 周和第 16 周肌内脂肪的半定量组织学分级结果，如油红 O 染色组织学切片所见。0= 无脂肪沉积，4= 大量脂肪沉积。正常肌肉中未见脂肪。无论是否切断神经，在切断冈上肌腱和冈下肌腱后，冈下肌（IS）比冈上肌（SS）具有更多的肌内脂肪。术后第 16 周的标本比第 8 周的标本含有更多的肌内脂肪。经允许引自 Kim HM, Galatz LM, Lim C, Havlioglu N, Thomopoulos S: The effect of tear size and nerve injury on rotator cuff muscle fatty degeneration in a rodent animal model. *J Shoulder Elbow Surg* 2012;21（7）:847-858.

模型中也可以看到，并且比在大鼠模型中更严重。在家兔模型中，切断肩胛下肌腱后肌肉湿重和肌纤维横截面面积均减小，脂肪含量增高。[36] 与大鼠模型相反，这些发现在切断肌腱和同时切断肌腱与神经的动物中是相似的。大鼠、小鼠和家兔模型研究表明，神经变性在肌肉脂肪变性的发展中发挥了作用。大鼠模型体内和体外细胞培养研究表明，抑制 Wnt 信号通路可增加脂肪生成标志基因的表达，导致脂肪在肩袖中堆积。[37]

撕裂对残余肩部结构的影响

最近的研究调查了肩袖撕裂对完整的肩袖肌腱、肱二头肌腱和喙肩韧带的影响。在大鼠模型中，冈上肌脱离导致冈下肌、肩胛下肌和肱二头肌腱的横截面面积增加，模量降低。[38-39] 两个肌腱撕裂比单个肌腱撕裂的危害性更大，并且随着时间的推移这种危害性更明显（图 2-5）。这些损伤可能是由剩余肌腱负荷方式改变造成的。在大鼠模型中通过剥离冈上肌 – 冈下肌进一步研究发现，肱二头肌的改变开始于肌腱的关节内部分，随后延伸到关节外部分。[40] 不同程度肩袖撕裂患者的活检标本中含有不同水平的基质金属蛋白酶（MMPs）和血管内皮生长因子（VEGF）。[41-42] MMPs 能降解细胞外基质蛋白，特别是胶原蛋白分子，而 VEGF 与血管生成有关。肩袖撕裂患者的 VEGF、MMP-1 和 MMP-9 表达增加，但 MMP-3 表达减少。关节侧部分撕裂与

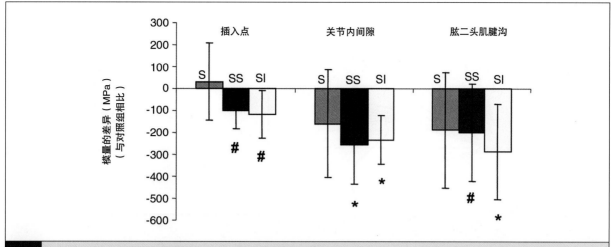

图 2-5　大鼠在冈上肌和肩胛下肌剥离（SS）或冈上肌和冈下肌剥离（SI）后 4~8 周内，与对照组大鼠相比肱二头肌腱模量下降。S= 冈上肌剥离，*= 与对照组有显著差异，#= 倾向于与对照组有差异。经允许引自 Peltz CD，Perry SM，Getz CL，Soslowsky LJ: Mechanical properties of the long-head of the biceps tendon are altered in the presence of rotator cuff tears in a rat model. *J Orthop Res* 2009;27（3）:416-420.

囊侧撕裂有差异。扫描声学显微镜显示，与对照组标本相比，有肩袖撕裂或骨赘的尸体标本的喙肩韧带弹性模量增加。[43]肩袖撕裂时肩的结构成分、组织学和力学性质的改变，对治疗策略具有指导意义。

肌腱变性的遗传学和生物学

虽然肌腱变性的组织学已得到广泛研究，但其生物学直到最近才得到关注。从肩袖疾病患者中采集的样本显示，随着退变的进展，出现了与血管生成和炎症相关的失衡。[44]肌腱变性后发生血管增生。炎症虽然不是慢性肌腱变性的特征，但可能存在于其早期阶段。对冈上肌腱撕裂患者的肩胛下肌腱进行活检发现，与患者撕裂的冈上肌腱或对照组的肩胛下肌腱的活检相比，其巨噬细胞、肥大细胞和 T 细胞染色增强。[45]冈上肌腱撕裂越大，炎症细胞浸润越少。冈上肌腱撕裂患者的肩胛下肌腱可能是早期肌腱病变的模型。

目前，细胞凋亡在肩袖疾病中的作用存在争议。肩袖疾病患者的活检显示，在撕裂的冈上肌标本和相应的肩胛下肌标本中，各处的凋亡细胞数量均增加。[46]大鼠和人类的退行性冈上肌腱标本的热休克蛋白和胱天蛋白酶增加，抗凋亡（热

休克蛋白）和促凋亡（胱天蛋白酶）基因之间存在不平衡。[47]然而，跑步训练长达 16 周的大鼠没有出现细胞凋亡或新生血管。这些大鼠确实有胰岛素样生长因子 -1 的增加，胰岛素样生长因子 -1 影响细胞增殖、细胞存活和软骨发生。[48]晚期肩袖疾病可发展为钙化性肌腱病，其基因表达的改变与骨的发育和吸收有关。[49]这些对肩袖疾病不同阶段之间的差异的认识将改进诊断和治疗方式。

机械负荷影响肌腱变性。大鼠冈上肌腱负荷的变化改变了 MMPs 和金属蛋白酶组织抑制剂（TIMPs）的表达。[50]肌腱病变的特点是 MMPs 和 TIMPs 不平衡。过度活动的大鼠冈上肌腱表达软骨标记物[51]（图 2-6）。这些软骨标记物和其他同样受短期过度活动调节的基因在休息后恢复到接近基线水平。[52]此外，蛋白聚糖和亲肝素调节肽（一种促进软骨发生的因子）的水平随着过度活动而增加[53]（表 2-1）。肩袖肌腱病中的肌腱细胞可能正在向软骨细胞表型转化。虽然机械负荷过高被认为是肩袖疾病的主要原因，但也存在遗传易感性的证据。[54]需要进一步研究，以阐明肩袖的机械力学、遗传学和生物学之间复杂的相互作用，以及它们在肩袖退变的发生和发展中的作用。

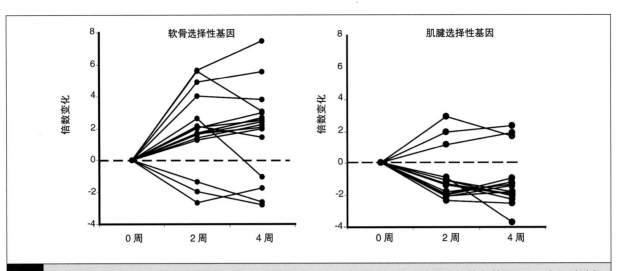

图 2-6 过度活动对经过跑步训练的大鼠的冈上肌腱的影响。17 个软骨选择性（软骨特征性）基因和 12 个肌腱选择性（肌腱特征性）基因，与未训练的对照组相比，发生了调节（表现为基因表达的倍数变化）。一般来说，过度活动上调软骨标记物，下调肌腱标记物。似乎过度活动会导致冈上肌腱变得更像软骨而不是更像肌腱。经允许引自 Archambault JM, Jelinsky SA, Lake SP: Rat supraspinatus tendon expresses cartilage markers with overuse. *J Orthop Res* 2007;25（5）:617-624.

表 2-1

与正常肌腱相比，经过 2 周或 4 周过度活动（跑步训练）后，大鼠冈上肌腱的遗传物质和蛋白质变化

	表达水平	
分子	2 周后	4 周后
胶原		
1α1 mRNA	-	--
2α1 mRNA	+	+
3α1 mRNA	+	=
6α1 mRNA	++	=
饰胶蛋白聚糖		
mRNA	+	++
蛋白质	=	++
双糖链蛋白聚糖		
mRNA	++	++
多能蛋白聚糖		
mRNA	++	++
蛋白质	=	++
聚集蛋白聚糖		
mRNA	++	++
蛋白质	++	++
SOX9		
mRNA	++	+
糖胺聚糖		
总量	=	++
硫酸皮肤素	=	++
硫酸乙酰肝素	=	=

表 2-1

与正常肌腱相比，经过 2 周或 4 周过度活动（跑步训练）后，大鼠冈上肌腱的遗传物质和蛋白质变化（续）

	表达水平	
分子	2 周后	4 周后
糖类磺基转移酶 -14（促进硫酸皮肤素合成）	++	=
亲肝素调节肽		
mRNA	=	=
蛋白质	+	++

注：-，表达降低；--，表达进一步降低；=，与对照组表达无差异；+，表达增加；++，表达进一步增加。经允许引自 Attia M, Scott A, Duchesnay A, Carpentier G, Soslowsky LJ, Huynh MB, Van Kuppevelt TH, Gossard C, Courty J, Tassoni MC, Marteli I: Alterations of overused supraspinatus tendon: A possible role of glycosaminoglycans and heparin affine regulatory peptide/pleiotrophin in early tendon pathology. *J Orthop Res* 2012;30（1）:61-71.

肌腱变性和撕裂的演变

　　肩袖退变可导致肩袖部分撕裂，进而发展为全层撕裂，并可扩大范围。这一演变的原因尚未完全确定。肌腱变性的不同阶段表达不同水平的低氧诱导因子 -1α（HIF-1α），随着变性的增加而呈现出细胞凋亡增加的趋势。[55] 促凋亡蛋白 BNip3 的表达也有类似的趋势。HIF-1α 的改变也

见于回缩的肩袖撕裂肌腱。[56]血管密度增加与回缩的量有关，表明新生血管可能是追踪演变的有用参数。这些退化的样本也有 MMP-1 和 MMP-9 水平的增高和 MMP-3 水平的降低。[57]MMP-9 表达增加与回缩量增高相关。与部分撕裂相比，全层撕裂的滑膜中促炎细胞因子和血管生长因子增加。[58]冈上肌腱活检显示全层撕裂的组织重塑和新生血管增加。此外，对肩关节冈上全层撕裂的肩胛下肌进行活检发现，与部分撕裂的肩部相比，前者的肩胛下肌变性和重塑增加。这些结果表明，更大的撕裂导致更严重的滑膜炎症、冈上肌腱基质变性和肩胛下肌腱变性（图 2-7）。

肌腱的愈合、修复和治疗

愈合

肌腱愈合被分为炎症、增殖（纤维增生）和重塑（成熟）三个基本阶段。最近的研究专注于分子愈合的基础科学、肌腱愈合的新成像技术以及在每个基本阶段可获得最佳结果的治疗方案。为了进一步了解肌腱愈合过程中的分子水平变化，研究者在术后多个时间点测量生长因子浓度进行了分析。在大鼠模型中，在手术分离和修复冈上肌腱后 1 周观察到生长因子的表达增加，第

16 周，生长因子浓度逐渐下降至对照组的水平或无法检测到的水平。最初的生长因子的增加可能归因于炎症反应，而术后第 8 周时中间物质的特异性增加可能归因于肌腱愈合时增加的负荷环境。这一发现提供了进一步的证据，即负荷影响肌腱愈合[59]（表 2-2）。

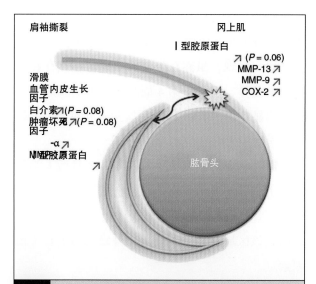

图 2-7 肩袖撕裂与滑膜炎症的关系。撕裂大小与滑膜中促炎反应呈正相关。绿色箭头表示增高。经允许引自 Shindle MK, Chen CC, Robertson C, et al: Full-thickness supraspinatus tears are associated with more synovial inflammation and tissue degeneration than partial-thickness tears. *J Shoulder Elbow Surg* 2011;20（6）: 917–927.

表 2-2

手术分离和修复冈上肌腱 1~16 周后，大鼠冈上肌腱的生长因子浓度（插入 / 中间物质）

生长因子	非手术对照组	术后时间（周）				
		1	2	4	8	16
碱性成纤维细胞生长因子	+/+	+++/+++	++/+++	+/+	++/++	+/-
骨形成蛋白 -12	+/+	+++/+++	+/++	+/+	++/++	+/-
骨形成蛋白 -13	+/-	++/+++	++/+	++/+	++/+	-/-
骨形成蛋白 -14	+/++	++/+++	+/+	+/+	+/++	+/-
软骨寡聚基质蛋白	+/+	+++/+++	++/+	+/+	+/+	+/-
结缔组织生长因子	+/+	+++/++	++/++	+/+	+/++	+/-
血小板衍生生长因子 -B	*/+	*/+++	*/++	*/+	*/+	*/+
转化生长因子 -β1	+/+	++/++	++/++	-/+	+/++	-/-

注：通过半定量染色强度的中位值表示生长因子浓度。+，低；++，中等；+++，高；-，痕量；*，未检测到。经允许引自 Würgler-Hauri CC, Dourte LM, Baradet TC, Williams GR, Soslowsky LJ: Temporal expression of 8 growth factors in tendon-to-bone healing in a rat supraspinatus model. *J Shoulder Elbow Surg* 2007;16（5, suppl）:S198-S203.

传统的石膏或吊带固定仅限制肩关节的大范围运动。然而，有研究者猜测暂时消除张力对早期愈合是有益的。有两项研究使用了大鼠冈上肌分离和修复模型来评估全肌麻痹对插入部位愈合的影响。其中一项研究检查了在手术修复冈上肌后注射 A 型肉毒毒素的效果，发现 A 型肉毒毒素对肌腱的力学特性和插入部位的愈合产生了负面影响，特别是在应用了石膏固定的大鼠中。[60]另一项研究发现，虽然在类似的早期时间点存在机械力学差异，但术后第 4 周时实验组的胶原纤维组织明显改善，术后 24 周后实验组和对照组的机械力学性能无明显差异。[61]

通过超声造影评估手术修复 3 个月后人类肩胛冈上肌腱的血供变化。有损伤的肌腱在插入部位的血管容积和静息灌注显著降低。[62]这一发现表明，该区域的血供质量是外科修复的重要考虑因素。

修复的效果

手术修复冈上肌腱撕裂通常是有效的，但仍有大约 25% 的修复是不成功的。目前，研究的一个热点是调查和更好地了解修复后体内的变化、影响这些变化的因素以及如何评估术后反应。研究者对可能用于预测修复后功能结果的因素进行了多元回归分析。根据既往的报道，患者的年龄是手术结果的决定性因素，但其未被证实是独立的因变量，而只是与一些重要变量（包括撕裂回缩、脂肪变性和肌肉力量等）相关的变量。[63]术前冈上肌和冈下肌的肌肉萎缩和脂肪浸润评分是功能结果的重要预测因子，二者相互关联，并且通常随着撕裂大小的增加而恶化（图 2-8）。肌肉萎缩和脂肪浸润在手术后 1 年不仅没有改善，相反，如果患者在手术时有这些情况，则还会恶化。修复不成功的肩部恶化更严重。因此，应尽早进行修复，以尽量减少脂肪浸润和肌肉萎缩的影响。[64]

研究者使用一种在麻醉大鼠中测量活体肩关节僵硬度的新设备时发现，大鼠的肩关节如果被固定，则僵硬度会增加，然而，这种差异是短暂的，并且在术后第 8 周后不再显著。将这种设备

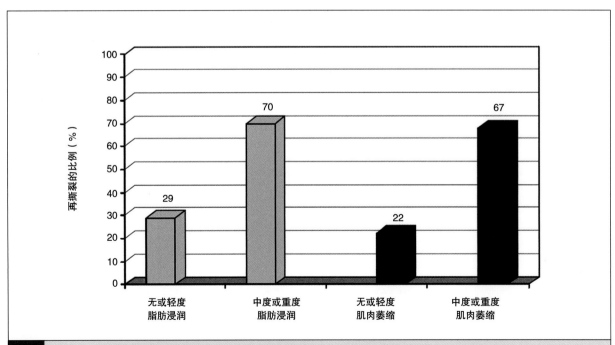

图 2-8　临床上不明显（或显著）的脂肪浸润或肌肉萎缩对肩袖再撕裂的影响（*P*<0.05）。经允许引自 Gladstone JN, Bishop JY, Lo IK Flatow EL: Fatty infiltration and atrophy of the rotator cuff do not improve after rotator cuff repair and correlate with poor functional outcome. *Am J Sports Med* 2007;35（5）:719–728.

的测量结论推广到人体，将有助于临床评估。考虑到对修复后插入部位特性的益处，在固定的情况下肩关节僵硬度的暂时增加是可以接受的。[65]

研究人员使用家兔模型发现，CT可以显示手术修复的肌腱－骨结合结构的强度。[66]在愈合过程中增加血流量导致一定程度的信号衰减，并且衰减在术后随时间增加。最重要的是，早期图像中出现的低衰减及更高的结合强度与降低失败的可能性相关。早期CT检查可能有助于预测手术成功的可能性。另一项研究使用X线立体摄影测量分析来测量标记物的迁移。在肩袖撕裂的开放性修复过程中，外科医师将金属珠植入肱骨大结节，并将钢丝缝合到患者的冈上肌腱中。1年后，标记物在完整修复的肌腱中平均移动6.3 mm；在完全失败的修复中平均移动23.7 mm。大部分移动发生在积极康复期（术后2~3个月），这意味着再撕裂最容易发生于这段时间内，这可能与物理治疗中的活动水平有关。而在手术后第3~4个月和1年后，迁移是最小的，可能是因为这一时期是修复的开始阶段，完全修复可以承受未来的负荷。[67]

早期的临床工作表明，在部分修复大面积（包括冈下肌和冈上肌）撕裂时，只有冈下肌被重新连接，才有可能恢复足够的功能。最近在大鼠模型的研究中使用了两种方法，即剥离和定量运动测量方法。部分和完全修复的结果与未修复的结果有显著差异，双肌腱复位的结果与单纯冈下肌腱复位的结果无显著差异。[68]这些发现支持通过部分修复来恢复足够功能的临床实践。一项旨在评估修复类型对冈上肌腱和冈下肌腱之间相互作用的特定影响的人体研究发现，经骨等效关节镜技术导致了高负荷时交互作用的减少，从而降低了冈下肌对冈上肌腱的作用。这一发现揭示，与传统的开放经骨修复相比，部分修复可能存在风险。[69]

术后治疗和非手术治疗

肩袖修复和退变治疗通常效果不佳，这促进了对治疗技术的研究。除了修复技术的细节之外，外科医师还可以通过制订康复方案来影响患者的预后。此外，新兴的治疗技术已经获得越来越多的关注。

一系列使用大鼠模型的实验研究了修复后多个时间点的固定和运动的效果：固定4周者胶原组织结构得到改善，但固定16周者未见改善；固定16周后机械力学性能较好，但固定4周后无明显变化。如此看来，长期固定使修复具有更强的组织性，这最终提高了机械性能。[70]一项随访研究将固定与两种不同的被动运动康复方案结合起来，这两种方案均可导致活动范围明显缩小，这可能是因为肩峰下瘢痕形成增加。[71]短期固定后令大鼠进行笼内活动或跑步机跑步。运动大鼠的物理和机械性能较差，表明组织紊乱、基质增加、瘢痕产生。[72]

临床研究试图确定积极的和较有限的早期被动运动康复方案的相对有效性。在一项研究中，接受积极的康复治疗的患者每天接受2次手法治疗，并在指导下每天进行3次摆动和伸展运动。[73]接受较有限的康复治疗的患者由运动机持续辅助运动，每天仅进行2次前屈伸展运动。以上方案持续6周，然后开始使用伸展和加强方案。接受积极治疗的患者在术后第3个月有更大的活动范围和更好的临床评估结果，但在术后1年时这些差异不显著。积极治疗组的30例患者中有7例发生再撕裂，而有限治疗组的34例患者中只有3例发生再撕裂。

研究者对非撕裂肩袖肌腱病患者进行自然疗法与运动锻炼治疗的效果进行了比较。自然疗法包括抗炎膳食咨询、使用膳食补充剂（phlogenzym）和每周针灸。两组均提供护理服务、物理治疗和一片药片（运动锻炼治疗组患者使用安慰剂）。两组患者在主观问卷上都表示症状明显改善，其中自然疗法治疗组的改善明显大于运动锻炼治疗组。运动范围的定量测量显示，与基线和运动锻炼治疗组患者相比，自然疗法治疗组的患者的情况明显改善；相反，运动锻炼治疗组患者在运动范围方面没有明显改善。[74]

总结

肩袖肌腱对肩关节的稳定至关重要，并使肩关节具有独特的运动范围，但这些结构容易退化和损伤。当前的研究持续探索着这些结构的分子解剖学和愈合生物学，并在识别和量化重要分子及详细描述插入位点方面取得了进展。对关节力学的建模提高了对相关结构之间的相互作用的理解，从而加深了对解剖功能的认识。肌腱病理演变的生物学正在慢慢被阐明，用于体内测量的新成像技术也已经取得了很大的进展。从手术技术和康复方案到遗传学和生活方式，研究者们正不断深入对影响退化和愈合的因素的理解。未来的研究将继续通过动物、人体和临床研究来阐明这些因素。生物增强技术和组织工程的进展可能为治疗这些肌腱提供新的方式。

参考文献

[1] Matuszewski PE, Chen YL, Szczesny SE, et al: Regional variation in human supraspinatus tendon proteoglycans: Decorin, biglycan, and aggrecan. *Connect Tissue Res* 2012;53(5):343-348.

Enzyme-linked immunosorbent assays of cadaver tissue revealed no regional difference in decorin concentrations, but aggrecan and biglycan were regionally variable.

[2] Wopenka B, Kent A, Pasteris JD, Yoon Y, Thomopoulos S: The tendon-to-bone transition of the rotator cuff: A preliminary Raman spectroscopic study documenting the gradual mineralization across the insertion in rat tissue samples. *Appl Spectrosc* 2008;62(12): 1285-1294.

Quantification of mineral content using Raman spectroscopy led to a challenge to the belief that the insertion site should be thought of in terms of distinct zones.

[3] Cashman PM, Baring T, Reilly P, Emery RJ, Amis AA: Validation of a new technique to monitor rotator cuff tears. *J Med Eng Technol* 2010;34(3):159-165.

Steel sutures were used as Roentgen stereophotogrammetric analysis markers to track rotator cuff tissue deformation in an ovine model. Although this technique was less accurate than bone motion tracking, it provided a method to measure soft-tissue migration in vivo.

[4] Derwin KA, Milks RA, Davidson I, Iannotti JP, Mc-Carron JA, Bey MJ: Low-dose CT imaging of radioopaque markers for assessing human rotator cuff repair: Accuracy, repeatability and the effect of arm position. *J Biomech* 2012;45(3):614-618.

This study investigated the accuracy and repeatability of distance measurement between markers in the rotator cuff using CT. Arm position and location of the bead within the rotator cuff affect measurements.

[5] Bey MJ, Kline SK, Baker AR, McCarron JA, Iannotti JP, Derwin KA: Estimation of dynamic, in vivo softtissue deformation: Experimental technique and application in a canine model of tendon injury and repair. *J Orthop Res* 2011;29(6):822-827.

Biplane radiographic analysis was used in a canine model to distinguish an intact infraspinatus repair, a failed repair, and a control.

[6] Kim YS, Kim JM, Bigliani LU, Kim HJ, Jung HW: In vivo strain analysis of the intact supraspinatus tendon by ultrasound speckles tracking imaging. *J Orthop Res* 2011;29(12):1931-1937.

Two-dimensional speckle tracking echocardiography showed differences in strain between deep and superficial regions of the supraspinatus tendon as well as differences in isometric and isotonic motions.

[7] Seki N, Itoi E, Shibuya Y, et al: Mechanical environment of the supraspinatus tendon: Three-dimensional finite element model analysis. *J Orthop Sci* 2008; 13(4):348-353.

Three-dimensional finite element model analysis of the supraspinatus tendon mechanical environment showed a maximal tensile stress on the articular side of the anterior edge of the supraspinatus tendon.

[8] Lake SP, Miller KS, Elliott DM, Soslowsky LJ: Effect of fiber distribution and realignment on the nonlinear and inhomogeneous mechanical properties of human supraspinatus tendon under longitudinal tensile loading. *J Orthop Res* 2009;27(12):1596-1602.

Longitudinally loaded cadaver supraspinatus tendon specimens varied in moduli values and collagen alignment, depending on the region tested.

[9] Lake SP, Miller KS, Elliott DM, Soslowsky LJ: Tensile

properties and fiber alignment of human supraspinatus tendon in the transverse direction demonstrate inhomogeneity, nonlinearity, and regional isotropy. *J Biomech* 2010;43(4):727-732.

This follow-up study investigated transverse loading on cadaver supraspinatus tendon specimens. Differences existed between bursal- and joint-side specimens, with values for the bursal specimens similar to those achieved in longitudinal loading.

[10] Chaudhury S, Holland C, Vollrath F, Carr AJ: Comparing normal and torn rotator cuff tendons using dynamic shear analysis. *J Bone Joint Surg Br* 2011;93(7): 942-948.

Dynamic shear analysis was used to determine the storage modulus of biopsy samples taken from healthy and torn rotator cuff tissue. Massive tears had a reduced storage modulus.

[11] Andarawis-Puri N, Ricchetti ET, Soslowsky LJ: Rotator cuff tendon strain correlates with tear propagation. *J Biomech* 2009;42(2):158-163.

In an ovine cadaver model, the principal infraspinatus tendon strains were correlated with tear propagation.

[12] Andarawis-Puri N, Ricchetti ET, Soslowsky LJ: Interaction between the supraspinatus and infraspinatus tendons: Effect of anterior supraspinatus tendon fullthickness tears on infraspinatus tendon strain. *Am J Sports Med* 2009;37(9):1831-1839.

In a human cadaver study, infraspinatus tendon strains increased with supraspinatus tear size and loading. There are mechanical interactions between these two tendons.

[13] Andarawis-Puri N, Kuntz AF, Ramsey ML, Soslowsky LJ: Effect of glenohumeral abduction angle on the mechanical interaction between the supraspinatus and infraspinatus tendons for the intact, partial-thickness torn, and repaired supraspinatus tendon conditions. *J Orthop Res* 2010;28(7):846-851.

In a human cadaver study, the abduction angle affected the interaction between the supraspinatus and infraspinatus tendons. Abduction at 30° decreased supraspinatus and infraspinatus tendon strain.

[14] Andarawis-Puri N, Kuntz AF, Kim SY, Soslowsky LJ: Effect of anterior supraspinatus tendon partialthickness tears on infraspinatus tendon strain through a range of joint rotation angles. *J Shoulder Elbow Surg* 2010;19(4):617-623.

In a human cadaver study, joint rotation angles affected the interaction between the supraspinatus and infraspinatus tendons.

[15] Andarawis-Puri N, Kuntz AF, Jawad AF, Soslowsky LJ: Infraspinatus and supraspinatus tendon strain explained using multiple regression models. *Ann Biomed Eng* 2010;38(9):2979-2987.

Regression models using data described in earlier studies revealed that the abduction angle and supraspinatus loading are significant predictors of strain in the infraspinatus and supraspinatus tendons. Supraspinatus tear size was not a predictor of infraspinatus strain.

[16] Abboud JA, Kim JS: The effect of hypercholesterolemia on rotator cuff disease. *Clin Orthop Relat Res* 2010;468(6):1493-1497.

Cholesterol levels were measured in 147 patents. Those with a rotator cuff tear were found to have higher cholesterol levels. Age, sex, and body mass index were not found to be predictive of rotator cuff tears.

[17] Beason DP, Abboud JA, Kuntz AF, Bassora R, Soslowsky LJ: Cumulative effects of hypercholesterolemia on tendon biomechanics in a mouse model. *J Orthop Res* 2011;29(3):380-383.

Hypercholesterolemia had a detrimental effect in a mouse model of tendon elastic modulus.

[18] Bedi A, Fox AJ, Harris PE, et al: Diabetes mellitus impairs tendon-bone healing after rotator cuff repair. *J Shoulder Elbow Surg* 2010;19(7):978-988.

Rats with streptozotocin-induced hyperglycemia had poor recovery from supraspinatus repair at 1- and 2-week postoperative time points.

[19] Cadet ER, Vorys GC, Rahman R, et al: Improving bone density at the rotator cuff footprint increases supraspinatus tendon failure stress in a rat model. *J Orthop Res* 2010;28(3):308-314.

Ovariectomy and bisphosphonate administration in rats were used to explore the effects of estrogen deficiency and bone mineral density on the supraspinatus tendon insertion site.

[20] Ichinose R, Sano H, Kishimoto KN, Sakamoto N, Sato M, Itoi E: Alteration of the material properties of the normal supraspinatus tendon by nicotine treatment in a rat model. *Acta Orthop* 2010;81(5):634-638.

The effect of nicotine on the mechanical properties of healthy tendons was investigated. Increased elastic moduli were found in the treated rats.

[21] Perry SM, Getz CL, Soslowsky LJ: Alterations in function after rotator cuff tears in an animal model. *J Shoulder Elbow Surg* 2009;18(2):296-304.

Supraspinatus detachment in a rat model altered gait and

range of motion. These effects were increased with the addition of a second rotator cuff tendon detachment.

[22] Sarver JJ, Dishowitz MI, Kim SY, Soslowsky LJ: Transient decreases in forelimb gait and ground reaction forces following rotator cuff injury and repair in a rat model. *J Biomech* 2010;43(4):778-782.

Step length and ground reaction forces are altered immediately after rotator cuff injury and repair in a rat model but return to control levels within 4 weeks.

[23] Grumet RC, Hadley S, Diltz MV, Lee TQ, Gupta R: Development of a new model for rotator cuff pathology: The rabbit subscapularis muscle. *Acta Orthop* 2009;80(1):97-103.

The rabbit subscapularis traverses a bony tunnel, in a manner similar to the human supraspinatus tendon. The mechanical properties of the native rabbit subscapularis tendon were quantified.

[24] Longo UG, Franceschi F, Ruzzini L, et al: Histopathology of the supraspinatus tendon in rotator cuff tears. *Am J Sports Med* 2008;36(3):533-538.

Supraspinatus tendon samples taken from patients with a tear had more degeneration than those taken from control subjects.

[25] Chaudhury S, Dicko C, Burgess M, Vollrath F, Carr AJ: Fourier transform infrared spectroscopic analysis of normal and torn rotator-cuff tendons. *J Bone Joint Surg Br* 2011;93(3):370-377.

Fourier transform infrared spectroscopy revealed differences in the chemical and structural composition of normal rotator cuffs and those with a partial, small, medium, large, or massive tear.

[26] Steinbacher P, Tauber M, Kogler S, Stoiber W, Resch H, Sänger AM: Effects of rotator cuff ruptures on the cellular and intracellular composition of the human supraspinatus muscle. *Tissue Cell* 2010;42(1):37-41.

Increased muscle degeneration and fatty tissue were found in massive rotator cuff tear muscle biopsy samples.

[27] Kim HM, Dahiya N, Teefey SA, Keener JD, Galatz LM, Yamaguchi K: Relationship of tear size and location to fatty degeneration of the rotator cuff. *J Bone Joint Surg Am* 2010;92(4):829-839.

Ultrasound of patients with a rotator cuff tear revealed that larger tears and tears located at the anterior portion of the supraspinatus tendon are more likely to result in fatty degeneration of the muscle. Level of evidence: III.

[28] Melis B, DeFranco MJ, Chuinard C, Walch G: Natural history of fatty infiltration and atrophy of the supraspinatus muscle in rotator cuff tears. *Clin Orthop Relat Res* 2010;468(6):1498-1505.

A retrospective review of patients with a rotator cuff tear found a moderate level of fatty infiltration 3 years after symptoms occurred and a severe level by 5 years. Level of evidence: IV.

[29] Oh JH, Kim SH, Kim JH, Shin YH, Yoon JP, Oh CH: The level of vitamin D in the serum correlates with fatty degeneration of the muscles of the rotator cuff. *J Bone Joint Surg Br* 2009;91(12):1587-1593.

A lower serum level of vitamin D was associated with increased fatty degeneration of the muscle in patients with a rotator cuff tear.

[30] Fuchs B, Zumstein M, Regenfelder F, et al: Upregulation of alpha-skeletal muscle actin and myosin heavy polypeptide gene products in degenerating rotator cuff muscles. *J Orthop Res* 2008;26(7):1007-1011.

Reverse transcription–polymerase chain reaction on patients' supraspinatus tendon biopsies showed upregulation of α-skeletal muscle actin and myosin heavy polypeptide-1 gene transcripts, correlating with fatty degeneration.

[31] Ward SR, Sarver JJ, Eng CM, et al: Plasticity of muscle architecture after supraspinatus tears. *J Orthop Sports Phys Ther* 2010;40(11):729-735.

Several changes in supraspinatus muscle occurred after supraspinatus tendon transection in rats. All changes except muscle mass and length returned to control levels within 9 weeks.

[32] Buchmann S, Walz L, Sandmann GH, et al: Rotator cuff changes in a full thickness tear rat model: Verification of the optimal time interval until reconstruction for comparison to the healing process of chronic lesions in humans. *Arch Orthop Trauma Surg* 2011; 131(3):429-435.

Muscle and tendon degeneration occurred after detachment of the rat supraspinatus tendon. The 3-week time point mimicked several characteristics of chronic tears in humans.

[33] Farshad M, Würgler-Hauri CC, Kohler T, Gerber C, Rothenfluh DA: Effect of age on fatty infiltration of supraspinatus muscle after experimental tendon release in rats. *BMC Res Notes* 2011;4:530.

Significant fatty infiltration could not be found 6 weeks after supraspinatus tendon transection in young and old rats.

[34] Dourte LM, Perry SM, Getz CL, Soslowsky LJ: Tendon properties remain altered in a chronic rat rotator cuff

model. *Clin Orthop Relat Res* 2010;468(6):1485- 1492.

Acute detachment of the supraspinatus and infraspinatus tendons in rats caused degenerative changes similar to those in chronic tears in humans. The severity of the injury ensured that these changes were not transient.

[35] Kim HM, Galatz LM, Lim C, Havlioglu N, Thomopoulos S: The effect of tear size and nerve injury on rotator cuff muscle fatty degeneration in a rodent animal model. *J Shoulder Elbow Surg* 2012;21(7):847-858.

The addition of a suprascapular nerve transection to supraspinatus and infraspinatus tendon transections increased the fatty degeneration of the muscles in rats and mice.

[36] Rowshan K, Hadley S, Pham K, Caiozzo V, Lee TQ, Gupta R: Development of fatty atrophy after neurologic and rotator cuff injuries in an animal model of rotator cuff pathology. *J Bone Joint Surg Am* 2010; 92(13):2270-2278.

Transection of the subscapularis tendon with the addition of subscapular nerve transection in rabbits resulted in fatty atrophy of the muscle and degeneration of the nerve.

[37] Itoigawa Y, Kishimoto KN, Sano H, Kaneko K, Itoi E: Molecular mechanism of fatty degeneration in rotator cuff muscle with tendon rupture. *J Orthop Res* 2011; 29(6):861-866.

Reverse transcription–polymerase chain reaction of rotator cuff muscles with a tendon rupture revealed decreased Wnt10b expression and increased adipogenic marker genes. Wnt signaling may play a role in fatty degeneration.

[38] Perry SM, Getz CL, Soslowsky LJ: After rotator cuff tears, the remaining (intact) tendons are mechanically altered. *J Shoulder Elbow Surg* 2009;18(1):52-57.

After detachment of one or two rotator cuff tendons in a rat model, the remaining rotator cuff tendons (infraspinatus, subscapularis) exhibited signs of degeneration.

[39] Peltz CD, Perry SM, Getz CL, Soslowsky LJ: Mechanical properties of the long-head of the biceps tendon are altered in the presence of rotator cuff tears in a rat model. *J Orthop Res* 2009;27(3):416-420.

After detachment of one or two rotator cuff tendons in a rat model, the long head of the biceps tendon exhibited signs of degeneration.

[40] Peltz CD, Hsu JE, Zgonis MH, Trasolini NA, Glaser DL, Soslowsky LJ: Intra-articular changes precede extra-articular changes in the biceps tendon after rotator cuff tears in a rat model. *J Shoulder Elbow Surg* 2012;21(7):873-881.

After detachment of the supraspinatus and infraspinatus tendons in a rat model, the long head of the biceps tendon first showed signs of degeneration in the intraarticular region. Over time, these changes extended the length of the tendon.

[41] Lakemeier S, Schwuchow SA, Peterlein CD, et al: Expression of matrix metalloproteinases 1, 3, and 9 in degenerated long head biceps tendon in the presence of rotator cuff tears: An immunohistological study. *BMC Musculoskelet Disord* 2010;11:271.

Biopsy specimens of the long head of the biceps tendon from patients with a rotator cuff tear showed increased expression of MMP-1 and MMP-9 as well as decreased expression of MMP-3.

[42] Lakemeier S, Reichelt JJ, Timmesfeld N, Fuchs-Winkelmann S, Paletta JR, Schofer MD: The relevance of long head biceps degeneration in the presence of rotator cuff tears. *BMC Musculoskelet Disord* 2010; 11:191.

Biopsy specimens of the long head of the biceps tendon from patients with a rotator cuff tear showed increased VEGF expression, vessel size, and vessel density.

[43] Kijima H, Minagawa H, Saijo Y, et al: Degenerated coracoacromial ligament in shoulders with rotator cuff tears shows higher elastic modulus: Measurement with scanning acoustic microscopy. *J Orthop Sci* 2009; 14(1):62-67.

Coracoacromial ligaments from cadavers with a rotator cuff tear showed increased elastic modulus as measured with scanning acoustic microscopy.

[44] Savitskaya YA, Izaguirre A, Sierra L, et al: Effect of angiogenesis-related cytokines on rotator cuff disease: The search for sensitive biomarkers of early tendon degeneration. *Clin Med Insights Arthritis Musculoskelet Disord* 2011;4:43-53.

Patients with a rotator cuff tear had increased levels of interleukin-1β, interleukin-8, and VEGF in their blood. Angiogenin and interleukin-10 were decreased. Rotator cuff disease causes imbalances in pro- and anti-inflammatory genes and angiogenesis.

[45] Millar NL, Hueber AJ, Reilly JH, et al: Inflammation is present in early human tendinopathy. *Am J Sports Med* 2010;38(10):2085-2091.

Subscapularis tendon biopsies from patients with a torn supraspinatus show increased macrophage, mast cell, and T-cell expression. Subscapularis tendons from patients with a torn supraspinatus may be a model for early tendinopathy, and inflammation is present.

[46] Lundgreen K, Lian OB, Engebretsen L, Scott A: Tenocyte apoptosis in the torn rotator cuff: A primary or secondary pathological event? *Br J Sports Med* 2011; 45(13):1035-1039.

Supraspinatus and subscapularis tendon biopsy samples from patients with a torn supraspinatus tendon showed an increased apoptotic index. Torn supraspinatus tendons showed an increase in p53, unlike subscapularis tendons, and this finding suggests different apoptotic pathways.

[47] Millar NL, Wei AQ, Molloy TJ, Bonar F, Murrell GA: Heat shock protein and apoptosis in supraspinatus tendinopathy. *Clin Orthop Relat Res* 2008;466(7): 1569-1576.

Heat shock protein and apoptotic genes are upregulated in biopsy specimens from patients with torn supraspinatus tendons as well as rats that have undergone a supraspinatus overuse protocol.

[48] Scott A, Cook JL, Hart DA, Walker DC, Duronio V, Khan KM: Tenocyte responses to mechanical loading in vivo: A role for local insulin-like growth factor 1 signaling in early tendinosis in rats. *Arthritis Rheum* 2007;56(3):871-881.

Supraspinatus tendons from rats that underwent an overuse protocol exhibited increased local insulin-like growth factor–1 expression and phosphorylation of downstream targets insulin receptor substrate–1 and extracellular signal–related kinases–1/2.

[49] Oliva F, Barisani D, Grasso A, Maffulli N: Gene expression analysis in calcific tendinopathy of the rotator cuff. *Eur Cell Mater* 2011;21:548-557.

Biopsy specimens from patients with calcific tendinopathy of the rotator cuff showed increased expression of tissue transglutaminase–2, osteopontin, and cathepsin K as well as decreased bone morphogenetic protein–4 and –6.

[50] Thornton GM, Shao X, Chung M, et al: Changes in mechanical loading lead to tendonspecific alterations in MMP and TIMP expression: Influence of stress deprivation and intermittent cyclic hydrostatic compression on rat supraspinatus and Achilles tendons. *Br J Sports Med* 2010;44(10):698-703.

Stress deprivation in excised rat tendons caused increased MMP-13, MMP-3, and TIMP-2 expression. Intermittent cyclic hydrostatic compression caused increased MMP-13 in the excised rat supraspinatus tendon.

[51] Archambault JM, Jelinsky SA, Lake SP, Hill AA, Glaser DL, Soslowsky LJ: Rat supraspinatus tendon expresses cartilage markers with overuse. *J Orthop Res* 2007;25(5):617-624.

Supraspinatus tendons from rats that underwent an overuse protocol exhibited increased expression of several cartilage genes.

[52] Jelinsky SA, Lake SP, Archambault JM, Soslowsky LJ: Gene expression in rat supraspinatus tendon recovers from overuse with rest. *Clin Orthop Relat Res* 2008; 466(7):1612-1617.

Rest for 2 or 4 weeks after 2 or 4 weeks of an overuse protocol returned gene expression and biochemical composition to near-normal levels in rats. Collagen content remained slightly decreased.

[53] Attia M, Scott A, Duchesnay A, et al: Alterations of overused supraspinatus tendon: A possible role of glycosaminoglycans and HARP/pleiotrophin in early tendon pathology. *J Orthop Res* 2012;30(1):61-71.

Sulfated glycosaminoglycans increased after an overuse protocol was used in rats. Heparin affine regulatory peptide, a cytokine that regulates developmental chondrocyte formation, also increased, indicating the change toward a chondrocyte phenotype.

[54] Tashjian RZ, Farnham JM, Albright FS, Teerlink CC, Cannon-Albright LA: Evidence for an inherited predisposition contributing to the risk for rotator cuff disease. *J Bone Joint Surg Am* 2009;91(5):1136-1142.

Review of the Utah Population Database revealed that patients diagnosed with rotator cuff disease before age 40 years had relatedness in close and distant relationships, suggesting a genetic predisposition. Level of evidence: III.

[55] Benson RT, McDonnell SM, Knowles HJ, Rees JL, Carr AJ, Hulley PA: Tendinopathy and tears of the rotator cuff are associated with hypoxia and apoptosis. *J Bone Joint Surg Br* 2010;92(3):448-453.

Biopsies from patients with different stages of rotator cuff impingement or tearing revealed alterations in HIF-1α and BNip3 expression and apoptosis, depending on the stage.

[56] Lakemeier S, Reichelt JJ, Patzer T, Fuchs-Winkelmann S, Paletta JR, Schofer MD: The association between retraction of the torn rotator cuff and increasing expression of hypoxia inducible factor 1α and vascular endothelial growth factor expression: An

immunohistological study. *BMC Musculoskelet Disord* 2010; 11:230.

Biopsies from patients with a torn rotator cuff revealed increased HIF and VEGF expression, fatty infiltration, and muscular atrophy. Vessel density was correlated with tendon retraction.

[57] Lakemeier S, Braun J, Efe T, et al: Expression of matrix metalloproteinases 1, 3, and 9 in differing extents of tendon retraction in the torn rotator cuff. *Knee Surg Sports Traumatol Arthrosc* 2011;19(10):1760-1765.

Biopsy samples from patients with a torn rotator cuff revealed increased MMP-1 and MMP-9 as well as decreased MMP-3. MMP-9 expression was correlated with tendon retraction.

[58] Shindle MK, Chen CC, Robertson C, et al: Fullthickness supraspinatus tears are associated with more synovial inflammation and tissue degeneration than partial-thickness tears. *J Shoulder Elbow Surg* 2011; 20(6):917-927.

Samples from patients' synovium, bursa, torn supraspinatus tendon, and subscapularis tendon revealed that synovial inflammation and tissue degeneration increased with tear size.

[59] Würgler-Hauri CC, Dourte LM, Baradet TC, Williams GR, Soslowsky LJ: Temporal expression of 8 growth factors in tendon-to-bone healing in a rat supraspinatus model. *J Shoulder Elbow Surg* 2007;16(5, suppl): S198-S203.

Examination of the differential temporal expression of growth factors revealed a peak 1 week postoperatively and a second surge of some factors during remodeling.

[60] Galatz LM, Charlton N, Das R, Kim HM, Havlioglu N, Thomopoulos S: Complete removal of load is detrimental to rotator cuff healing. *J Shoulder Elbow Surg* 2009;18(5):669-675.

In a rat model, the use of botulinum toxin A and casting was found to be inferior to botulinum toxin A alone, which was inferior to casting alone.

[61] Hettrich CM, Rodeo SA, Hannafin JA, Ehteshami J, Shubin Stein BE: The effect of muscle paralysis using Botox on the healing of tendon to bone in a rat model. *J Shoulder Elbow Surg* 2011;20(5):688-697.

Botulinum toxin A had a positive effect on early collagen alignment but a negative effect on later crosssectional area and load to failure.

[62] Gamradt SC, Gallo RA, Adler RS, et al: Vascularity of the supraspinatus tendon three months after repair: Characterization using contrast-enhanced ultrasound. *J*

Shoulder Elbow Surg 2010;19(1):73-80.

A new technique was successful in characterizing blood flow to the region of interest and suggests the importance of vascular considerations during surgery.

[63] Oh JH, Kim SH, Kang JY, Oh CH, Gong HS: Effect of age on functional and structural outcome after rotator cuff repair. *Am J Sports Med* 2010;38(4):672-678.

Multivariate regression was used to show that age is merely correlated with poor surgical outcomes and is not necessarily a causal factor. Level of evidence: IV.

[64] Gladstone JN, Bishop JY, Lo IK, Flatow EL: Fatty infiltration and atrophy of the rotator cuff do not improve after rotator cuff repair and correlate with poor functional outcome. *Am J Sports Med* 2007;35(5): 719-728.

Multivariate analysis revealed the influence and persistence of fatty deposits and reduced muscularity. Level of evidence: II.

[65] Sarver JJ, Peltz CD, Dourte L, Reddy S, Williams GR, Soslowsky LJ: After rotator cuff repair, stiffness—but not the loss in range of motion—increased transiently for immobilized shoulders in a rat model. *J Shoulder Elbow Surg* 2008;17(1, suppl):S108-S113.

A novel device was created for measuring joint stiffness, and the effects of plaster casts were evaluated.

[66] Trudel G, Ramachandran N, Ryan SE, Rakhra K, Uhthoff HK: Supraspinatus tendon repair into a bony trough in the rabbit: Mechanical restoration and correlative imaging. *J Orthop Res* 2010;28(6):710-715.

CT was found useful for predicting restoration of mechanical properties shortly after surgery. Given the importance of the rapid healing reaction, minimal postoperative loading is recommended.

[67] Baring TK, Cashman PP, Reilly P, Emery RJ, Amis AA: Rotator cuff repair failure in vivo: A radiostereometric measurement study. J Shoulder Elbow Surg 2011; 20(8):1194-1199.

Metallic bone and tendon marker migration provides new insight into temporal and activity-based rates of retearing.

[68] Hsu JE, Reuther KE, Sarver JJ, et al: Restoration of anterior-posterior rotator cuff force balance improves shoulder function in a rat model of chronic massive tears. *J Orthop Res* 2011;29(7):1028-1033.

A new in vivo model of two-tendon repair suggests that in a massive tear, surgical repair of the infraspinatus may be sufficient only for restoring functionality.

[69] Andarawis-Puri N, Kuntz AF, Ramsey ML, Soslowsky

LJ: Effect of supraspinatus tendon repair technique on the infraspinatus tendon. *J Biomech Eng* 2011;133(3): 031008.

Cadaver shoulders revealed a decreased recruitment of the infraspinatus at high loads when arthroscopic repair was used, compared with open transosseous repair.

[70] Gimbel JA, Van Kleunen JP, Williams GR, Thomopoulos S, Soslowsky LJ: Long durations of immobilization in the rat result in enhanced mechanical properties of the healing supraspinatus tendon insertion site. *J Biomech Eng* 2007;129(3):400-404.

Immobilization was found to lead to early improvement in collagen organization and later improvement in mechanical properties.

[71] Peltz CD, Dourte LM, Kuntz AF, et al: The effect of postoperative passive motion on rotator cuff healing in a rat model. *J Bone Joint Surg Am* 2009;91(10):2421-2429.

The negative effect of passive motion on range of motion was attributed to increased scar formation.

[72] Peltz CD, Sarver JJ, Dourte LM, Würgler-Hauri CC, Williams GR, Soslowsky LJ: Exercise following a short immobilization period is detrimental to tendon properties and joint mechanics in a rat rotator cuff injury model. *J Orthop Res* 2010;28(7):841-845.

This study provided cautionary evidence about postoperative exercise.

[73] Lee BG, Cho NS, Rhee YG: Effect of two rehabilitation protocols on range of motion and healing rates after arthroscopic rotator cuff repair: Aggressive versus limited early passive exercises. *Arthroscopy* 2012; 28(1):34-42.

Early aggressive exercise led to improvement in scores after 3 months but not after 1 year, and it may increase the risk of retearing. Level of evidence: II.

[74] Szczurko O, Cooley K, Mills EJ, Zhou Q, Perri D, Seely D: Naturopathic treatment of rotator cuff tendinitis among Canadian postal workers: A randomized controlled trial. *Arthritis Rheum* 2009;61(8):1037- 1045.

Acupuncture, diet, and supplements were found to benefit patients with rotator cuff tendinitis. Level of evidence: I.

第三章　肩袖愈合的生物强化

Kathleen A. Derwin, PhD; David Kovacevic, MD; Myung-Sun Kim, MD, PhD; Eric T. Ricchetti, MD

引言

肩袖撕裂至少影响 40% 的 60 岁以上人群，是导致肩部疼痛、功能减退和无力的常见原因。在美国，每年进行超过 25 万次的肩袖修复。[1]尽管对疾病过程的理解更加深入了，手术治疗也取得了进展，但肩袖修复后的愈合仍然是一项重大的临床挑战。文献报道的修复失败的发生率为 20%~70%，与患者的年龄、撕裂范围、撕裂迁延程度、肌肉萎缩、肌肉变性、肌腱质量、修复技术和术后康复有关。[2-4]需要通过机械强化来促进修复，增强肌腱内在的生物学愈合潜力。为了改善肩袖修复的愈合情况和（或）诱导功能性组织再生，研究者们已经对支架、富血小板血浆（platelet-rich plasma，PRP）、特定生长因子和细胞种植等组织工程策略进行了探索。

支架

在过去的 10 年中，来自哺乳动物细胞外基质

Dr. Derwin or an immediate family member has received royalties from the Musculoskeletal Transplant Foundation; has received nonincome support (such as equipment or services), commercially derived honoraria, or other non-research-related funding (such as paid travel) from the Musculoskeletal Transplant Foundation; and serves as a board member, owner, officer, or committee member of the Orthopaedic Research Society. None of the following authors or any immediate family member has received anything of value from or has stock or stock options held in a commercial company or institution related directly or indirectly to the subject of this chapter: Dr. Kovacevic, Dr. Kim, and Dr. Ricchetti.

（ECM）和（或）由合成聚合物构成的支架已被 FDA 批准作为用于人体肩袖修复的医疗设备上市。使用支架进行肩袖修复的基本原理包括支架可在修复后使肩袖即刻承担机械负荷并可在术后愈合阶段增加修复肌腱的机械强度，或通过提高肌腱愈合的速度和质量来增强肌腱的机械强度。特别是细胞外基质衍生的支架被认为可通过其自然组成、三维结构和重塑生物分子为宿主细胞提供化学和结构上的引导性环境。[5-6]虽然合成聚合物支架可能不会影响修复愈合的生物学，但它可以长时间保持其机械性能，机械性地稳定修复构筑物，直到宿主组织愈合完成。

商用支架

合成聚合物支架和非人类来源的细胞外基质支架通过了 FDA 的 510（K）监管程序，在人体中使用没有明显的风险，已被批准作为医疗设备使用。FDA 的 510（K）监管程序证明，这些支架在性能、生物相容性、安全性、稳定性、无菌性和包装方面均与所宣称的相符。不需要强制要求通过临床前研究或受控的人体临床研究证实疗效。这些支架已被 FDA 批准为增强装置，用于加强肩袖手术期间的缝合或缝合锚钉修复。与以上两种支架相反，人类来源的细胞外基质支架被划入用于移植的人体组织（21 CFR，Pt. 1270），并且不需要 FDA 批准即可使用。表 3-1 列出了具有 FDA 认证的用于肩袖修复的商用支架。

支架使用的基础科学研究

应用支架修复肩袖的基础科学研究通过体外

表 3-1

具有 FDA 认证的、用于肩袖修复的商用支架

产品	支架类型	支架材料	供货商家
Restore Orthobiologic Implant	细胞外基质	猪小肠黏膜下层	DePuy（Warsaw, IN）
CuffPatch	细胞外基质	猪小肠黏膜下层（交联）	Organogenesis（Canton, MA）
GraftJacket	细胞外基质	人真皮	Wright Medical（Arlinton, TX）
ArthroFlex	细胞外基质	人真皮	Arthrex（Naples, FL）
Conexa	细胞外基质	猪真皮（α 半乳糖还原）	Tornier（Montbonnot, France）
Zimmer Collagen Repair	细胞外基质	猪真皮（交联）	Zimmer（Warsaw, IN）
TissueMend	细胞外基质	牛真皮（胎牛）	Stryker（Mahwah, NJ）
BioBLanket	细胞外基质	牛真皮（交联）	Kensey Nash（Exton, PA）
OrthADAPT Bioimplant	细胞外基质	马心包膜（交联）	Pegasus Biologics（Irvine, CA）
OrthADAPT PR Bioimplant	细胞外基质 + 合成聚合物	马心包膜（交联）含聚醚醚酮纤维	Pegasus Biologics
SportMesh Soft Tissue Reinforcement	合成聚合物	聚氨酯	Biomet Sports Medicine（Warsaw, IN）
X-Repair	合成聚合物	聚 –L– 丙交酯	Synthasome（San Diego, CA）
Biomerix RCR Patch	合成聚合物	聚碳酸酯聚氨酯 – 尿素	Biomerix（Fremont, CA）

实验和动物模型评估支架的宿主反应、重塑特征、生物力学及实际适用性等。[7] 细胞外基质支架在宿主中引起不同的组织学和形态学反应。这些反应取决于支架的物种来源、组织来源、加工方法、终端灭菌方法和机械负载环境等。宿主对细胞外基质支架的免疫反应主要由巨噬细胞成分参与。巨噬细胞成分似乎是一个关键的决定因素，它也许是小肠黏膜下层（SIS）应用成功并产生结构性重塑的预测因子，SIS 是一种可被快速（在几天到几周内）吸收的细胞外基质。目前，对于使用细胞外基质材料（如真皮）时的免疫细胞的作用知之甚少，这些材料经历较慢的重塑过程，并且在一定程度上可被宿主的组织侵入。应用交联细胞外基质支架会出现异物巨细胞、慢性炎症和（或）致密的不良的纤维组织累积。宿主对合成聚合物支架的反应的持续时间和强度由合成聚合物支架的生物材料组成和形态（大小、形状、孔隙度和粗糙度）决定，并且也可能由植入部位的生物学

和机械因素决定。细胞外基质支架或合成聚合物支架修复肩袖的动物模型研究普遍报道了良好的组织学结果和肌腱样重塑。

支架的材料、形状和缝合保持性能影响其在手术植入后对被修复肌腱的机械性能的增强程度。支架应用的注意事项，包括固定缝线的数量、类型和位置，以及修复时的支架预张紧，均与支架的性能表现相关。重要的是要注意，支架降解预计在手术植入后的几天到几周内发生，降解的速度和程度取决于支架的类型和重塑特征。降解导致机械强度损失，但宿主组织的沉积和重塑可以强化修复。大多数支架在重塑过程中的各个细节，包括支架降解、融合和宿主组织沉积的速度和程度等，目前还没有完全明确。

应用支架修复肩袖的临床研究

细胞外基质支架中的第一批临床研究对象是非交联猪 SIS（Restore Orthobiologic Implant, DePuy）[8-11]。在两项研究中，20%~30% 的患者术

后出现严重的非细菌性炎症反应[10-11]。基于这种并发症，美国骨科医师学会（AAOS）不推荐使用非交联猪 SIS（Restore Orthobiologic Implant，Depay）治疗人类肩袖撕裂。[12] 使用非交联人真皮支架（例如，GraftJacket，Wright Medical）作为增强和介入装置的回顾性随访研究报道，患者的术后情况与术前情况相比有所改善，但这些研究未设置实验组与对照组（接受非加强修复的患者）进行比较（表3-2）。[13-17] 两个小的回顾性病例研究报道了交联真皮支架（Zimmer Collagen Repair，Zimmer）的临床使用效果，结果存在差异（表3-2）。[18-19] 一项前瞻性随机对照研究调查了 GraftJacket 用于加强慢性双肌腱撕裂修复的情况。研究发现，肩袖加强修复患者的美国肩肘外科协会（ASES）肩关节疼痛和功能障碍评分及 Constant 肩关节评分的得分明显优于非加强修复患者的得分，并且治愈率也明显高于非加强修复患者。[20] 在术后第1年或第2年随访时，钆增强磁共振关节造影显示 85% 的加强修复是完整的，而仅有 40% 的非加强修复是完整的。未观察到与人脱细胞真皮基质相关的不良事件。这些研究结果支持对用于治疗肩袖撕裂的非交联真皮衍生支架的进一步研究。

只有一项使用合成聚合物支架修复肩袖的临床研究被报道[2]。将聚碳酸酯聚氨酯 - 尿素 Biomerix RCR Patch（Biomerix）作为一种增强装置用于 10 例接受冈上肌腱或冈下肌腱全层撕裂（平均撕裂大小为 2 cm）开放性修复的患者，并对这种合成聚合物支架的术后效果进行了评价。[21] 在术后 1 年的随访中，结果评分有显著改善。超声和 MRI 显示 10% 的修复失败。然而，该研究缺乏用于比较的对照组，特别是仅有少数患者发生修复失败，这意味着很难确定移植物的确切效果。本研究中的平均撕裂大小为小到中等大小的撕裂，这种程度的撕裂可能不像大的或大量撕裂那样通常需要加强修复。

目前有几种支架可供骨科医师用于肩袖修复。无论是何种肩袖修复支架，其独特的物理、化学和（或）生物学特征及使用方式均对支架的有效性具有关键作用。只有两项前瞻性随机对照研究采用了一部分商用支架[10,20]，目前，许多支架都没有可用的同行评议的临床数据可以参考。由于缺乏临床

表3-2

肩袖修复支架的临床研究

产品	研究发表（年份）	证据等级和研究类型	撕裂程度（病例数）	手术类型/支架应用技术
GraftJacket	Burkhead 等[13]（2007）	Ⅳ级，回顾性病例研究	大量（17）	开放/加强
	Dopirak 等[14]（2007）	Ⅳ级，回顾性病例研究	大量，非修复性（16）	关节镜/中间放置
	Bond 等[15]（2008）Wong 等[16]（2010）（Bond 等[15]更新）	Ⅳ级，回顾性病例研究	大量，非修复性（45）	关节镜/中间放置
	Barber 等[20]（2012）	Ⅱ级，前瞻性随机对照研究	慢性双肌腱撕裂 > 3 cm（加强，22；非加强，20）	关节镜/加强
Acellular human dermal matrix	Rotini 等（2011）	Ⅳ级，回顾性病例研究	大或大量（2）大或大量（3）	关节镜/加强和中间放置开放/加强和中间放置
Zimmer Collagen Repair	Soler 等[18]（2007）	Ⅳ级，回顾性病例研究	大量（4）	开放/中间放置
	Badhe 等[19]（2008）	Ⅳ级，回顾性病例研究	大或大量（10）	开放/中间放置
Biomerix RCR Patch	ENcalada-Diaz 等[21]（2011）	Ⅳ级，回顾性病例研究	小或中等，平均 2 cm（10）	开放/加强

表 3-2

肩袖修复支架的临床研究（续）

随访时间	MRI 或超声失败率	评分系统及平均分数	结果
14 个月	3/12	UCLA: 术前 9.06, 随访 26.12	无不良事件报告 评分、力量和运动范围有所改善 17 例患者中有 14 例对结果满意 再撕裂的范围较术前 MRI 小
12~38 个月	3/16	UCLA: 术前 18.4, 随访 30.4 Constant: 术前 53.8, 随访 84	无不良事件报告 评分、疼痛、力量和运动范围有所改善 16 例患者中有 15 例对结果满意 13 例患者的 MRI 显示移植物完全侵入正常组织
24~68 个月		UCLA: 术前 18.4, 随访 27.5 WORC: 随访 75.2 ASES: 随访 84.1	1 例患者出现深部伤口感染（免疫力下降）需要进行关节镜灌洗、清创和抗生素治疗 1 例患者长期存在神经失用症状，症状在 1 年后消失 手术时间均小于 3 小时
12~38 个月	加强组 3/20 非加强组 9/15	UCLA: 加强组随访 28.2, 非加强组随访 28.3 Constant: 加强组随访 91.9, 非加强组随访 85.3 ASES: 加强组随访 98.9, 非加强组随访 94.8	无不良事件报告 与非加强组相比较，加强组患者的 Constant 和 ASES 及 MRI 下关节愈合率均显著增加
12~18 个月	2/5	Constant: 术前 64, 随访 88	无不良事件报告 修复后的 MRI 显示移植物完全侵入天然组织
3~6 个月	4/4	未报告	老年患者（71~82 岁） 所有患者在术后 3~6 个月均出现移植物脱离 所有患者均出现炎症反应，并且在翻修手术时被发现存在移植物崩解和组织坏死
3~5 年	2/10	Constant: 术前 42, 随访 62	无不良事件报告 评分、疼痛、运动范围有改善 10 例患者中有 9 例对结果满意
12 个月	1/10	ASES: 术前 44, 随访 73 UCLA: 随访 29.2 SST: 术前 3.6, 随访 7.7	相对小的撕裂（冈上肌单腱撕裂或冈下肌单腱撕裂） 无不良事件报告 评分、疼痛和运动范围有所改善

注：ASES=ASES 肩关节疼痛和功能障碍评分（100 分），Constant=Constant 肩关节评分（100 分），SST= 肩关节简明测试（12 分），UCLA= 美国加利福尼亚大学洛杉矶分校肩关节评分（35 分），WORC= 加拿大西安大略肩袖指数（100 分）。

证据，AAOS 尚未提出支持或反对使用同种软组织移植物或异种软组织移植物治疗肩袖撕裂患者的建议。[12] 要回答与这些设备相关的许多问题，如它们的适应证、手术应用、安全性、作用机制和疗效等，需要设计良好的随机对照研究。

PRP

临床对血小板浓缩物的关注可以追溯到 1954 年，当时有证据表明 PRP 中存在凝血因子拮抗剂。[22] 目前，美国国家医学图书馆（PubMed）数据库中有超过 6000 条关于 PRP 的引文，并且在这些文献中几乎有一半是在过去十几年内发表的。最近的重点是血小板浓缩物在愈合中的生物学潜力。这种血液制品已在牙科、口腔颌面外科、整形外科和矫形外科中用于促进损伤后和修复后的愈合。[23-26] 广泛使用 PRP 的基本原理是，浓缩促进愈合的生长因子，并将它们重新引入损伤部位，从而增强组织再生中的细胞募集、增殖和分化。[27]

定义和制备注意事项

PRP 是一种自体血液衍生制品，每微升 PRP 至少含有 100 万个血小板，比正常血液基线水平高 4~7 倍。[28] 然而，这个简单的定义并不能准确地反映不同类型的 PRP 配方之间的差异。一种新的定性分类系统比较了血小板浓缩物，并依据组成提出了一些术语。[29] 根据白细胞含量、外源性血小板活化情况和是否存在强力纤维蛋白网架，可定义 6 类血小板浓缩物（表 3-3）。白细胞的存在意味着制备的血小板浓缩物不仅含有促进损伤部位愈合的生长因子，还含有炎症细胞因子和 MMPs。[30]

表 3-3

血小板浓缩物定性分类系统

血小板浓缩物	是否含有白细胞	是否出现外源性血小板活化	是否存在强力纤维蛋白网架
纯富 PRP	否	否	否
富白细胞富 PRP	是	否	否
纯富 PRP 凝胶	否	是	否
富白细胞血小板血浆凝胶	是	是	否
纯富血小板纤维蛋白	否	是	是
富白细胞血小板纤维蛋白	是	是	是

注：经允许引自 Dohan Ehrenfest DM, Bielecki T, Mishra A, et al: In search of a consensus terminology in the field of platelet concentrates for surgical use: Platelet-rich plasma（PRP），platelet-rich fibrin（PRF），fibrin gel polymerization and leukocytes. *Curr Pharm Biotechnol* 2012;13（7）:1131-1137.

在损伤部位外源性应用氯化钙或凝血酶后立即注射血小板浓缩物，通过 α 颗粒使血小板活化、凝块形成和生长因子释放。[28] 普遍认为大约 70% 的存储生长因子在 10 分钟内释放，并且接近 100% 的生长因子在 1 小时内释放。[31] 生长因子的释放可以通过产生富血小板纤维蛋白（PRF）基质来延迟。氯化钙存在下的第二次离心可将纤维蛋白原转化为纤维蛋白。致密的纤维蛋白基质捕获完整的血小板，以使生长因子缓慢释放 5~7 天。[28] 了解血小板浓缩物的细胞组成、生长因子浓度和基质结构有助于临床医师和研究者评估商业制剂配方及其临床应用情况。例如，某种类型的血小板浓缩物可能对治疗特定的肌肉骨骼疾病最为有效。

商用血小板浓缩物制备系统

血小板浓缩物是通过离心患者的外周静脉血获得的，是悬浮在一定体积血浆中的血小板浓缩制剂。[32] 目前有超过 16 种商用血小板浓缩物制备系统。[33] 这些系统在制备方案、血小板捕获效率、白细胞含量、激活剂的使用和生长因子含量（表 3-4）等方面各不相同，所以它们制备的血小板浓缩物的配方存在明显不同。患者之间固有的生物差异性可能导致在使用同一个系统生产的血小板浓缩物时效果存在显著差异。[34] 在用同一制备系统制备的来自同一个体的血小板浓缩物中有可能白细胞和血小板数量存在着显著的变化，并且也有可能出现一些患者的血小板不能被某一个制备系统浓缩，但能被另一个制备系统成功浓缩的情况。[30,34] 血小板浓缩物制备质量和患者反应的广泛差异无疑会影响血小板浓缩物对组织愈合的生物效应。研究人员和临床医师必须设法识别、量化和记录每位患者的血小板浓缩物中存在的成分，以便研究其在结缔组织愈合再生疗法中的效果。

表 3-4

商用血小板浓缩物制备系统的特性

系统（商家）	血液量（ml）	方法	离心时间 / 速度	PRP（ml）
Cascade Medical FIBRINET（Musculoskeletal Transplant Foundation, Edison,NJ）	9~18	PRP: 单离心 PRFM: 双离心	PRP:6 min/1100×g PRFM:6 min/1100×g+ 15 min/1450×g	4~9
Gravitational Platelet Separation（GPS）Ⅲ（Biomet）	27~110	单离心	15 min/1900×g	3~12
Autologous Conditioned Plasma-Double Syringe（ACP-DS）（Arthrex）	9	单离心	5 min/1500 rpm	3
SmartPReP（Harvest Technologies,Plymouth,MA）	20~120	双离心	14 min/1000×g	3~20
Magellan（Medtronic, Minneapolis,MN）	30~60	双离心	4~6 min/1200×g	6
Plasma Rich in Growth Factors-Endoret（PRGF-Endoret）;（BTI Biotechnology, Blue Bell,PA）	9~72	单离心	8 min/580×g	4~32

注：PRFM= 富血小板纤维蛋白基质或膜（取决于全血容量和第二次离心的持续时间）。离心设备的速度参数常用"每分钟转数（单位：rpm）"或"离心力（常以重力加速度的倍数形式表示）"来表示。

使用血小板浓缩物的基础科学研究

在手术时应用血小板浓缩物有助于加强修复组织的局部生物学行为，因为血小板通常在愈合的早期炎症阶段参与组织稳态调节和血栓形成。血小板含有 α 颗粒，脱颗粒时会释放黏附蛋白、凝血因子和生长因子。血浆由许多蛋白质、电解质和激素组成。[27,30]血小板浓缩物含有高浓度的生长因子（如血小板衍生生长因子、血管源性生长因子、转化生长因子 –β1、碱性成纤维细胞生长因子、表皮生长因子、肝细胞生长因子和胰岛素样生长因子 –1），这些生长因子已知在细胞的增殖、分化和趋化，血管的生成以及细胞外基质的产生中发挥作用。此外，这些生长因子可以影响肌腱愈合（表 3-4）。[27,32-33,35]

关于血小板浓缩物对肌腱愈合的影响，已有几个关键的基础科学发现。体外研究均发现血小板浓缩物对培养的肌腱细胞的基因表达和基质合成有积极影响。[36-38]动物模型研究发现，使用血小板浓缩物可以促进肌腱愈合。在大鼠跟腱切除模型中，与应用缺乏血小板的血浆或生理盐水相比，在损伤部位应用同种异体 PRP 凝胶可使损伤部位有更好的机械性能。[39-40]在家兔模型中，与对照组相比，使用 PRP 凝胶加强髌腱缺损修复可使新生的血管化组织更加成熟和致密。[41]在犬模型中，用富血小板纤维蛋白（platelet-rich fibrin, PRF）加强损伤修复并不能提高损伤部位的组织愈合率或组织学质量。[42]虽然基础科学文献总体上支持血小板浓缩物具有增强肌腱愈合的潜力这一观点，但是，要发挥血小板浓缩物的潜在疗效，在其使用时间、浓度和配方的合理选择方面，还有很多问题需要解决。

血小板浓缩物用于肩袖修复的临床研究

对美国国家医学图书馆和 Cochrane 协作数据库进行电子搜索，使用搜索词"PRP"和"肩袖"检出了 8 项临床研究，这些研究报道了血小

表 3-4

商用血小板浓缩物制备系统的特性（续）

最终血小板浓度	是否含有白细胞	激活剂	抗凝剂	生长因子水平
1~1.5 倍	否	氯化钙	柠檬酸钠	PDGF：N/A EGF：5~10 倍 VEGF：5~10 倍 TGF-β1：5~10 倍 IGF-1：5~10 倍
3~8 倍	是	氯化钙 / 自体凝血酶	ACD-A	PDGF：N/A EGF：3.9 倍 VEGF：6.2 倍 TGF-β1：3.6 倍 IGF-1：1 倍
2~3 倍	否	无	ACD-A	PDGF：25 倍 EGF：5 倍 VEGF：11 倍 TGF-β1：4 倍 IGF-1：1 倍
4~6 倍	是	氯化钙 / 牛凝血酶	ACD-A	PDGF：4.4 倍 EGF：4.4 倍 VEGF：4.4 倍 TGF-β1：4.4 倍 IGF-1：N/A
3~7 倍	是	氯化钙	ACD-A	—
2~3 倍	否	氯化钙	柠檬酸钠	—

注：ACD-A= 抗凝剂柠檬酸葡萄糖溶液 A；EGF= 表皮生长因子；IGF-1= 胰岛素样生长因子 -1；N/A= 未知；PDGF= 血小板衍生生长因子；TGF-β1= 转化生长因子 -β1；VEGF= 血管内皮生长因子。经允许引自 Hall MP, Band PA, Meislin RJ, Jazrawi LM, Cardone DA: Platelet-rich plasma: Current concepts and application in sports medicine. *J Am Acad Orthop Surg* 2009;17（10）: 602-608. 及 Castillo TN, Pouliot MA, Kim HJ, Dragoo JL: Comparison of growth factor and platelet concentration from commercial platelet-rich plasma separation systems. *Am J Sports Med* 2011;39（2）: 266-271; Lopez-Vidriero E, Goulding KA, Simon DA, Sanchez M, Johnson DH: The use of platelet-rich plasma in arthroscopy and sports medicine: Optimizing the healing environment. *Arthroscopy* 2010;26（2）: 269-278.

板浓缩物在肩袖修复中的使用。其中 6 项研究提供了 Ⅰ级、Ⅱ级或Ⅲ级证据。这些研究的设计和结果总结于表 3-5 中。这 6 项研究中有 4 项使用了 Cascade Medical FIBRINET 系统（美国肌肉骨骼移植基金会）创建 PRF 矩阵，在关节镜下修复小到大的肩袖撕裂期间将该 PRF 矩阵插入肌腱 - 骨界面。[43-46] 与未接受 PRF 治疗的患者相比，没有一项研究报道接受 PRF 治疗的患者在最后的随访中有更好的功能结果。有两项研究使用 MRI 或超声检查来评估肌腱愈合，发现无论患者是否接受 PRF 治疗，再撕裂率没有差异。[43,46] 有一项研究发现，接受 PRF 治疗的患者的再撕裂率明显较高[45]，也有一项研究发现，在未接受 PRF 治疗的患者中，再撕裂率明显较高。[44] 而另一项研究却发现，两组患者在最终再撕裂率上没有组间差异，但接受 PRF 治疗的患者的肌腱信号强度确实有显著改善，且在接受 PRF 治疗的患者中，完全修复者的肌腱有增大的趋势。[43] 这些结果表明 PRF 对肩袖愈合有积极作用。[47] 相反，另一项研究发现 PRF 治疗是修复术后第 12 周时肌腱缺损的重要预测因子，这一发现表明 PRF 对肩袖肌腱愈合有负面影响。[46]

表 3-5

血小板浓缩物用于肩袖修复的临床研究

系统（厂商）	研究发表（年份）	证据等级和研究类型	手术修复类型/撕裂大小和类型	血小板浓缩物应用（病例数）
Cascade Medical FIBRINET（Musculoskeletal Transplant Foundation）	Castricini 等[43]（2011）Arnoczky[47]（2011）	Ⅰ级，前瞻性随机对照研究	关节镜双列 小到中等冈上肌撕裂	对照组（45）将 PRF 置于肌腱 - 骨界面（43）
	Bergeson 等[45]（2012）	Ⅲ级，病例对照研究	关节镜，单列或双列 1~3 个肌腱撕裂≥ 2 cm	对照组（21）将 2 个 PRF 构件置于肌腱 - 骨界面（16）
	Barber 等[44]（2011）	Ⅲ级，病例对照研究	关节镜，单列 /1~2 个肌腱撕裂，1~5 cm	对照组（20）将 2 个 PRF 构件置于肌腱 - 骨界面（20）
	Rodeo 等[46]（2012）	Ⅰ级，前瞻性随机对照研究	关节镜，单列或双列 / 小到大撕裂	对照组（39）将 PRF 构件置于肌腱 - 骨界面（40）
Gravitational Platelet Separation（GPS）Ⅲ（Biomet）	Randelli 等[48]（2011）	Ⅰ级，前瞻性随机对照研究	关节镜，单列 /1~3 个肌腱撕裂	对照组（27）将 PRF 注射于肌腱 - 骨修复位点（26）
COBE Spectra LRS Turbo（CaridianBCT, Lakewood,CO）	Jo 等[49]（2011）	Ⅱ级，前瞻性队列研究	关节镜缝合桥技术 / 小到巨大撕裂	对照组（23）将 3 个贫白细胞 PRP 凝胶置于肌腱 - 骨界面（19）

6 项研究中有 2 项使用了血小板浓缩物配方，而不是 Cascade Medical FIBRINET 系统。在一项随机研究中，在关节镜下修复 1~3 个肌腱撕裂时，将重力血小板分离（GPS）Ⅲ系统（Biomet）制备的 PRF 注射于肌腱 – 骨界面[48]。接受 PRF 治疗的患者疼痛的改善早于未接受 PRF 治疗的患者。接受 PRF 治疗的患者在术后第 3 个月时的力量和功能结果评分较好，但在术后第 6 个月时则不然。MRI 显示两组在术后 2 年的再撕裂率没有差异。一项前瞻性队列研究评估了用 COBE Spectra LRS Turbo 系统（CaridianBCT，Lakewood，CO）制备的 PRP 凝胶[49]。该研究在关节镜下修复小到大的肌腱撕裂时，于肌腱 – 骨界面植入 3 种 PRP 凝胶。对照组患者在术后第 3 个月时功能结果评分有所改善，但术后第 3 个月后两组患者在力量、活动范围或功能结果评分方面无组间差异。在术后平均 20 个月的随访中，两组患者在总体满意度或治愈率方面没有组间差异。

现有的临床数据没有提供血小板浓缩物用于肩袖修复再生疗法的有效性的确凿证据。在早期随访中，没有发现使用血小板浓缩物治疗的患者的功能结果或愈合率与对照组存在差异。从现有的临床数据中得出关于血小板浓缩物疗效的结论尚有困难，因为不同的研究在撕裂大小、修复技术、血小板浓缩特性（血小板浓度、白细胞含量、纤维蛋白结构和生长因子水平）、应用技术和康复方案等方面存在很大差异。现有的研究受到样本量相对较小、成像结果具有主观性，功能结果评估方法多样以及血小板浓缩物表征有限或缺失的限制。需要适度强化Ⅰ级或Ⅱ级研究，对以上变量进行记录并在可行的范围内控制变量。在肩袖修复领域，关于血小板浓缩物的使用时机、剂量、应用方式和配方的影响，仍有许多问题有待研究。

虽然临床研究报道使用血小板浓缩物的并发症很少，但有一项研究报道了 2 例需要再次手术的切口深部感染患者，这 2 例患者在肩袖修复期

表 3-5

血小板浓缩物用于肩袖修复的临床研究（续）

平均随访时间（月）	MRI 或超声失败率	评分系统：末次随访平均分	结果
20.2（范围 16~30）	4/38（10.5%） 1/40（2.5%）	Constant:PRF 88.4, C 88.4	与再撕裂率组的常量评分无显著差异 完全修复组的 MRI 信号强度评分显著改善
27（范围 18~45）	8/21（38.1%） 9/16（56.3%）	ASES:PRF 87,C 84 Constant:PRF 73,C 76	所有测量结果均无组间差异 PRF 治疗组的再撕裂率显著升高
13（范围 3~19）		UCLA:PRF 29,C 29 WORC:PRF 80,C 82 SANE:PRF 89,C 87	2 例 PRF 治疗患者发生痤疮丙酸杆菌深部感染，需要灌洗切口和清创
33（范围 24~44）	12/20（60%） 6/20（30%）	ASES:PRF 95.7,C 94.7 Constant:PRF 88.1,PC 84.7	PRF 治疗组的 ROWE 显著升高，但其他评分在组间无显著差异
28.3（范围 24~44）		SST:PRF 11.3,C 11.4 SANE:PRF 94.5,C 93.7 ROWE:PRF 94.9,C 84.8	对照组的再撕裂率显著升高
12	6/31（19.4%） 12/36（33.3%）	ASES:PRF 91.30,C 96.43 L'Insalata:PRF 90.39, C 94.11	所有力量评估结果均无组间差异 再撕裂率无显著组间差异 PRF 回归分析是再撕裂的显著预测指标
24	12/23（52.2%） 9/22（40.9%）	Constant:PRF 82.4,C 78.7 UCLA:PRF 33.3,C 31.2 SST:PRF 11.3,C 10.9	PRF 治疗组术后 1 个月内疼痛显著减轻，3 个月时外旋力和所有评分均显著增高 第 6、12 和 24 个月随访时的外旋力均无组间差异 小撕裂患者使用 PRF 治疗，第 3、6、12 和 24 个月随访时的外旋力均显著增加 再撕裂率无组间差异 修复程度与年龄、撕裂形状和回缩显著相关
20.3 ± 1.89 18.94 ± 1.63	7/17（41.2%） 4/15（26.7%）	ASES:PRP 87.61, C 89.92 Constant:PRP 79.12, C 82.00 UCLA:PRP 31.78, C 30.83 DASH:PRP 13.19, C 8.48 SST:PRP 9.83, C 10.57 SPADI:PRP 12.03, C 10.08	对照组患者第 3 个月随访时的 ASES、常量评分和 SPADI 显著升高 3 个月后所有测量指标均无组间差异 满意度和再撕裂率无显著组间差异

注：ASES=ASES 肩关节疼痛和功能障碍评分（100 分）；Constant=Constant 肩关节评分（100 分）；C= 对照组；DASH= 上肢功能问卷（100 分）；L'Insalata=L'Insalata 肩关节等级评定问卷（100 分）；PRP= 富血小板血浆；PRF= 富血小板纤维蛋白；ROWE=ROWE 肩关节评分（100 分）；SANE= 单纯数字化评估（100 分）；SPADI= 肩关节疼痛和功能障碍指数（100 分）；SST= 肩关节简明测试（12 分）；UCLA= 美国加利福尼大学洛杉矶分校肩关节评分（35 分）；WORC= 加拿大西安大略肩袖指数（100 分）。

间接受了 PRF 治疗。[45] 未确定 PRF 治疗和感染之间存在因果关系，其他回顾性研究也未见报道与使用血小板浓缩物有关的并发症或感染。需要进一步研究以更好地明确与应用血小板浓缩物加强肩袖修复愈合相关的感染风险。

总结

肩关节外科医师正在使用多种类型的支架和血小板浓缩物来加强肩袖修复后的愈合。这些策略在概念上具有吸引力，并得到了基础科学研究的支持，但支持它们在提高治愈率和患者功能结果方面的有效性的临床证据有限。这些产品可能只对特定的患者群体和（或）手术适应证有效。它们的功效可能取决于它们的制备或交付的方式。为了挖掘支架装置和血小板浓缩物的全部治疗潜力，必须考虑这些产品的复杂性，研究人员和临床医师必须继续对其作用机制、最佳适应证和使用方法进行严格的科学研究。

参考文献

[1] Colvin AC, Egorova N, Harrison AK, Moskowitz A, Flatow EL: National trends in rotator cuff repair. *J Bone Joint Surg Am* 2012; 94(3):227-233.

Between 1996 and 2006 there was a significant shift from inpatient to outpatient rotator cuff repair surgery in the United States. The increase in rates of rotator cuff repair was dramatic, particularly for arthroscopically assisted repair.

[2] Tashjian RZ, Hollins AM, Kim HM, et al: Factors affecting healing rates after arthroscopic double-row rotator cuff repair. *Am J Sports Med* 2010; 38(12):2435-2442.

A retrospective case study found that older age and longer duration of follow-up were associated with lower healing rates after double-row rotator cuff repair. The biologic limitation at the repair site appears to be the most important factor influencing tendon healing, even with a double-row construct. Level of evidence: IV.

[3] Toussaint B, Schnaser E, Bosley J, Lefebvre Y, Gobezie R: Early structural and functional outcomes for arthroscopic double-row transosseous-equivalent rotator cuff repair. *Am J Sports Med* 2011; 39(6):1217-1225.

Short-term results of a retrospective case study suggested that the clinical outcomes and structural integrity of transosseous-equivalent double-row rotator cuff repairs compare favorably with those reported for other double-row suture anchor techniques in rotator cuff repair. Level of evidence: IV.

[4] Koh KH, Kang KC, Lim TK, Shon MS, Yoo JC: Prospective randomized clinical trial of single- versus double-row suture anchor repair in 2- to 4-cm rotator cuff tears: Clinical and magnetic resonance imaging results. *Arthroscopy* 2011; 27(4):453-462.

A prospective randomized controlled study found that the clinical results and retear rates of double-row repair with one additional medial suture anchor were not significantly different from those of single-row repair with two lateral suture anchors in patients with a medium to large rotator cuff tear. Level of evidence: I.

[5] Reing JE, Zhang L, Myers-Irvin J, et al: Degradation products of extracellular matrix affect cell migration and the proliferation. *Tissue Eng Part A* 2009; 15(3):605-614.

ECM degradation products had chemotactic and mitogenic activities for multipotential progenitor cells, and the same degradation products inhibited both chemotaxis and proliferation of differentiated endothelial cells.

[6] Badylak SF, Freytes DO, Gilbert TW: Extracellular matrix as a biological scaffold material: Structure and function. *Acta Biomater* 2009; 5(1):1-13.

An overview of the composition and the structure of selected ECM scaffold materials includes the effects of manufacturing methods on structural properties and resulting mechanical behavior of the material and the in vivo degradation and remodeling of ECM scaffolds, with an emphasis on tissue function.

[7] Ricchetti ET, Aurora A, Iannotti JP, Derwin KA: Scaffold devices for rotator cuff repair. *J Shoulder Elbow Surg* 2012; 21(2):251-265.

The basic science and clinical understanding of commercially available synthetic and ECM scaffolds for rotator cuff repair are reviewed, with an emphasis on host response and scaffold remodeling, mechanical and suture-retention properties, and preclinical and clinical studies.

[8] Metcalf MH, Savoie FH III, Kellum B: Surgical technique for xenograft (SIS) augmentation of rotator-cuff repairs. *Oper Tech Orthop* 2002; 12:204-208.

[9] Sclamberg SG, Tibone JE, Itamura JM, Kasraeian S: Six-month magnetic resonance imaging follow-up of large and massive rotator cuff repairs reinforced with porcine small intestinal submucosa. *J Shoulder Elbow Surg* 2004; 13(5):538-541.

[10] Iannotti JP, Codsi MJ, Kwon YW, Derwin K, Ciccone J, Brems JJ: Porcine small intestine submucosa augmentation of surgical repair of chronic two-tendon rotator cuff tears: A randomized, controlled trial. *J Bone Joint Surg Am* 2006; 88(6):1238-1244.

[11] Walton JR, Bowman NK, Khatib Y, Linklater J, Murrell GA: Restore Orthobiologic Implant: Not recommended for augmentation of rotator cuff repairs. *J Bone Joint Surg Am* 2007; 89(4):786-791.

A retrospective case-control study reported the open repair of large or massive rotator cuff tears using Restore Orthobiologic Implant. Overall satisfaction and range of motion were not significantly different between groups, but patients who did not receive augmentation had significantly greater strength and sports participation. Four patients who received Restore had a severe postoperative reaction requiring surgical treatment. Level of evidence: III.

[12] Pedowitz RA, Yamaguchi K, Ahmad CS, et al; American Academy of Orthopaedic Surgeons: Optimizing the management of rotator cuff problems. *J Am Acad Orthop Surg* 2011; 19(6):368-379.

Of 31 recommendations for the optimal management of rotator cuff issues, 19 were determined to be inconclusive, 4 were classified as moderate grade, 6 as weak, and 2 as consensus statements of expert opinion.

[13] Burkhead WZ, Schiffern SC, Krishnan SG: Use of Graft Jacket as an augmentation for massive rotator cuff tears. *Semin Arthroplasty* 2007; 18:11-18.

A retrospective case-control study reported the open repair of massive rotator cuff tears using GraftJacket. Strength, range of motion, and outcome scores were improved, and no complications were observed. Level of evidence: IV.

[14] Dopirak R, Bond JL, Snyder SJ: Arthroscopic total rotator cuff replacement with an acellular human dermal allograft matrix. *Int J Shoulder Surg* 2007; 1(1):7-15.

A retrospective case-control study reported the technique and short-term results of arthroscopic repair of irreparable rotator cuff tears using GraftJacket. Strength, pain, range of motion, and outcome scores were improved, and no complications were observed. Level of evidence: IV.

[15] Bond JL, Dopirak RM, Higgins J, Burns J, Snyder SJ: Arthroscopic replacement of massive, irreparable rotator cuff tears using a GraftJacket allograft: Technique and preliminary results. *Arthroscopy* 2008; 24(4):403-409, e1.

A retrospective case-control study reported the technique and short-term results of arthroscopic repair of irreparable rotator cuff tears using GraftJacket. Strength, pain, range of motion, and outcome scores were improved, and no complications were observed. Level of evidence: IV.

[16] Wong I, Burns J, Snyder S: Arthroscopic GraftJacket repair of rotator cuff tears. *J Shoulder Elbow Surg* 2010; 19(2, suppl):104-109.

A retrospective case-control study reported the arthroscopic repair of irreparable rotator cuff tears using GraftJacket. Outcome scores were improved, and two complications were observed. The procedure was considered safe and associated with high patient satisfaction, without the morbidity of tendon transfer or arthroplasty. Level of evidence: IV.

[17] Rotini R, Marinelli A, Guerra E, et al: Human dermal matrix scaffold augmentation for large and massive rotator cuff repairs: Preliminary clinical and MRI results at 1-year follow-up. *Musculoskelet Surg* 2011; 95(1, suppl):S13-S23.

A retrospective case-control study reported the arthroscopic or open repair of large or massive rotator cuff tears using GraftJacket. Outcome scores were improved, and no adverse events reported. Level of evidence: IV.

[18] Soler JA, Gidwani S, Curtis MJ: Early complications from the use of porcine dermal collagen implants (Permacol) as bridging constructs in the repair of massive rotator cuff tears: A report of 4 cases. *Acta Orthop Belg* 2007; 73(4):432-436.

A retrospective case-control study reported the open repair of massive rotator cuff tears using Zimmer Collagen Repair. Graft disruption occurred 3 to 6 months postoperatively in all patients. Inflammatory reaction was seen in all patients, with graft disintegration and tissue necrosis observed at revision surgery. Level of evidence: IV.

[19] Badhe SP, Lawrence TM, Smith FD, Lunn PG: An assessment of porcine dermal xenograft as an augmentation graft in the treatment of extensive rotator cuff tears. *J Shoulder Elbow Surg* 2008; 17(1, suppl): S35-S39.

A retrospective case-control study reported the open repair of large or massive rotator cuff tears using Zimmer Collagen Repair. Outcome scores, pain, range of motion, and abduction power improved, and no adverse events were reported. Level of evidence: IV.

[20] Barber FA, Burns JP, Deutsch A, Labbé MR, Litchfield RB: A prospective, randomized evaluation of acellular human dermal matrix augmentation for arthroscopic rotator cuff repair. *Arthroscopy* 2012; 28(1):8-15.

A prospective randomized controlled study reported the arthroscopic repair of chronic two-tendon rotator cuff tears with or without GraftJacket augmentation. Patients treated with augmentation had significantly better outcome scores and a significantly better healing rate on magnetic resonance arthrography, compared with those treated without augmentation. No adverse events were reported. Level of evidence: II.

[21] Encalada-Diaz I, Cole BJ, Macgillivray JD, et al: Rotator cuff repair augmentation using a novel polycarbonate polyurethane patch: Preliminary results at 12 months' follow-up. *J Shoulder Elbow Surg* 2011; 20(5):788-794.

A retrospective case-control study reported the open

repair of small to medium rotator cuff tears using Biomerix RCR Patch. Pain, range of motion, and outcome scores were improved, and no complications were observed. Level of evidence: IV.

[22] Kingsley CS: Blood coagulation: Evidence of an antagonist to factor VI in platelet-rich human plasma. *Nature* 1954; 173(4407):723-724.

[23] Del Fabbro M, Bortolin M, Taschieri S, Weinstein R: Is platelet concentrate advantageous for the surgical treatment of periodontal diseases? A systematic review and meta-analysis. *J Periodontol* 2011; 82(8): 1100-1111.

PRP may exert a positive adjunctive effect when used in combination with graft materials for the treatment of intrabone defects. No significant benefit of platelet concentrates was found for the treatment of gingival recession.

[24] Marx RE, Carlson ER, Eichstaedt RM, Schimmele SR, Strauss JE, Georgeff KR: Platelet-rich plasma: Growth factor enhancement for bone grafts. *Oral Surg Oral Med Oral Pathol Oral Radiol Endod* 1998; 85(6):638-646.

[25] Knighton DR, Ciresi KF, Fiegel VD, Austin LL, Butler EL: Classification and treatment of chronic nonhealing wounds: Successful treatment with autologous platelet-derived wound healing factors (PDWHF). *Ann Surg* 1986; 204(3):322-330.

[26] Sheth U, Simunovic N, Klein G, et al: Efficacy of autologous platelet-rich plasma use for orthopaedic indications: A meta-analysis. *J Bone Joint Surg Am* 2012; 94(4):298-307.

A meta-analysis of the efficacy of PRP for orthopaedic applications found that PRP provided no significant benefit as late as 24 months across randomized or prospective cohort studies in patients with an orthopaedic injury.

[27] Foster TE, Puskas BL, Mandelbaum BR, Gerhardt MB, Rodeo SA: Platelet-rich plasma: From basic science to clinical applications. *Am J Sports Med* 2009; 37(11):2259-2272.

The basic science of PRP is examined, with a description of current clinical applications in sports medicine. Human studies published in the orthopaedic surgery and sports medicine literature are reviewed and evaluated. The use of PRP in amateur and professional sports is reviewed, and the regulation of PRP by anti- doping agencies is discussed.

[28] Civinini R, Macera A, Nistri L, Redl B, Innocenti M: The use of autologous blood-derived growth factors in bone regeneration. *Clin Cases Miner Bone Metab* 2011; 8(1):25-31.

This review describes the biologic properties of platelets and their factors, as well as the methods used for producing PRP, to provide a basic science background and an overview of evidence-based medicine on the clinical application of PRP in bone healing.

[29] Dohan Ehrenfest DM, Bielecki T, Mishra A, et al: In search of a consensus terminology in the field of platelet concentrates for surgical use: Platelet-rich plasma (PRP), platelet-rich fibrin (PRF), fibrin gel polymerization and leukocytes. *Curr Pharm Biotechnol* 2012; 13(7):1131-1137.

A consensus terminology is proposed for characterizing products derived from platelet concentrates.

[30] Boswell SG, Cole BJ, Sundman EA, Karas V, Fortier LA: Platelet-rich plasma: A milieu of bioactive factors. *Arthroscopy* 2012; 28(3):429-439.

In addition to platelets, a role is described for growth factors, soluble proteins, electrolytes, plasma hormones, leukocytes, and erythrocytes in the clinical response to PRP. Depending on the specific constituents of a PRP preparation, the clinical use theoretically can be matched to the pathology to improve clinical efficacy.

[31] Marx RE: Platelet-rich plasma: Evidence to support its use. *J Oral Maxillofac Surg* 2004; 62(4):489-496.

[32] Hall MP, Band PA, Meislin RJ, Jazrawi LM, Cardone DA: Platelet-rich plasma: Current concepts and application in sports medicine. *J Am Acad Orthop Surg* 2009; 17(10):602-608.

Current concepts and the use of PRP in sports medicine are reviewed.

[33] Castillo TN, Pouliot MA, Kim HJ, Dragoo JL: Comparison of growth factor and platelet concentration from commercial platelet-rich plasma separation systems. *Am J Sports Med* 2011; 39(2):266-271.

Three commercially available PRP separation systems produced single-donor PRP with different compositions and different concentrations of growth factors and white blood cells.

[34] Mazzocca AD, McCarthy MB, Chowaniec DM, et al: Platelet-rich plasma differs according to preparation method and human variability. *J Bone Joint Surg Am* 2012; 94(4):308-316.

The levels of platelets, growth factors, red blood cells, and white blood cells were quantified across patients using commercially available one-step and two-step separation systems, and intraindividual variability in

PRP was determined. Within the evaluated procedures, platelet numbers and the numbers of white blood cells differed significantly in and between individuals.

[35] Kobayashi M, Itoi E, Minagawa H, et al: Expression of growth factors in the early phase of supraspinatus tendon healing in rabbits. *J Shoulder Elbow Surg* 2006; 15(3):371-377.

[36] Schnabel LV, Mohammed HO, Miller BJ, et al: Platelet rich plasma (PRP) enhances anabolic gene expression patterns in flexor digitorum superficialis tendons. *J Orthop Res* 2007; 25(2):230-240.

Tendon explants cultured in 100% PRP had enhanced gene expression of three matrix molecules, with no concomitant increase in the catabolic molecules metalloproteinase-3 and -13.

[37] de Mos M, van der Windt AE, Jahr H, et al: Can platelet-rich plasma enhance tendon repair? A cell culture study. *Am J Sports Med* 2008; 36(6):1171-1178.

In human tenocyte cultures, platelet-rich clot releasate and platelet-poor clot releasate stimulate cell proliferation and total collagen production. Platelet-rich clot releasate, not platelet-poor clot releasate, slightly increases the expression of matrix-degrading enzymes and endogenous growth factors.

[38] Jo CH, Kim JE, Yoon KS, Shin S: Platelet-rich plasma stimulates cell proliferation and enhances matrix gene expression and synthesis in tenocytes from human rotator cuff tendons with degenerative tears. *Am J Sports Med* 2012; 40(5):1035-1045.

PRP promoted cell proliferation and enhanced gene expression as well as the synthesis of tendon matrix in tenocytes from human rotator cuff tendons with degenerative tears.

[39] Virchenko O, Grenegård M, Aspenberg P: Indepen- dent and additive stimulation of tendon repair by thrombin and platelets. *Acta Orthop* 2006; 77(6): 960-966.

[40] Aspenberg P, Virchenko O: Platelet concentrate injection improves Achilles tendon repair in rats. *Acta Orthop Scand* 2004; 75(1):93-99.

[41] Lyras D, Kazakos K, Verettas D, et al: Immunohistochemical study of angiogenesis after local administration of platelet-rich plasma in a patellar tendon defect. *Int Orthop* 2010; 34(1):143-148.

PRP gel was applied to a central full-thickness patellar tendon defect in rabbits. Neovascularization was significantly higher in rabbits treated with PRP during the first 2 weeks and was significantly lower during the third and fourth weeks compared with control rabbits. The tissue formed in the PRP-treated rabbits was more mature and dense with less elastic fibers remaining.

[42] Visser LC, Arnoczky SP, Caballero O, Gardner KL: Evaluation of the use of an autologous platelet-rich fibrin membrane to enhance tendon healing in dogs. *Am J Vet Res* 2011; 72(5):699-705.

PRF membrane was applied to a central full-thickness patellar tendon defect in dogs. There was no significant difference in the histologic quality of the repair tissue in between the control (empty) defects and the PRF membrane–treated defects at 4 or 8 weeks.

[43] Castricini R, Longo UG, De Benedetto M, et al: Platelet-rich plasma augmentation for arthroscopic rotator cuff repair: A randomized controlled trial. *Am J Sports Med* 2011; 39(2):258-265.

A prospective randomized controlled study reported the arthroscopic repair of small to medium rotator cuff tears with or without PRF matrix. There were no between-group differences in outcome scores or retear rates. The MRI signal intensity score improved in those treated with PRF. Level of evidence: I.

[44] Barber FA, Hrnack SA, Snyder SJ, Hapa O: Rotator cuff repair healing influenced by platelet-rich plasma construct augmentation. *Arthroscopy* 2011; 27(8): 1029-1035.

A case-control study reported the arthroscopic repair of one- or two-tendon rotator cuff tears with or without PRF matrix. There were no differences in outcome scores between groups, other than Rowe scores. The retear rate was significantly lower in those treated with PRF. Level of evidence: III.

[45] Bergeson AG, Tashjian RZ, Greis PE, Crim J, Stoddard GJ, Burks RT: Effects of platelet-rich fibrin matrix on repair integrity of at-risk rotator cuff tears. *Am J Sports Med* 2012; 40(2):286-293.

A case-control study reported the arthroscopic repair of one- to three-tendon rotator cuff tears with or without PRF matrix. There were no between-group differences in outcome scores. The retear rate was significantly higher in those treated with PRF. Level of evidence: III.

[46] Rodeo SA, Delos D, Williams RJ, Adler RS, Pearle AD, Warren RF: The effect of platelet-rich fibrin matrix on rotator cuff tendon healing: A prospective, randomized clinical study. *Am J Sports Med* 2012; 40(6):1234- 1241.

A prospective randomized controlled study reported the arthroscopic repair of small to large rotator cuff tears with or without PRF matrix. There were no between-group differences in strength, outcome scores, or retear rate. PRF was a significant predictor of a tendon defect at 12 weeks. Level of evidence: I.

[47] Arnoczky SP: Platelet-rich plasma augmentation of rotator cuff repair: Letter. *Am J Sports Med* 2011; 39(6): NP8-NP9, author reply NP9-NP11.

A letter to the editor and author reply commented on the MRI findings and conclusions published in Castricini R, Longo UG, De Benedetto M, et al, *Sports Med* 2011; 39(2)258-265.

[48] Randelli P, Arrigoni P, Ragone V, Aliprandi A, Cabitza P: Platelet rich plasma in arthroscopic rotator cuff repair: A prospective RCT study, 2-year follow- up. *J Shoulder Elbow Surg* 2011; 20(4):518-528.

A prospective randomized controlled study reported the arthroscopic repair of one- to three-tendon rotator cuff tears with or without PRF matrix. There were no between-group differences in healing rates or scores after 6, 12, and 24 months. Subanalysis of small tears showed that patients treated with PRF had increased strength at 3, 6, 12, and 24 months. Level of evidence: I.

[49] Jo CH, Kim JE, Yoon KS, et al: Does platelet-rich plasma accelerate recovery after rotator cuff repair? A prospective cohort study. *Am J Sports Med* 2011; 39(10):2082-2090.

A prospective cohort study reported the arthroscopic repair of small to massive rotator cuff tears with or without leukocyte-poor PRP gels. There were no between-group differences in range of motion or outcome scores, in satisfaction, or retear rates after 3 months. Level of evidence: II.

第四章 反肩关节置换术的运动学和生物力学

Christopher P. Roche, MSBE, MBA; Lynn Crosby, MD

盂肱关节解剖学

盂肱关节是人体最灵活的关节，但关节面曲率的不匹配导致盂肱关节存在一定的不稳定性。盂肱关节的运动形式分为转动（仅限于旋转）、滑动（仅限于平移）和滚动（旋转加平移）。[1-2]在其整个运动范围内，盂肱关节的稳定性是由肌肉收缩的协调作用辅助实现的，并受韧带和关节囊收紧的控制，肌肉、韧带和关节囊的状态都会因为关节位置和运动类型的不同而不同。肩部的肌肉对于肩部的灵活性和稳定性很重要。[3]

三角肌是肩带上最大的，也是最重要的肌肉。三角肌作为肩部主动肌在肩胛骨平面上产生向前抬高的力。三角肌有 3 个头部，分别是三角肌前部（前肩峰和锁骨）、中部（肩峰的外侧边缘）和后部（肩胛棘）。这几个头部加在一起的质量约占肩部肌肉质量的 20%。[4]在轻度外展时，肱骨头大结节周围的三角肌中部产生稳定的压缩力，但这种压缩力比此时肩袖产生的肱骨头压缩

力小。[5-6]

肩袖产生肱骨围绕盂窝旋转所需的扭矩，同时将肱骨头压入肩胛盂。[7]肩袖围绕肱骨近端分布，以便在盂肱关节的所有位置进行有效的关节加压，令肩袖在动态中保持关节平衡，从而补偿盂肱关节骨性约束的缺乏。[8-10]具体来说，肩袖前侧（肩胛下肌）和后侧（冈下肌和小圆肌）的解剖分布产生了一对横向力偶，使得在关节的所有位置上，肱骨头在前向和后向运动时始终近乎位于肩胛盂窝的中心。[11-13]

肩袖撕裂关节病

肩袖完整性的破坏，最常见的是肩袖肌腱的撕裂，可能对盂肱关节的稳定性产生破坏性的后果。当肩袖既不能将肱骨头压入肩胛盂内，也不能平衡肩部其他肌肉（主要是三角肌）的力量时，肱骨头倾向于向上移动并撞击肩峰的下表面。这种撞击可能导致肩袖的进一步撕裂及肩袖口肌肉的脂肪浸润，进而导致继发于摩擦力增加和软骨营养缺乏的关节炎性改变。持续撕裂导致肱骨头进一步撞击肩峰下表面，并最终导致肱骨头塌陷、肱二头肌腱脱位，以及肩胛盂上部、肩峰和喙突的磨损。[14-15]Neer 使用术语"肩袖撕裂关节病"来描述由于大量全层肩袖撕裂导致的长时间的、渐进性的肩峰下撞击，所造成的盂肱关节的关节炎和磨损或塌陷的情况。[14]

Mr. Roche or an immediate family member serves as a paid consultant to or is an employee of Exactech; and has stock or stock options held in Exactech. Dr. Crosby or an immediate family member serves as a board member, owner, officer, or committee member of the American Orthopaedic Association and the American Shoulder and Elbow Surgeons; has received royalties from Exactech; is a member of a speakers' bureau or has made paid presentations on behalf of Exactech; serves as a paid consultant to or is an employee of Exactech; and has received research or institutional support from Exactech.

反肩关节置换术的哲学史和设计史

反肩关节假体是在 20 世纪 70 年代早期被设计出来的，用于治疗肩袖撕裂关节病患者。该装置可通过抵抗肱骨头的上行移位来减轻疼痛并预防肩峰、喙突和肩胛盂的进行性侵蚀。[16]反肩关节假体可反转解剖凹陷，使肩胛盂关节部件凸起，并且使肱骨关节部件凹陷，从而形成可防止肱骨头向上移动的固定的关节。由于关节结构匹配性的限制，反肩关节假体的运动方式仅限于旋转。目前，有 Fenlin、Reeves-Leeds、Kessel 和 Neer-Averill 这几种反肩关节假体。[17-23]这些假体都有一个受限且匹配的关节，其旋转中心位于肩胛盂外侧。这些设计的缺点是在关节盂骨 - 植入物界面上产生了过大的扭矩，会影响固定并导致机械故障。这些早期的产品已被美国市场淘汰。[16,23]

在 1987 年，Grammont 推出了一种反肩关节假体，包括一个直径 42mm 的凸起的肩胛盂组件，其厚度约为球体的 2/3，以及一个凹陷的肱骨头组件，其深度约为球体的 1/3。这种早期的设计也与肩胛盂失效有关，1991 年，这种假体被改良为使用固定的中心钉进行非骨水泥固定，以便同时万向锁定和使用加压螺钉。此外，凸起的肩胛盂的厚度被减少到球体直径的一半，以便将关节旋转中心放置在肩胛盂窝的内侧。[16,24-26]

Grammont 型反肩关节假体使关节旋转中心居中，从而将关节盂骨 - 植入物界面上的扭矩降至最低，并增加外展肌的力臂长度。现在市场上的反肩关节假体全部改良自 Grammont 型反肩关节假体。虽然侧移旋转中心（相对于 Grammont 型反肩关节假体）已被建议作为降低肩胛骨切迹风险的一种方法，但首选的缓解方法（首先由 Nyffeler 等[27]推荐）是沿着肩胛盂下缘定位肩胛盂组件，观察有无下倾斜。这种定位还有一个好处，那就是可以下移关节旋转中心，从而拉长三角肌并改善其静息时的紧张度和张力。

反肩关节置换术的生物力学和运动学

肌肉产生力线，这些力线转换为扭矩时，与关节旋转中心和肌肉产生的力线之间的垂直距离成比例。[3,28]这个垂直距离被称为力臂，力臂加大 50% 以上意味着肌肉仅需要低于 50% 的力来产生特定的扭矩或运动。力臂相对于关节旋转中心的位置决定了肌肉接下来的运动形式。肩部的运动形式包括外展内收（在肩胛面、冠状面或横断面）、内旋外旋（围绕肱骨长轴）和屈伸（在矢状面）。肌肉只能在紧张时产生张力，肌肉的紧张可以通过收缩（肌肉缩短）或超出静止长度的伸展（肌肉延长）产生。因此，肌肉缩短、肌肉延长和肌肉长度不变时皆可形成运动。当力线与关节旋转中心重合时，肌肉长度不变的运动就发生了。[28]换句话说，肌肉的收缩可以使关节稳定或运动，这取决于肌肉相对于旋转中心的力线。肌肉可以起主动肌（引起运动）、拮抗肌（稳定运动）和两者兼有的作用（双相功能，同时起主动肌和拮抗肌的作用，这取决于关节在运动范围内的特定位置）。[3,28]肌肉的力臂越大，肌肉产生运动和支撑外部负载所需的扭矩的能力就越大。更大的力臂要求肌肉更大程度的收缩（需要更多的肌肉缩短来产生给定的运动）。肌肉的力臂只是其产生扭矩的能力的一个组成部分，其他组成部分包括肌肉的生理横截面面积、结构、神经活动和长度 - 张力关系。[3]

目前反肩关节假体中的解剖凹陷倒置和旋转中心的下移与内移显著改变了肩部每块肌肉与其正常生理功能的关系。内移旋转中心会拉长三角肌并增加其前、中、后部外展力臂的长度，使它们在外展时发挥更大的作用。[5,29-32]这些外展力臂的增大，增强了三角肌在肩胛骨和冠状面上抬起手臂的能力，代偿了冈上肌、肩胛下肌上部及冈下肌等肩袖肌肉（这些肌肉通常发生病变）的功能受损。向内侧移动旋转中心也会使肱骨向内侧平移，加大剩余肩袖肌肉的松弛程度，并在肩

胛颈处于轻度抬举位时导致肱骨撞击（肩胛骨切迹）。[33-34]

　　与正常肩关节相比，行反肩关节置换术后的关节，其旋转中心的下移拉长了三角肌。将三角肌延长 10%~20%，可改善其静息紧张度和张力，并可增加其收缩强度，改善肩关节的整体稳定性。当手臂处于 0° 外展位时，不同设计的反式肩部移植物可将三角肌拉长 13%~17%（与正常肩部相比）。[5,29] 最佳张力取决于肱骨的延长程度，建议延长超过 2.5 cm，因为延长肱骨可增加主动抬高高度。[35-36] 相比之下，肱骨缩短可导致脱位风险增加。然而，三角肌的延长改变了正常的三角肌外形，这减小了其围绕大结节的包绕角度，降低了肩关节稳定性。此外，三角肌延长会影响美观度。[5-6,33] 肱骨延长增加可能导致肩峰应力性骨折和臂丛神经病变。[37-38] 恢复肱骨结节的外侧位置，

对于以相对自然的生理方式拉伸剩余的肩袖肌肉以恢复旋转强度是重要的。[33-34] 虽然过度拉伸这些肌肉可以改善其静息紧张度和张力，但也可能增加肩胛下肌腱切断术后的修复难度。旋转中心下移也改变了肩胛下肌和冈下肌从低抬举位时的内收肌转换为高抬举位时的外展肌的转换临界点。在正常肩关节中，肩胛下肌腱和冈下肌腱会跨越旋转中心。当反肩关节置换术的旋转中心下移时，肩胛下肌腱和冈下肌腱位于关节旋转中心下方，因此，在整个手臂抬高过程中，肩胛下肌主要充当内收肌（图 4-1）。在一些患者中，这些肌肉可能完全丧失其双相功能，这对肩关节的灵活性和稳定性都有重要影响。[30,33]

　　反肩关节假体的设计参数和其在肩胛骨及肱骨中的位置，会影响关节旋转中心相对于正常肩关节的变化（表 4-1）。一些研究报道使用 Grammont 型

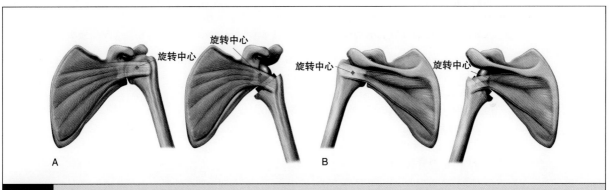

图 4-1　肩胛下肌腱（A）和冈下肌腱（B）相对于旋转中心的位置的比较图。正常肩关节（左）和反肩关节假体（右）

表 4-1

反肩关节假体旋转中心的研究

研究发表（年份）	反肩关节假体	旋转中心的移位（相对于正常肩关节）	
		向内侧（mm）	向下方（mm）
Boileau 等[26]（2005）	36-mm Grammont（DePuy,Warsaw,IN）	19.0 ± 9.9	未见报道
Henninger 等[37]（2012）	36-mm Grammont（Tornier, Montbonnot,France）	17.3 ± 1.8	9.7 ± 3.5
Saltzman 等[39]（2010）	36-mm Grammont（DePuy）	28.3	11.1
	Reverse（DJO Medical,Austin,TX）	17.2	15.3
Jobin 等[29]（2011）	Grammont（DePuy 和 Tornier）和 Zimmer（Warsaw,IN）	18 ± 7	未见报道
Ackland 等[32]（2010）	Zimmer	20.9 ± 3.9	9.5 ± 4.1
DeWilde 等[5]（2004）	Grammont（DePuy）	28.6	未见报道
	Reverse（DJO Medical）	16.5	未见报道

假体伴有关节旋转中心 18 mm 的内移，还有一些研究报道了 28 mm 的内移。[5,26,29,32,37,39] 这种明显的差异主要反映了测量技术上的差异，报道关节旋转中心较小内移的研究一般直接在患者术前和术后的 X 线片上测量，而发现较大内移距离的研究多使用计算机模型。虽然直接从患者的 X 线片获得的测量结果考虑了肱骨近端的自然解剖变异（如肱骨头的直径、颈角、偏移量和厚度），但数据可能会被经常与肩袖撕裂关节病相关的肱骨头塌陷及手术准备和植入方法的不同（例如，肱骨颈切割和关节窝成形术）所影响。[34] 表 4-2 显示了当肱骨在肩胛骨平面内外展时，正常肩关节和反肩关节假体外展力臂的比较研究，正力臂值表示外展，负力臂值表示内收。

表 4-2

肱骨在肩胛骨平面内外展时，正常肩关节和反肩关节假体外展力臂的比较研究

研究发表（年份）	力臂	
	正常肩关节	反肩关节假体
Poppen 和 Walker[50]（1978）	从外展 30° 至外展 150°，三角肌中部的外展力臂从 18 mm 增加至 30 mm	未做比较或评估
	从外展 30° 至外展 150°，三角肌前部的外展力臂从 5 mm 增加至 45 mm	
	在外展 60° 时，三角肌后部从内收肌转换为外展肌，在外展至 150° 时，三角肌后部外展力臂达到最大值 20 mm	
	肩胛下肌在外展 90° 时，从内收肌转换为外展肌，在外展至 120° 时达到外展力臂最大值 10 mm	
Otis 等[28]（1994）	三角肌中部在外展 0° 时，力臂为 18 mm，在外展 60° 时，力臂为 30 mm	未做比较或评估
	三角肌前部在外展 0° 时，力臂为 –8 mm，在外展 15° 时，从内收肌转换为外展肌，在外展 60° 时，力臂为 21 mm	
	三角肌后部在外展 0° 时，力臂为 –55 mm，在外展 60° 时，力臂为 15 mm	
Jobin 等[29]（2012）	三角肌中部在外展 0° 时，力臂为（18±6）mm	三角肌中部在外展 0° 时的外展力臂为（36±6）mm [平均值，Grammont 型假体（DePuy/Tornier）和 Zimmer 假体]
Kontaxis 和 Johnson[30]（2009）	三角肌中部在外展 0° 时，外展力臂达最大值 35 mm	三角肌中部在外展 0° 时，外展力臂为 40 mm，在外展 90° 时，力臂为 55 mm（Grammont 型假体）
	三角肌前部在外展 0° 时，力臂为 –30 mm，在外展 40° 时，从内收肌转换为外展肌，在外展 150° 时，外展力臂达最大值 40 mm	三角肌前部在外展 5° 时，从内收肌转换为外展肌，在外展 150° 时，外展力臂达最大值 40 mm
	三角肌后部在外展 0° 时，力臂为 –25 mm，在外展 75° 时从内收肌转换为外展肌，在外展 150° 时，外展力臂达最大值 20 mm	三角肌后部在外展 15° 时，从内收肌转换为外展肌，在外展 150° 时，外展力臂达最大值 21 mm
	冈下肌在外展 25° 时，从内收肌转换为外展肌，在外展 0°~150° 时，力臂范围为 –3.6~17.9 mm	冈下肌在全部运动范围内均为内收肌，在外展 0°~150° 时，力臂范围为 –16.8~–1.5 mm
	肩胛下肌在外展 25° 时，从内收肌转换为外展肌，在外展 0°~150° 时，力臂范围为 –4.0~15.7 mm	肩胛下肌在外展 120° 时，从内收肌转换为外展肌，在外展 0°~150° 时，力臂范围为 –20.2~4.5 mm

表 4-2

肱骨在肩胛骨平面内外展时，正常肩关节和反肩关节假体外展力臂的比较研究（续）

研究发表（年份）	力臂	
	正常肩关节	反肩关节假体
Terrier 等[31]（2008）	三角肌中部在外展 15° 时，外展力臂达最大值 35 mm	三角肌中部在外展 15° 时，外展力臂为 38 mm，在外展 110° 时，力臂达最大值 48 mm，在外展 90° 时，力臂较正常肩长 20 mm（36-mm Grammont 型假体）
	三角肌前部在外展 15° 时，力臂为 0 mm，在外展 150° 时，外展力臂达最大值 28 mm	三角肌前部的伸展力臂在外展 15° 时，为 20 mm，在外展 150° 时达最大值 38 mm
	三角肌后部在外展 15° 时，力臂为 –25 mm，在外展 90° 时，从内收肌转换为外展肌，在外展 150° 时，力臂达最大值 25 mm	三角肌后部在外展 15° 时，力臂为 –10 mm，在外展 45° 时从内收肌转换为外展肌，在外展 150° 时达最大值 30 mm
Ackland 等[32]（2010）	解剖学全肩关节置换术，三角肌中部的外展力臂在外展 0° 时为 9 mm，在外展 80°~100° 时达最大值 26 mm	三角肌中部的外展力臂在外展 0° 时为 30 mm，在外展 90° 时达最大值 45 mm（Zimmer 假体）
	三角肌前部的外展力臂在外展 0° 时为 1 mm，在外展 95° 时达最大值 27 mm	三角肌前部的外展力臂在外展 0° 时为 16 mm，95° 时达最大值 35 mm
	三角肌后部的外展力臂在外展 0° 时为 –18 mm，在外展 120° 时达最大值 2 mm	三角肌后部的外展力臂在外展 0° 时为 0 mm，在外展 120° 时达最大值 12 mm

Grammont 型反肩关节假体（以下简称 Grammont 型假体）在恢复主动外展和前屈方面是有帮助的，但对肩袖缺损和三角肌功能正常的患者来说，在恢复主动的内外旋功能方面的效果较差。[40-42] 将 Grammont 型假体的旋转中心外移，已被证明可改善肩关节的主动内外旋、强度和稳定性。[33] 通过侧移关节旋转中心，侧移肱骨，拉紧剩余的肩袖肌肉，并将肱骨组件的肩胛颈下撞击减轻至最小。侧移关节旋转中心也增加了关节盂骨 - 植入物界面上的扭矩，并缩短了三角肌外展力臂的长度。[5,37] 三角肌外展力臂随着旋转中心的侧移而减短，三角肌作为外展肌的作用减弱，并且需要更大的力在肩胛骨或冠状面内抬起手臂。[37] 这些升高的载荷和扭矩可能对假体固定、患者康复有负面影响并导致肌肉疲劳和应力性骨折。肱骨可以在不侧移关节旋转中心的情况下侧移。这样做的好处是可以在恢复肩袖肌肉的解剖长度和张力的同时，保持 Grammont 型假体外展肌力臂长度，并使肩胛盂 - 骨界面上的扭矩最小化。可以侧移肱骨以使大结节尽量位于

更接近正常的解剖学位置，同时最大限度地减轻肩胛颈下的肱骨衬垫撞击[43-44]，这可以通过减小 Grammont 型假体的接近 155° 的肱骨颈角，成比例地增加 Grammont 型假体的肱骨小结节的直径和厚度，减少肱骨衬垫约束，或增加肱骨衬垫 - 肱骨干的内侧偏移量来实现。在全肩关节置换术中，增加肱骨干的内侧偏移量可以增加三角肌中部力臂以及三角肌中部对较大结节的包绕角度，从而通过将肱骨头压入肩胛盂来帮助稳定关节。[6] 图 4-2 通过比较三种反肩关节假体和正常肩关节，显示了反肩关节置换术设计对肱骨定位的影响。

力臂较小的肌肉的代偿作用和由位于关节周围的两条相反的肌肉力线产生的合力，都可以增加关节的稳定性，但二者均会增加总的关节反作用力。[45] 由于这些原因，在反肩关节置换术中，关于肩胛下肌 - 小结节的修复是有争议的。当肩胛下肌起内收肌作用时，其力线与肩胛面和冠状面内、肱骨低位和中位抬高时的三角肌相反，这种反作用力要求三角肌产生更大的力来实现给

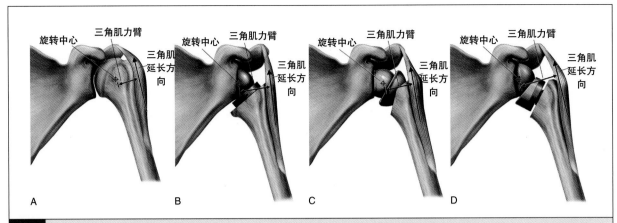

图 4-2　正常肩关节（A）和三种反肩关节假体在肩胛盂下缘 0° 倾斜时的旋转中心、三角肌力臂、三角肌延长方向（三角肌肌力）和肱骨位置的比较。所有图示在肩胛骨平面内外展至 15°。B. 36-mm Grammont（DePuy；旋转中心内移和肱骨组件内移）。C. 32-mm Reverse（DJO Medical；旋转中心外移和肱骨组件内移）。D. 38-mm Equinoxe（Exactech, Gainesville, FL；旋转中心内移和肱骨组件外移）

定的运动。[30,32,46] 这些反作用力增加了关节稳定性，并可能抵消三角肌在关节盂骨 – 植入物界面上产生的扭矩。患者外旋肌较弱时，更应该进行肩胛下肌 – 小结节的修复。一项使用肩关节控制器的研究发现，肩胛下肌松解后，三角肌和后肩袖仅需产生较小的力便可以使肩关节外展。[46] 肩胛下肌 – 小结节修复后，关节的反作用力增加426%，肩关节外展 15° 时所需的三角肌肌力增加 132%，所需后肩袖产生的力增加 460%。由于许多患者的后肩袖因撕裂或脂肪浸润而受损，因此后肩袖可能无法支持高负荷。一些研究者建议尽可能修复肩胛下肌 – 小结节，因为其可降低使用 Grammont 型假体时的脱位率。[47] 这种观察可能不适用于反肩关节假体的使用，因为这些假体不会使肱骨向内平移（增加其余肩袖肌肉的松弛）。[33-34] 在准备通过反肩关节置换术修复肩胛下肌 – 小结节时，这些因素都应该被考虑，因为可能不是所有假体或所有临床情况都需要进行肩胛下肌 – 小结节的修复。

失去外旋和极度内旋能力会损害患者在手臂抬高时保持手臂中立旋转位的能力（司号员体征阳性）。患者不能进行许多日常活动，如饮水、吃饭、洗发和握手。[40-42] 功能正常的肩部，内旋肌占主导地位。人类肩关节有 4 个内旋肌（肩胛下肌，大圆肌、胸大肌和背阔肌），只有 2 个外旋肌（冈下肌和小圆肌）。因此，外旋缺陷对日常活动的影响比内旋缺陷大，特别是在抬起手臂时。[40-41] 仅三角肌正常不足以恢复肩关节的主动外旋功能，即使采用侧移的反肩关节假体也是如此。因此，如果患者有外旋功能障碍，通常建议在反肩关节置换术中进行肌肉移位。通常将附着于肱骨前侧的 1 个或多个内旋肌经旋转中心转移到肱骨后侧，在那里它们的收缩将导致肩关节外旋。背阔肌是反肩关节置换术中最常转移的肌肉，它被从肱骨干前侧分离并重新连接到大结节。[48] 另一种常见的肌肉移位方法是改进后的 L'Episcopo 方法，该方法是将背阔肌和大圆肌都转移到大结节。虽然肌肉移位已被证明可以恢复肩关节主动外旋功能，但如果小圆肌功能正常，则不进行肌肉移位。[40-41] 此外，应该认识到这种肌肉移位手术限制了肩关节的主动内旋功能，并进一步改变了各肩部肌肉的正常生理功能及其关系。

肩胛骨形态改变了反肩关节置换术后的运动学。异常的肩胛盂磨损模式，以及为了减少肩胛盂下撞击并发症而设计的肩胛盂术前准备和放置假体的策略（例如，10°~15° 下倾），会影响旋转中心、肌肉力臂、肌肉长度和肌肉力线。随着假体的进一步内移和向下倾斜，三角肌中部对大结节的包绕急剧减少。此外，严重的肩胛盂磨损使关节线内移，增加了肩带肌肉的松弛。肩胛骨磨损达到一定程度后，肱骨将严重内移，以至于三角肌产生一种偏向力，从而导致肩关节不稳定。[49]

总结

　　反肩关节置换术对于肩袖缺损和三角肌功能正常的患者，可有效地缓解肩部疼痛，恢复肩部的主动外展和前屈功能。解剖学凹陷的倒置恢复了肩部的稳定性，旋转中心的下移和内移（与正常肩相比）延长了外展力臂并拉长了三角肌，从而促进了肩关节的功能和灵活性的改善。肩关节反向运动学可能受到假体设计参数、假体在肩胛骨上的定位以及异常的肩胛骨形态 – 肩胛盂磨损模式的影响。未来的研究应该集中于优化这些运动学参数的方法，以提高肩部的整体功能，帮助改善患者的日常活动能力。

致谢

　　作者感谢 MattHamilton 博士和 PhongDiep 对手稿的贡献。

参考文献

［1］ Morrey BF: *The Shoulder*, ed 2. Philadelphia, PA, WB Saunders, 1998, pp 233-276.

［2］ Yu J, McGarry MH, Lee YS, Duong LV, Lee TQ: Biomechanical effects of supraspinatus repair on the glenohumeral joint. *J Shoulder Elbow Surg* 2005;14(1, suppl S):65S-71S.

［3］ Kuechle DK, Newman SR, Itoi E, Morrey BF, An KN: Shoulder muscle moment arms during horizontal flexion and elevation. *J Shoulder Elbow Surg* 1997;6(5):429-439.

［4］ Lee SB, An KN: Dynamic glenohumeral stability provided by three heads of the deltoid muscle. *Clin Orthop Relat Res* 2002;400:40-47.

［5］ De Wilde LF, Audenaert EA, Berghs BM: Shoulder prostheses treating cuff tear arthropathy: A compara- tive biomechanical study. *J Orthop Res* 2004;22(6):1222-1230.

［6］ Lemieux PO, Hagemeister N, Tétreault P, Nuño N: Influence of the medial offset of the proximal humerus on the glenohumeral destabilising forces during arm elevation: A numerical sensitivity study. *Comput Methods Biomech Biomed Engin* 2013;16(1):103-111.
A computer model study assessed the influence of humeral head medial offset on joint stability. Varying the medial offset influenced the destabilizing action of the middle deltoid, where a larger medial offset increased the middle deltoid wrapping around the tuberosity.

［7］ Lippitt SB, Vanderhooft JE, Harris SL, Sidles JA, Harryman DT II, Matsen FA III: Glenohumeral stability from concavity-compression: A quantitative analysis. *J Shoulder Elbow Surg* 1993;2(1):27-35.

［8］ Sharkey NA, Marder RA: The rotator cuff opposes superior translation of the humeral head. *Am J Sports Med* 1995;23(3):270-275.

［9］ Parsons IM, Apreleva M, Fu FH, Woo SL: The effect of rotator cuff tears on reaction forces at the glenohumeral joint. *J Orthop Res* 2002;20(3):439-446.

［10］ Mura N, O'Driscoll SW, Zobitz ME, et al: The effect of infraspinatus disruption on glenohumeral torque and superior migration of the humeral head: A biomechanical study. *J Shoulder Elbow Surg* 2003;12(2):179-184.

［11］ Burkhart SS, Nottage WM, Ogilvie-Harris DJ, Kohn HS, Pachelli A: Partial repair of irreparable rotator cuff tears. *Arthroscopy* 1994;10(4):363-370.

［12］ Halder AM, Zhao KD, O'Driscoll SW, Morrey BF, An KN: Dynamic contributions to superior shoulder stability. *J Orthop Res* 2001;19(2):206-212.

［13］ Labriola JE, Lee TQ, Debski RE, McMahon PJ: Stability and instability of the glenohumeral joint: The role of shoulder muscles. *J Shoulder Elbow Surg* 2005;14(1, suppl S):S32-S38.

［14］ Neer CS II, Craig EV, Fukuda H: Cuff-tear arthropathy. *J Bone Joint Surg Am* 1983;65(9):1232-1244.

［15］ Visotsky JL, Basamania C, Seebauer L, Rockwood CA, Jensen KL: Cuff tear arthropathy: Pathogenesis, classification, and algorithm for treatment. *J Bone Joint Surg Am* 2004;86-A(2, suppl 2):35-40.

［16］ Flatow EL, Harrison AK: A history of reverse total shoulder arthroplasty. *Clin Orthop Relat Res* 2011;469(9):2432-2439.
A literature review described the evolution of reverse

shoulder prosthesis design, focusing on the challenges of historical designs and describing the influence of the Grammont prosthesis on current designs.

[17] Fenlin JM Jr: Semi-constrained prosthesis for the rotator cuff deficient patient. *Orthop Trans* 1985;9:55.

[18] Redfern TR, Wallace WA: *Joint Replacement in the Shoulder and Elbow.* Oxford, United Kingdom, Butterworth and Heinemann, 1998, pp 6-16.

[19] Reeves B, Jobbins B, Dowson D, Wright V: A total shoulder endoprosthesis. *Eng Med* 1974;1:64-67.

[20] Bayley I, Kessel L: *The Kessel Total Shoulder Replacement: Shoulder Surgery.* New York, NY, Springer Verlag, 1982.

[21] Broström LA, Wallensten R, Olsson E, Anderson D: The Kessel prosthesis in total shoulder arthroplasty: A five-year experience. *Clin Orthop Relat Res* 1992;277:155-160.

[22] Wretenberg PF, Wallensten R: The Kessel total shoulder arthroplasty: A 13- to 16-year retrospective followup. *Clin Orthop Relat Res* 1999;365:100-103.

[23] Neer CS II: *Shoulder Reconstruction.* Philadelphia, PA, WB Saunders, 1990.

[24] Grammont P, Trouillod P, Laffay JP, Deries X: Etude et Realisation D'une Novelle Prosthese D'Paule. *Rhumatologie* 1987;39:17-22.

[25] Grammont PM, Baulot E: Delta shoulder prosthesis for rotator cuff rupture. *Orthopedics* 1993;16(1):65-68.

[26] Boileau P, Watkinson DJ, Hatzidakis AM, Balg F: Grammont reverse prosthesis: Design, rationale, and biomechanics. *J Shoulder Elbow Surg* 2005;14(1, suppl S):147S-161S.

[27] Nyffeler RW, Werner CM, Gerber C: Biomechanical relevance of glenoid component positioning in the reverse Delta III total shoulder prosthesis. *J Shoulder Elbow Surg* 2005;14(5):524-528.

[28] Otis JC, Jiang CC, Wickiewicz TL, Peterson MG, Warren RF, Santner TJ: Changes in the moment arms of the rotator cuff and deltoid muscles with abduction and rotation. *J Bone Joint Surg Am* 1994;76(5):667-676.

[29] Jobin CM, Brown GD, Bahu MJ, et al: Reverse total shoulder arthroplasty for cuff tear arthropathy: The clinical effect of deltoid lengthening and center of rotation medialization. *J Shoulder Elbow Surg* 2012;21(10):1269-1277.
Forty-nine consecutive patients who underwent reverse shoulder arthroplasty for cuff tear arthropathy were prospectively studied to correlate functional outcomes with deltoid lengthening and center of rotation medi-

alization. Deltoid lengthening was found to be correlated with active forward elevation.

[30] Kontaxis A, Johnson GR: The biomechanics of reverse anatomy shoulder replacement—a modelling study. *Clin Biomech (Bristol, Avon)* 2009;24(3):254-260.
A computer modeling study quantified deltoid abductor moment arm and muscle forces associated with a normal shoulder and a Delta reverse shoulder prosthesis. Impingement and scapular notching were simulated under various conditions.

[31] Terrier A, Reist A, Merlini F, Farron A: Simulated joint and muscle forces in reversed and anatomic shoulder prostheses. *J Bone Joint Surg Br* 2008;90(6):751-756.
A computer modeling study quantified deltoid abductor moment arms and forces in the reverse shoulder prosthesis compared with an anatomic prosthesis. The reverse prosthesis was evaluated under two conditions: with only a deficient supraspinatus and with no rotator cuff.

[32] Ackland DC, Roshan-Zamir S, Richardson M, Pandy MG: Moment arms of the shoulder musculature after reverse total shoulder arthroplasty. *J Bone Joint Surg Am* 2010;92(5):1221-1230.
Cadaver shoulders were used to measure muscle moment arms with anatomic and reverse shoulder arthroplasty. Increases in the length of the moment arms were observed for the major abductors, flexors, adductors, and extensors with reverse shoulder arthroplasty.

[33] Frankle M, Siegal S, Pupello D, Saleem A, Mighell M, Vasey M: The Reverse Shoulder Prosthesis for glenohumeral arthritis associated with severe rotator cuff deficiency: A minimum two-year follow-up study of sixty patients. *J Bone Joint Surg Am* 2005;87(8):1697-1705.

[34] Herrmann S, König C, Heller M, Perka C, Greiner S: Reverse shoulder arthroplasty leads to significant biomechanical changes in the remaining rotator cuff. *J Orthop Surg Res* 2011;6:42.
Subscapularis and teres minor rotation moment arms and muscle lengths were calculated from CT reconstructions of seven cadavers with reverse shoulder arthroplasty. The rotation moment arms and muscle lengths were decreased compared with those of the anatomic shoulder.

[35] Lädermann A, Walch G, Lubbeke A, et al: Influence of arm lengthening in reverse shoulder arthroplasty. *J Shoulder Elbow Surg* 2012;21(3):336-341.

Radiographic measurements of humeral lengthening were made from 183 reverse shoulder arthroplasties. At a minimum 1-year follow-up, lengthening of the humerus was evaluated relative to the contralateral side. Shortening of the arm reduced active anterior elevation.

[36] Lädermann A, Williams MD, Melis B, Hoffmeyer P, Walch G: Objective evaluation of lengthening in reverse shoulder arthroplasty. *J Shoulder Elbow Surg* 2009;18(4):588-595.

A technique was proposed to preoperatively plan adequate deltoid tensioning using radiographic measurements from the contralateral arm.

[37] Henninger HB, Barg A, Anderson AE, Bachus KN, Burks RT, Tashjian RZ: Effect of lateral offset center of rotation in reverse total shoulder arthroplasty: A biomechanical study. *J Shoulder Elbow Surg* 2012;21(9):1128-1135.

A shoulder controller was used to evaluate cadaver shoulders before and after reverse shoulder arthroplasty, with spacers added to laterally shift the center of rotation. Center of rotation lateralization had no influence on adduction or external rotation but increased abduction and dislocation forces because of smaller moment arms.

[38] Gallo RA, Gamradt SC, Mattern CJ, et al: Instability after reverse total shoulder replacement. *J Shoulder Elbow Surg* 2011;20(4):584-590.

After 57 reverse shoulder arthroplasties, instability occurred in 9 shoulders within the first 6 months. All 9 patients had a compromised subscapularis tendon, and 5 had a questionable glenosphere position.

[39] Saltzman MD, Mercer DM, Warme WJ, Bertelsen AL, Matsen FA III: A method for documenting the change in center of rotation with reverse total shoulder arthroplasty and its application to a consecutive series of 68 shoulders having reconstruction with one of two different reverse prostheses. *J Shoulder Elbow Surg* 2010;19(7):1028-1033.

The change in center of rotation on preoperative and postoperative radiographs is quantified using two different reverse shoulder implants. The position of the center of rotation was found to be significantly different after surgery and between the two implant designs.

[40] Boileau P, Chuinard C, Roussanne Y, Bicknell RT, Rochet N, Trojani C: Reverse shoulder arthroplasty combined with a modified latissimus dorsi and teres major tendon transfer for shoulder pseudoparalysis associated with dropping arm. *Clin Orthop Relat Res* 2008;466(3):584-593.

A prospective study of 11 patients with a combined loss of active elevation and external rotation found that reverse shoulder arthroplasty and latissimus dorsi and teres major transfer restored both active elevation and external rotation.

[41] Boileau P, Rumian AP, Zumstein MA: Reversed shoulder arthroplasty with modified L'Episcopo for combined loss of active elevation and external rotation. *J Shoulder Elbow Surg* 2010;19(2, suppl):20-30.

A study of 17 patients with a combined loss of active elevation and external rotation found that reverse shoulder arthroplasty and latissimus dorsi and teres major transfer restored both active elevation and external rotation.

[42] Favre P, Loeb MD, Helmy N, Gerber C: Latissimus dorsi transfer to restore external rotation with reverse shoulder arthroplasty: A biomechanical study. *J Shoulder Elbow Surg* 2008;17(4):650-658.

A biomechanical analysis quantified external rotation moment arms after latissimus dorsi transfer and reverse shoulder arthroplasty using two different humeral cup designs.

[43] Roche C, Flurin PH, Wright T, Zuckerman J: An evaluation of the relationship between prosthetic design parameters and clinical failure modes. *Proceedings of the 19th Annual Symposium.* Auburn, CA, International Society for Technology in Arthroplasty, 2006, p. 288. http://www.instaonline.org. Accessed July 19, 2012.

[44] Roche C, Flurin PH, Wright T, Crosby LA, Mauldin M, Zuckerman JD: An evaluation of the relationships between reverse shoulder design parameters and range of motion, impingement, and stability. *J Shoulder Elbow Surg* 2009;18(5):734-741.

A computer modeling study modified the Grammont reverse shoulder prosthesis and made recommendations to minimize impingement and improve stability. Subtle changes in design parameters were found to minimize impingement and offer potential for dramatic functional improvements in range of motion and jump distance.

[45] Bergmann G, Graichen F, Bender A, Kääb M, Rohlmann A, Westerhoff P: In vivo glenohumeral contact forces—measurements in the first patient 7 months postoperatively. *J Biomech* 2007;40(10):2139-2149.

Glenohumeral forces and moments were presented at 7-month follow-up of a patient who received an instrumented shoulder implant with telemetric data transmission. The maximum reported force was 150% of body weight.

[46] Onstot BR, Suslak AG, Colley R, Jacofsky MC, Otis JC, Hansen ML: Consequences of concomitant subscapularis repair with reverse total shoulder arthroplasty. *Transactions of the 58th Annual Meeting.* Rosemont, IL, Orthopaedic Research Society, 2012, paper 297.

A shoulder controller study evaluated the impact of subscapularis repair on reverse shoulder biomechanics in a cadaver scapula. Repair of the subscapularis increased the deltoid force, the joint reaction force, and the posterior rotator cuff force compared with an unrepaired cadaver specimen.

[47] Edwards TB, Williams MD, Labriola JE, Elkousy HA, Gartsman GM, O'Connor DP: Subscapularis insufficiency and the risk of shoulder dislocation after reverse shoulder arthroplasty. *J Shoulder Elbow Surg* 2009; 18(6):892-896.

A prospective study of Grammont reverse shoulder arthroplasty in 138 patients found that the subscapularis was reparable in 62 patients and irreparable in 76 patients. All 7 dislocations occurred in patients whose subscapularis was irreparable. Repair of the subscapularis is recommended whenever possible.

[48] Gerber C, Maquieira G, Espinosa N: Latissimus dorsi transfer for the treatment of irreparable rotator cuff tears. *J Bone Joint Surg Am* 2006;88(1):113-120.

[49] Norris TR, Kelly JD: Management of glenoid bone defects in revision shoulder arthroplasty: A new application of the reverse total shoulder prosthesis. *Tech Shoulder Elbow Surg* 2007;8(1):37-46.

A one-stage method is presented for treating patients with severe glenoid wear who are in need of reverse shoulder arthroplasty. Clinical challenges and surgical technique are discussed.

[50] Poppen NK, Walker PS: Forces at the glenohumeral joint in abduction. *Clin Orthop Relat Res* 1978;135: 165-170.

第五章 肘关节置换术的生物力学

James A. Johnson, PhD; Graham J. W. King, MD, MSc, FRCSC

引言

已经可以确定的是，肘关节可以承受超过身体重量的力。过去几十年对肘关节置换术的生物力学研究着眼于移植物－骨结构的负荷转移和压力分析。重点关注移植物重建肱尺关节和肱桡关节的动力学及稳定性。通过最近的研究进展，骨科医师可以更好地理解桡骨头置换术的生物力学，尤其是桡骨头假体的形状和放置位置，以及移植物的设计和假体柄的固定。由于移植物力线对于负荷转移非常重要，尤其是在肱尺关节侧，因此计算机辅助技术通常被用来优化手术中移植物的放置。最近的研究热点还包括涉及肱骨小头和冠突的半关节置换术。

桡骨头置换术

从生物力学角度看，桡骨头置换术置入假体的两个原则是使假体替代桡骨头的关节区域和使假体柄插入桡骨颈髓腔以使假体与天然骨相固定。

Dr. King or an immediate family member serves as a board member, owner, officer, or committee member of the American Shoulder and Elbow Surgeons; has received royalties from Wright Medical Technology, Tornier, and Tenet Medical; is a member of a speakers' bureau or has made paid presentations on behalf of Wright Medical Technology; and serves as a paid consultant to or is an employee of Wright Medical Technology. Neither Dr. Johnson nor any immediate family member has received anything of value from or has stock or stock options held in a commercial company or institution related directly or indirectly to the subject of this chapter.

动力学和稳定性

逐渐明确的是，桡骨头假体的设计对于重建肘关节的稳定性至关重要。为了确定双极桡骨头假体（以下简称双极假体）与单极桡骨头假体（以下简称单极假体）生物力学特征的区别，已经开展了大量研究。通过尸体模型比较双极和单极假体的肱桡关节稳定性，单极假体所提供的防止半脱位的稳定性与天然肘关节相近，双极假体容易出现半脱位，可能是因为后者减少了凹陷压迫的稳定作用。[1]在一个肘关节不稳定模型中，通过相似的实验模型检测天然肘关节、单极假体、双极假体的形状和设计对向后方移位的抵抗作用。[2]尽管双极假体的倾斜能力被认为有利于关节运动和关节接触，但研究者发现桡骨头的倾斜减少了发生半脱位所需的力，因此双极假体的稳定性低于单极假体或天然肘关节。有趣的是，具有解剖学形态的桡骨头假体与天然桡骨头具有相似的稳定性，比有更浅的凹陷关节面的环状桡骨头假体更加稳定，这可以解释该发现。一项实验研究发现双极假体的适应性很好，可确保关节面接触不受关节位置的影响，但是会有假体位置异常的趋势。[3]在另一项体外实验中，双极假体可自控力线，而更易固定的单极假体无法自控力线。[4]这一实验结果对于在手术中没有获得合适的假体力线的病例尤为重要，而这类病例并不少见。

研究者还着眼于对桡骨头假体关节盘的几何学特征的研究。在一项针对单极假体关节盘的曲率半径和深度对稳定性的影响的研究中，关节盘更深的解剖型假体与天然桡骨头相匹配，而具有更大曲率半径的关节盘浅的环状桡骨头假体与天然桡骨头并不匹配[5]（图5-1）。目前，研究者们正在不断革新桡骨头假体关节面形状的设计，努力获得更优化的负荷转移，减轻肱骨小头软骨磨损。

软组织为天然肘关节和肘关节假体提供了重要的约束力。肱桡关节的稳定性主要源于置入的关节盘的凹陷压迫作用，以及侧副韧带、环状韧带和关节囊提供的稳定性。桌面模型用于确定软组织在负荷下抵抗向后移位的作用。[6] 软组织的约束力在双极假体中是最重要的。在天然桡骨头或单极假体中，软组织的作用较小，其稳定性主要依靠桡骨假体关节盘和肱骨小头的凹陷压迫作用。

应用金属桡骨头置换改善了肘关节的动力学和稳定性，但并没有使之回归正常，这可能是因为通过传统的手术技术很难同时恢复关节的协调性和轴向高度。[7] 如果假体的厚度小于天然结构，则肯定会增加关节松弛度。相反，如果假体的厚度大于天然结构，则关节松弛度会降低并可能增加有害的关节接触应力以及改变肱骨小头磨损程度和肱尺关节协调性。最近有研究报道了诊断桡骨头假体过长的困难性。[8] 一项尸体标本研究通过肌肉负荷和X线片评估了桡骨头假体厚度每增加2 mm时对肱尺关节协调性的影响。当假体厚度超出天然结构6 mm时即可在影像学上发现明显的肱尺关节不协调（图5-2）。关节面接触应力及关节运动轨迹的改变可能导致关节厚度发生很小的改变，但这些观点都尚未得以确定。要确定

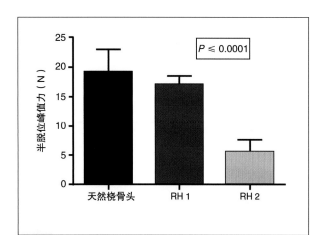

图 5-1 天然桡骨头和两种桡骨头假体的平均半脱位峰值力比较图。RH 1= 解剖型桡骨头假体，RH 2= 环状桡骨头假体。经允许引自 Chanlalit C, Shukla DR, Fitzsimmons JS, An KN, O'Driscoll SW: Influence of prosthetic design on radiocapitellar concavity-compression stability. *J Shoulder Elbow Surg* 2011;20:885-890.

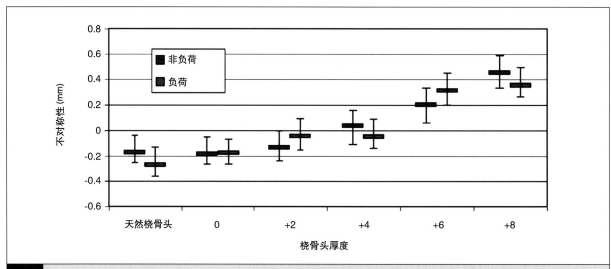

图 5-2 随着桡骨头假体厚度的增加（过长），内侧肱尺关节不对称性也增加。0= 正确型号的移植物。经允许引自 Frank SG, Grewal R, Johnson J, Faber KJ, King GJ, Athwal GS: Determination of correct implant size in radial head arthroplasty to avoid overlengthening. *J Bone Joint Surg Am* 2009;91（7）:1738-1746.

更优的桡骨头的关节面设计和桡骨头假体的放置，以恢复外侧柱高度并确保更好的肱尺关节和肱桡关节之间的负荷转移，尚需进一步的研究。

固定

桡骨头置换术中对于假体柄的最优固定方法尚未确定。假体柄的固定方法很大程度上取决于桡骨头的形态。已经确定的是，天然桡骨头是偏椭圆形的，并偏心于桡骨颈中心。因此，非骨水泥固定可用于轴对称的假体，使假体柄与髓腔紧密结合，或可使用双极假体以确保桡骨盘状关节面与肱骨小头的运动轨迹相协调。一款商用假体的设计尝试复制桡骨近端的不对称形状。假体柄的准确固定是设计的前提条件，以确保正确的假体方向并避免肱骨小头上的运动轨迹出现错误。可以通过使用骨水泥固定假体柄或通过适合骨长入的孔隙表面准确地固定。

若使用非骨水泥，则还需要在放置假体后最大程度地减少界面间的微动，以保证骨成功长入。对于这种桡骨头假体的固定模式知之甚少，尽管

骨科医师普遍认同采用相对于髓腔更大的假体柄以获得可靠的压配。然而，就像在股骨髓腔或肱骨髓腔内插入非骨水泥柄一样，这一操作存在骨折的危险。这一危险因假体柄和（或）宿主髓腔的锥形形态而增加。一项针对假体柄的型号对初始稳定性影响的尸体模型研究关注过由大号假体柄及由环形应力（hoop stresses）所致的骨折。[9]研究者得出的结论是，环形应力所致的皮质小骨折不会导致明显的微动和失去稳定性，这在临床上是可以接受的。有一项研究发现半喷砂装置的初始稳定性与全喷砂装置的初始稳定性相当。[10]这一发现提示半喷砂装置可能更好，因为半喷砂装置在假体柄取出和应力遮挡方面更具优势。有研究者通过尸体模型研究了假体柄的型号、长度和形状（直柄或锥形柄）在接受偏心轴向负荷时对桡骨头假体稳定性的影响。[11]完全填充髓腔被发现是影响桡骨头假体初始稳定性的最关键因素，而假体柄的长度和形状并没有明显影响初始稳定性（图5–3）。有

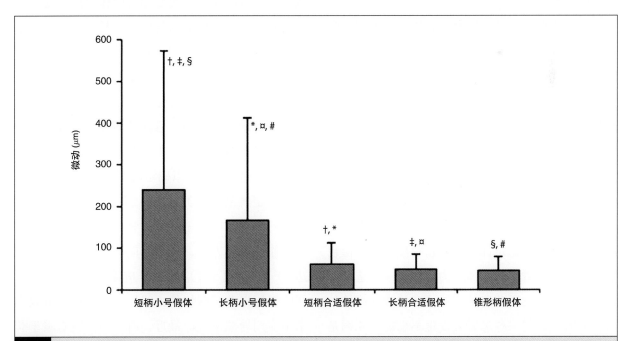

图 5–3 图表显示被测试的 5 种假体的活动（混合数据）。应用小号假体时活动明显增加（P<0.02）。短柄小号假体和长柄小号假体之间没有明显差异，而短柄合适假体、长柄合适假体和锥形柄假体之间也没有明显差异。图中标注相同符号的组之间存在显著性差异。经允许引自 Ferreira LM, Stacpoole RA, Johnson JA, King GJ: Cementless fixation of radial head implants is affected by implant stem geometry: An in vitro study. *Clin Biomech (Bristol, Avon)* 2010;25（5）:422–426.

研究通过桌面模型确定压配桡骨头假体柄的微动以及研究锉的型号及插入力度。[12]通过这些研究发现扩大髓腔和采用更大直径的假体柄可以最大程度地减少微动发生。用力插入假体柄可以减少微动，而插入柄的力量大小可作为术中判断假体柄固定程度的有效度量标准。总之，这些研究提示非骨水泥压配桡骨头假体的最佳初始固定可以通过选择改善髓腔填充的假体柄的型号来实现，尤其是假体柄的直径。尚需开展临床研究以确定假体柄的型号对假体固定和其表现的长期影响。

全肘关节置换术

全肘关节置换术最常见的失败原因是假体松动和材料磨损。几乎所有的假体都是通过丙烯酸骨水泥与周围骨皮质固定。运动模式和跨关节负荷改变可以导致假体－骨水泥界面或骨水泥－骨界面失去固定。关节特征和力线是影响肱骨和尺骨假体－骨水泥－骨复合物结构负荷和应力的两个最重要因素。

肱尺关节

铰链式全肘关节置换术的假体常被称为半限制关节或松弛铰链关节，因为其允许小范围的次级运动（如尺骨内外翻或内外旋）和初级屈伸运动。次级运动的允许活动量是一项被考虑到的设计特点，大多数全肘关节置换术假体存在一些内外翻和旋转松弛度。连接装置的过度限制会导致负荷通过骨－假体界面转移，从而造成机械性松动，而限制不足会导致肘关节不稳定。

连接全肘关节假体为尺骨和肱骨组成部分之间的限制增加了稳定性，可阻止脱位发生，但也可能是假体－骨水泥界面应力增加的一个重要原因。理论上，应用非连接装置可有效减少假体的负荷和磨损，但一些患者会发生不稳定，原因是很难实现确切的韧带固定或应用抗风湿药物所导致的延迟愈合。

最近的一项实验研究及一项有限元分析检测了非连接 iBP 假体（Biomet,Warsaw,IN）的骨应力。[13]在人工肱骨和人工尺骨上应用应变测试仪，在行肘关节置换术前后进行测量，毗邻假体尖端的骨应变明显增加。与完整骨相比，人工肱骨和尺骨骨骺部的骨松质应变减小。可以得出的结论是，非连接性肘关节假体可能存在骨疲劳失效的风险，尤其是在尺骨。并且，在骨骺部的应力遮挡可能会促进骨吸收。这一作用可能与连接性假体相近。可以考虑通过改进假体柄的形状、长度和材料减轻应力遮挡的程度并改善对骨的负荷转移。

假体力线

如果假体的肱骨和尺骨组件的力线不理想，会对连接装置增加更多的限制，磨损和假体－骨水泥界面的应力均会增加，可能导致组件松动和机械性失效。动力学和负荷转移方面发生改变的首要原因是关节的位置和力线不合适。对于肱尺关节，组件的机械轴与解剖学屈伸轴不相符会改变关节正常的运动特征。这些异常的运动路径会改变韧带和关节囊的张力以及肌肉的力臂和活动轨迹。关节的动力学改变导致假体力的改变及继发的假体－骨结构的力的异常。最近的全肘关节置换术的生物力学研究着眼于肱尺关节力线，注重重建解剖学屈伸轴。

肱骨假体柄的位置受控于铰链关节的力线与肘关节解剖学屈伸轴。目前的研究已证实铰链关节的力线可以通过肱骨小头和滑车形态确定，明确每一结构的中心可以确定解剖学屈伸轴。然而，术中确定解剖学屈伸轴并不容易。3 位经过专业培训的骨科医师在一系列肱骨远端病例中预判解剖学屈伸轴的方向，各个方向的力线偏差最高可达 10°[14]（图 5-4）。因此，应该研究更好的手术切除引导以改善假体的力线，或者在肘关节置换术中应用导航系统。最近，有一项研究着眼于获得满意的尺骨假体力线的方法。[15]对桡骨头假体位置和中心方位的认知的逐渐深入，不仅有助于改善尺骨大乙状切迹（引导嵴）中心突的中点和方向与相应尺骨关节解剖屈伸轴的匹配的准确性，

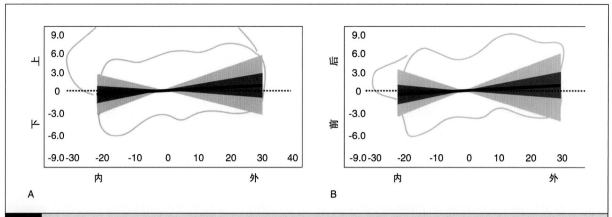

图 5-4　图表显示屈伸轴测定中的内外翻和内外旋误差。根据每一标本的单位矢量分析得出内外翻（额状面）（A）以及内外旋（冠状面）（B）的结果。虚线 = 水平轴（0°）；实线 = 平均角度（1.5°外翻，1.6°外旋）；深灰区域 = 平均线 1 个标准差内的区域（4.5°外翻至 1.5°内翻，4.9°外旋至 1.7°内旋）；浅灰区域 = 剩余值（9.6°外翻至 6.3°内翻，10.2°外旋至 8.3°内旋）。近端、前方及内侧为正向。经允许引自 Brownhill JR, Furukawa K, Faber KJ, Johnson JA, King GJ: Surgeon accuracy in the selection of the flexion–extension axis of the elbow: An in vitro study. *J Shoulder Elbow Surg* 2006;15（4）:451–456.

也可以改善预判动力学屈伸轴的准确性。这一发现提示骨科医师（或计算机导航系统）在肘关节置换术中应当在确定尺骨假体方向时考虑桡骨头的位置和方向。尺骨切除引导还应当考虑桡骨头的特征，以提高尺骨假体放置的准确性。

最近，一项体外生物力学实验研究了肱骨假体力线不良对于负荷的影响。[16] 位置良好的假体上的负荷明显低于位置靠前或异常旋转的假体上

的负荷（图 5-5）。这些增加的负荷，特别是内外翻和内外旋，更可能导致聚乙烯连接装置磨损，从而增加松动的可能性。

用假体重建关节的天然解剖位置对减少负荷和损伤非常重要，但这可能很难在现有的假体系统中获得，因为假体柄支撑于髓腔内。最近的研究检测了骨的形态及关节位置与髓腔内假体柄的位置偏离的关系。一项基于 CT 的研究检测了 40

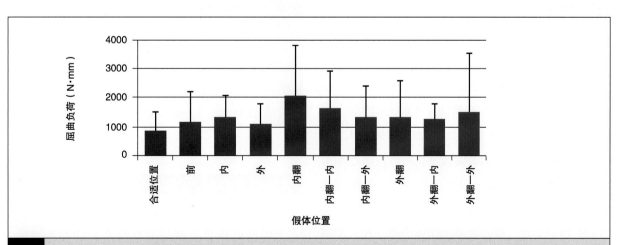

图 5-5　图表显示旋后位主动屈曲的平均弯曲负荷。逐一显示了 10 个假体在测试位置屈曲活动时的弯曲负荷（平均值 + 标准差）。经允许引自 Brownhill JR, Pollock JW, Ferreira LM, Johnson JA, King GJ: The effect of implant malalignment on joint loading in total elbow arthroplasty: An in vitro study. *J Shoulder Elbow Surg* 2012;21（8）:1032–1038.

例病例的肱骨远端髓腔轴线和屈伸轴的关系。[17]研究者量化了向前偏离及两条轴线间的肘关节角度。屈伸轴从髓腔轴线向前偏离的距离与髓腔长度成比例。关节面宽度、肘关节角度及前后径长度和髓腔曲率之间没有关系。研究者认为，使用组配式肱骨侧假体以适应肱骨远端自然前弓和关节面偏心的变异，肘关节屈伸轴可能会恢复得更好。这些研究人员最近的一项研究通过对31例病例的尺骨近端的CT检查确定了接近关节面的髓腔形状。[18]研究发现，向后及向外侧的偏离从关节中心向远端增加。男性的平均外翻角度为8°（±4°），女性为7.2°（±3.1°）。研究者得出的结论是，可能需要使用模块化的尺骨假体及更长的柄，以适应髓腔相对于关节轴线的偏离变异。

近些年，研究者们在探索影像学和计算机辅助下的全肘关节置换术方面取得了实质性的进展。这一基于逻辑的方法可以在很大程度上减少通过视觉识别标志导致的假体放置错误。该方法在髋关节置换术和膝关节置换术中的成功促进了对上肢应用相似技术的探索。一项早期研究探讨了使用基于表面的配准技术的可能性。[19]通过应用手持镭射扫描仪和传统的应用于尸体标本远端关节面的双点标记，可使标记误差保持在1~2 mm。在确定靶轴时，应用基于表面的标记会比医师的视觉预判更准确。通过尸体标本对肱骨远端标志选择和骨缺损对于图像引导标记准确性的影响进行了研究。[20]研究发现即使存在实质的骨缺损，仍可以通过仅存的解剖学标志准确地在术前CT图像上标记，误差约为1 mm（移位）和0.5°（旋转）。CT下的良好力线及在术中的表面数字化可以仅通过相对较小的肱骨远端关节周围区域获得。适当轨迹技术和影像学技术的应用可以基于对侧未受损肘关节的影像学表现，保证准确的假体力线。在一项研究中，研究者证实双侧肱骨远端的解剖学差异大概为0.5 mm（移位）和1.0°（旋转），在通过对侧进行影像学技术和计算机辅助的假体重建中可以

接受。[21]最近有研究通过尸体标本评估了计算机辅助肱骨假体柄力线测量的准确性。[22]将假体进行缩短（以减少髓腔撞击），其力线误差为1.3 mm（±0.5 mm）移位和1.2°（±0.4°）旋转。在常规假体中，力线误差为1.9 mm（±1.1 mm）移位和3.6°（±2.1°）旋转（图5-6）。结论是，具有固定外翻角度的肱骨假体难以准确放置，因此恢复屈伸轴力线较困难；可能需要提供更多外翻角度变异的假体。

目前，对肱尺关节体外假体力线的认知已经有很多，进一步的工作是将这些认知应用于患者假体放置的改进。

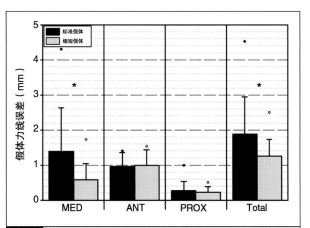

图5-6 图表显示移位中的假体力线误差（平均值＋标准差）。针对每一误差都提供了三向的误差［内外（MED），前后（ANT），远近（PROX）］和总误差（Total）。圆点＝每一移位中的最大误差（mm）；＊=明显差异（P<0.05）。经允许引自McDonald CP, Peters TM, Johnson JA, King GJ: Stem abutment affects alignment of the humeral component in computer-assisted elbow arthroplasty. *J Shoulder Elbow Surg* 2011;20（6）:891-898.

其他假体系统

近期的研究关注点是研发针对关节炎、骨折或剥脱性骨软骨炎所致的肱骨小头缺损的假体。一项基于CT的50例尸体标本的形态学研究量化了肱骨小头关节面的矢状面和横断面。[23]矢状面和横断面的曲率半径分别为11.6 mm（±1.4 mm）

和 14 mm（±3 mm；范围为 9.6~20.9 mm）。这些发现提示肱骨小头并不是呈球形的。通过不同的形态学测量发现了大量的肱骨头变异；这一发现提示采用非定制的假体可能不是好的选择。半关节置换术的重要关注点在于与天然软骨表面接触力学特性的改变。这类研究是通过比较球形金属肱骨小头假体和椭球形金属肱骨小头假体与尸体标本的天然桡骨头的关节接触面积进行。[24] 用一种特殊的印记材料量化接触面积，从而评估关节的压力负荷。解剖型假体和球形假体的接触面积（分别为 59% 和 51%）明显低于天然关节。同一研究还发现在单间室置换中，两种肱骨小头假体与超高分子量聚乙烯桡骨头的接触面积相似。这一发现提示虽然天然肱骨小头是椭球形的，但是球形肱骨小头假体仍可以满足临床假体设计需要。关节接触面积变小可能与金属假体的硬度相

关，需要进一步研究新型的半关节置换假体。研究者在尸体上肢中模拟肘关节活动以研究不同活动中的球形和椭球形假体。[25] 切除肱骨小头导致肘关节内外翻松弛度增加 3.1° 及尺侧外旋增加 1.5°；假体的设计可以修正肘关节不稳定。总之，这些研究支持以球形假体治疗肱骨小头缺损的效果。

最近出现了对冠突假体的探索。[26] 金属冠突假体基于人体测量学研究发展而来。研究者应用上肢关节运动模拟装置量化了冠突完整、冠突缺损及假体重建的尸体标本的肘关节内外翻松弛度。标准型号和更大型号的冠突假体都可以恢复关节稳定性，且与完整状态相近（图 5-7）。在侧副韧带缺损时，使用更大型号的冠突假体可以获得比使用标准型号假体更好的稳定性。这一发现提示冠突假体虽然没有商业可用性，但可能在未来治

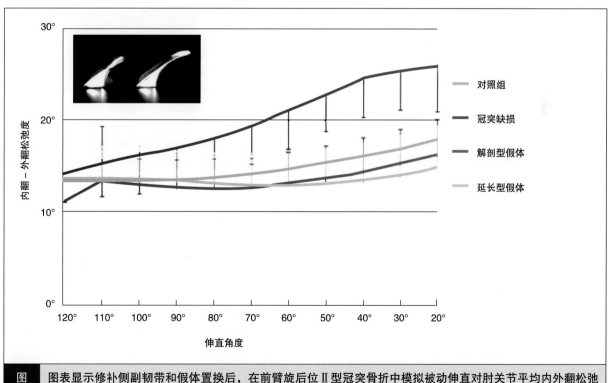

图 5-7 图表显示修补侧副韧带和假体置换后，在前臂旋后位 Ⅱ 型冠突骨折中模拟被动伸直对肘关节平均内外翻松弛度的影响。天然冠突 40% 缺损可增加肘关节松弛度。解剖型假体或延长型假体与天然冠突相似，可提高肘关节稳定性。误差条图指示标准差。嵌入图：解剖型假体侧位观（左），延长型假体侧位观（右）。经允许引自 Alolabi B, Gray A, Ferreira LM, Johnson JA, Athwal GS, King GJ: Reconstruction of the coronoid using an extended prosthesis: An in vitro biomechanical study. *J Shoulder Elbow Surg* 2012;21（7）:969-976.

疗无法重建的粉碎性冠突骨折中具有重要意义。

虽然对这些半关节置换假体的研究还处在初始阶段，但是即将实现在设计和发展上的巨大进展。未来还可能出现其他微创假体设计。

总结

在过去的 5 年，关于桡骨头假体的设计和型号，以及髓腔固定的研究取得了明显的进展。尤其是对桡骨头置换解剖学特征的重要新知识，以及对稳定性和动力学的关注。针对全肘关节置换假体的设计和力线的研究强调在影像学和计算机辅助下进行手术以改善假体放置。目前，愈加明确的是，肘关节假体的设计需要适应肱骨和尺骨髓腔的特征，并有较大的选择范围，尤其在为了恢复解剖学形态而将肘关节假体放置于关节时。已有一些关于肱骨小头和特殊小型冠突假体的早期研究的报道，在将来很有可能会发展出更多的半关节置换假体和微创手术方法。

参考文献

[1] Moon JG, Berglund LJ, Zachary D, An KN, O'Driscoll SW: Radiocapitellar joint stability with bipolar versus monopolar radial head prostheses. *J Shoulder Elbow Surg* 2009;18(5):779-784.

An experimental cadaver study examined the stability of radial head components. A monopolar prosthesis is more effective in stabilizing the radiocapitellar joint than a bipolar prosthesis. The bipolar device has a compromising effect on the concavity compression stability of the radiocapitellar joint.

[2] Chanlalit C, Shukla DR, Fitzsimmons JS, An KN, O'Driscoll SW: The biomechanical effect of prosthetic design on radiocapitellar stability in a terrible triad model. *J Orthop Trauma* 2012;26(9):539-544.

In an in vitro model of a terrible triad injury, two monopolar radial head implants conferred greater radiocapitellar stability than bipolar implants. The anatomic prosthesis provided more stability than the nonanatomic prosthesis.

[3] Moungondo F, El Kazzi W, van Riet R, Feipel V, Rooze M, Schuind F: Radiocapitellar joint contacts after bipolar radial head arthroplasty. *J Shoulder Elbow Surg* 2010;19(2):230-235.

Molding techniques were used to determine radiocapitellar contact before and after radial head replacement, using the bipolar design of the Judet device. Contact area averaged 44% and 33% in the intact and implant-reconstructed elbows, respectively. Because of intraprosthetic mobility, contact areas were not dependent on elbow position when the bipolar implant was used. This factor led to abnormal positioning of the prosthesis with supination, causing subluxation over the trochlea lateral margin.

[4] Yian E, Steens W, Lingenfelter E, Schneeberger AG: Malpositioning of radial head prostheses: An in vitro study. *J Shoulder Elbow Surg* 2008;17(4):663-670.

An in vitro study analyzed the ability to perform anatomic radial head replacement and to study radiocapitellar prosthetic subluxation under unstable conditions. Anatomic alignment of radial head implants was difficult to consistently achieve. Bipolar implants offer better self-alignment, which can be difficult to achieve with rigid implants. Posterolateral stress produced radiocapitellar subluxation in the rigid but not the bipolar implants.

[5] Chanlalit C, Shukla DR, Fitzsimmons JS, An KN, O'Driscoll SW: Influence of prosthetic design on radiocapitellar concavity-compression stability. *J Shoulder Elbow Surg* 2011;20(6):885-890.

An experimental study examined the influence of the shape of the articular dish of a monopolar radial head implant on joint stability. An implant that more closely matches the normal anatomy is more effective than a shallow implant with a longer-than-normal radius of curvature.

[6] Chanlalit C, Shukla DR, Fitzsimmons JS, Thoreson AR, An KN, O'Driscoll SW: Radiocapitellar stability: The effect of soft tissue integrity on bipolar versus monopolar radial head prostheses. *J Shoulder Elbow Surg* 2011;20(2):219-225.

An in vitro model was used to measure the effects of the soft tissues on radiocapitellar stability in monopolar and bipolar radial head prostheses. Stability was better with a monopolar radial head prosthesis, particularly in the absence of soft-tissue support.

[7] Beingessner DM, Dunning CE, Gordon KD, Johnson JA, King GJ: The effect of radial head excision and arthroplasty on elbow kinematics and stability. *J Bone Joint Surg Am* 2004;86-A(8):1730-1739.

[8] Frank SG, Grewal R, Johnson J, Faber KJ, King GJ, Athwal GS: Determination of correct implant size in

radial head arthroplasty to avoid overlengthening. *J Bone Joint Surg Am* 2009;91(7):1738-1746.

The purpose of this biomechanical study was to identify clinical and radiographic features that may be used to diagnose overlengthening of the radius intraoperatively and on postoperative radiographs. Radial head implants of different thicknesses were implanted into cadaver specimens and assessed radiographically. Incongruity of the medial ulnohumeral joint can be radiographically assessed only after overlengthening of the radius by at least 6 mm.

[9] Chanlalit C, Shukla DR, Fitzsimmons JS, An KN, O'Driscoll SW: Effect of hoop stress fracture on micro-motion of textured ingrowth stems for radial head replacement. *J Shoulder Elbow Surg* 2012;21(7):949-954.

Grit-blasted radial head prosthetic stems of increasing sizes were implanted into cadaver specimens. Insertion forces and implant micromotion were measured. A small radial neck fracture occurred with a stem oversized by 1 mm, but it did not compromise stability or micromotion.

[10] Chanlalit C, Fitzsimmons JS, Moon JG, Berglund LJ, An KN, O'Driscoll SW: Radial head prosthesis micro-motion characteristics: Partial versus fully grit-blasted stems. *J Shoulder Elbow Surg* 2011;20(1):27-32.

This in vitro study found that the stability of a radial head stem partially grit blasted at the proximal end was similar to that of a stem grit blasted along the full length.

[11] Ferreira LM, Stacpoole RA, Johnson JA, King GJ: Cementless fixation of radial head implants is affected by implant stem geometry: An in vitro study. *J Shoulder Elbow Surg* 2010;25(5):422-426.

This experimental study examined the effects of radial head stem geometry on the initial stability of uncemented implants of various geometries and lengths. Filling the diameter of the canal was found to be more relevant than filling the length. A canal-filling stem reduced implant micromotion to less than 50 microns.

[12] Moon JG, Berglund LJ, Domire Z, An KN, O'Driscoll SW: Stem diameter and micromotion of press fit radial head prosthesis: A biomechanical study. *J Shoulder Elbow Surg* 2009;18(5):785-790.

This experimental study determined the effect of the stem diameter and insertion force on stability with a press-fit radial head designed for bone ingrowth. The greatest stability in the press-fit implant was achieved by maximizing sizing in the neck canal.

[13] Completo A, Pereira J, Fonseca F, Ramos A, Relvas C, Simões J: Biomechanical analysis of total elbow replacement with unlinked iBP prosthesis: An in vitro and finite element analysis. Clin Biomech (Bristol, Avon) 2011;26(10):990-997.

This experimental and computational study quantified strains and stresses in bone and cement around humeral and ulnar implant stems. In the epiphyseal region, a strain reduction was observed relative to the intact bones, but strains increased markedly at the tip.

[14] Brownhill JR, Furukawa K, Faber KJ, Johnson JA, King GJ: Surgeon accuracy in the selection of the flexion-extension axis of the elbow: An in vitro study. *J Shoulder Elbow Surg* 2006;15(4):451-456.

[15] Brownhill JR, Ferreira LM, Pichora JE, Johnson JA, King GJ: Defining the flexion-extension axis of the ulna: Implications for intra-operative elbow alignment. J Biomevh Eng 2009;131(2):021005.

An in vitro study determined the relationship of vari- ous kinematically and anatomically derived flexion axes of the ulna, with a focus on the accuracy of implant positioning. The most accurate technique was found to be an anatomic-based measurement that used the guiding ridge of the greater sigmoid notch of the ulna and the radial head.

[16] Brownhill JR, Pollock JW, Ferreira LM, Johnson JA, King GJ: The effect of implant malalignment on joint loading in total elbow arthroplasty: An in vitro study. *J Shoulder Elbow Surg* 2012;21(8):1032-1038.

An in vitro study used load sensors in the ulnohumeral articulation to determine the effect of implant alignment on joint loading in cadaver-based testing. Loading increased with malaligned implant positions, but combinations of internal-external and varus-valgus malrotations that tended to preserve the line of action of the elbow flexors were less aggressive.

[17] Brownhill JR, King GJ, Johnson JA: Morphologic analysis of the distal humerus with special interest in elbow implant sizing and alignment. *J Shoulder Elbow Surg* 2007;16(3, suppl):S126-S132.

The relationship between the medullary canal axis and the flexion-extension axis of the distal humerus was examined as they relate to implant selection and design for elbow arthroplasty. The anterior offset of the flexion-extension axis relative to the medullary canal axis was proportional to the length of canal proximally that was used to determine the alignment of the stem.

[18] Brownhill JR, Mozzon JB, Ferreira LM, Johnson JA, King GJ: Morphologic analysis of the proximal ulna with special interest in elbow implant sizing and alignment. *J Shoulder Elbow Surg* 2009;18(1):27-32.

A CT-based study assessed the shape of the medullary

canal relative to the articular surface. Both the posterior and lateral offsets increased distally from the articulation center. The average valgus angulation was 8° in men and 7.2° in women. It was suggested that longer stemmed ulnar implants may require a modular design to meet anatomic constraints during implant positioning.

[19] McDonald CP, Brownhill JR, King GJ, Johnson JA, Peters TM: A comparison of registration techniques for computer- and image-assisted elbow surgery. Comput Aided Surg 2007;12(4):208-214.

An experimental study compared the alignment of the flexion-extension axis of a surface-based registration technique (using a handheld laser scanner) to a con- ventional paired-point registration. Registration was better by a factor of approximately 2 for the surface- based technique.

[20] McDonald CP, Beaton BJ, King GJ, Peters TM, Johnson JA: The effect of anatomic landmark selection of the distal humerus on registration accuracy in computer-assisted elbow surgery. J Shoulder Elbow Surg 2008;17(5):833-843.

An in vitro study determined the anatomic landmarks needed to successfully register surface digitizations to a preoperative image of the distal humerus. It was shown that close alignment can be achieved using a portion of the distal humerus that is measurable intraoperatively, even with major loss of articular structures.

[21] McDonald CP, Peters TM, King GJ, Johnson JA: Computer assisted surgery of the distal humerus can employ contralateral images for preoperative planning, registration, and surgical intervention. 2009;18(3):469-477.

A study determined whether the contralateral side can be used to determine implant position in the setting of bone loss. In CT scans of paired distal humeri, the anthropometric features were similar, with side-to-side differences in the range of 1.0° and 0.5 mm. The geometry found on preoperative imaging of the contralateral normal elbow may be used for referencing anatomic landmarks on the surgical side.

[22] McDonald CP, Peters TM, Johnson JA, King GJ: Stem abutment affects alignment of the humeral component in computer-assisted elbow arthroplasty. J Shoulder Elbow Surg 2011;20(6):891-898.

An in vitro study used computer-assisted alignment (based on a preoperative image) of the implant axis with the humeral flexion-extension axis for a regular and a reduced-length humeral implant. Implant alignment was markedly improved in the reduced-length stem. Because of impingement with the regular stems, it was concluded that a humeral component with a fixed valgus angulation cannot be reproducibly positioned if maintenance of the flexion-extension axis is required.

[23] Sabo MT, McDonald CP, Ng J, Ferreira LM, Johnson JA, King GJ: A morphological analysis of the humeral capitellum with an interest in prosthesis design. J Shoulder Elbow Surg 2011;20(6):880-884.

The purpose of this CT-based study was to quantify the anthropometric features of the capitellum in an effort to enhance implant design. The capitellum was found not to be spherical in shape, and there is substantial variability in the relationship between its height and width and between the radii of curvature in the sagittal and transverse planes. These variations may result in challenges in the design of implants that match the anatomic characteristics.

[24] Sabo MT, Shannon H, Ng J, Ferreira LM, Johnson JA, King GJ: The impact of capitellar arthroplasty on elbow contact mechanics: Implications for implant design. J Shoulder Elbow Surg 2011;26(5):458-463.

An experimental study used a casting technique to as- sess the contact mechanics of both a spherical and an anatomic-based capitellar implant against the native radius and a unicompartmental design. Relative to the native state, both capitellar implants resulted in large decreases in contact area, suggesting that the radial head cartilage would have increased contact pressures. The contact areas for the anatomic and spherical hemiarthroplasties were not significantly different, nor were those for the unicompartmental devices.

[25] Sabo MT, Shannon HL, Deluce S, et al: Capitellar excision and hemiarthroplasty affects elbow kinematics and stability. J Shoulder Elbow Surg 2012;21(8):1024, e4.

An evaluation of the effect of capitellar excision, with and without implant replacement, on stability using cadaver specimens in a testing simulator found that the capitellum has a role as a stabilizer to valgus and external rotation ulnohumeral articulation. These instabilities were corrected by capitellar hemiarthroplasty.

[26] Alolabi B, Gray A, Ferreira LM, Johnson JA, Athwal GS, King GJ: Reconstruction of the coronoid using an extended prosthesis: An in vitro biomechanical study. J Shoulder Elbow Surg 2012;21(7):969-976.

Using an elbow simulator and cadaver limbs, varus- valgus laxity was measured in intact, coronoid- deficient, and coronoidrestored states using both an anatomic and an extended prosthesis. The anatomic device with ligament repair restores stability to the in- tact state relative to the coronoid-deficient state. With ligament insufficiency, the extended device produces greater stability than the anatomic implant, although stability remains less than that of the intact elbow.

第二部分

不稳定与运动损伤

栏目编委：
Patrick J. McMahon, MD

第六章　盂肱关节不稳定的临床评估、影像学表现和分型

Brett D. Owens, MD

引言

盂肱关节不稳定常见于运动员及年轻有活力的患者。在运动员群体中，盂肱关节不稳定的发生率仅次于肩锁关节损伤，会导致更严重的残疾，并且与其他肩部损伤相比，盂肱关节不稳定的治疗可能需要更多的外科干预。[1-3] 对于年龄在25岁以下的具有盂肱关节症状的患者，在确诊为其他疾病之前，其默认的诊断就应当是不稳定。

对于肩关节不稳定的治疗取决于适当的分型及患者易感因素评级。对不稳定的判定需要有盂肱关节活动范围超过生理限度的主观感受，同时检查者可以通过客观地测量关节活动范围以判断松弛度。有症状的不稳定，生理性松弛和（或）病理性松弛及影像学表现是确定适当治疗方式的关键。

临床评估

患者病史

获得高质量的患者病史对于评估可疑的肩关节不稳定至关重要。盂肱关节完全脱位比盂肱关节半脱位更容易诊断，因为绝大多数盂肱关节完全脱位患者会经历人工复位过程。通常患者是在急诊室接受复位，因此复位前及复位后的影像学照片常可用于评估。在急诊室以外的地方进行复位的情况很常见，如在运动场进行复位，与复位者进行交流可以得知损伤情况和复位难易程度等信息。慢性不稳定患者可能会告知医师他们是自行复位的。

对于半脱位的报告会有更多变数，因为半脱位并不需要人工复位。患者常描述他们的肩关节"滑出去后又回来"。这个过程可能包括脱位后自行复位（称为短暂脱位事件）。[4] 不稳定的另一种极端情况是，投掷或做其他过顶操作的运动员会描述相似的微小的不稳定。因此，获得尽可能多的细节以评估患者的受伤机制及活动状态非常重要。患者如果同时具有前方不稳定和后方不稳定可能会报告伸展上臂时摔倒；后方不稳定者常在上臂90°前屈时受伤，前方不稳定者常在上臂快速移动至极度前屈和（或）外展位时受伤。

如果患者具有慢性复发性不稳定，应当尝试确定早前脱位的次数。早前多次脱位提示可能存在骨缺损。确定脱位时所处的活动状态可以获得更多信息。自发性脱位提示关节囊严重松弛。[5] 睡眠时出现盂肱关节不稳定可能与盂肱关节的骨缺损或软组织缺陷相关。

在翻修手术前，应当获得完整的手术史，包括手术记录及任何可用的关节镜照片。前期使用热探针行关节囊缝合术的病例，应注意术中遇到软组织缺陷的可能性，可能需要行关节囊加强术。

患者的病史应包括患者的运动目标。计划重返校际体育活动的年轻运动员患者的复发风险明

Dr. Owens or an immediate family member serves as a paid consultant to the Musculoskeletal Transplant Foundation and serves as a board member, owner, officer, or committee member of the American Orthopaedic Society for Sports Medicine and the Society of Military Orthopaedic Surgeons.

显比欠活跃的患者高。应告知患者复发的风险及可选择的手术治疗方式。

体格检查

患者的病史可以引导检查者将注意力集中于体格检查的具体方面，但是全面的上肢检查对避免遗漏病史中没有提到的可能的病理机制是重要的。对于肩关节不稳定的体格检查遵循常规的骨骼肌肉检查程序，包括视诊、触诊、关节活动范围评估、肌力检查、神经血管检查及特殊检查。应充分暴露双侧肩关节。每一项检查都应从健侧肩关节开始以了解患者肩关节的正常松弛度并使患者对检查者建立信心。

对于肩胛带的视诊，评估肌肉轮廓以确定三角肌、冈上肌或冈下肌萎缩所致的不对称。肩关节外侧缘变方及肩峰突出可能提示腋神经损伤所致的三角肌萎缩。评估肩胛体位置，排除翼状肩胛。视诊肩关节周围皮肤以评估之前的手术切口，检查是否存在萎缩的皮肤或提示胶原异常的变宽增生的瘢痕。触诊整个肩胛带有助于排除并发症并确定是否需要特殊检查和影像学检查。

活动范围

在记录压痛点后，进行肩关节全方位活动范围检查，这有助于记录最大主动前屈、内收和90°外展时的内旋角度，以及内收和90°外展时的外旋角度。内收内旋的记录方式是记录相应的椎体水平。投掷运动员的主力肢体的外旋能力常增强，并伴有内旋功能缺失，导致其整体活动弧与对侧肢体相称。当整体活动弧小于对侧25°以上时提示盂肱关节内旋缺陷，患者可能出现内侧撞击或盂唇病变。

检查者应确定主动活动障碍的患者是否存在完全被动活动。重要的是，存在关节交锁的肩关节后脱位患者的主动和被动外旋功能是否同时功能缺失。大范围的肩袖损伤初始时可表现为主动外旋功能缺失，而存在完全的被动活动。在肩关节前屈和外展时从后方观察患者，以判断肩胛骨是否对称或在活动时有无翼状肩胛。内侧或外侧翼状肩胛可能是胸长神经或第Ⅺ对脑神经麻痹所致，也可能发生于投掷运动员或肩关节多向不稳定的肩胛骨动力障碍患者。

肌力检查

在主动活动检查时，记录肩关节外展、屈伸肘关节和屈伸腕关节时的肌力是很重要的。也应记录手内在肌的肌力。肌力分级是有缺点的，因为检查具有主观性并且只能测量静态肌力，但是肌力分级可以为检查者提供基线参考，以便将患侧肢体与对侧肢体进行比较。

应该对肩袖肌肉的肌力进行特别评估。Jobe空罐试验可以仅检测冈上肌的肌力。做这一检查时，患者上臂屈曲90°至肩胛骨水平，拇指指向下方，检查者施加向下的力。患者在对抗向下的力时出现疼痛或无力提示冈上肌肌肉－肌腱单元病变。可通过对抗外旋和外展90°检测后方肩袖的肌力。

对于不稳定的患者，尤其是有开放性手术史的患者，单独评估肩胛下肌功能是非常重要的。可进行背后推离试验：患者将手放置于腰椎部，检查者将患者的手从背部举起移开并嘱患者维持体位。如不能维持体位，则提示肩胛下肌功能不全。当内旋出现疼痛使患者无法舒适地将手置于腰椎部时会给此检查带来困难。患者使用肱三头肌将手从背部移开可能使该试验出现假阴性结果。患者因内旋挛缩无法完成背后推离试验时可行压腹试验（belly-press test）。患者将手放置于腹部，腕关节处于中立位，肘关节与躯干同平面。如果肩胛下肌完好，患者可以通过内旋肩关节向腹部施加压力。肩胛下肌功能不全者无法内旋肱骨及屈腕或向后移动肘关节以按压腹部。还有一种压腹试验（belly-off test）与之相似，检查者一只手维持固定患者的患侧肘关节，使其肩关节轻度屈曲内旋，另一只手将患者的手放于腹部，嘱患者维持最大内旋位。检查者松手后，患者的手从腹部抬起离开为检查结果阳性，提示肩胛下肌功能不全。熊抱试验时患者上臂前屈90°，肘关节屈曲并抬起以尽可能地远离躯体前方，手放置于对侧肩关节。检查者尝试在患者的对抗下将患者的手从肩关节提起。肌电图检查显示，通过熊抱试验、背后推离试验、压腹试验可检查肩胛下肌的所有部分。[6]

神经血管检查

神经损伤在肩关节脱位中常见，记录初始神经检查的情况很重要。近期一项研究发现，在3633例脱位患者中，神经损伤的发生率为13.5%。[7]可以通过肩关节外侧感觉评估腋神经。腋神经的运动功能可通过观察患者对抗肩关节外展时的表现及感受三角肌收缩的情况进行检查。腋神经损伤在肩关节脱位中最常见，还应当对正中神经、尺神经、桡神经及肌皮神经的检查进行记录。

血管检查应从简单的肢体视诊开始，注意是否有皮肤苍白、营养改变、静脉充血和毛发缺失。触诊桡动脉及尺动脉搏动，观察毛细血管充盈情况并进行双侧对比。

前方不稳定

创伤性前方不稳定最常见于年轻运动员，但通常不单独发生。因此，发现复合性不稳定非常重要。诊断前方不稳定最常用的检查是恐惧试验，传统方法是患者取坐位或平卧位，使床沿支撑肩胛骨，[8]上臂外展90°，屈肘，检查右肩关节时检查者的右手扶着患者的右肘关节。令患者上臂外旋，检查者左手拇指在患者的肱骨头后方施加向前的力。在进行此操作时患者产生的疼痛和恐惧感与前方盂唇损伤有关。在恐惧试验的结果可疑并怀疑前方不稳定时，可行增强试验。行增强试验时，患者取与恐惧试验相同的体位，上臂外展并极度外旋，检查者对患者的肱骨近端施加向前的力。再复位试验的体位与恐惧试验体位相同，上臂位置同恐惧试验，对患者的肱骨近端施加向后的力，恐惧感减弱和疼痛缓解是阳性结果。[9]再复位试验的肩关节疼痛缓解与上盂唇复合体病变相关。再复位试验完成后行释放试验（或恐惧试验），将施加于肱骨近端的向后的力移除。[10]阳性结果是肩关节疼痛和恐惧感再度出现。

加载－移位试验是确定肱骨头在肩胛盂上被动移位的首选方法。患者取坐位或平卧位，上臂外展20°且维持与肩胛骨同平面并轻度屈曲。检查右肩关节时，检查者用右手握住患者右前臂，通过肩胛盂向肱骨头中心施加压力。检查者将左手拇指和示指置于肱骨头处以控制肱骨近端并施加向前的力。然后，施加向后及向下的力。加载－移位试验根据肱骨头移位程度以改良的Hawkins评分分级，Ⅰ级时肱骨头沿肩胛盂白微小移位，Ⅱ级时肱骨头移位至肩胛盂缘或超出肩胛盂缘，作用力移除后可复位，Ⅲ级时肱骨头移位超出肩胛盂缘，作用力移除后维持脱位状态。[11]

可通过Gagey过度外展试验评估盂肱下韧带的完整性。[12]检查时患者取坐位，检查者坐于患者后方。患者的肘关节呈90°位，上臂为旋转中立位。检查者一只手向下推肩胛带，另一只手提拉放松的上肢。肩关节被动外展超过105°提示盂肱下韧带松弛（图6-1）。在初始报告中，肩关

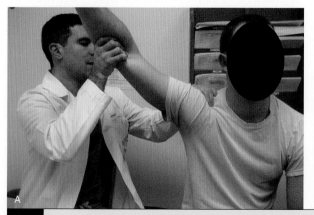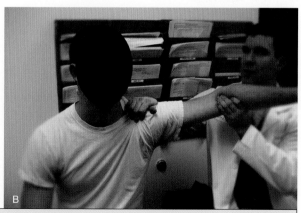

图6-1 前下方不稳定的20岁男性患者的临床照片。右侧肘关节Gagey过度外展试验阳性（A），左侧肘关节正常（B）。MRI显示该患者的盂肱韧带肱骨侧撕脱

节不稳定患者中有 85% 出现肩关节被动外展超过 105°，而剩余 15% 的患者因出现恐惧感和疼痛而表现为肩关节外展受限。[12]

后方不稳定

后方加载－移位试验在患者上臂与肩胛骨位于同一平面、外展 45° 并处于旋转中立位时进行。检查者站在取坐位或平卧位的患者的一旁，一只手握住患者肘关节以控制上臂，并对肱骨施加向肩胛盂方向的力，另一只手在患者三角肌止点附近握住肱骨并施加向后的力。患者上臂逐渐内旋以增加后方关节囊和韧带结构的张力并减少移位。评分系统与加载－移位试验相同。肱骨头移位不超过 50% 被认为是正常的，但试验结果经常需要同对侧肩关节比较以确定有无不对称的移位。

后方应力试验（或后方恐惧试验）在患者取坐位或平卧位时进行，上臂前屈 90° 并极度内旋。[10] 检查者的一只手在患者的肘关节上施加向后的力，另一只手控制肩关节后方以触诊肱骨头。阳性结果为触诊到肱骨头半脱位或脱位、患者对即将发生的脱位有恐惧感、患者出现疼痛症状。抖动试验，患者取坐位，上臂前屈 90° 并保持极度内收和内旋位。检查者对患者的肘关节施加向后的力。如果此时上臂出现脱位或半脱位提示后方不稳定。维持向后施加的力的同时，检查者缓慢地外展患者的肩关节，此时伴随肱骨头复位出现咔嗒声或抖动感。

下方及多向不稳定

下方松弛的程度可以通过凹陷征量化，患者取坐位，上肢放松并置于一侧呈旋转中立位。检查者向肱骨远端施加向下的牵引力，同时观察肩峰外缘。如下方不稳定则可形成深沟，并能在肩峰外侧下方的三角肌表面测量凹陷的宽度。在极度外旋位重复该检查，使前方关节囊和肩袖间隙产生张力。在外旋时持续出现凹陷征提示肩袖间隙功能不全。

多向不稳定的患者可出现任何与不稳定相关的体格检查结果。不少患者具有包括对侧肩关节在内的多关节韧带松弛的体征。全身关节活动范围可以通过 Beighton 评分系统（0~9 分）评估，骨骼发育成熟的成年人的评分高于 4 分即为全身关节活动过度。[13] 如果患者可以做到以下 9 项中的某一项，即得 1 分：左侧和（或）右侧小指掌指关节过伸超过 90°，左侧和（或）右侧拇指触及前臂掌侧，左侧和（或）右侧肘关节过伸超过 10°，左侧和（或）右侧膝关节过伸超过 10°，完全伸膝时手掌可以水平放置于地面。评分为 4 分或高于 4 分者可以诊断为全身韧带松弛。评分为 2 分或高于 2 分者可能有盂肱关节不稳定史。[14]

肱二头肌和上盂唇复合体病变

上盂唇分离可能与盂肱关节不稳定相关，并常见于其他关节内病变。对肩关节的全面评估应包括对上盂唇的检查。主动挤压试验，检查者站在患者后方，患者上臂前屈 90°，内收 15°，极度内旋肩关节并将拇指指向地面。[15] 患者对抗检查者施加的向下的力并报告疼痛部位。在极度旋后位重复该检查。当手掌朝上可缓解肩关节深部疼痛时为阳性结果，提示存在上盂唇病变。普遍认为主动挤压试验是诊断上盂唇复合体病变时敏感性最高的检查（47%）。[16] 肩关节上方疼痛可能提示肩锁关节损伤或撞击综合征。所谓的上盂唇病变试验也是通过牵拉肱二头肌止点，在胸前内收患侧肩关节，伸肘并内旋前臂完成的。该试验的阳性结果是肱二头肌腱沟处疼痛，可听到关节弹响，或出现恐惧感。摇转试验，患者上肢上举至 160°，与肩胛骨位于同一平面，检查者对患者上肢轴向加压，并使患者肩关节被动地从极度内旋转换至极度外旋。有盂肱关节脱位史的患者的摇转试验结果存在不确定性，因为该试验的肩关节的位置与恐惧试验的位置相似。前方滑动试验，患者将手置于臀部，拇指向后。检查者站于患者后方，将一只手放于患者肩关节上方，另一只手放于患者肘关节。然后，检查者向肩关节施加轻度的向前上方的作用力，使肱二头肌止点受力。[19] 阳性结果包括肩关节前方疼痛、肩关节前方区域可有弹响和再次出现过顶活动时的症状。前方滑动试验被认为是诊断上盂唇复合体病变时特异性最高的检查（84%）。[16] 上盂唇复合体撕裂的患者在经典的肱二头肌激惹试验（如Speed 试验和 Yergason 试验）中也可能出现疼痛。Speed 试验，患者前屈上臂，屈肘 30°，前臂旋后。Yergason 试验，患者在屈肘 90° 时对抗旋后。对于这两个试验，肱二头肌腱沟处出现疼痛为阳性结果。

影像学检查

X 线片

影像学检查对肩关节不稳定的有效治疗至关重要（表 6-1）。通常，首选的影像学检查是 X 线片。标准前后位和腋位是肩关节的经典 X 线透视体位。西点腋位（West Point axillary view）片用于更好地显示肩胛盂前下缘及评估骨性撕脱[18]（图 6-2）。前后内旋位片或 Stryker 切迹位片用于更好地显示 Hill-Sachs 损伤（图 6-3）。Bernageau 位片

表 6-1

肩关节病变 X 线透视体位

肩关节病变	最佳 X 线透视体位	X 线透视技巧
骨性 Bankart 损伤	西点腋位	患者俯卧，上臂外展 90°，旋转中立位，暗盒置于肩关节上方，向头侧倾斜 25°，从腋窝投射（图 6-2）
	Bernageau 位	患者站立，上臂外展，手置于头部，暗盒置于腋窝处，向尾侧倾斜 30°，向肩关节后方投射
	Garth 位	患者站立，暗盒置于肩关节后方，向尾侧倾斜 45° 投射
盂肱关节脱位	外侧腋位	患者平卧，上臂外展，暗盒置于肩关节上方，向腋窝投射
Hill-Sachs 损伤	前后内旋位	患者站立或平卧，上臂内旋，暗盒置于肩关节后方，从肩关节前方向后方投射
	Garth 位	患者站立，暗盒置于肩关节后方，向尾侧倾斜 45° 投射
	Stryker 切迹位	患者平卧，手置于头部，肘关节指向上方，暗盒置于肩关节后方，向头侧倾斜 10° 投射，靶心位于喙突（图 6-3）

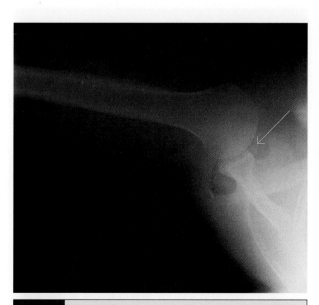

图 6-2　西点腋位片可见骨性 Bankart 损伤（箭头）

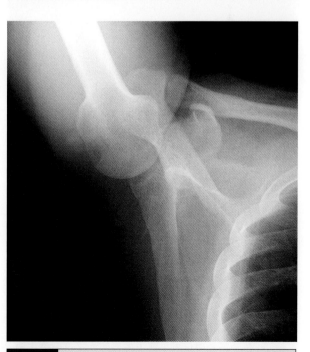

图 6-3　Stryker 切迹位片可见 Hill-Sachs 损伤

有助于肩胛盂骨缺损的鉴别。[19]

MRI 检查

肩关节不稳定的患者均有行 MRI 检查的指征。MRI 检查的质量因设备不同而有差异，间接钆增强或直接钆增强有助于评估不同损伤类型的盂唇和关节囊，以及关节囊容积。Bankart 损伤在发生创伤性盂肱关节脱位或半脱位的年轻运动员中的比例很高。这一病变常在轴位和冠状位清楚显示，但也可以在外展外旋位显示[4, 20]（图 6-4）。前方盂唇骨膜套袖样撕脱（ALPSA 病变）可在 MRI 图像上显示。ALPSA 病变与慢性复发性不稳定相关，其手术修复效果不佳。[21-22]

盂肱韧带肱骨侧撕脱（HAGL 损伤）最佳显示于冠状位的钆增强扫描。HAGL 损伤难以单纯从影像学结果进行分型，但辨别盂肱下韧带前后束是否完整至关重要，因为这是影响修复方法的选择的一个因素。[23]

CT 检查

尽管 MRI 检查可以显示骨缺损，但是如果怀疑骨缺损或考虑行翻修手术，大多数医师还是推荐使用 CT 检查。当前通过三维 CT 重建协助测量骨缺损，可以将肱骨头去除以便于肩胛盂评估。

肩胛盂骨缺损

肩胛盂骨缺损越来越多地被认为是导致肩关节不稳定的因素。骨缺损的出现可能与单纯关节镜修复后复发率高相关。[24]骨缺损甚至可见于只报告有半脱位情况的患者（图 6-5）。骨缺损可能是磨损性的或发生于骨性 Bankart 损伤。近期的一项研究发现，在接受固定手术的肩关节不稳定患者中，有 72% 出现骨缺损，严重骨缺损者（缺损大于 20%）占 7.5%。[25]对于需要行骨性结构加强手术的骨缺损量仍存在争论。然而，普遍认为 0~15% 的缺损是可接受的，而 20%~30% 是显著缺损，推荐行骨性结构加强手术。[26]

通过影像学手段测量肩胛盂骨缺损的困难在于缺少正常肩胛盂的形态学数据。一些研究者推荐将患侧肩关节影像与健侧肩关节影像做对比。[27]肩胛盂骨缺损可以通过同侧三维 CT 重建，在正面观上以最佳匹配圆圈覆盖测量。[28]通过专用的计算机软件，研究者可以数字化建立骨缺损区域并计算骨缺损比例。其他报道的用于测量骨缺损的方法涉及三维 CT 的应用，减除肱骨头

| 图
6-4 | 患有复发性半脱位的 21 岁学校足球运动员的 MRI 影像。在轴位和冠状位未见盂唇病变，但在外展外旋位可见前下盂唇的无移位撕裂（箭头）。关节镜下检查结果证实了这一发现 |

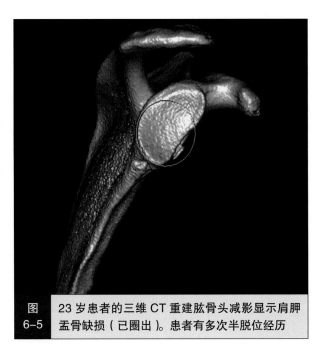

| 图
6-5 | 23 岁患者的三维 CT 重建肱骨头减影显示肩胛盂骨缺损（已圈出）。患者有多次半脱位经历 |

并于肩胛盂正面观的下部添加圆圈，如图 6-6 所示。[26] 有一项测量技术可以直接将病变直径与肩胛盂下部的半径进行比较。当病变直径大于肩胛盂下部的半径时，该关节抵抗脱位的能力低于正常关节的 70%。

最佳的测量方法和有意义的骨缺损量都尚未确定。术前评估骨缺损的 CT 检查的指征范围应当放宽。如果测量的骨缺损量超过 20%，医师应当考虑在行关节镜下 Bankark 修复和行加强手术之间做出选择，并且应当告知患者复发风险。

肱骨头骨缺损

肱骨头骨缺损既可能单独存在，亦有可能与肩胛盂骨缺损同时存在。Hall 测量技术仍是评估骨缺损比例的绝佳方法。起初 Hall 测量技术是用于 X 线片的，现在也用在轴位 MRI 和 CT 上。测量骨缺损形成的角度，将其以关节面形成的 180°圆弧分割。[30] 25% 的 Hill-Sachs 损伤可能不需要治疗。[31-32] 除了损伤的大小，是否嵌顿也很重要。嵌顿的 Hill-Sachs 损伤在生理活动范围内与肩胛盂前下

图
6-6　三维 CT 重建测量裸区（点）至骨缺损边缘的距离（A）及骨缺损后缘至裸区（B）的距离。骨缺损量的计算公式是（B-A）/2Bx100%

部接触，这将导致关节镜下软组织修补失败。[24] 关节镜检查时处理嵌顿的 Hill-Sachs 损伤是最合适的。

分型

有很多针对肩关节不稳定的分型系统，但并没有一个被广泛接受的分型系统。大多数分型系统都是根据不稳定方向、创伤与非创伤性以及韧带松弛度分型的。

早期，根据肩关节不稳定方向，大多数脱位为前脱位。在早期的研究中，后脱位在所有脱位中仅占 4%。[33] 骨科医师在一段时间内始终使用这种仅基于不稳定方向的分型系统，最近的一项前瞻性队列研究报道，在年轻运动员的脱位中，有 5% 是后脱位。[34] 完全性后方不稳定（后脱位）少见，但向后半脱位常见，占所有半脱位的 11%[34]。

区分脱位和半脱位的最常用方法是依据受伤机制。最初将脱位按创伤性和非创伤性分型时，非创伤性脱位患者的复发率更高。[35] 将半脱位按创伤性、非创伤性和自发性分型时，非创伤性和自发性半脱位采用非手术治疗可以获得较好的结果。[36-37] 在应用最广泛的分型系统中，两类肩关节不稳定广泛决定了诊断和治疗。第一大类为非创伤性、多方向、双侧肩关节不稳定（AMBRI 类），初始进行康复或下关节囊紧缩术。第二大类包括创伤性脱位、单一方向脱位及常见的需手术治疗的 Bankart 损伤（TUBS 类）。AMBRI 类和 TUBS 类准确地描述了不稳定谱的两极，但并没有体现二者之间的过渡。[38]

另一分型系统基于肩关节不稳定是静态的、动态的还是自发的。[29] 静态型根据脱位方向分出亚型，动态型根据有无韧带松弛分出亚型。最近有一种科学的对不稳定进行分型的方法。[39] 该系统的 4 个分型依据如下：1 年内不稳定的次数（1 次、2~5 次或多于 5 次）、病因学（创伤性或非创伤性）、不稳定方向（前、下或后）以及严重程度（半脱位或脱位）。这一分型系统称为 FEDS 综合分型系统，涵盖了不稳定的所有 36 种可能的情况，可以在同一机构中重复使用。[40]

这些分型系统可能成为重要的研究工具，但对于做出合适的治疗决策帮助并不大。近期有一项研究根据发表的复发数据对初始前脱位治疗决策进行了分析，该分析结果可能有助于外科医师告知患者预期风险。[41]近期引入的不稳定严重性指数评分将一些患者相关变量纳入考虑之中，如年龄、活动水平及病理改变，并对 6 项特定危险因素进行了评分。如果总分低于或等于 6 分，则预期关节镜下修复术后的复发率为 10%，如果总分高于或等于 7 分则预期复发率为 70%[42]（表 6–2）。

表 6–2

不稳定严重指数评分

预后因素	评分
年龄	
小于 20 岁	2
大于 20 岁	0
术前运动参与水平	
竞技水平	2
业余水平或无	0
术前运动类型	
接触性或超过头顶的用力运动	1
其他	0
肩关节过度松弛	
前方或下方过度松弛	1
松弛度正常	0
前后位片上 Hill–Sachs 损伤	
外旋位可见	2
外旋位不可见	0
前后位片上肩胛盂轮廓	
轮廓缺失	2
无轮廓缺失	0
总分	10

注：如果总分≤ 6 分，则预期关节镜下修复术后的复发率为 10%，如果总分≥ 7 分，则预期关节镜下修复术后的复发率为 70%。经允许引自 Balg F, Boileau P: The instability severity index score: A simple pre-operative score to select patients for arthroscopic or open shoulder stabilization. *J Bone Joint Surg Br* 2007;89（11）:1470–1477.

总结

肩关节不稳定常见于年轻运动员。对于这类患者，在确诊为其他疾病之前，肩关节的症状就代表了存在不稳定。诊断时需结合完整的病史、体格检查和影像学检查结果。X 线检查和 MRI 检查常规用于鉴别常见于完全脱位和半脱位的盂唇和骨软骨损伤。如果怀疑肩胛盂骨缺损，需行 CT 检查，该缺损与单纯关节镜下软组织固定后效果不佳相关。不稳定可通过多种方式分型，对不稳定的方向、严重程度与创伤属性的理解有助于分析风险及计划理想的手术固定方式。

参考文献

[1] Zacchilli MA, Owens BD: Epidemiology of shoulder dislocations presenting to emergency departments in the United States. *J Bone Joint Surg Am* 2010;92(3):542-549.

An epidemiologic study of emergency department visits for glenohumeral dislocation found an incidence that was higher than previously reported in the United States but consistent with European literature. The highest incidence was in men and boys in the second or third decade of life.

[2] Kaplan LD, Flanigan DC, Norwig J, Jost P, Bradley J: Prevalence and variance of shoulder injuries in elite collegiate football players. *Am J Sports Med* 2005;33(8):1142-1146.

[3] Headey J, Brooks JH, Kemp SP: The epidemiology of shoulder injuries in English professional rugby union. *Am J Sports Med* 2007;35(9):1537-1543.

An epidemiologic study of English rugby union players found that glenohumeral dislocation led to more time lost from sport (81 days) than any other shoulder injury.

[4] Owens BD, Nelson BJ, Duffey ML, et al: Pathoanatomy of first-time, traumatic, anterior glenohumeral subluxation events. *J Bone Joint Surg Am* 2010;92(7):1605-1611.

A high rate of Bankart and Hill-Sachs lesions was found in patients who underwent early imaging after a first traumatic anterior glenohumeral subluxation. The term transient luxation was introduced for subluxation with significant pathology. A high index of suspicion and early imaging were recommended for young athletes.

[5] Neer CS II, Foster CR: Inferior capsular shift for involuntary inferior and multidirectional instability of the shoulder: A preliminary report. *J Bone Joint Surg Am*

1980;62(6):897-908.

［6］ Pennock AT, Pennington WW, Torry MR, et al: The influence of arm and shoulder position on the bearhug, belly-press, and lift-off tests: An electromyographic study. *Am J Sports Med* 2011;39(11):2338-2346.

An electromyelographic study of tests for subscapularis function found that all tests are effective for determining subscapularis deficiency but do not allow differentiation between upper and lower subscapularis function.

［7］ Robinson CM, Shur N, Sharpe T, Ray A, Murray IR: Injuries associated with traumatic anterior glenohumeral dislocations. *J Bone Joint Surg Am* 2012;94(1):18-26.

Review of a large trauma database found 3,633 patients with anterior glenohumeral dislocation, of whom 13.5% had a neurologic deficit after reduction and 33.4% had a rotator cuff tear or an avulsion fracture.

［8］ Rowe CR, Zarins B: Recurrent transient subluxation of the shoulder. *J Bone Joint Surg Am* 1981;63(6):863-872.

［9］ Jobe FW, Kvitne RS, Giangarra CE: Shoulder pain in the overhand or throwing athlete: The relationship of anterior instability and rotator cuff impingement. *Orthop Rev* 1989;18(9):963-975.

［10］ Silliman JF, Hawkins RJ: Classification and physical diagnosis of instability of the shoulder. *Clin Orthop Relat Res* 1993;291:7-19.

［11］ McFarland EG, Tanaka MJ, Papp DF: Examination of the shoulder in the overhead and throwing athlete. *Clin Sports Med* 2008;27(4):553-578.

Current shoulder examination techniques and their clinical efficacy are described.

［12］ Gagey OJ, Gagey N: The hyperabduction test. *J Bone Joint Surg Br* 2001;83(1):69-74.

［13］ Moriatis Wolf J, Cameron KL, Owens BD: Impact of joint laxity and hypermobility on the musculoskeletal system. *J Am Acad Orthop Surg* 2011;19(8):463-471.

Ligamentous laxity is reviewed, with its effect on the musculoskeletal system and shoulder-specific concerns. The routine use of a Beighton score assessment is recommended.

［14］ Cameron KL, Duffey ML, DeBerardino TM, Stoneman PD, Jones CJ, Owens BD: Association of general-ized joint hypermobility with a history of glenohumeral joint instability. *J Athl Train* 2010;45(3):253-258.

A correlation was found between an elevated Beighton score for ligamentous laxity and a history of glenohumeral instability in young athletes.

［15］ O'Brien SJ, Pagnani MJ, Fealy S, McGlynn SR, Wilson JB: The active compression test: A new and effective test for diagnosing labral tears and acromioclavicular joint abnormality. *Am J Sports Med* 1998;26(5):610-613.

［16］ McFarland EG, Kim TK, Savino RM: Clinical assessment of three common tests for superior labral anterior-posterior lesions. *Am J Sports Med* 2002;30(6):810-815.

［17］ Kibler WB, McMullen J: Scapular dyskinesis and its relation to shoulder pain. *J Am Acad Orthop Surg* 2003; 11(2):142-151.

［18］ Rokous JR, Feagin JA, Abbott HG: Modified axillary roentgenogram: A useful adjunct in the diagnosis of recurrent instability of the shoulder. *Clin Orthop Relat Res* 1972;82:84-86.

［19］ Bernageau J, Patte D, Debeyre J, Ferrane J: Intérêt du profil glénoïdien dans les luxations récidivantes de l'épaule. *Rev Chir Orthop Reparatrice Appar Mot* 1976;62(2, suppl)142-147.

［20］ Taylor DC, Arciero RA: Pathologic changes associated with shoulder dislocations: Arthroscopic and physical examination findings in first-time, traumatic anterior dislocations. *Am J Sports Med* 1997;25(3):306-311.

［21］ Ozbaydar M, Elhassan B, Diller D, Massimini D, Higgins LD, Warner JJ: Results of arthroscopic capsulolabral repair: Bankart lesion versus anterior labroligamentous periosteal sleeve avulsion lesion. *Arthroscopy* 2008;24(11):1277-1283.

Patients with an ALPSA lesion had a higher rate of recurrent instability after arthroscopic soft-tissue repair than those with a Bankart lesion.

［22］ Kim DS, Yoon YS, Yi CH: Prevalence comparison of accompanying lesions between primary and recurrent anterior dislocation in the shoulder. *Am J Sports Med* 2010;38(10):2071-2076.

A review found a higher rate of Bankart lesions, ALPSA lesions, Hill-Sachs lesions, and glenoid bone loss after arthroscopic soft-tissue repair in patients with recurrent anterior instability than in patients with a single anterior dislocation.

［23］ Bui-Mansfield LT, Banks KP, Taylor DC: Humeral avulsion of the glenohumeral ligaments: The HAGL lesion. *Am J Sports Med* 2007;35(11):1960-1966.

The literature on HAGL lesions is reviewed, and a comprehensive classification system is presented.

［24］ Burkhart SS, De Beer JF: Traumatic glenohumeral bone defects and their relationship to failure of arthroscopic Bankart repairs: Significance of the invertedpear glenoid and the humeral engaging Hill-Sachs lesion. *Arthroscopy* 2000;16(7):677-694.

[25] Milano G, Grasso A, Russo A, et al: Analysis of risk factors for glenoid bone defect in anterior shoulder instability. *Am J Sports Med* 2011;39(9):1870-1876.

CT evaluation of patients with instability showed that glenoid bone loss was correlated with the number of dislocation events.

[26] Piasecki DP, Verma NN, Romeo AA, Levine WN, Bach BR Jr, Provencher MT: Glenoid bone deficiency in recurrent anterior shoulder instability: Diagnosis and management. *J Am Acad Orthop Surg* 2009; 17(8): 482-493.

A comprehensive review of glenoid bone deficiency includes the relevant literature and guidelines for the clinician. A method of bone loss measurement is presented for use in CT or arthroscopy.

[27] Baudi P, Righi P, Bolognesi D, et al: How to identify and calculate glenoid bone deficit. *Chir Organi Mov* 2005; 90(2): 145-152.

[28] Sugaya H, Moriishi J, Dohi M, Kon Y, Tsuchiya A: Glenoid rim morphology in recurrent anterior glenohumeral instability. *J Bone Joint Surg Am* 2003; 85(5): 878-884.

[29] Gerber C, Nyffeler RW: Classification of glenohumeral joint instability. *Clin Orthop Relat Res* 2002;400:65-76.

[30] Hall RH, Isaac F, Booth CR: Dislocations of the shoulder with special reference to accompanying small fractures. *J Bone Joint Surg Am* 1959;41(3):489-494.

[31] Sekiya JK, Jolly J, Debski RE: The effect of a Hill-Sachs defect on glenohumeral translations, in situ capsular forces, and bony contact forces. *Am J Sports Med* 2012;40(2):388-394.

A cadaver laboratory study found that the presence of a 25% humeral head defect did not significantly increase glenohumeral translation if the capsule was intact.

[32] Skendzel JG, Sekiya JK: Diagnosis and management of humeral head bone loss in shoulder instability. *Am J Sports Med* 2012; 40(11):2633-2644.

A thorough overview of the literature on humeral head bone loss in patients with shoulder instability is presented, with clinical treatment guidelines.

[33] McLaughlin HL, MacLellan DI: Recurrent anterior dislocation of the shoulder: II. A comparative study. *J Trauma* 1967;7(2):191-201.

[34] Owens BD, Duffey ML, Nelson BJ, DeBerardino TM, Taylor DC, Mountcastle SB: The incidence and characteristics of shoulder instability at the United States Military Academy. *Am J Sports Med* 2007;35(7):1168-1173.

A prospective study of shoulder instability epidemiology in a high-risk population found that 85% of all events were subluxations and confirmed earlier findings that 80% of events were anterior.

[35] Rowe CR: Prognosis in dislocations of the shoulder. *J Bone Joint Surg Am* 1956;38-A(5):957-977.

[36] Rockwood CA Jr: Subluxation of the shoulder: The classification, diagnosis, and treatment. *Orthop Trans* 1979;3:306.

[37] Burkhead WZ Jr, Rockwood CA Jr: Treatment of instability of the shoulder with an exercise program. *J Bone Joint Surg Am* 1992;74(6):890-896.

[38] Thomas SC, Matsen FA III: An approach to the repair of avulsion of the glenohumeral ligaments in the management of traumatic anterior glenohumeral instability. *J Bone Joint Surg Am* 1989;71(4):506-513.

[39] Kuhn JE: A new classification system for shoulder instability. *Br J Sports Med* 2010;44(5):341-346.

The FEDS classification system was introduced. This comprehensive system has 36 possible categories of instability and may be better suited to research than clinical use.

[40] Kuhn JE, Helmer TT, Dunn WR, Throckmorton V TW: Development and reliability testing of the frequency, etiology, direction, and severity (FEDS) system for classifying glenohumeral instability. *J Shoulder Elbow Surg* 2011;20(4):548-556.

The FEDS system was found to be reproducible in a single-institution evaluation.

[41] Mather RC III, Orlando LA, Henderson RA, Lawrence JT, Taylor DC: A predictive model of shoulder instability after a first-time anterior shoulder dislocation. *J Shoulder Elbow Surg* 2011;20(2):259-266.

A decision-tree analysis based on published recurrence rates was intended to provide clinicians with a means of counseling patients on recurrence risk based on their demographic characteristics.

[42] Balg F, Boileau P: The instability severity index score: A simple pre-operative score to select patients for arthroscopic or open shoulder stabilisation. *J Bone Joint Surg Br* 2007;89(11):1470-1477.

The instability severity index score is a clinical tool for risk stratifying patients with instability based on their age, activity level, and clinical presentation. This tool appears to be best for guiding clinicians as to the risk of recurrence after soft-tissue repair and determining whether a patient can benefit from an augmented repair.

第七章　急性和慢性肩关节脱位

Geoffrey S. Van Thiel, MD, MBA; Wendell Heard, MD; Anthony A. Romeo, MD, CDR;
Matthew T. Provencher, MD, MC, USN

引言

盂肱关节具有相当大的活动范围，因此是最常脱位的大关节。盂肱关节的稳定依靠静态和动态的限制、关节内负压以及朝向关节凹面的压迫。真正的盂肱关节脱位是完全的不稳定，肱骨头与肩胛盂之间的接触完全丧失。肱骨头位于脱位处，需要手法复位以恢复解剖关系。自发地复位是有可能的，尤其是当存在肩胛盂骨缺损或合并有肱骨头骨缺损时。

美国 2010 年的肩关节脱位的发生率为 23.9/100 000。[1]在所有脱位的患者中男性占 72%，15~29 岁者占 47%。脱位患者的年龄分布呈双峰分布，峰值位于年轻人和 70 岁以上者。在一项纳入 4141 例学生的研究中，有 18 例发生脱位，其中 17 例为前脱位。[2]这一结果与之前报道的数值相符。

Dr. Romeo or an immediate family member has received royalties from Arthrex; is a member of a speakers' bureau or has made paid presentations on behalf of Arthrex, DJ Orthopaedics, and the Joint Restoration Foundation; serves as a paid consultant to Arthrex; has received research or institutional support from Arthrex and DJ Orthopaedics; has received nonincome support (such as equipment or services), commercially derived honoraria, or other non–research-related funding (such as paid travel) from Arthrex and DJ Orthopaedics; and serves as a board member, owner, officer, or committee member of the American Orthopaedic Society for Sports Medicine, American Shoulder and Elbow Surgeons, and the Arthroscopy Association of North America. Dr. Provencher or an immediate family member serves as a board member, owner, officer, or committee member of the American Academy of Orthopaedic Surgeons; American Orthopaedic Society for Sports Medicine; American Shoulder and Elbow Surgeons; Arthroscopy Association of North America; International Society of Arthroscopy, Knee Surgery, and Orthopaedic Sports Medicine; San Diego Shoulder Institute, and the Society of Military Orthopaedic Surgeons. Neither of the following authors nor any immediate family member has received anything of value from or owns stock in a commercial company or institution related directly or indirectly to the subject of this chapter: Dr. Van Thiel and Dr. Heard.

急性肩关节前脱位

病理解剖学和相关损伤

患者的年龄是预期肩关节前脱位病理解剖、可能的并发症及预后的最重要因素。年龄小于 40 岁的患者更有可能出现盂唇和关节囊韧带损伤。年龄等于或大于 40 岁的患者更有可能伴有肩袖、肱骨近端或周围神经血管结构的损伤。

急性肩关节前脱位后，通过关节镜检查可以观察到关节囊盂唇损伤，如前盂唇撕裂、前方关节囊缺损或盂肱韧带肱骨止点撕脱损伤（图 7-1）。在 1990 年定义了 3 种损伤形态：无盂唇损伤的关节囊撕裂，见于 13% 的患者，是一种稳定的损伤；关节囊撕裂合并盂唇部分分离，见于 24% 的患者，存在轻度不稳定；关节囊撕裂合并盂唇完全分离，见于 62% 的患者，极不稳定。[3]一项生物力学研究发现，单纯前下盂唇分离并不导致盂肱关节脱位。[4]在外旋外展位，Bankart 损伤需延伸至后上盂唇，才会导致张力机制失效并发生前脱位。

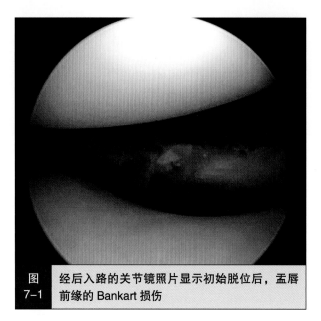

图
7-1　经后入路的关节镜照片显示初始脱位后，盂唇前缘的 Bankart 损伤

随着患者年龄的增长，肩袖损伤愈加常见。肩关节前脱位可以导致肩袖后上方撕脱或肩胛下肌腱撕裂。在年龄大于 60 岁的肩关节前脱位患者中，肩袖撕裂可见于 49% 的患者。[5] 在对肩关节前脱位患者进行体格检查时，应当对肩袖进行评估。进一步的影像学检查可以协助诊断。

肩胛盂、肱骨近端或喙突骨折均可以发生于肩关节前脱位。肩胛盂前缘骨折通常是前下方关节囊盂唇结构的骨性撕脱。大结节骨折发生于 1/3 的脱位中，且更常见于年长患者。肩关节前脱位常合并 Hill-Sachs 损伤，但其真正的临床意义和处理方式尚存在争论。

患者病史

患者在发生急性肩关节前脱位后，通常在训练场地内或急诊室接受评估。常见的损伤原因是外展、伸展及来自后方的力作用于上臂的复合作用。需要确定患者的肩关节受伤史。在随访过程中获得病史是十分必要的，包括损伤原因、是否需要复位、复位的时间和地点、复位前和复位后的影像学检查结果、初始脱位后的复发情况。

体格检查

对于肩关节前脱位的患者，系统的上肢检查对发现可能合并的病理情况非常有用。患者常以另一侧上臂将患侧上臂托住并使其抵住躯干。视诊肩胛带肌肉轮廓，肩峰突出或肱骨头出现于前方提示前脱位未复位。触诊部位应包括胸锁关节、喙突、肱二头肌长头腱、肩锁关节及大结节。此外，确诊肩峰下缘可以评估肱骨头相对于肩胛盂的位置。若盂肱关节前脱位，可触及肩峰外缘下方空虚感。检查时，应当触诊整个肩胛骨。

肩关节脱位复位后应当评估主动和被动活动范围，巨大肩袖撕裂者外旋功能丧失，但具有完整的被动活动范围。站在患者背后观察患者主动前屈外展时的肩胛骨运动。此外，应当对患肢进行肌力检查并与对侧比较。进行完整的肌力检查非常重要，检查范围应包括手内在肌、屈腕肌、伸腕肌、屈肘肌、伸肘肌、肩外展肌以及组成肩袖的每一块肌肉。

进行完整的神经血管检查并仔细记录。神经损伤最常见于老年患者及合并骨折的患者。腋神经拴系于盂肱关节前后方且可活动范围小，因此容易受损。如需进行手法复位，则必须在复位前及复位后进行神经血管检查。

对于近期复位的肩关节，针对前方不稳定行特殊检查会比较困难且并不必要。恐惧试验、增强试验以及再复位试验阳性都可以提示前方盂唇损伤。此外，可通过加载 - 移位试验评估肱骨头在肩胛盂上的被动移动，通过 Gagey 过度外展试验评估盂肱下韧带的完整性。

闭合复位

对于急性脱位的患者，负责治疗的医师必须尽快做出复位决定。是否可以不拍摄 X 线片就进行复位，例如，在训练场地内直接进行复位，尚存在争论。一些医师相信，立即复位肩关节更好，因为此时肌肉尚未出现痉挛，故复位时不需要镇静。在比赛场地内进行复位后，绝不允许运动员回场继续比赛，为确认复位及评估骨性结构，需要在复位后拍摄 X 线片。对于在急诊室的患者，若肌肉保护机制已经启动，如不给予镇静或关节内麻醉，疼痛会阻碍复位。

Stimson 法复位肩关节前脱位是安全有效的。[6]在患者患处关节腔内注射利多卡因。患者取俯卧位，上臂下垂，医师牵引旋转患者肱骨以复位肩关节。牵引–对抗牵引法，患者平卧，医师顺患肢畸形方向施加牵引，同时将床单围于患者胸部进行对抗牵引。Milch 法，医师一只手置于患者肩关节脱位侧腋窝，另一只手握住患侧手，并对其进行外旋，然后施加牵引以复位肱骨头。对 40 例患者行小剂量术前给药下外旋法肩关节前脱位闭合复位，其中 29 例患者的手术成功了。[7]所谓的 FARES（快速、可靠和安全）在不应用麻醉药物时依然有效。[8]患者取仰卧位，前臂位于旋转中立位，伸肘，上臂置于体侧。医师站在患侧并轻缓地施加轴向牵引，逐渐移动上臂以加大外展，同时对上臂进行持续的短程垂直振荡。在上臂外展 90°时，外旋上臂。大多数复位发生于约 120°外展时。[8]

影像学检查

通过复位前影像可以确定脱位方向及相关骨折。通过复位后影像可以确认复位情况及显示复位前影像未见的相关损伤。肩关节轻度内旋位的前后位 X 线片可以显示大结节骨折。真正的前后位 X 线片可以显示肩胛盂骨折。Bankart 损伤，即肩胛盂前方缺损或盂肱下韧带附着处的骨性撕脱，可以通过西点改良腋位片（West Point modified axillary view）显示。Stryker 切迹位 X 线片可以显示肱骨头后上部的 Hill-Sachs 缺损。如需要进一步的骨影像学检查，CT 尤其有助于评估肩胛盂前方骨缺损或 Hill-Sachs 损伤。MRI 有助于评估肩关节前脱位相关病理改变。Bankart 损伤、盂唇撕裂、肩袖撕裂、盂肱韧带肱骨止点撕脱损伤或关节软骨缺损可以通过 MRI 确诊。

非手术治疗

肩关节前脱位复位后的治疗方式因人而异。通常，将肩关节置于内旋位吊带制动是一种被接受的针对初次肩关节前脱位患者的治疗方式。在不适感消失后去除吊带。有一项纳入 25 例患者的研究通过关节镜评估了将上臂制动于外旋位的效果。[9]该研究报道，盂唇的最佳复位为将上臂制动于外展 30°并外旋 60°位时，并认为将肩关节制动于内旋位会增加复发性不稳定的发生率。一项前瞻性随机研究对 40 名患者进行了制动于内旋位和外旋位的效果比较。[10]在随访的 15 个月中，制动于外旋位的患者没有复发，但制动于内旋位的患者有 30% 的复发率。然而，对随访的分析并不支持这一发现。[11]

在赛季中发生脱位的运动员希望继续比赛，这为治疗带来了困难。30 例肩关节前脱位的运动员患者中有 26 例可以通过非手术治疗包括无限制的早期活动、使用重物加强以及肩关节支具限制外展外旋的治疗方法返回赛场继续完成赛季剩下的比赛。[12]当患者的患肢肌力和功能活动范围对称，允许完全参与特定的运动时，就可以被允许重回体育活动。另外 4 例患者中，有 2 例篮球运动员患者和 1 例曲棍球运动员患者无法回归体育运动。此外，还有 1 例患者回归了体育运动，但由于复发性不稳定而再次退出了赛场。两位患者在复位后即刻回归运动，没有耽误任何比赛。在 26 例完整完成赛季比赛的患者中，有 12 例（46%）在赛季末接受手术固定。最初的 30 例患者中的 16 例（53%）在某一时间点接受了手术固定。[12]

总体上，采用非手术治疗的肩关节前脱位患者可在主动活动范围完全恢复和双侧上肢肌力正常的情况下回归体育运动。如果患者要回归接触性或碰撞性的体育运动，可用可调节的支具保护易损伤的肩关节。

手术治疗

年轻患者的脱位复发率高，而且关节镜下修复的成功率逐步提高，因此人们对于手术治疗急性肩关节前脱位的兴趣逐步增加。一项针对非手术治疗肩关节前脱位的 25 年的随访研究报道，12~22 岁患者的复发率为 72%，23~29 岁患者的复发率为

56%，大于 30 岁者为 27%。[13]一项针对急性肩关节前脱位的涉及 5 项研究共 239 名患者的荟萃分析发现，尽管体育运动的要求很高，但经手术治疗的年轻患者的复发性不稳定和脱位或半脱位的发生率显著低于经非手术治疗的年轻患者。[14]

一项针对年轻患者（其中大部分是橄榄球运动员）的关节镜下治疗和非手术治疗急性创伤性肩关节前脱位的前瞻性非随机对照研究发现，手术治疗可获得更好的结果。[15]初次急性创伤性肩关节前脱位后 18 个月内的脱位复发率在非手术治疗者中为 94.5%；在手术治疗的患者中，只有 1 例患者发生复发性脱位，96% 的患者获得了非常好的结果。一项小型前瞻性随机对照研究比较了关节镜下治疗和非手术治疗初次急性创伤性肩关节前脱位的效果，发现接受关节镜下治疗的 9 例患者中有 1 例出现复发性脱位，而接受非手术治疗的 12 例患者中有 9 例出现复发性脱位。[16]

在某些情况下，关节镜下治疗前方不稳定属于禁忌，应行切开手术治疗，如出现明显的骨缺损。[17-18]一些医师建议在关节镜下修复盂肱韧带肱骨止点撕脱伤（创伤性前方不稳定的少见情况），但大多数医师建议行切开手术。对于合并肩胛下肌腱断裂的原始脱位和前期手术失败的翻修手术，也是切开手术更为有效。

肩关节前脱位合并骨缺损

盂肱关节不稳定合并肩胛盂骨缺损的治疗难度大，正确诊断是十分重要的。盂肱关节的生物力学稳定性在肩胛盂表面骨缺损达 15%~20% 时出现改变。[19]目前，治疗肩胛盂前方骨缺损的技术包括几种喙突移位术、新鲜胫骨远端异体骨软骨移植及自体髂骨移植。[20-23]

一些研究描述了 Hill-Sachs 损伤对复发性不稳定的影响。关节镜下损伤修复手术失败和术后的复发性不稳定与肱骨头大面积缺损相关。[24-25]一项生物力学研究提示，肱骨头骨缺损达到 12.5% 就可以影响关节稳定性，37.5%~50% 的缺损可通过异体骨软骨移植恢复盂肱关节的稳定性。[26]

急性肩关节后脱位

肩关节后脱位相对少见，占所有创伤性盂肱关节脱位的 2%~5%。[27]并且，后脱位在肩关节脱位漏诊中所占比例更高，因为其不容易被发现，并且与会分散诊断注意力的高能量创伤和惊厥相关。[28-29]高达 79% 的后脱位会在初诊时被医师忽视。[30]最近有研究发现，50% 的后脱位在初诊时被漏诊。[31]一篇纳入所有符合筛选条件的文献的综述则认为这一漏诊率仅为 24%。[32]初诊时漏诊可导致诊断的延后并最终影响治疗方案的实施。

一项关于急性肩关节后脱位的流行病学研究报道，发生率为 1.1/100 000，20~49 岁的男性和年龄大于 70 岁者的发生率更高。[33]在导致后脱位的病因中，创伤性病因占 67%，由癫痫或物质戒断所致的惊厥占 31%。6% 的脱位患者伴有肩袖撕裂，常累及肩胛下肌。这些患者年龄为 54~75 岁，其中有 2 例患者需要修复肩袖。小的反 Hill-Sachs 损伤（小于 1.5 cm³）可见于 58% 的患者，大的 Hill-Sachs 损伤可见于 42% 的患者。

一些骨科文献报道了复发性不稳定的发生率，但后脱位较为少见影响了这些数据的质量。2 年的随访中，19% 的肩关节出现复发性不稳定。[33]在 23 例肩关节中，16 例原始脱位的原因是惊厥，且绝大多数于原始损伤后的 8 个月内复发。已确定的复发危险因素包括年龄小于 40 岁（复发率 30%）、惊厥（复发率 42%），以及 Hill-Sachs 损伤大于 1.5 cm³（复发率 50%）。这些危险因素可以同时存在，每一项都可增加一定复发风险。对于不存在危险因素的患者，再脱位率仅为 3%。

相关损伤在急性后脱位的治疗中起到重要作用。报道称后脱位相关损伤的发生率为 65%。[32]34% 的脱位出现骨折，29% 的脱位出现反 Hill-Sachs 损伤，13% 出现肩袖撕裂。进一步的分析显示，存在后脱位但没有骨折或 Hill-Sachs 损伤时，肩袖撕裂的发生率增加 5 倍。后脱位的发生常与其他相关病理改变及更严重的损伤相关。

患者病史

后脱位可发生于严重的创伤，有研究报道，后脱位可以同时合并肱骨干骨折和肱骨远端骨折。有 3 例患者在用髓内针治疗肱骨干骨折时漏诊了后脱位。[34] 后脱位的诊断存在困难，不仅受分散医师注意力的其他创伤的影响，而且也与悬吊上臂的吊带位置有关。

在惊厥状态，相对强大的后方肩袖肌肉强烈收缩导致肩关节脱位。有研究报道，惊厥或电击可导致双侧肩关节脱位。患者提供的病史可能并不包括已知脱位的相关创伤史，反而可能包括与肩关节无关的单一重大事件。

体格检查

典型的肩关节后脱位的体格检查结果包括无法外旋盂肱关节以及屈曲和外展受限。上臂可以置于吊带位，因为肱骨头固定于肩胛盂后方。然而，在慢性脱位患者中，屈曲和外展可达 80°~90°。同时，也可见到肩关节前方变平坦及喙突突出。

影像学检查

当存在后脱位时，患者因疼痛而很难取腋位，但腋位通常是最有价值的 X 线透视体位。如果考虑损伤累及骨性结构，CT 图像可以提供指导治疗的必要信息。尽管早期研究报道了 50%~79% 的漏诊率，但是某一创伤中心的研究却只报道了 9% 的漏诊率。[33] 研究中应用的诊断方法是通过 Velpeau 位或改良腋位垂直肩关节进行 X 线透视。

前后位片可显示一些后脱位的特征性改变，包括灯泡征（内旋导致丧失正常的结节轮廓）（图 7-2）和 Moloney 线（与髋关节的 Shenton 线相似）中断。这些有可能只是微小的改变。为了提高显示能力，在一项纳入 2 例患者的研究中，因患者无法忍受腋位摄影，故通过超声诊断后脱位。[35] 这一技术在推广使用前还需要进一步在可控的环境中进行分析。

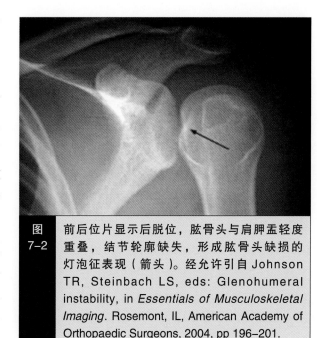

图 7-2　前后位片显示后脱位，肱骨头与肩胛盂轻度重叠，结节轮廓缺失，形成肱骨头缺损的灯泡征表现（箭头）。经允许引自 Johnson TR, Steinbach LS, eds: Glenohumeral instability, in *Essentials of Musculoskeletal Imaging*. Rosemont, IL, American Academy of Orthopaedic Surgeons, 2004, pp 196–201.

MRI 图像可以为后脱位患者提供更多信息。一项纳入 36 例初次肩关节后脱位患者的 MRI 回顾性综述发现，其中 31 例（86%）存在反 Hill-Sachs 损伤，11 例（31%）存在反骨性 Bankart 损伤[36]，12 例（19%）存在肩袖全层撕裂（4 例冈上肌撕裂、3 例冈下肌撕裂、5 例肩胛下肌撕裂），且 21 例（58%）存在后方关节囊盂唇复合体撕裂（10 例后方盂唇套袖样撕脱、11 例反 Bankart 损伤）（图 7-3）。

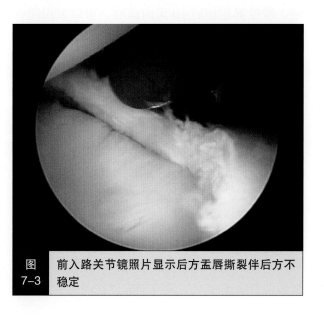

图 7-3　前入路关节镜照片显示后方盂唇撕裂伴后方不稳定

治疗决策

对后脱位的治疗选择多样。可基于以下几个问题的答案做出决策：脱位是否已复位？肩关节复位多久了？肩关节脱位的频率？脱位是如何发生的？是否有肱骨头或盂唇的骨性损伤？患者上肢的功能状态？

一些患者的个体原因可以影响治疗决策和治疗结果。例如，接触性体育运动员后方不稳定的复发率较均值高。[37] 一项回顾性综述发现与脱位 4 周后接受治疗的患者相比，在脱位 4 周内接受治疗的患者具有明显更好的结果评分。[31] 这一发现强调了早期诊断和早期治疗的必要性，目前，早期治疗的定义并不明确。一些专家定义急性脱位和早期治疗为 3 周内，其他人则认为 6 周是更合适的节点。必须基于不同的病例情况做出治疗决策。

闭合或关节镜下复位

复位是治疗肩关节后脱位的重要第一步。必要时实施全身麻醉。应在复位前确定是否存在骨性损伤。在为 7 位肱骨头骨缺损量达 30% 的患者在全身麻醉下施行闭合复位，手术非常成功。[38] 肩关节后脱位的复位技术包括在屈曲位内收和内旋位跨躯干牵引上臂。轻柔地从后方推肱骨头可引导其越过肩胛盂后方。研究中的所有（120例）脱位都在伤后 10 天内诊断，可以采用闭合复位。[33]

如果闭合复位没有成功，可以尝试关节镜下复位。[39] 将交换棒从关节镜后方置入并放置于肱骨头内上方。肩胛盂前缘作为支点，力作用于肩袖而非肱骨关节面。

非手术治疗

在没有明显骨性病理改变或患者对功能要求较低时，可以选择非手术治疗。一项纳入 35 例后脱位患者的回顾性综述发现，与接受手术治疗的患者相比，6 例接受非手术治疗的患者具有明显更高的结果评分。[31] 这项研究存在固有偏倚，部分患者因为严重的损伤接受了手术治疗，尽管如此，非手术治疗的患者获得了好的结果评分，也提供了一些信息。

对于急性肩关节脱位患者，非手术治疗应当是一线治疗方式。对于肩关节后脱位已复位的患者的治疗，吊带维持于轻度外展和旋转中立位。[33] 在复位后 4 周内每天进行 20 分钟钟摆练习，之后去除吊带，开始物理治疗。复位 2 年后随访时患者只有轻度的内旋受限。

手术治疗

如果肩关节后脱位的非手术治疗失败，则需要考虑手术干预。先对肱骨头和肩胛盂骨缺损进行分析。肱骨头缺损在后脱位所致复发性不稳定中比在前脱位中更重要。必须评估骨缺损的大小以决定合适的治疗方式。如果患者有症状或后脱位复发且没有骨缺损，可行初步的软组织重建，前脱位时也是如此。此时，行关节镜下肩关节后方稳定手术（包括后方关节囊垂直移位和盂唇解剖修复）可以获得好的结果。[40] 然而，存在骨缺损时通常必须通过以下技术治疗：顶起肱骨缺损、异体骨移植替代缺损、肌腱加强或关节置换术。

顶起肱骨缺损

肱骨头骨缺损在病理性后脱位不稳定中起到重要作用。基于肱骨头骨缺损比例的不同选择治疗方式。一些研究者建议骨缺损小于 25% 的患者通过将肱骨头缺损顶起进行治疗，而骨缺损比例为 25%~40% 者可以通过异体骨移植重建治疗。更大的骨缺损应行关节置换术治疗。然而，并没有具有确定性的研究支持治疗方式的选择。病例研究报道应用不同的治疗模式通过多种技术治疗病变范围迥异的骨缺损，包括关节镜、肩胛下肌切断和通过肩袖间隙暴露。例如，报道称对于骨缺损比例大于 40% 且无其他病理改变的患者，开放手术可获得满意结果。[41] 复位累及 50% 肱骨头的压缩骨折后，通过切开肩袖间隙暴露下行经肱骨可吸收生物螺钉固定。[42]2 例患者获得好的临床效果，在平均 26 个月的随访中没有骨关节炎或坏死的影像学表现。

然而，这些针对大的骨缺损的复位技术有失败的可能性。一例存在后脱位的患者，关节镜下将 40% 的肱骨头缺损顶起，以异体骨填塞并用 2 枚松质骨螺钉固定。[43]术后影像学检查提示肱骨关节面恢复满意；然而，在术后第 6 个月随访时，发生了移植骨吸收和骨缺损处塌陷，需要行肱骨头置换术。

在顶起并复位关节面碎块后，多种结构可以用于维持复位。自体髂骨移植可以用于维持急性交锁性后脱位的不稳定的关节复位。[44]关节处小块软骨通过可吸收针和纤维蛋白胶水固定。在 6 例肩关节后脱位且压缩骨折为 20%~40% 的患者中，将软骨整块顶起，用松质骨（单纯取自髂骨或与异体松质骨合并使用）填充缺损。[45]软骨以置于受累区的缝合锚固定。在 63 个月的随访中，2 例患者获得极好的结果，4 例患者获得好的结果。1 例患者再脱位并以相同的方法治疗。其他维持关节碎块的选择包括使用松质骨螺钉、使用可吸收生物螺钉、异体骨移植和使用骨水泥。

异体骨移植替代缺损

异体骨移植替代物是在肱骨头尚可恢复时，对大的肱骨缺损或粉碎关节面的治疗选择。将受累区域楔形切除，并用异体肱骨或异体股骨头来源的匹配的楔形骨块替代切除区域。有 6 例患者接受异体骨重建 40% 的肱骨头缺损，其中 3 例患者因惊厥而脱位，另外 3 例患者因创伤而脱位。[46]有 5 例脱位患者最初复位但出现复发。受伤 7~8 周后，所有患者均使用异体肱骨头骨块治疗。在术后第 62 个月的最终随访时，没有患者出现复发性不稳定。4 例患者可以全方位无痛活动，2 位患者出现关节范围下降并伴有疼痛。

尽管在后脱位中肱骨头骨缺损更常见，但肩胛盂骨缺损也可以通过异体骨移植以类似前方不稳定时的骨阻挡技术成功治疗。8 例患者通过开放手术，经后入路离断三角肌暴露肩胛盂，以三皮质髂骨移植至后下肩胛盂。[47]在 34 个月的随访中，没有患者出现复发性不稳定，但所有患者尚存间断性疼痛。3 例患者需要进行第二次手术以取出螺钉或缝合三角肌止点。关节镜技术已经用于通过肩袖间隙放置后方骨阻挡物。[48]根据需要，异体骨移植既可用于肱骨骨缺损，亦可用于肩胛盂骨缺损。

肌腱加强

在肱骨头前方存在骨缺损时进行肩胛下肌腱加强在 1952 年第一次被提出。[49-50]通过多年来的数次改良，这一技术已演化为关节镜下操作，无须横断肩胛下肌。然而，由于骨重建技术的成功，这些操作在近几年的应用明显减少。一项回顾性比较研究发现，在肌腱加强的同时行异体骨解剖重建或自体骨解剖重建会得到一致的不良结果，这一发现与之前的研究结果相同。[31]

关节置换术

肱骨头有大的骨缺损或年龄大于 60 岁且活动水平较低的肩关节脱位患者，可选择行肩关节置换术。这些患者术后可获得明显的功能改善，但对于骨关节炎患者，关节置换术的结果依然不佳。[51]

患者可能存在多个区域的病理改变。一例 77 岁的非创伤性肩关节后脱位的男性患者有 40% 的肱骨头骨缺损和 30% 的肩胛盂后下部骨缺损。他接受了半肩关节置换术，肩胛盂后方的骨性阻挡物取材于被切除的肱骨头，通过胸大肌三角肌入路，经皮拧入后方螺钉。[52]

慢性肩关节脱位

研究者用不同的时间点定义慢性脱位，从初始脱位后 24 小时至 6 周不等。建议的时间点是初始脱位后 3 周。[53]未发现的盂肱关节脱位所致的慢性脱位相对不常见，尽管通常有骨折发生。一项纳入 61 例慢性脱位病例的综述发现 50% 的病例合并骨折，33% 的病例存在神经损伤，28% 的病例为后脱位。[54] 其他研究发现，在从业 5~10 年的骨科医师中有 50% 见过慢性脱位，在从业 10~20 年者中有 70% 见过慢性脱位，而在从业超过 20 年者中有 90% 见过慢性脱位。[30,54] 尽管慢性脱位少见，但骨科医师应当了解其诊断与治疗选择。

任何伴随慢性脱位的肩关节病理改变都应当能辨认。通常肱骨头关节软骨会发生退变。在前脱位，有可能发展为明显的软组织挛缩，伴有肱骨头和邻近神经血管结构粘连。同时发生的肩袖撕裂（有时巨大）可能影响肩关节稳定性，肩胛下肌断裂和肱二头肌腱脱位也有可能发生。盂肱关节骨缺损可以明显影响关节稳定性，肩胛盂前下部骨缺损常见于前脱位，肱骨前上部骨缺损常见于后脱位。这些肱骨头骨缺损和肩胛盂骨缺损所致的病变组织嵌入会导致复位困难。总体上，对慢性肩关节脱位的治疗具有挑战性。治疗方案可根据患者的功能状态、同时存在的病理改变等因素来决定。

慢性后脱位

很多慢性后脱位患者有酒精依赖或年龄超过

70 岁。患者难以提供清楚的病史，可能导致初诊漏诊。存在惊厥病史或多发创伤的患者也应当彻底评估。患者的其他医疗情况、功能状态及期望都应当明确，这些都会影响最终的治疗方案。患者可能描述：起初肩关节疼痛，之后疼痛缓解并且恢复平腰水平活动。然而，患者肩关节持续无法外旋。体格检查结果与急性后脱位相似。在慢性后脱位中，为了获取一定的功能活动范围，肱骨头可能已经明显变形（图 7-4）。

慢性后脱位的影像学检查结果与急性后脱位相同。外侧腋位片提供肩胛盂累及范围及肱骨头压缩与否等重要的信息。压缩的程度可以通过估计缺损大小以及与关节表面弧度对比来量化。所有的影像学检查都应当检查骨折的可能。如果发现累及骨性结构，推荐 CT 检查评估骨性结构破坏的量与位置。

治疗

虽然存在解剖畸形及严重的盂肱关节旋转受限，但是慢性后脱位可以很好地耐受，尤其是年龄超过 70 岁的患者或衰弱患者。这样的患者可能重获一定的关节活动范围以满足日常活动需要并很少出现疼痛。找到手术和预期结果之间的平衡是很重要的。惊厥无法控制的患者，不接受术后

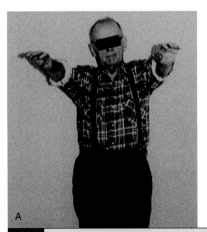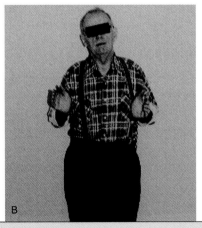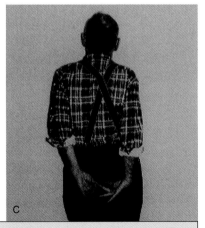

图 7-4　双侧慢性后脱位的 60 岁男性患者。前屈（A）、外旋（B）及内旋（C）活动受限。经允许引自 Zuckerman JD: *Comprehensive Care of Orthopaedic Injuries in the Elderly*. Baltimore, MD, Urban & Schwarzenberg, 1990, pp 287–288.

康复训练的患者或没有疼痛且功能需求低的患者，应当考虑行非手术治疗。对于这些患者，手术风险超过了改善结果的潜在收益。

对于能够从手术干预中获益的患者，有多种软组织、骨性结构和假体手术可供选择。具体选择受一些患者因素和伴发的病理改变影响：患者的年龄、功能需求、受伤后时间、肩胛盂骨质量和骨缺损以及肱骨骨质量和骨缺损。受伤后时间和手术方式被认为是最重要的结果预期因素。[31]患者在原始脱位4周内接受治疗有相对高的结果评分，接受恢复解剖结构治疗者同样获得了相对高的结果评分（肱骨头顶起或异体植骨）。然而，这项研究具有固有偏倚，损伤严重的患者通常接受半肩关节置换术，因此并不是行异体骨移植重建的合适人选。

闭合复位

如果脱位时间短于3周、肱骨头压缩程度小于25%且没有其他肱骨骨折，可以行闭合复位。一些研究者认为脱位后6周内且肱骨头骨缺损小于关节面的20%时都可以尝试复位。[55]在一项研究中，脱位后4周内复位，30例患者中有19例复位成功，而复位时间晚于4周，10例患者中只有1例成功。[54]

对于慢性损伤，复位时应当动作轻柔。为了获得彻底的松弛，应当行全身麻醉。控制内旋可以协助牵拉后方关节囊，向外侧牵引以使肱骨头从肩胛盂缘解锁。之后即可在控制外旋下复位盂肱关节。上臂在轻度外旋位（约20°）用支具固定。应当注意发生不稳定的点，应用支具时应避免此位置。在复位后的早期就可允许患者开始外旋活动。

手术选择

如果患者的损伤是相对急性的，肱骨头受累小于50%且关节软骨尚可恢复，可以考虑将肱骨头骨缺损的压缩解除并植骨。[56]这需要通过手术开窗顶起关节面骨块并以自体骨移植或异体骨移植作为支撑。

如果患者的肱骨骨缺损相对小（小于40%），可考虑应用当前的肩胛下肌腱移位方法，保留其在小结节止点。[57-58]因为患者接受骨性重建可以获得较好的预后，因此上述操作不再被经常用到。

异体骨移植重建是被认可的治疗尚可恢复的肱骨头骨缺损的方法，尤其是对于相对年轻的患者。大小匹配的新鲜冰冻肱骨或异体股骨头用于重建。在一项平均54个月的随访中，13例缺损为25%~50%的患者获得了较好的预后。[56]

肩关节置换术的适应证包括肱骨头骨缺损大于50%，严重的软骨损伤以及显著的骨量减少。需要根据病例情况选择全肩关节置换术、半肩关节置换术或表面置换。一项针对13例通过肩关节置换术治疗的肩关节慢性交锁性后脱位的研究发现，其中11例患者的术后关节活动范围得以改善，但Constant肩关节评分的平均分为59.4。[51]1例患者需要接受翻修手术，另1例患者出现严重的肱骨头上移。

慢性前脱位

对于慢性前脱位的患者，通过视诊患侧及健侧肩关节可以发现患侧肩关节的三角肌隆起消失、肩峰后部变方。慢性前脱位常明显限制旋转。上臂在外旋时远离躯干。慢性前脱位的疼痛感因人而异，患者可能长期处于脱位状态却只有轻微疼痛。完善全套神经血管检查并记录以评估腋神经损伤和动脉损伤。

对于后脱位患者，有一些因素影响着手术适应证，包括是否存在骨缺损。在后脱位中，肩胛盂常保持结构完整，而慢性前脱位与之相反，常合并肩胛盂前下部骨缺损。在脱位的同时可发生骨折，也可在之后逐渐磨损形成骨缺损。前方关节囊结构常撕裂，为了达到肩关节稳定的效果，需要将其重新修复附着。

手术治疗

应在慢性前脱位的手术入路中仔细评估神经

血管结构。通常，这些结构与瘢痕组织粘连，分离困难。术中需要辨识腋神经并加以保护，发生腋动脉损伤时可以请血管外科医师处理。对于慢性后脱位有很多治疗选择。

盂唇修补在急性前脱位的处理中一直是焦点所在，在慢性前脱位中也十分重要。一项研究评估了 8 例未复位的慢性肩关节脱位合并 Hill-Sachs 损伤小于 40% 的患者，平均伤后 10 周。[59] 所有患者均接受开放手术经肩胛盂盂唇缝线修补。在最终随访中，这些患者的平均 Rowe-Zarin 评分为 86 分，平均前屈受限为 18°，平均外旋受限为 17.5°。关节镜下完成相同修补获得了满意的结果。[60]

慢性前脱位中肩胛盂常受累。如果肩胛盂骨缺损小于 20%，可以行 Bankart 修补，实施或不实施骨性加强均可。骨性加强应当在肩胛盂骨缺损超过 20% 时实施。可通过自体骨移植、异体骨移植或喙突移位实现。

肱骨头缺损小于 25% 时，如果肩关节保持稳定，复位后则不需要进一步治疗。如果肱骨头缺损大于 25%，则应当在复位后进一步治疗。如果肱骨头缺损小于 50%，关节软骨尚可恢复，且骨量满意，可以考虑解除缺损压缩。如果关节软骨无法恢复，可考虑行异体骨移植重建。[61] 脱位大于 6 个月时，骨的质量常很差，可考虑行关节置换术。从前入路行异体骨移植重建肱骨头后外部骨缺损时常需要暴露很大的范围（图 7-5）。肩胛

下肌必须完全离断，离断时应保护营养肱骨头的旋肱前动脉。

任何超过 6 个月的脱位都可能对关节面造成不可逆的损伤。因此，如果这类脱位患者合并大于 50% 的肱骨头骨缺损、较差的骨质量，或患者的功能需求较低，应当考虑行关节镜手术。医师应当确保维持适当的肩关节后伸（约 30°）以防止进一步的前方不稳定。越来越多的文献支持通过反肩关节置换术治疗急性肱骨近端骨折，可以考虑将反式全肩关节置换术应用于慢性前脱位。对于明显的肩胛盂前部骨缺损和肩胛下肌功能不全，假体的治疗效果明显。然而，目前尚没有关于通过这一方法治疗慢性前脱位的结果报道。

总体上，慢性脱位的治疗方法复杂，需要考虑患者个体和与损伤相关的多种因素。如何选择对某一患者来说的最佳治疗方案尚无定论。现有的治疗慢性后脱位或慢性前脱位的策略是基于目前可用的证据做出的（图 7-6，7-7）。

总结

急性和慢性肩关节脱位的情况复杂，没有适用于所有情况的解决方法。然而，有一些基本点可以确定。有研究证据支持年龄小于 25 岁的患者初始前脱位后的复发率高，因此一些专家推荐在初始脱位后进行修复，但也有一些研究者报道经非手术治疗，如多种康复和制动治疗，可获得满

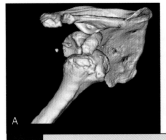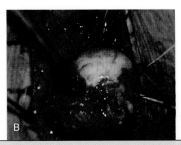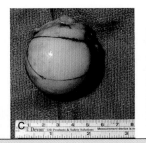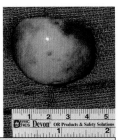

图 7-5　A. 三维 CT 重建显示交锁的前脱位。B. 术中照片显示大的 Hill-Sachs 损伤。C. 异体肱骨头。D. 异体肱骨头节段

意的结果。如果想要对前方不稳定行手术治疗，则必须评估肩胛盂前部和肱骨头骨缺损的情况。如果骨缺损明显，单纯行关节镜下软组织手术有可能失败，还需要处理骨性病变。

　　对于慢性肩关节脱位的可用治疗选择各异。

需要考虑骨缺损比例以及肱骨头和肩胛盂可恢复的程度。如果剩余骨组织可以恢复并对移植骨起到支持作用，可考虑行异体骨移植替代。许多这样的关节损伤需要行假体置换以改善关节功能。

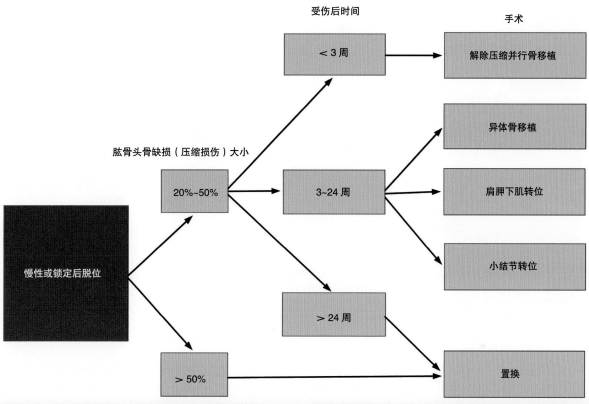

手术		指征
重建	异体骨移植	压缩损伤为 20%~50% 所有年轻患者 骨和软骨情况好的所有老年患者
	肩胛下肌腱转位	肱骨头骨缺损（压缩损伤）<25% 且持续不稳定
	小结节转位	肱骨头骨缺损（压缩损伤）为 20%~45% 且软骨情况好，但是骨量差；患者不愿意异体骨移植
置换	全肩关节置换术	压缩损伤 >50%，任何年龄 老年患者，骨量差，压缩损伤 <50% 任何软骨情况差的患者
	半肩关节置换术	肩胛盂软骨情况好的半肩关节置换术

图 7-6 慢性或锁定后脱位的处理流程

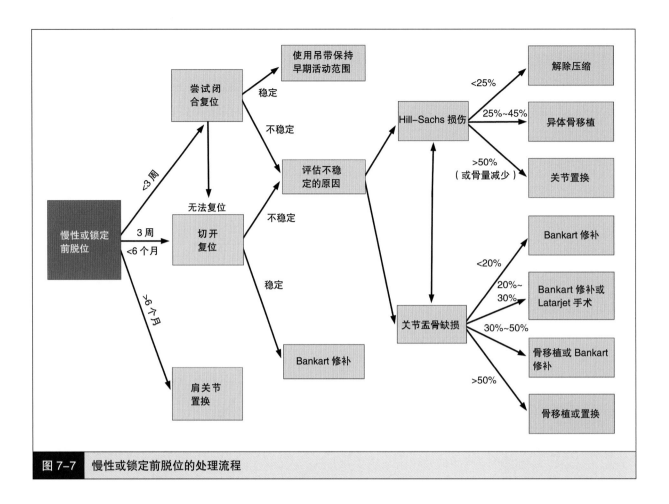

图 7-7　慢性或锁定前脱位的处理流程

参考文献

［1］ Zacchilli MA, Owens BD: Epidemiology of shoulder dislocations presenting to emergency departments in the United States. *J Bone Joint Surg Am* 2010;92(3):542-549.
The overall incidence of shoulder dislocations seen in US emergency departments was 23.9 per 100,000. Male sex and young age were the most important risk factors for injury.

［2］ Owens BD, Duffey ML, Nelson BJ, DeBerardino TM, Taylor DC, Mountcastle SB: The incidence and characteristics of shoulder instability at the United States Military Academy. *Am J Sports Med* 2007;35(7):1168-1173.
A descriptive epidemiologic study found that traumatic glenohumeral instability events are common in young athletes, and 85% of these events are subluxations.

［3］ Baker CL, Uribe JW, Whitman C: Arthroscopic evaluation of acute initial anterior shoulder dislocations. *Am J Sports Med* 1990;18(1):25-28.

［4］ Pouliart N, Marmor S, Gagey O: Simulated capsulolabral lesion in cadavers: Dislocation does not result from a bankart lesion only. *Arthroscopy* 2006;22(7):748-754.

［5］ Shin SJ, Yun YH, Kim DJ, Yoo JD: Treatment of traumatic anterior shoulder dislocation in patients older than 60 years. *Am J Sports Med* 2012;40(4):822-827.
More than half of the patients older than 60 years with traumatic anterior shoulder dislocation had a rotator cuff tear or an anterior capsulolabral injury. Clinical outcomes were satisfactory with early detection of abnormalities and treatments tailored to associated injuries.

［6］ Miller SL, Cleeman E, Auerbach J, Flatow EL: Comparison of intra-articular lidocaine and intravenous sedation for reduction of shoulder dislocations: A randomized, prospective study. *J Bone Joint Surg Am* 2002;84(12):2135-2139.

［7］ Eachempati KK, Dua A, Malhotra R, Bhan S, Bera JR: The external rotation method for reduction of acute anterior dislocations and fracture-dislocations of the shoulder. *J Bone Joint Surg Am* 2004;86(11):2431-2434.

［8］ Sayegh FE, Kenanidis EI, Papavasiliou KA, Potoupnis ME, Kirkos JM, Kapetanos GA: Reduction of acute anterior dislocations: A prospective randomized study comparing a new technique with the Hippocratic and Kocher methods. *J Bone Joint Surg Am* 2009; 91(12):2775-2782.

The authors introduced the FARES method for reducing an anterior shoulder dislocation and compared it with the Hippocratic and Kocher methods in 154 patients. The FARES method was found to be more effective, less time consuming, less painful, and effective when performed by one person. Level of evidence: I.

[9] Hart WJ, Kelly CP: Arthroscopic observation of capsulolabral reduction after shoulder dislocation. *J Shoulder Elbow Surg* 2005;14(2):134-137.

[10] Itoi E, Hatakeyama Y, Kido T, et al: A new method of immobilization after traumatic anterior dislocation of the shoulder: A preliminary study. *J Shoulder Elbow Surg* 2003;12(5):413-415.

[11] Liavaag S, Brox JI, Pripp AH, Enger M, Soldal LA, Svenningsen S: Immobilization in external rotation after primary shoulder dislocation did not reduce the risk of recurrence: A randomized controlled trial. *J Bone Joint Surg Am* 2011;93(10):897-904.

Anterior shoulder dislocation in 188 patients was treated with bracing in internal or external rotation. The rate of recurrence was not lower with immobilization in external rotation. Level of evidence: I.

[12] Buss DD, Lynch GP, Meyer CP, Huber SM, Freehill MQ: Nonoperative management for in-season athletes with anterior shoulder instability. *Am J Sports Med* 2004;32(6):1430-1433.

[13] Hovelius L, Olofsson A, Sandström B, et al: Nonoperative treatment of primary anterior shoulder dislocation in patients forty years of age and younger: A prospective twenty-five-year follow-up. *J Bone Joint Surg Am* 2008;90(5):945-952.

At 25-year follow-up, half of the 257 nonsurgically treated anterior shoulder dislocations in patients age 12 to 25 years had not recurred or had become stable.

[14] Handoll HH, Almaiyah MA, Rangan A: Surgical versus non-surgical treatment for acute anterior shoulder dislocation. *Cochrane Database Syst Rev* 2004;1: CD004325.

[15] Larrain MV, Botto GJ, Montenegro HJ, Mauas DM: Arthroscopic repair of acute traumatic anterior shoulder dislocation in young athletes. *Arthroscopy* 2001; 17(4):373-377.

[16] Bottoni CR, Wilckens JH, DeBerardino TM, et al: A prospective, randomized evaluation of arthroscopic stabilization versus nonoperative treatment in patients with acute, traumatic, first-time shoulder dislocations. *Am J Sports Med* 2002;30(4):576-580.

[17] Balg F, Boileau P: The instability severity index score: A simple pre-operative score to select patients for arthroscopic or open shoulder stabilisation. *J Bone Joint Surg Br* 2007;89(11):1470-1477.

In a prospective study of 131 consecutive patients with recurrent anterior shoulder instability who underwent arthroscopic Bankart repair, the risk factors for recurrent instability after surgery were age younger than 20 years, competitive or contact athletic participation, hyperlaxity, a Hill-Sachs lesion, or loss of the sclerotic inferior glenoid contour. A scoring system helped determine whether arthroscopic treatment would be sufficient.

[18] Porcellini G, Campi F, Pegreffi F, Castagna A, Paladini P: Predisposing factors for recurrent shoulder dislocation after arthroscopic treatment. *J Bone Joint Surg Am* 2009;91(11):2537-2542.

In a study of 385 patients who underwent a single arthroscopic Bankart repair, 13% of the patients younger than 22 years and 6.3% of the older patients had a recurrence at 36-month follow-up. The risk factors were age at the time of the first dislocation, male sex, and the time from the first dislocation until surgery. Level of evidence: II.

[19] Itoi E, Lee SB, Berglund LJ, Berge LL, An KN: The effect of a glenoid defect on anteroinferior stability of the shoulder after Bankart repair: A cadaveric study. *J Bone Joint Surg Am* 2000;82(1):35-46.

[20] Provencher MT, Ghodadra N, LeClere L, Solomon DJ, Romeo AA: Anatomic osteochondral glenoid reconstruction for recurrent glenohumeral instability with glenoid deficiency using a distal tibia allograft. *Arthroscopy* 2009;25(4):446-452.

A novel technique for the management of glenoid bone loss used a fresh osteochondral distal tibia allograft. The advantages included improved graft availability compared with fresh glenoid specimens, a cartilaginous interface, excellent conformity of the graft, and no requirement for presurgical sizing. Studies are needed to evaluate long-term efficacy.

[21] Warner JJ, Gill TJ, O'Hollerhan JD, Pathare N, Millett PJ: Anatomical glenoid reconstruction for recurrent anterior glenohumeral instability with glenoid deficiency using an autogenous tricortical iliac crest bone graft. *Am J Sports Med* 2006;34(2):205-212.

[22] Hovelius L, Sandström B, Olofsson A, Svensson O, Rahme

H: The effect of capsular repair, bone block healing, and position on the results of the Bristow- Latarjet procedure (study III): Long-term follow-up in 319 shoulders. *J Shoulder Elbow Surg* 2012;21(5):647-660.

The results of the May modification of the Bristow-Latarjet procedure were evaluated in 319 shoulders. The procedure yielded consistently good results, with bony fusion in 83%. Recurrent instability was more likely if the coracoid was placed 1 cm or more medial to the rim. The addition of a horizontal capsular shift to the coracoid transfer improved the recurrence rate and the subjective results.

[23] Hovelius L, Vikerfors O, Olofsson A, Svensson O, Rahme H: Bristow-Latarjet and Bankart: A comparative study of shoulder stabilization in 185 shoulders during a seventeen-year follow-up. *J Shoulder Elbow Surg* 2011;20(7):1095-1101.

Subjective patient evaluations and postoperative stability were better after Bristow-Latarjet repair in 88 consecutive shoulders than after Bankart repair with anchors in 97 shoulders.

[24] Boileau P, Villalba M, Héry JY, Balg F, Ahrens P, Neyton L: Risk factors for recurrence of shoulder instability after arthroscopic Bankart repair. *J Bone Joint Surg Am* 2006;88(8):1755-1763.

[25] Burkhart SS, De Beer JF: Traumatic glenohumeral bone defects and their relationship to failure of arthroscopic Bankart repairs: Significance of the invertedpear glenoid and the humeral engaging Hill-Sachs lesion. *Arthroscopy* 2000;16(7):677-694.

[26] Sekiya JK, Wickwire AC, Stehle JH, Debski RE: Hill- Sachs defects and repair using osteoarticular allograft transplantation: Biomechanical analysis using a joint compression model. *Am J Sports Med* 2009;37(12):2459-2466.

A controlled laboratory study quantified data on the critical defect size of Hill-Sachs lesions requiring surgical repair and the ability of allograft transplantation to restore joint stability. Defects measuring 12.5% of the humeral head have biomechanical effects that may affect joint stability, and defects of 37.5% may benefit from osteoarticular allografting.

[27] Kowalsky MS, Levine WN: Traumatic posterior glenohumeral dislocation: Classification, pathoanatomy, diagnosis, and treatment. *Orthop Clin North Am* 2008; 39(4):519-533, viii.

The classification, pathoanatomy, diagnosis, and treatment of traumatic posterior glenohumeral dislocation were reviewed in detail.

[28] Cicak N: Posterior dislocation of the shoulder. *J Bone Joint Surg Br* 2004;86(3):324-332.

[29] Kayali C, Agus H, Kalenderer O, Turgut A, Imamoglu T: Overlooked posterior shoulder dislocation: Preoperative and postoperative CT studies (a case report). *Ortop Traumatol Rehabil* 2009;11(2):177-182.

A sustained posterior shoulder dislocation initially was overlooked. The patient later was treated with a modified McLaughlin procedure.

[30] Rowe CR, Zarins B: Chronic unreduced dislocations of the shoulder. *J Bone Joint Surg Am* 1982;64(4): 494-505.

[31] Schliemann B, Muder D, Gessmann J, Schildhauer TA, Seybold D: Locked posterior shoulder dislocation: Treatment options and clinical outcomes. *Arch Orthop Trauma Surg* 2011;131(8):1127-1134.

In a review of 35 patients with a locked posterior shoulder dislocation, the shoulder remained stable after closed reduction in 6 patients, and the treatment was nonsurgical. The treatment was surgical in 29 patients. The patients treated nonsurgically had a slightly better outcome. There was a high correlation between the time to correct diagnosis and outcome.

[32] Rouleau DM, Hebert-Davies J: Incidence of associated injury in posterior shoulder dislocation: Systematic review of the literature. *J Orthop Trauma* 2012;26(4): 246-251.

Of 475 patients (543 shoulders) with posterior shoulder dislocation, 34% had seizures. Injury was associated with 65% of dislocations. Fractures were most common, followed by reverse Hill-Sachs injuries and rotator cuff tears. In the absence of fracture or a reverse Hill-Sachs injury, the risk of rotator cuff tear increased almost fivefold.

[33] Robinson CM, Seah M, Akhtar MA: The epidemiology, risk of recurrence, and functional outcome after an acute traumatic posterior dislocation of the shoulder. *J Bone Joint Surg Am* 2011;93(17):1605-1613.

Posterior glenohumeral dislocations were retrospectively reviewed in 112 patients treated nonsurgically. Survival analysis revealed that recurrent instability occurred within the first year in 17.7%. On multivariable analysis, age younger than 40 years, dislocation during a seizure, and a reverse Hill-Sachs lesion larger than 1.5 cm^3 were predictive of recurrent instability.

[34] Singh S, Tan CK, Sinopidis C, Frostick S, Brownson P: Missed posterior dislocation of the shoulder after intramedullary fixation of humeral fractures: A report of

three cases. *J Shoulder Elbow Surg* 2009;18(3): e33-e37. Three patients had a posterior shoulder dislocation after humeral nailing.

[35] Yuen CK, Chung TS, Mok KL, Kan PG, Wong YT: Dynamic ultrasonographic sign for posterior shoulder dislocation. *Emerg Radiol* 2011;18(1):47-51.
Bedside ultrasonography was used for diagnosing posterior shoulder dislocation. The dynamic ultrasonographic sign of posterior shoulder dislocation is described.

[36] Saupe N, White LM, Bleakney R, et al: Acute traumatic posterior shoulder dislocation: MR findings. *Radiology* 2008;248(1):185-193.
MRI of traumatic posterior shoulder dislocation revealed a reverse Hill-Sachs lesion in 86% of the patients and a posterocaudal labrocapsular lesion in almost 60%. A full-thickness rotator cuff tear occurred in approximately 20%.

[37] Bradley JP, Baker CL III, Kline AJ, Armfield DR, Chhabra A: Arthroscopic capsulolabral reconstruction for posterior instability of the shoulder: A prospective study of 100 shoulders. *Am J Sports Med* 2006;34(7): 1061-1071.

[38] Duralde XA, Fogle EF: The success of closed reduction in acute locked posterior fracture-dislocations of the shoulder. *J Shoulder Elbow Surg* 2006;15(6):701-706.

[39] Verma NN, Sellards RA, Romeo AA: Arthroscopic reduction and repair of a locked posterior shoulder dislocation. *Arthroscopy* 2006;22(11):e1-e5.

[40] Savoie FH III, Holt MS, Field LD, Ramsey JR: Arthroscopic management of posterior instability: Evolution of technique and results. *Arthroscopy* 2008;24(4): 389-396.
In 136 shoulders surgically treated for primary posterior instability, no essential lesion was found for posterior instability. Multiple varied pathologies can be present in a shoulder with posterior instability.

[41] Gerber C, Lambert SM: Allograft reconstruction of segmental defects of the humeral head for the treatment of chronic locked posterior dislocation of the shoulder. *J Bone Joint Surg Am* 1996;78(3):376-382.

[42] Assom M, Castoldi F, Rossi R, Blonna D, Rossi P: Humeral head impression fracture in acute posterior shoulder dislocation: New surgical technique. *Knee Surg Sports Traumatol Arthrosc* 2006;14(7):668-672.

[43] Moroder P, Resch H, Tauber M: Failed arthroscopic repair of a large reverse Hill-Sachs lesion using bone allograft and cannulated screws: A case report. *Arthroscopy* 2012;28(1):138-144.
A reverse Hill-Sachs lesion affecting more than 40% of the articulating surface was treated arthroscopically using retrograde elevation, bone allografting, and cannulated screw insertion. Postoperative radiographs showed successful reduction of the impacted articulating surface of the humeral head. At 6-month follow-up, the patient had pain and symptoms of a frozen shoulder. Cross-sectional imaging showed necrosis, partial absorption, and loss of reduction of the formerly elevated segment, requiring humeral head replacement.

[44] Khayal T, Wild M, Windolf J: Reconstruction of the articular surface of the humeral head after locked posterior shoulder dislocation: A case report. *Arch Orthop Trauma Surg* 2009;129(4):515-519.
An acute locked posterior shoulder dislocation was successfully treated by reconstructing the articular surface of the humeral head with autologous bone graft from the iliac crest.

[45] Bock P, Kluger R, Hintermann B: Anatomical reconstruction for reverse Hill-Sachs lesions after posterior locked shoulder dislocation fracture: A case series of six patients. *Arch Orthop Trauma Surg* 2007;127(7): 543-548.
In six patients at an average 62-month follow-up, anatomic head reconstruction using spongiotic autograft or allograft proved to be valid for restoring shoulder function and stability.

[46] Martinez AA, Calvo A, Domingo J, Cuenca J, Herrera A, Malillos M: Allograft reconstruction of segmental defects of the humeral head associated with posterior dislocations of the shoulder. *Injury* 2008;39(3): 319-322.
Six men with posterior dislocation of the humeral head underwent surgical allograft treatment for a defect involving at least 40% of the articular surface. At discharge, four patients had no pain, instability, clicking or catching; two had pain, clicking, catching, and stiffness.

[47] Barbier O, Ollat D, Marchaland JP, Versier G: Iliac bone-block autograft for posterior shoulder instability. *Orthop Traumatol Surg Res* 2009;95(2):100-107.
Eight patients with recurrent posterior shoulder instability were treated with a posterior iliac bone-block procedure. All patients recovered normal joint range of motion in abduction and anterior elevation. In three patients, external rotation was limited an average of 20° compared with the opposite side. Only four patients were able to return to their preoperative sports activity level. At a mean 3-year follow-up, 80% had a satisfactory result.

[48] Barth J, Grosclaude S, Lädermann A, Denard PJ, Graveleau N, Walch G: Arthroscopic posterior bone

graft for posterior instability: The transrotator interval sparing cuff technique. *Tech Shoulder Elbow Surg* 2011;12(3):67-71.

In a new arthroscopic technique, the bone graft is passed through an anatomic portal, that is, the rotator cuff interval. One patient had a good result after bone graft was passed through the rotator cuff interval before being secured to the posterior glenoid.

[49] McLaughlin HL: Posterior dislocation of the shoulder. *J Bone Joint Surg Am* 1952;24-A(3):584-590.

[50] McLaughlin HL: Locked posterior subluxation of the shoulder: Diagnosis and treatment. *Surg Clin North Am* 1963;43:1621-1622.

[51] Gavriilidis I, Magosch P, Lichtenberg S, Habermeyer P, Kircher J: Chronic locked posterior shoulder dislocation with severe head involvement. *Int Orthop* 2010;34(1):79-84.

Retrospective review of 12 shoulder arthroplasties (11 patients) for a locked dislocation found a significant improvement in range of motion for flexion, abduction, and external rotation at a mean 37-month follow-up. There was a negative correlation between the Constant Shoulder Score and number of previous operations, pain, and duration of symptoms.

[52] Riggenbach MD, Najarian RG, Bishop JY: Recurrent, locked posterior glenohumeral dislocation requiring hemiarthroplasty and posterior bone block with humeral head autograft. *Orthopedics* 2012;35(2):e277-e282.

A 77-year-old man with a recurrent posterior shoulder dislocation was treated with humeral hemiarthroplasty and reconstruction of a large posteroinferior glenoid defect using a bone block created from humeral head autograft.

[53] Griggs SM, Holloway B, Williams GR Jr, Iannotti JP: *Disorders of the Shoulder Diagnosis and Management.* Philadelphia, PA, Lippincott, Williams & Wilkins, 2006, pp 461-486.

Chronic dislocations of the shoulder and associated techniques are described.

[54] Schulz TJ, Jacobs B, Patterson RL Jr: Unrecognized dislocations of the shoulder. *J Trauma* 1969;9(12): 1009-1023.

[55] Loebenberg MI, Cuomo F: The treatment of chronic anterior and posterior dislocations of the glenohumeral joint and associated articular surface defects. *Orthop Clin North Am* 2000;31(1):23-34.

[56] Diklic ID, Ganic ZD, Blagojevic ZD, Nho SJ, Romeo

AA: Treatment of locked chronic posterior dislocation of the shoulder by reconstruction of the defect in the humeral head with an allograft. *J Bone Joint Surg Br* 2010;92(1):71-76.

At a mean 54-month follow-up after humeral head reconstruction with femoral head allograft, 9 of 13 patients (10 men, 3 women; mean age, 42 years) had no pain or restriction of activities of daily living. No patient had symptoms of shoulder instability. The mean Constant-Murley Shoulder Score was 86.8 (range, 43 to 98).

[57] Spencer EE Jr, Brems JJ: A simple technique for management of locked posterior shoulder dislocations: Report of two cases. *J Shoulder Elbow Surg* 2005;14(6): 650-652.

[58] Delcogliano A, Caporaso A, Chiossi S, Menghi A, Cillo M, Delcogliano M: Surgical management of chronic, unreduced posterior dislocation of the shoulder. *Knee Surg Sports Traumatol Arthrosc* 2005;13(2): 151-155.

[59] Rouhani A, Navali A: Treatment of chronic anterior shoulder dislocation by open reduction and simultaneous Bankart lesion repair. *Sports Med Arthrosc Rehabil Ther Technol* 2010;2:15.

Eight patients with a chronic anterior shoulder dislocation underwent open reduction and capsulolabral complex repair an average 10 weeks after injury. Four shoulders were graded as excellent, three as good, and one as fair. All patients were able to perform daily activities with mild or no pain. Outcomes were found to be more favorable than with earlier methods.

[60] Galano GJ, Dieter AA, Moradi NE, Ahmad CS: Arthroscopic management of a chronic primary anterior shoulder dislocation. *Am J Orthop (Belle Mead NJ)* 2010;39(7):351-355.

A 70-year-old woman underwent arthroscopic reduction and labral fixation of a chronically dislocated shoulder.

[61] Mehta V: Humeral head plasty for a chronic locked anterior shoulder dislocation. *Orthopedics* 2009; 32(1):52.

A 52-year-old man had a chronic anterior shoulder dislocation with a massive Hill-Sachs lesion. The Hill-Sachs lesion was managed with humeral headplasty performed with an 8-mm anterior cruciate ligament guide adjacent to the lesser tuberosity. The Hill-Sachs lesion was tamped out to restore the contour of the humeral head and backfilled with allograft.

第八章 复发性肩关节前方不稳定

Brian D. Dierckman, MD; Neil Ghodadra, MD; Daniel J. Solomon, MD; Mark D. Stanley, MD;
John W. McNeil II , BA, CDR; Matthew T. Provencher, MD, MC, USN

引言

　　盂肱关节是人体最易脱位的关节。盂肱关节的骨性限制较少，因此关节活动范围大但同时也存在不稳定的危险。盂肱关节的静态限制和动态限制通过复杂的骨骼肌肉相互作用提供稳定性，某一限制结构或更多限制结构的损伤可导致肩关节由稳定发展为不稳定。很多患者在初次肩关节前脱位复位后，不再出现肩关节不稳定。[1]也有一部分患者发展为复发性肩关节前方不稳定，年轻的男性接触性项目运动员是最易受累的患者群体。

　　近些年，骨缺损在复发性不稳定中的关键作用已被证实。本章将讨论复发性肩关节前方不稳定的病理生理学、临床评估、影像学检查以及治疗和结果，着重于讨论肩胛盂和肱骨骨缺损。肩胛盂和（或）肱骨骨缺损在复发性肩关节不稳定中的准确意义尚需研究。

病理生理学

　　初次肩关节前脱位后，常见的损伤是前下盂唇和关节囊从肩胛盂缘附着处撕脱（Bankart 损伤）[2]（图 8-1）。同时，由于肱骨头与肩胛盂前下缘硬质骨的大力撞击，大多数患者存在肱骨头后外上部的压缩骨折（Hill-Sachs 损伤）。[3]然而，大多数初次 Hill-Sachs 损伤的特点是小、浅且临床表现不明显（图 8-2）。

　　在复发性肩关节不稳定中，进一步的肩关节静态和动态限制装置受损造成了骨和软骨缺损加剧，通常会导致退变发生。除了典型的 Bankart 损伤，还有一些因素在不同程度上导致了复发性肩关节不稳定。肩胛盂和肱骨头骨缺损被认为是大多数复发性肩关节不稳定患者的关键病理特征。在肩关节脱位中，肱骨头与肩胛盂前部撞击，导致

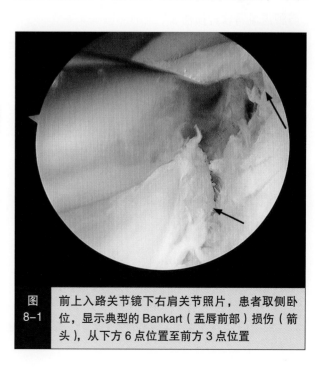

图 8-1　前上入路关节镜下右肩关节照片，患者取侧卧位，显示典型的 Bankart（盂唇前部）损伤（箭头），从下方 6 点位置至前方 3 点位置

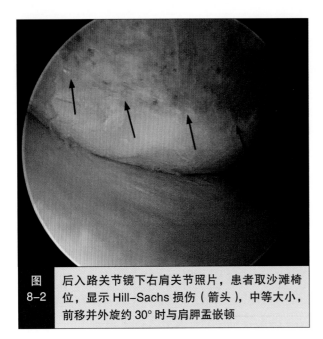

图 8-2　后入路关节镜下右肩关节照片，患者取沙滩椅位，显示 Hill-Sachs 损伤（箭头），中等大小，前移并外旋约 30° 时与肩胛盂嵌顿

肩胛盂磨损性骨缺损，并扩大了 Hill-Sachs 损伤范围。盂肱下韧带（IGHL）复合体因进一步受到牵拉而变薄，导致肩关节的静态限制装置弹性变形并受损。[4]

在对复发性肩关节前方不稳定患者进行影像学评估和关节镜探查时，可以相对频繁地见到一些不常见的解剖结构，包括 ALPSA 病变、HAGL 损伤、环状撕裂或盂唇广泛撕裂以及 GLAD 病变（肩胛盂盂唇软骨损伤）。

ALPSA 病变

肱骨头向前脱位，关节囊盂唇复合体从肩胛盂前下部剥离。在典型的 Bankart 损伤中，关节囊盂唇复合体从周围骨膜分离，但在 ALPSA 病变中，关节囊盂唇复合体仍然附着于骨膜，整个组织套袖沿肩胛盂颈内侧剥离。损伤的软组织沿肩胛盂颈在更内侧愈合（图 8-3）。[5]

ALPSA 病变在初次肩关节脱位中并不常见。一项研究发现在急性肩关节脱位病例中有 78% 存在 Bankart 损伤，在复发性肩关节脱位病例中有 97% 存在 Bankart 损伤或 ALPSA 病变。[6] ALPSA 病变只见于复发性肩关节脱位患者。

HAGL 损伤

在绝大多数肩关节脱位病例中，IGHL 和盂唇作为关节囊盂唇复合体从肩胛盂分离。不常见的是，IGHL 从肱骨颈附着处撕脱。[7] HAGL 损伤常被漏诊，因而没有得到适当的治疗。这一情况在近期被认识到是关节镜下固定手术失败的一个相对常见的原因（图 8-4）。

盂唇广泛撕裂

复发性肩关节前脱位可以导致盂唇广泛撕裂，撕裂可因反复创伤延伸至肩胛盂。[8] 不常见的是，这些广泛的病变是前方和后方不稳定同时发生的

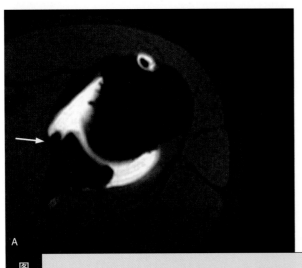

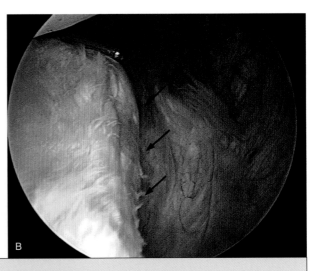

图 8-3　轴位 MRA 及前上入路关节镜下照片，显示同一 ALPSA 病变（箭头）

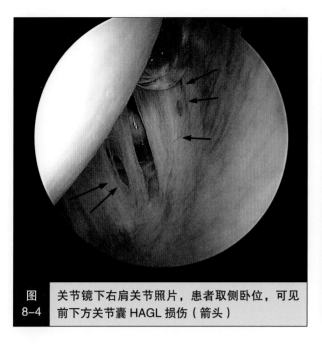

图 8-4　关节镜下右肩关节照片，患者取侧卧位，可见前下方关节囊 HAGL 损伤（箭头）

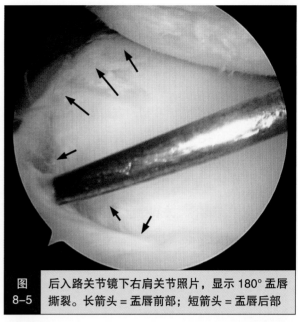

图 8-5　后入路关节镜下右肩关节照片，显示 180° 盂唇撕裂。长箭头 = 盂唇前部；短箭头 = 盂唇后部

结果。初始后方不稳定也可以导致盂唇周围撕裂。这些撕裂甚至可以延伸至肩胛盂周围并最终累及盂唇上部，或者在初始损伤时可发生上盂唇复合体病变（SLAP 损伤）（图 8-5）。

GLAD 病变

一些医师认为 GLAD 病变形成于早期前下方盂唇骨软骨损伤时。如果存在充足的内收力，肱骨头会向前脱位，并压迫肩胛盂，导致肩胛盂缘骨折。GLAD 病变主要使软骨盂唇连接处产生剪切力而非压力，因此其结果是软骨缺损而非骨折（图 8-6）。最初描述的 GLAD 病变是前方盂唇关节软骨损伤，不合并肩关节前方不稳定。重要的是，如果肩关节稳定，应当避免行关节囊缝合术，建议行前方盂唇修补并治疗软骨损伤。

骨缺损

复发性肩关节不稳定患者通常存在肩胛盂和（或）肱骨头的骨性损伤，这对于完全修复盂肱关节不稳定，理解盂肱关节不规则的骨性结构以及适当的治疗非常重要。对于复发性肩关节前方不稳定，必须要考虑骨缺损的两极现象，因为大多数患者在肩胛盂和肱骨头同时存在不同程度的骨缺损。

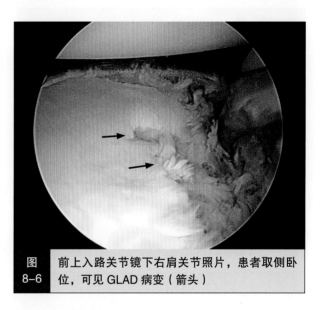

图 8-6　前上入路关节镜下右肩关节照片，患者取侧卧位，可见 GLAD 病变（箭头）

肩胛盂骨缺损

肩胛盂骨性结构的完整与否是影响肩关节不稳定手术结果的重要因素之一。肩胛盂前下部骨缺损使肱骨头与肩胛盂的接触面积减小，肩胛盂抵抗肱骨头剪切力的能力变小。[9] 前方骨缺损也可以降低肩胛盂的凹陷程度，进一步降低凹陷 - 压缩稳定力及减弱肩胛盂的支撑作用。[9-10]

已有研究报道一些不同的肩胛盂损伤形式，但没有建立明确的肩胛盂骨缺损模型。急性肩胛盂损伤的范围涵盖了明显轴向负荷损伤所致的大的骨折到在旋转剪切损伤中盂唇韧带复合体从肩胛盂移位所致的小骨性撕脱。慢性的磨损性骨缺损同样可以通过多种方式发生，从压缩损伤后变钝、变光滑的肩胛盂前缘到肩胛盂前方边缘的反复剪切和侵蚀。一项研究报道超过 50% 的患者在初始肩关节脱位后仅 15 个月就出现了侵蚀性肩胛盂骨缺损，但未见骨折块。[11]

无论是何种损伤机制，复发性肩关节脱位均加重了肩关节活动受限的程度。一些研究发现肩胛盂骨缺损是关节镜下肩关节稳定手术失败的最常见原因。[9, 12] 这一发现强调了辨别肩胛盂骨缺损在制订和执行适当的手术计划时的重要性。反复损伤可以导致肩胛盂凹陷变平甚至凸起，并形成肩胛盂的

反梨形表现（图 8-7）。一项研究报道，在具有反梨形肩胛盂的患者中，关节镜下修补的失败率明显增加。[9] 失败率在年轻接触性项目运动员组为 89%。

Hill-Sachs 损伤

Hill-Sachs 损伤发生于肩关节前方不稳定时肱骨头后外上部相对质软的松质骨与质硬的肩胛盂前下部皮质骨接触处。Hill-Sachs 损伤常见于复发性肩关节前脱位，一项研究发现 100% 的复发性肩关节前脱位患者都存在该损伤。大多数 Hill-Sachs 损伤无临床意义，但少数 Hill-Sachs 损伤会导致不稳定。病变大小和嵌顿是被广泛认可的治疗 Hill-Sachs 损伤时应考虑的两个重要因素。[9]

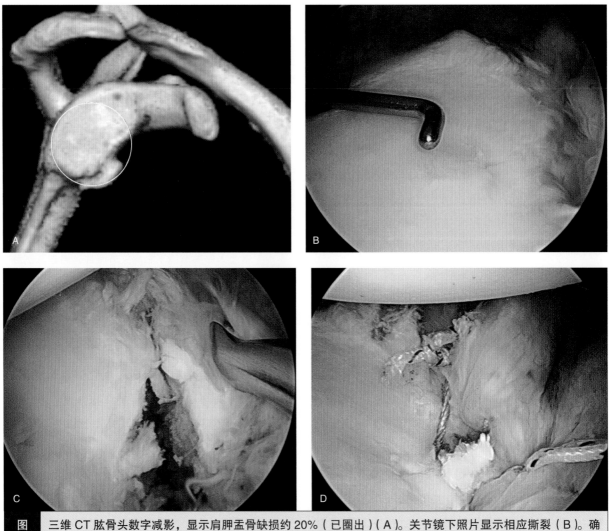

图 8-7　三维 CT 肱骨头数字减影，显示肩胛盂骨缺损约 20%（已圈出）（A）。关节镜下照片显示相应撕裂（B）。确定关节囊被完整地从盂唇提起以预处理撕裂，可见肩胛下肌腱（C）。在修补过程中见一骨性碎片（D）

深部的病变和（或）广泛的病变大多需要治疗。[3]必须清楚病变的位置和方向（图 8-8）。虽然，目前已有一些分型系统被提出，但尚无被临床医师广泛认可的（表 8-1）。

最近有研究者提出了肩胛盂轨迹的概念。[13]在一个尸体模型中，计算了在不同的外展角度和外旋角度下肱骨头与肩胛盂的接触面积。根据结果，研究者描述了在外展和外旋时肱骨头与肩胛盂接触的区域。如果 Hill-Sachs 损伤在肩胛盂轨迹范围内，其将与肩胛盂接触，不会发生嵌顿。肩胛盂骨缺损时，肩胛盂轨迹减小，Hill-Sachs 损伤更可能在轨迹以外，增加了发生嵌顿的风险，导致不稳定。尚需临床研究验证这一理论。

临床评估

全面了解患者的病史对于确定肩关节不稳定

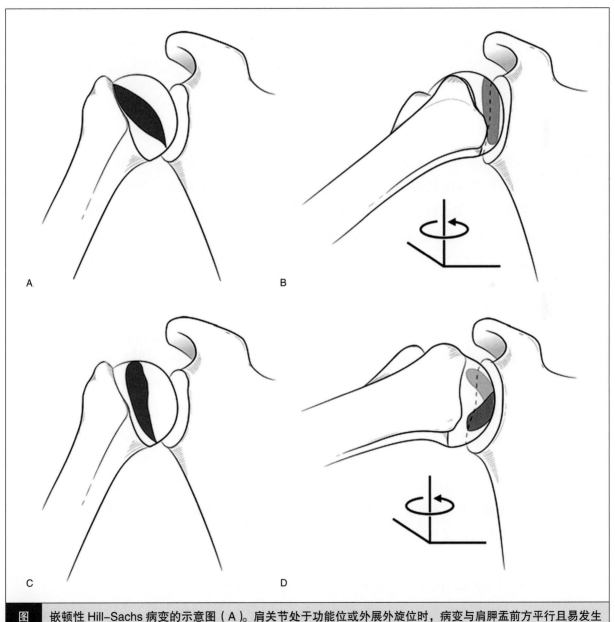

图 8-8　嵌顿性 Hill-Sachs 病变的示意图（A）。肩关节处于功能位或外展外旋位时，病变与肩胛盂前方平行且易发生嵌顿（B）。在非功能位受损，无嵌顿（C）。肩关节处于外展外旋位时，病变与肩胛盂不平行，不易发生嵌顿（D）。深灰色 = 前方病变；浅灰色 = 后方病变；实线 = 旋转轴和平面

表 8-1

Hill-Sachs 病变分型系统

系统	显示方法	描述
Rowe 等[53]	腋位片	轻度：长度为 2 cm，深度 ≤ 0.3 cm 中度：长度为 2~4 cm，深度为 0.3~1 cm 重度：长度为 4 cm，深度 ≥ 1 cm
Calandra 等[54]	直视	Ⅰ度：局限于关节软骨 Ⅱ度：延伸至软骨下骨 Ⅲ度：大的软骨下缺损
Franceschi 等[55]	直视	Ⅰ度：软骨性 Ⅱ度：骨磨损 Ⅲ度：hatchet 骨折
Flatow 等[29]	直视	Ⅰ度：无临床意义，病变占比 <20% Ⅱ度：可能有临床意义，病变占比为 20%~40% Ⅲ度：有临床意义，病变占比 >40%
Hall 等[56]	Stryker 切迹位	关节活动弧度的受累程度（百分比）
Richards 等[57]	腋部 MRI	腋部打开角度的受累程度（关节前缘 = 0°）

的病因和选择理想的治疗方式至关重要。通过确定不稳定的解剖学原因、初始损伤的严重程度、后续的不稳定事件及其趋势（是否变得更频繁或最初是否由低能量机制造成）、受伤时上臂的位置和复位的难易度（是否可以自行复位或是否需要到急诊室复位）以获得线索。初始肩关节脱位发生于足球比赛中，而现在却在睡觉时就可发生脱位的患者，或在肩关节活动中出现不稳定症状的患者，很可能存在明显的肩胛盂和（或）肱骨骨缺损。

病史

年龄相对年轻是脱位复发的重要危险因素之一。年龄小于 30 岁的患者较年长患者有明显更高的脱位复发率。[14]一项研究报道，在 252 例 15~35 岁的患者中，初始脱位后 2 年内复发率为 55.7%，15 岁男性患者的复发率可能达到 86%。[15]一项纳入 105 名患者的研究发现在脱位复位后 6 年内，年龄小于 20 岁的患者中有 64% 发生再脱位，而年龄大于 40 岁的患者中，只有 6% 发生再脱位。[16]Markov 决定模型最近被用来预测初始肩关节前脱位后的肩关节稳定性。[17]这一模型相对于高水平临床研究而言，在内旋位和外旋位有效，

预测 18 岁男性患者 1 年内发展为复发性不稳定的概率是 77%、10 年内保持稳定的概率是 32%。接受手术治疗的患者被包括在这一模型中。

一些活动可以从本质上增加肩关节脱位的危险，包括：①接触性运动，如足球、橄榄球、篮球、曲棍球、武术；②军事训练，如手拉手训练和障碍训练；③攀爬；④激流皮划艇；⑤其他上臂可能用力外展或外旋的体育活动。[18]人群研究报道年发生率区间为（0.82~28.30）/1000。在一项有选择性地针对年轻活跃个体（现役美国军人）的研究中，脱位的年发生率为 1.69/1000。[19]男性的脱位年发生率为 1.82/1000，女性的为 0.90/1000。更早针对美国军事学院学员的研究发现，不稳定事件（半脱位或脱位）的发生率为 28.3/1000。[14]对美国明尼苏达州奥姆斯特德县的所有初始肩关节前脱位患者情况的记录时间都超过 10 年，年发生率为 8.2/100 000[20]。

体格检查

应当行标准的针对肩关节松弛度和稳定性的检查。对于提示明显不稳定或骨缺损的发现应给予特别重视，包括活动时恐惧（外旋并外展 45°）、

外旋超过 30° 且轻度外展时恐惧、麻醉下检查时肩关节易脱位但需用力复位、可触及的扳机感（提示 Hill-Sachs 嵌顿）以及肩关节外旋超过 90° 上臂置于体侧（常为两侧，并合并广泛韧带松弛）。

很多患者在反复肩关节损伤后，肩胛骨控制能力变差，因此需要认真评估肩胛骨的动力机制。如果肩胛骨动力机制没有得以保留，则手术治疗是无效的。必须辨认位置性脱位和自主脱位，因为手术修复可能无法承受肌肉本身的力量，进而导致肩关节不稳定。

肩关节松弛度高于正常范围的患者有可能发生肩关节不稳定，这常由小的损伤引起。这些患者在初始脱位后有相对高的复发风险。医师应当提高警惕，评估常由微小创伤引起初始脱位的具有高松弛度（通常为双侧）的患者。[12] 在行手术前，患者应当接受合适的康复治疗，重点是加强动力稳定结构的力量，包括肩袖和肩胛旁肌群。医师可以考虑通过 Gagey 过度外展试验评估，以发现复发性脱位所致的下方关节囊薄弱。[21]

影像学检查

肩胛盂和（或）肱骨头骨缺损通常可见于复发性肩关节不稳定患者，也是导致关节镜下固定手术失败的最常见原因。可以通过影像学方法和关节镜评估肩胛盂骨缺损量。建议在术前通过 X 线片及更先进的影像学方法评估肩胛盂骨缺损量，以保证合适的术前计划和治疗合作。如果发现了明显的骨缺损，手术计划应改为骨性结构恢复手术（如 Latarjet 手术、胫骨远端异体骨移植和髂嵴异体骨移植）。

X 线片

应当为每一例患者拍摄标准的 X 线片（前后位、腋位和肩胛骨 Y 位）。西点位片和 Stryker 切迹位片也可能有助于诊断。西点位片增强了对前下方肩胛盂的显示。一些医师认为 X 线片足以显示肩胛盂骨缺损。[18] 如有任何异常，则需通过进一步的检查评估。肱骨骨缺损也可以通过 X 线片评估，尤其是在肩关节外旋位拍摄前后位片。[12] Stryker 切迹位片可以更好地显示 Hill-Sachs 损伤（图 8-9）。

MRI 检查

高质量的 MRI，无论是否包括磁共振关节造影（MRA），都有助于显示关节囊、盂唇和肩袖。关节囊的特定病变，包括 HAGL 损伤和关节囊冗余同样可以通过高质量的 MRI 发现。在怀疑 SLAP 损伤、广泛盂唇撕裂、固定手术失败或脱位复发时，MRA 具有明显优势（图 8-10）。虽然肩胛盂和肱骨头骨缺损可以在 MRI 上显示，但通过 CT 检查评估更为准确。[22]

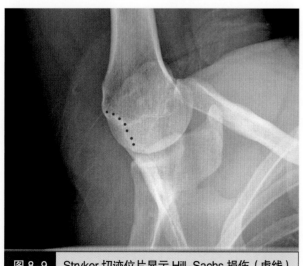

图 8-9　Stryker 切迹位片显示 Hill-Sachs 损伤（虚线）

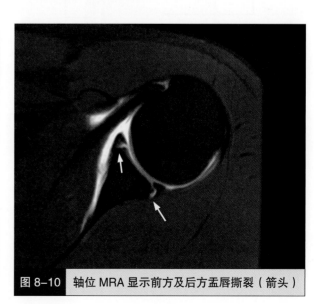

图 8-10　轴位 MRA 显示前方及后方盂唇撕裂（箭头）

CT 检查

三维重建 CT 及肱骨头减影是评估肩胛盂骨缺损的影像学检查金标准。[23] 医师可能无法通过 MRI 和 MRA 很好地分辨盂唇和骨，导致骨缺损量被低估。CT 还可更为准确地评估肩胛盂倾斜和发育不良，这两种情况也可导致肩关节不稳定，但不常见。当患者手术失败或存在双侧不稳定时应当进行 CT 检查。

一些描述通过 CT 和关节镜评估肩胛盂骨缺损的方法的文献已经发表，但是没有任何一种方法被广为接受。重要的是要理解这些方法的局限性。关节镜下评估骨缺损限制了医师制订精确的术前计划，因为医师必须做好准备随时在关节镜下或以开放手术的方式治疗病变。

一项尸体研究发现肩胛盂下 2/3 是真正的圆形，对骨缺损的测量方法基于这一发现。[24] 该圆形的圆心与解剖学上的裸点大致重合。最精确的测量肩胛盂骨缺损百分比的方法是基于表面积测量的[25]（图 8-11）。应用数字影像学软件，可以通过圆的整体表面积计算出骨性缺损的面积。尽管准确，但这一方法并不常用。大多数医师（包括本章的作者在内）更愿意采用 CT 和关节镜下肩胛盂缘测量的方法[26]（图 8-12）。测量从裸点到前缘的距离和到后缘的距离，用到后缘的距离减去到前缘的距离。将此值除以圆的半径以确定骨缺损的百分比。近期的工作揭示裸点较准确的圆心稍偏前，所以这一方法可能会过度估计骨缺损。[27] 其他的技术正在研究中，包括基于正弦理论的模型。[28]

对肱骨头缺损的测量和分类的透彻研究较少。最常见的体系将病变的严重程度根据累及关节面百分比分级。[29] Ⅰ 度病变累及小于 20% 的关节面，Ⅱ 度病变累及 20%~40% 的关节面，Ⅲ 度病变累及大于 40% 的关节面。

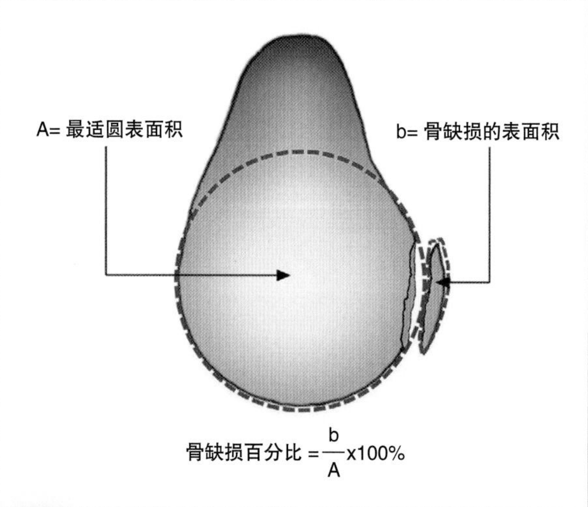

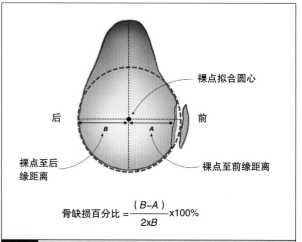

骨缺损百分比 $= \dfrac{b}{A} \times 100\%$

图 8-11 基于表面积估算肩胛盂骨缺损的示意图。在肩胛盂关节面的图像上，测量骨缺损的表面积 (b)，将适当的圆附加于肩胛盂下 2/3(A)。骨缺损的百分比可以量化为 b/A×100%。经允许引自 Provencher MT, Bhatia S, Ghodadra NS, et al: Recurrent shoulder instability. Current concepts for evaluation and management of glenoid bone loss. *J Bone Joint Surg Am* 2010;92(suppl 2);133–151.

裸点拟合圆心

后　前

裸点至后缘距离

裸点至前缘距离

骨缺损百分比 $= \dfrac{(B-A)}{2 \times B} \times 100\%$

图 8-12 基于肩胛盂缘距离估算肩胛盂骨缺损的示意图。在肩胛盂关节面的 CT 图像上，在肩胛盂隐窝处（即肩胛盂长轴与肩胛盂前后径最宽处的交点处）估计近似裸点的位置。以近似裸点为圆心画适当的圆匹配肩胛盂下 2/3。测量裸点至前缘的距离（A）及裸点至后缘的距离（B），骨缺损的百分比可以通过以下公式计算 $\dfrac{(B-A)}{2 \times B} \times 100\%$。经允许引自 Provencher MT, Bhatia S, Ghodadra NS, et al: Recurrent shoulder instability. Current concepts for evaluation and management of glenoid bone loss. *J Bone Joint Surg Am* 2010;92(suppl 2);133–151.

治疗和结果

手术治疗的最终目标是恢复患者肩关节的稳定和功能以及降低关节病变的风险，使患者关节病变的风险降低并安全地回归预期的活动。患者的年龄、预期术后活动水平，以及肩胛盂和（或）肱骨骨缺损的程度是在为患者制订特异性治疗方案时需要考虑的最重要的 3 个因素。

非手术治疗

对于大多数复发性肩关节不稳定患者，非手术治疗的效果有限。然而，如果患者年龄大于 50 岁且活动需求低、有严重的合并症（例如，无法控制的惊厥）或无法完成长期的术后康复锻炼，手术并非好的治疗选择。评估 40 岁以上肩关节不稳定患者的肩袖撕裂情况非常重要。非手术治疗主要着眼于肩关节动力稳定结构的加强，包括肩袖和肩胛旁肌肉。

赛季中的运动员是特殊且具有治疗挑战的患者群体。这些患者通常渴望尽快回归比赛并且愿意承担再脱位的风险。对于这类患者可以通过支具限制存在风险的外旋体位治疗，并将手术延后至赛季结束。[30]

手术治疗

针对复发性脱位的广泛病理改变尚无清楚的治疗策略，但常规的指南有助于医师根据患者的病史、体格检查结果和影像学检查结果选择特定的治疗方式。肩胛盂和肱骨头骨缺损所致的肩关节不稳定被认为是一种连续统一事件，因为这些情况通常同时发生。患者可能存在小而浅的 Hill-Sachs 损伤合并磨损性肩胛盂骨缺损达 30%；也可能仅存在小的肩胛盂骨缺损合并大的嵌顿性 Hill-Sachs 损伤；还可能存在 20% 的肩胛盂骨缺损合并中等大小的嵌顿性 Hill-Sachs 损伤。必须仔细地单独评估发生复发性肩关节前方不稳定的每一例患者，以确定不稳定的原因，所获得的线索可以协助医师为患者制订个体化的手术方案。这一路径可以优化治疗结果，同时避免了应用非特异性治疗策略时的过度治疗或治疗不到位。所有患者都应当在麻醉下接受全面、仔细的体格检查。医师应当仔细地评估肱骨头在向前、向下及向后各方向的移动范围。

大多数医师更愿意使用关节镜而非通过开放手术对大多数患者进行治疗。[31-33]关节镜可以更好地显露手术视野以及进行关节囊折叠缝合和前后方向上的移位。使用关节镜还避免了与切开手术相关的并发症和其他事件发生。近期的研究发现关节镜手术和传统切开手术相比，术后复发率持平或更低。[31-33]但应该注意，上述结果与近期的关节镜研究将伴有更大块骨缺损的患者排除有关。现已明确使用关节镜治疗这样的患者具有很高的失败风险。

一些医师推荐应用不稳定严重指数评分以协助判断是否应考虑以切开手术代替关节镜手术。[18]不稳定严重指数评分是基于对复发性肩关节前方不稳定患者危险因素的前瞻性判断而做出的，危险因素包括接受手术时年龄小于 20 岁、参与比赛性或接触性体育运动或涉及用力过顶活动的体育运动、肩关节过度松弛以及存在 Hill-Sachs 损伤和（或）在肩关节外旋前后位片上可见下方肩胛盂骨质轮廓缺失。将这些因素整合为总分 10 分的评分表并在相同的人群做回顾性试验。术前评分高于 6 分者存在无法接受的 70% 的复发风险（$P<0.001$）。

翻修手术

关节镜下固定手术可能因为各种原因失败，医师必须明确失败原因并制订适当的翻修手术方案。肩胛盂或肱骨头骨缺损是关节镜下固定手术失败的首要原因。其他原因包括年轻患者回归接触性运动、肩关节过度松弛、用力的过顶活动以及在手术中应用了 3 个或更少的锚。[12,18,34]

如果患者单独存在嵌顿性 Hill-Sachs 损伤，关节镜 Bankart 修补和 Remplissage 术可能足以满足治疗需求。[35]一些医师相信对于这些患者，不直接处理肱骨头骨缺损，而采用切开手术恢复肩胛盂骨性结构可以恢复更多的活动功能及肩关节稳定性。[36]目前尚无清晰的治疗策略。医师应当仔细判断所有的病理改变并选择最安全、最有效可行的手段。

特殊病变

辨识 ALPSA 病变是治疗的关键。没有专门鉴别 ALPSA 病变和 Bankart 病变的体格检查方法。影像学检查很难清楚地显示盂唇，因为其偏内侧并与肩胛盂颈相连。关节镜下必须定位盂唇（通过前上入路显示最佳）并将其谨慎地移动回肩胛盂缘以恢复其解剖位置。关节囊折叠缝合并将盂唇置于偏内侧未复位的位置会导致很高的失败风险。一些医师认为 ALPSA 病变是复发性肩关节脱位的结果，关节镜下修补 ALPSA 病变的预期成功率低于修补典型的 Bankart 损伤。[37]

HAGL 损伤也很难通过病史或体格检查与 Bankart 损伤相鉴别。MRI 尤其是 MRA 有助于辨识 HAGL 损伤。最可靠的影像学检查结果是冠状位 MRI 上关节囊呈泪滴状以及 IGHL 消失（图 8-13）。治疗 HAGL 损伤时，患者最好取侧卧位，关节镜通过平衡的牵引以进入盂肱关节下部。关节镜治疗 HAGL 损伤具有挑战性，医师应该做好关节镜手术不可行时行 HAGL 切开修补的准备。

GLAD 病变的临床意义尚不明确，但多数专家认为应当尽量有效地移动盂唇以覆盖裸露的骨面或以微骨折技术诱导骨缺损区域出现纤维软骨。

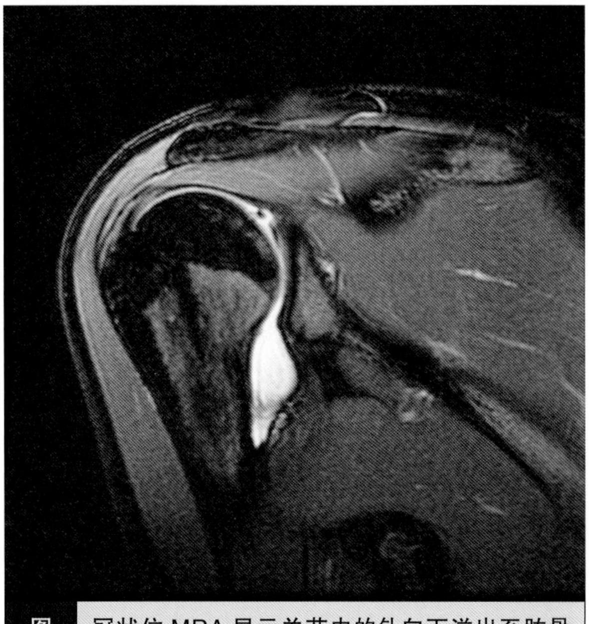

复发性肩关节前脱位可以导致广泛盂唇撕裂，撕裂可延伸至肩胛盂周围。患者常描述有数起低能量脱位发生以及明显疼痛，这在单纯盂唇撕裂中少见。撞击诱发试验可以显示后方和前方恐惧或不稳定，提示可能存在 SLAP 损伤。MRA 可以提高诊断的特异性，尤其是对于 SLAP 损伤，这对于在手术干预前制订最佳的治疗计划至关重要。由于需要对肩胛盂全周缘进行显露，建议患者取侧卧位。必须谨慎计划这一具有挑战性的手术，确定锚的使用数量以及对全周盂唇进行修补的工具。[8, 38]

骨缺损

在治疗复发性肩关节前方不稳定时，必须要考虑双极骨缺损。治疗一处病变而不考虑另一处会导致手术失败。大多数同时存在肩胛盂和肱骨头骨缺损的患者，可以单纯直接治疗肩胛盂骨缺损。恢复了肩胛盂前部相对正常的形态后，肩胛盂轨迹弧度有效地延长了，也防止了 Hill-Sachs 损伤导致的嵌顿。[4]

肩胛盂骨缺损

在复发性肩关节不稳定中，肩胛盂骨缺损可以通过一些已经被清晰阐明的技术进行手术治疗。当选择合适的骨性恢复手段时，需要考虑一些因素。尽管还没有有效的临床决策策略，但关于复发性肩关节前方不稳定中肩胛盂骨缺损的综述提供了一些总的指导性意见，即治疗方案决定于骨缺损的量。[22]基于其他研究者所做的生物力学和临床研究，综述的结论是前方肩胛盂骨缺损大于 25% 将显著提高不稳定事件发生的危险。[9, 39-41]骨缺损小于 15% 的临床意义不大，15%~25% 的骨缺损必须根据个体情况仔细评估。

喙突转位（Latarjet 手术）

喙突转位是恢复肩胛盂骨结构最常见的手术。在美国，如果患者存在超过 25% 的肩胛盂骨缺损或骨缺损小于 25% 但关节镜下固定手术不成

图 8-13　冠状位 MRA 显示关节内的钆向下溢出至肱骨干，提示 HAGL 损伤

功，常会施行该手术。肩胛盂和肱骨头同时出现骨缺损时，一些医师仍然认为肱骨头骨缺损在肩胛盂骨性形态恢复后不会导致嵌顿。[36]一些临床研究发现 Latarjet 手术在同时存在肩胛盂和肱骨头骨缺损的情况下效果极佳。[42-44]一项研究甚至建议 Latarjet 手术可以使存在大的嵌顿性 Hill-Sachs 损伤而没有肩胛盂骨缺损的患者获得稳定的肩关节。[36]这些研究者阐述骨性阻挡延长了肩胛盂轨迹弧度，使肱骨头不会外旋和前移，这样 Hill-Sachs 损伤不会在骨性阻挡物前方发生嵌顿。

喙突转位是有创操作，并非没有并发症。[44]如果移植物位置改变，会导致进一步的软骨损伤。[45]最近报道的关节镜下喙突转位具有操作难度，需要医师有充足的初始实验室经验。[46-47]

可供选择的针对肩胛盂骨缺损的骨移植物也在研究之内，因为喙突转位并不能完全重建正常的前方肩胛盂解剖轮廓。这些骨移植选择包括自体或异体髂骨移植、异体肩胛盂以及最近出现的异体胫骨远端骨移植[48]（图 8-14）。

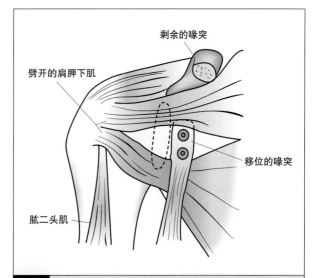

剩余的喙突

劈开的肩胛下肌

移位的喙突

肱二头肌

图 8-14　Latarjet 手术包括将喙突经劈开的肩胛下肌转位至肩胛盂内侧。喙突通过增强肩胛盂前缘为盂肱关节提供稳定性，联合腱在上臂外展和外旋时是稳定装置。经允许引自 Burns JP, Snyder SJ: Shoulder instability, in Fischgrund JS, ed: *Orthopaedic Knowledge Update 9*. Rosemont, IL, American Academy of Orthopaedic Surgeons, 2008, pp 301-311.

肱骨头骨缺损（Hill-Sachs 损伤）

大多数 Hill-Sachs 损伤是小（小于关节面20%）、浅且没有临床意义的。大于关节面40%的病变通常有临床表现并且必须接受治疗。挑战是确定累及关节面 20%~40% 的病变是否具有足够的临床治疗意义或因通过适当的治疗肩胛盂骨缺损而不具有明显的意义。

治疗应着眼于恢复稳定的运动弧。在许多患者中，仅恢复肩胛盂侧运动弧可能就足够了，因为恢复了正常的肩胛盂轨迹并减少了 Hill-Sachs 损伤发生嵌顿的风险。尤其重要的是要理解骨缺损是一个双极现象；在肩胛盂骨缺损的同时可能有潜在的中等大小的 Hill-Sachs 损伤，这增加了不稳定的风险。没有肩胛盂骨缺损时，Hill-Sachs 损伤可能不会与前方肩胛盂嵌顿。肩胛盂骨缺损时，发生肱骨头病变嵌顿所需的前移距离和外旋角度变小。已经有一些治疗肱骨头骨缺损的技术

被介绍，所有的技术都有一定的用途。

Remplissage 术

关节镜下 Remplissage 术（从法语"填充"衍变而来）从关节外填充肱骨头骨缺损治疗病变以防止嵌顿发生。该操作的开放手术方式称为 Connolly 手术，于 1972 年被报道，包括使部分大结节连同冈下肌腱转位到骨缺损处。关节镜技术于 2007 年被报道，包括后方关节囊固定及冈下肌腱固定。[49]尽管确切的 Remplissage 术指征并没有明确定义，但这一手术最宜用于中等或较大且浅表的 Hill-Sachs 损伤以及肩胛盂骨缺损小于20% 的患者。

关节镜下 Remplissage 术的早期满意效果已经被报道，一项研究报道了 98% 的稳定性。[35, 50]需要注意的是，该研究中的患者需要经过严格挑选，肩胛盂骨缺损有限且 Hill-Sachs 损伤较大。单纯 Remplissage 术可能不足以治疗肩胛盂缺损大于 25% 的患者，对于这些患者应当尽量考虑行针

对肩胛盂的骨性手术。

骨移植

骨移植用于恢复肱骨头的骨性结构，可预防嵌顿性 Hill-Sachs 损伤。通常不常见的大的 Hill-Sachs 损伤（超过关节面 40%）合并小的肩胛盂骨缺损是骨移植的指征。填充缺损并恢复正常解剖以重新建立肱骨头的关节弧，防止 Hill-Sachs 损伤嵌顿。自体骨移植和异体骨移植骨栓技术多采用新鲜冰冻异体骨软骨。[4, 51] 已有可信的结果被报道，尽管一项研究报告 18 名患者中有 8 名出现并发症。[52] 这些手术从技术上具有挑战性，必须要考虑到应用异体骨所致的疾病传播风险。

解除 Hill-Sachs 损伤所致的压缩骨折的手术是一种相对新的手术，可用的临床和生物力学数据很少。有一些不同的技术被报道，所有这些技术都涉及顶起压缩骨折块以及应用骨移植物以支撑抬起的骨块。这一技术的临床应用并没有规范，可能最适用于累及关节面小于 40% 的急性病变。

表面置换术

部分表面置换术、全表面置换术和半关节置换术用于恢复更正常的肱骨头弧度。这些手术均不适用于年轻、活动量大的患者，因为存在植入物松动和肩胛盂磨损的风险。其适应证尚不明确，但植入物最适用于年老、体力活动需求低或病变大于关节面 40% 者。最终，手术治疗通常应用于年龄大于 50 岁的患者，在这些患者中半肩关节置换术和全肩关节置换术的结果优于表面置换术。

总结

一些因素常导致复发性肩关节前方不稳定的发生。和大多数骨科疾病类似，完整的病史和体格检查为正确地诊断提供了重要的依据。进一步的影像学检查对于每一个复发性肩关节不稳定患者都是必要的。MRA 有助于描述 SLAP 损伤和更为广泛的或微小的肩胛盂病变。如果怀疑有肩胛盂骨缺损或明显的 Hill-Sachs 损伤，三维 CT 是更好的检查方法。肩胛盂和（或）肱骨头骨缺损存在于几乎所有的复发性肩关节不稳定患者，必须辨识并给予合适的治疗，以减少对关节的进一步损伤。先正确地诊断，再与患者进行恰当的沟通并给出合理的建议，最后选择理想的治疗方案。

参考文献

[1] Hovelius L, Augustini BG, Fredin H, Johansson O, Norlin R, Thorling J: Primary anterior dislocation of the shoulder in young patients: A ten-year prospective study. *J Bone Joint Surg Am* 1996;78(11):1677-1684.

[2] Taylor DC, Arciero RA: Pathologic changes associated with shoulder dislocations: Arthroscopic and physical examination findings in first-time, traumatic anterior dislocations. *Am J Sports Med* 1997;25(3):306-311.

[3] Armitage MS, Faber KJ, Drosdowech DS, Litchfield RB, Athwal GS: Humeral head bone defects: Remplissage, allograft, and arthroplasty. *Orthop Clin North Am* 2010;41(3):417-425.
A comprehensive literature review was provided for remplissage, allograft reconstruction, and arthroplasty in the treatment of Hill-Sachs lesions, with a useful algorithm based on lesion size and patient factors.

[4] Provencher MT, Frank RM, Leclere LE, et al: The Hill-Sachs lesion: Diagnosis, classification, and management. *J Am Acad Orthop Surg* 2012;20(4):242-252.
The diagnosis, classification, and management of the Hill-Sachs lesion in anterior shoulder instability were discussed.

[5] Neviaser TJ: The anterior labroligamentous periosteal sleeve avulsion lesion: A cause of anterior instability of the shoulder. *Arthroscopy* 1993;9(1):17-21.

[6] Yiannakopoulos CK, Mataragas E, Antonogiannakis E: A comparison of the spectrum of intra-articular lesions in acute and chronic anterior shoulder instability. *Arthroscopy* 2007;23(9):985-990.
A case study compared arthroscopic findings during treatment of acute and chronic instability. ALPSA lesions, Bankart lesions, and inverted pear glenoids were found significantly more often in patients with chronic instability.

[7] Wolf EM, Cheng JC, Dickson K: Humeral avulsion of glenohumeral ligaments as a cause of anterior shoulder instability. *Arthroscopy* 1995;11(5):600-607.

[8] Tokish JM, McBratney CM, Solomon DJ, Leclere L,

Dewing CB, Provencher MT: Arthroscopic repair of circumferential lesions of the glenoid labrum. *J Bone Joint Surg Am* 2009;91(12):2795-2802.

Thirty-nine shoulders with a circumferential labral lesion were prospectively followed for a mean 31.8 months. Significant improvements in functional and pain scores were reported, and only two shoulders developed recurrent instability.

[9] Burkhart SS, De Beer JF: Traumatic glenohumeral bone defects and their relationship to failure of arthroscopic Bankart repairs: Significance of the invertedpear glenoid and the humeral engaging Hill-Sachs lesion. *Arthroscopy* 2000;16(7):677-694.

[10] Lazarus MD, Sidles JA, Harryman DT II, Matsen FA III: Effect of a chondral-labral defect on glenoid con- cavity and glenohumeral stability: A cadaveric model. *J Bone Joint Surg Am* 1996;78(1):94-102.

[11] Mologne TS, Provencher MT, Menzel KA, Vachon TA, Dewing CB: Arthroscopic stabilization in patients with an inverted pear glenoid: Results in patients with bone loss of the anterior glenoid. *Am J Sports Med* 2007; 35(8):1276-1283.

Outcomes of arthroscopic stabilization were reviewed in 21 patients with significant glenoid bone loss. Three patients developed recurrent instability, and patients with attritional bone loss had lower outcomes scores than those with a bony fragment.

[12] Boileau P, Villalba M, Héry JY, Balg F, Ahrens P, Neyton L: Risk factors for recurrence of shoulder instability after arthroscopic Bankart repair. *J Bone Joint Surg Am* 2006;88(8):1755-1763.

[13] Yamamoto N, Itoi E, Abe H, et al: Contact between the glenoid and the humeral head in abduction, exter- nal rotation, and horizontal extension: A new concept of glenoid track. *J Shoulder Elbow Surg* 2007;16(5): 649-656.

The authors present a novel concept known as the glenoid track, based on cadaver data. The glenoid track represents the area on the humeral head that makes contact with the glenoid when the shoulder is in various abduction–external rotation positions.

[14] Owens BD, Duffey ML, Nelson BJ, DeBerardino TM, Taylor DC, Mountcastle SB: The incidence and characteristics of shoulder instability at the United States Military Academy. *Am J Sports Med* 2007;35(7):1168-1173.

All shoulder instability events at the US Military Academy were prospectively captured during an 8-month period. In 4,141 students, 117 events occurred, yielding a 1-year incidence of 2.8%.

[15] Robinson CM, Howes J, Murdoch H, Will E, Graham C: Functional outcome and risk of recurrent instability after primary traumatic anterior shoulder dislocation in young patients. *J Bone Joint Surg Am* 2006;88(11): 2326-2336.

[16] te Slaa RL, Wijffels MP, Brand R, Marti RK: The prognosis following acute primary glenohumeral dislocation. *J Bone Joint Surg Br* 2004;86(1):58-64.

[17] Mather RC III, Orlando LA, Henderson RA, Lawrence JT, Taylor DC: A predictive model of shoulder instability after a first-time anterior shoulder dislocation. *J Shoulder Elbow Surg* 2011;20(2):259-266.

A Markov decision model was created to predict the long-term outcome of initial anterior shoulder dislocation, with internal and external validation.

[18] Balg F, Boileau P: The instability severity index score: A simple pre-operative score to select patients for arthroscopic or open shoulder stabilisation. *J Bone Joint Surg Br* 2007;89(11):1470-1477.

Several factors were correlated with the recurrence of instability in initial anterior dislocation and were combined into a 10-point preoperative Instability Severity Index Score. A score greater than 6 was correlated with a recurrence rate of 70%.

[19] Owens BD, Dawson L, Burks R, Cameron KL: Incidence of shoulder dislocation in the United States military: Demographic considerations from a high-risk population. *J Bone Joint Surg Am* 2009;91(4): 791-796.

The overall incidence of anterior shoulder instability in military personnel was 1.69 dislocations per 1,000 person-years. White men younger than 30 years with a junior rank in the US Army were identified as being at highest risk.

[20] Simonet WT, Melton LJ III, Cofield RH, Ilstrup DM: Incidence of anterior shoulder dislocation in Olmsted County, Minnesota. *Clin Orthop Relat Res* 1984;186: 186-191.

[21] Gagey OJ, Gagey N: The hyperabduction test. *J Bone Joint Surg Br* 2001;83(1):69-74.

[22] Piasecki DP, Verma NN, Romeo AA, Levine WN, Bach BR Jr, Provencher MT: Glenoid bone deficiency in recurrent anterior shoulder instability: Diagnosis and management. *J Am Acad Orthop Surg* 2009; 17(8):482-493.

A detailed review was presented of the diagnosis and management of glenoid bone loss in recurrent anterior shoulder instability.

[23] Rerko MA, Pan X, Donaldson C, Jones GL, Bishop JY: Comparison of various imaging techniques to quantify glenoid bone loss in shoulder instability. *J Shoulder Elbow Surg* 2012.

Radiographs, MRI, CT, and three-dimensional CT were compared for the detection of various-size glenoid defects in cadaver shoulders. Three-dimensional CT was found to be the most accurate of the four modalities.

[24] Huysmans PE, Haen PS, Kidd M, Dhert WJ, Willems JW: The shape of the inferior part of the glenoid: A cadaveric study. *J Shoulder Elbow Surg* 2006;15(6): 759-763.

[25] Sugaya H, Moriishi J, Dohi M, Kon Y, Tsuchiya A: Glenoid rim morphology in recurrent anterior glenohumeral instability. *J Bone Joint Surg Am* 2003; 85(5):878-884.

[26] Sugaya H, Kon Y, Tsuchiya A: Arthroscopic repair of glenoid fractures using suture anchors. *Arthroscopy* 2005;21(5):635.

[27] Kralinger F, Aigner F, Longato S, Rieger M, Wambacher M: Is the bare spot a consistent landmark for shoulder arthroscopy? A study of 20 embalmed glenoids with 3-dimensional computed tomographic reconstruction. *Arthroscopy* 2006;22(4):428-432.

[28] Detterline AJ, Provencher MT, Ghodadra N, Bach BR Jr, Romeo AA, Verma NN: A new arthroscopic technique to determine anterior-inferior glenoid bone loss: Validation of the secant chord theory in a cadaveric model. *Arthroscopy* 2009;25(11):1249-1256.

The traditional method of measuring glenoid bone loss based on distance from the bare spot was compared with a new model based on secant chord theory in cadaver specimens. The secant chord theory model was more accurate but required more complex mathematical calculations.

[29] Flatow EL, Warner JI: Instability of the shoulder: Complex problems and failed repairs. Part I: Relevant biomechanics, multidirectional instability, and severe glenoid loss. *Instr Course Lect* 1998;47:97-112.

[30] Buss DD, Lynch GP, Meyer CP, Huber SM, Freehill MQ: Nonoperative management for in-season athletes with anterior shoulder instability. *Am J Sports Med* 2004;32(6):1430-1433.

[31] Archetti Netto N, Tamaoki MJ, Lenza M, et al: Treatment of Bankart lesions in traumatic anterior instability of the shoulder: A randomized controlled trial comparing arthroscopy and open techniques. *Arthroscopy* 2012;28(7):900-908.

Forty-two patients were randomly assigned to open or arthroscopic treatment of anterior shoulder instability with an isolated Bankart lesion. At 37.5-month follow-up, there was no clinical difference in recurrence or outcome scores between the two groups.

[32] Zaffagnini S, Marcheggiani Muccioli GM, Giordano G, et al: Long-term outcomes after repair of recurrent post-traumatic anterior shoulder instability: Comparison of arthroscopic transglenoid suture and open Bankart reconstruction. *Knee Surg Sports Traumatol Arthrosc* 2012;20(5):816-821.

The outcomes of 110 consecutive patients treated with open or arthroscopic stabilization for recurrent anterior shoulder instability were retrospectively reviewed. There were no differences in recurrence rates or outcomes scores between groups.

[33] Petrera M, Patella V, Patella S, Theodoropoulos J: A meta-analysis of open versus arthroscopic Bankart repair using suture anchors. *Knee Surg Sports Traumatol Arthrosc* 2010;18(12):1742-1747.

This meta-analysis found no overall difference in recurrence rates between open and arthroscopic stabilization for recurrent anterior shoulder instability. When studies more recent than 2002 were compared, arthroscopically treated patients were found to have lower recurrence rates.

[34] Calvo E, Granizo JJ, Fernández-Yruegas D: Criteria for arthroscopic treatment of anterior instability of the shoulder: A prospective study. *J Bone Joint Surg Br* 2005;87(5):677-683.

[35] Boileau P, O'Shea K, Vargas P, Pinedo M, Old J, Zumstein M: Anatomical and functional results after arthroscopic Hill-Sachs remplissage. *J Bone Joint Surg Am* 2012;94(7):618-626.

The authors' early experience with remplissage was reported for the treatment of Hill-Sachs lesions as part of anterior shoulder instability. At a mean 24-month follow-up, 98% of the patients had a stable shoulder, and 74% of the patients had more than 75% filling of the defect.

[36] Burkhart SS, De Beer JF, Barth JR, Cresswell T, Roberts C, Richards DP: Results of modified Latarjet reconstruction in patients with anteroinferior instability and significant bone loss. *Arthroscopy* 2007;23(10): 1033-1041.

The results of the Latarjet procedure in patients with recurrent anterior shoulder instability and an inverted pear glenoid were presented. The overall recurrence rate was 4.9% at a mean 59-month follow-up.

[37] Ozbaydar M, Elhassan B, Diller D, Massimini D, Higgins LD, Warner JJ: Results of arthroscopic capsulolabral repair: Bankart lesion versus anterior labroligamentous periosteal sleeve avulsion lesion. *Arthroscopy* 2008;24(11):1277-1283.

A retrospective study found that patients with an ALPSA lesion were more likely to have dislocation before arthroscopic capsulolabral repair and had a higher recurrence rate after surgery than those with a traditional Bankart lesion.

[38] Lo IK, Burkhart SS: Triple labral lesions: Pathology and surgical repair technique-report of seven cases. *Arthroscopy* 2005;21(2):186-193.

[39] Itoi E, Lee SB, Berglund LJ, Berge LL, An KN: The effect of a glenoid defect on anteroinferior stability of the shoulder after Bankart repair: A cadaveric study. *J Bone Joint Surg Am* 2000;82(1):35-46.

[40] Greis PE, Scuderi MG, Mohr A, Bachus KN, Burks RT: Glenohumeral articular contact areas and pressures following labral and osseous injury to the anteroinferior quadrant of the glenoid. *J Shoulder Elbow Surg* 2002;11(5):442-451.

[41] Lo IK, Parten PM, Burkhart SS: The inverted pear glenoid: An indicator of significant glenoid bone loss. *Arthroscopy* 2004;20(2):169-174.

[42] Neyton L, Young A, Dawidziak B, et al: Surgical treatment of anterior instability in rugby union players: Clinical and radiographic results of the Latarjet-Patte procedure with minimum 5-year follow-up. *J Shoulder Elbow Surg* 2012;21(12):1721-1727.

Retrospective review of 34 rugby players (37 shoulders) found that no patients reported recurrence of instability at a mean 12-year follow-up after the Latarjet-Patte procedure for recurrent anterior shoulder instability.

[43] Hovelius L, Vikerfors O, Olofsson A, Svensson O, Rahme H: Bristow-Latarjet and Bankart: A comparative study of shoulder stabilization in 185 shoulders during a seventeen-year follow-up. *J Shoulder Elbow Surg* 2011;20(7):1095-1101.

Retrospective review of 185 consecutive patients who underwent Bankart repair or the Bristow-Latarjet procedure for recurrent shoulder instability found that patients treated with the Bristow-Latarjet procedure reported better functional outcomes and lower recurrence rates at a mean 17-year follow-up.

[44] Shah AA, Butler RB, Romanowski J, Goel D, Karada-gli D, Warner JJ: Short-term complications of the Latarjet procedure. *J Bone Joint Surg Am* 2012;94(6): 495-501.

Short-term complications associated with the Latarjet procedure were studied in 45 patients (48 shoulders). Five procedures (10%) resulted in neurologic injury, four procedures (8%) in recurrent instability, and three procedures (6%) in a superficial infection.

[45] Ghodadra N, Gupta A, Romeo AA, et al: Normalization of glenohumeral articular contact pressures after Latarjet or iliac crest bone-grafting. *J Bone Joint Surg Am* 2010;92(6):1478-1489.

A cadaver study evaluated the effect of iliac crest bone graft or coracoid piece positioning on level and location of peak contact pressures in a Latarjet procedure. Placing the graft flush with the native glenoid and using the inferior portion of the coracoid as the glenoid face are recommended.

[46] Boileau P, Mercier N, Roussanne Y, Thélu CÉ, Old J: Arthroscopic Bankart-Bristow-Latarjet procedure: The development and early results of a safe and reproducible technique. *Arthroscopy* 2010;26(11):1434-1450.

Retrospective review of an all-arthroscopic Latarjet procedure in 47 consecutive patients found good results in most patients, although there were seven migrations and one bone block fracture.

[47] Lafosse L, Boyle S: Arthroscopic Latarjet procedure. *J Shoulder Elbow Surg* 2010;19(2, suppl):2-12.

Of the first 100 patients treated with an all-arthroscopic Latarjet procedure, 91 had an excellent result, but 11 had a complication.

[48] Provencher MT, Bhatia S, Ghodadra NS, et al: Recurrent shoulder instability: Current concepts for evaluation and management of glenoid bone loss. *J Bone Joint Surg Am* 2010;92(suppl 2):133-151.

A comprehensive review of the evaluation and the management of recurrent anterior shoulder instability focused on the role of glenoid bone loss.

[49] Purchase RJ, Wolf EM, Hobgood ER, Pollock ME, Smalley CC: Hill-Sachs "remplissage": An arthroscopic solution for the engaging Hill-Sachs lesion. *Arthroscopy* 2008;24(6):723-726.

An arthroscopic technique based on the Connolly open infraspinatus tenodesis technique was described for the treatment of an engaging Hill-Sachs lesion in patients with anterior shoulder instability.

[50] Franceschi F, Papalia R, Rizzello G, et al: Remplissage repair—new frontiers in the prevention of recurrent

shoulder instability: A 2-year follow-up comparative study. *Am J Sports Med* 2012;40(11):2462-2469.

Retrospective review of 50 patients with an engaging Hill-Sachs lesion found recurrent instability in 20% of the patients treated with a traditional arthroscopic Bankart repair alone but none in patients treated with arthroscopic Bankart repair combined with remplissage.

[51] Diklic ID, Ganic ZD, Blagojevic ZD, Nho SJ, Romeo AA: Treatment of locked chronic posterior dislocation of the shoulder by reconstruction of the defect in the humeral head with an allograft. *J Bone Joint Surg Br* 2010;92(1):71-76.

Retrospective review of 13 patients treated with humeral head allograft reconstruction for a locked chronic posterior shoulder dislocation found that 9 patients had no pain or restriction of activities of daily living. Good overall functional outcomes were reported.

[52] Miniaci A, Gish MW: Management of anterior glenohumeral instability associated with large Hill-Sachs defects. *Tech Shoulder Elbow Surg* 2004;5:170-175.

[53] Rowe CR, Zarins B, Ciullo JV: Recurrent anterior dislocation of the shoulder after surgical repair: Apparent causes of failure and treatment. *J Bone Joint Surg Am* 1984;66(2):159-168.

[54] Calandra JJ, Baker CL, Uribe J: The incidence of Hill-Sachs lesions in initial anterior shoulder dislocations. *Arthroscopy* 1989;5(4):254-257.

[55] Franceschi F, Longo UG, Ruzzini L, Rizzello G, Maffulli N, Denaro V: Arthroscopic salvage of failed arthroscopic Bankart repair: A prospective study with a minimum follow-up of 4 years. *Am J Sports Med* 2008;36(7):1330-1336.

A prospective study of 10 carefully selected patients found that arthroscopic revision surgery for a Bankart lesion was successful at an average 68-month follow-up.

[56] Hall RH, Isaac F, Booth CR: Dislocations of the shoulder with special reference to accompanying small fractures. *J Bone Joint Surg Am* 1959;41(3):489-494.

[57] Richards RD, Sartoris DJ, Pathria MN, Resnick D: Hill-Sachs lesion and normal humeral groove: MR imaging features allowing their differentiation. *Radiology* 1994;190(3):665-668.

第九章　肩关节后方及多向不稳定

Fotios P. Tjoumakaris, MD; James P. Bradley, MD

引言

肩关节后方不稳定和多向不稳定的症状是重叠的。大多数患者症状不明确，并且诊断也困难。在过去的数年中，肩关节后方或多向不稳定的处理有了明显的改进。随着影像学及肩关节镜技术的进步，外科处理有了明显的改善，且文献报道患者的预后也较之前更佳。

临床评估

病史

后方或多向不稳定的患者较少有报道是创伤性脱位的。肩关节后脱位经典的机制是触电、癫痫发作或向后的力直接作用于肩关节（典型的是接触性体育运动或摩托车碰撞）。患者主诉肩关节活动时疼痛、外旋困难并且需要在急诊科行闭合复位。通常令患肢处于内旋位并置于吊带中是最舒服的。后方不稳定患者较后脱位患者症状轻，并且难以将症状联系于某一特定事件或损伤。这类患者可能在将手臂置于某些特定位置或做某些动作时引发症状或疼痛，如经身体前方内收手臂或过顶投

Dr. Tjoumakaris or an immediate family member is a member of a speakers' bureau or has made paid presentations on behalf of Ferring Pharmaceuticals. Dr. Bradley or an immediate family member serves as a board member, owner, officer, or committee member of the American Orthopaedic Society for Sports Medicine; has received royalties from Arthrex; and has received research or institutional support from Arthrex.

掷。很多患者可能出现经常性的后方半脱位；患者可能主诉肩关节疼痛、乏力或投掷速度降低。当症状变得持续时，患者会主诉上肢麻木或感觉患肢"濒死"。多向不稳定患者也会主诉肩关节疼痛、日常生活中手臂活动困难，并且经常有双侧肩关节症状。确定患肢确切的活动范围及症状的诱发机制是很困难的，因为患者的症状通常比较隐匿且会与肩袖撞击相混淆（表9-1）。

表 9-1
复发后方不稳定患者的常见症状
肩关节疼痛
肩关节乏力
投掷速度降低
无力（"死臂"感）
上肢麻木、感觉异常

体格检查

医师应该仔细地评估患者的颈椎及颈椎压迫引起的肩关节和上肢疼痛。通过颈椎的评估，包括触诊、关节活动范围评估和激发试验（Spurling试验），以判断有无神经根性颈椎病，该病也可能导致肩关节和肩胛骨周围的疼痛。全面的肩关节检查对每个肩关节疼痛和功能障碍者来说都是必要的检查。肌力、肌肉萎缩与否、主被动活动范围和肩胛骨节奏及同步性都应该作为检查的内容，这些可能有助于发现并发症。例如，Jerk试验和Kim试验等激发试验能帮助发现肱骨头滑过关节盂后缘时的不稳定和疼痛[1-2]。

Jerk 试验是真正的后方不稳定试验，需在患者坐位时进行。稳定患者肩胛骨，在患者手臂从外展内旋位水平经过躯干的同时施加向后的推力。听到肩关节弹响（类似当嘟声）提示肩关节出现后方半脱位。当手臂被放回起始位置后，肱骨头复位时可以听到第二声弹响。Kim 试验需患者坐位上臂 90° 外展，检查者握住近端上臂并在前臂上举 45° 时向后施加作用力。该操作诱发疼痛则提示后下方盂唇损伤，这也是导致后方不稳定的原因（图 9-1）。应力轴移试验可以评估肩关节松弛程度，而恐惧试验被用来评估前方不稳定。复位后恐惧感消失，可以进一步评估不稳定的方向。手术中发现肱骨头后方半脱位很常见，而且只有很大程度的松弛才会引起临床不稳定。[3] 韧带松弛常通过肘关节和膝关节过伸、髌骨活动范围、掌指关节过伸和向下方施加应力以观察肩峰前外侧缘的深沟征来检查。深沟征是指存在肩关节外旋时不会消失的凹陷宽度大于 2 cm 的凹陷，在有症状的患者中被视为病理现象并提示可能有肩袖间隙松弛。在最近的一个断面研究中，健康患者的深沟征与肩关节不稳定的病史有关。[4] 通过对比双侧上肢整体的神经血管检查结果评估脉搏或神经功能的差异，如有不同则可能提示胸廓出口综合征或臂丛病变。肩关节多向不稳定患者可能表现

为应力轴移试验时移位增大、深沟征阳性、恐惧试验阳性以及 Jerk 试验和 Kim 试验阳性。多项试验阳性提示肩关节囊整体松弛。后方不稳定的患者在后方关节囊受力（后方应力轴移试验、Jerk 试验或 Kim 试验）时最可能会出现这些情况，提示一个单独的损伤。很多的重叠因素可能存在，而这可能会让患者的最佳治疗方案的制订遇到困难。

流行病学

肩关节后方不稳定的发病率占整个肩关节不稳定的发病率的 5%。[5] 大约 50% 的肩关节后方不稳定有创伤的因素。大多数脱位的病因是创伤；其他的病因则是癫痫或电击。据报道，肩关节后脱位的年发病率为 1.1/100 000，发病年龄高峰是 20~49 岁和大约 70 岁。首次脱位的年龄小、合并癫痫及大的反 Hill-Sachs 损伤者容易复发。大约有 20% 的患者在首次后脱位发生后的 1 年内复发。[6]

多向不稳定更常见于 20~30 岁的人群，并且最容易发生于反复过肩活动的运动员，例如，排球、游泳和体操运动员。[7] 两个方向上的不稳定应诊断为多向不稳定，诊断通常具有挑战性，且被误诊为单一方向的不稳定可能导致初始治疗失败。这些患者的流行病学特点通常难以量化，因为在目前的骨科文献中并不存在诊断标准。是否

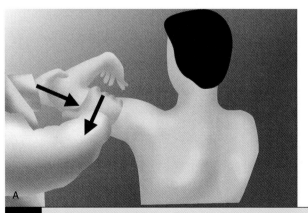
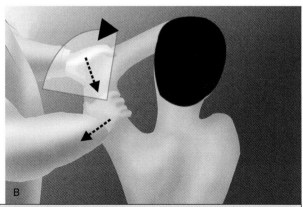

图 9-1　Kim 试验。A. 上臂 90° 外展，检查者对近端上臂施加轴向和向下的力（箭头）。B. 当外展的手臂上举 45°，检查者在手臂内收经过躯干时施加向后的力和轴向压力（虚线箭头）。如果出现疼痛，则为阳性并高度提示后下方盂唇损伤

将有一个方向的脱位但是其他平面松弛的患者纳入诊断尚存在争议。

解剖学

盂肱关节的稳定依赖于静态稳定（关节囊、盂唇、肩胛盂和软骨盂唇倾角）及动态稳定（肩袖、肩胛骨和胸廓肌肉，以及神经肌肉控制）（表9-2）。在创伤或癫痫导致后脱位的患者中，肩胛盂或肱骨头的骨性结构可能受损，从而导致后方肩胛盂骨折（或缺损）或肱骨头前方压缩骨折（反Hill-Sachs损伤）。在这些患者中，骨缺损的程度可能会很大程度上与不稳定的发生有关系。因为肱骨头内旋，损伤部位可能嵌顿并导致半脱位和脱位复发。肩胛盂和软骨盂唇后倾可能是复发性不稳定和半脱位的一个危险因素（或其结果）。由后方反复受力或不稳定导致的盂唇损伤可能从后方盂唇裂缝发展到Kim损伤（非完全的、隐匿的后下方盂唇撕裂），再发展到反Bankart损伤。可能发生关节囊撕裂、后方盂唇关节囊骨膜套袖样撕脱或盂肱后下韧带肱骨侧撕裂并导致后方不稳定复发。[8-12]前锯肌活动减少、斜方肌活动增强和胸小肌静息长度缩短等导致的肩胛骨动力学改变被证实能改变盂肱关节的稳定性；尸体研究发现当肩胛骨后倾超过15°时，后方不稳定增加。[13-14]肩袖在动态稳定中也起到了很关键的作用，并且肩袖撕裂可能存在于任何年龄的肩关节后脱位患者。凹面压力缺失和复发性不稳定可能发生在骨性结构和韧带结构正常的情况下。复发性后方半脱位可能与异常盂肱关节移位导致的肩袖病变相关。临床医师的警惕心及仔细的影像学筛查对准确诊断和制订治疗计划非常重要。

影像学检查

常规的影像学检查通常对创伤或可疑的急性脱位具有诊断性。通常拍摄这3个位置（前后位、肩胛骨Y位和腋位）的X线片。拍摄后脱位患者

表9-2
肩关节后方和多向不稳定的解剖学因素

解剖学因素	病理
静态稳定	
肱骨头	反Hill-Sachs损伤
	肱骨头后倾角度增加
肩胛盂	后方肩胛盂骨折（或缺损）
盂唇	盂唇撕裂
	软骨盂唇后倾角度增加
	Kim损伤
	后方盂唇关节囊骨膜套袖样撕脱
关节囊	关节囊撕裂
	关节囊薄弱或松弛
	盂肱下韧带后方撕裂和盂肱韧带后方肱骨侧撕裂
动态稳定	
肌肉控制	肩袖撕裂
	稳定肩胛骨的肌肉（菱形肌、胸小肌和前锯肌）肌力弱
神经肌肉控制	癫痫或电击时强力内旋

的腋位片可能有困难，因为上臂外旋不稳定。这类患者的正位X线片可能出现肩胛窝空虚征和灯泡征（肱骨近端内旋后出现灯泡形状）（图9-2）。如果不能拍摄传统的腋位片，Velpeau腋位片有时会有帮助。需要在X线片上检查后方肩胛盂缘的

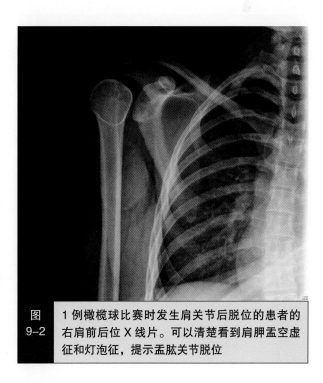

图 9-2　1例橄榄球比赛时发生肩关节后脱位的患者的右肩前后位X线片。可以清楚看到肩胛盂空虚征和灯泡征，提示盂肱关节脱位

骨缺损和肱骨头前方的反 Hill-Sachs 损伤。此外，还需要检查合并的大小结节、外科颈或肱骨头骨折，任何类型的骨性损伤都可能影响外科治疗。[15]CT 可能对确认骨性损伤的类型有帮助，尤其是在 X 线片不能诊断时。CT 有利于确认 Hill-Sachs 损伤的大小、后方肩胛盂的骨缺损程度以及肩胛盂后倾的角度，该角度可能与复发性不稳定有关。

MRA 和 MRI 是检查后方关节囊盂唇复合体损伤最好的影像学方法。轴向图像能显示肱骨头相对肩胛盂后方移位、后方盂唇关节囊撕裂、后方盂唇撕裂形成的盂唇旁囊肿以及盂肱后下韧带复合体肱骨侧撕裂。[16]隐匿损伤（Kim 损伤或不完全及近于完全的盂唇裂隙）、后方骨膜套袖样撕裂和软骨盂唇后倾的增加也能通过轴向 MRI 或 MRA 图像观察和量化（图 9-3）。肩袖撕裂、骨水肿、压缩骨折和关节软骨异常可以通过 MRI 评估并且见于很多患者。一项最近的研究发现在 MRA 检查过程中使手臂屈曲、内收和内旋能进一步确认后下方关节盂损伤的患者是否合并更为隐匿的后方关节囊和盂唇异常。[17]多向不稳定的患者一般不具有特别的盂唇病变，但是可能具有不稳定的骨性形态改变，例如，软骨盂唇后倾增加和后方关节囊扩张。[18]

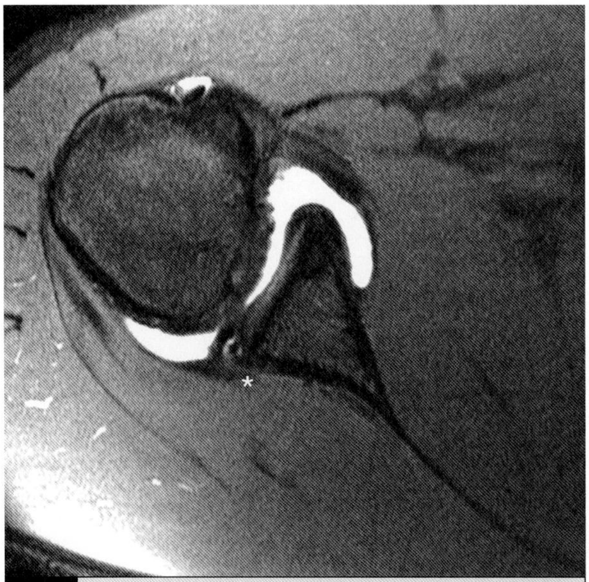

治疗

非手术治疗

肩关节后方和多向不稳定的治疗在过去的十几年中有了长足的进步。对于急性脱位和骨折导致不稳定的患者，通常闭合复位和骨折固定以恢复盂肱关节的稳定性。对于复发后方不稳定或多向不稳定的患者，物理治疗是一线治疗。即使进行了积极的治疗和力量练习，仍有很多患者的非手术治疗失败，因此需要手术治疗。[19]近期一项关于多向不稳定患者的研究发现，对于恢复盂肱关节正常动力学和肌肉活动，关节囊轴移和物理治疗结合的效果要优于单纯物理治疗。[20]这项发现强调了非手术方法治疗不稳定患者的难度。然而，很多患者受益于最初的非手术治疗并可能避免手术干预，尤其是那些肩胛骨周围肌肉功能不佳的患者。

手术治疗

关节镜手术已经是不合并骨性缺损的肩关节后方或多向不稳定治疗的金标准（图 9-4）。曾经有很多后方不稳定患者通过开放手术稳定后方来治疗，复发率为 0~40%。很少有患者能够恢复到之前的活动或运动水平。[21-27]开放手术的高复发率和患者的不满意使得对关节镜治疗的研究增多。在使用了现代关节镜技术后，平均复发率接近 5%，绝大多数研究的复发率为 0~10%。很大比例的患者恢复到之前的活动或运动水平。[28]一项关节镜手术和开放手术的对比研究发现采用关节镜手术治疗的患者功能结果更好。[29]一项尸体生物力学研究发现，切开骨阻挡技术过分纠正后方平移，并且恢复下方稳定性的效果比关节镜下后方 Bankart 修复差。[30]运用现代关节镜技术，在高需求投掷运动员中的失败率相对较低（5%~10%）。[31-35]在这些回顾性研究中，未能

图 9-3　T2 加权成像轴向 MRA 图像显示后方关节盂裂隙合并 Kim 损伤。患者的症状是持续的复发性后方半脱位。* = 盂唇裂隙区域

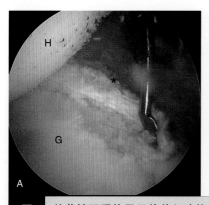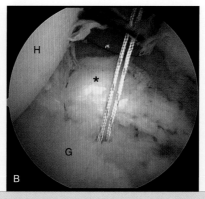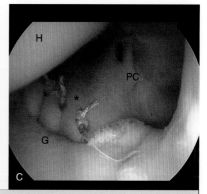

图
9-4
关节镜下照片显示从前入路修补后方盂唇。患者侧卧。A. 后方盂唇从肩胛盂后缘撕裂，同时由于复发性后方半脱位出现肩胛盂关节软骨缺损。B. 放置缝合锚以确保后方盂唇和关节囊复位于关节盂缘。C. 最终修补。后入路已修补以防止因缺损部位出现关节囊功能不足。*= 盂唇；G= 肩胛盂；H= 肱骨头；PC= 后方关节囊

使用缝合锚折叠后方关节囊可能是少数不成功的一个技术因素。[36]

关节囊轴移开放手术为大多数多向不稳定的患者提供了长期的稳定。最近的研究发现，关节镜手术的成功率与其相当，且有趋势显示通过关节镜手术治疗的患者恢复体育活动的结果更佳。[37]最近的尸体研究发现关节镜折叠较传统的开放手术对关节囊的容量缩小更多，进一步证实了关节镜手术优于开放手术。[38]一项关于高需求运动员的多向不稳定研究显示，91% 的患者完全恢复或具有满意的关节活动范围，而 86% 的患者能够进行之前水平的竞技活动。[39]与传统开放手术相比，关节镜手术的优势包括能够处理合并的病变（如上盂唇前后向撕裂、全关节囊松弛和肩袖撕裂）和前后方关节囊松弛，且并发症比开放手术少。[36]

对于合并骨缺损锁定肩关节后脱位、病理性关节盂后倾、骨缺损或盂肱韧带肱骨侧撕裂的患者，开放手术可能是更好的治疗方法。对于具有巨大肱骨头骨缺损的反 Hill-Sachs 损伤患者，更好的选择可能是异体骨软骨重建、肱骨头成形术或小结节移位（McLaughlin 技术）。[40]对于肩胛盂或肱骨头后倾增加的患者，肩胛盂和肱骨截骨能提供稳定性，但是这些治疗方法近年来逐渐不再流行。

关节镜下治疗后方不稳定

对于大多数后方不稳定或复发性后方半脱位患者，关节镜技术对后方盂唇或关节囊的修补能达到完美的效果，复发率和并发症的发生率很低。在这里描述的推荐技术可能会有差异但是仍然能达到一个不错的效果。通常患者取侧卧位，垫沙袋以防止压伤，采用斜角肌间阻滞或全身麻醉使肌肉完全放松。患肢 45° 外展和轻度前屈位置于牵引架上，使用 4.6~6.8 kg 的重量牵引。

先建立后方单一入路放置锚和处理缝线，于肩峰外侧缘沿线定位。这个入路允许锚放置的轨迹相对肩胛盂关节面的角度成 45°（图 9-5）。如果后入路未提供下方锚置入的最佳轨迹，则外侧辅助入路可能在肩胛盂 7 点位置提供更好的轨迹。于肱二头肌腱下方的肩袖旋转间隙建立前入路。前方放置一个直径 5.75 mm 的空套管以提供关节镜视野，后方放置一个直径 8.25 mm 的空套管作为工作通道。确认盂唇和关节囊病变后，用骨膜剥离器将盂唇从后方肩胛盂边缘掀起。使用电钻和刨刀清理肩胛盂后缘（图 9-6）。通常将骨膜剥离器和刨刀从前入路置入比从后入路置入更有用。关节镜可经前入路放置锚和处理缝线。前入路放置 70° 关节镜有利于观察后方及下方肩胛盂缘。缝合锚一般沿肩胛盂后缘置入，从下方

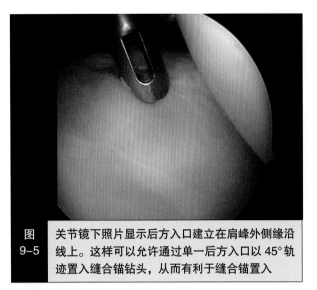

图 9-5 关节镜下照片显示后方入口建立在肩峰外侧缘沿线上。这样可以允许通过单一后方入口以 45° 轨迹置入缝合锚钻头，从而有利于缝合锚置入

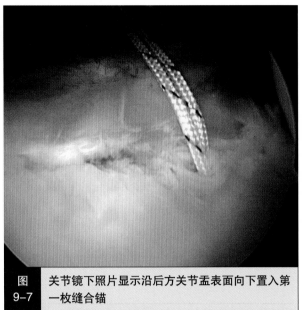

图 9-7 关节镜下照片显示沿后方关节盂表面向下置入第一枚缝合锚

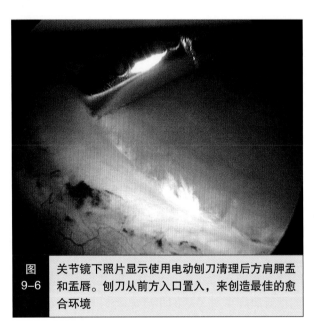

图 9-6 关节镜下照片显示使用电动刨刀清理后方肩胛盂和盂唇。刨刀从前方入口置入，来创造最佳的愈合环境

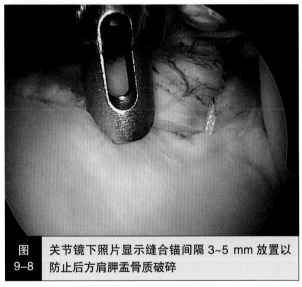

图 9-8 关节镜下照片显示缝合锚间隔 3~5 mm 放置以防止后方肩胛盂骨质破碎

开始根据需要向上方延伸（图 9-7）。推荐使用 2.0~2.4 mm 直径生物兼容性锚，放置间隔为 3~5 mm，以避免外侧肩胛盂骨折（图 9-8）。锚定后的线脚（距肩胛盂最远）于缝合锚稍下方及外侧穿过盂唇和关节囊以折叠关节囊。对不应该折叠关节囊的患者（如高水平投掷运动员），缝线可于锚位置穿过周围的盂唇以防止后方关节囊过度收紧。使用一缝合钩以辅助过线，缝线按从下至上的方向打结（图 9-9）。当通过后方入口过线时，同时取出缝线和过线器以避免绕线（图 9-10）。随后收紧缝线，为使线结远离盂肱关节，

将已经穿过关节囊和盂唇的缝线（距关节盂最远）用作后线脚（图 9-11）。对于延伸至盂唇上方的撕裂，可使用带 1 号线的 2 mm 锚或无结的 2.9 mm 锚来避免线结在盂肱关节活动时磨损后上方肩袖。当所有的锚放置后，关闭后入路以防止后方关节囊中应力集中。盂唇解剖复位于后方肩胛盂缘后，在关闭关节囊的同时还可以让术者检测修复效果。将后方套筒撤至后方关节囊水平。用一新月形缝合钩带线穿过入路的一侧，然后用一穿刺抓钳从另一侧取出缝线（图 9-12）。缝线随后可打结至后方关节囊旁（图 9-13）。改变缝线

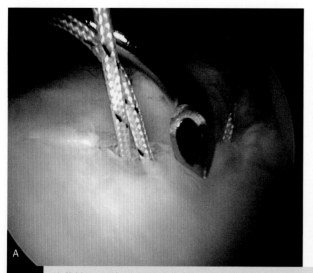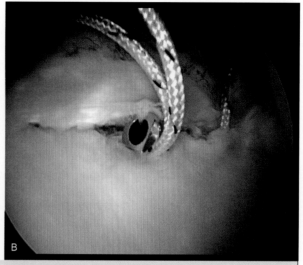

图
9-9　关节镜下照片显示用缝合钩经后方盂唇和关节囊复合体穿过缝线，前方观察入路。A. 通过后入路置入一个短缝合弯钩。B. 缝合钩在缝合锚水平穿过盂唇和关节囊复合体，如果行关节囊折叠，则于缝合锚稍下方穿过

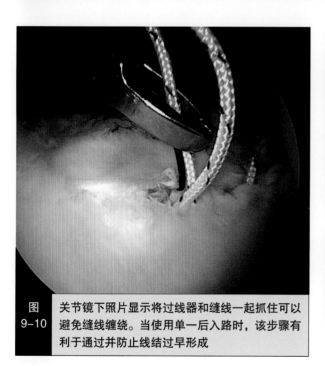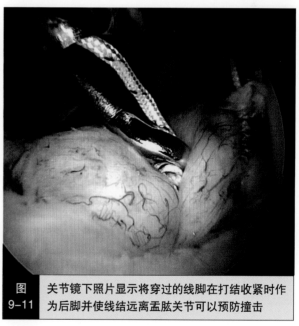

图
9-10　关节镜下照片显示将过线器和缝线一起抓住可以避免缝线缠绕。当使用单一后入路时，该步骤有利于通过并防止线结过早形成

图
9-11　关节镜下照片显示将穿过的线脚在打结收紧时作为后脚并使线结远离盂肱关节可以预防撞击

到入口的距离可以为后方关节囊提供更多的张力。当所有缝线打结后修补完成，关闭后方关节囊，防止病理性盂肱关节后方移位（图9-14）。

术后使用外展吊带，被动活动范围训练可于术后次日开始，中立位外旋和90°前屈于术后第4周开始。术后第6周时可去除吊带，患者从辅助下主动活动范围训练缓慢过渡到无限制主动活动

训练。术后第4个月时，通常肩关节疼痛消失并基本恢复正常的活动范围，同时开始肩袖力量和功能训练。术后第5个月时，开始等速和等张训练。根据具体活动的性质，患者可于术后第6个月时评估是否恢复活动。过顶运动运动员或投掷运动员可以在该时期开始恢复活动。

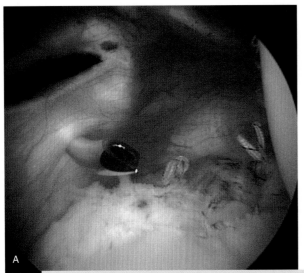

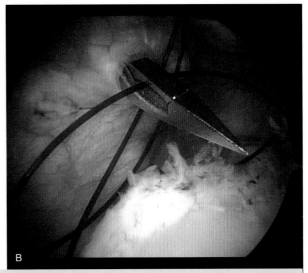

图 9-12 关节镜下照片显示盂唇修复后关闭后入路。A. 将后方套管置于后入路稍后方备用。在入路的一侧,用一个新月形缝合钩穿过后方关节囊。B. 穿刺抓钳在后入路的另一侧抓住穿过的蓝色缝线以关闭入路

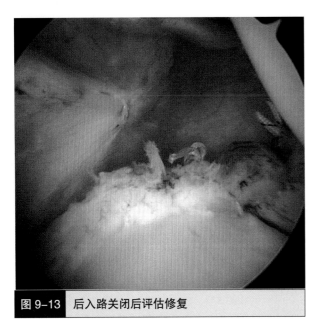

图 9-13 后入路关闭后评估修复

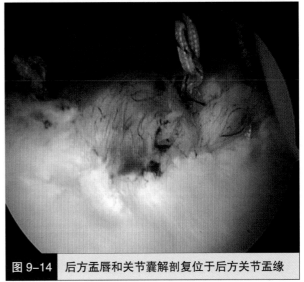

图 9-14 后方盂唇和关节囊解剖复位于后方关节盂缘

总结

肩关节后方和多向不稳定代表了一组损伤的类型,常由多因素造成。肩胛盂和肱骨后倾的解剖学变异、关节囊缺失、盂唇损伤、急性外伤造成的骨缺损和肌肉动态控制也与不稳定的类型有关。MRI 和 MRA 可提高诊断这类情况的敏感性和特异性。影像学的发现应结合体格检查结果以用于制订个体化的治疗方案。如果非手术治疗效果不理想,则行关节镜手术。关节镜手术通常作为一线的手术方法,并且能够处理很多病理类型,同时具有较低的复发率和较高的患者满意度。

参考文献

[1] Kim SH, Park JC, Park JS, Oh I: Painful jerk test: A predictor of success in nonoperative treatment of posteroinferior instability of the shoulder. *Am J Sports Med* 2004;32(8):1849-1855.

[2] Kim SH, Park JS, Jeong WK, Shin SK: The Kim test: A

novel test for posteroinferior labral lesion of the shoulder. A comparison to the jerk test. *Am J Sports Med* 2005;33(8):1188-1192.

[3] Jia X, Ji JH, Petersen SA, Freehill MT, McFarland EG: An analysis of shoulder laxity in patients undergoing shoulder surgery. *J Bone Joint Surg Am* 2009;91(9): 2144-2150.

Shoulder laxity was correlated with pathologic instability in patients undergoing surgery. Greater laxity while under anesthesia was significantly correlated with shoulder instability.

[4] Owens BD, Duffey ML, Deberardino TM, Cameron KL: Physical examination findings in young athletes correlate with history of shoulder instability. *Orthopedics* 2011;34(6):460.

A cross-sectional study evaluated more than 700 healthy patients using physical examination techniques. Patients with a history of instability were more likely to have increased posterior translation, an apprehension sign, a sulcus sign, and a positive relocation sign.

[5] Robinson CM, Aderinto J: Recurrent posterior shoulder instability. *J Bone Joint Surg Am* 2005;87(4): 883-892.

[6] Robinson CM, Seah M, Akhtar MA: The epidemiology, risk of recurrence, and functional outcome after an acute traumatic posterior dislocation of the shoulder. *J Bone Joint Surg Am* 2011;93(17):1605-1613.

A retrospective review defined the epidemiology of posterior shoulder dislocation. Recurrence was found in 17.7% of the patients within the first year after injury. Recurrence of instability was associated with age younger than 40 years, a seizure-associated dislocation, and a large reverse Hill-Sachs lesion.

[7] Gaskill TR, Taylor DC, Millett PJ: Management of multidirectional instability of the shoulder. *J Am Acad Orthop Surg* 2011;19(12):758-767.

The authors discuss the diagnosis and treatment of multidirectional shoulder instability.

[8] Kim SH, Noh KC, Park JS, Ryu BD, Oh I: Loss of chondrolabral containment of the glenohumeral joint in atraumatic posteroinferior multidirectional instability. *J Bone Joint Surg Am* 2005;87(1):92-98.

[9] Kim SH, Ha KI, Yoo JC, Noh KC: Kim's lesion: An incomplete and concealed avulsion of the posteroinferior labrum in posterior or multidirectional posteroinferior instability of the shoulder. *Arthroscopy* 2004;20(7): 712-720.

[10] Safran O, Defranco MJ, Hatem S, Iannotti JP: Poste-

rior humeral avulsion of the glenohumeral ligament as a cause of posterior shoulder instability: A case report. *J Bone Joint Surg Am* 2004;86-A(12):2732-2736.

[11] Shah AA, Butler RB, Fowler R, Higgins LD: Posterior capsular rupture causing posterior shoulder instability: A case report. *Arthroscopy* 2011;27(9):1304-1307.

A 20-year-old man had successful arthroscopic repair of a posterior capsular rupture that resulted in posterior instability of the shoulder.

[12] Bokor DJ, Fritsch BA: Posterior shoulder instability secondary to reverse humeral avulsion of the glenohumeral ligament. *J Shoulder Elbow Surg* 2010;19(6): 853-858.

A retrospective review of 19 patients diagnosed with posterior capsular disruption after a traumatic injury to the shoulder found a high number of associated lesions: labral tear (more than 50%), reverse Bankart lesion (26%), chondral injury (21%), rotator cuff tear (21%), and extension of the tear into the posterior band of the inferior glenohumeral ligament (11%).

[13] Ludewig PM, Reynolds JF: The association of scapular kinematics and glenohumeral joint pathologies. *J Orthop Sports Phys Ther* 2009;39(2):90-104.

The role of scapular kinematics specific to shoulder pathology is outlined. Reduced serratus activation and pectoralis minor contracture were associated with rotator cuff impingement and instability in the cited studies.

[14] Kikuchi K, Itoi E, Yamamoto N, et al: Scapular inclination and glenohumeral joint stability: A cadaveric study. *J Orthop Sci* 2008;13(1):72-77.

Nine cadavers were studied by loading the glenohumeral joint in different directions with alterations in scapular inclination. Posterior and inferior stability increased with an anterior tilt of more than 5° and a superior tilt of 10°. This study shows the importance of the scapular position in maintaining glenohumeral joint stability.

[15] Robinson CM, Akhtar A, Mitchell M, Beavis C: Complex posterior fracture-dislocation of the shoulder: Epidemiology, injury patterns, and results of operative treatment. *J Bone Joint Surg Am* 2007;89(7):1454-1466.

Epidemiologic data were obtained from a study of 26 patients with complex posterior fracture-dislocation of the shoulder. The incidence of this injury was determined to be 0.6 per 100,000 per year. Most injuries occurred secondary to a seizure or a fall from height in middle-aged men. Surgical results and outcomes generally are favorable after open reduction and internal fixation.

[16] Tung GA, Hou DD: MR arthrography of the posterior labrocapsular complex: Relationship with glenohumeral joint alignment and clinical posterior instability. *AJR Am J Roentgenol* 2003;180(2):369-375.

[17] Chiavaras MM, Harish S, Burr J: MR arthrographic assessment of suspected posteroinferior labral lesions using flexion, adduction, and internal rotation positioning of the arm: Preliminary experience. *Skeletal Radiol* 2010;39(5):481-488.

Diagnostic confidence for detecting posterior labral pathology was increased in nine patients when MRA in flexion, adduction, and internal rotation was used.

[18] Jana M, Gamanagatti S: Magnetic resonance imaging in glenohumeral instability. *World J Radiol* 2011;3(9): 224-232.

MRI findings consistent with instability are outlined. Cited studies of multidirectional instability show that labral pathology often is absent. Increased chondrolabral retroversion is a more characteristic finding in these patients.

[19] Misamore GW, Sallay PI, Didelot W: A longitudinal study of patients with multidirectional instability of the shoulder with seven- to ten-year follow-up. *J Shoulder Elbow Surg* 2005;14(5):466-470.

[20] Nyiri P, Illyés A, Kiss R, Kiss J: Intermediate biomechanical analysis of the effect of physiotherapy only compared with capsular shift and physiotherapy in multidirectional shoulder instability. *J Shoulder Elbow Surg* 2010;19(6):802-813.

In a prospective study, the kinematic patterns in patients with multidirectional instability who were treated with physical therapy only or with physical therapy and capsular shift were compared with those of healthy control subjects. Surgery and physical therapy led to the more close approximation of normal shoulder kinematics, with a durable outcome at 4 years.

[21] Tibone JE, Bradley JP: The treatment of posterior subluxation in athletes. *Clin Orthop Relat Res* 1993;291: 124-137.

[22] Hawkins RJ, Janda DH: Posterior instability of the glenohumeral joint: A technique of repair. *Am J Sports Med* 1996;24(3):275-278.

[23] Bigliani LU, Pollock RG, McIlveen SJ, Endrizzi DP, Flatow EL: Shift of the posteroinferior aspect of the capsule for recurrent posterior glenohumeral instability. *J Bone Joint Surg Am* 1995;77(7):1011-1020.

[24] Fronek J, Warren RF, Bowen M: Posterior subluxation

of the glenohumeral joint. *J Bone Joint Surg Am* 1989; 71(2):205-216.

[25] Misamore GW, Facibene WA: Posterior capsulorrhaphy for the treatment of traumatic recurrent posterior subluxations of the shoulder in athletes. *J Shoulder Elbow Surg* 2000;9(5):403-408.

[26] Meuffels DE, Schuit H, van Biezen FC, Reijman M, Verhaar JA: The posterior bone block procedure in posterior shoulder instability: A long-term follow-up study. *J Bone Joint Surg Br* 2010;92(5):651-655.

At 18-year follow-up after the posterior bone block procedure for posterior shoulder instability, 36% of the patients had a recurrence of dislocation, and almost 50% would not have the surgery a second time. More than one third of the patients had evidence of osteoarthritis, with deteriorating outcomes over the study period.

[27] Rhee YG, Lee DH, Lim CT: Posterior capsulolabral reconstruction in posterior shoulder instability: Deltoid saving. *J Shoulder Elbow Surg* 2005;14(4):355-360.

[28] Bahk MS, Karzel RP, Snyder SJ: Arthroscopic posterior stabilization and anterior capsular plication for recurrent posterior glenohumeral instability. *Arthroscopy* 2010;26(9):1172-1180.

At midterm follow-up, 29 patients had a good result after arthroscopic posterior stabilization with a balanced capsular plication. However, patients with supplemental anterior plication reported more pain, and this adjunctive procedure probably is unnecessary.

[29] Bottoni CR, Franks BR, Moore JH, DeBerardino TM, Taylor DC, Arciero RA: Operative stabilization of posterior shoulder instability. *Am J Sports Med* 2005; 33(7):996-1002.

[30] Wellmann M, Bobrowitsch E, Khan N, et al: Biomechanical effectiveness of an arthroscopic posterior Bankart repair versus an open bone block procedure for posterior shoulder instability. *Am J Sports Med* 2011; 39(4):796-803.

A cadaver study compared an arthroscopic posterior repair to a capsular repair with a bone block procedure after the creation of a posterior capsulolabral injury. The bone block procedure was found to overcorrect posterior translation and did not reduce inferior translation. The arthroscopic technique more effectively restored normal joint kinematics.

[31] Williams RJ III, Strickland S, Cohen M, Altchek DW, Warren RF: Arthroscopic repair for traumatic posterior shoulder instability. *Am J Sports Med* 2003;31(2): 203-209.

［32］ Mair SD, Zarzour RH, Speer KP: Posterior labral injury in contact athletes. *Am J Sports Med* 1998;26(6): 753-758.

［33］ Radkowski CA, Chhabra A, Baker CL III, Tejwani SG, Bradley JP: Arthroscopic capsulolabral repair for posterior shoulder instability in throwing athletes compared with nonthrowing athletes. *Am J Sports Med* 2008;36(4):693-699.

A prospective study compared the results of arthroscopic posterior repair for athletes in throwing and nonthrowing sports. The overall results were favorable and comparable in approximately 90% of patients. Nonthrowing athletes were more likely to return to their previous level of sport (71%) than throwing athletes (55%).

［34］ Seroyer S, Tejwani SG, Bradley JP: Arthroscopic capsulolabral reconstruction of the type VIII superior labrum anterior posterior lesion: Mean 2-year follow-up on 13 shoulders. *Am J Sports Med* 2007; 35(9):1477-1483.

All patients with a type VIII superior labrum anterior and posterior lesion were able to return to sports at a minimum 2-year follow-up, and 69% were able to compete at their previous level of play.

［35］ Bradley JP, Baker CL III, Kline AJ, Armfield DR, Chhabra A: Arthroscopic capsulolabral reconstruction for posterior instability of the shoulder: A prospective study of 100 shoulders. *Am J Sports Med* 2006;34(7): 1061-1071.

［36］ Tjoumakaris FP, Bradley JP: The rationale for an arthroscopic approach to shoulder stabilization. *Arthroscopy* 2011;27(10):1422-1433.

A rationale is presented for using arthroscopic techniques for most incidences of shoulder instability. The results of recent studies of arthroscopic results are similar or superior to those of earlier studies.

［37］ Jacobson ME, Riggenbach M, Wooldridge AN, Bishop JY: Open capsular shift and arthroscopic capsular plication for treatment of multidirectional instability. *Arthroscopy* 2012;28(7):1010-1017.

A systematic review of level IV studies found that the results of arthroscopic surgery and open capsular shift were similar for the treatment of multidirectional shoulder instability with regard to recurrent instability, loss of external rotation, return to sport, and overall complications.

［38］ Sekiya JK, Willobee JA, Miller MD, Hickman AJ, Willobee A: Arthroscopic multi-pleated capsular plication compared with open inferior capsular shift for reduction of shoulder volume in a cadaveric model. *Arthroscopy* 2007;23(11):1145-1151.

A study of seven cadavers assessed the extent of volume reduction with arthroscopic capsular plication compared with an open capsular shift. The authors found that capsular volume was reduced with both techniques, but the arthroscopic technique was slightly superior (58% versus 45% reduction).

［39］ Baker CL III, Mascarenhas R, Kline AJ, Chhabra A, Pombo MW, Bradley JP: Arthroscopic treatment of multidirectional shoulder instability in athletes: A retrospective analysis of 2- to 5-year clinical outcomes. *Am J Sports Med* 2009;37(9):1712-1720.

After arthroscopic surgery for multidirectional instability in 43 patients, 91% had full or satisfactory range of motion, 98% had normal or slightly decreased strength, and 86% were able to return to their previous level of sport.

［40］ Hawkins RJ, Neer CS II, Pianta RM, Mendoza FX: Locked posterior dislocation of the shoulder. *J Bone Joint Surg Am* 1987;69(1):9-18.

第十章　复发性肩关节不稳定的关节镜下重建

Robert A. Arciero, MD; D. Nicholas Reed, MD

引言

盂肱关节是最灵活的关节，其稳定性依赖于动态稳定和静态稳定的精细平衡。任何限制结构的损伤都能引起一系列情况，从完全脱位到反复微小不稳定或非创伤性不稳定都有可能。大多数肩关节不稳定是前方不稳定，早期、适当的治疗对预防复发通常是必要的。了解其病理、影像学和手术技术才能通过关节镜下重建成功治疗复发性不稳定，以上所有对一个有经验的骨科医师来说都是必要的。

临床评估

患者病史

在制订术前和术中计划前，应全面了解患者病史（表10-1）。患者的年龄、性别、优势手、医疗情况（如癫痫、过度松弛和酒精依赖）、职业、活动水平和手术预期等都需要了解。应注意初次脱位的年龄，因为年龄较小则复发的风险会增加。[1]确切的病因应通过了解患者的创伤史、微创伤、过度松弛及创伤的程度来确定；任何这些情况之一都可能影响术前计划。为确认不稳定的方向，应

Dr. Arciero or an immediate family member is a member of a speakers' bureau or has made paid presentations on behalf of Arthrex; has stock or stock options held in Soft Tissue Regeneration; and has received research or institutional support from Arthrex. Neither Dr. Reed nor any immediate family member has received anything of value from or owns stock in a commercial company or institution related directly or indirectly to the subject of this chapter.

明确手臂在脱位或半脱位时的确切位置以及诱发类似症状的手臂位置。应询问患者不稳定症状的发生频率、症状复发的难易程度、睡眠中是否存在不稳定。患者的答案可能有助于医师了解软组织损伤和骨缺损的严重程度。初次脱位是否需要手法复位也很重要。需要手法复位通常意味着主要是软组织损伤，可能合并骨性损伤。之前治疗相关的手术记录和影像学资料可能影响手术计划，也应该进行研究。如有自发不稳定或心理障碍的病史，则应记录下来，因为该类患者最好采用非手术治疗。

体格检查

应该进行详细的体格检查和双侧体格检查结果对比（表10-2）。患侧和健侧都应从前方和后方两个方向观察，以发现不对称和手术瘢痕。主动及被动活动范围以及肩袖力量都应记录。肩袖薄弱与复发前方不稳定相关。[2]如果患者接受过开放手术，应该通过压腹试验和lift-off试验来记录肩胛下肌的完整性。应该记录诱发不稳定时手臂的位置。外展外旋位不稳定提示前方不稳定。应记录外展和外旋的确切角度，如果外展外旋角度相对较小则提示骨性缺损。前屈、内收和内旋导致疼痛或不稳定提示后方不稳定。如果内旋或外旋出现深沟征，则应该记录并与对侧对比。进行详细的神经检查，尤其注意腋神经。

初始检查完成后，应进行激发试验。前方不稳定采用恐惧试验和复位试验评估，后方不稳定

表 10-1

与不稳定相关的病史

发现	意义
初次脱位的年龄	年龄越小则复发的风险越高（尤其是小于 25 岁的患者）
医疗情况（如癫痫或电击）	后脱位或后方不稳定的风险增加
创伤或手法复位	明确的创伤或手法复位提示相对严重的软组织损伤或可能存在肩胛盂或肱骨头的骨性损伤
活动水平（如参与的体育活动）	参加接触性对抗运动的运动员复发风险增加
初次脱位时的手臂位置	外展和外旋提示前方不稳定。前屈、内收和内旋提示后方不稳定
过度松弛	应考虑多向不稳定
脱位的频率	频率高可能提示骨缺损
睡眠时不稳定	应考虑骨缺损
激发症状或不稳定的难易程度	引起症状的外展和外旋的角度逐渐变小提示累及的骨性结构增加

表 10-2

与不稳定相关的体征

发现	意义
瘢痕和双侧不对称	手术瘢痕可以提供与之前的手术或创伤相关的信息。双侧不对称提示继发于肌肉损伤、肌腱损伤或神经损伤的肌肉萎缩
肩关节活动范围	与对侧相比关节活动范围减小提示粘连性关节炎或骨软组织阻挡
肩袖检查	40 岁以上的脱位患者常合并肩袖损伤。肩袖薄弱可能与复发性不稳定并发。应仔细评估肩胛下肌
激发症状或不稳定的手臂位置	外展和外旋提示前方不稳定。前屈、内收和内旋提示后方不稳定
激发试验（恐惧试验、再复位、Jerk 试验）	检查结果提示不稳定方向
神经检查	应检查腋神经和肌皮神经，这两条神经可能因为之前的手术或创伤受到损伤
过度松弛（肘关节反屈、拇指触前臂试验及深沟征）	过度松弛提示多向不稳定
颈椎评估	全面地评估以排除颈部损伤引起的肩关节疼痛

采用 Jerk 试验评估。应力轴移试验可用来评估前方不稳定和后方不稳定。有复发性不稳定病史的患者更有可能出现恐惧试验阳性、再复位、深沟征和后方移位的增加。[3]关于肘关节反屈、掌指关节过度松弛和拇指触前臂试验阳性提示关节过度松弛，存在此类体征的患者应进行锻炼而不是手术。详细的肩关节体格检查应该包含全面的颈椎评估，以排除颈椎疾病造成的肩关节症状。

影像学检查

初始影像学的检查应包含一系列标准的创伤 X 线片，包括前后位片、肩胛骨 Y 位片和腋位片。此外，还应包含特殊体位如西点腋位（改良腋位）和 Stryker 切迹位，前者用于观察肩胛盂骨损伤，后者用于观察肱骨头（Hill-Sachs）损伤[4]（图 10-1）。

对于软组织的检查，MRI 比其他检查更具优势，因此 MRI 有助于评估复发性不稳定。创伤性前脱位患者最常见的损伤是 Bankart 损伤，即前下方关节囊盂唇撕裂。[5]

与初次脱位的患者相比，复发性不稳定患者后方盂唇撕裂、SLAP 损伤和肩袖损伤的发生率更高。[6]MRI 还能观察盂肱韧带肱骨侧撕裂、关

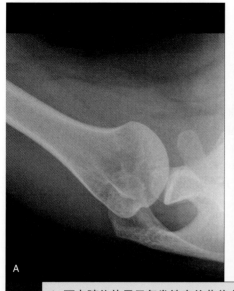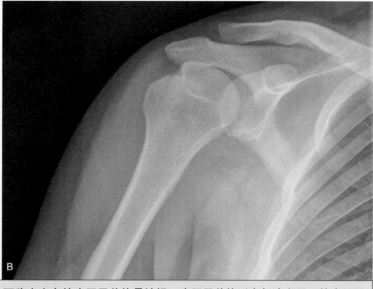

图 10-1　A. 西点腋位片显示复发性肩关节前方不稳定患者的肩胛盂前缘骨缺损。肩胛盂前缘形态与清晰显示的肩胛盂后缘相比是异常的。B. Stryker 切迹位片显示创伤性肩关节脱位患者的右侧肱骨头存在 Hill-Sachs 损伤，外侧可见肱骨头的异常形态

节囊撕裂或薄弱以及骨水肿。术前发现合并的病变能让医师对手术的准备更加充分，从而改善预后。[7-8]

对于观察骨缺损，MRI 不如 CT 有用。CT 能够准确地评估盂唇和肱骨头的骨损伤。辨别和正确治疗骨缺损是很重要的，因为只处理软组织病变会导致关节镜下稳定的失败率增加。[9-10] 重要的是，应该认识到多达 90% 的复发性不稳定患者存在肩胛盂缘缺损，而存在 Hill-Sachs 损伤者高达 100%。[11-12] 三维 CT 能准确评估 Hill-Sachs 损伤，肱骨头数字减影技术能从正面观察肩胛盂来发现肩胛盂骨缺损[13]（图 10-2）。有很多技术可用来计算肱骨侧和肩胛盂侧的骨缺损比例，医师应该完整地掌握其中一种技术[14-16]（表 10-3，图 10-3）。复发性不稳定患者的术前三维 CT 检查指征应予以放宽。术前 CT 对于以下情况也是必要的：初次脱位有明显创伤、影像学检查提示有骨改变、有数次复位史、不稳定频率增加和造成不稳定的应力减少、轻微外展和外旋引起不稳定、睡眠时不稳定、肩胛盂发育不良、倾角异常以及术后不稳定。

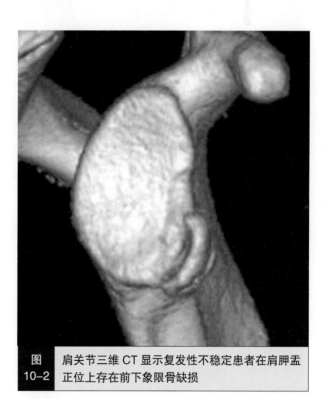

图 10-2　肩关节三维 CT 显示复发性不稳定患者在肩胛盂正位上存在前下象限骨缺损

表 10-3

评估关节盂骨缺损的常用方法

方法	原理
X 线检查，包括创伤系列片和特殊体位相（西点位、顶斜位）	手术瘢痕可以提供与之前的手术或创伤相关的信息。不对称提示继发于肌肉损伤、肌腱损伤或神经损伤的肌肉萎缩
MRI 检查	有助于评估软组织损伤，但不能评估骨缺损的比例
三维 CT 检查	有助于测量肩胛盂的骨缺损。最简单的方式如下 · 测量肩胛盂的骨缺损，缺损的最大径 6~8 mm 大约等于骨缺损 25% · 在肩胛盂正面测量裸点（裸点位于下方真肩胛盂环的中心，到前缘和后缘的距离相等）。裸点到完整关节盂前缘的距离（A）和裸点到肩胛盂后缘的距离（B），骨缺损的比例为〔(B–A)/2B〕× 100%
关节镜检查	应在肩关节镜手术术前估算肩胛盂骨缺损，也可以在术中观察裸点到肩胛盂前缘的距离（A）和裸点到肩胛盂后缘的距离（B），然后用公式〔(B–A)/2B〕× 100% 来计算

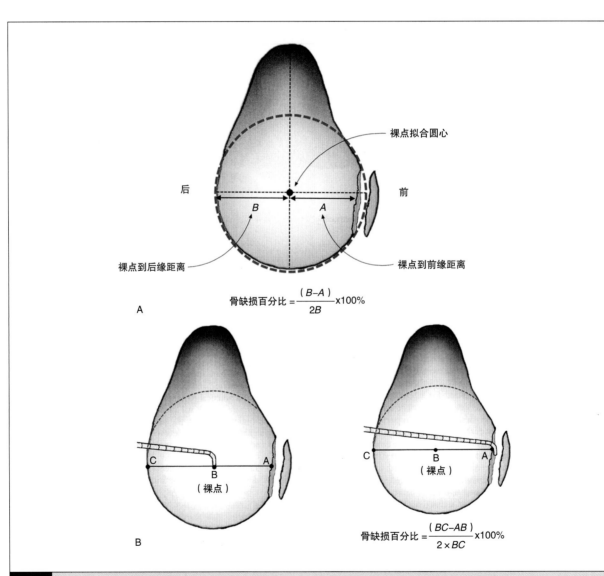

$$骨缺损百分比 = \frac{(B-A)}{2B} \times 100\%$$

$$骨缺损百分比 = \frac{(BC-AB)}{2 \times BC} \times 100\%$$

图 10-3　**图示基于肩胛盂缘距离（A）和肩胛盂裸点（B）的骨缺损估算方法。经允许引自** Provencher MT, Bhatia S, Ghodadra NS, et al: Recurrent shoulder instability: current concepts for evaluation and management of glenoid bone loss. *J Bone Joint Surg Am* 2010;92（Suppl 2）:133–151.

病理解剖学

骨缺损

如果骨缺损处理不当，则治疗肩关节不稳定的手术不太可能成功。[9-10]患者的病史和体格检查应提供肩胛盂或肱骨侧骨缺损的信息。反复脱位会增加肩胛盂骨缺损的发生率和扩大肩胛盂骨缺损的范围。

脱位的次数越多、患者初次脱位的年龄越年轻，严重缺损（累及超过 20% 的下方肩胛盂）的可能性越高。[17]合理的术前影像学检查可以确认骨缺损，这可能影响术前计划。

盂唇和盂肱韧带

盂唇是一个环绕肩胛盂的纤维软骨结构，可增加肩胛盂的表面积和深度以限制肱骨头在肩胛盂的平移。盂肱下韧带（IGHL）复合体是包含一组前束和一组后束并由关节囊袋连接而成的大韧带。盂肱下韧带复合体与盂唇汇集，在关节镜下很容易辨认。盂肱下韧带复合体的作用是在手臂 90° 外展和外旋时阻止肱骨头相对于肩胛盂前移。前下方盂唇和 IGHL 分离被称为 Bankart 损伤。持续的 Bankart 损伤会导致肩关节前方不稳定（图 10-4）。复发性不稳定的患者，IGHL 会出现异常和薄弱。成功的关节镜修复需要将盂唇与肩胛盂和 IGHL 复合体缝合以恢复张力。

在复发性不稳定的患者中，撕裂的盂唇和 IGHL 复合体可在偏内侧的肩胛盂颈处愈合。这种情况被称为 ALPSA 病变（图 10-5）。ALPSA 病变会导致 IGHL 复合体张力和盂唇的缓冲作用丧失，导致持续的不稳定。与单纯 Bankart 损伤的患者相比，复发性不稳定患者和 ALPSA 病变患者通常有更多的脱位次数和较低的手术成功率。[18]

复发性不稳定患者可能还存在向上延伸的盂唇病变，导致 SLAP 损伤。在术前，SLAP 损伤患者脱位次数通常较单纯 Bankart 损伤患者多。与 ALPSA 病变患者不同，SLAP 损伤患者在术后复发率和功能方面与单纯 Bankart 损伤患者没有区别。[19]HAGL 损伤或 IGHL 外侧撕裂也可能是复发性不稳定的原因（图 10-6）。术前必须辨认出 HAGL 损伤，并在开放手术或关节镜手术中予以处理。绝大多数复发性不稳定会导致关节囊的形态异常或薄弱。关节囊张力恢复失败会导致手术失败。关节囊沿 IGHL 前束连线折叠 1 cm 可减轻松弛并恢复关节囊的正常张力。[20]

肩袖间隙

肩袖间隙由盂肱上韧带、盂肱中韧带、肱二头肌长头腱、喙肱韧带和关节囊组成。关闭肩袖间隙对前方不稳定患者的利弊尚有争议。关闭肩袖间隙能够改善前方稳定性但是会导致外旋活动减少，

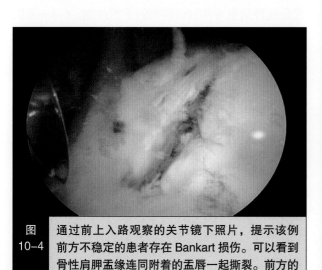

图 10-4　通过前上入路观察的关节镜下照片，提示该例前方不稳定的患者存在 Bankart 损伤。可以看到骨性肩胛盂缘连同附着的盂唇一起撕裂。前方的 IGHL 与盂唇相连

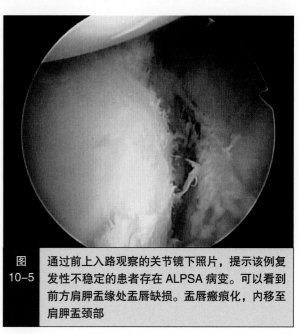

图 10-5　通过前上入路观察的关节镜下照片，提示该例复发性不稳定的患者存在 ALPSA 病变。可以看到前方肩胛盂缘处盂唇缺损。盂唇瘢痕化，内移至肩胛盂颈部

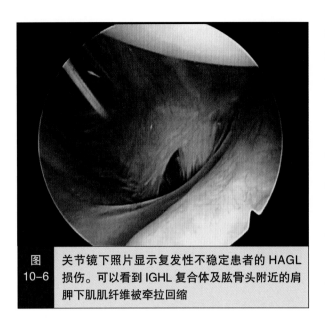

图 10-6　关节镜下照片显示复发性不稳定患者的 HAGL 损伤。可以看到 IGHL 复合体及肱骨头附近的肩胛下肌肌纤维被牵拉回缩

可能会引起活动减少及进展为关节炎。[21-22]

肩袖

肩袖损伤很少发生在年龄小于 40 岁的肩关节脱位患者。如果肩关节脱位患者的年龄大于 40 岁，则肩袖损伤风险增加，如果患者的脱位后疼痛和力量减弱超过 3 个星期，则应考虑存在肩袖损伤。

治疗计划

非手术治疗

大多数复发性不稳定患者需要手术干预，除非患者存在多向不稳定，因为这类患者需要考虑非手术治疗。非手术治疗可能也更适合于具有明显合并症、功能要求低、癫痫、精神原因故意脱位不能够配合术后康复以及不愿配合术后康复的患者。非手术治疗通常需要在一段时间制动后进行肩袖和肩胛骨周围肌肉的力量锻炼。

进行非手术治疗的现役运动员可以在一段时间的制动后使用支具或挽具保护并进行力量锻炼。在这些运动员中，复发率为 37%，50% 需要手术干预。[23]

使用吊带治疗急性脱位的争议集中在最初脱位后使用什么类型的吊带上。一些研究发现外旋位制动能减少脱位后复发前方不稳定的风险，但是还有一些研究质疑这个结论。[24] 最近一项荟萃分析发现制动超过 1 周没有益处，小于 30 岁的患者的复发率更高，采用传统吊带制动和采用外旋位吊带制动的复发率无区别。[24]

手术治疗

关节镜下重建治疗复发性肩关节不稳定的地位在持续上升。一项基于美国骨科手术委员会的研究数据显示，有倾向于关节镜固定而非切开修复的趋势，以及所有关节镜治疗患者的并发症数量更少。[25] 如果术者能完全辨认合并的软组织和骨缺损并运用现代技术和器械正确处理，关节镜手术的成功率与开放手术的成功率相当。[26] 两项最近的荟萃分析发现在治疗 Bankart 损伤的早期关节镜下缝合锚修补的成功率与切开修复的成功率相当。[27-28] 然而，切开修复 Bankart 损伤依然是经时间检验能使肩关节恢复稳定和良好功能的标准治疗方式。[5] 成功的关节镜下重建要求医师能够发现并治疗骨缺损及所有软组织病变、采用合理的手术步骤和技术以及识别复发风险较高的患者。

肩胛盂骨缺损

无论是开放手术还是关节镜手术，在术前能够发现肩胛盂骨缺损对手术成功至关重要。如果在术前没有发现肩胛盂骨缺损，那么术者可以在术中通过肩胛盂裸点测量骨缺损。但是，术前还是应该尽一切努力来识别肱骨和肩胛盂的骨缺损，这样才能充分地评估患者并制订确切的手术计划。6~8 mm 的前方骨缺损提示 25% 的肩胛盂骨缺损，手术计划必须进行相应的改变。如果存在肩胛盂前下方骨缺损，则手术的失败率高达 80%。[9] 骨缺损严重到什么程度需要进行切开修复是存在争议的，大多数研究者同意切开修复适合骨缺损程度大于 20% 的患者。[29-30] 然而，所有关节镜下修复的骨性 Bankart 损伤，只要保留并修复受损骨折块，则治疗结果就能接受（失败率小于 10%）。[31-32] 如果骨缺损 20%~25% 且骨折块不存在，则需要行开放手术恢复肩胛盂的功能弧。

开放手术处理复发性不稳定的结果良好，例

如髂骨嵴移植、异体胫骨移植、Bristow 手术（喙突尖移位）及 Latarjet 手术（整个喙突基底及喙肱韧带和联合腱移位）。最近一篇综述报道 Bristow-Latarjet 手术能得到持续满意的结果，骨性愈合率为 83%，将喙突放在肩胛盂缘内侧 1 cm 以内并附带关节囊水平轴移的方法的复发率更低。[33]

肱骨头损伤

肱骨头关节面的缺损（Hill-Sachs 损伤）几乎存在于每一个复发性不稳定患者。大多数缺损很小且对稳定性的影响也很小。手术治疗 Hill-Sachs 损伤合并肩胛盂骨缺损或外展外旋嵌顿于肩胛盂缘（称为嵌顿性 Hill-Sachs 损伤）时，如果只处理软组织则很容易导致失败。[9,12]大多数这样的损伤只需要处理肩胛盂骨缺损，这样能增加旋转的弧度并预防嵌顿性 Hill-Sachs 损伤及其引起的复发。大（大约 30%）的肱骨头骨缺损仍需要进行处理。[34]三维 CT 可以用来定量肱骨头的缺损。术中可将患者手臂置于外展外旋位以确认 Hill-Sachs 损伤是否存在嵌顿，如果存在则必须处理。

关节镜下填充（将后方关节囊和肩胛下肌腱填充入 Hill-Sachs 损伤的关节囊肌腱固定）是一种新的治疗选择，可以避免开放手术可能带来的并发症和防止肱骨头嵌顿于肩胛盂。很多研究显示大的或嵌顿性 Hill-Sachs 损伤能够通过关节镜下 Bankart 修复和填充治疗，并且不会减小活动范围，关节镜手术的复发率与开放手术的复发率相当。[35-37]然而，多达 33% 的患者在填充术后经历过后上方的疼痛。[38]开放手术治疗 Hill-Sachs 损伤仍然被广泛应用且比较可靠。这些手术包括抬高缺损、骨移植、异体关节面移植、金属表面置换、旋转截骨和半肩关节置换术。

软组织病理

关节镜重建可以直接观察所有的骨性损伤和软组织损伤。长期存在复发性不稳定的患者一般都有广泛的软组织损伤，必须予以正确的治疗以保证治疗成功。对于 Bankart 损伤，盂唇和盂肱下韧带复合体必须恢复合适的张力及正确的位置。仔细地观察整个盂唇并处理后方损伤或 SLAP 损伤是非常重要的。对于 ALPSA 损伤，最好是通过前上方入路观察，必须予以松解并复位于肩胛盂，恢复正常的位置和张力以确保手术成功。HAGL 损伤通常能在术前 MRI 发现，但也可以通过关节镜检查发现。虽然有经验的医师可以通过关节镜修复 HAGL，但是也应该考虑采用肩胛下肌保留入路行开放手术治疗。由反复肩关节不稳定导致的或手术史导致的关节囊缺损在治疗时非常具有挑战性。两年随访研究显示，异体移植重建前关节囊盂唇结构能达到确切的治疗效果，并且对于年轻患者，该方法可以作为关节融合的替代方法。[39]

对于关节镜下不稳定手术，一直存在是否关闭旋转间隙的争议。关闭旋转间隙可减少外旋，改善前方不稳定。肩袖间隙闭合的指征包括：过度松弛、复发性不稳定、与对侧不对称且不能通过外旋纠正的深沟征翻修手术和从事对抗性运动的运动员（稳定比活动范围更重要）。[40]旋转间隙关闭也用于后方不稳定，然而不关闭旋转间隙也能改善后方稳定性，这使得该方法受到质疑。[22]

患者筛选

为了增加手术的成功率，需要正确的病史和体格检查以筛选适合行关节镜下重建的患者。如果患者满足以下条件则手术成功的可能性增加：初次脱位骨缺损小于 20%、无嵌顿性 Hill-Sachs 损伤、Bankart 损伤组织条件良好、无其他合并的软组织损伤以及无过度松弛。对于参加过顶运动的运动员或参加非碰撞运动的年龄小于 20 岁的运动员，倾向于手术治疗。

手术技术

术前应该有准确的诊断和术前计划。术前，每一例患者都应该在麻醉下进行检查以确认诊断及保证无漏诊。患者体位根据术者习惯，侧卧位下纵向牵引能够得到下方肩胛盂最好的视野和入路。入路的建立对于不稳定的修复是很重要的。后入路应该建立在肩胛盂平面的连线上，这个位置比传统的后入路更靠外侧。前入路的建立需要使用由外向内的技术来确保正确的定位和防止关节面损伤。前上入路的定位应该在旋转间隙的高度，而前下入路应建于肩胛下肌稍上方。入路应该允许到达下隐窝。

观察所有骨性结构和软组织是至关重要的。必须处理所有并发的损伤。通过后入路可以看到Bankart损伤，而通过前上入路可以确保ALPSA病变不被遗漏。松解Bankart损伤以准备恢复张力和修复。当术者可看到肩胛下肌纤维时，提示关节囊盂唇已充分松解。松解拟进行修复区域的肩胛盂周围的所有软组织。在松解和准备以后，术者决定是否放置缝合锚及缝线。应该将锚钉在关节软骨水平放置于肩胛盂平面和肩胛颈连接处。锚钉一定不能

过度向内放置，因为这样会造成张力不正常，而且一定不能太靠近肩胛盂表面以防损伤关节软骨和继发关节囊盂唇复合体复位不良。

锚钉放置的正确位置是，从肩胛盂平面的5点和6点位置之间开始，最少放置3枚锚钉。[9,41] 术者应该确保锚钉被放置到合适的位置以防止术后肱骨头撞击。有多项研究评估过不同的锚钉和缝线。最近的研究发现无论是传统的还是新型的无线结系统，都可以恢复关节囊盂唇的高度且愈合结果相似。[42-46] 下一步是恢复IGHL复合体的张力。张力线应该放置于相应的锚钉尾侧5~10 mm处以提供合适的张力。例如，将一枚锚钉放置在5点位置则需将张力线放置在关节囊盂唇和IGHL复合体周围1 cm的6点位置。所有的软组织都应该被牵拉至5点位置的锚钉位置，将张力线内所有软组织向头侧移动5~10 mm以建立合适的张力（图10-7）。

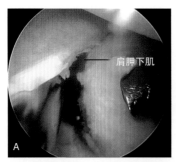
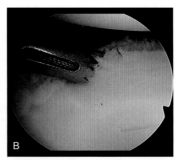
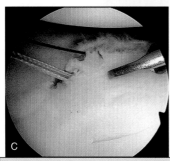
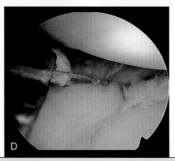
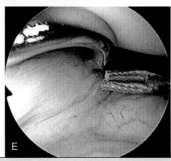

图 10-7　关节镜照片显示治疗前方不稳定的手术技术和锚钉的放置。A. 当看到肩胛下肌肌纤维则说明松解充分。探钩位于肩胛盂缘和盂唇之间，肩胛下肌肌腹位于深层。B. 锚钉于松解完成后放置。锚钉位于前肩胛盂平面的5点和6点位置之间。C. 过线器于缝线下方穿出。关节囊穿刺点位于出口下方1 cm处可确保IGHL复合体恢复合适的张力。D. 缝线双脚已经穿过并以水平褥式方式收紧。线结远离关节面，通过初始缝合锚恢复缓冲作用和IGHL复合体的张力。E. 缝线于下方打结，新月形缝合钩正将组织移至下一枚锚钉，并置于上一枚锚钉上方。可以看到用于恢复张力的关节囊盂唇组织的张力数量。经允许引自 Arciero RA, Mazzocca A: Arthroscopic treatment of anterior instability: Surgical technique, in Provencher MT, Romeo AA, eds: *Shoulder Instability: A Comprehensive Approach*. Philadelphia, PA, Elsevier-Saunders, 2012, pp 126-146 .

术前和术中看到多余的关节囊需要处理以防止复发。关节囊组织应该包含在修复区域中，通过修复盂唇的锚钉将缝线置于盂唇外侧 1 cm 处的关节囊内。关节囊的打磨能促进关节囊与盂唇的愈合。

修复完成后需进行检查以确保恢复 IGHL 的张力和缓冲作用（图 10-8）。如果有必要，可以在后方盂唇放置锚钉修复后方撕裂，或术者可决定关闭肩袖间隙。然而肩袖间隙的关闭不应作为常规操作（图 10-9）。

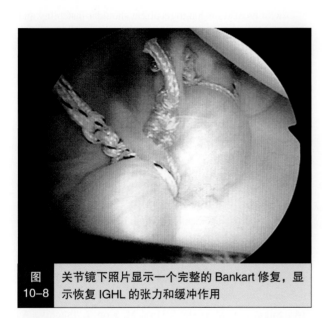

图 10-8　关节镜下照片显示一个完整的 Bankart 修复，显示恢复 IGHL 的张力和缓冲作用

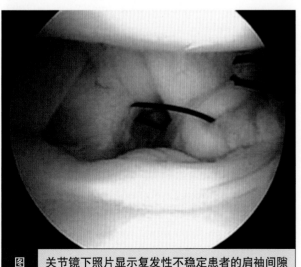

图 10-9　关节镜下照片显示复发性不稳定患者的肩袖间隙关闭

并发症和争议

遵循术前及术中的建议和使用良好的技术可以大大降低包括复发性不稳定在内的关节镜下稳定后的各种并发症风险。存在骨或软组织缺损的患者，如果条件更适合开放手术，则不要行关节镜手术治疗。如果只处理损伤的组织并实施严格的术后康复计划，术后僵硬等并发症是可以避免的。软骨溶解的风险可以通过避免热灼伤和留置止疼泵来降低。

高风险患者

术前必须要识别出复发风险较高的患者。术者可用术前不稳定量化评分来帮助识别这样的患者。评分系统为 10 分制，以下各项存在 1 项则计 2 分：小于 20 岁，职业为竞技运动员，外旋位正位可见 Hill-Sachs 损伤和正位 X 线片可见关节盂形态改变；以下各项存在 1 项则计 1 分：存在过度松弛，从事接触性或过顶运动。如果患者的总分高于 6 分，则复发风险高于 70%，而小于或等于 6 分则复发风险为 10%。[10] 其他研究发现患者的性别为男性、年龄小于 22 岁和存在复发性不稳定是关节镜手术失败的风险因素，这些患者也应密切评估。[47-48]

争议

关于对不稳定肩关节行关节镜手术治疗存在很多争议。尤其是在治疗接触性运动的运动员中。一些医师支持对这类运动员采用开放手术，而有的医师支持关节镜下治疗。两方的观点都有研究证据支持。[49-52]

总结

复发性肩关节不稳定的关节镜下重建的指征范围一直在扩大。如果能仔细地关注术前和术中的各方面情况，那么关节镜下重建可以得到非常满意的结果。

参考文献

［1］Robinson CM, Howes J, Murdoch H, Will E, Graham C: Functional outcome and risk of recurrent instability after primary traumatic anterior shoulder dis- location in young patients. *J Bone Joint Surg Am* 2006;88(11):2326-2336.

［2］ Edouard P, Degache F, Beguin L, et al: Rotator cuff strength in recurrent anterior shoulder instability. *J Bone Joint Surg Am* 2011;93(8):759-765.

Internal and external rotator cuff weakness was associated with recurrent anterior instability.

［3］ Owens BD, Duffey ML, Deberardino TM, Cameron KL: Physical examination findings in young athletes correlate with history of shoulder instability. *Orthopedics* 2011;34(6):460.

One hundred patients with a history of shoulder instability were compared with healthy control subjects. The patients were more likely to have increased posterior translation and positive apprehension, relocation, and sulcus signs.

［4］ Itoi E, Lee SB, Amrami KK, Wenger DE, An KN: Quantitative assessment of classic anteroinferior bony Bankart lesions by radiography and computed tomography. *Am J Sports Med* 2003;31(1):112-118.

［5］ Gill TJ, Micheli LJ, Gebhard F, Binder C: Bankart repair for anterior instability of the shoulder: Long-term outcome. *J Bone Joint Surg Am* 1997;79(6):850-857.

［6］ Gutierrez V, Monckeberg JE, Pinedo M, Radice F: Arthroscopically determined degree of injury after shoulder dislocation relates to recurrence rate. *Clin Orthop Relat Res* 2012;470(4):961-964.

Patients with recurrent shoulder dislocation had more soft-tissue injury, including posterior labral tears, SLAP tears, and rotator cuff pathology, compared with patients having a first episode of shoulder dislocation. Level of evidence: II.

［7］ Porcellini G, Paladini P, Campi F, Paganelli M: Shoulder instability and related rotator cuff tears: Arthroscopic findings and treatment in patients aged 40 to 60 years. *Arthroscopy* 2006;22(3):270-276.

［8］ Rhee YG, Ha JH, Park KJ: Clinical outcome of anterior shoulder instability with capsular midsubstance tear: A comparison of isolated midsubstance tear and midsubstance tear with Bankart lesion. *J Shoulder Elbow Surg* 2006;15(5):586-590.

［9］ Burkhart SS, De Beer JF: Traumatic glenohumeral bone defects and their relationship to failure of arthroscopic Bankart repairs: Significance of the invertedpear glenoid and the humeral engaging Hill-Sachs lesion. *Arthroscopy* 2000;16(7):677-694.

［10］ Balg F, Boileau P: The instability severity index score: A simple pre-operative score to select patients for arthroscopic or open shoulder stabilisation. *J Bone Joint Surg Br* 2007;89(11):1470-1477.

A 10-point preoperative instability severity index was created and evaluated through retrospective review of 131 patients. Points were assigned for age, sports participation, hyperlaxity, and bony deficiency. Patients with a score higher than 6 had a recurrence risk of 70%.

［11］ Piasecki DP, Verma NN, Romeo AA, Levine WN, Bach BR Jr, Provencher MT: Glenoid bone deficiency in recurrent anterior shoulder instability: Diagnosis and management. *J Am Acad Orthop Surg* 2009; 17(8):482-493.

An excellent review of glenoid bone loss is presented, with its relationship to recurrent shoulder instability and an algorithm for diagnosis and treatment.

［12］ Cetik O, Uslu M, Ozsar BK: The relationship between Hill-Sachs lesion and recurrent anterior shoulder dislocation. *Acta Orthop Belg* 2007;73(2):175-178.

In 30 patients with recurrent anterior dislocation, a positive correlation was found between a greater number of dislocations and greater extent and depth of a Hill-Sachs lesion.

［13］ Provencher MT, Bhatia S, Ghodadra NS, et al: Recurrent shoulder instability: Current concepts for evaluation and management of glenoid bone loss. *J Bone Joint Surg Am* 2010;92(suppl 2):133-151.

An update is provided on the evaluation, diagnosis, and treatment of patients with glenoid bone loss and recurrent shoulder instability.

［14］ Sugaya H, Moriishi J, Dohi M, Kon Y, Tsuchiya A: Glenoid rim morphology in recurrent anterior glenohumeral instability. *J Bone Joint Surg Am* 2003; 85(5):878-884.

［15］ Cho SH, Cho NS, Rhee YG: Preoperative analysis of the Hill-Sachs lesion in anterior shoulder instability: How to predict engagement of the lesion. *Am J Sports Med* 2011;39(11):2389-2395.

A review of 107 shoulders after arthroscopic Bankart repair for traumatic anterior shoulder instability used three-dimensional CT to evaluate Hill-Sachs lesions. Engaging Hill-Sachs lesions were larger and more horizontally oriented. Level of evidence: II.

［16］ Chuang TY, Adams CR, Burkhart SS: Use of preoperative three-dimensional computed tomography to quantify glenoid bone loss in shoulder instability. *Arthroscopy* 2008;24(4):376-382.

Recurrent instability and glenoid bone loss were reviewed with three-dimensional CT in 25 patients. Patients could be identified as needing an open procedure based on glenoid bone loss.

[17] Milano G, Grasso A, Russo A, et al: Analysis of risk factors for glenoid bone defect in anterior shoulder instability. *Am J Sports Med* 2011;39(9):1870-1876.

In a review of 161 patients with anterior shoulder instability, the number of dislocations and age at first dislocation were the most significant predictors of glenoid bone loss in anterior shoulder instability.

[18] Ozbaydar M, Elhassan B, Diller D, Massimini D, Higgins LD, Warner JJ: Results of arthroscopic capsulolabral repair: Bankart lesion versus anterior labroligamentous periosteal sleeve avulsion lesion. *Arthroscopy* 2008;24(11):1277-1283.

In a review of 93 shoulders with recurrent anterior shoulder instability, patients with an ALPSA lesion had more recurrent dislocations and a higher failure rate after arthroscopic capsulolabral repair than patients with a Bankart lesion alone.

[19] Hantes ME, Venouziou AI, Liantsis AK, Dailiana ZH, Malizos KN: Arthroscopic repair for chronic anterior shoulder instability: A comparative study between patients with Bankart lesions and patients with combined Bankart and superior labral anterior posterior lesions. *Am J Sports Med* 2009;37(6):1093-1098.

A review of 63 patients with anterior shoulder instability found no difference at 2-year follow-up in stability or function based on whether the patient had Bankart repair alone or combined Bankart and SLAP repair. Level of evidence: II.

[20] Shapiro TA, Gupta A, McGarry MH, Tibone JE, Lee TQ: Biomechanical effects of arthroscopic capsulorrhaphy in line with the fibers of the anterior band of the inferior glenohumeral ligament. *Am J Sports Med* 2012;40(3):672-680.

A cadaver study evaluated intact shoulders, shoulders with anterior instability, and arthroscopically plicated shoulders. A 10-mm arthroscopic plication in line with the fibers of the anterior band of the IGHL complex effectively reduced capsular laxity without overconstraining the joint.

[21] Randelli P, Arrigoni P, Polli L, Cabitza P, Denti M: Quantification of active ROM after arthroscopic Bankart repair with rotator interval closure. *Orthopedics* 2009;32(6):408.

Rotator cuff interval closure can provide anterior stability but results in a reduction of external rotation.

[22] Mologne TS, Zhao K, Hongo M, Romeo AA, An KN, Provencher MT: The addition of rotator interval closure after arthroscopic repair of either anterior or posterior shoulder instability: Effect on glenohumeral translation and range of motion. *Am J Sports Med* 2008;36(6):1123-1131.

Rotator cuff interval closure can improve anterior shoulder stability, but posterior stability is not improved.

[23] Buss DD, Lynch GP, Meyer CP, Huber SM, Freehill MQ: Nonoperative management for in-season athletes with anterior shoulder instability. *Am J Sports Med* 2004;32(6):1430-1433.

[24] Paterson WH, Throckmorton TW, Koester M, Azar FM, Kuhn JE: Position and duration of immobilization after primary anterior shoulder dislocation: A systematic review and meta-analysis of the literature. *J Bone Joint Surg Am* 2010;92(18):2924-2933.

A meta-analysis found no benefit to conventional sling immobilization of longer than 1 week for the treatment of primary anterior shoulder dislocation in relatively young patients. Bracing in external rotation may be less effective than believed.

[25] Owens BD, Harrast JJ, Hurwitz SR, Thompson TL, Wolf JM: Surgical trends in Bankart repair: An analysis of data from the American Board of Orthopaedic Surgery certification examination. *Am J Sports Med* 2011;39(9):1865-1869.

Data show that the number of arthroscopic shoulder stabilization procedures is increasing and the number of open repairs is decreasing. The overall rate of complications was lower overall after arthroscopic stabilization.

[26] Mahirogulları M, Ozkan H, Akyüz M, Ug̃ras, AA, Güney A, Kus,kucu M: Comparison between the results of open and arthroscopic repair of isolated traumatic anterior instability of the shoulder. *Acta Orthop Traumatol Turc* 2010;44(3):180-185.

Open and arthroscopic Bankart repairs for recurrent anterior shoulder instability were compared. The average follow-up was 26.1 months, and metal anchors were used in all patients. The results of both were similar in terms of recurrence and patient satisfaction.

[27] Petrera M, Patella V, Patella S, Theodoropoulos J: A meta-analysis of open versus arthroscopic Bankart repair using suture anchors. *Knee Surg Sports Traumatol Arthrosc* 2010;18(12):1742-1747.

A meta-analysis found that arthroscopic Bankart repair had better results than open repair in terms of recurrence in studies published later than 2002.

[28] Hobby J, Griffin D, Dunbar M, Boileau P: Is arthroscopic surgery for stabilisation of chronic shoulder instability as effective as open surgery? A systematic review and meta-analysis of 62 studies including 3044 arthroscopic operations. *J Bone Joint Surg Br* 2007;89(9):1188-1196.

A systematic literature search identified 62 studies of Bankart lesions treated arthroscopically or open. When the newest and most effective techniques were used, failure rates were similar at 2-year follow-up.

[29] Yamamoto N, Itoi E, Abe H, et al: Effect of an anterior glenoid defect on anterior shoulder stability: A cadaveric study. *Am J Sports Med* 2009;37(5):949-954.

In a laboratory cadaver study, 2-mm increments of glenoid bone were removed and stability was checked. A 20% loss at the 3-o'clock position significantly decreased anterior stability.

[30] Sugaya H, Moriishi J, Kanisawa I, Tsuchiya A: Arthroscopic osseous Bankart repair for chronic recurrent traumatic anterior glenohumeral instability: Surgical technique. *J Bone Joint Surg Am* 2006;88(suppl 1, Pt 2):159-169.

[31] Zhu YM, Jiang CY, Lu Y, Xue QY: Clinical results after all arthroscopic reduction and fixation of bony Bankart lesion. *Zhonghua Wai Ke Za Zhi* 2011;49(7): 603-606.

Forty patients with a bony Bankart lesion were treated all-arthroscopically using suture anchors, and the bony lesion was included in the repair. The recurrence rate was 8.9%.

[32] Ikeda H: "Rotator interval" lesion. Part 1: Clinical study. *Nihon Seikeigeka Gakkai Zasshi* 1986;60(12): 1261-1273.

[33] Hovelius L, Sandström B, Olofsson A, Svensson O, Rahme H: The effect of capsular repair, bone block healing, and position on the results of the Bristow-Latarjet procedure (study III): Long-term follow-up in 319 shoulders. *J Shoulder Elbow Surg* 2012;21(5): 647-660.

A review of the open Bristow-Latarjet procedure with long-term follow-up found consistently good results, with fusion in 83% of the patients. A medially placed coracoid (more than 1 cm) led to relatively poor re- sults.

[34] Millett PJ, Clavert P, Warner JJ: Open operative treatment for anterior shoulder instability: When and why? *J Bone Joint Surg Am* 2005;87(2):419-432.

[35] Park MJ, Tjoumakaris FP, Garcia G, Patel A, Kelly JD IV: Arthroscopic remplissage with Bankart repair for the treatment of glenohumeral instability with Hill- Sachs defects. *Arthroscopy* 2011;27(9):1187-1194.

A review of 20 patients who underwent arthroscopic Bankart repair with remplissage for recurrent anterior glenohumeral instability and a Hill-Sachs defect involving more than 25% of the humeral head found that 85% of the patients had a satisfactory result. Level of evidence: IV.

[36] Haviv B, Mayo L, Biggs D: Outcomes of arthroscopic "remplissage": Capsulotenodesis of the engaging large Hill-Sachs lesion. *J Orthop Surg Res* 2011;6:29.

A review of 11 patients who underwent arthroscopic surgery with remplissage for recurrent instability with a large engaging Hill-Sachs lesion found that the technique was effective with respect to recurrence, motion, and function.

[37] Zhu YM, Lu Y, Zhang J, Shen JW, Jiang CY: Arthroscopic Bankart repair combined with remplissage technique for the treatment of anterior shoulder instability with engaging Hill-Sachs lesion: A report of 49 cases with a minimum 2-year follow-up. *Am J Sports Med* 2011;39(8):1640-1647.

A review of 49 patients with an engaging Hill-Sachs lesion who underwent arthroscopic Bankart repair and remplissage found a failure rate of 8.2% at a mean 29-month follow-up, with no significant impairment of shoulder function. Level of evidence: IV.

[38] Nourissat G, Kilinc AS, Werther JR, Doursounian L: A prospective, comparative, radiological, and clinical study of the influence of the "remplissage" procedure on shoulder range of motion after stabilization by arthroscopic Bankart repair. *Am J Sports Med* 2011; 39(10):2147-2152.

Patients with Bankart repair alone and patients with Bankart repair and remplissage had identical recurrence rates and no difference in shoulder range of motion. One third of the patients had posterosuperior pain. Level of evidence: II.

[39] Dewing CB, Horan MP, Millett PJ: Two-year outcomes of open shoulder anterior capsular reconstruction for instability from severe capsular deficiency. *Arthroscopy* 2012;28(1):43-51.

Allograft reconstruction of anterior capsulolabral structures for capsular deficiency was performed on 22 shoulders. Outcomes were satisfactory in terms of recurrence and function. Level of evidence: IV.

[40] Chechik O, Maman E, Dolkart O, Khashan M, Shabtai L, Mozes G: Arthroscopic rotator interval closure in

shoulder instability repair: A retrospective study. *J Shoulder Elbow Surg* 2010;19(7):1056-1062.

There was an additive effect on shoulder stability in 37 patients who underwent arthroscopic rotator cuff interval closure in addition to arthroscopic Bankart repair. Systemic hyperlaxity was associated with recurrent dislocation and poor outcome.

[41] van der Linde JA, van Kampen DA, Terwee CB, Dijksman LM, Kleinjan G, Willems WJ: Long-term results after arthroscopic shoulder stabilization using suture anchors: An 8- to 10-year follow-up. *Am J Sports Med* 2011;39(11):2396-2403.

Sixty-eight shoulders treated for anterior instability with arthroscopic Bankart repair were followed for 8 to 10 years. The presence of a Hill-Sachs defect and the use of more than three anchors increased the risk of recurrence. Level of evidence: IV.

[42] Milano G, Grasso A, Santagada DA, Saccomanno MF, Deriu L, Fabbriciani C: Comparison between metal and biodegradable suture anchors in the arthroscopic treatment of traumatic anterior shoulder instability: A prospective randomized study. *Knee Surg Sports Traumatol Arthrosc* 2010;18(12):1785-1791.

Arthroscopic stabilization was performed in 78 patients with recurrent anterior shoulder instability. Patients were compared based on the use of metal or biodegradable anchors. At 2-year follow-up, there was no difference in recurrence rates.

[43] Slabaugh MA, Friel NA, Wang VM, Cole BJ: Restoring the labral height for treatment of Bankart lesions: A comparison of suture anchor constructs. *Arthroscopy* 2010;26(5):587-591.

The Bio-Suture Tak (Arthrex, Naples, FL) and Push-Lock (Arthrex) suture anchors were compared for Bankart lesion restoration in 10 cadaver glenoids. A three-dimensional digitizer was used to measure re- stored labral height after fixation. No difference was noted.

[44] Oh JH, Lee HK, Kim JY, Kim SH, Gong HS: Clinical and radiologic outcomes of arthroscopic glenoid labrum repair with the BioKnotless suture anchor. *Am J Sports Med* 2009;37(12):2340-2348.

Arthroscopic glenoid labral repair was performed with the BioKnotless anchor (DePuy, Warsaw, IN) in 97 patients who were followed for a mean 34.1 months. The anchors were found to be comparable to standard metal anchors without knot tying. Level of evidence: IV.

[45] Thal R, Nofziger M, Bridges M, Kim JJ: Arthroscopic Bankart repair using Knotless or BioKnotless suture anchors: 2- to 7-year results. *Arthroscopy* 2007;23(4): 367-375.

Arthroscopic Bankart repair was performed in 73 patients using knotless or BioKnotless suture anchors. At a minimum 2-year follow-up, the recurrence rate was 6.9%, and all patients had a reliable return of function.

[46] Monteiro GC, Ejnisman B, Andreoli CV, de Castro Pochini A, Cohen M: Absorbable versus nonabsorbable sutures for the arthroscopic treatment of anterior shoulder instability in athletes: A prospective randomized study. *Arthroscopy* 2008;24(6):697-703.

Anchors with absorbable and nonabsorbable suture were compared in the treatment of arthroscopic Bankart repair. No differences were found between the two types of anchors at a minimum 24-month follow-up.

[47] Yan H, Cui GQ, Wang JQ, Yin Y, Tian DX, Ao YF: Arthroscopic Bankart repair with suture anchors: Results and risk factors of recurrence of instability. *Zhonghua Wai Ke Za Zhi* 2011;49(7):597-602.

Arthroscopic Bankart repair with suture anchors was performed in 259 patients with recurrent shoulder instability. At a minimum 1-year follow-up, patients younger than 20 years and athletes were at high risk for recurrence.

[48] Porcellini G, Campi F, Pegreffi F, Castagna A, Paladini P: Predisposing factors for recurrent shoulder dislocation after arthroscopic treatment. *J Bone Joint Surg Am* 2009;91(11):2537-2542.

A review of 385 patients who underwent arthroscopic Bankart repair for unidirectional instability found that age younger than 22 years, age at time of first dislocation, and male sex were risk factors for recurrence at 36-month follow-up.

[49] Uhorchak JM, Arciero RA, Huggard D, Taylor DC: Recurrent shoulder instability after open reconstruction in athletes involved in collision and contact sports. *Am J Sports Med* 2000;28(6):794-799.

[50] Pagnani MJ, Dome DC: Surgical treatment of traumatic anterior shoulder instability in American football players. *J Bone Joint Surg Am* 2002;84-A(5):711-715.

[51] Ide J, Maeda S, Takagi K: Arthroscopic Bankart repair using suture anchors in athletes: Patient selection and postoperative sports activity. *Am J Sports Med* 2004; 32(8):1899-1905.

[52] Mazzocca AD, Brown FM, Carreira DS, Hayden J, Romeo AA: Arthroscopic anterior shoulder stabilization of collision and contact athletes. *Am J Sports Med* 2005;33(1):52-60.

第十一章 投掷运动员的肩关节损伤

John Tokish, MD; Kelly Fitzpatrick, DO

引言

对投掷运动员肩关节损伤的治疗一直是一个挑战。由于存在很高的应力和力学要求，投掷运动员肩关节的病理生理学非常特殊。投掷运动员的肩关节旋转角速度可达到 7000°/s，这是所有体育活动中被报道的最快角速度。[1] 投掷运动员的肩关节通过外旋增加、内旋减少、肱骨及肩胛盂后倾增加和前方关节囊松弛来适应功能要求。在每一次投掷中，肩关节周围的软组织都受到应力影响，投掷肩的继发改变和功能要求导致其更容易发生以下病变，如部分肩袖撕裂、前方关节囊松弛或假性松弛、后上方关节囊挛缩、后方或后上方盂唇损伤、肱二头肌腱病变以及肩胛带肌功能异常。[2]

治疗肩关节投掷活动障碍的主要挑战是区分病理性改变和正常适应性改变。"全处理"会导致投掷活动不能恢复到之前的水平。因此，整个手术团队应该进行谨慎的术前评估、细致的手术操作并制订合理的术后康复计划，以治疗功能恢复需求高的运动员。

Neither of the following authors nor any immediate family member has received anything of value from or has stock or stock options held in a commercial company or institution related directly or indirectly to the subject of this chapter: Dr. Tokish and Dr. Fitzpatrick.

生物力学

投掷运动员必须尽力追求更快的投掷速度。肩关节不仅需要在最大的活动范围、最大的应力条件下达到最快的速度，还必须有足够的稳定性来保证其位于中心并为活动提供稳定的杠杆。投掷动作分为 6 个时期（图 11-1，表 11-1）。第一期为准备期，身体通过腿部、躯干和核心开始把力量传递到肩关节。该期盂肱关节所受应力很小。挥臂早期手臂外展和外旋。挥臂晚期，手臂达到最大外旋后开始向目标移动，前方结构紧张并且肩袖产生的应力高达 650 N。[3] 加速期始于前臂开始内旋时，结束于球脱手的瞬间。这一期的特点是上肢产生最快的速度。大部分能量于此期传递到球，而盂肱关节所受应力很小。球脱手之后立即进入减速期，此时肩关节及其周围软组织须承受不同方向上的应力。肩关节所受的牵张力可高达 950 N，压力高于 1000 N，且后方剪切力可高达 400 N。[3-4] 在跟随期，应力开始恢复至正常，同时压力减小至 400 N。

年轻的普通人在自然状态下关节囊的失效负荷是 800~1200 N。这样就可以理解为什么投掷运动员容易受伤，以及为什么优化投掷力学非常重要。一项针对年轻投掷运动员的研究发现，与力学环境不佳的投掷者相比，正常的力学环境可以减少肱骨内旋扭矩，并降低肘关节外翻负荷。[5]

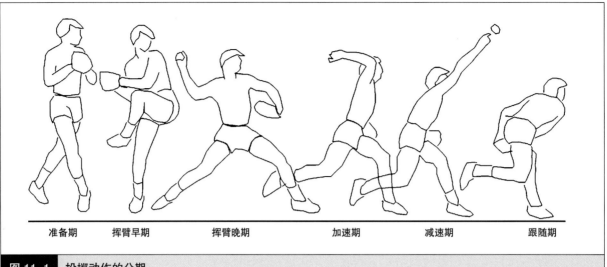

| 准备期 | 挥臂早期 | 挥臂晚期 | 加速期 | 减速期 | 跟随期 |

图 11-1 投掷动作的分期

表 11-1

投掷动作的分期（右手投掷运动员）

分期	描述	评价
准备期	双手握球，身体保持平衡。左脚沿本垒之间的连线向后退一小步，右脚随后平行于投手板（一些教练让投掷运动员将脚楔入投手板以便使躯体外侧位于投手板上方）。左下肢处于一个受控的、活跃的状态，并且髋关节仍处于水平并指向本垒。当髋关节开始活动，会构成一个以髋关节为尖，躯干和右脚为两边的 V 字形。髋关节指向击球手。然后，脱下右手手套并握住球	这是所有成功投掷的要素，投掷运动员挥臂期会根据个人习惯提高重心 在该分期，肩关节相对不参与运动。双肩移动缓慢，双手合拢，肌肉活动性差
挥臂早期	手从上方抓住球。肩关节随后在肩胛骨平面抬高大约 100° 并外旋大约 45°。随着髋关节继续朝本垒活动，V 字形变得更加明显。髋关节保持水平，并尽可能推迟旋转。对击球者隐藏球，使其不能判断投掷的方向。左腿缓慢而轻松地放下，直至脚触及土堆	手的起始位置使肩关节位于内旋位，该位置对盂肱关节而言是一个安全的位置 三角肌和冈上肌共同作用外展肱骨。其他肩袖肌肉不活动
挥臂晚期	左脚与土堆接触，落于右脚的宽度之内并指向本垒。降低核心，释放能量，将重量均匀分布于两脚之间。躯干于直立位保持平衡，尽量延迟躯干旋转	目标是让肱骨最大程度外旋。肱骨保持高于肩胛骨平面水平并从 46° 外旋至 170° 三角肌和冈上肌活动减少，但是其他肩袖肌肉活动增加以稳定关节。斜方肌中部、菱形肌、肩胛提肌和前锯肌活动，使肩胛骨为肱骨头提供有效的支撑
加速期	加速期始于肱骨内旋，大约为 0.05 s，球以 161 km/h 的速度离开手掌。两脚位于土堆 手臂的加速和身体其余部分的减速相配合，将能量传递至上肢和球	该活动需在双脚稳定的基础上进行 盂肱关节和肩胛胸壁关节相关肌肉的协同收缩使上肢稳定且能够快速地活动
减速期	球脱手后右髋关节被带至左腿上方。右脚离地，身体核心则在控制下降低	从手臂活动开始，将未传递至球的动能传递至大的肌肉
跟随期	放下手臂	作用于手臂的力量减小

注：经允许引自 McMahon PJ, Tibone JE, Pink MM: Functional anatomy and biomechanics of the shoulder, in Delee JC, Drez D Jr, Miller MD, eds: *Delee and Drez's Orthopaedic Sports Medicine*: Principles and Practice, ed 2. Philadelphia, PA, Saunders, 2003, p 850.

肩关节投掷障碍

　　阐述肩关节投掷障碍的假说有很多。对于其相关病理学因素的认识一直在发展，同时诊断和手术技术也随时间在改进。1959年，肩胛盂后下方骨软骨瘤被描述为职业投掷运动员肩关节疼痛的病因，激发于后方关节囊和肱三头肌腱的反复牵拉。[6]这个假说随后逐渐不被认同，尽管最近后方关节囊病变的重要性再次被认识到。撞击综合征于1972年被报道并且最初作为肩关节投掷疼痛的一个病因。[7]肩关节投掷疼痛的症状和体征与撞击综合征的表现有重叠，并且肩袖也经常被累及。然而，1985年一项针对接受肩峰成形术治疗撞击患者的研究发现，即使疼痛缓解效果不错，但是18名运动员中只有4名重返投掷运动。[8]

　　20世纪90年代，继发撞击假说得到发展，该假说认为撞击的原因是反复的前方关节囊牵拉造成的前方肩关节不稳定。通过肩胛下肌劈开入路减少关节囊容量能使疼痛显著缓解，但是术后能否重返高水平的投掷运动仍然是不确切的。[9]

　　到20世纪90年代后期，关节镜逐渐变成评估投掷肩的一个重要辅助工具。后上方肩胛盂的肩袖撞击称为内撞击，被认为是由前方松弛或反复外展外旋应力导致的微小不稳定造成的。前方不稳定常存在于投掷运动员中并与内撞击相关。[10-11]然而，关节镜检查16名存在内撞击但无不稳定的投掷运动员后发现，外展外旋位肩袖撞击导致部分肩袖撕裂和后方关节囊损伤。[12]一项关于网球运动员的研究发现有症状的内撞击可以发生于没有前方不稳定或松弛的主力侧肩关节。[13]松弛一直是肩关节投掷障碍的一个影响因素并且最近也被认为是血管损伤的一个可能因素。[14]在投球50次后评估投掷对上肢血流的作用，合并松弛的专业运动员只有35%的血流增加，而无松弛征象的运动员血流增加115%。

　　在2003年，有研究者对内撞击本身是一个继发于后上方关节囊挛缩的病理而非生理现象这一观点提出质疑。[2]后方关节囊增厚最近被发现是投掷肩的一种适应性改变。[15]后上方关节囊挛缩被认为能使肱骨向后上方移动，新形成的接触方式会导致在有投掷障碍的肩关节中所见的肩袖和盂唇病变。[2]盂肱关节内旋障碍（GIRD）是投掷肩的特点。其他研究证实了投掷肩中GIRD的高发病率，以及纠正GIRD能缓解症状。[2,16-17]然而，对于这个概念的支持证据也存在争议。在2006年，最初支持GIRD的生物力学研究者修正了他们的模型，发现移位及与此同时的关节囊挛缩实际上是在前下方发生的，并且发生于跟随期而不是挥臂期。[18]另外，GIRD被发现存在于大概40%的无症状投掷运动员。[19]最近的研究证据提示过度的水平外展是内撞击的关键原因。[20]实际上，肩关节投掷障碍可能代表的是当个体的解剖和生理为适应超过正常生理极限的情况而产生的一系列改变。

常见的病理后遗症

　　无论何种病因，投掷肩都会有一些常见的后遗症，包括SLAP损伤、近端肱二头肌病变、部分肩袖损伤及肩胛运动障碍。投掷肩的最早描述见于1985年，当时肱二头肌抗张力失效被假设为其损伤机制，并且最初的治疗方式是清理。[21]然而，还有一种理论认为SLAP损伤产生于脱壳机制，即外旋肩关节产生肱二头肌起点的应力导致的撕裂，被称为对投掷肩损伤的致命一击。[2,22]

　　肩袖损伤可能是投掷肩最常见的病理改变。全层撕裂不常见，但是关节面侧的部分撕裂普遍存在于投掷运动员并被认为是由急性张力和（或）反复偏心活动的微损伤所导致的。这些撕裂被描述为发生在后上方的冈上肌和冈下肌止点的结合点，并被认为是内撞击的结果。[12,23]

　　随着对肩关节力学的认识进步，肩胛盂的位置成为评估投掷运动员肩关节疼痛的一个重要内容。对肩胛运动障碍概念进行大量临床研究发现，肩胛盂的位置对撞击和前方不稳定很重要。[24]SICK

肩胛骨综合征指的是肩胛骨位置异常（scapular malposition）、内下缘凸起（inferior medial border prominence）、喙突疼痛和位置异常（coracoid pain and malposition）以及肩胛骨活动的力学异常（dyskinesis of scapular movement）。[25]肩胛骨活动的力学异常可能源于肩胛骨周围肌肉的不平衡、肌力弱或神经损伤，最近的一些研究提示在肩关节投掷障碍中，肌肉功能不足是肩胛骨动力障碍的危险因素之一。在有投掷相关疼痛史的青少年投球运动员中发现，其中部分投球运动员的斜方肌和冈上肌较没有疼痛的投球运动员的更薄弱。[26]另外的研究发现在专业投球者中也有类似的情况。赛季前存在外旋肌和冈上肌肌力弱的投掷运动员与不存在该情况的投掷运动员相比，前者出现赛季中投掷相关损伤并需要手术干预的风险要更高。[27]采用单性能疲劳模型发现投掷运动员的外旋肌受主观意志控制的力量减弱。[28]这项研究的结论是预防疲劳和增强神经肌肉刺激的康复策略有可能预防投掷运动的相关损伤。

临床评估

病史和体格检查

肩关节投掷障碍的患者绝大多数都在挥臂期或跟随期存在后方肩关节疼痛。很多患者可能描述一种肩关节失控、失速感或一种"死臂"感。体格检查可能出现压痛、外旋增加和内旋减少、不稳定或松弛、后方撞击试验阳性以及更多的传统撞击征象。[29-30]内旋较对侧减少超过20°（于盂肱关节外展90°测量），尤其是在活动范围减小的情况下，则提示GIRD（图11-2）。对于这样的患者，检查者必须关注运动员的核心力量、肩胛骨和任何相关的肩关节病变。在SICK肩胛骨综合征或肩胛骨动力障碍中，可以经常看到当患者反复抬起和放下手臂或启动肩胛骨动态稳定结构时，肩胛骨静态的或动态的位置异常。[25]其他关键的体格检查包括疼痛复位试验阳性（提示肩关节微不稳定）、主动挤压试验阳性（提示SLAP损伤）以及睡眠伸展时疼痛。

影像学检查

肩关节投掷障碍的影像学检查应包括标准系列X线片，但是X线片表现经常是正常的。最重要的检查还是MRI和MRA，这两种检查对于发现盂唇病变、肩袖和肱二头肌病变、关节囊增厚、滑囊病变以及骨水肿有更高的准确性。CT不是常规检查，但是如果在最初的X线片中有骨性异常则可能需要进行CT检查。

治疗

非手术治疗

因为投掷运动员有很强的适应性和很大程度

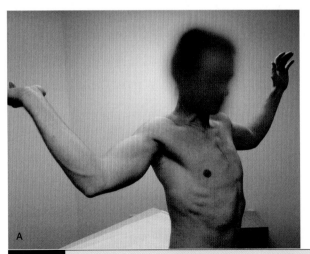
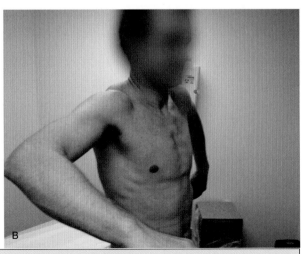

图11-2　临床照片显示盂肱关节内旋减少。A. 与对侧相比，右侧肩关节的外旋增加。B. 右侧肩关节内旋受限角度与盂肱关节内旋受限角度一致

的病理性改变，所以很难为投掷肩患者设计良好的对照研究。对很多运动员来说，非手术治疗可以帮助他们成功地避免手术。投掷动作是一条从近端向远端传递能量的运动链（表11-2）。任何此链中的缺陷都可能会转变为一个更远端的损伤。因此，肩关节投掷障碍的成功非手术治疗需要包括修复运动链的每一个环节，包括肩关节本身。髋和腿的力量必须加以维持，且核心力量决不能忽视。肩胛平台必须优化，因为这是核心力量转换成肩关节速度的关键点。肩关节的康复包括肩胛骨、动态稳定结构和后方关节囊的治疗。SICK肩胛骨综合征可以通过保留肩胛骨的力学环境得到有效治疗。[25]

肩袖肌力弱在投掷肩疼痛中非常常见，并且肩袖的力量增强是任何非手术治疗的关键点。大多数投掷类运动员存在肩关节后方关节囊紧张，其症状可以通过伸展锻炼来缓解，例如睡眠者伸展（图11-3）。与参与短期伸展项目的投球运动员相比，参与内旋伸展项目数年的投球运动员具有更好的内旋和总的活动范围。[31]

在大多数患者中，这个综合的方法是有效的。一项最近的研究报道了研究者跟踪一个职业联盟棒球队超过3年的经历。[17]其中，很多投球运动员有

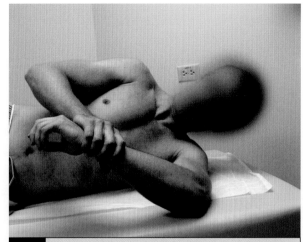

| 图 11-3 | 睡眠者伸展。患者侧卧，患侧在下，将手臂推向地面。对于GIRD患者，这个动作强调对后方关节囊的拉伸 |

GIRD的体征和症状，但是绝大多数经过严密的康复锻炼后得到了缓解。患有GIRD的40个投球运动员中只有3个需要手术。另一个研究发现采用睡眠者伸展和肩胛胸壁关节康复为主的非手术治疗对96个投掷运动员的恢复效果是100%。[25]

手术治疗

如果经过充分的非手术治疗没有效果，患者则应考虑接受手术治疗。在手术治疗之前应该制订与损伤相关的康复计划（表11-3）。患侧和健

表11-2

投掷力学和非手术治疗的缺陷

运动链断裂点	结果	治疗
在准备期或跨步时过早地向前活动	手臂滞后于躯体	加强核心肌肉
双腿并拢	减少骨盆-躯体旋转 投掷运动员必须经过身体投掷，减少运动链的动力生成	增强髋关节外旋肌群的力量
双腿分开	骨盆过早旋转 不匹配的运动链 手臂滞后于躯体 肩部必须产生更多的力量以维持速度	增强髋关节内旋肌群的力量
直立位投掷（躯干前倾缺失）	加速力量作用于球的距离变短 产生的速度减慢	加强核心肌群的力量
出球时引导膝的屈曲增加	躯干前方屈曲和旋转产生的动力减少	拉伸腘绳肌
内旋消失	加速力量作用于球的距离变短	睡眠者伸展
肩胛骨动力异常	挥臂晚期的肱骨外旋消失（肩胛骨回撤减少） 肩峰下撞击	稳定肩胛骨

表 11-3

投掷运动员的综合处理

诊断	体格检查发现	非手术治疗	手术治疗
微小不稳定	恐惧试验阳性	稳定肩胛骨	有限的关节囊轴移
内撞击	撞击征阳性	稳定肩胛骨 增强肩袖 睡眠者伸展	肩袖清理（±SLAP 清理）或修复
SLAP 损伤	主动挤压试验阳性	休息	SLAP 清理或修复
GIRD	疼痛伴内旋减少	睡眠者伸展	有限的后方关节囊松解
关节侧部分肩袖撕裂	肩袖检查时疼痛或肌力弱	增强肩袖	清理或修复

侧的肩关节都应在麻醉下进行检查。着重观察松弛的类型和活动范围的差异。特别要注意的是在90°外展位下稳定肩胛骨进行内旋和外旋检查，因为该检查能够发现 GIRD。检查完后再进行体位摆放和肩关节铺单。

标准的后入路位于肩峰后外侧边缘下方和内侧约 2 cm 处。标准的前入路于直视下建立于肩袖间隙。将这个通道置于肩袖间隙可方便后上方肩胛盂和肩袖的显露。用探针评估投掷肩常见的病变。注意观察肱二头肌腱及其附着点，以及上方盂唇。鉴别正常的盂唇隐窝和 SLAP 损伤很重要。如果怀疑存在不稳定，则应该用探针仔细检查前后盂唇（图 11-4）。应该仔细观察冈上肌和冈下肌的下表面，因为部分肩袖损伤是投掷肩损伤中很典型的表现。必须反复对肩关节进行动态检查，包括外展外旋位（内撞击的位置）。后上方盂唇和肩袖后方的接触通常是病

理性的，并且需要仔细检查是否存在由后剥效应导致的肱二头肌从后上方盂唇剥脱。内撞击可通过清理或修复治疗，主要依据损伤的程度选择治疗方式。

关节面侧的部分撕裂较经典的肩袖撕裂更偏后，可通过将手臂的牵引去除并将其置于外展外旋位观察。虽然有研究报道原位修复治疗运动员恢复投掷的结果良好，但是最常用的方法是切除创面（图 11-5）。[11] 全层损伤的修复并不一定能让投掷运动员恢复投掷，并且需要注意不要过分激进地切除创面或将部分损伤转变为全层撕裂修复。有研究报道，恢复投掷的比例为 25%~87%，治疗合并的病变具有更好的结果[21,32-33]（表 11-4）。

SLAP 损伤延伸至后方肱二头肌腱根部的情况常见于投掷肩障碍。必须注意区分真正的 SLAP 病理性撕裂和在后剥效应下适应性改变所致的盂唇分离。SLAP 损伤的产生仍然存在争论，但是

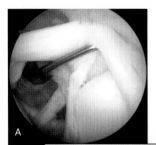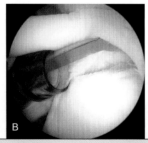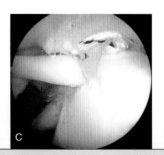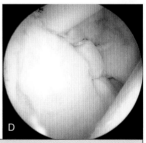

图 11-4　关节镜照片显示 SLAP 修复。A. 肱二头肌异常脱落和活动性异常。B. 采用 liberator 或刨刀进行上方肩胛盂的准备以促进出血。C. 修复的后方视角，线结远离肩胛盂以避免肩关节活动时磨损软骨。D. 修复的前方视角。经允许引自 Keener KD, Brophy RH: Superior labral tears of the shoulder: Pathogenesis, evaluation, and treatment. *J Am Orthop Surg* 2009;17:627-637.

这可能是疼痛产生的原因，可造成不稳定的感觉，并影响投掷的速度和准确性。

　　有很多 SLAP 损伤修复的手术技巧可收到很好的效果。基本的方法包括关节镜诊断（图 11-4）。用一枚探针评估上方盂唇的完整性并区分盂唇隐窝和真正的 SLAP 损伤。真正的 SLAP 损伤会向内延伸至肩胛盂的软骨部分且会导致活动性异常。使用关节镜刨刀或 liberator 去除纤维软骨以获得正常出血的基底，从而促进修复的愈合。过线器或类似的

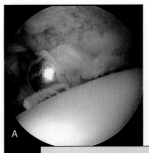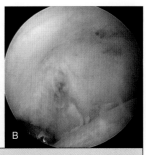

图 11-5　关节镜照片显示关节面侧的部分肩袖撕裂伴磨损。A. 有限清理前。B. 有限清理后。进行有限清理是为了避免影响肩袖完整性

表 11-4

投掷运动员肩袖病变的研究

研究发表（年份）	患者类型（数量）	处理	结果
Reynolds 等[33]（2008）	竞技性棒球投球者（82 例）	清理部分肩袖撕裂	55% 恢复至之前的竞技水平
Andrews 等[21]（1985）	投掷运动员（36 例，包括 23 例棒球投球者）	清理关节侧部分肩袖撕裂	85% 重返比赛；76% 恢复至之前的竞技水平
Conway[11]（2001）	棒球运动员（9 例）	修复肌腱内的肩袖撕裂	89% 恢复至之前的竞技水平或更高的竞技水平
Ferrari 等[32]（1994）	竞技性棒球投球者（7 例）	清理肩袖撕裂（包括或不包括盂唇）	85% 重返运动

器械用于上方盂唇的简单缝合或褥式缝合。不稳定的 SLAP 损伤应该修复，但是必须避免修复过紧导致的肱二头肌腱嵌顿。不要试图将肱二头肌锚定于肩胛盂表面，这项操作可能出现于修复盂唇治疗不稳定时。术者应该考虑移除小部分撞击肩胛盂的结构并使用低切迹技术，例如，无线结或褥式修复。这些方法如果不能成功可能会导致缝线与肩袖止点接触。

　　过顶投掷运动员的 SLAP 损伤修复目前只有零星的报告（表 11-5）。最初的研究报道了 100% 的修复率，87% 的运动员恢复了之前的竞技水平，但是这样的结果并未在其他研究中出现。[34-35] 最近，一篇系统性综述收集了包含棒球投球者的 5 项研究，其报道 SLAP 损伤修复后恢复竞技的比

表 11-5

过顶投掷运动员肩袖病变的研究

研究发表（年份）	患者类型（数量）	处理	结果
Morgan 等[35]（1998）	投掷运动员（102 例，包括 37 例棒球投球者）	SLAP 修复	87% 恢复至之前的竞技水平
Kim 等[37]（2002）	过顶投掷运动员（18 例）	SLAP 修复	只有 22% 恢复至之前的竞技水平
Reinold 等[38]（2003）	投掷运动员（130 例，包括 105 例棒球投球者）	SLAP 修复及关节囊热挛缩	87% 重返比赛；修复加关节囊热挛缩的结果优于单纯修复
Ide 等[39]（2005）	棒球投球者（19 例）	SLAP 修复	63% 恢复至之前的竞技水平；棒球投球者的结果较其他过顶投掷运动员的结果差
Neuman 等[40]（2011）	过顶投掷运动员（30）	SLAP 修复	84% 恢复至之前的竞技水平；满意率为 93%

例为 22%~64%。[34]

如果非手术治疗对 GIRD 患者无效，则应该在关节镜下仔细评估其后方关节囊的增厚（图 11-6）。极少数的患者可以考虑采用后方关节囊松解来维持部分的内旋。电刀能提供一个安全的边界，因为电刀靠近神经会引起肌肉收缩从而警示术者。关节镜钻头也可以被小心地使用于关节囊盂唇交界处选择性的关节囊松解。无论使用什么方法，

都需要靠近肩胛盂松解，因为该部位能为腋神经提供最好的缓冲。对投掷运动员的 GIRD 采用后方关节囊松解很少见于同行评审的文献中。如采用该方法，则疼痛缓解较可靠，但恢复投掷的效果相对可靠性较低。[36]16 例运动员中的 11 例（69%）恢复到伤前的竞技水平。只有 4 例存在单纯后下方关节囊紧张，这些发现提示投掷肩的病理复杂性。[36]

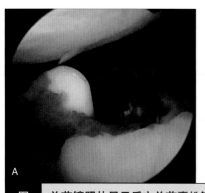 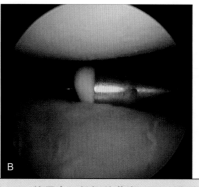 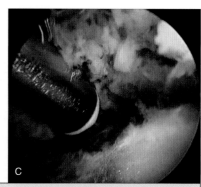

图 11-6　关节镜照片显示后方关节囊松解。A. 使用电刀松解关节囊，可以看到后方关节囊特征性增厚。B. 可用探钩进行更准确的松解。C. 紧贴肩胛盂近端松解以防止腋神经损伤

康复

投掷肩手术必须要有术后计划。术者必须与运动员训练员沟通，以保证软组织在早期活动中以及肌肉节奏与力量训练中得到保护。运动员核心力量的维持计划应不受手术影响。术后应立刻开始对肩胛骨平台的再训练，应该包含肩胛骨的前后伸展、上下活动和内外旋转（图 11-7）。如果手术纠正不包含修复，那么应鼓励患者尽快恢复手臂的主被动活动范围。活动需加以管理以保证正确地稳定肩胛骨肌肉。在正确的节奏下完成早期活动后，过渡至力量和速度训练并重新建立肩胛骨平台和躯体核心的连接。从低负荷、低速锻炼开始过渡至模拟竞技体育的多平面、高负荷、高速活动。不能忽视耐力因素，因为疲劳会导致不良的力学机制并对恢复竞技不利。

当运动员恢复牢固的核心力量、全范围活动、

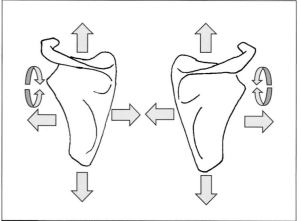

图 11-7　肩胛骨平台的再训练过程中主要肩胛骨周围肌肉活动的示意图。外侧和内侧箭头分别代表前锯肌、胸小肌、斜方肌和菱形肌作用下的前后活动。上下箭头分别代表菱形肌、肩胛提肌、胸小肌和背阔肌作用下的上下活动。环形箭头示斜方肌、前锯肌、肩胛提肌、菱形肌和胸小肌作用下的上下旋转

有效的力量和合适的肩胛骨节奏时，可以在专业运动员训练员的管理下开始恢复投掷的康复计划。最开始，运动员需描述自己在低速下启动投掷的能力、活动范围恢复的程度、核心力量以及肩胛骨稳定性。

恢复投掷的训练计划与早期活动的过渡原则一致。投掷从低速开始，采用重量较轻的球，投掷相对短的距离。如果投掷活动中存在任何缺陷则停止进一步的康复。随着运动员的恢复，距离、速度和重复次数可以逐渐增加至竞技要求的完整活动水平。此时，增加活动次数以适应竞技要求。康复计划必须个体化，对任何盂唇或肩袖的修复都需要加以保护直至愈合，并施以必要的制动措施。

总结

投掷肩的治疗一直是一个挑战。投掷肩通常合并多种病变，包括盂唇和肩袖的撕裂、病理性松弛以及后方关节囊紧张。非手术治疗对大多数患者是有效的。当有必要进行手术治疗时，术者必须仔细鉴别适应性的解剖改变和病理变化。恢复投掷绝不是仅通过手术治疗就能完成的。需要团队精细合作，术后肩关节应进行合理的运动链康复以适应投掷运动极端的功能要求。

参考文献

［1］ Fleisig GS, Andrews JR: *The Athlete's Shoulder*. New York, NY, Churchill Livingstone, 1994, pp 360-365.

［2］ Burkhart SS, Morgan CD, Kibler WB: The disabled throwing shoulder: Spectrum of pathology. Part I: Pathoanatomy and biomechanics. *Arthroscopy* 2003; 19(4):404-420.

［3］ Fleisig GS, Andrews JR, Dillman CJ, Escamilla RF: Kinetics of baseball pitching with implications about injury mechanisms. *Am J Sports Med* 1995;23(2): 233-239.

［4］ Kuhn J, Lindholm SR, Huston LJ: Failure of the biceps superior labral complex (SLAP lesion) in the throwing athlete: A biomechanical model comparing maximal cocking to early deceleration. *J Shoulder Elbow Surg* 2000;9(463):463.

［5］ Davis JT, Limpisvasti O, Fluhme D, et al: The effect of pitching biomechanics on the upper extremity in youth and adolescent baseball pitchers. *Am J Sports Med* 2009;37(8):1484-1491.

Quantitative motion analysis and high-speed video were used to assess baseball pitching mechanics based on biomechanical parameters (hip, hand, arm, shoulder, and foot position) in 169 pitchers age 9 to 18 years. Pitchers with three or more correct parameters had lower humeral internal rotation torque, lower elbow valgus load, and greater pitching efficiency.

［6］ Bennett GE: Elbow and shoulder lesions of baseball players. *Am J Surg* 1959;98:484-492.

［7］ Neer CS II: Anterior acromioplasty for the chronic impingement syndrome in the shoulder: A preliminary report. *J Bone Joint Surg Am* 1972;54(1):41-50.

［8］ Tibone JE, Jobe FW, Kerlan RK, et al: Shoulder impingement syndrome in athletes treated by an anterior acromioplasty. *Clin Orthop Relat Res* 1985;198: 134-140.

［9］ Jobe FW, Giangarra CE, Kvitne RS, Glousman RE: Anterior capsulolabral reconstruction of the shoulder in athletes in overhand sports. *Am J Sports Med* 1991; 19(5):428-434.

［10］ Paley KJ, Jobe FW, Pink MM, Kvitne RS, ElAttrache NS: Arthroscopic findings in the overhand throwing athlete: Evidence for posterior internal impingement of the rotator cuff. *Arthroscopy* 2000;16(1):35-40.

［11］ Conway JE: Arthroscopic repair of partial-thickness rotator cuff tears and SLAP lesions in professional baseball players. *Orthop Clin North Am* 2001;32(3): 443-456.

［12］ Walch G, Boileau P, Noel E, Donell ST: Impingement of the deep surface of the supraspinatus tendon on the posterosuperior glenoid rim: An arthroscopic study. *J Shoulder Elbow Surg* 1992;1(5):238-245.

［13］ Sonnery-Cottet B, Edwards TB, Noel E, Walch G: Results of arthroscopic treatment of posterosuperior glenoid impingement in tennis players. *Am J Sports Med* 2002;30(2):227-232.

［14］ Bast SC, Weaver FA, Perese S, Jobe FW, Weaver DC, Vangsness CT Jr: The effects of shoulder laxity on upper extremity blood flow in professional baseball pitchers. *J Shoulder Elbow Surg* 2011;20(3):461-466.

Eighteen male professional baseball pitchers were examined for signs of shoulder laxity (positive sulcus sign or relocation test), and a vascular examination was performed before and after a 50-pitch session. The 10 pitchers without a sign of laxity had an average arterial volume flow increase of 115%, but the pitchers who had a laxity sign had only a 35% increase in blood flow.

[15] Thomas SJ, Swanik CB, Higginson JS, et al: A bilateral comparison of posterior capsule thickness and its correlation with glenohumeral range of motion and scapular upward rotation in collegiate baseball players. *J Shoulder Elbow Surg* 2011;20(5):708-716.
Posterior capsular thickness was measured in both shoulders of baseball players. The authors found a significantly greater thickness in the dominant throwing arm, which was negatively correlated with internal rotation.

[16] Verna C: Shoulder flexibility to reduce impingement. *3rd PBATS Book of Abstracts.* Ellicott City, MD, Professional Baseball Athletic Trainer Society, 1991, abstract 18.

[17] Wilk KE, Macrina LC, Fleisig GS, et al: Correlation of glenohumeral internal rotation deficit and total rotational motion to shoulder injuries in professional baseball pitchers. *Am J Sports Med* 2011;39(2):329-335.
Signs of GIRD were assessed in 122 professional pitchers in three consecutive preseasons. The 40 pitchers with GIRD were almost twice as likely to be injured as those without GIRD (= 0.17).

[18] Huffman GR, Tibone JE, McGarry MH, Phipps BM, Lee YS, Lee TQ: Path of glenohumeral articulation throughout the rotational range of motion in a thrower's shoulder model. *Am J Sports Med* 2006;34(10): 1662-1669.

[19] Tokish J, Curtin MS, Kim YK, Hawkins RJ: Glenohumeral internal rotation deficit in the asymptomatic professional pitcher and its relationship to humeral retroversion. *J Sports Sci Med* 2008;7:78-83.

[20] Mihata T, Gates J, McGarry MH, Lee J, Kinoshita M, Lee TQ: Effect of rotator cuff muscle imbalance on forceful internal impingement and peel-back of the superior labrum: A cadaveric study. *Am J Sports Med* 2009;37(11):2222-2227.
A cadaver study assessed the rotator cuff and the effect of muscle imbalance during the late cocking phase of throwing. Decreased subscapularis muscle strength resulted in increased maximum external rotation and increased glenohumeral contact pressure, possibly leading to rotator cuff or labral pathology.

[21] Andrews JR, Broussard TS, Carson WG: Arthroscopy of the shoulder in the management of partial tears of the rotator cuff: A preliminary report. *Arthroscopy* 1985;1(2):117-122.

[22] Burkhart SS, Morgan CD, Kibler WB: The disabled throwing shoulder: Spectrum of pathology. Part II: Evaluation and treatment of SLAP lesions in throwers. *Arthroscopy* 2003;19(5):531-539.

[23] Jobe CM: Posterior superior glenoid impingement: Expanded spectrum. *Arthroscopy* 1995;11(5):530-536.

[24] Warner JJ, Micheli LJ, Arslanian LE, Kennedy J, Kennedy R: Scapulothoracic motion in normal shoulders and shoulders with glenohumeral instability and impingement syndrome: A study using Moiré topographic analysis. *Clin Orthop Relat Res* 1992;285: 191-199.

[25] Burkhart SS, Morgan CD, Kibler WB: The disabled throwing shoulder: Spectrum of pathology. Part III: The SICK scapula, scapular dyskinesis, the kinetic chain, and rehabilitation. *Arthroscopy* 2003;19(6): 641-661.

[26] Trakis JE, McHugh MP, Caracciolo PA, Busciacco L, Mullaney M, Nicholas SJ: Muscle strength and range of motion in adolescent pitchers with throwing-related pain: Implications for injury prevention. *Am J Sports Med* 2008;36(11):2173-2178.
Adolescent pitchers with or without shoulder pain were compared with respect to range of motion and posterior muscular strength. There was no significant difference in range of motion, but pitchers with pain had significantly weaker posterior musculature.

[27] Byram IR, Bushnell BD, Dugger K, Charron K, Harrell FE Jr, Noonan TJ: Preseason shoulder strength measurements in professional baseball pitchers: Identifying players at risk for injury. *Am J Sports Med* 2010;38(7): 1375-1382.
Shoulder strength in prone internal and external rotation and seated external rotation was examined in professional pitchers during spring training over 5 years. A statistically significant correlation was found between weakened supraspinatus strength in external rotation and in-season throwing injury requiring surgery.

[28] Gandhi J, ElAttrache NS, Kaufman KR, Hurd WJ: Voluntary activation deficits of the infraspinatus present as a consequence of pitching-induced fatigue. *J Shoulder Elbow Surg* 2012;21(5):625-630.
High school baseball pitchers' external rotation strength was measured before and after simulated pitching. Significant fatigue and weakness were noted. Voluntary infraspinatus muscle activation appears to contribute to external rotation muscle weakness in a fatigued pitcher.

[29] Myers JB, Laudner KG, Pasquale MR, Bradley JP,

Lephart SM: Glenohumeral range of motion deficits and posterior shoulder tightness in throwers with pathologic internal impingement. *Am J Sports Med* 2006;34(3):385-391.

[30] Meister K, Buckley B, Batts J: The posterior impinge-ment sign: Diagnosis of rotator cuff and posterior labral tears secondary to internal impingement in overhand athletes. *Am J Orthop (Belle Mead NJ)* 2004; 33(8):412-415.

[31] Lintner D, Mayol M, Uzodinma O, Jones R, Labos-siere D: Glenohumeral internal rotation deficits in professional pitchers enrolled in an internal rotation stretching program. *Am J Sports Med* 2007;35(4): 617-621.

The effectiveness of the sleeper stretch was assessed by comparing pitchers based on length of participation in a stretching program. Pitchers with at least 3 years' participation had 20° more internal rotation and a 23° greater total arc of motion compared with those hav- ing less lengthy participation.

[32] Ferrari JD, Ferrari DA, Coumas J, Pappas AM: Poste-rior ossification of the shoulder: The Bennett lesion. Etiology, diagnosis, and treatment. *Am J Sports Med* 1994;22(2):171-176.

[33] Reynolds SB, Dugas JR, Cain EL, McMichael CS, Andrews JR: Débridement of small partial-thickness rotator cuff tears in elite overhead throwers. *Clin Orthop Relat Res* 2008;466(3):614-621.

Data obtained for 67 of 82 professional pitchers after débridement of a partial-thickness rotator cuff tear re-vealed a 76% rate of return to competition and a 55% rate of return to the same or a higher level of compe-tition.

[34] Gorantla K, Gill C, Wright RW: The outcome of type II SLAP repair: A systematic review. *Arthroscopy* 2010;26(4):537-545.

A systematic review assessed the arthroscopic repair of type II SLAP lesions at a minimum 2-year follow-up. Outcomes varied dramatically, with return to play ranging from 20% to 94% (from 22% to 64% in baseball players). No prospective studies have assessed these outcomes. The repair of type II SLAP lesions does not appear to have a predictable outcome.

[35] Morgan CD, Burkhart SS, Palmeri M, Gillespie M: Type II SLAP lesions: Three subtypes and their rela- tionships to superior instability and rotator cuff tears. *Arthroscopy* 1998;14(6):553-565.

[36] Yoneda M, Nakagawa S, Mizuno N, et al: Arthro-scopic capsular release for painful throwing shoulder with posterior capsular tightness. *Arthroscopy* 2006; 22(7):e1-e5.

[37] Kim SH, Ha KI, Kim SH, Choi HJ: Results of arthro-scopic treatment of superior labral lesions. *J Bone Joint Surg Am* 2002;84-A(6):981-985.

[38] Reinold MM, Wilk KE, Hooks TR, Dugas JR, An-drews JR: Thermal-assisted capsular shrinkage of the glenohumeral joint in overhead athletes: A 15- to 47-month follow-up. *J Orthop Sports Phys Ther* 2003; 33(8):455-467.

[39] Ide J, Maeda S, Takagi K: Sports activity after arthro-scopic superior labral repair using suture anchors in overhead-throwing athletes. *Am J Sports Med* 2005; 33(4):507-514.

[40] Neuman BJ, Boisvert CB, Reiter B, Lawson K, Ciccotti MG, Cohen SB: Results of arthroscopic repair of type II superior labral anterior posterior lesions in overhead athletes: Assessment of return to preinjury playing level and satisfaction. *Am J Sports Med* 2011; 39(9):1883-1888.

A retrospective review of arthroscopically repaired SLAP tears in throwing athletes found that at midterm follow-up, patients believed they had returned to ap-proximately 84.1% of preinjury level of function. The overall satisfaction rate was 93%.

第十二章 肩关节不稳定修复手术的并发症

James G. Distefano, MD; Albert Lin, MD; Jon J.P. Warner, MD; Laurence D. Higgins, MD

引言

盂肱关节不稳定是一个宽泛的概念，包含多种不同的病理过程和情况。患者可能合并有一系列症状，原因可能是肩关节创伤或先天性肩关节松弛。手术的目标是恢复动态和静态的平衡以允许日常活动、恢复工作和参加竞技体育活动。需要考虑的重要因素包括年龄、主利手、吸烟史、总体活动范围、过顶运动的参与情况和遗传病史，如埃勒斯 – 当洛斯综合征或马方综合征。[1-3] 解剖异常可能包含不同范围和不同程度的软组织和骨性损伤。术者必须综合患者情况和手术因素以预测肩关节不稳定手术并发症的风险，并选择风险最小的治疗策略。

Dr. Warner or an immediate family member has received nonincome support (such as equipment or services), commercially derived honoraria, or other non–research-related funding (such as paid travel) from Arthrocare, DJ Orthopaedics, Arthrex, Mitek, and Bret, Smith & Nephew: Fellowship Support. Dr. Higgins or an immediate family member serves as a board member, owner, officer, or committee member of the American Shoulder and Elbow Surgeons Value Committee, Membership Committee, and Program Planning Committee; the Arthroscopy Association of North America Education Committee; the American Academy of Orthopaedic Surgeons Patient Safety and Value Committee; and Advocacy for Improvement in Mobility (AIM); and has received nonincome support (such as equipment or services), commercially derived honoraria, or other non–research-related funding (such as paid travel) from Arthrex Smith & Nephew: Fellowship Support, Breg, and DePuy. Neither of the following authors nor any immediate family member has received anything of value from or has stock or stock options held in a commercial company or institution related directly or indirectly to the subject of this chapter: Dr. Distefano and Dr. Lin.

解剖学因素

导致肩关节临床不稳定的损伤可能有很多种。理解患者的解剖异常对于掌握疾病进展和治疗失败的原因极其重要。在创伤性肩关节前脱位中，典型的破裂是 Bankart 损伤，即前下方盂唇的撕裂（图 12-1）。然而，尸体研究发现手术单纯分离前下方盂唇并不会出现不稳定。完全的不稳定需要有其他盂肱韧带、关节囊或骨性结构的损伤。[4]

关节盂的骨性缺损和（或）肱骨头 Hill–Sachs 损伤或反 Hill–Sachs 损伤，经常形成于脱位的时候。与初次脱位的患者相比，盂肱下韧带或盂肱中韧带损伤、Hill–Sachs 损伤在复发性不稳定患者前方不稳定脱位的手术治疗中被发现的概率很高。[5]

为减少复发性不稳定的风险，治疗前必须正确地认识病变。例如，后方盂唇撕裂、关节囊撕裂、肩胛盂缘缺损或反 Hill–Sachs 损伤可能合并存在于后方不稳定中。检查合并存在的 SLAP 损伤或肩袖病变非常重要，这可能与不稳定相关。生物力学研究发现人为制造一个 SLAP 损伤会增加肱骨的前移，在修复 Bankart 损伤的同时修复 SLAP 损伤的效果良好。[6-7] 关于肩袖间隙在治疗肩关节不稳定中的地位仍然存在争议，研究者间观点不同。

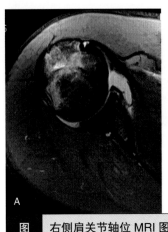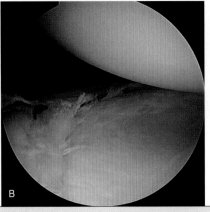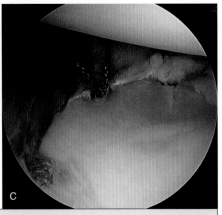

图 12-1　右侧肩关节轴位 MRI 图像显示 Bankart 损伤及前方盂唇脱落（A）。后入路下的关节镜照片显示缝合锚修补之前（B）和之后（C）的 Bankart 损伤

手术治疗

手术治疗的策略主要可以分为仅针对软组织结构、仅针对骨缺损和针对这两者三种。每种策略中都有关节镜手术及开放手术的方案。软组织方案包括盂唇修复、盂肱韧带修复、肩袖修补和关节囊折叠。骨性方案包括 Bankart 修补、Bristow 手术、Latarjet 手术、Putti-Platt 手术以及其他自体或异体移植重建的方案。

肩关节不稳定手术的并发症可能发生在术中、术后即刻、围手术期或随后数年。复发是不稳定手术最常见的并发症。此外，也会发生内固定断裂或失效、术后肩关节僵硬、残留疼痛、神经损伤、感染和骨性关节炎。

不稳定复发的原因

不稳定术后复发半脱位或脱位的原因有很多。术者必须全面彻底地了解肩关节的正常解剖和解剖学变异，正确地诊断所有患者的病理损伤并选择合理的治疗方案。[8] 手术失败可能与很多原因有关，如诊断和治疗选择、手术技术或其他不可避免的原因。

诊断和治疗选择

不稳定手术术后失败的常见原因之一就是没有发现所有的临床特点和解剖异常。全面的术前准备应始于通过询问患者病史来了解不稳定的方

向、频率和症状严重性。病理性松弛导致的疼痛或功能障碍必须与不影响正常活动的体育运动（如体操）导致的功能性的超生理活动范围相鉴别。此外，对患者的心理疾病、用药或为求关注而故意脱位的情况也应加以甄别。

体格检查应该着重关注整体的韧带松弛或多向不稳定，二者均会影响治疗选择和治疗结果。活动范围能提供有关继发病理过程的信息。例如，外旋较对侧增大可能提示肩胛下肌功能不良。必须进行全面的神经血管检查，尤其需要关注腋神经和肌皮神经。

当诊断为病理性松弛时，则应将注意力转向确认受累的肩关节结构及其程度。常用的影像学检查体位包括 Grashey 肩胛骨前后位、肩胛骨 Y 位、腋位、西点位、Hill-Sachs 位和 Stryker 切迹位（表 12-1）。这些体位的影像学检查可确认肩关节是否匹配并提供关于肩胛盂和肱骨的骨性压缩及骨缺损信息。

与不稳定相关的病理性损伤在影像学检查和术中都有可能被忽视。不能正确地认识关节囊结构不良、软组织或骨性 Bankart 损伤、盂肱关节断裂、翼状肩胛、骨缺损或肩袖损伤等情况会导致预后不良。未发现及治疗盂肱韧带的病变是不稳定复发的一个显著原因。在 64 例肩关节前方不稳定的患者中盂肱

表 12-1

肩关节复发性不稳定的影像学检查

影像学体位	投照技术	关键特征
肩关节前后位	X 线球管与躯体冠状面垂直	肩关节的总体影像
肩胛骨前后位（Grashey、真前后位）	患者以患侧为轴外旋 35°~40°，球管与肩胛体垂直	下方肩胛盂缘缺损（代表骨缺损）
肩胛骨 Y 位（肩胛骨侧位）	患者侧方肩关节面对胶片盒站立，并向前旋转 35°~40°。球管正对肩胛骨内侧面	肩峰及喙突呈 Y 形
腋位	胶片盒位于肩关节上方，上肢外展。球管正对腋窝	前、后方半脱位或脱位 Hill-Sachs 损伤或反 Hill-Sachs 损伤 肩胛骨倾角
西点位	患者俯卧。球管与头侧及内侧与喙突各成 25°	前下肩胛盂缘
Stryker 切迹位	患者仰卧，手位于头后方且肘关节指向天花板。球管向头侧倾斜 10°	后方肱骨压缩 Hill-Sachs 损伤

注：经允许引自 Egol K, Koval K, Zuckerman J: *The Handbook of Fractures*, ed 4. Philadelphia, PA, Lippincott, Williams, and Wilkins, 2010.

韧带肱骨侧（HAGL）撕脱的发生率为 9.3%。[4]最近的研究发现了更多的韧带损伤，包括反 HAGL 撕脱、骨性 HAGL 撕脱和肩胛盂侧撕脱。[9-10]HAGL 损伤和 Bankart 损伤同时发生的情况称为悬浮损伤。

另一个影响肩关节复发性不稳定的病理包括区分 Bankart 损伤和 ALPSA 病变（图 12-2）。在一项对 93 例创伤性前关节前脱位肩关节镜下缝合锚固定后至少 2 年的随访发现，复发率在单纯 Bankart 损伤中为 7.4%，而在 ALPSA 病变中为 19.2%。[11]脱位-半脱位事件的平均次数在 ALPSA 病变患者中为 12.3 次，而在 Bankart 损伤患者中为 4.9 次，这就提示复发事件会导致组织质量下降和修复牢固性降低。

虽然大多数患者的肩关节不稳定是发生在前方，但是后方不稳定也确实存在。后方不稳定的术后复发率为 0~12%。[12]一项关于 27 例接受肩关节镜下后方盂唇修补的患者的回顾性研究发现在平均 5.1 年的随访中，92% 的患者疼痛缓解，且未发生不稳定的复发。[13]后方手术的失败原因包括未能成功发现其他不稳定的方向或未处理多余的或质量不佳的关节囊。在后方不稳定手术后，过顶投掷运动员恢复竞技的比例相对低，并且接触对抗性运动员存在再脱位的风险。[2]从这个结果来看，建议术者在过顶投掷运动员中关节囊可稍松而在接触性对抗运动员中可稍紧。[12]

未能识别出与前方松弛并发的后方和（或）下方不稳定会导致预后不良。造成多向不稳定术后

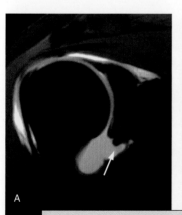 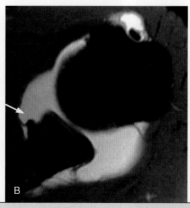 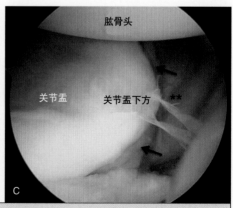

图 12-2 右侧肩关节 ALPSA 病变（箭头）的冠状位（A）和轴位（B）MRI 图像。关节镜照片显示右侧肩关节 ALPSA 病变（箭头），以及盂唇脱落和内侧移位（C）。**= 盂肱下韧带

复发率相对较高的因素包括并发多发韧带松弛、肩胛盂发育不良、肩袖损伤和周围盂唇撕裂。[14] 虽然切开行全关节囊移位是肩关节多向不稳定的经典治疗模式，但是关节镜手术已越来越受欢迎并与开放手术结果相当。[15]

通过肩袖间隙关闭来治疗不稳定的手术效果存在很多争议。肩袖间隙关闭可通过关节镜手术或开放手术完成。开放手术通常是从内向外的组织折叠，这可以改善后方和下方盂肱关节平移。一项对比关节镜和切开行肩袖间隙关闭的尸体研究发现，两种方法均不会改善后方平移，并且只有切开折叠可以改善下方稳定性。[16] 然而，对于前方平移，两种办法均能改善。切开折叠主要改善中立位的平移。关节镜下关闭主要改善手臂外展和外旋位的平移。

很多研究主要通过影像学检查确定骨缺损程度。如果怀疑有骨缺损，则推荐使用肩胛盂和肱骨头的三维 CT。量化肩胛盂骨缺损一般是在 CT 上将下方 2/3 的肩胛盂看作一个圆形，并将直接测量骨缺损的不同参数用于与对侧肩关节比较。三维 CT 重建预测骨缺损的准确性为 96%[17]（图 12-3）。

关节镜下评估肩胛盂骨缺损可能较困难。需要对一个近似椭圆形的不规则表面进行描述。利用裸点进行测量的方法包括把肩胛盂裸点作为中线并比较前方和后方的骨量。然而，一项解剖学研究质疑了裸点是否可以作为肩胛盂的解剖中点。[18] 在尸体肩关节的肩胛盂长轴 0° 和 45° 处建立骨缺损模型。[19] 关节镜下裸点模型在 0° 模型中能准确描述骨缺损，但是在 45° 模型中会过高估计骨缺损。弦切理论方法测量肩胛盂骨缺损，即将下方肩胛盂看作一个圆形，再通过关节镜测量受影响及未受影响的区域，并以几何测算对比。[20] 该方法被认为较裸点法更准确，但仍然有 4% 的误差。

假如所有解剖学因素均能被正确识别，则很容易分析及做出治疗选择。很多解剖学因素与肩关节不稳定相关，但是确定它们各自的问题尤其困难。例如，有研究明确显示在无肩胛盂或肱骨缺损且有足够组织的情况下，一个正确的切开或关节镜下软组织操作能获得好的结果（表 12-2）。肩胛盂和肱骨缺损可以独自或一起出现，且两者的严重性具有差异。因此，对严重骨缺损的诊断和是否根据搜集的缺损程度信息改变该诊断都显得更加困难。

肱骨侧的骨缺损发生在脱位时肱骨头与肩胛盂缘的撞击。反复的半脱位或脱位后，缺损逐渐侵蚀并增大。随访 194 例关节镜下 Bankart 修复患者发现，如果没有明显的骨缺损，则复发率为 4%，但是如果肩胛盂为倒梨形或存在嵌顿性 Hill-Sachs 损伤，则复发率为 67%[21]（图 12-4）。肱骨

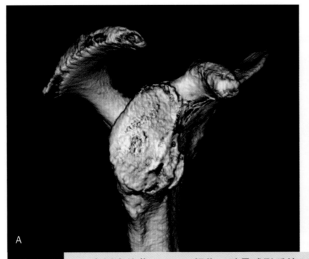
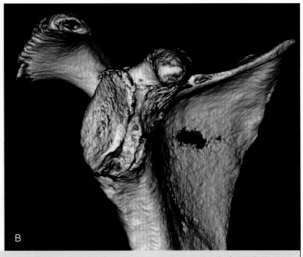

图 12-3　A. 右侧肩关节 Bankart 损伤，肱骨减影后的三维 CT 重建。B. 斜位三维 CT 重建显示损伤内侧移位

表 12-2					
肩关节不稳定复发率的近期相关研究报道					
研究发表（年份）	手术方式	病例数	平均随访（年）	体育相关	复发率
Bonnevialle 等[77]（2009）	切开手术	79	7.1	83%	12.6%
Elmlund 等[78]（2008）	关节镜手术	84	8.2	87%	11%
Fabre 等[79]（2010）	切开手术	50	28	73%	16%
Law 等[80]（2008）	关节镜手术	38	2.3	100%	5.2%
Ogawa 等[56]（2010）	切开手术	167	8.7	—	4.8%
Oh 等[38]（2009）	关节镜手术	37	3	40.5%	5.4%
Porcellini 等[81]（2009）	关节镜手术	385	3	—	8.1%
Thal 等[82]（2007）	关节镜手术	73	> 2	—	6.9%
Thomazeau 等[42]（2010）	关节镜手术	125	1.5	73%	3.2%
Voos 等[23]（2010）	关节镜手术	83	2.75	46%	18%

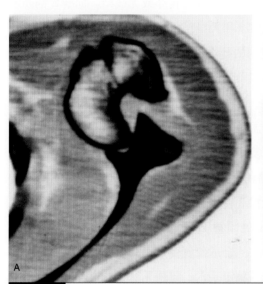
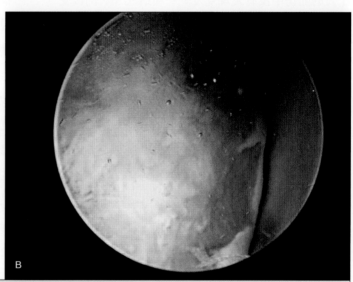

图 12-4　A. 左侧肩关节巨大 Hill-Sachs 损伤轴位 CT。B. 同一肩关节的关节镜照片显示嵌顿性 Hill-Sachs 损伤

缺损可根据缺损的面积、累及肱骨头的比例、缺损的深度或缺损的体积进行分类。明显的累及肱骨头的比例超过 25% 的骨缺损需要手术治疗。[22]一项纳入 83 例关节镜下 Bankart 修补的前瞻性研究发现，术后 2 年以上患者的复发率为 18%。[23] Hill-Sachs 损伤大于 250 mm³、患者年龄大于 20 岁及韧带松弛与复发明显相关。通过尸体研究在最大外旋位上不同外展角度下嵌顿于肩胛盂缘的 Hill-Sachs 损伤的面积。[24]如果肩袖边缘至内侧骨性损伤的距离大于肩胛盂宽度的 84%，则会发生嵌顿。

明显的嵌顿性 Hill-Sachs 损伤通常通过开放手术治疗。异体骨移植、骨软骨移植、表面置换及关节镜下填充都可以采用。填充包括将后方肩袖肌腱固定于肱骨缺损处以防止嵌顿。该方法允许关节镜下治疗复发性不稳定或合并肱骨缺损的不稳定。[25]

生物力学研究将严重肩胛盂骨缺损定义为骨缺损 20%~30%。[26-27]前方缺损的研究较后方缺损多。[28]复发性不稳定的肩胛盂骨缺损的重建方法包括自体髂骨移植、部分或全部喙突移位以及异体骨移植。关节镜技术在肩胛盂骨移植和 Latarjet 手术中均有了很大发展。[29]关节镜下手术技术要求较高且并未发现优于开放手术，但是具有关节镜手术固有的优势。[27]采用异体胫骨远端来进行肩胛盂缺损骨移植，可以很好地匹配肩胛盂的自然弧度。

Bristow 手术和 Latarjet 手术治疗肩胛盂骨缺损均能提供良好的结果。[30-31] 45°缺损模型的尸体研究显示，在多个位置下 Latarjet 肩袖较骨移植对盂肱关节平移的限制作用更佳。[32] Latarjet 肩袖的稳定性可能包括肩胛盂骨缺损的增强、关节囊的关闭和外展外旋位下联合腱的悬吊作用。[33]骨的阻挡作用在一项纳入 26 例接受 Latarjet 手术的患者的前瞻性研究中受到质疑。[30] CT 用于评估移植物骨溶解。虽然大约 60% 的喙突会出现骨溶解，但是在平均 17.5 个月的随访中没有发现复发。一项纳入 319 例接受 Bristow 手术的患者的回顾性研究发现了 5% 的再脱位率和 13% 的半脱位率[31]。内移或相对于肩胛盂缘移位超过 1 cm 会导致再脱位的发生率增加。

即使喙突转位可能改善肩关节稳定性，但还是有出现复发的报道。一项纳入 46 例行髂骨移植翻修 Latarjet 手术后失败（称为改良 Eden-Hybinette 术）的患者的研究发现，在平均 6.8 年的随访中有 4 例复发。[34]

骨结构的 Bankart 损伤指肩胛盂缘前方骨折（骨性 Bankart 损伤）或后方骨折（反骨性 Bankart 损伤），根据导致脱位的暴力方向是前方还是后方确定具体的骨折类型。在这些肩胛盂骨缺损中，盂唇和关节囊常与骨折块相连。骨性 Bankart 损伤经典的治疗方法是切开修补，并且根据骨折块的大小，可能需要行骨移植术。有研究报道使用关节镜技术能得到良好结果。对比 41 例 3 个月内治疗的急性损伤患者及 27 例 3 个月后治疗的慢性损伤患者，只有 3 例患者在 4 年的随访中失联。[35]虽然每个组中只有 1 例再脱位，术前及术后 Rowe 评分在慢性损伤患者中显著降低。

手术技术

术者技巧的缺乏和术前计划（决定采用开放手术还是关节镜手术）的不合理会导致复发。最初，开放手术是治疗肩关节不稳定的主流治疗方式，但目前使用关节镜治疗的趋势逐渐增加。[35]关节镜技术在骨锚技术、组织病理理解和手术技术上已有改进。已证明关节镜手术的效果与开放手术的效果相当。

使用经肩胛盂缝线和不同类型的骨锚在关节镜下修复盂唇和关节囊。影响失败率的因素包括缝合锚的设计、数量、材料、大小和位置。肩胛盂缝合锚采用金属材料、生物复合材料和生物可吸收材料制造。使用生物可吸收锚及金属锚可能导致骨溶解。[36]邻近缝合锚的骨吸收会导致创伤条件下（如接触性竞技运动中损伤）的肩胛盂缘骨折。[37]

锚可预置缝线材料亦或无线结。标准骨锚固定的再脱位率和无线结骨锚固定的再脱位率相当。[38]如果使用的缝合锚数量少于 3 枚，则更容易复发脱位。[39]充分松解关节囊盂唇组织对准备骨床非常重要。必须折叠关节囊的扩张部分和多余部分以恢复盂唇的缓冲作用。

修复盂唇的锚置于盂缘下方偏内侧不能恢复合适的盂唇缓冲作用。对于单纯的创伤性不稳定，一种技术是将 3 枚锚钉置于 3 点位置下方，在距肩胛盂缘 2 mm 处倾斜 45°进入骨面。[40]是否能将锚置入肩胛盂下方的合适位置受通道位置的影响。虽然套管常用于不稳定手术，但是无套管通道可经肩胛下肌建立，以便将缝合锚放置于更靠近下方的 5 点位置与 6 点位置之间。尤其重要的是，要确认将锚钉埋入软骨表面以防止肱骨头的软骨损伤（图 12-5）。

对于手术固定后不稳定复发的患者，如果没有明显骨缺损可考虑软组织手术。理想的适应证包括成功手术后的创伤性再脱位以及存在初次手术未处理的病变。关节镜可能与开放手术失败相关。一项纳入 22 例开放手术失败后接受关节镜手术的患者的回顾性研究中，患者接受过 Latarjet 手术、Eden-Hybinette 或 Bankart 修复和关节囊移位，这些患者接受了关节镜下软组织修复、选择性的内固定取出，4 例患者还接受了肩袖间隙关闭。[41]在平均 43 个月的随访中，1 例出现复发半

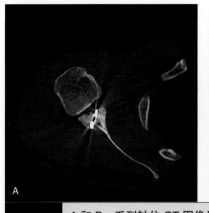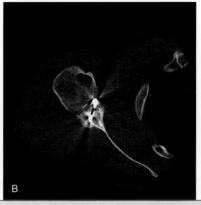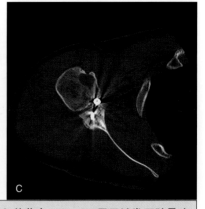

图 12-5　A 和 B. 系列轴位 CT 图像显示右侧肩关节 Latarjet 手术固定螺钉置入关节内。C. CT 显示继发了肱骨头缺损

脱位，2 例存在主观的恐惧感但是对结果尚满意。

不可避免的因素

即使有完美的诊断和手术技术，仍有很多手术因术者不可控的因素而失败。一个更具挑战性的因素是患者不配合，包括不能耐受术后佩戴吊带、活动、理疗和随访等术后处理。结果可能是 Bankart 损伤、关节囊再撕裂、小结节截骨修复肩胛下肌修复失败、经喙突移位或骨移植物的切出。很多患者相关的因素是不能避免的，例如，摔倒、癫痫抽搐、感染或过于激进的理疗所致的断裂。

无论是术者还是患者都不能控制患者的基因成分。患者存在埃勒斯 - 当洛斯综合征、马方综合征或关节过度松弛等组织弹性变化会导致术后反复的关节过度松弛。相反，如果术后出现大量的瘢痕组织，则患者容易出现关节僵硬。术前能够认识到这些因素可帮助在必要时调整术前计划的制订和术后康复。

再脱位的风险预测

一项病例对照研究包含 131 例关节镜下 Bankart 修复复发性肩关节不稳定的患者。[3] 这些患者 31 个月的总体复发率是 13%。根据 6 个因素制订了 10 分制不稳定严重性评分（表 12-3）。如果患者的分数高于 6 分，则提示需要行切开非软组织手术来降低复发风险。

一项前瞻性多中心观察性研究报道的前方关

表 12-3

评估软组织修复术后前方不稳定复发风险的不稳定严重性评分

术前的风险因素	分数
小于 20 岁	2 分
参与竞技性体育活动	2 分
参与接触性或过顶类体育活动	1 分
前方或下方过度松弛	1 分
影像学可见的 Hill-Sachs 损伤	2 分
影像学可见的正常关节盂内轮廓异常	2 分
总分	10 分
分数	复发风险
＜3 分	5%
3~6 分	10%
＞6 分	70%

注：经允许引自 Balg F, Boileau P: The instability severity index score: A simple pre-operative score to select patients for arthroscopic or open shoulder stabilisation. *J Bone Joint Surg Br* 2007;89(11):1470-1477.

节镜固定治疗不稳定评分小于或等于 4 分的患者的短期结果显示，在 18 个月的随访中，符合纳入标准的 125 例患者中有 4 例（3.2%）存在复发。[42]

并发症

僵硬

不稳定手术的目标是重建肩关节稳定性并维持功能性活动范围。影响术后肩关节活动的因素有很多，包括手术类型、肩关节制动时长、理疗方案和瘢痕组织形成的潜在能力。手术固定后的复发创伤性前方不稳定的肩关节通常较对侧肩关节存在活动受限。其中，外旋受限最为常见，体侧外旋受限为 8°~33.6°，在手臂 90° 外展位外旋平均受限 6°~24.4°。[43]一项研究显示在 90° 外展位内旋受限平均为 19.2°。这些活动受限并未发现会独立影响长期肩关节病变的发展。[44]

先进行术后处理，包括吊带制动肩关节 4~6 周，随后逐渐过渡到辅助下的主动活动锻炼。目标通常是在术后 2~3 个月内达到全范围被动活动。[38]一种方案是在术后 3 个月内限制肩关节上举 – 外展超过 90° 及外旋超过 30°，然后过渡到全范围活动。[45]另一个方案是在早期使用枪手型支具，上臂内旋置于体前。[46]

关节囊折叠和盂唇修复的后方固定手术占不稳定手术的比例小于 10%。术后方案类似前方不稳定，包括吊带制动 6 周限制最大内旋和减少后方修复部位的应力。[47]经外展吊带制动后，开始轻柔的被动和主动活动，然后过渡到术后 4~6 个月的力量锻炼。一项纳入 112 例关节镜下固定后方肩关节脱位患者的回顾性研究发现，与对侧上臂相比，患侧上臂在 90° 外展位内旋减少 12%，术后 1 年内的再脱位率为 17.7%。[48]患侧上臂在体侧和 90° 外展位的外旋分别减少 8.7% 和 5.4%。

填充手术最主要的缺点在于生物力学研究中发现存在外旋受限。[49]一项研究对比了联合和不联合填充手术的关节镜下 Bankart 修复，发现二者术后活动范围无区别。[50]然而，33% 的接受Bankart 修补及填充手术的患者反映术后 2 年存在后上方疼痛，这可能与部分或不完全的缺损愈合有关。目前，对于肩袖肌腱固定于骨缺损是否能获得满意的功能结果还不能确定。

疼痛

疼痛是肩关节术后的一个常见并发症。[40,43]一项对 60 例 Bankart 修复后患者超过 10 年的随访研究报道，疼痛的发生率达 50%。[51]肩关节固定后的疼痛既可能是病理组织残留的一个征象，也可能是术中未处理或术后固定失败的结果。术后疼痛大多数是多因素的。可能是继发于并发的病变，例如，肩袖或肱二头肌腱病变、软骨损伤、术后特发性关节囊炎、肌力和肌耐力减退，或合并其他因素。[52]

早期疼痛可能也会发生于盂肱关节退行性关节炎及关节内缝合锚突出，以及关节囊灼烧或与使用关节内止痛导管等相关的软骨溶解。[53-55]感染较为少见，但是可能是早期或晚期疼痛的一个原因。治疗术后疼痛可能是令人苦恼的挑战，尤其是一些患者没有持续的不稳定且反复的体格检查及影像学检查未显示结构性的相关因素。在这种状况下，首选的治疗方式是非手术治疗。物理治疗结合抗炎药物可以维持活动范围和力量。

一项纳入 282 例创伤性肩关节前方不稳定患者的研究发现，关节炎性改变可见于 11.3% 的 X 线片及 31.2% 的 CT 图像。[56]大多数的关节炎是轻微的或 X 线片难以发现的。这项研究改进了固定手术中对基线改变的认识。在关节镜固定手术中发现，87 例患者中有 55 例（63%）存在软骨损伤。[57]在 20 年的随访研究中发现，关节炎改变的范围为 35%~71%。[58-59]关节炎发病的可能性与脱位时年龄大、手术前脱位次数多、盂唇的退变重等相关。[53,60]一项对 257 例肩关节不稳定术后 25 年随访的研究显示，44% 的病例肩关节影像学正常，29% 有轻度改变，9% 有中度改变，而 17% 有重度改变。[61]

肱骨或肩胛盂缺损的切开重建手术包括结构骨移植，在匹配缺损的曲率的技术上是一种挑战。尸体肩关节前下方肩胛盂缺损的模型通过 Latarjet手术或髂骨移植重建。[62]确认接触压力的 Tekscan压力感受器最好在骨移植物埋入表面和 Latarjet 手术移植物被旋转时放置，以便下表面与肩胛盂匹配。接触压力的长期改变可能会导致关节炎的发展并严重损伤放置于外侧的凸起的移植骨。

神经损伤

神经损伤可发生于脱位时或肩关节稳定手术。

在 3633 例创伤性前方盂肱关节脱位的患者中，复位后神经损伤的发生率为 13.5%。[63] 在 210 例神经损伤的患者中，腋神经受累的比例为 73.8%，尺神经受累的比例为 10.5%，正中神经受累的比例为 3.8%，桡神经受累的比例为 1.4%，而肌皮神经受累的比例为 1%。多神经或臂丛神经损伤的发生率为 9.5%。合并肩袖撕裂或大结节骨折的患者发生神经损伤的可能性最大。

神经损伤可能发生于开放手术或关节镜手术中，虽然大多数研究报道的神经损伤是在开放手术之后发生的。神经损伤的发生率为 1%~8%，而一项纳入 282 例前方切开固定手术的研究报道，感觉运动神经损伤的发生率为 8.2%。[64-65] 因为手术部位在盂肱关节近端，所以开放手术和关节镜手术中最常见的受累神经是腋神经和肌皮神经。[40] 尸体解剖研究发现，腋神经在盂肱下韧带下方 1~1.5 cm 处，感觉支最靠近肩胛盂缘，而肌皮神经约在喙突下方 5 cm 处穿出喙肱肌。[66-67] 这些位置可能与前方稳定及下方关节囊移位手术密切相关，存在腋神经损伤风险，而在开放手术中放置

拉钩和手术器械则对两条神经都有损伤的风险（图 12-6）。关节镜下神经损伤可能源于不适当的下方入路的建立，患者体位摆放不当，对手臂的不当操作或牵拉导致的臂丛神经牵拉。[40,68] 一项解剖研究发现臂丛神经在一些患者中仅距离肩胛盂缘 5 mm，而沿肩胛颈放置的拉钩可能与臂丛神经接触。[69] 然而多数神经损伤是牵拉所致的短暂性神经麻痹，极少数是因为直接撕裂。[69]

喙突移位和骨阻挡手术治疗肩胛盂骨缺损的广泛应用引起了研究者对其他神经损伤并发症的注意，例如，肩胛上神经损伤。除了臂丛神经牵拉损伤和肌皮神经麻痹，有研究报道，Latarjet 手术后的肩胛上神经麻痹，可能是因为肩胛上神经位于后方肩胛盂缘近端，使得螺钉置入时尤其危险。[70] 这种风险存在于所有需要穿过后方肩胛盂置入螺钉的骨性手术。

很多研究集中于在关节镜下或切开固定中预防神经损伤。在 128 例使用肩胛下肌劈开入路行前方切开固定治疗的患者中，只有 1 例（0.8%）存在腋神经支配区麻痹并自行完全恢复。[71] 一项前瞻

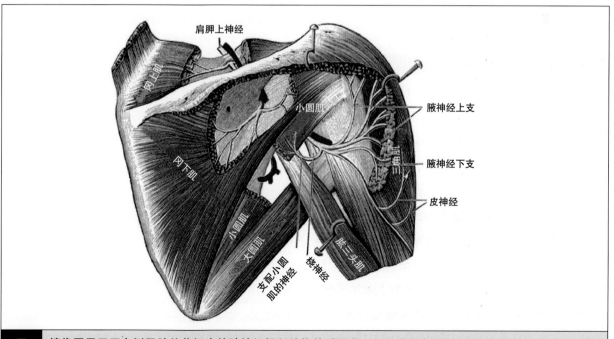

肩胛上神经　腋神经上支　腋神经下支　皮神经　冈上肌　小圆肌　冈下肌　小圆肌　大圆肌　支配小圆肌的神经　桡神经　肱三头肌

| 图 12-6 | 镜像图显示了右侧盂肱关节相应的腋神经解剖结构的后面观。经允许引自 Gray H, Mayo Goss C: Gray's anatomy of the human body. *Am J Surg* 1955:90（4）:810. |

性研究连续随访了 20 例在关节镜手术中接受神经监测的患者。[72] 在 11 例接受关节囊热灼烧的患者中，有 4 例因为监测到可能出现神经损伤而改变了手术方式。没有患者存在临床症状。虽然这是一项关于关节囊热灼烧的研究，但是研究中使用的似乎逐渐被淡化的神经监测技术可能对预防神经损伤有帮助，尤其是在 Latarjet 手术这类可能需要关注靠近器械和拉钩近端的神经的开放手术中。

感染

虽然感染可能发生在任何手术中，但是在肩关节固定术后相对少见。[40] 感染的发病率在开放手术后是 0~6%，关节镜术后为 0.04%~0.23%。[73-74] 在一项超过 21 年的研究中，只有 6 例肩关节固定患者术后因感染痤疮丙酸杆菌接受治疗，这也是最常见的致病菌。[75] 对不可吸收缝线周围的晚期感染窦道应保持高度警惕。有少数病例报道了少见感染，其中 1 例是发生在关节镜下 Bankart 修复的金属缝合锚周围。[76] 当感染发生在肩关节不稳定手术后，应遵循积极探查、彻底清创和冲洗以及静脉滴注抗生素等骨科治疗原则。如果肩关节固定后出现术后感染，必须适当延长培养时间着重寻找培养困难的痤疮丙酸杆菌。[75]

总结

不稳定术后最常见的并发症包括复发、肩关节僵硬、疼痛、神经血管损伤和感染，可由很多因素引起，例如，术前未能发现病变或未能发现所有病变。必须进行全面的临床和影像学检查以确认不稳定的方向、软组织的质量和是否存在大量肩胛盂和（或）肱骨缺损。选择合理的手术方式后，不合适的操作可能导致固定物凸起、固定失败、软骨损伤或邻近神经血管结构损伤。术后处理必须兼顾僵硬和肩关节松弛复发之间的平衡。与所有其他的骨科疾病一样，患者依从性差和继发的创伤事件会严重影响治疗结果。

参考文献

[1] Cho NS, Hwang JC, Rhee YG: Arthroscopic stabilization in anterior shoulder instability: Collision athletes versus noncollision athletes. *Arthroscopy* 2006;22(9): 947-953.

[2] Balg F, Boileau P: The instability severity index score: A simple pre-operative score to select patients for arthroscopic or open shoulder stabilisation. *J Bone Joint Surg Br* 2007;89(11):1470-1477.

A prospective case control study of 131 patients with recurrent anterior shoulder instability who underwent suture anchor stabilization found a 14.5% recurrence rate. Significant factors were used to create a 10-point predictive scoring system.

[3] Radkowski CA, Chhabra A, Baker CL III, Tejwani SG, Bradley JP: Arthroscopic capsulolabral repair for posterior shoulder instability in throwing athletes compared with nonthrowing athletes. *Am J Sports Med* 2008;36(4):693-699.

In a cohort study, 107 shoulders in athletes with isolated posterior shoulder instability underwent arthroscopic stabilization. The results were comparable in throwing and nonthrowing athletes, except there was a lower rate of return to preinjury competition level in throwing athletes (55% versus 71%).

[4] Wolf EM, Cheng JC, Dickson K: Humeral avulsion of glenohumeral ligaments as a cause of anterior shoulder instability. *Arthroscopy* 1995;11(5):600-607.

[5] Spatschil A, Landsiedl F, Anderl W, et al: Posttraumatic anterior-inferior instability of the shoulder: Arthroscopic findings and clinical correlations. *Arch Orthop Trauma Surg* 2006;126(4):217-222.

[6] Cho HL, Lee CK, Hwang TH, Suh KT, Park JW: Arthroscopic repair of combined Bankart and SLAP lesions: Operative techniques and clinical results. *Clin Orthop Surg* 2010;2(1):39-46.

A retrospective cohort study compared arthroscopic repair of an isolated Bankart tear and a combined Bankart and SLAP tear in 47 patients. Both groups had improvement, but return of range of motion was slower after the combined repair.

[7] Hantes ME, Venouziou AI, Liantsis AK, Dailiana ZH, Malizos KN: Arthroscopic repair for chronic anterior shoulder instability: A comparative study between patients with Bankart lesions and patients with combined Bankart and superior labral anterior posterior lesions. *Am J Sports Med* 2009;37(6):1093-1098.

A prospective cohort study of 38 patients with arthroscopic isolated Bankart tear repair and 25 with combined Bankart and SLAP tear repair found comparably improved Constant and Rowe scores. There was a single redislocation in each group at 2-year follow-up.

［8］ Tischer T, Vogt S, Kreuz PC, Imhoff AB: Arthroscopic anatomy, variants, and pathologic findings in shoulder instability. *Arthroscopy* 2011;27(10):1434-1443.

The literature on normal, pathologic, and variant arthroscopic anatomy is reviewed.

［9］ Hill JD, Lovejoy JF Jr, Kelly RA: Combined posterior Bankart lesion and posterior humeral avulsion of the glenohumeral ligaments associated with recurrent posterior shoulder instability. *Arthroscopy* 2007;23(3): e1-e3.

In a case report of recurrent of posterior glenohumeral instability caused by a posterior Bankart lesion and a posterior HAGL lesion, both were treated arthroscopically with suture anchors.

［10］ Wolf EM, Siparsky PN: Glenoid avulsion of the glenohumeral ligaments as a cause of recurrent anterior shoulder instability. *Arthroscopy* 2010;26(9):1263-1267.

Three patients with recurrent anterior shoulder instability caused by avulsion of the glenohumeral ligaments had arthroscopic repair.

［11］ Ozbaydar M, Elhassan B, Diller D, Massimini D, Higgins LD, Warner JJ: Results of arthroscopic capsulolabral repair: Bankart lesion versus anterior labroligamentous periosteal sleeve avulsion lesion. *Arthroscopy* 2008;24(11):1277-1283.

Of 99 patients with anterior instability who underwent arthroscopic stabilization, the 67 with an isolated Bankart tear had a recurrence rate of 7.4% at an average 5-year follow-up, compared with a 19.2% rate in the 26 patients with an ALPSA lesion.

［12］ Bradley JP, Tejwani SG: Arthroscopic management of posterior instability. *Orthop Clin North Am* 2010; 41(3):339-356.

The literature on posterior instability was reviewed, with pathoanatomy, history, physical examination factors, imaging, treatment options, and postoperative rehabilitation.

［13］ Williams RJ III, Strickland S, Cohen M, Altchek DW, Warren RF: Arthroscopic repair for traumatic posterior shoulder instability. *Am J Sports Med* 2003;31(2): 203-209.

［14］ Schenk TJ, Brems JJ: Multidirectional instability of the shoulder: Pathophysiology, diagnosis, and management. *J Am Acad Orthop Surg* 1998;6(1):65-72.

［15］ Alpert JM, Verma N, Wysocki R, Yanke AB, Romeo AA: Arthroscopic treatment of multidirectional shoulder instability with minimum 270 degrees labral repair: Minimum 2-year follow-up. *Arthroscopy* 2008; 24(6):704-711.

A retrospective study of 13 patients who underwent arthroscopic stabilization for multidirectional instability involving labral tears larger than 270° found a 15% recurrence rate. Eighty-five percent of the patients were completely or mostly satisfied with the results at average 56-month follow-up.

［16］ Provencher MT, Mologne TS, Hongo M, Zhao K, Tasto JP, An KN: Arthroscopic versus open rotator interval closure: Biomechanical evaluation of stability and motion. *Arthroscopy* 2007;23(6):583-592.

A basic science biomechanical study tested stability and range of motion after arthroscopic and open rotator cuff interval closure. Neither technique improved posterior stability, and both resulted in significant loss of external rotation. Only the open rotator cuff interval closure improved sulcus stability.

［17］ Chuang TY, Adams CR, Burkhart SS: Use of preoperative three-dimensional computed tomography to quantify glenoid bone loss in shoulder instability. *Arthroscopy* 2008;24(4):376-382.

The glenoid index was calculated in a retrospective study of 25 patients with anterior instability who underwent bilateral preoperative CT. A level of 0.75 corresponded to arthroscopic findings guiding toward a soft-tissue or bony stabilization procedure.

［18］ Kralinger F, Aigner F, Longato S, Rieger M, Wambacher M: Is the bare spot a consistent landmark for shoulder arthroscopy? A study of 20 embalmed glenoids with 3-dimensional computed tomographic reconstruction. *Arthroscopy* 2006;22(4):428-432.

［19］ Provencher MT, Detterline AJ, Ghodadra N, et al: Measurement of glenoid bone loss: A comparison of measurement error between 45 degrees and 0 degrees bone loss models and with different posterior arthroscopy portal locations. *Am J Sports Med* 2008;36(6): 1132-1138.

A basic science study of 14 cadaver shoulders evaluated the ability of the arthroscopic bare spot method to determine the extent of anterior-inferior bone loss in 12.5% and 25% models and at two angles relative to the long axis of the glenoid. The bare spot method was found to be accurate in the 0° model and overestimated bone loss in the 45° model.

[20] Detterline AJ, Provencher MT, Ghodadra N, Bach BR Jr, Romeo AA, Verma NN: A new arthroscopic technique to determine anterior-inferior glenoid bone loss: Validation of the secant chord theory in a cadaveric model. *Arthroscopy* 2009;25(11):1249-1256.

A basic science study of seven cadaver shoulders compared the ability of the arthroscopic bare spot and secant chord theory methods to evaluate glenoid bone loss. Regardless of the amount of bone loss or the portal position, the scant chord theory was more accurate, 157 although more extensive mathematical calculations were required.

[21] Burkhart SS, De Beer JF: Traumatic glenohumeral bone defects and their relationship to failure of arthroscopic Bankart repairs: Significance of the invertedpear glenoid and the humeral engaging Hill-Sachs lesion. *Arthroscopy* 2000;16(7):677-694.

[22] Cetik O, Uslu M, Ozsar BK: The relationship between Hill-Sachs lesion and recurrent anterior shoulder dislocation. *Acta Orthop Belg* 2007;73(2):175-178.

A correlation was found between the number of dislocations and the extent and the depth of a Hill-Sachs lesion. A patient with recurrent anterior shoulder dislocation should receive early surgical treatment to prevent lesion progression.

[23] Voos JE, Livermore RW, Feeley BT, et al; HSS Sports Medicine Service: Prospective evaluation of arthroscopic bankart repairs for anterior instability. *Am J Sports Med* 2010;38(2):302-307.

A study of 83 patients with anterior shoulder instability who underwent arthroscopic Bankart repair found an 18% recurrence rate. The identified risk factors included age younger than 25 years, general ligamentous laxity, and a Hill-Sachs lesion larger than 250 mm³.

[24] Yamamoto N, Itoi E, Abe H, et al: Contact between the glenoid and the humeral head in abduction, exter- nal rotation, and horizontal extension: A new concept of glenoid track. *J Shoulder Elbow Surg* 2007;16(5): 649-656.

A basic science biomechanical study of nine cadaver shoulders tested stability after simulated Hill-Sachs lesions at maximal external rotation and with 0°, 30°, and 60° of abduction. There was an increased risk of engagement when the width of the lesion was more than 84% of the glenoid width.

[25] Park MJ, Tjoumakaris FP, Garcia G, Patel A, Kelly JD IV: Arthroscopic remplissage with Bankart repair for the treatment of glenohumeral instability with Hill- Sachs

defects. *Arthroscopy* 2011;27(9):1187-1194.

A case study of 20 patients with recurrent anterior shoulder instability and a large Hill-Sachs defect who underwent arthroscopic Bankart repair with remplissage found a 15% recurrence rate at a mean 2-year follow-up. Range of motion was not reported.

[26] Itoi E, Lee SB, Berglund LJ, Berge LL, An KN: The effect of a glenoid defect on anteroinferior stability of the shoulder after Bankart repair: A cadaveric study. *J Bone Joint Surg Am* 2000;82(1):35-46.

[27] Provencher MT, Ghodadra N, LeClere L, Solomon DJ, Romeo AA: Anatomic osteochondral glenoid reconstruction for recurrent glenohumeral instability with glenoid deficiency using a distal tibia allograft. *Arthroscopy* 2009;25(4):446-452.

This is a case study and a description of the technique for using fresh distal tibial osteochondral allograft for reconstructing three shoulders with anterior instability and glenoid bone loss averaging 30%.

[28] Yamamoto N, Muraki T, Sperling JW, et al: Stabilizing mechanism in bone grafting of a large glenoid defect. *J Bone Joint Surg Am* 2010;92(11):2059-2066.

A basic science biomechanical study used 13 cadaver shoulders to create anterior-inferior glenoid defects at increasing 2-mm increments. There was a significant decrease in the force required to translate the humeral head at defects larger than 19% of the glenoid length.

[29] Lafosse L, Lejeune E, Bouchard A, Kakuda C, Gobezie R, Kochhar T: The arthroscopic Latarjet procedure for the treatment of anterior shoulder instability. *Arthroscopy* 2007;23(11):e1-e5.

The background and the indications for the Latarjet procedure are reviewed, with the technique for the arthroscopic procedure. At 8-month follow-up of 62 patients, the results were 98% excellent or good, with an average return to sport 10 weeks after surgery.

[30] Di Giacomo G, Costantini A, de Gasperis N, et al: Coracoid graft osteolysis after the Latarjet procedure for anteroinferior shoulder instability: A computed tomography scan study of twenty-six patients. *J Shoulder Elbow Surg* 2011;20(6):989-995.

In a prospective study, 26 patients underwent Latarjet reconstruction followed by CT. At a mean 17.5-month follow-up, an average of 60% of the coracoid had undergone osteolysis, but 69.2% of the patients had an excellent Rowe score.

[31] Hovelius L, Sandström B, Olofsson A, Svensson O, Rahme H: The effect of capsular repair, bone block

healing, and position on the results of the Bristow-Latarjet procedure (study III): Long-term follow-up in 319 shoulders. *J Shoulder Elbow Surg* 2012;21(5): 647-660.

A combined retrospective and prospective study in- volved 319 patients treated with the Bristow-Latarjet procedure, in three groups. The overall recurrence rate was 5%. Placement of the coracoid more than 1 cm medial to the glenoid rim predisposed the shoulder to redislocation. Bony fusion occurred in 83% of the pa- tients.

[32] Wellmann M, Petersen W, Zantop T, et al: Open shoulder repair of osseous glenoid defects: Biomechanical effectiveness of the Latarjet procedure versus a contoured structural bone graft. *Am J Sports Med* 2009;37(1):87-94.

A basic science biomechanical study compared shoulder stability after Latarjet and bone-grafting procedures in cadavers. The Latarjet procedure better restricted anterior and anteroinferior translation, particularly at 60°of abduction.

[33] Wellmann M, de Ferrari H, Smith T, et al: Biomechanical investigation of the stabilization principle of the Latarjet procedure. *Arch Orthop Trauma Surg* 2012; 132(3):377-386.

A basic science biomechanical study of 12 cadaver shoulders tested the contributions of the Latarjet procedure to humeral translation. The conjoined tendon, the coracoacromial ligament, capsular reconstruction, and subscapularis integrity all contribute to the stabilizing mechanism of the Latarjet reconstruction.

[34] Lunn JV, Castellano-Rosa J, Walch G: Recurrent anterior dislocation after the Latarjet procedure: Outcome after revision using a modified Eden-Hybinette operation. *J Shoulder Elbow Surg* 2008;17(5):744-750.

In a study of 46 patients after a failed Latarjet procedure reconstructed with the Eden-Hybinette operation, 34 patients were followed for a mean 6.8 years. There were four redislocations, and 13 patients had persistent apprehension. Nonetheless, 79% of the patients had a good or an excellent result at final follow-up.

[35] Owens BD, Harrast JJ, Hurwitz SR, Thompson TL, Wolf JM: Surgical trends in Bankart repair: An analysis of data from the American Board of Orthopaedic Surgery certification examination. *Am J Sports Med* 2011;39(9):1865-1869.

In a descriptive epidemiology study, American Board of Orthopaedic Surgery data showed a trend toward arthroscopic shoulder stabilization over time, compared with open repair. The overall reported complications were lower after arthroscopic stabilization than after open surgery.

[36] Athwal GS, Shridharani SM, O'Driscoll SW: Osteolysis and arthropathy of the shoulder after use of bioabsorbable knotless suture anchors: A report of four cases. *J Bone Joint Surg Am* 2006;88(8):1840-1845.

[37] Banerjee S, Weiser L, Connell D, Wallace AL: Glenoid rim fracture in contact athletes with absorbable suture anchor reconstruction. *Arthroscopy* 2009;25(5): 560-562.

A rim fracture was reported in three athletes with recurrent dislocation after labral repair using absorbable sutures. Fractures in the area of the sutures were noted as well as the possibility of absorbable sutures playing a role in weakening bone substance at the fracture site.

[38] Oh JH, Lee HK, Kim JY, Kim SH, Gong HS: Clinical and radiologic outcomes of arthroscopic glenoid labrum repair with the BioKnotless suture anchor. *Am J Sports Med* 2009;37(12):2340-2348.

Clinically and radiologically, the knotless anchor appears to be an acceptable alternative for arthroscopic labral repair, and it avoids certain drawbacks of the conventional knot-tying suture anchor. Level of evidence: IV.

[39] Boileau P, Villalba M, Héry JY, Balg F, Ahrens P, Neyton L: Risk factors for recurrence of shoulder instability after arthroscopic Bankart repair. *J Bone Joint Surg Am* 2006;88(8):1755-1763.

[40] Kang RW, Frank RM, Nho SJ, et al: Complications associated with anterior shoulder instability repair. *Arthroscopy* 2009;25(8):909-920.

A review categorized complications of anterior shoulder instability surgery and summarized the treatment options.

[41] Boileau P, Richou J, Lisai A, Chuinard C, Bicknell RT: The role of arthroscopy in revision of failed open anterior stabilization of the shoulder. *Arthroscopy* 2009; 25(10):1075-1084.

Arthroscopic revision of failed open anterior shoulder stabilization provided satisfactory results in a selected patient population. The main advantage of the arthroscopic approach is avoiding of anterior dissection and axillary nerve injury, although persistent pain and osteoarthritis progression remain concerns. Level of evidence: IV.

[42] Thomazeau H, Courage O, Barth J, et al; French Arthroscopy Society: Can we improve the indication for

Bankart arthroscopic repair? A preliminary clinical study using the ISIS score. *Orthop Traumatol Surg Res* 2010;96(8, suppl):S77-S83.

A multicenter study found that an Instability Severity Index Score equal to or less than 4 can be predictive of a successful outcome after arthroscopic Bankart repair. Level of evidence: IV.

[43] Pelet S, Jolles BM, Farron A: Bankart repair for recurrent anterior glenohumeral instability: Results at twenty-nine years' follow-up. *J Shoulder Elbow Surg* 2006;15(2):203-207.

[44] Hovelius L, Saeboe M: Neer Award 2008: Arthropathy after primary anterior shoulder dislocation—223 shoulders prospectively followed up for twenty-five years. *J Shoulder Elbow Surg* 2009;18(3):339-347.

A 25-year prospective study of 227 patients with radiographic imaging of 225 shoulders found that age at primary dislocation, recurrence, high-energy sports, and alcohol abuse were associated with the development of arthropathy. The absence of a recurrence also was associated with arthropathy.

[45] Robinson CM, Jenkins PJ, White TO, Ker A, Will E: Primary arthroscopic stabilization for a first-time anterior dislocation of the shoulder: A randomized, double-blind trial. *J Bone Joint Surg Am* 2008;90(4): 708-721.

A prospective randomized double-blind study compared primary arthroscopic stabilization for a first-time anterior dislocation with arthroscopy and lavage. There was a marked treatment benefit from primary arthroscopic repair of a Bankart lesion. Level of evidence: I.

[46] Savoie FH III, Holt MS, Field LD, Ramsey JR: Arthroscopic management of posterior instability: Evolution of technique and results. *Arthroscopy* 2008;24(4): 389-396.

No essential lesion is present in posterior instability. Attention and treatment of all contributing lesions leads to successful outcomes after arthroscopic repair of posterior instability. Level of evidence: IV.

[47] Bradley JP, Forsythe B, Mascarenhas R: Arthroscopic management of posterior shoulder instability: Diagnosis, indications, and technique. *Clin Sports Med* 2008; 27(4):649-670.

The diagnosis, evaluation, and management of posterior instability are reviewed, with nonsurgical and surgical treatment approaches.

[48] Robinson CM, Seah M, Akhtar MA: The epidemiology, risk of recurrence, and functional outcome after an acute traumatic posterior dislocation of the shoulder. *J Bone Joint Surg Am* 2011;93(17):1605-1613.

A retrospective study found that the prevalence of posterior dislocation was relatively low. The most common complication was recurrent instability, which occurred in 17.7% of shoulders within the first year after dislocation. The risk was highest in patients who were younger than 40 years, sustained the dislocation during a seizure, and had a large humeral head defect. Level of evidence: IV.

[49] Giles JW, Elkinson I, Ferreira LM, et al: Moderate to large engaging Hill-Sachs defects: An in vitro biomechanical comparison of the remplissage procedure, allograft humeral head reconstruction, and partial resurfacing arthroplasty. *J Shoulder Elbow Surg* 2012;21(9):1142-1151.

A biomechanical study of cadaver shoulders found that all procedures improved stability. Shoulders that had undergone humeral head or partial-resurfacing arthroplasty resembled intact shoulders, but those that had undergone remplissage did not. Remplissage improved stability and eliminated engagement but caused a reduction in range of motion. Humeral head and partial-resurfacing arthroplasty reestablished full range of motion, but partial-resurfacing arthroplasty could not fully prevent engagement.

[50] Nourissat G, Kilinc AS, Werther JR, Doursounian L: A prospective, comparative, radiological, and clinical study of the influence of the "remplissage" procedure on shoulder range of motion after stabilization by arthroscopic Bankart repair. *Am J Sports Med* 2011; 39(10):2147-2152.

A prospective cohort study compared arthroscopic Bankart repair alone and in conjunction with remplissage. The remplissage technique did not alter the range of motion of the shoulder compared with the Bankart procedure alone. One third of the patients experienced posterosuperior pain. Level of evidence: II.

[51] Gill TJ, Micheli LJ, Gebhard F, Binder C: Bankart repair for anterior instability of the shoulder: Long-term outcome. *J Bone Joint Surg Am* 1997;79(6):850-857.

[52] Wall MS, Warren RF: Complications of shoulder instability surgery. *Clin Sports Med* 1995;14(4):973-1000.

[53] Franceschi F, Papalia R, Del Buono A, Vasta S, Maffulli N, Denaro V: Glenohumeral osteoarthritis after arthroscopic Bankart repair for anterior instability. *Am J Sports Med* 2011;39(8):1653-1659.

Degenerative joint disease of the glenohumeral joint was associated with older age at first dislocation, increased time from the first episode to surgery, increased number of preoperative dislocations, increased number of anchors used at surgery, and more degenerated labrum at surgery. The number of anchors and the state of the labrum were most associated with a risk of radiographic degenerative changes. Level of evidence: IV.

[54] Good CR, Shindle MK, Kelly BT, Wanich T, Warren RF: Glenohumeral chondrolysis after shoulder arthroscopy with thermal capsulorrhaphy. *Arthroscopy* 2007; 23(7):e1-e5.

In a retrospective study, eight patients had chondrolysis after shoulder arthroscopy. Five had undergone thermal capsulorrhaphy. Level of evidence: IV.

[55] Rapley JH, Beavis RC, Barber FA: Glenohumeral chondrolysis after shoulder arthroscopy associated with continuous bupivacaine infusion. *Arthroscopy* 2009;25(12):1367-1373.

A retrospective study compared patients receiving a continuous infusion of 0.5% bupivacaine without epinephrine at different rates and into the glenohumeral joint or the subacromial space. The risk of developing chondrolysis depended on the device and rate, location, and length of infusion. Level of evidence: III.

[56] Ogawa K, Yoshida A, Ikegami H: Osteoarthritis in shoulders with traumatic anterior instability: Preoperative survey using radiography and computed tomography. *J Shoulder Elbow Surg* 2006;15(1):23-29.

[57] Hayes ML, Collins MS, Morgan JA, Wenger DE, Dahm DL: Efficacy of diagnostic magnetic resonance imaging for articular cartilage lesions of the glenohumeral joint in patients with instability. *Skeletal Radiol* 2010;39(12):1199-1204.

A retrospective MRI study used intraoperative findings as the gold standard. MRI had high sensitivity and specificity for diagnosing articular cartilage injury in patients with glenohumeral instability and was equally reliable with or without intra-articular contrast medium. Level of evidence: IV.

[58] Ogawa K, Yoshida A, Matsumoto H, Takeda T: Outcome of the open Bankart procedure for shoulder instability and development of osteoarthritis: A 5- to 20- year follow-up study. *Am J Sports Med* 2010;38(8): 1549-1557.

A prospective study examined the risk of progression to osteoarthritis after open Bankart surgery. Most postoperatively detected osteoarthritis had developed before surgery. The role of surgery in osteoarthritis was inconclusive. Level of evidence: III.

[59] Castagna A, Markopoulos N, Conti M, Delle Rose G, Papadakou E, Garofalo R: Arthroscopic Bankart suture-anchor repair: Radiological and clinical outcome at minimum 10 years of follow-up. *Am J Sports Med* 2010;38(10):2012-2016.

A study of the long-term outcomes of arthroscopic Bankart suture-anchor repair found that the recurrence rate declined over time. Involvement in contact sports or overhead activities appeared to be a risk factor. Degenerative changes of the glenohumeral joint were noted but had no significant effect on clinical outcomes. Level of evidence: IV.

[60] Cameron ML, Kocher MS, Briggs KK, Horan MP, Hawkins RJ: The prevalence of glenohumeral osteoarthrosis in unstable shoulders. *Am J Sports Med* 2003; 31(1):53-55.

[61] Hovelius L, Saeboe M: Documentation of dislocation arthropathy of the shoulder "area index": A better method to objectify the humeral osteophyte? *J Shoulder Elbow Surg* 2008;17(2):197-201.

A radiographic study defined a method of interpreting and quantifying dislocation arthropathy of the glenohumeral joint.

[62] Ghodadra N, Gupta A, Romeo AA, et al: Normalization of glenohumeral articular contact pressures after Latarjet or iliac crest bone-grafting. *J Bone Joint Surg Am* 2010;92(6):1478-1489.

A biomechanical cadaver study examined the effect on articular contact pressures of graft position in iliac crest bone grafting of the glenoid and the Latarjet procedure. Glenohumeral contact pressure was optimally restored with a flush iliac crest bone graft or a flush Latarjet bone block in which the inferior aspect of the coracoid became the glenoid surface.

[63] Robinson CM, Shur N, Sharpe T, Ray A, Murray IR: Injuries associated with traumatic anterior glenohumeral dislocations. *J Bone Joint Surg Am* 2012;94(1): 18-26.

A prospective study analyzed traumatic anterior glenohumeral dislocation in 3,633 patients. Rotator cuff tears, greater tuberosity fractures, and neurologic deficits were found to be more common than previously believed.

[64] Boardman ND III, Cofield RH: Neurologic complications of shoulder surgery. *Clin Orthop Relat Res* 1999; 368:44-53.

[65] Ho E, Cofield RH, Balm MR, Hattrup SJ, Rowland CM: Neurologic complications of surgery for anterior shoulder instability. *J Shoulder Elbow Surg* 1999;8(3): 266-270.

[66] Loomer R, Graham B: Anatomy of the axillary nerve and its relation to inferior capsular shift. *Clin Orthop Relat Res* 1989;243:100-105.

[67] Eglseder WA Jr, Goldman M: Anatomic variations of the

musculocutaneous nerve in the arm. *Am J Orthop (Belle Mead NJ)* 1997;26(11):777-780.

[68] Carter CW, Moros C, Ahmad CS, Levine WN: Arthroscopic anterior shoulder instability repair: Techniques, pearls, pitfalls, and complications. *Instr Course Lect* 2008;57:125-132.

Arthroscopic techniques for anterior shoulder instability were outlined, with complications and tips for avoiding them.

[69] McFarland EG, Caicedo JC, Guitterez MI, Sherbondy PS, Kim TK: The anatomic relationship of the brachial plexus and axillary artery to the glenoid: Implications for anterior shoulder surgery. *Am J Sports Med* 2001; 29(6):729-733.

[70] Maquieira GJ, Gerber C, Schneeberger AG: Suprascapular nerve palsy after the Latarjet procedure. *J Shoulder Elbow Surg* 2007;16(2):e13-e15.

After a Latarjet procedure, a patient had suprascapular nerve palsy resulting from a posteriorly proud screw entering the suprascapular notch.

[71] McFarland EG, Caicedo JC, Kim TK, Banchasuek P: Prevention of axillary nerve injury in anterior shoulder reconstructions: Use of a subscapularis muscle-splitting technique and a review of the literature. *Am J Sports Med* 2002;30(4):601-606.

[72] Esmail AN, Getz CL, Schwartz DM, Wierzbowski L, Ramsey ML, Williams GR Jr: Axillary nerve monitoring during arthroscopic shoulder stabilization. *Arthroscopy* 2005;21(6):665-671.

[73] McFarland EG, O'Neill OR, Hsu CY: Complications of shoulder arthroscopy. *J South Orthop Assoc* 1997; 6(3):190-196.

[74] Mair SD, Hawkins RJ: Open shoulder instability surgery; Complications. *Clin Sports Med* 1999;18(4): 719-736.

[75] Sperling JW, Cofield RH, Torchia ME, Hanssen AD: Infection after shoulder instability surgery. *Clin Orthop Relat Res* 2003;414:61-64.

[76] Ticker JB, Lippe RJ, Barkin DE, Carroll MP: Infected suture anchors in the shoulder. *Arthroscopy* 1996; 12(5):613-615.

[77] Bonnevialle N, Mansat P, Bellumore Y, Mansat M, Bonnevialle P: Selective capsular repair for the treatment of anterior-inferior shoulder instability: Review of seventy-nine shoulders with seven years' average follow-up. *J Shoulder Elbow Surg* 2009;18(2): 251-259.

A retrospective study found a 90% satisfaction rate and 80% good to excellent results at midterm follow-up of patients who underwent selective capsular repair for posttraumatic anterior glenohumeral instability. Level of evidence: IV.

[78] Elmlund A, Kartus C, Sernert N, Hultenheim I, Ejerhed L: A long-term clinical follow-up study after arthroscopic intra-articular Bankart repair using absorbable tacks. *Knee Surg Sports Traumatol Arthrosc* 2008;16(7):707-712.

At a mean 8-year follow-up, arthroscopic repair with absorbable tacks led to a stable shoulder with good function in most of the 73 patients. Dislocation or subluxation had occurred in 19%.

[79] Fabre T, Abi-Chahla ML, Billaud A, Geneste M, Durandeau A: Long-term results with Bankart procedure: A 26-year follow-up study of 50 cases. *J Shoulder Elbow Surg* 2010;19(2):318-323.

At a follow-up more than 20 years in 49 patients, including 36 contact athletes, after an open Bankart procedure for recurrent shoulder instability, most patients had a stable shoulder and had returned to their previous level of sports activity. Radiographic osteoarthritis was found in 69% of the patients.

[80] Law BK, Yung PS, Ho EP, Chang JJ, Chan KM: The surgical outcome of immediate arthroscopic Bankart repair for first time anterior shoulder dislocation in young active patients. *Knee Surg Sports Traumatol Arthrosc* 2008;16(2):188-193.

At a mean 28-month follow-up, an immediate Bankart repair and accelerated rehabilitation program were found to be an effective method of treating young, active patients with traumatic anterior shoulder dislocation.

[81] Porcellini G, Campi F, Pegreffi F, Castagna A, Paladini P: Predisposing factors for recurrent shoulder dislocation after arthroscopic treatment. *J Bone Joint Surg Am* 2009;91(11):2537-2542.

A 36-month study found that the risk of redislocation after arthroscopic repair of an anterior shoulder dislocation can be determined based on patient sex, age, and elapsed time from first dislocation to surgery.

[82] Thal R, Nofziger M, Bridges M, Kim JJ: Arthroscopic Bankart repair using Knotless or BioKnotless suture anchors: 2- to 7-year results. *Arthroscopy* 2007;23(4): 367-375.

A retrospective study of 73 patients found a 6.9% recurrence rate 2 to 7 years after arthroscopic Bankart repair using knotless suture anchors. There were minimal loss of motion and good function, even among contact athletes. Level of evidence: IV.

第三部分

骨科核心知识

栏目编委：
Sumant G. Krishnan, MD

第十三章　肩袖疾病的解剖、病理机制、自然病程和非手术治疗

Hiroyuki Sugaya, MD

引言

肩袖疾病包括肩袖部分撕裂、肩袖全层撕裂及肩袖肌腱炎。判断患者的肩关节疼痛和功能障碍是否由肩袖疾病本身引起并不容易。在年龄大于 65 岁的患者中经常能够通过 MRI 和超声检查发现肩袖组织病变。一些有肩关节疼痛的患者并没有肩袖组织病变的证据，而有些患者虽没有症状但影像学检查有肩袖撕裂的表现。[1] 肩关节症状的存在与否同时受生理因素和心理因素的影响，例如，会最终索赔并得到赔偿的患者，其手术效果通常较其他患者差。[2-3]

外科医师必须同时评估功能因素和结构因素。肩袖功能、肩胛骨的位置和活动范围、姿势、脊柱活动范围、骨盆倾斜程度以及下肢的功能都是影响肩关节症状的因素。肩关节对功能性疾病的易感性在很大程度上取决于肩胛带的独特性质。肩袖、关节囊和肱二头肌腱连接肩胛骨和肱骨头。肩胛骨和上肢作为一个功能单元仅通过肩锁关节和胸锁关节与躯干相连。换言之，连接肩胛骨 – 上肢单元和躯干的主要结构为肩胛骨周围肌肉。肩胛骨的位置会极大地影响姿势和下肢功能，不正确的姿势同样会限制肩胛骨的活动。肩胛骨功能减退很容易导致肩胛带周围出现症状。[4] 对于有肩关节症状的患者的非手术治疗，纠正受损的

Dr. Sugaya or an immediate family member is a member of a speakers' bureau or has made paid presentations on behalf of Mitek and Smith & Nephew and serves as an unpaid consultant to Mitek and Smith & Nephew.

肩胛胸廓功能是首选。[5]

解剖学

肩胛带的解剖相对较复杂。肩胛骨前方通过前锯肌和胸小肌，后方通过上斜方肌、下斜方肌、菱形肌、肩胛提肌和背阔肌与躯干相连。上述组织的肌张力和弹性很大程度上影响着肩胛功能。[4] 三角肌包绕着肩关节，其前方起自锁骨内侧 1/2 和肩峰前外侧部，向后延伸至肩胛冈，远端止于肱骨近端 1/3 的三角肌结节。因此，三角肌在肩袖的协助下，是肩关节外展的主要力量来源。

冈上肌和冈下肌

肩袖由肩胛下肌、冈上肌、冈下肌和小圆肌的腱性止点构成。传统观点认为，冈上肌起自肩胛上窝，止于大结节的上部；冈下肌起自肩胛窝，止于肱骨头的后部，大结节的中部。[5-7] 但是，近年来肩关节外科医师和解剖学家的研究表明，冈上肌止于大结节上部最前方的局限区域，甚至部分止于小结节，而冈下肌止于大结节中部接近上 1/2 处 [8-9]（图 13-1）。这些研究发现冈下肌分为两束：斜行纤维，起自肩胛窝，止于大结节中上部；横行纤维，起自肩胛冈下部，止于斜行纤维的腱性部分 [10]（图 13-2）。盂肱关节关节囊有宽大的附着点，尤其是在冈下肌和小圆肌的腱性止点之间 [11]（图 13-3）。据推测，这一增厚的关节囊可以沿着冈下肌和小圆肌的腱性止点发挥肌腱的功能，可能跟手术中经常见到的巨大肩袖撕裂的分层有关。[11]

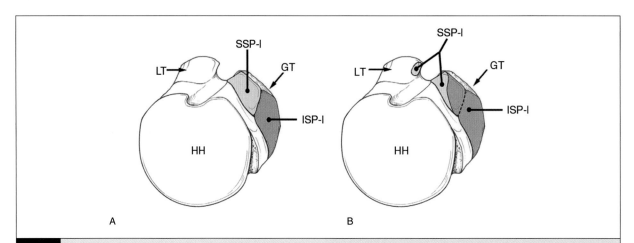

图 13-1　右侧肱骨上部示意图，显示冈上肌和冈下肌的止点。A. 普遍认为冈上肌止于大结节的最上方区域，冈下肌止于大结节中部。B. 近期的研究表明，冈下肌的止点占一半左右的最上方区域及全部的中间区域，冈上肌止于最上方区域的前内侧，有时可止于小结节。GT= 大结节；HH= 肱骨头；ISP-I= 冈下肌止点；LT= 小结节；SSP-I= 冈上肌止点。经允许引自 Mochizuki T, Sugaya H, Uomizu M, et al: Humeral insertion of the supraspinatus and infraspinatus: New anatomical findings regarding the footprint of the rotator cuff. *J Bone Joint Surg Am* 2008;90（5）:962-969.

肩胛下肌

肩胛下肌既是唯一位于前方的肩袖肌肉，也是肩袖中体积最大的肌肉。近年来关节镜技术的发展使研究者们认识到了肩胛下肌腱撕裂的重要性。其发病率也明显比早期报道的高。[12-14]

肩胛下肌内有数条肌腱，最头侧的肌腱较其他肌腱更长、更厚，肩胛下肌腱最近端的附着点亦由此长厚肌腱发出，附着点位于小结节最近端上部，其余肩胛下肌腱附着于小结节前内侧部。[12]远端肩胛下肌附着点变窄，肌纤维更靠近肱骨，而腱性组织非常短（图 13-4）。最近端的肩胛下肌腱延伸成一条较薄的腱滑，附着于肱骨头凹。此腱滑的主要功能是为肩胛下肌腱提供更大的附着区域，并为结节间沟提供光滑的基底，稳定肱二头肌长头腱（LHB），防止其脱位（图 13-5）。[15]最头侧的肌腱附着点最强大，在临床上也最重要，其连同腱滑一起形成最宽大的附着区域。[15]

肩胛下肌的某些腱性纤维被发现跨过 LHB 止于小结节，这些纤维通过 LHB 增强了最头侧肩胛下肌的附着。[8-9]止于小结节的纤维与逗号征联系密切，逗号征是前上方肩袖全层撕裂的重要标志。[16]

手术中，强烈推荐对止点进行修复重建以增强初始固定的强度，尤其是对头侧的肩胛下肌撕裂。

小圆肌

小圆肌比其他肩袖肌肉体积小，其紧邻冈下肌止点下方，止于大结节[11]（图 13-3）。即使在巨大三肌腱撕裂时，小圆肌的腱性止点通常也会保持完整。小圆肌的体积常左右手术决策，因为其可预测巨大肩袖撕裂手术治疗的预后。小圆肌同三角肌一起受腋神经支配。而肩胛上神经穿过肩胛上结节支配冈上肌，随后向下走行支配肩胛下肌。

体格检查

详细的病史采集对于准确诊断肩部症状的病因非常重要。医师应询问患者症状出现的情况、持续时间和特点，同时注意外伤性因素、症状加重和缓解因素、早期治疗情况及对治疗的反应。如果疼痛为主要症状，则必须弄清楚疼痛是否在夜间或上肢处于休息位置时出现。静息痛很有可能是由盂肱关节或肩峰下滑囊炎症造成的。[17]

常规进行普通 X 线检查，有助于确定肩袖撕

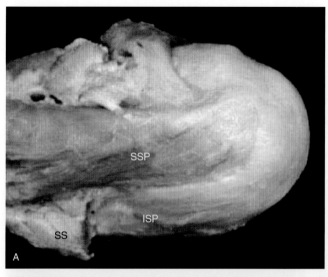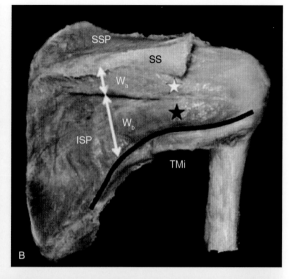

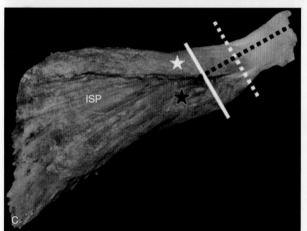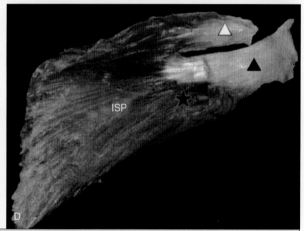

图 13-2　冈上肌和冈下肌的肌肉、肌腱形态图。A. 右肩上面观，显示冈上肌和冈下肌的肌肉、肌腱。B. 右肩背面观，显示冈下肌的肌肉、肌腱，包括横行部分（白色五角星）和斜行部分（黑色五角星）。黑线显示冈下肌与小圆肌的边界。C. 冈下肌从肩胛骨和肱骨大结节分离后的背面观，很容易辨别横行部分（白色五角星）和斜行部分（黑色五角星）。黑线和白线分别显示纵行组织节段和横行组织节段。D. 冈下肌背面观，横行部分（黑色五角星）已从斜行部分分离。斜行纤维有长且厚的腱性部分（黑色三角），附着于大结节，横行纤维仅存在短且薄的腱膜（白色三角），附着于斜行纤维的腱性部分，而不附着于大结节。ISP= 冈下肌，SS= 肩胛冈，SSP= 冈上肌，TMi= 小圆肌，W$_a$= 肩胛冈中点处横行纤维的宽度，W$_b$= 肩胛冈中点处斜行纤维的宽度。经允许引自 Arai R, Mochizuki T, Yamaguchi K, et al: Functional anatomy of the superior glenohumeral and coracohumeral ligaments and the subscapularis tendon in view of stabilization of the long head of the biceps tendon. *J Shoulder Elbow Surg* 2010;19（1）:58-64.

裂的关节病变和其他肩关节疾病，如钙化性肌腱炎、原发性骨关节炎和单纯肱骨头上移。应基于病史和普通 X 线片上获得的信息进行体格检查。肩袖疾病患者的体格检查分为 4 部分：①视诊、触诊和力量检查；②肩胛胸廓功能检查；③主被动活动范围；④肩胛骨活动检查。

　　进行肩胛胸廓的动力学检查时，应令患者取

站立位，检查患者的姿势和肩胛骨位置。肩胛骨位置不良，包括伸长、前倾、向下旋转及下沉（与对侧对比），均是肩胛动力障碍的重要表现。[4-5]此类肩关节疾病患者通常喙突压痛明显。同样在站立位时，对主被动活动范围进行评估，由疼痛弧检查开始。如果患侧肩关节无法完全抬起，医师一定要评估活动受限的原因，包括疼痛、僵硬和肩胛功能

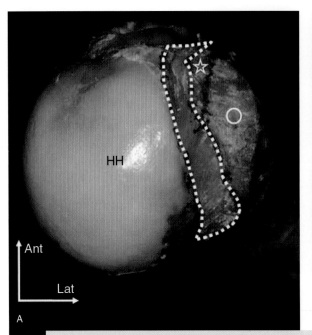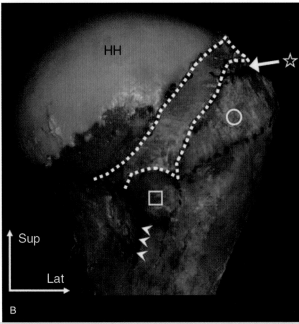

图
13-3
肱骨的上面观（A）和背面观（B），显示关节囊的附着区域（白色虚线），冈上肌（五角星、黑色虚线）和冈下肌（圆圈）的附着部位以及小圆肌的腱性附着区域（矩形）和肌性附着区域（箭头）。HH= 肱骨头，Ant= 前，Lat= 外侧，Sup= 上。经允许引自 Nimura A, Kato A, Yamaguchi K, et al: The superior capsule of the shoulder joint complements the insertion of the rotator cuff. *J Shoulder Elbow Surg* 2012;21（7）:867-872.

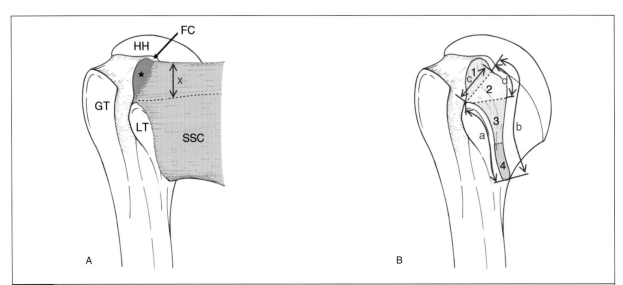

图
13-4
右肩肩胛下肌止点范围示意图。A. 最上方的肩胛下肌腱止于小结节最上缘，其余肌腱止于小结节的前内侧。最上方止点［头侧肌腱的外侧部分（*）］和腱滑组成的结构在拐角处与肱二头肌长头腱的下表面直接接触。头侧肌腱的纵径（x）有足够的长度以减小肱二头肌腱的弧度。B. 肩胛下肌附着区域由腱滑的附着区域构成：肌腱最上方止点（1）；另一肌腱止点（2）；肌肉止点（3）；肩胛下肌附着范围的边界（4），即外缘（a）、内缘（b）、外上缘（c）和内上缘（d）。外上缘（c）具有足够的长度支撑肱二头肌腱。HH= 肱骨头；FC= 肱骨头凹；GT= 大结节；LT= 小结节；SSC= 肩胛下肌。经允许引自 Arai R, Sugaya H, Mochizuki T, Nimura A, Moriishi J, Akita K: Subscapularis tendon tear: An anatomic and clinical investigation. *Arthroscopy* 2008;24（9）:997-1004.

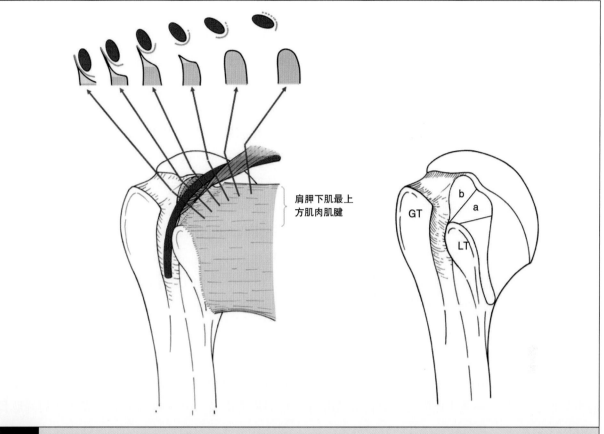

肩胛下肌最上
方肌肉肌腱

图 13-5	示意图显示肱二头肌长头腱（红色）、肩胛下肌最上方肌腱（灰色）、盂肱上韧带（SGHL，绿色）和肩胛下肌止点腱滑（黄色）的位置关系。肩胛下肌最上方止点是肩胛下肌最上方肌腱在小结节上缘的宽大附着区（a），该附着区向肱骨头凹延伸成一腱滑（b）。SGHL 在盂肱关节内侧壁靠近关节盂处折叠并向外侧延伸，螺旋形包绕肱二头肌长头，并附着于肩胛下肌腱滑。SGHL 的起始点并不明确，肩胛下肌最上方止点在 SGHL 后方支撑 LHB，SGHL 与喙肱韧带连续，喙肱韧带覆盖整个盂肱关节，目前认为其张力可传递至 SGHL，因为这两条韧带形成了同一疏松结缔组织。这种张力可能对 SGHL 对抗 LHB 的脱位有益。GT= 大结节；LT= 小结节。经允许引自 Arai R, Sugaya H, Mochizuki T, Nimura A, Moriishi J, Akita K: Subscapularis tendon tear: An anatomic and clinical investigation. *Arthroscopy* 2008;24（9）:997-1004.

障碍。评估双侧肩关节前屈、外展、在侧方时外旋、肩关节外展 90° 时外旋和内旋的范围，以及拇指可触及到的脊柱的最高水平。尤其在肩关节由前屈或外展 90° 内旋位下降的反向期，医师可能观察到患者疼痛加重和肩胛骨异常活动。不论患者是否存在肩袖撕裂，这种现象在肩峰下疼痛患者中都很典型。

对怀疑有肩袖疾病而无肩关节僵硬的患者，需在患者坐位或站立位时对其双侧肩关节常规进行以下几项力量检查：在肩胛骨平面肩关节外展 30° 和 90° 时的外展力量检查（Jobe 试验）、

水平位肩关节屈曲 90° 和 120° 时的前屈力量检查（Whipple 试验）、上臂在侧方时的外旋力量检查。外旋力量减弱和（或）外旋迟滞征是后上方肩袖巨大撕裂的特征性表现。此外，所有患者均应接受熊抱试验和腹部加压试验以进行肩胛下肌力量检查，因为据研究报道，肩胛下肌撕裂的发生率高达 27%~37%。[12-14]

患者仰卧位外展和水平位屈曲联合试验可用于评估肩胛运动障碍。[18] 对于特定的肩关节问题有很多诱发试验，但是为了提高检查效率，临床医师必须清楚最有效的检查方法。

肩袖撕裂的病理机制

尽管肌腱纤维断裂是所有肩袖撕裂的最终病理表现，但是目前对于非创伤性肩袖疾病，仍没有统一的病因学和病理机制解释。致病因素是多方面的，通常可以分为内源性因素和外源性因素。内源性因素包括年龄相关性肌腱退变，外源性因素以机械撞击最为典型。[19]

内源性因素

有症状的和无症状的肩袖撕裂的发病率均随着年龄的增长而增高。一个年龄大于66岁的单侧肩关节疼痛患者，有50%的可能性存在双侧肩袖撕裂。[20]这一现象表明随着年龄的增长，肌腱会出现进行性退变。最近的组织病理学研究发现了早已存在的年龄相关性肌腱退变征象。在平均年龄60岁的关节侧肩袖部分撕裂患者中，关节镜下完整的残留肌腱组织同样存在中等程度的组织病理学退变。[21]一项关于撕裂肩袖肌腱组织内侧残端的研究报道，薄而排列杂乱的胶原纤维、黏液样退变和玻璃样变性的发生频率和分布表明撕裂肌腱存在早期退变。肩袖撕裂的主要原因是轻微创伤和中层、深层肌腱已经存在的退行性改变。[22]一项研究通过在静脉内注射造影剂后进行强化超声检查比较了肩袖撕裂患者和无肩袖撕裂患者的肌腱内血供情况，发现不管是否存在肩袖撕裂，年长患者肌腱内的血流均明显低于年轻患者。[23]

年龄相关性肌腱退变导致肌腱肿胀和增厚，使得本就因年龄相关性骨刺形成和滑囊增厚而狭窄的肩峰下间隙变得更狭小。上肢活动很容易就可以引起滑囊侧肩袖撕裂，尤其是在肩胛胸壁关节僵硬导致的肩胛骨活动性较差的患者中。部分关节侧肩袖撕裂可能主要由内源性肩袖退变导致，没有过多外源性因素的参与。[24]在全层肩袖撕裂的患者中，随着撕裂面积的增大，成纤维细胞和炎症细胞的数目逐渐减少，这反映了撕裂的肩袖愈合能力的改变。[25]同时，随着肩袖撕裂面积的增加，血管数目和血管化能力也表现出进行性降低。[25-26]吸烟也可以降低肩袖肌腱形成血管的能力。[27]肩袖撕裂与吸烟的剂量和时间相关，这表明吸烟是肩袖撕裂发展中重要的危险因素。[28]

肩袖病变和肩关节症状与遗传有一定关系。[20,29]一项研究发现，肩袖疾病呈家族聚集性，并存在家族谱系。[30]患者的近亲和远亲的发病风险均明显升高。这些研究强烈支持肩袖疾病存在遗传倾向。现在越来越多的证据表明有数条基因通路与肩袖肌腱的构成有关，在肩袖发生病变时这些基因通路出现改变，影响细胞外基质、脉管系统和细胞内信号传递。[31]将来仍需进一步研究以明确与肩袖撕裂相关的遗传学和生物学因素。

外源性因素

外源性因素包括解剖变异和周围软组织直接压迫，解剖变异包括肩峰形态改变、肩峰骨和肩峰骨刺，肩峰骨刺通过骨性撞击压迫肩袖。原发性肩峰撞击最初由Neer报道，其发生于肩峰肱骨间隙变窄或突出的前外侧钩状肩峰或喙肩韧带肥大的患者，他们在上臂抬起时会磨损肩袖。肩峰的形态特点看似不太容易导致肩袖撕裂。实际上，近期的研究表明，肩峰形态和肩峰指数（大的肩峰外侧延伸被认为是肩袖全层撕裂的显著致病因素[32]）与肩袖疾病无关，而肩峰骨刺在有症状和无症状的患者中均与肩袖全层撕裂高度相关。[33]肩胛骨运动障碍导致的肩胛功能减退是最可能导致肩袖撕裂的外源性因素，尤其是当存在年龄相关性肩峰骨刺形成时。[4-5,33]外科医师应该了解动态因素，例如，上臂活动时由于肩胛骨位置不良或运动障碍导致的肩胛骨代偿性运动消失。与静态的形态学改变相比，动态因素是肩袖撕裂的重要外源性因素。

另一个导致肩袖病变的外源性因素是反复微创伤导致的内在撞击。这一情况发生于反复做空中投掷动作的患者，该动作会导致关节侧肩袖部分撕裂，尤其是当患者存在肩胛骨运动障碍时更容易发生。尽管病因还存在争议，但是存在内在撞击的患者，其后方关节囊通常较紧，或盂肱韧带前束松弛而后方肌肉紧张，从而导致大结节内侧肩袖止点与关节盂后上方在上举后期和投掷加速期出现撞击。这种反复活动导致冈上肌后方和冈下肌前方出现关节侧部分撕裂，同时合并后上方盂唇撕裂。

肩袖撕裂的自然病程

尽管部分肩袖撕裂或小的撕裂具有自发愈合的潜力，但是通常认为撕裂会随着时间进展。不过，有些肩袖撕裂并不会出现肩关节症状。在年龄大于 65 岁的患者中，由于胸椎活动范围缩小及后凸畸形导致肩胛胸廓功能改变，有时必然会出现肩袖损伤。外科医师在选择治疗方式时必须了解无症状肩袖撕裂的自然病程。

无症状撕裂的症状改变

目前，尚未清楚有症状和无症状的肩袖撕裂的区别。[34-35]但是，在无症状全层肩袖撕裂出现症状变化时，撕裂加重是其中的一个原因。[36]一项研究使用超声检查对 58 例一侧肩关节有症状而另一侧肩关节无症状的肩袖撕裂患者进行了超过 5 年的纵向自然病史研究，[37]发现 51% 的之前无症状的肩关节在平均 2.8 年以后出现了症状，撕裂大小的进展与症状的进展相关，包括疼痛的显著增加和进行日常活动的能力减退。双侧肩袖疾病（包括有症状和无症状的）在最初有单侧肩关节疼痛的患者中很常见。[20]

有症状的撕裂的进展

在一项前瞻性研究中，年龄小于或等于 60 岁的全层肩袖撕裂范围相对较小的患者接受了非手术治疗。[38]在平均 29 个月的随访中，49% 的患者撕裂范围增加，43% 的患者无变化，8% 的患者范围缩小。随访时出现明显疼痛与超声检查发现撕裂加重存在相关性。一项回顾性研究发现，肩袖撕裂进展的危险因素包括年龄大于 60 岁、全层撕裂和肩袖肌肉脂肪浸润。[39]但是，一项针对

24 例患者的肩部结构的临床研究发现，小的、有症状的全层撕裂在一定的时期内并不会全部出现进展。[40]这些患者拒绝对有症状的单纯全层冈上肌撕裂进行手术修复。在诊断后平均 42 个月的随访中，撕裂的平均大小在标准 MRI 上没有变化。患者对结果的满意度也极高。

对于小的、有症状的肩袖撕裂，影响非手术治疗效果的最重要因素是撕裂加重。研究者深入研究了 123 例通过含显微线圈的高分辨率 MRI 诊断的全层肩袖撕裂患者，并对影响他们所接受的非手术治疗效果的相关因素进行了研究。[41]研究发现冈上肌肌肉内肌腱的完整性是影响治疗效果的最显著因素。在冈上肌的解剖切迹中，冈上肌肌肉内肌腱的主要部分止于上关节面的最前方，撕裂加重可能与这一部分是否撕裂（即使是很小的撕裂）有关[8-9,11]（图 13-1，13-3）。如果最前方肌肉内肌腱止点损伤，撕裂就会进展，无症状的肩关节最终也会出现症状，而有症状的肩关节的症状会持续存在。

脂肪浸润和巨大肩袖撕裂

脂肪浸润会随着撕裂范围的增加、受累肌腱数量的增加或肌腱断裂后时间的推移而进展。在一项纳入 1688 例行手术修复的肩袖撕裂患者的回顾性研究中，中度（Goutallier 2 级）冈上肌脂肪浸润在出现症状之后的平均第 3 年出现，重度脂肪浸润（Goutallier 3 或 4 级）在平均第 5 年出现。[42]切线征在症状出现后的平均第 4.5 年出现。在同一组患者中，出现多发肌腱撕裂时，冈下肌脂肪浸润明显增加；同样随着年龄的增长，脂肪浸润也显著加重。[43]Goutallier 2 级冈下肌脂肪浸润在症状出现后的平均第 2.5 年出现，Goutallier 3 级或 4 级脂肪浸润在平均第 4 年出现。Goutallier 2 级肩胛下肌脂肪浸润在症状出现后的平均第 2.5 年出现，Goutallier 3 级或 4 级在平均第 5 年出现。[44]该研究的作者认为应该在中度（Goutallier 2 级）脂肪浸润和萎缩（切线征阳性）出现之前

进行手术修复，尤其是对于多发肌腱撕裂患者。

部分多发肌腱撕裂患者仍无症状或仅有中度症状。但是，撕裂和脂肪浸润最终会发展到无法修复的程度。在一项对 19 例巨大肩袖撕裂患者的非手术治疗研究中，尽管在至少 4 年的随访中患者的肩关节出现了明显的退行性改变，包括盂肱关节骨关节炎和脂肪浸润，但患者仍能保持满意的关节功能。[45]

非手术治疗

目前，研究者们对肩袖撕裂的最佳治疗方案仍未达成共识。治疗方案的选择应基于患者的症状。[46] 有症状的肩袖撕裂患者可能存在炎症性疼痛、功能受限（如肩胛运动障碍）和解剖结构完整性受损。手术仅能解决解剖学因素。考虑到目前对于有症状的和无症状的肩袖撕裂的区别缺少合理定义，因此在实施手术之前，尝试缓解患者疼痛和改善功能受限非常重要。

疼痛治疗

疼痛是大多数患者的初始症状。在治疗时早期控制疼痛非常重要，尤其是与上臂姿势无关、休息时或夜间都存在的炎症性疼痛。尽管冰敷、休息、NSAIDs 类药物和改变活动方式是炎症性疼痛的一线治疗方式，但是盂肱关节或肩峰下滑囊激素注射可能是最有效、最可靠的治疗方式。[17,47-48] 与特定关节活动相关的疼痛（疼痛弧或撞击征）为机械性或功能性疼痛，选择手术治疗或物理治疗以纠正肩胛功能障碍。在治疗时，及早缓解炎症性疼痛对提高物理治疗或手术治疗的治疗效果尤其重要。

物理治疗

在中老年肩袖撕裂患者中，由于肌肉和周围组织弹性下降，胸椎出现后凸畸形，肩胛骨活动通常受限。[4-5] 因此，在进行肩袖功能恢复和肩胛骨稳定治疗之前，最重要的第一步治疗是恢复肩胛骨和躯干的活动范围。正常肩胛带机械功能的

恢复从肩袖功能上举和前伸以及肩胛骨稳定性训练开始，然后进行躯干和下肢核心稳定性训练以进行更复杂的活动。尽管肩袖及周围肌肉的拉伸和力量的自我导向性训练也有效，但是如果患者胸椎僵硬，仍强烈推荐进行专业的物理治疗。[49-50]

参考文献

[1] Yamamoto A, Takagishi K, Kobayashi T, Shitara H, Osawa T: Factors involved in the presence of symptoms associated with rotator cuff tears: A comparison of asymptomatic and symptomatic rotator cuff tears in the general population. *J Shoulder Elbow Surg* 2011; 20(7):1133-1137.

In 211 patients, 283 shoulders had a full-thickness ro- tator cuff tear, but approximately two thirds of the shoulders did not have symptoms. The factors in symptomatic shoulders with a rotator cuff tear were a positive impingement sign, weakness in external rotation, and a tear in the dominant arm.

[2] Holtby R, Razmjou H: Impact of work-related compensation claims on surgical outcome of patients with rotator cuff related pathologies: A matched casecontrol study. *J Shoulder Elbow Surg* 2010;19(3): 452-460.

The surgical outcomes of patients with a work-related compensation claim were compared with those of a historical control group based on age, sex, and level of pathology. Both groups improved significantly. At baseline and 1 year after surgery, the patients with a claim had a significantly higher level of disability.

[3] Cuff DJ, Pupello DR: Prospective evaluation of postoperative compliance and outcomes after rotator cuff repair in patients with and without workers' compensation claims. *J Shoulder Elbow Surg* 2012;21(12): 1728-1733.

Compliance and outcomes of rotator cuff repair were compared in patients with or without a workers' compensation claim. Patients with a claim had a higher rate of postoperative noncompliance (52% versus 4%). Patients with a claim who had no evidence of noncompliance had significantly more improvement and a more favorable outcome than patients with a claim who were noncompliant.

[4] Kibler WB, Sciascia A, Wilkes T: Scapular dyskinesis and its relation to shoulder injury. *J Am Acad Orthop Surg* 2012;20(6):364-372.

The scapula plays a key role in almost every aspect of normal shoulder function. Patients with shoulder impingement, rotator cuff disease, labral injury, clavicle fracture, acromioclavicular joint injury, or multidirectional instability should be evaluated for scapular dyskinesis and treated accordingly.

[5] Kibler WB: The scapula in rotator cuff disease. *Med Sport Sci* 2012;57:27-40.

The scapula serves as the platform or the base for the muscles of the rotator cuff, and scapular dyskinesis is frequently identified in rotator cuff disease. Careful examination for scapular dyskinesis and its causative mechanisms should be part of the comprehensive evaluation of patients with rotator cuff disease.

[6] Curtis AS, Burbank KM, Tierney JJ, Scheller AD, Curran AR: The insertional footprint of the rotator cuff: An anatomic study. *Arthroscopy* 2006;22(6):e1.

[7] Dugas JR, Campbell DA, Warren RF, Robie BH, Millett PJ: Anatomy and dimensions of rotator cuff insertions. *J Shoulder Elbow Surg* 2002;11(5):498-503.

[8] Mochizuki T, Sugaya H, Uomizu M, et al: Humeral insertion of the supraspinatus and infraspinatus: New anatomical findings regarding the footprint of the rotator cuff. *J Bone Joint Surg Am* 2008;90(5):962-969.

In 113 cadaver specimens, the footprint of the supraspinatus on the greater tuberosity was found to be much smaller than previously believed. This area of the greater tuberosity is occupied by a substantial amount of the infraspinatus.

[9] Mochizuki T, Sugaya H, Uomizu M, et al: Humeral insertion of the supraspinatus and infraspinatus: New anatomical findings regarding the footprint of the rotator cuff. Surgical technique. *J Bone Joint Surg Am* 2009;91(suppl 2, pt 1):1-7.

Surgical techniques were recommended based on anatomic study of the footprint of the supraspinatus and the infraspinatus in 113 cadaver specimens.

[10] Kato A, Nimura A, Yamaguchi K, Mochizuki T, Sugaya H, Akita K: An anatomical study of the transverse part of the infraspinatus muscle that is closely related with the supraspinatus muscle. *Surg Radiol Anat* 2012;34(3):257-265.

A cadaver study found that the infraspinatus is composed of oblique and transverse parts according to muscle fiber direction. Both parts have a partially independent morphology. The transverse part inserts into the main tendinous portion of the oblique part as a thin tendinous membrane.

[11] Nimura A, Kato A, Yamaguchi K, et al: The superior capsule of the shoulder joint complements the insertion of the rotator cuff. *J Shoulder Elbow Surg* 2012; 21(7):867-872.

The attachment of the articular capsule of the shoulder joint was found to occupy a substantial area of the greater tuberosity. At the border between the infraspinatus and the teres minor, the very thick attachment of the articular capsule compensated for the lack of attachment of muscular components.

[12] Arai R, Sugaya H, Mochizuki T, Nimura A, Moriishi J, Akita K: Subscapularis tendon tear: An anatomic and clinical investigation. *Arthroscopy* 2008;24(9): 997-1004.

The subscapularis insertion anatomy was investigated in view of the stabilizing function of the long head of the biceps tendon. The prevalence of subscapularis tendon tears was evaluated by reviewing surgical records and videotapes.

[13] Adams CR, Schoolfield JD, Burkhart SS: Accuracy of preoperative magnetic resonance imaging in predicting a subscapularis tendon tear based on arthroscopy. *Arthroscopy* 2010;26(11):1427-1433.

The diagnostic accuracy of MRI of subscapularis tendon tears was studied by comparing preoperative MRI interpretations by radiologists with arthroscopic evaluations of the same shoulders.

[14] Garavaglia G, Ufenast H, Taverna E: The frequency of subscapularis tears in arthroscopic rotator cuff repairs: A retrospective study comparing magnetic resonance imaging and arthroscopic findings. *Int J Shoulder Surg* 2011;5(4):90-94.

A medical chart review of 348 consecutive arthroscopic rotator cuff repairs found subscapularis tears in 129 (37%). Good agreement was found with supraspinatus MRI results, but MRI often failed to reveal subscapularis and infraspinatus tears.

[15] Arai R, Mochizuki T, Yamaguchi K, et al: Functional anatomy of the superior glenohumeral and coracohumeral ligaments and the subscapularis tendon in view of stabilization of the long head of the biceps tendon. *J Shoulder Elbow Surg* 2010;19(1):58-64.

Twelve cadaver shoulders were used to study the anatomy of the lateral rotator cuff interval and the most cranial subscapularis tendon insertion area.

[16] Lo IK, Burkhart SS: The comma sign: An arthroscopic guide to the torn subscapularis tendon. *Arthroscopy* 2003;19(3):334-337.

［17］Gialanella B, Prometti P: Effects of corticosteroids injection in rotator cuff tears. *Pain Med* 2011;12(10):1559-1565.

A randomized controlled study found that intra-articular injection of triamcinolone improved pain relief for 3 months. The drug action was not prolonged or potentiated by two injections at a 21-day interval.

［18］Pappas AM, Zawacki RM, McCarthy CF: Rehabilitation of the pitching shoulder. *Am J Sports Med* 1985;13(4):223-235.

［19］Maffulli N, Longo UG, Berton A, Loppini M, Denaro V: Biological factors in the pathogenesis of rotator cuff tears. *Sports Med Arthrosc* 2011;19(3):194-201.

The biologic factors involved in the pathogenesis of rotator cuff tears were investigated. An understanding of the mechanism of rotator cuff pathology could guide the design, the selection, and the implementation of treatment strategies, such as biologic modulation and preventive measures.

［20］Yamaguchi K, Ditsios K, Middleton WD, Hildebolt CF, Galatz LM, Teefey SA: The demographic and morphological features of rotator cuff disease: A comparison of asymptomatic and symptomatic shoulders. *J Bone Joint Surg Am* 2006;88(8):1699-1704.

［21］Yamakado K: Histopathology of residual tendon in high-grade articular-sided partial-thickness rotator cuff tears (PASTA lesions). *Arthroscopy* 2012;28(4): 474-480.

More than 90% of the macroscopically intact residual tendon tissue of partial articular-surface tendon avulsion tears in 30 patients (mean age, 60 years) had moderate histopathologic degeneration.

［22］Hashimoto T, Nobuhara K, Hamada T: Pathologic evidence of degeneration as a primary cause of rotator cuff tear. *Clin Orthop Relat Res* 2003;415:111-120.

［23］Funakoshi T, Iwasaki N, Kamishima T, et al: In vivo visualization of vascular patterns of rotator cuff tears using contrast-enhanced ultrasound. *Am J Sports Med* 2010;38(12):2464-2471.

Enhanced ultrasound images were used to investigate the vascularity of intact and torn rotator cuffs. There was a significant age-related decrease in blood flow in the intratendinous region but not in bursal tissue. Blood flow in ruptured rotator cuffs did not differ from that in intact rotator cuffs.

［24］Modi CS, Smith CD, Drew SJ: Partial-thickness articular surface rotator cuff tears in patients over the age of 35: Etiology and intra-articular associations. *Int J Shoulder Surg* 2012;6(1):15-18.

Partial-thickness articular-side tears were common in patients older than 35 years who required arthroscopic surgery for rotator cuff pathology, probably reflecting injury to an already-degenerated rotator cuff. This finding supports the theory of intrinsic degeneration of the tendon in this age group and probably represents an etiology different from that of young athletes.

［25］Longo UG, Berton A, Khan WS, Maffulli N, Denaro V: Histopathology of rotator cuff tears. *Sports Med Arthrosc* 2011;19(3):227-236.

Tendon abnormalities of the rotator cuff include alteration of collagen fiber structure, tenocytes, cellularity, and vascularity. Ruptured tendons have marked collagen degeneration and disordered arrangement of collagen fibers. Fibroblast population decreases as the size of the rotator cuff tear increases.

［26］Hegedus EJ, Cook C, Brennan M, Wyland D, Garrison JC, Driesner D: Vascularity and tendon pathology in the rotator cuff: A review of literature and implications for rehabilitation and surgery. *Br J Sports Med* 2010;44(12):838-847.

Studies reflecting recent improvements in design and technology support that increased vascularity is a normal response to a small tear. As tear size increases, the healing response fails and vascularity decreases.

［27］Carbone S, Gumina S, Arceri V, Campagna V, Fagnani C, Postacchini F: The impact of preoperative smoking habit on rotator cuff tear: Cigarette smoking influences rotator cuff tear sizes. *J Shoulder Elbow Surg* 2012;21(1):56-60.

A correlation was found among cigarette smoking, rotator cuff tearing, and tear size. Increasing tear size corresponded to increasing numbers of daily and lifetime cigarettes smoked.

［28］Baumgarten KM, Gerlach D, Galatz LM, et al: Cigarette smoking increases the risk for rotator cuff tears. *Clin Orthop Relat Res* 2010;468(6):1534-1541.

A questionnaire was administered to 586 consecutive patients age 18 years or older with a diagnostic shoulder ultrasound for unilateral, atraumatic shoulder pain and no history of shoulder surgery. A dosage- and time-dependent relationship was found between smoking and rotator cuff tears.

［29］Gwilym SE, Watkins B, Cooper CD, et al: Genetic influences in the progression of tears of the rotator cuff. *J Bone Joint Surg Br* 2009;91(7):915-917.

Genetic factors were found to have a role in the development and the progression of full-thickness rotator cuff tears in a comparison study involving patients' siblings.

[30] Tashjian RZ, Farnham JM, Albright FS, Teerlink CC, Cannon-Albright LA: Evidence for an inherited predisposition contributing to the risk for rotator cuff disease. *J Bone Joint Surg Am* 2009;91(5):1136-1142.

A population-based resource combining genealogic data and clinical data was used in finding a significantly elevated risk of rotator cuff disease in second- and third-degree relatives of patients diagnosed with rotator cuff disease before age 40 years.

[31] Chaudhury S, Carr AJ: Lessons we can learn from gene expression patterns in rotator cuff tears and tendinopathies. *J Shoulder Elbow Surg* 2012;21(2): 191-199.

Genetic predisposition to rotator cuff tears was reviewed, with gene changes related to rotator cuff tears, cellular dysregulation, metaplasia, and modulation or manipulation of gene expression.

[32] Nyffeler RW, Werner CM, Sukthankar A, Schmid MR, Gerber C: Association of a large lateral extension of the acromion with rotator cuff tears. *J Bone Joint Surg Am* 2006;88(4):800-805.

[33] Hamid N, Omid R, Yamaguchi K, Steger-May K, Stobbs G, Keener JD: Relationship of radiographic acromial characteristics and rotator cuff disease: A prospective investigation of clinical, radiographic, and sonographic findings. *J Shoulder Elbow Surg* 2012; 21(10):1289-1298.

The presence of an acromial spur was associated with the presence of a full-thickness rotator cuff tear. The acromial morphology classification system is an unreliable method of assessing the acromion, and the acromial index shows no association with the presence of rotator cuff disease.

[34] Keener JD, Steger-May K, Stobbs G, Yamaguchi K: Asymptomatic rotator cuff tears: Patient demographics and baseline shoulder function. *J Shoulder Elbow Surg* 2010;19(8):1191-1198.

When asymptomatic, a rotator cuff tear is associated with a clinically insignificant loss of shoulder function compared with an intact rotator cuff. The presence of pain is important for creating a measurable loss of shoulder function in rotator cuff–deficient shoulders. Hand dominance appears to be an important risk factor for pain.

[35] Moosmayer S, Tariq R, Stiris MG, Smith HJ: MRI of symptomatic and asymptomatic full-thickness rotator cuff tears: A comparison of findings in 100 subjects. *Acta Orthop* 2010;81(3):361-366.

Tear characteristics were compared in 50 patients with an asymptomatic full-thickness rotator cuff tear and 50 patients with a symptomatic tear. Statistically significant associations were found between symptoms and tear size exceeding 3 cm in the mediolateral plane, a positive tangent sign, and fatty degeneration exceeding grade 1 in the supraspinatus and infraspinatus muscles.

[36] Mall NA, Kim HM, Keener JD, et al: Symptomatic progression of asymptomatic rotator cuff tears: A prospective study of clinical and sonographic variables. *J Bone Joint Surg Am* 2010;92(16):2623-2633.

Pain in a shoulder with an asymptomatic rotator cuff tear is associated with an increase in tear size. A large tear is more likely to become painful in the short term than a small tear.

[37] Yamaguchi K, Tetro AM, Blam O, Evanoff BA, Teefey SA, Middleton WD: Natural history of asymptomatic rotator cuff tears: A longitudinal analysis of asymptomatic tears detected sonographically. *J Shoulder Elbow Surg* 2001;10(3):199-203.

[38] Safran O, Schroeder J, Bloom R, Weil Y, Milgrom C: Natural history of nonoperatively treated symptomatic rotator cuff tears in patients 60 years old or younger. *Am J Sports Med* 2011;39(4):710-714.

In a prospective study, patients age 60 years or younger were treated nonsurgically for a relatively small full-thickness rotator cuff tear. No correlation was found between considerable pain at the time of the follow-up ultrasound (mean, 29 months) and a clinically significant increase in tear size.

[39] Maman E, Harris C, White L, Tomlinson G, Shashank M, Boynton E: Outcome of nonoperative treatment of symptomatic rotator cuff tears monitored by magnetic resonance imaging. *J Bone Joint Surg Am* 2009;91(8): 1898-1906.

A retrospective study of 54 patients (mean age, 58.8 years) with a nonsurgically treated rotator cuff tear found that the factors associated with progression were age older than 60 years, a full-thickness tear, and fatty infiltration of the rotator cuff muscles.

[40] Fucentese SF, von Roll AL, Pfirrmann CW, Gerber C, Jost B: Evolution of nonoperatively treated symptomatic isolated full-thickness supraspinatus tears. *J Bone Joint Surg Am* 2012;94(9):801-808.

Twenty-four consecutive patients were offered repair of an isolated, symptomatic, small, full-thickness supraspinatus tear. Those who refused surgical treatment had surprisingly high satisfaction. There was no increase in the average rotator cuff tear size 3.5 years after surgical repair was recommended.

[41] Tanaka M, Itoi E, Sato K, et al: Factors related to successful outcome of conservative treatment for rotator cuff tears. *Ups J Med Sci* 2010;115(3):193-200.

The success of nonsurgical treatment was significantly affected by the integrity of the intramuscular tendon of the supraspinatus, as determined by high-resolution MRI with a microscopy coil, supraspinatus muscle atrophy, the impingement sign, and the external rotation angle.

[42] Melis B, DeFranco MJ, Chuinard C, Walch G: Natural history of fatty infiltration and atrophy of the supraspinatus muscle in rotator cuff tears. *Clin Orthop Relat Res* 2010;468(6):1498-1505.

A retrospective review of 1,688 patients with a rotator cuff tear found that moderate supraspinatus fatty infiltration, a positive tangent sign, and severe fatty infiltration appeared at an average of 3 years, 4.5 years, and 5 years, respectively, after the onset of symptoms.

[43] Melis B, Wall B, Walch G: Natural history of infraspinatus fatty infiltration in rotator cuff tears. *J Shoulder Elbow Surg* 2010;19(5):757-763.

Moderate and severe infraspinatus fatty infiltration appeared an average of 2.5 years and 4 years, respectively, after the onset of symptoms. A relatively large tendon tear, a longer delay after tendon rupture, and older patient age were associated with more common and severe fatty infiltration.

[44] Melis B, Nemoz C, Walch G: Muscle fatty infiltration in rotator cuff tears: Descriptive analysis of 1688 cases. *Orthop Traumatol Surg Res* 2009;95(5): 319-324.

The mean time from tendon rupture to grade 2 fatty infiltration was 3 years for the supraspinatus and 2.5 years for the infraspinatus or the subscapularis. The mean time to grade 3 or 4 fatty infiltration was 5, 4, or 3 years for the supraspinatus, the infraspinatus, or the subscapularis, respectively.

[45] Zingg PO, Jost B, Sukthankar A, Buhler M, Pfirrmann CW, Gerber C: Clinical and structural outcomes of nonoperative management of massive rotator cuff tears. *J Bone Joint Surg Am* 2007;89(9):1928-1934.

At a mean 48-month follow-up after nonsurgical treatment of 19 consecutive patients with a massive rotator cuff tear, shoulder function, including active range of motion, was almost maintained despite significant progression of degenerative structural joint changes.

[46] Longo UG, Franceschi F, Berton A, Maffulli N,

Droena V: Conservative treatment and rotator cuff tear progression. *Med Sport Sci* 2012;57:90-99.

There is no definite consensus on the best management for patients with a rotator cuff tear. Few randomized controlled studies are available on nonsurgical management.

[47] Hong JY, Yoon SH, Moon J, Kwack KS, Joen B, Lee HY: Comparison of high- and low-dose corticosteroid in subacromial injection for periarticular shoulder disorder: A randomized, triple-blind, placebo-controlled trial. *Arch Phys Med Rehabil* 2011;92(12):1951-1960.

The efficacy of corticosteroid (triamcinolone acetonide) was compared at the two most widely used dosages (40 mg and 20 mg) for subacromial injection in patients with a periarticular shoulder disorder. Because no significant difference was found, the initial use of the lower dosage was preferred.

[48] Zufferey P, Revaz S, Degailler X, Balague F, So A: A controlled trial of the benefits of ultrasound-guided steroid injection for shoulder pain. *Joint Bone Spine* 2012;79(2):166-169.

Local steroid injection for shoulder pain led to significant improvement in pain and function for as long as 12 weeks. Ultrasound examination to define the origin of shoulder pain and guide injection can provide as much as 6 weeks of significant additional benefit.

[49] Bennell K, Wee E, Coburn S, et al: Efficacy of standardised manual therapy and home exercise programme for chronic rotator cuff disease: Randomised placebo controlled trial. *BMJ* 2010;340:c2756.

A standard program of manual therapy and home exercise did not confer immediate improvement in pain and function compared with a realistic placebo treatment in middle-aged and older adults with chronic rotator cuff disease. Greater improvement was apparent at follow-up, however, particularly in shoulder function and strength. This finding suggests that the benefit of active treatment requires time to manifest.

[50] Bas¸kurt Z, Bas¸kurt F, Gelecek N, Özkan MH: The effectiveness of scapular stabilization exercise in the patients with subacromial impingement syndrome. *J Back Musculoskelet Rehabil* 2011;24(3):173-179.

A randomized study found that adding scapular stabilization exercises to stretching and strengthening exercises increased the effectiveness of physical therapy in increasing muscle strength, developing joint position sense, and decreasing scapular dyskinesis in patients with subacromial impingement syndrome.

第十四章　部分肩袖撕裂

Ian K.Y. Lo, MD, FRCSC

引言

尽管部分肩袖撕裂（PTRCT）很常见，但是关于其最佳的治疗方案仍存在争议。大部分关于肩袖撕裂的文献都是描述全层肩袖撕裂（FTRCT）的，而且大部分关于 PTRCT 的研究集中在手术治疗效果或手术技术上。几乎没有针对 PTRCT 的病因学及非手术治疗的研究。对于该疾病的自然病史的理解相对较少是导致对最佳治疗方案存在争议的原因之一。

解剖学

肩袖肌腱是由冈上肌、冈下肌、小圆肌和肩胛下肌联合构成的多层次复杂结构，其止于肱骨头内侧。[1]一些尸体研究确定了肩袖肌腱止点的大致解剖。其中一项研究测量了每个肌腱止点由内向外的宽度和由前向后的长度，发现各肌腱止点的宽度和长度的变化范围很大[2]（表 14-1）。还有一项研究发现冈上肌腱止点的平均宽度为

Dr. Lo or an immediate family member serves as a board member, owner, officer, or committee member of the Arthroscopy Association of North America; has received royalties from Arthrex, Arthrocare, and Lippincott; is a member of a speakers' bureau or has made paid presentations on behalf of Arthrocare and Arthrex; serves as a paid consultant to or is an employee of Arthrocare; serves as an unpaid consultant to Tenet Medical and Smith & Nephew; has received research or institutional support from Arthrocare, Arthrex, Linvatec, and Smith & Nephew; and has stock or stock options held in Tenet Medical.

12.1 mm（范围：9~15 mm），平均长度为 25 mm（范围：19~27 mm）。[3]

一项尸体研究提出了对肩袖肌腱止点的另一种观点（图 14-1）。[4]该研究描述，冈下肌腱止点呈向前弯曲的梯形，占据了大结节上关节面外侧的大部分，这一区域既往被认为是冈上肌的止点。冈上肌腱的止点小，呈三角形，位于大结节最前方区域；在 21% 的标本中发现冈上肌部分肌纤维止于小结节。这些解剖学发现需要进一步证实。应该注意，PTRCT（定义为撕裂不超过肌腱厚度的 50%）的临床治疗流程仍然是基于肩袖肌腱止点的传统描述。

发病率、病因学和发病机制

尸体研究和影像学研究发现，PTRCT 的发病率为 13%~32%。[5-8]一项针对无症状患者的 MRI 研究发现其整体发病率为 20%。[8]发病率与年龄高度相关；26% 的年龄大于 60 岁的患者有 PTRCT，年龄小于 40 岁的患者只有 4% 有 PTRCT。很多 PTRCT 是无症状的，很可能是年龄相关的继发的退行性改变。因此，将临床表现与影像学发现联系起来非常重要。

一些病因学因素单独作用或共同作用可导致肩袖的解剖学损伤。内源性因素包括与年龄相关的显微解剖学改变（例如，细胞数目减少、纤维变薄或断裂、肉芽组织形成）、代谢解剖学改变和血管解剖学改变（例如，血供减少或出现乏血管

表 14-1

肩袖肌腱止点的宽度和长度

肩袖肌腱止点	平均宽度 /mm（范围）	平均长度 /mm（范围）
冈上肌腱止点	16 (12~20)	23 (18~33)
冈下肌腱止点	18 (12~24)	28 (20~45)
小圆肌腱止点	21 (10~33)	29 (20~40)
肩胛下肌腱止点	20 (15~25)	40 (35~55)

注：经允许引自 Curtis AS, Burbank KM, Tierney JJ, Scheller AD, Curran AR: The insertional footprint of the rotator cuff: An anatomic study. *Arthroscopy* 2006;22（6）:603–609.

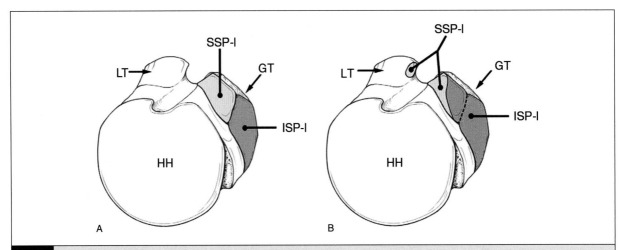

图 14-1 右肱骨上部示意图，显示冈上肌和冈下肌在肱骨上的止点。A. 一种普遍观点是冈上肌止于大结节最高区域，冈下肌止于大结节中间区域。B. 另一种观点是冈下肌止点包括大结节近一半的最高区域及全部的中间区域，冈上肌的止点为大结节最高区域的前内侧部分，有时还包括小结节的最上方区域。GT= 大结节；HH= 肱骨头；ISP-I= 冈下肌止点；LT= 小结节；SSP-I= 冈上肌止点。经允许引自 Mochizuki T, Sugaya H, Uomizu M, et al: Humeral insertion of the supraspinatus and infraspinatus: New anatomic findings regarding the footprint of the rotator cuff. *J Bone Joint Surg Am* 2008;90:962–969.

区）。这些因素使肩袖在剪切应力下容易出现肌腱内退行性撕裂。导致 PTRCT 的外源性因素包括经典的肩峰下（出口）撞击、内部撞击和盂肱关节不稳定或松弛。单次或反复外伤（例如，反复过顶投掷）会导致拉伸超负荷和纤维断裂。

目前，已经确定了一些普遍性病因学因素，还有一些特定的因素可能跟某些特殊类型肩袖撕裂的易感性有关。老年患者的 PTRCT 通常发生在紧邻肱二头肌腱后方的关节面，继发于年龄相关的退行性改变。相反，经常投掷的年轻运动员的 PTRCT 通常发生在冈上肌和冈下肌腱交汇处附近。这一特点表明，经常投掷的年轻运动员存在不同的病因学因素

（例如，肩袖纤维过度扭曲、存在扭转应力、存在内部撞击），出现更后方的关节面撕裂。[9]

PTRCT 的自然病程仍不清楚，相关的研究也极少。在平均 1.1 年的随访中，80% 的 PTRCT 患者撕裂范围增加，28% 的患者进展为全层撕裂。[10] 近些年几项研究表明，PTRCT 的自然病程并非如此之差。[11-13] 总体而言，连续的超声检查表明，在 30 例 PTRCT 患者中，4 例进展为 FTRCT（13%）。[11] 在 20 例仍无症状的患者中，所有 PTRCT 均未进展为 FTRCT。近来有一项研究通过 MRI 或者核磁共振关节造影（MRA）对 37 例 PTRCT 患者进行了分析。在平均 4.4 年的随访

中，28 例（76%）患者的撕裂无明显进展，6 例（16%）患者的撕裂范围增大，3 例（8%）患者进展为 FTRCT。累及肌腱厚度超过 50% 的 PTRCT 很有可能加重，55% 累及肌腱厚度超过 50% 的患者出现进展，而累及肌腱厚度少于 50% 的患者仅 14% 出现进展。

影像学检查

超声检查用于诊断和定量 PTRCT 及 FTRCT 的价值正在不断提高。其用于诊断 FTRCT 的准确性与 MRI 相似，但其在社区医院用于诊断和定量 PTRCT 的准确性仍存在争议。[14-15] 超声检查仍受限于超声医师的经验及其诊断明显的盂肱关节病变的能力。一项包括 65 项研究的评价肩袖撕裂影像学诊断的荟萃分析表明，超声检查用于诊断 PTRCT 的敏感性（66.7%）和特异性（93.5%）与 MRI（敏感性是 63.6%，特异性是 91.7%）类似。[16]

MRA 也是一种诊断 PTRCT 的影像学手段，尤其是用于关节面撕裂的诊断。MRA 的平均敏感性为 85.9%，平均特异性为 96%。MRA 用于诊断 PTRCT 的准确性明显优于超声或 MRI。附加外展外旋位检查可以进一步增加 MRA 诊断关节面 PTRCT 的敏感性。[17-18]

分型

PTRCT 通常可以根据解剖部位（囊部、关节面或实质部）、受累肌腱（冈上肌、冈下肌、小圆肌或肩胛下肌）以及受累面积和深度（肌腱撕裂厚度的百分比）进行分型。[19-20] 最常用的分型是基于解剖部位和肌腱撕裂深度的分型[19]（表 14-2）。该分型系统不能区分某些因素，例如，矢状面撕裂范围、撕裂面积、组织结构质量和撕裂原因。

最近有学者对肩袖撕裂分型系统的观察者间信度提出了质疑。10 名经过培训的肩关节外科医师对 27 例手术证实存在肩袖撕裂的患者的 MRI 进行了分析。[21] 结果发现对于区分 FTRCT

表 14-2

部分肩袖撕裂的分型

部位

关节面
囊部
肌腱内

级别	撕裂大小（占肩袖厚度百分比）
Ⅰ 级	< 3 mm（< 25%）
Ⅱ 级	3~6 mm（25%~50%）
Ⅲ 级	> 6 mm（> 50%）

注：经允许引自 Ellman H: Diagnosis and treatment of incomplete rotator cuff tears. *Clin Orthop Relat Res* 1990;254:64-74.

和 PTRCT 及确定 PTRCT 的部位（囊部或者关节面），观察者间的一致性高，但对于确定 PTRCT 的分型，观察者间的一致性较差。另一项使用关节镜录像带的类似研究也发现 PTRCT 分级的观察者间一致性较差。[22]

非手术治疗

PTRCT 可采取多种非手术治疗，包括物理治疗、激素注射、抗炎治疗和使用镇痛药等。与 FTRCT 相比，PTRCT 患者更常接受非手术治疗，因为 PTRCT 的肌肉萎缩、脂肪浸润和严重撕裂加重的风险很低。[13] 最近的一项研究专门对 76 例 PTRCT 患者的非手术治疗效果进行了分析，发现约 50% 的患者非手术治疗成功，在平均 46 个月的随访中，91% 的患者对治疗满意。非主力侧非外伤患者及撕裂小于 50% 的患者非手术治疗成功的可能性更高。

手术治疗

适应证

PTRCT 手术治疗的适应证并不明确，主要根据患者因素（年龄、活动水平、职业和运动情况）、临床因素（外伤史、疼痛严重程度、虚弱程度和非手术治疗效果）和病理因素（囊部或关节面撕裂和撕裂厚度百分比）决定。慢性撕裂且仅有轻度症状的患者最初通常选择非手术治疗。年轻患者、外伤导致撕裂超过 50% 的患者或经过充分非手术治疗无效的患者应选择手术治疗。

50% 规则的基本原理

手术治疗 PTRCT 的方式包括清理和修复，可同时进行（或不进行）肩峰下减压。一般而言，清理［同时进行（或不进行）肩峰下减压］可用于撕裂小于 50% 的 PTRCT 患者。对于撕裂大于 50% 的 PTRCT 患者，应考虑进行肩袖修复［同时进行（或不进行）肩峰下减压］。对撕裂深度大于 50% 的 PTRCT 患者进行手术修复的原理主要基于一项对 65 例撕裂深度大于 50% 的 PTRCT 患者的回顾性研究。[23] 32 例患者进行了关节镜下肩峰成形术，其余 33 例患者除肩峰成形术外，还进行了小切口肩袖修复。治疗方式的选择不是随机的，而是基于术前与患者的讨论。在 2~7 年的随访中，仅行关节镜下肩峰成形术的患者美国加利福尼亚大学洛杉矶分校（UCLA）肩关节评分平均为 22.7 分，而同时进行了小切口肩袖修复的患者平均为 31.6 分。

该研究有一些缺陷（如非随机和回顾性研究），但几项生物力学研究同样支持 50% 规则。在一项尸体研究中，对不同损伤程度的关节面 PTRCT 施加周期性应力。[24] 结果仅撕裂深度大于 50% 的关节面 PTRCT 的剩余邻近肩袖纤维的张力显著增加，对 PTRCT 进行修复后张力回到正常水平。另一项尸体研究制作了逐渐增大的冈上肌腱囊部 PTRCT 模型。[25] 当囊部撕裂深度大于 50% 时，完整肌腱的张力增加。随着撕裂深度的增加，剩余完整肌腱的应力非线性增加。

肌腱撕裂的深度是决定手术方式的一个因素，另外，在决定治疗方案时，也应考虑其他一些显著的因素（患者因素、临床因素和病理因素）。

关节镜清理和肩峰下减压

关节镜清理通常用于肌腱撕裂厚度小于 50% 的 PTRCT（Ⅰ 度或 Ⅱ 度撕裂），肩关节特异评分证

实可取得良到好的结果。[26-32] 额外进行肩峰下减压并不能显著改善患者症状。[33] 尽管关节镜清理［同时进行（或不进行）肩峰成形术］可以获得良好的结果，但是一项研究发现，对于某些特定的撕裂，关节镜清理相对容易失败。[27] 在平均 52 个月的随访中，超过 90% 的患者取得了良好的效果，8% 的患者治疗失败，其中大部分为囊部 PTRCT。囊部 PTRCT 患者进行关节镜清理和肩峰成形术的失败风险为 29%，其中更大的囊部撕裂的失败风险为 38%。该研究结果表明，对于囊部 PTRCT，即使撕裂小于 50%，也应该考虑进行修复。

关节镜清理的长期效果并不清楚。在平均 101 个月的随访中，治疗侧肩关节的 Constant 肩关节评分平均为 65 分，约比对侧低 20 分。[26] 关节镜清理术后，仅有 57% 的患者可以恢复到伤前运动水平且没有症状；20% 的患者可以恢复到低一级别的运动水平，因为存在持续疼痛；22% 的患者无法进行运动。[26] 即使在高水平的投掷运动员中，也仅有 55% 可以恢复到伤前运动水平或达到更高的运动水平。[31]

关节镜清理［同时进行（或不进行）肩峰下减压］并不能使 PTRCT 愈合或阻止其进展。在关节镜下肩峰成形和清理术后平均 8.4 年的随访中，在 26 例患者中有 9 例患者超声检查证实进展为 FTRCT。[28] 与之相似，在一篇对 46 例关节面 PTRCT 行关节镜下肩峰成形术和清理术的报道中，在平均 4.2 年的随访中，超声检查证实 3 例患者（6.5%）进展为 FTRCT。[29] 但是，仅 1 例患者临床效果较差。

关节镜修复

目前有多种手术技术用于 PTRCT 的修复，包括原位技术和将 PTRCT 转变成 FTRCT 的技术。PTRCT 转变成 FTRCT 具有一定优势，因为其允许使用标准的关节镜下修复。原位技术，如经肌腱或完全经关节内修复，可以保留部分肩袖的完整性。原位技术更适用于关节面 PTRCT，可以保

留外侧肩袖的完整性。保留外侧正常肌腱可能有助于对肩袖切迹进行更接近解剖学的重建。

多项研究对 PTRCT 修复技术的生物力学性能进行了报道。一项研究比较了经肌腱修复和转变为全层撕裂后进行双排修复用于治疗 50% 关节面 PTRCT 的效果。[34] 在循环载荷下，经肌腱修复的间隙形成明显更小，最终失效所需应力也明显更大。[35] 在一个 PTRCT 的绵羊模型中，研究者比较了不同修复技术的肩袖切迹的接触压力及修复强度，发现经肌腱修复和双排修复的接触压力相似，但经肌腱修复最终失效所需应力明显更高。

尽管保留部分肩袖的完整性在理论上具有优势，但是临床研究并未证实经肌腱修复比转变为 FTRCT 后进行修复更具优势（表 14-3）。[36-47] 大部分临床研究发现将 PTRCT 转变为 FTRCT 取得了良好效果，患者的满意率超过 90%。[36-39] 在将 PTRCT 转变为 FTRCT 修复后，大部分肩袖撕裂愈合。在一项对 42 例患者（平均年龄 53 岁）进行的平均 39 个月的随访研究中，患者的 ASES 肩

关节疼痛和功能障碍评分由平均 46.1 分增加至平均 82.1 分。[38] 术后平均 11 个月的超声检查证实 88% 的修复保持完整。在出现再次撕裂和实现愈合的患者之间，临床效果无明显差异。与完全修复的患者相比，再次撕裂的患者年龄更大。

在一项对 22 例经转变为全层撕裂治疗的患者至少 2 年的随访研究中，患者的 UCLA 肩关节评分由 19.4 分改善为 32.9 分。[39] MRI 证实 18 例患者（82%）的肩袖完整，4 例患者（18%）再次出现全层或接近全层的撕裂。虽然肌腱的完整性与术后 UCLA 肩关节评分无关，但是与肩袖仍撕裂的患者相比，肌腱完整的患者临床功能评分的改善更明显。

经肌腱修复也可取得良好的临床效果，肩关节特异性评分明显改善，患者满意率高于 90%（表 14-3）。[40-44] 但是，经过仔细地临床评估后发现，很多患者（包括肩关节特异性分级评分评为"极好"的患者）存在残留症状。在一项纳入 54 例经肌腱肩袖修复的患者平均 2.7 年的随访

表 14-3

关节镜修复治疗部分肩袖撕裂的临床与解剖效果

研究者	病例数	修复类型	临床效果		解剖结果（影像学方法）
			术前评分→术后随访评分（评分系统）	患者满意率	
Porat 等[36]	36	转变为 FTRCT	17.2 → 31.5（UCLA）		
Deutsch[37]	41	转变为 FTRCT	42 → 93（ASES）	98%	
Kamath 等[38]	42	转变为 FTRCT	46.1 → 82.1（ASES）	93%	88% 完整（超声）
Lyengar 等[39]	22	转变为 FTRCT	19.1 → 32.9（UCLA）		82% 完整（MRI）
Waibl 和 Buess[40]	22	经肌腱修复	17.1 → 31.2（UCLA）	91%	
Ide 等[41]	17	经肌腱修复	17.3 → 32.9（UCLA）		
Castagna 等[42]	54	经肌腱修复	45.3 → 90.6（Constant）14.1 → 32.9（UCLA）	98%	
Castricini 等[43]	31	经肌腱修复	44.4 → 91.6（Constant）	93%	100% 完整（MRI）
Seo 等[44]	24	经肌腱双排修复	38 → 89（ASES）	92%	
Tauber 等[45]	16	经骨修复	15.8 → 32.8（UCLA）	94%	
Spencer[46]	20	经关节修复	74 → 92（Penn）		

注：FTRCT= 全层肩袖撕裂；ASES=ASES 肩关节疼痛和功能障碍评分；UCLA=UCLA 肩关节评分；Penn=Penn 肩关节评分；Constant=Constant 肩关节评分。

研究中，98%的患者对治疗结果满意，UCLA 评分、Constant 肩关节评分和肩关节简明测试评分明显改善。[42]进一步仔细评估发现，41%的患者在肩关节极度活动时偶尔存在肩部不适，尤其是在日常活动或运动需要外展和内收肩关节时。对于肌腱回缩严重，仅有小的切迹裸露的患者，尤其是老年非外伤性损伤的此类患者，残留症状发生的可能性明显增加。尽管在此项研究中缺少对照组和替代治疗组，但该研究仍表明经肌腱修复不是此类患者最佳的治疗方法。

一项研究报道了 31 例经肌腱肩袖修复患者平均 33 个月随访的临床与解剖效果。[43]Constant 肩关节评分由平均 44.4 分增加到平均 91.6 分，93%的患者获得良好结果。随访 MRI 证实无再发肩袖撕裂，所有患者的结节区域覆盖良好。患者可以在术后平均第 3.5 个月重返工作岗位。

仅有一项研究比较了关节镜下经肌腱肩袖修复和转换为 FTRCT 后修复的临床效果。[47]74 例患者随机分为经肌腱修复组和转变为 FTRCT 修复组。在至少 2 年的随访中，两组患者的 Constant 肩关节评分（经肌腱修复组由 62.5 分增加至 87.6 分；转变为 FTRCT 修复组由 57.8 分增加至 86.9 分）和疼痛视觉模拟评分（经肌腱修复组由 8.6 分改善至 5.4 分；转变为 FTRCT 修复组由 9.1 分改善至 5.4 分）均明显改善，两组间无显著差别。但是，亚组分析发现转变为 FTRCT 修复组患者术后力量的改善明显优于经肌腱修复组患者。

总结

尽管目前已经有一些对 PTRCT 的研究报道，但是其最佳的治疗方案仍存在争议。这有可能是因为不同类型的 PTRCT 存在不同的病因、具有不同的自然病程，所以非手术治疗或手术治疗有不同的成功率。对于撕裂小于 50%的患者，进行关节镜清理不论是否同时进行肩峰下减压均可取得良好的短期效果，但其长期疗效尚不清楚。对于撕裂大于 50%的患者，通常考虑手术修复，可取得良好效果。目前有多种修复技术被报道，但尚缺乏足够的证据证实某种技术优于其他技术。

参考文献

[1] Clark JM, Harryman DT II: Tendons, ligaments, and capsule of the rotator cuff: Gross and microscopic anatomy. 1992;74(5):713-725.

[2] Curtis AS, Burbank KM, Tierney JJ, Scheller AD, Curran AR: The insertional footprint of the rotator cuff: An anatomic study. 2006;22(6):e1.

[3] Ruotolo C, Fow JE, Nottage WM: The supraspinatus footprint: An anatomic study of the supraspinatus insertion. 2004;20(3):246-249.

[4] Mochizuki T, Sugaya H, Uomizu M, et al: Humeral insertion of the supraspinatus and infraspinatus: New anatomical findings regarding the footprint of the rotator cuff. 2008;90(5):962-969.
A cadaver study described an alternative interpretation of the supraspinatus and infraspinatus tendon insertions. The supraspinatus inserted into the most anterior aspect of the greater tuberosity; in 21% of the specimens, it also inserted into the lesser tuberosity. The infraspinatus curved anteriorly to occupy the lateral aspect of the greater tuberosity.

[5] Sano H, Ishii H, Trudel G, Uhthoff HK: Histologic evidence of degeneration at the insertion of 3 rotator cuff tendons: A comparative study with human cadaveric shoulders. 1999;8(6):574-579.

[6] Fukuda H: Partial-thickness rotator cuff tears: A modern view on Codman's classic. 2000;9(2):163-168.

[7] Lohr JF, Uhthoff HK: The pathogenesis of degenerative rotator cuff tears. 1987;11:237.

[8] Sher JS, Uribe JW, Posada A, Murphy BJ, Zlatkin MB: Abnormal findings on magnetic resonance images of asymptomatic shoulders. 1995; 77(1):10-15.

[9] Burkhart SS, Morgan CD, Kibler WB: The disabled throwing shoulder: Spectrum of pathology. Part I: Pathoanatomy and biomechanics. 2003; 19(4):404-420.

[10] Yamanaka K, Matsumoto T: The joint side tear of the rotator cuff: A follow-up study by arthrography. 1994;304:68-73.

[11] Mall NA, Kim HM, Keener JD, et al: Symptomatic progression of asymptomatic rotator cuff tears: A prospective study of clinical and sonographic variables. 2010;92(16):2623-2633.

In a prospective evaluation of 195 patients with an asymptomatic rotator cuff tear, 4 of 30 patients with a PTRCT had full-thickness progression with symptoms. No patient progressed while remaining asymptomatic. Level of evidence: III.

[12] Maman E, Harris C, White L, Tomlinson G, Shashank M, Boynton E: Outcome of nonoperative treatment of symptomatic rotator cuff tears monitored by magnetic resonance imaging. 2009;91(8):1898-1906.

At a mean 20-month follow-up, 26 of 30 patients (86%) with a PTRCT remained stable as determined by serial MRI. Level of evidence: IV.

[13] Lo IK, Denkers MR, More KD, Hollinshead R, Boorman RS: Paper No. 75—Partial thickness rotator cuff tears: Observe or operate? CD-ROM, Rosemont, IL, American Acadamy of Orthopaedic Surgeons, 2012, pp 883-884.

The nonsurgical treatment of PTRCTs was reviewed in 74 patients. The success rate was approximately 50%. Patients with an atraumatic onset involving the non-dominant extremity and a tear of less than 50% were most likely to have a successful result. Level of evidence: IV.

[14] Teefey SA, Rubin DA, Middleton WD, Hildebolt CF, Leibold RA, Yamaguchi K: Detection and quantification of rotator cuff tears: Comparison of ultrasonographic, magnetic resonance imaging, and arthroscopic findings in seventy-one consecutive cases. 2004;86(4):708-716.

[15] Teefey SA, Middleton WD, Payne WT, Yamaguchi K: Detection and measurement of rotator cuff tears with sonography: Analysis of diagnostic errors. 2005;184(6):1768-1773.

[16] de Jesus JO, Parker L, Frangos AJ, Nazarian LN: Accuracy of MRI, MR arthrography, and ultrasound in the diagnosis of rotator cuff tears: A meta-analysis. 2009;192(6):1701-1707.

A meta-analysis of 65 articles evaluating MRI, MRA, and ultrasonography for diagnosing rotator cuff tears found that MRA was significantly more accurate for detecting PTRCTs. Level of evidence: I.

[17] Jung JY, Jee WH, Chun HJ, Ahn MI, Kim YS: Magnetic resonance arthrography including ABER view in diagnosing partial-thickness tears of the rotator cuff: Accuracy, and inter- and intra-observer agreements. 2010;51(2):194-201.

The addition of the abduction–external rotation view increased sensitivity as well as interobserver and intra-observer agreement when MRA was used to detect ar-throscopically confirmed PTRCTs. Level of evidence: I.

[18] Herold T, Bachthaler M, Hamer OW, et al: Indirect MR arthrography of the shoulder: Use of abduction and external rotation to detect full- and partial- thickness tears of the supraspinatus tendon. 2006;240(1):152-160.

[19] Ellman H: Diagnosis and treatment of incomplete rotator cuff tears. 1990;254: 64-74.

[20] Snyder SJ: Arthroscopic classification of rotator cuff lesions and surgical decision making, in , ed 2. Philadelphia, PA, Lippincott, Williams & Wilkins, 2003, pp 201-207.

[21] Spencer EE Jr, Dunn WR, Wright RW, et al: Interobserver agreement in the classification of rotator cuff tears using magnetic resonance imaging. 2008;36(1):99-103.

An evaluation by 10 fellowship-trained orthopaedic shoulder specialists led to high interobserver agreement for distinguishing between FTRCTs and PTRCTs and determining the location of PTRCTs but poor interobserver agreement for determining PTRCT grade. Level of evidence: II.

[22] Kuhn JE, Dunn WR, Ma B, et al: Interobserver agreement in the classification of rotator cuff tears. 2007;35(3):437-441.

Interobserver agreement by 12 orthopaedic surgeons was high for distinguishing between FTRCTs and PTRCTs and the location of the PTRCT but poor for PTRCT grade when observing videotaped arthroscopic surgery. Level of evidence: II.

[23] Weber SC: Arthroscopic debridement and acromio-plasty versus mini-open repair in the treatment of significant partial-thickness rotator cuff tears. 1999;15(2):126-131.

[24] Mazzocca AD, Rincon LM, O'Connor RW, et al: Intra-articular partial-thickness rotator cuff tears: Analysis of injured and repaired strain behavior. 2008;36(1):110-116.

A biomechanical study evaluated the effect on adjacent rotator cuff strain of varying depths and repairs of articular-surface PTRCTs. Rotator cuff strain was significantly increased in tears of 50% or more of tendon thickness and was restored to close to normal after repair.

[25] Yang S, Park HS, Flores S, et al: Biomechanical analysis of bursal-sided partial thickness rotator cuff tears. 2009;18(3):379-385.

A biomechanical study evaluated the effect of increasingly deeper bursal-side PTRCTs on adjacent rotator cuff strain. Strain in the adjacent posterior portion was significantly higher if the tear was at least 60% of tendon thickness.

[26] Budoff JE, Rodin D, Ochiai D, Nirschl RP: Arthroscopic rotator cuff debridement without decompression for the treatment of tendinosis. 2005;21(9):1081-1089.

[27] Cordasco FA, Backer M, Craig EV, Klein D, Warren RF: The partial-thickness rotator cuff tear: Is acromioplasty without repair sufficient? 2002;30(2):257-260.

[28] Kartus J, Kartus C, Rostgård-Christensen L, Sernert N, Read J, Perko M: Long-term clinical and ultrasound evaluation after arthroscopic acromioplasty in patients with partial rotator cuff tears. 2006; 22(1):44-49.

[29] Liem D, Alci S, Dedy N, Steinbeck J, Marquardt B, Möllenhoff G: Clinical and structural results of partial supraspinatus tears treated by subacromial decompression without repair. 2008;16(10):967-972.

The clinical results of arthroscopic débridement and decompression were evaluated at a mean 50.3-month follow-up of 46 consecutive patients. ASES scores significantly improved, and only 6.5% of the patients had progressed to an FTRCT on ultrasonography. Level of evidence: IV.

[30] Park JY, Yoo MJ, Kim MH: Comparison of surgical outcome between bursal and articular partial thickness rotator cuff tears. 2003;26(4):387-390.

[31] Reynolds SB, Dugas JR, Cain EL, McMichael CS, Andrews JR: Débridement of small partial-thickness rotator cuff tears in elite overhead throwers. 2008;466(3):614-621.

After arthroscopic débridement of a PTRCT, 76% of the elite overhead-throwing athletes were able to return to competitive pitching at a professional level, and 55% were able to return to the same or higher level of competition. Level of evidence: IV.

[32] Snyder SJ, Pachelli AF, Del Pizzo W, Friedman MJ, Ferkel RD, Pattee G: Partial thickness rotator cuff tears: Results of arthroscopic treatment. 1991;7(1):1-7.

[33] Strauss EJ, Salata MJ, Kercher J, et al: Multimedia article: The arthroscopic management of partial-thickness rotator cuff tears. A systematic review of the literature. 2011;27(4):568-580.

A systematic review of 16 studies on the arthroscopic management of PTRCTs led to recommendations for surgical treatment. Level of evidence: IV.

[34] Gonzalez-Lomas G, Kippe MA, Brown GD, et al: In situ transtendon repair outperforms tear completion and repair for partial articular-sided supraspinatus tendon tears. 2008;17(5):722-728.

A biomechanical study found that in situ transtendon rotator cuff repair of articular-side PTRCTs led to significantly less gap formation and a higher ultimate failure strength than full-thickness conversion followed by double-row repair.

[35] Peters KS, Lam PH, Murrell GA: Repair of partial-thickness rotator cuff tears: A biomechanical analysis of footprint contact pressure and strength in an ovine model. 2010;26(7):877-884.

A biomechanical study found that transtendon and double-row rotator cuff repair had greater footprint contact pressures than tension-band single-row repair for articular-surface PTRCTs. The ultimate load to failure was higher after a transtendon repair than a double-row or single-row repair.

[36] Porat S, Nottage WM, Fouse MN: Repair of partial thickness rotator cuff tears: A retrospective review with minimum two-year follow-up. 2008;17(5):729-731.

A retrospective study evaluated the success of full-thickness conversion and repair of PTRCTs at a mean 42.4-month follow-up. Thirty of 36 patients had a good to excellent result using UCLA criteria. Level of evidence: IV.

[37] Deutsch A: Arthroscopic repair of partial-thickness tears of the rotator cuff. 2007; 16(2):193-201.

A retrospective study evaluated the success of full-thickness conversion and repair of PTRCTs. At a mean 38-month follow-up, there was significant improvement in the ASES score, and 98% of the patients were satisfied. Level of evidence: IV.

[38] Kamath G, Galatz LM, Keener JD, Teefey S, Middleton W, Yamaguchi K: Tendon integrity and functional outcome after arthroscopic repair of high-grade partial-thickness supraspinatus tears. 2009;91(5):1055-1062.

Full-thickness conversion and repair of PTRCTs led to a mean ASES score of 82.1 and intact repair on ultrasonography in 88% of the patients. Patients with an intact rotator cuff repair were younger than those with a recurrent tear. Level of evidence: IV.

[39] Iyengar JJ, Porat S, Burnett KR, Marrero-Perez L, Hernandez VH, Nottage WM: Magnetic resonance imaging tendon integrity assessment after arthroscopic partial-thickness rotator cuff repair. 2011;27(3):306-313.

The anatomic results of full-thickness conversion and repair of PTRCTs were evaluated on MRI. In 82% of the patients, there was no evidence of a recurrent FTRCT, but 18% had a persistent defect. Integrity was not correlated with outcome. Level of evidence: IV.

[40] Waibl B, Buess E: Partial-thickness articular surface supraspinatus tears: A new transtendon suture technique. 2005;21(3):376-381.

[41] Ide J, Maeda S, Takagi K: Arthroscopic transtendon repair of partial-thickness articular-side tears of the rotator cuff: Anatomical and clinical study. 2005;33(11):1672-1679.

[42] Castagna A, Delle Rose G, Conti M, Snyder SJ, Borroni M, Garofalo R: Predictive factors of subtle residual shoulder symptoms after transtendinous arthroscopic cuff repair: A clinical study. 2009;37(1):103-108.
At a minimum 2-year follow-up after transtendon repair of a PTRCT, 41% of the 54 patients had some residual symptoms at the extremes of range of motion during activities of daily living or sports, despite excellent shoulder scores. Level of evidence: IV.

[43] Castricini R, Panfoli N, Nittoli R, Spurio S, Pirani O: Transtendon arthroscopic repair of partial-thickness, articular surface tears of the supraspinatus: Results at 2 years. 2009;93(suppl 1):S49-S54.
The clinical and anatomic results of 33 patients were reviewed at a mean 33-month follow-up after transtendon repair of a PTRCT. The mean Constant score was 91.6, with no recurrent tears on MRI. Level of evidence: IV.

[44] Seo YJ, Yoo YS, Kim DY, Noh KC, Shetty NS, Lee JH: Trans-tendon arthroscopic repair for partial-thickness articular side tears of the rotator cuff. 2011;19(10):1755-1759.
A modified transtendon bridging repair technique using medial and lateral anchors led to a mean ASES score of 89, and 22 of 24 patients were satisfied with the procedure. Level of evidence: IV.

[45] Tauber M, Koller H, Resch H: Transosseous arthroscopic repair of partial articular-surface supraspinatus tendon tears. 2008;16(6):608-613.
The use of an in situ transosseous technique for repair of articular-surface PTRCTs led to a mean UCLA score of 32.8, and 15 of 16 patients were satisfied with the procedure. Level of evidence: IV.

[46] Spencer EE Jr: Partial-thickness articular surface rotator cuff tears: An all-inside repair technique. 2010;468(6):1514-1520.
A technique for all intra-articular repair of articular-surface PTRCTs was described. At a mean 29-month follow-up, the mean Penn Shoulder Score improved to 92, and 19 of 20 patients were able to return to sports at the same or a higher level. Level of evidence: IV.

[47] Castagna A, Gumina S, Borroni M, Delle Rose G, Conti M, Garofalo R: Partial articular-sided supraspinatus tear: A comparison between transtendon repair and tear completion and repair. White Sulpher Springs, VA, American Shoulder and Elbow Surgeons, 2011, paper 30.
Seventy-four patients with an articularsurface PTRCT were randomly assigned to conversion to an FTRCT and repair or to transtendon repair. Mean Constant and visual analog scale scores improved in both groups of patients, with no significant between-group differences. Patients assigned to conversion had signif- icantly more improvement in strength. Level of evidence: II.

第十五章　全层肩袖撕裂的手术治疗

Sumant G. Krishnan, MD; Glen H. Rudolph, MD; Raffaele Garofalo, MD

引言

肩袖撕裂是导致肩关节疼痛和功能障碍的常见原因之一。肩袖病变的患病人群广泛，从年轻的高水平投掷运动员的部分肩袖撕裂到老年患者的巨大不可修复性全层撕裂。肩袖撕裂中，还可能出现多条肌腱同时撕裂，其中冈上肌腱撕裂最常见。全层撕裂的发生率随着年龄的增加而增高，在年龄大于 50 岁的患者中，发生率接近 50%。[1]

随着人口老龄化的到来，骨科医师必然会遇到越来越多的老年全层肩袖撕裂病例。全层肩袖撕裂无法自行愈合。随着时间的推移，撕裂会逐渐稳定或加重。此外，受累的肌肉 – 肌腱单位随着时间的推移也会出现不可逆性脂肪浸润和肌肉萎缩，从而影响治疗效果。手术修复适用于非手术治疗后仍存在持续疼痛的患者。肩袖修复最流

Dr. Krishnan or an immediate family member serves as a board member, owner, officer, or committee member of the American Shoulder and Elbow Surgeons and the Arthroscopy Association of North America; has received royalties from Tornier, TAG Medical, and Ossur; is a member of a speakers' bureau or has made paid presentations on behalf of Tornier; serves as a paid consultant to or is an employee of Tornier and TAG Medical; and has received nonincome support (such as equipment or services), commercially derived honoraria, or other non–researchrelated funding (such as paid travel) from DePuy Mitek and Tornier. Neither of the following authors nor any immediate family member has received anything of value from or has stock or stock options held in a commercial company or institution related directly or indirectly to the subject of this chapter: Dr. Rudolph and Dr. Garofalo.

行的手术方式经历了开放手术、小切口手术和关节镜手术的演变。肩袖修复的主要目标是通过将撕裂的肌腱重新修复至肱骨近端切迹来重建解剖结构，进而改善患者的疼痛和功能。遗憾的是，并非所有手术修复的肌腱都能愈合。目前，对影响手术修复肩袖愈合的生物学和生物力学因素尚未完全明确，并且对最佳的修复方法和术后康复手段也未达成统一意见。

分型

肩袖撕裂可以根据病因、病程长短、范围、形状、受累肌腱数目和部位进行分型。由于肩袖撕裂的特点各异，目前尚无标准的分型。目前，多个肩袖撕裂分型都旨在指导治疗。这些分型通常基于从一个维度测量撕裂的最大宽度或计算受累肌腱的数目。关于撕裂类型和最优修复方法的正式确定需要考虑三维结构信息，可通过术前 MRI 和关节镜检查获得。

近来提出的一个使用冠状面（长度）和矢状面（宽度）信息进行的肩袖撕裂几何分型可以指导治疗及判断预后。[2] I 型撕裂呈新月形（短而宽），可将撕裂修复到切迹上。II 型撕裂呈纵行（L 形或 U 形，长而窄），通常也可修复至切迹，部分需要边对边修复。III 型撕裂巨大且肌腱回缩（撕裂长而宽），通常需要边缘重叠修复。III 型撕裂大于 $2 \ cm^2$ 者有可能可以部分修复，也可能需要肌腱转移。IV 型撕裂发生在既往存在肩袖关节病变的

患者中，患者无肩峰下间隙和盂肱关节间隙。V型撕裂通常无法修复，应行关节置换术。

合并病变

忽视被肩袖撕裂掩盖的其他肩关节合并病变是影响手术效果的一个常见因素。肱二头肌腱、盂肱关节、肩锁关节、肩胛上神经和肩峰小骨均可影响肩袖撕裂的症状表现。想要获得好的效果需要在检查阶段对每一个病变进行诊断并恰当治疗。

盂肱关节退行性病变患者通常主诉肩关节深部疼痛，有时有捻发音或夜间痛。可通过普通 X 线片诊断。存在严重盂肱关节退行性病变时不能进行肩袖修复，因为术后制动会加重已存在的关节炎。肩锁关节关节炎在肩袖疾病患者中非常常见。特殊的表现包括影像学退行性改变、肩锁关节区压痛，以及交叉前臂内收或进行主动加压试验时疼痛。手术时可行切开或关节镜下锁骨远端切除。8% 的人群中存在肩峰骨，术前可以通过标准的腋位 X 线片确定。手术治疗包括复位和固定或切除未融合的骨块。肩胛上神经受压可导致肩关节疼痛、无力，与全层冈上肌和（或）冈下肌撕裂的表现类似。这种情况可以和冈上肌撕裂和回缩（至少 2 cm）同时存在。如怀疑存在肩胛上神经病变，应进行肌电图或神经传导试验检查。

为诊断患者所有疼痛的来源，必须对与症状相关的病变进行评估。对怀疑导致疼痛的部位注射 1% 利多卡因是一个简单而有效的诊断方法。该技术方便快捷，可以为制订治疗计划提供宝贵的信息。

手术治疗

肩袖撕裂的修复方法应该根据患者的个体情况而选择，需要考虑撕裂的大小、类型、肌腱质量及肌腱回缩程度。肩袖撕裂可通过开放手术、关节镜辅助手术、小切口手术或全关节镜手术成功治疗。[3-5] 所有肩袖修复手术技术的目标均为使肌

腱在其止点上牢固固定，并使其在接触面之间实现解剖愈合。为了达到这个目的，修复必须具有高固定强度，修复时骨与肌腱的间隙要尽可能小，并且在周期性负荷下始终具备力学稳定性。

经骨缝合肩袖修复技术被认为是所有外科技术的金标准[6]（图 15-1）。不管采用何种手术入路，都必须谨慎处理喙肩弓和三角肌。肩峰和喙肩韧带可部分限制肱骨头向前上方移位。三角肌是盂肱关节同步化运动的动力结构。三角肌附着点分离和喙肩弓功能障碍是肩袖修复的严重并发症，可导致严重的肩关节功能障碍。肩峰成形术和肩峰下减压在肩袖手术中有确切的治疗价值。其目标是通过打磨肩峰下表面使之变光滑，以在不损伤三角肌起点和不影响喙肩弓稳定性的情况下，减少肩袖的压力和磨损。

切开修复

计划进行切开修复肩袖前应该进行诊断性关节镜检查。关节镜可以让外科医师在切开修复肩袖前观察并治疗合并病变。对于大或巨大撕裂，关节镜观察到的盂肱关节炎可能比术前影像学表现得更加严重。根据病变情况，治疗计划也可能改变，不再进行肩袖修复，而进行关节镜下清理、肩峰下减压和肱二头肌切断或固定。关节镜下肱二头肌腱切断或固定可以有效治疗无法修复的肩袖撕裂以及肱二头肌腱完整时的肩关节疼痛和功能障碍。如果小圆肌萎缩或缺如，可出现肩关节假性麻痹。肩关节假性麻痹和严重肩袖关节病变是单独进行关节镜下肱二头肌腱切断或固定的禁忌证。[7]

在完成诊断性关节镜检查后，切开修复肩袖之前，需关闭关节镜检查通道，重新进行肩关节消毒、铺单，以预防感染。仔细设计手术切口，并考虑到行翻修手术的可能性。在进行切开修复大或巨大撕裂时，术前规划尤其重要。由肩锁关节后缘向肩峰前外侧角做斜切口，在三角肌前中部的缝隙向远端延伸 2~3 cm，可以为肩袖修复提

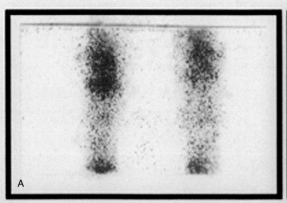
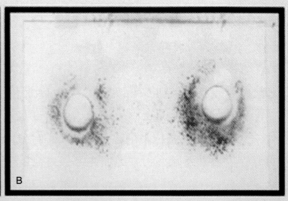

图
15-1 压力敏感性图像显示经骨缝合修复后（A）和缝合锚修复后（B）肩袖肌腱－骨接触部位的压力。经允许引自 Park MC, Cadet ET, Levine WN, Bigliani LU, Ahmad CS: Tendon–to–bone pressure distributions at a repaired rotator cuff footprint using transosseous suture and suture anchor fixation techniques. *Am J Sports Med* 2005;33:1154–1159.

供良好的视野，还可经该切口进入前上方行反肩关节置换术。

锁骨远端切除和两步肩峰成形术可以更好地显露肩峰下间隙，而无须进行三角肌劈开。切除肩峰下黏液囊可以更好地显露肩袖，并有助于旋转上臂。肩关节外旋内收时触摸喙肱韧带，如紧张则进行松解。显露肩袖并进行评估、松解和修复。近年来随着技术的进步，关节镜下肩袖修复的效果已经非常接近切开修复的效果。单排、双排、经骨和类似经骨技术将在关节镜肩袖修复部分介绍。

将三角肌重新缝合到肩峰上是肩袖切开修复的关键步骤，该步骤对术后康复也有重要影响。必须仔细地、牢固地重建以避免康复期裂开。使用不可吸收缝线单纯间断缝合劈开的三角肌，三角肌与骨的重建通常采用锁骨远端周围缝合或经肩峰骨道缝合。研究报道切开修复肩袖后 5 年和 10 年的整体成功率（定义为无须进行额外手术治疗）分别为 94% 和 83%。[8] 2 年内无须进行再次手术干预的修复通常在第 10 年时也可保持完整。肩袖修复的成功率与修复肌腱的数量有关。

小切口肩袖修复的提出是为了减少三角肌相

关并发症，但研究结果表明其与切开修复的效果类似。[9] 在一项随机对照研究中，术后第 3 个月随访时小切口肩袖修复的效果明显优于切开修复，但在第 2 年随访时，两组无明显差异。[3]

关节镜下修复

关节镜下肩袖修复越来越流行，成功、有效的修复需要有条理地逐步进行。患者的体位由手术医师决定。普遍选择改良的沙滩椅位，使用带关节臂的上肢固定器以便术中调整上臂的位置。通常会采用 4 个入路（后入路、后外侧入路、前外侧入路和前上入路）。关节镜下的三维成像有助于识别撕裂类型，帮助手术医师选择恰当的修复方式。通过外侧入路观察撕裂的类型和大小的效果最佳，后外侧入路更适合观察肩峰下间隙和肩袖解剖。通过切除软组织和骨性突起行两步肩峰成形术。在修复大或巨大撕裂时可保留喙肩韧带。一项试验证据为 I 级的研究表明肩袖修复时进行肩峰下减压无益处，患者功能无进一步改善。[10] 关节镜下修复组和小切口修复组在平均 24 个月的随访中，活动范围和临床功能评分均无差异。小切口修复组的术后翻修和并发症（包括关节纤维化和撞击）的发生率更高。当然，研究中小切口修复组的随访时间相对更长，这也可能是并发症发生率高的原因。一项回顾性队列研究报道小切口修复后翻修和关节纤维化的发生风险增加了近 2 倍。[9]

单排修复和双排修复

缝合锚在切开修复和关节镜下肩袖修复中均被用于将撕裂肌腱重新固定到肩袖切迹上。在过去的 20 年，单排修复是标准的修复技术。单排修复时，缝合锚根据医师的习惯和肌腱的活动范围置于切迹的内侧或外侧，呈线性排列。单排修复最常见的失败原因是缝线从肌腱中切出（图 15-2）。目前有很多种方法用于增加组织的把持力。改良 Mason-Allen 缝合（Alex 缝合）在术后第 2 年随访时被超声证实撕裂率为 38%。[11]通过改良的缝合方式进行单排重建可以得到比单纯缝合修复更高的生物力学性能，并达到与双排修复类似的生物力学强度。[12-13]一项前瞻性研究比较了大量缝合和简单缝合用于关节镜下小或中等全层肩袖撕裂的临床效果，两种缝合方式无明显差异，但超声检查证实大量缝合对于修复完整性的保持效果比简单缝合更好。[14]在单排修复中，每个缝合锚进行多重缝合可以提高固定效果。3 倍应力缝合应用于单排修复比双排修复在生物力学上更具优势，但是尚无临床研究证实。[15]

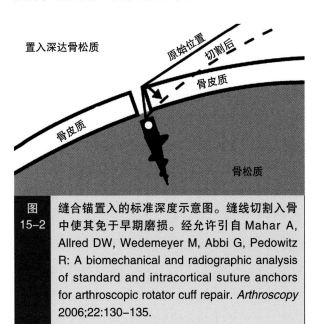

置入深达骨松质

原始位置

切割后

骨皮质

骨皮质

骨松质

图 15-2　缝合锚置入的标准深度示意图。缝线切割入骨中使其免于早期磨损。经允许引自 Mahar A, Allred DW, Wedemeyer M, Abbi G, Pedowitz R: A biomechanical and radiographic analysis of standard and intracortical suture anchors for arthroscopic rotator cuff repair. *Arthroscopy* 2006;22:130–135.

缝合锚有多种不同的材质，目前尚无科学证据表明某种材料的缝合锚优于另一种材料的。一项关于全层肩袖撕裂的前瞻性随机对照研究发现金属缝合锚和生物可降解缝合锚之间功能上无差别。[16]缝合锚置入的角度会影响缝线 - 肌腱间的固定强度。一项对实验用肩袖模型的研究发现缝合锚与切迹表面呈 90° 置入时，软组织固定效果优于标准的 45° 置入。[17]骨 - 缝合锚处力学稳定性的丢失会导致缝合锚松动、移位和拔出，文献报道该并发症发生率约为 0.3%。[18]

单排修复和双排修复在治疗肩袖撕裂时，何者效果更佳目前尚未达成共识。双排修复费用更高且费时，关节镜下操作的难度更大。生物力学研究表明双排修复优于单排修复，固定强度更大，切迹修复更好，间隙和应力更低。[12,19-22]但是，一项对牛的动物实验研究却发现两者在生物力学方面无差别。[23]

近年来几项前瞻性随机对照研究发现单排修复和双排修复在短期随访时，患者的临床功能和活动范围无差别。[24-30]一项研究通过术后 MRI 观察了肩袖在切迹上的愈合情况，另一项研究发现两种修复方式的再撕裂率相似。其他研究均发现单排修复比双排修复更容易出现再撕裂。[26-27]

撕裂的大小可能是选择修复方式的一个决定因素。[28]对撕裂大于 3 cm 的患者采用双排修复，术后第 2 年随访时患者的功能评分更高。[31]一项研究也发现双排修复大的撕裂效果更佳。[32]在对关节镜下肩袖修复患者至少 2 年的随访中，撕裂大于 3 cm 的患者，采用双排缝合锚修复及菱形缝合修复者的力量比采用单排缝合锚修复者的力量更强。[33]但是，对于各种不同大小的撕裂，两者术后第 6 个月和第 24 个月的 MRI 检查显示修复的愈合情况无差别。大部分资料认为，对于大的陈旧性撕裂，双排修复更适合，而对于小的撕裂（小于 3 cm），单排修复已足够。患者的长期效果不仅取决于肌腱 - 骨的固定强度，还与肌腱的生物性能有关，因为年龄小于 40 岁的患者采用关节镜下单排修复中等或大的全层肩袖撕裂也能取得良好效果。[34]

经骨修复

切开经骨缝合肩袖修复被认为是肩袖手术的金标准。最初的经骨通道修复技术，缝线起自切迹最内侧的骨通道，然后在距离肩袖游离缘 1 cm 处穿过肩袖。经骨修复除了能提供更大的接触面积外，还具有更高的平均切迹压力。一项三维有限元分析采用 23 种常用技术和缝合方式（单排、双排和经骨）模拟冈上肌修复并测定了应力分布。单排修复和双排修复的应力集中区在缝合锚置入处。肌肉收缩过程中，应力集中区转移到肌腱的囊表面。这些资料有可能可以解释再撕裂的形式为缝线从肌腱切出，而且支持缝合锚修复最薄弱的区域在缝线 – 肌腱连接处的假设。经骨缝合的应力集中区在骨 – 肌腱连接处，肌腱部位不是应力集中区。这表明经骨修复的最薄弱点在缝线 – 骨连接处。[35]

为将原始的经骨修复复制到关节镜手术中，研究者们进行了多次尝试。有研究者尝试使用前交叉韧带胫骨导向钻在大结节钻孔，缝线从通道穿过后使用套管针或过线器穿过肩袖。[36] 还有一种关节镜下经骨肩袖修复技术使用关节镜骨针改良缝线穿过的方法。[37] 专门用于关节镜下经骨通道修复的工具已经被使用了数年，取得了良好效果 [18]。使用一次性非缝合锚经骨固定，外科医师可以重复地在关节镜下制作出经骨缝合入路，并取得可靠的结果。[18]

经骨等效修复

经骨等效修复（又称为缝合桥接技术）的出现是为了在获得双排修复力学性能的同时，获得经骨修复的切迹覆盖。其良好的压力性能归功于斜的桥接缝合臂。类似经骨修复通过将外侧肌腱的边缘压平获得边缘稳定性，并防止与肩峰 – 喙肩韧带弓接触，后者被认为与固定失败有关。[38] 类似经骨修复可以获得与关节镜下双排修复相似的患者

满意度、临床功能和再撕裂率。明显影响肌腱愈合的唯一因素是患者年龄大于 60 岁。再撕裂的方式有两种：肌腱未愈合和切迹处愈合而内侧再撕裂。[39] 一项研究比较了单排修复、双排修复和双排修复联合经骨等效修复的效果，发现双排修复联合经骨等效修复术后再撕裂率最低，该技术尤其适用于大或巨大撕裂。[40]

近年来关节镜技术在肩袖修复方面发展迅速。生物力学及临床研究表明经骨修复和经骨等效肩袖修复的骨 – 肌腱接触面活动范围小，切迹重建效果佳，失败所需的周期应力高，修复部位的应力分布好。[35,41-43] 尽管这些技术很吸引人，但目前尚无临床研究证实某种技术明显优于另一种或哪种技术最佳。

总结

全层肩袖撕裂现在可通过多种开放手术或关节镜手术完成。近年来也有很多重大进展，比如关节镜下经骨修复或经骨等效修复的发展，但是没有文献证据证实哪种技术具有明确优势。手术医师应该熟悉每一种技术的优缺点，让每一位患者获得最好的功能恢复。后续的研究应进一步提高这些手术技术的成功率，包括损伤肌腱的愈合率。

参考文献

［1］ Yamaguchi K, Tetro AM, Blam O, Evanoff BA, Teefey SA, Middleton WD: Natural history of asymptomatic rotator cuff tears: A longitudinal analysis of asymptomatic tears detected sonographically. *J Shoulder Elbow Surg* 2001;10(3):199-203.

［2］ Davidson J, Burkhart SS: The geometric classification of rotator cuff tears: A system linking tear pattern to treatment and prognosis. *Arthroscopy* 2010;26(3):417-424.

A useful classification system for rotator cuff tears assigns a prognostic value for each type, after appropriate treatment.

［3］ Mohtadi NG, Hollinshead RM, Sasyniuk TM, Fletcher JA, Chan DS, Li FX: A randomized clinical trial comparing open to arthroscopic acromioplasty with miniopen rotator cuff repair for full-thickness rotator cuff tears: Disease-specific quality of life outcome at an average 2-year follow-up. *Am J Sports Med* 2008;36(6):1043-1051.

No difference in long-term outcomes was found after open or miniopen rotator cuff repair. Arthroscopic acromioplasty with a miniopen approach to the rotator cuff led to improved outcome scores at 3-month postoperative follow-up. Level of evidence: I.

[4] Zumstein MA, Jost B, Hempel J, Hodler J, Gerber C: The clinical and structural long-term results of open repair of massive tears of the rotator cuff. *J Bone Joint Surg Am* 2008;90(11):2423-2431.

Patients had improvement 3 to 10 years after massive rotator cuff tears were treated in an open fashion, despite a 57% rate of retearing and an increase in tear size and fatty infiltration.

[5] Morse K, Davis AD, Afra R, Kaye EK, Schepsis A, Voloshin I: Arthroscopic versus mini-open rotator cuff repair: A comprehensive review and meta-analysis. *Am J Sports Med* 2008;36(9):1824-1828.

A meta-analysis compared the results of arthroscopic and miniopen rotator cuff repairs at a minimum 1-year and average 2-year follow-up. There was no statistical difference in functional outcomes or complications.

[6] Ramsey ML, Getz CL, Parsons BO: What's new in shoulder and elbow surgery. *J Bone Joint Surg Am* 2009;91(5):1283-1293.

A review of 2007 and 2008 articles highlighted new and emerging evidence and trends in treating shoulder and elbow disease.

[7] Boileau P, Baqué F, Valerio L, Ahrens P, Chuinard C, Trojani C: Isolated arthroscopic biceps tenotomy or tenodesis improves symptoms in patients with massive irreparable rotator cuff tears. *J Bone Joint Surg Am* 2007;89(4):747-757.

After isolated biceps tenotomy in selected patients with an irreparable rotator cuff tear, 78% were satisfied with the result and had an overall statistical improvement in Constant score. An intact teres minor was an important factor for success. Level of evidence:III.

[8] Millett PJ, Horan MP, Maland KE, Hawkins RJ: Long-term survivorship and outcomes after surgical repair of full-thickness rotator cuff tears. *J Shoulder Elbow Surg* 2011;20(4):591-597.

At 5- or 10-year follow-up after open treatment of ro- tator cuff tears, survivorship was 94% or 83%, re-

spectively. Survivorship rates and outcomes scores were higher after repair of single-tendon tears than after chronic tears and tears involving the subscapularis. Level of evidence: IV.

[9] Nho SJ, Shindle MK, Sherman SL, Freedman KB, Lyman S, MacGillivray JD: Systematic review of arthroscopic rotator cuff repair and mini-open rotator cuff repair. *J Bone Joint Surg Am* 2007;89(suppl 3):127-136.

A systematic review found no statistically significant differences in functional or clinical outcomes or complication rates after arthroscopic or miniopen rotator cuff repairs at a mean 24-month follow-up. There was a slightly higher percentage of complications after miniopen repair.

[10] Milano G, Grasso A, Salvatore M, Zarelli D, Deriu L, Fabbriciani C: Arthroscopic rotator cuff repair with and without subacromial decompression: A prospective randomized study. *Arthroscopy* 2007;23(1):81-88.

In the short term, there was no statistical difference in the outcomes of rotator cuff repair with or without subacromial decompression, with consideration of age, gender, dominance, location, shape, area, retraction, reducibility, and fatty infiltration. Level of evidence: I.

[11] Castagna A, Conti M, Markopoulos N, et al: Arthroscopic repair of rotator cuff tear with a modified Mason-Allen stitch: Mid-term clinical and ultrasound outcomes. *Knee Surg Sports Traumatol Arthrosc* 2008;16(5):497-503.

At a minimum 24-month follow-up of 29 patients treated arthroscopically for an isolated supraspinatus tear with a single anchor and modified Mason-Allen stitch, Constant scores improved significantly, and the retear rate was 38%.

[12] Lorbach O, Bachelier F, Vees J, Kohn D, Pape D: Cyclic loading of rotator cuff reconstructions: Single-row repair with modified suture configurations versus double-row repair. *Am J Sports Med* 2008;36(8):1504-1510.

A biomechanical study of single- and double-row suture configurations for rotator cuff repair in a porcine model found that double-row repair with corkscrew anchors had the greatest pull-out strength.

[13] Nelson CO, Sileo MJ, Grossman MG, Serra-Hsu F: Single-row modified Mason-Allen versus double-row arthroscopic rotator cuff repair: A biomechanical and surface area comparison. *Arthroscopy* 2008;24(8):941-948.

A biomechanical study comparing the strength and the

contact surface area of a single-row modified Mason-Allen suture configuration and a double-row arthroscopic configuration found no difference in strength. The surface area was better with the double-row technique.

[14] Ko SH, Friedman D, Seo DK, Jun HM, Warner JJ: A prospective therapeutic comparison of simple suture repairs to massive cuff stitch repairs for treatment of small- and medium-sized rotator cuff tears. *Arthroscopy* 2009;25(6):583-589, e1-e4.

Clinical outcomes were not significantly different in single row rotator cuff repairs using a massive rotator cuff stitch or a simple stitch. The massive rotator cuff stitch had superior integrity on follow-up ultrasound examination. Level of evidence: III.

[15] Barber FA, Herbert MA, Schroeder FA, Aziz-Jacobo J, Mays MM, Rapley JH: Biomechanical advantages of triple-loaded suture anchors compared with double- row rotator cuff repairs. *Arthroscopy* 2010;26(3):316-323.

A biomechanical study of two single-row and three double-row repair techniques found that a single row of triple-loaded anchors was more resistant to gap formation than any double-row repair. The addition of a ripstop stitch enhanced stretch resistance.

[16] Milano G, Grasso A, Salvatore M, Saccomanno MF, Deriu L, Fabbriciani C: Arthroscopic rotator cuff repair with metal and biodegradable suture anchors: A prospective randomized study. *Arthroscopy* 2010;26(9, suppl):S112-S119.

No difference was found between metal and biodegradable suture anchors when individual patient variables were accounted for. Level of evidence: I.

[17] Strauss E, Frank D, Kubiak E, Kummer F, Rokito A: The effect of the angle of suture anchor insertion on fixation failure at the tendon-suture interface after rotator cuff repair: Deadman's angle revisited. *Arthroscopy* 2009;25(6):597-602.

A biomechanical study compared pull-out strength and gap formation in suture anchors inserted at 45° and 90°. Anchors inserted at 90° had better cyclic load to failure and gap formation.

[18] Garofalo R, Castagna A, Borroni M, Krishnan SG: Arthroscopic transosseous (anchorless) rotator cuff repair. *Knee Surg Sports Traumatol Arthrosc* 2012;20(6):1031-1035.

Dedicated single-use instrumentation was used to reliably and reproducibly create bone tunnels and pass su- tures through the greater tuberosity for a purely arthroscopic transosseous rotator cuff repair. Preliminary results were reported. Level of evidence: V.1

[19] Ahmad CS, Kleweno C, Jacir AM, et al: Biomechanical performance of rotator cuff repairs with humeral rotation: A new rotator cuff repair failure model. *Am J Sports Med* 2008;36(5):888-892.

A biomechanical study compared gap formation in single-row and double-row repairs in neutral, 45° internal, and 45° external rotation. Gapping was less in double-row than single-row repairs. Gapping was greater in internal rotation than in external rotation and was least in neutral.

[20] Baums MH, Buchhorn GH, Gilbert F, Spahn G, Schultz W, Klinger HM: Initial load-to-failure and failure analysis in single- and double-row repair techniques for rotator cuff repair. *Arch Orthop Trauma Surg* 2010;130(9):1193-1199.

A biomechanical study compared single-row repair (Mason-Allen stitches) and double-row repair (single-row repair plus medial horizontal mattress stitches) using polyester or polyblend suture material. The double-row technique was superior with both suture types.

[21] Baums MH, Spahn G, Steckel H, Fischer A, Schultz W, Klinger HM: Comparative evaluation of the tendon-bone interface contact pressure in different single- versus double-row suture anchor repair techniques. *Knee Surg Sports Traumatol Arthrosc* 2009;17(12):1466-1472.

A biomechanical study examined time-zero contact pressures for three single-row and two double-row suture configurations. Contact pressures and footprint coverage were superior with the double-row techniques and the use of arthroscopic Mason-Allen sutures in a single-row construct.

[22] Milano G, Grasso A, Zarelli D, Deriu L, Cillo M, Fabbriciani C: Comparison between single-row and double-row rotator cuff repair: A biomechanical study. *Knee Surg Sports Traumatol Arthrosc* 2008;16(1):75-80.

A biomechanical study compared single-row and double-row rotator cuff repairs with or without tension on the tendon. Single-row repair under tension was significantly inferior to the other repairs in displacement under cyclic loading.

[23] Mahar A, Tamborlane J, Oka R, Esch J, Pedowitz RA: Single-row suture anchor repair of the rotator cuff is biomechanically equivalent to double-row repair in a bovine model. *Arthroscopy* 2007;23(12):1265-1270.

A biomechanical study in a bovine model that compared single-row and double-row repairs found no statistical differences in repair elongation or load to failure.

[24] Grasso A, Milano G, Salvatore M, Falcone G, Deriu L, Fabbriciani C: Single-row versus double-row arthroscopic rotator cuff repair: A prospective randomized clinical study. *Arthroscopy* 2009;25(1):4-12.

A short-term comparison of clinical outcomes after double-row or single-row arthroscopic repair found no statistical differences between the two groups at 2 years when individual patient factors were considered. Level of evidence: I.

[25] Burks RT, Crim J, Brown N, Fink B, Greis PE: A prospective randomized clinical trial comparing arthroscopic single- and double-row rotator cuff repair: Magnetic resonance imaging and early clinical evaluation. *Am J Sports Med* 2009;37(4):674-682.

At 1-year follow-up, a comparison of arthroscopic double-row and single-row rotator cuff repairs found no difference in clinical outcomes or on MRI. One retear occurred in each patient group. Level of evidence: I.

[26] Franceschi F, Ruzzini L, Longo UG, et al: Equivalent clinical results of arthroscopic single-row and double-row suture anchor repair for rotator cuff tears: A randomized controlled trial. *Am J Sports Med* 2007;35(8):1254-1260.

At 2-year follow-up, there were no differences in clinical results or healing rates after single-row or double- row arthroscopic rotator cuff repair. The double-row repairs had greater integrity on MRI. Level of evidence: I.

[27] Charousset C, Grimberg J, Duranthon LD, Bellaiche L, Petrover D: Can a double-row anchorage technique improve tendon healing in arthroscopic rotator cuff repair? A prospective, nonrandomized, comparative study of double-row and single-row anchorage techniques with computed tomographic arthrography tendon healing assessment. *Am J Sports Med* 2007;35(8):1247-1253.

At 6-month follow-up, clinical results and healing (assessed on CT) were compared after double-row or single-row rotator cuff repair. There were no differences, except the double-row repair had superior healing. Level of evidence: II.

[28] Sugaya H, Maeda K, Matsuki K, Moriishi J: Repair integrity and functional outcome after arthroscopic double-row rotator cuff repair: A prospective outcome study. *J Bone Joint Surg Am* 2007;89(5):953-960.

At an average 14-month follow-up, healing of double- row rotator cuff repairs was evaluated using MRI. Retearing rates were 5% for small to medium-sized tears and 40%

for large to massive tears. Level of evidence:IV.

[29] Aydin N, Kocaoglu B, Guven O: Single-row versus double-row arthroscopic rotator cuff repair in small- to medium-sized tears. *J Shoulder Elbow Surg* 2010;19(5):722-725.

At a minimum 2-year follow-up, the clinical outcomes of single-row and double-row rotator cuff repairs were compared. All shoulders had functional improvement, with no significant difference in clinical outcomes. Level of evidence: II.

[30] Koh KH, Kang KC, Lim TK, Shon MS, Yoo JC: Prospective randomized clinical trial of single- versus double-row suture anchor repair in 2- to 4-cm rotator cuff tears: Clinical and magnetic resonance imaging results. *Arthroscopy* 2011;27(4):453-462.

Clinical and MRI outcomes of large to massive rotator cuff tears were compared after single-row or double- row repair. There were no differences in clinical outcomes or rates of retearing on MRI. Level of evidence: I.

[31] Park JY, Lhee SH, Choi JH, Park HK, Yu JW, Seo JB: Comparison of the clinical outcomes of single- and double-row repairs in rotator cuff tears. *Am J Sports Med* 2008;36(7):1310-1316.

A comparison of clinical outcomes after single-row or double-row rotator cuff repair found no significant differences in scores on three measures at 2-year follow-up. Level of evidence: II.

[32] Pennington WT, Gibbons DJ, Bartz BA, et al: Comparative analysis of single-row versus double-row repair of rotator cuff tears. *Arthroscopy* 2010;26(11):1419-1426.

No clinical difference was found in a comparison of clinical outcomes and MRI-assessed healing after double-row rotator cuff repair or single-row repair using a massive cuff stitch. The healing of similar-size tears was better after double-row repair. Level of evidence: III.

[33] Ma HL, Chiang ER, Wu HT, et al: Clinical outcome and imaging of arthroscopic single-row and double-row rotator cuff repair: A prospective randomized trial. *Arthroscopy* 2012;28(1):16-24.

Clinical outcome, muscle strength, and repair integrity were compared after single-row or double-row rotator cuff repair. At 6-month and 2-year follow-up, the strength of larger tears was significantly better after double-row repair. No other differences were found. Level of evidence: II.

[34] Krishnan SG, Harkins DC, Schiffern SC, Pennington SD, Burkhead WZ: Arthroscopic repair of full- thickness

tears of the rotator cuff in patients younger than 40 years. *Arthroscopy* 2008;24(3):324-328.

At a minimum 2-year follow-up, clinical outcomes of rotator cuff repair were evaluated in patients younger than 40 years. Almost all of the tears were traumatic. All of the tears improved, with 90% of the patients returning to their previous level of activity. Level of evidence: IV.

[35] Sano H, Yamashita T, Wakabayashi I, Itoi E: Stress distribution in the supraspinatus tendon after tendon repair: Suture anchors versus transosseous suture fixation. *Am J Sports Med* 2007;35(4):542-546.

A biomechanical study compared stress distribution within the tendon after single-row, double-row, or transosseous repair. The concentrations of stress were significantly higher with suture anchor repair than with transosseous repair.

[36] Kim KC, Rhee KJ, Shin HD, Kim YM: Arthroscopic transosseous rotator cuff repair. *Orthopedics* 2008;31 (4):327-330.

A technique was described for using an anterior cruci- ate ligament guide to pass transosseous sutures through the greater tuberosity to repair the rotator cuff. The technique is recommended in the presence of osteoporotic bone that is unable to hold an anchor.

[37] Frick H, Haag M, Volz M, Stehle J: Arthroscopic bone needle: A new, safe, and cost-effective technique for rotator cuff repair. *Tech Shoulder Surg* 2010;11:107-112.

A technique for arthroscopic use of a bone needle to pass sutures transosseously reduced the cost of surgery by 80%. The mean Constant score normalized for age and sex was 92% at 1-year follow-up.

[38] Park MC, Tibone JE, ElAttrache NS, Ahmad CS, Jun BJ, Lee TQ: Part II: Biomechanical assessment for a footprint-restoring transosseous-equivalent rotator cuff repair technique compared with a double-row re- pair technique. *J Shoulder Elbow Surg* 2007;16(4):469-476.

A biomechanical study compared transosseous-equivalent and double-row techniques by measuring stiffness, gap formation, and ultimate load to failure. Stiffness and gap formation were not significantly different. The transosseous-equivalent repair had a greater load to failure.

[39] Voigt C, Bosse C, Vosshenrich R, Schulz AP, Lill H: Arthroscopic supraspinatus tendon repair with suture-bridging technique: Functional outcome and magnetic resonance imaging. *Am J Sports Med* 2010;38(5):983-991.

Suture bridge treatment of rotator cuff tears led to clinical outcomes and retearing rates similar to those of published double-row repair studies at 4-month, 1-year, and mean 2-year follow-up. Level of evidence:IV.

[40] Mihata T, Watanabe C, Fukunishi K, et al: Functional and structural outcomes of single-row versus double-row versus combined double-row and suture-bridge repair for rotator cuff tears. *Am J Sports Med* 2011;39(10):2091-2098.

A large study comparing the functional and structural outcomes of three anchor-based techniques for rotator cuff repair found that the combined double-row and suture bridge technique had a significantly lower re-tearing rate for massive cuff tears compared with single-row and double-row repairs. Level of evidence: III.

[41] Zheng N, Harris HW, Andrews JR: Failure analysis of rotator cuff repair: A comparison of three double-row techniques. *J Bone Joint Surg Am* 2008;90(5):1034-1042.

A biomechanical study of double-row repair using anchors medially with three different techniques for the lateral row found a significantly higher failure rate with the anchor lateral techniques than the Mason- Allen transosseous technique.

[42] Frank JB, ElAttrache NS, Dines JS, Blackburn A, Crues J, Tibone JE: Repair site integrity after arthroscopic transosseous-equivalent suture-bridge rotator cuff repair. *Am J Sports Med* 2008;36(8):1496-1503.

Healing after suture bridge rotator cuff repair was evaluated on MRI at a minimum 1-year follow-up. Supraspinatus tears had healed in 89% of patients, supraspinatus-infraspinatus tears had healed in 86%, and massive tears had healed in 100%. Level of evidence: IV.

[43] Tocci SL, Tashjian RZ, Leventhal E, Spenciner DB, Green A, Fleming BC: Biomechanical comparison of single-row arthroscopic rotator cuff repair technique versus transosseous repair technique. *J Shoulder Elbow Surg* 2008;17(5):808-814.

A biomechanical study compared arthroscopic single-row repair and Mason-Allen transosseous repair in rotator cuff tears of different sizes. Gapping was greater in massive tears and occurred posteriorly. There were no technique-based differences in gapping.

第十六章 巨大肩袖撕裂

Daniel M. Hampton, MD; Ruth A. Delaney, MB BCh, MRCS; Laurence D. Higgins, MD

引言

巨大肩袖撕裂尽管有很多种定义和分类，但并没有一个精确的定义。一些研究者将其定义为最大撕裂的前后径超过 5 cm，另一些研究者则将其定义为至少两根肌腱完全断裂。[1-2] 由于定义不同，所以很难对不同研究进行直接比较。巨大肩袖撕裂仅偶尔由急性损伤引起，大部分由慢性肩袖撕裂进展而来。慢性基础上的急性巨大撕裂是在已存在的小撕裂的基础上由外伤导致的撕裂范围增大。[3] 巨大肩袖撕裂的发生率为 10%~40%。[1]

慢性肩袖撕裂通常合并明显的肌肉脂肪浸润和肌腱回缩，这使修复过程变得十分复杂，某些巨大撕裂甚至无法修复。并不是所有的巨大肩袖撕裂都无法修复，也不是所有无法修复的肩袖撕裂都是巨大撕裂。大部分巨大肩袖撕裂患者因功能障碍而有明显的无力。年轻患者的功能障碍比老年患者更严重。文献报道后上方巨大撕裂（累及冈上肌和冈下肌）比前上方撕裂（累及冈上肌和肩胛下肌）更常见。[4]

Dr. Higgins or an immediate family member has received nonincome support (such as equipment or services), commercially derived honoraria, or other nonresearch related funding (such as paid travel) from Arthrex, Smith & Nephew, Breg, and DePuy and serves as a board member, owner, officer, or committee member of the American Shoulder and Elbow Surgeons, the Arthroscopy Association of North America, the American Academy of Orthopaedic Surgeons, and the Advocacy for Improvement in Mobility. Neither of the following authors nor any immediate family member has received anything of value from or has stock or stock options held in a commercial company or institution related directly or indirectly to the subject of this chapter: Dr. Hampton and Dr. Delaney.

生物力学

肩袖的生物力学功能是在活动时维持肱骨头位于关节盂的中心。[5-7] 但是，目前尚不清楚活动时正常应力下的不同时期生物力学的改变。最近的一项尸体标本研究表明，从冈上肌完全撕裂发展到冈下肌撕裂是一个关键期，肱骨头的动力学发生明显变化。[8] 冈上肌完全撕裂但冈下肌未受累时，高负荷下标本的外展功能受限，但肱骨头的动力学性能不受影响。这些研究表明，单纯冈上肌撕裂时平衡力偶仍得以维持。

自然病程

巨大肩袖撕裂的自然病程并未被完全阐明。研究者的经验大部分来自对非手术治疗患者的检查结果，包括药物治疗和理疗的患者。这些结果可能无法真实反应巨大肩袖撕裂的自然病程，可能存在明显偏倚，因为患者选择不进行手术治疗，或者患者存在不可修复的撕裂。但是，MRI 研究表明，非手术治疗患者撕裂的大小平均增加了 3.29 cm。[2-3] 脂肪浸润明显增加，冈上肌、冈下肌和肩胛下肌的 Goutallier 分级增加，可修复撕裂进展为不可修复撕裂。一项研究发现，由于脂肪浸润增加和肩峰肱骨间隙减小至 7 mm 以下，50% 的可修复撕裂变为不可修复撕裂，肩峰肱骨间隙平均减少了 2.6 mm。此外，巨大肩袖撕裂生物力学性能的改变还导致盂肱关节炎的影像学分期进展。目前发现了数个导致病情加重的危险因素：撕裂肌腱的数量、撕裂大小、外展无力、盂肱关节炎的严重程度、脂肪浸润分级及肩峰肱骨间隙。[9]

临床评估

患者通常主诉疼痛和无力。有症状的撕裂患者通常在夜间和日常活动时出现疼痛。根据撕裂大小的不同，患者还可能出现假性麻痹。假性麻痹的定义为盂肱关节被动活动不受限且无神经损伤时主动上举不超过 90°。[10]不同患者肩关节无力和活动受限的范围差别很大。确定患者的疼痛是否确实由肩袖撕裂引起非常重要。粘连性关节囊炎、颈椎疾病、肱二头肌腱疾病和肩锁关节炎导致的疼痛与肩袖撕裂导致的疼痛非常相似。典型肩袖撕裂的疼痛位于肩关节前外侧，疼痛通常向三角肌止点放射。疼痛放射至肘关节以下甚至到手部时应怀疑颈椎疾病或周围神经受压。

体格检查应从双侧肩关节的视诊开始，暴露要充分。巨大肩袖撕裂常存在明显的冈上肌萎缩和（或）冈下肌凹陷，视诊很容易发现，触诊更容易发现。应记录患侧肩的主动和被动活动，并与健侧对比。主动和被动活动的差别可以为肩袖功能的诊断提供重要线索。主动活动时观察肩胛骨的动态活动也十分重要。巨大撕裂患者通常存在肩胛骨代偿，体格检查时应该注意到。应进行肩袖肌肉力量测试，并评估各种迟滞征（Lag signs）。前上方撕裂可导致内旋无力和上举疼痛、无力。后上方撕裂可导致上举和外旋无力。

有几个临床征象提示修复的预后较差。肱骨头在静态时前上方半脱位是巨大前上方撕裂无法修复的征象。对抗外展时的动态前上方半脱位也预示着修复的预后不良。假性瘫痪和真垂肩征是冈下肌严重病变、脂肪浸润的表现，Goutallier 分

级 2 级或以上。[11-12]Hornblower 征阳性提示小圆肌严重脂肪浸润，无法成功修复。[13]

总之，静态或动态半脱位和慢性迟滞征提示肩袖撕裂无法修复。尽管临床医师可以测量无力的程度及功能障碍的水平，但是必须由患者决定是否接受治疗。只有患者不能接受现有的功能或者现有功能受限很有可能出现进展时，才可以选择进一步治疗。

影像学检查

普通 X 线片是肩痛患者的首选影像学检查。X 线片可以显示盂肱关节和肱骨头的位置、肩锁关节和肩峰形态。评估怀疑存在肩袖疾病的患者时，需要的标准 X 线片包括一张真正的肩关节正位（Grashey 位）片、一张肩胛骨 Y 位（出口位）片和一张腋位片。在 Grashey 位上可以观察肱骨头上移的情况，并进行定量分析。[1]

肩峰肱骨间隙用于定量肱骨头上移程度，健康人的正常范围为 7~14 mm。[14]肩峰肱骨间隙与肩袖撕裂的大小有关。Hamada 分型将肩峰肱骨间隙分为 1~5 级，其中第 4 级又被改良，分为两个亚级[15-16]（表 16-1）。随着肩峰肱骨间隙的减小（分级升高），肩袖肌肉脂肪浸润的程度增高。最近的一项综述发现接受了修复手术的 1 级和 2 级巨大撕裂患者中，2 级巨大撕裂患者的再撕裂率更高，没有患者进展为 3 级或更高级别。[17]

表 16-1

肩峰肱骨间隙的 Hamada 分型

分级	肩峰肱骨间隙的状态
1 级	正常（7~14 mm）
2 级	变窄
3 级	变窄，合并肩峰凹变
4 级	变窄，合并肩峰凹变及盂肱关节间隙变窄 a
5 级	变窄，合并肩峰凹变及肱骨头塌陷

注：a 在改良的分型系统（Walch 分型）中，4A 为盂肱关节炎，无肩峰下关节炎；4B 为盂肱关节炎合并肩峰下关节炎。

CT 或 MRI 检查可以准确地确定撕裂大小、撕裂肌腱数量、肌腱回缩情况、组织质量、骨性结构形态和肌腹脂肪浸润情况。MRI 已经成为肩关节软组织评估的主要手段。MRI 可以可靠地反映肩袖撕裂的特征。如果患者无法进行 MRI 检查，CT 关节造影检查也可以提供非常有价值的信息。CT 关节造影检查可用于观察肌肉的脂肪浸润情况以进行 Goutallier 分级[18]（表 16-2）。MRI 也可以用于评估脂肪浸润，在矢状位 T1 像观察肌肉内脂肪含量最佳，但是切面必须足够偏内以观察肌腹[19]（图 16-1）。严重的肌肉回缩会导致肌肉汇聚，可能导致医师低估脂肪浸润的程度。最近有研究对分型系统的观察者内和观察者间的可信度提出了质疑。[20]

脂肪浸润程度是修复效果的重要预后因素。3 级或 4 级脂肪浸润患者的修复效果很可能比轻度浸润患者的差。[12,20]一项对 22 例 3 级或 4 级脂肪浸润患者的研究发现，部分患者在修复后临床功能有改善。[21]但是，大部分学者仍认为高度脂肪浸润患者手术修复后的临床及影像学结果较差。大部分研究也发现脂肪浸润为 2 级或更低级别的患者修复效果更佳。[22-23]

肌腱回缩加重也与脂肪浸润的分级增加相关（图 16-2）。最近的研究发现，在脂肪浸润分级小于或等于 3 级时大部分肌肉肌腱的回缩是由肌纤维本身导致的。肌腱回缩仅发生于脂肪浸润分级为 2 级及以上的患者，3 级或 4 级脂肪浸润患者的所有肌腱回缩均源自于肌腱。这一发现表明，解剖修复肌腱并不能解剖重建高度脂肪浸润患者的肌肉 - 肌腱单元。[24]

超声检查现在也可用于肩袖检查。肩关节便携式超声的优点为花费低、无创、无副作用，可以在生理性活动时动态观察肩袖，且结果随时可得。超声不能穿透骨骼，因此，如果巨大肩袖撕裂患者的肌腱回缩到肩峰内侧，超声就无法提供

表 16-2	
Goutallier 脂肪浸润分级	
分级	脂肪浸润程度
0 级	正常肌肉
1 级	可见一些脂肪条纹
2 级	脂肪含量小于肌肉含量
3 级	脂肪含量与肌肉含量相当
4 级	脂肪含量大于肌肉含量

图 16-1	肩胛骨 Y 位 MRI 矢状位 T1 加权图像上显示冈下肌严重脂肪浸润

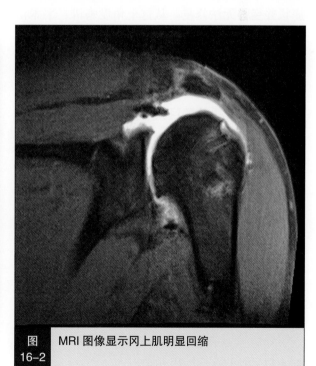

图 16-2	MRI 图像显示冈上肌明显回缩

很多信息。检查的准确性很大程度上依赖检查者的经验和技术水平。[25] 近期的研究表明,有经验的超声医师阳性预测值为 96%,阴性预测值为 95%。撕裂根据大小分为小撕裂(前后径小于 1 cm)、中等撕裂(前后径 1~3 cm)、大或巨大撕裂(前后径大于 3 cm),撕裂越大,检查的准确性越高。[26]

非手术治疗

非手术治疗在某些情况下也适用于巨大肩袖撕裂。[3,27] 一项研究回顾性分析了 19 例巨大肩袖撕裂患者的自然病程,所有患者均接受了标准的康复治疗。[3] 这些患者对功能要求低或者拒绝手术。在平均 4 年的随访中,患者平均相对 Constant 肩关节评分为 83 分,平均主观肩关节评分为 68 分,肩关节活动范围得以维持。盂肱关节炎加重,肩峰肱骨间隙减小,撕裂增大,脂肪浸润加重。50% 在诊断时可修复的撕裂在最后随访时变得不可修复。该研究的作者认为,有中等程度症状的巨大肩袖撕裂患者尽管非手术治疗后结构性病变出现进展,但仍可以获得令人满意的关节功能。作者还指出,可修复的撕裂有可能出现症状并变得无法修复。从这个角度来讲,手术治疗方式的选择可能仅限于对手术技术要求高的肌腱转移、成功率有限的切开或关节镜下清理及反肩关节置换。

无法耐受手术的巨大肩袖撕裂患者推荐进行规律的前三角肌康复治疗。[27] 一项纳入 17 例巨大肩袖撕裂、冈上肌和冈下肌 Goutallier 4 级脂肪浸润患者的前瞻性研究发现,患者在经过规范的前三角肌康复治疗后,平均 Constant 肩关节评分由 26 分增加至 63 分。肩关节各个方向的活动均改善,尤其是前屈上举。大部分患者前三角肌的稳定使得患者的肩关节功能和疼痛得到充分改善。该研究的作者认为,规律的前三角肌功能锻炼联合镇痛药物应该是高龄、合并严重疾病的巨大肩袖撕裂患者的首选治疗方式。

清理和肩峰下减压

以缓解巨大、不可修复肩袖撕裂患者疼痛为目标的手术引起了学者们对巨大撕裂进行清理的兴趣,可以在清理的同时行肩峰成形术或肩峰下减压。这些技术可能对肩关节力量和活动范围的改善无益,但是可以明显缓解疼痛,尤其是对功能要求比较低的患者。由于疼痛缓解,患者还可能获得其他功能的改善,尤其是对于疼痛还有其他来源的患者,其他病变也得到了治疗,例如,肱二头肌腱疾病。[16]

一项研究报道了 31 例不可修复肩袖撕裂患者(平均年龄 70.6 岁),这些患者均接受了关节镜下清理。[28] 其中,24 例患者同时进行了肱二头肌腱切断。为了保留喙肩弓,没有行肩峰成形术。在平均 47 个月的随访中,患者 Constant 肩关节评分明显改善,由平均 24 分改善至平均 69.8 分,视觉模拟疼痛评分由 7.8 分降为 2.9 分,Constant 肩关节评分手术侧明显低于对侧。10 例(32%)患者的结果归为优,7 例(23%)良,9 例(29%)一般,5 例(16%)差。由于没有进行手术干预,随访时患者的影像学表现变差:10 例(32%)患者盂肱关节炎加重,肩峰肱骨间隙由 8.3 mm 降至 7.0 mm。总体而言,虽然影像学退行性变加重,但患者的临床功能明显改善。

前下部分肩峰成形术最初由 Neer 报道,目前已经成为一项关节镜手术。[4,29] 随着对该手术技术经验的增加,学者们已经认识到喙肩弓的重要性,同时认识到对巨大肩袖撕裂行肩峰成形术的一个潜在并发症是肱骨头上移。一项对 7 例肩关节尸体标本的研究设置了 5 种情况:喙肩韧带完整、喙肩韧带骨膜下松解、标准的肩峰成形术、喙肩韧带重建和改良的 Neer 肩峰成形术。研究者持续向前上方施加 150 N 的应力,测量肱骨头前上方移位情况。[30] 与前方肩峰成形术和改良 Neer 肩峰成形术相比,喙肩韧带重建后肱骨头前上移位明显减少。该研究的作者推测喙肩韧带重建或许能为巨大肩袖撕裂提供必要的稳定性，防止肱骨头前上方过度移位或从喙肩弓脱出。行肩峰成形术时仅需切除少量骨质，应尽可能保留喙肩韧带。学者们建议，如果喙肩韧带不能保留，应进行内侧束的解剖重建。一项研究报道了 16 例巨大肩袖损伤患者，通过将喙肩韧带骨性缝合至喙突进行了修复。[31] 在 10 例完整随访的患者中，8 例获得了满意的效果并可进行过顶上举活动，2 例效果不满意。没有患者发生肱骨头前上方半脱位。尽管该研究中撕裂无法修复，但是保留或者重建喙肩韧带的肩峰成形术可以保留喙肩弓的部分被动稳定效应。

2002 年，有学者报道了一种在治疗巨大、不可修复肩袖撕裂的同时保留喙肩韧带的手术技术。该技术被称为结节成形术，即去除肱骨的骨赘，重塑大结节外形，使其与肩峰更吻合，不进行肩峰成形术。在确定肩袖是否可修复前保留完整的肩峰和喙肩韧带。在确定肩袖是否可修复前保持喙肩弓不被破坏非常重要。20 例患者接受了该手术治疗，患者术前有疼痛症状，肩袖撕裂同时累及冈上肌和冈下肌，且撕裂大小至少为 5 cm，2 例患者同时存在部分肩胛下肌撕裂。所有患者在进行了松解后，均由于肌腱过度回缩和（或）组织质量过差放弃了肩袖修复手术。19 例患者接受了至少 27 个月的随访，其中 12 例患者结果为优，6 例为良，1 例为一般。13 例（68%）患者疼痛完全缓解，无夜间痛。同时，所有患者均残留外旋无力。研究结果表明，患者疼痛缓解且功能有改善，但是改善的程度还是不如肩峰成形术和肩袖修复。该研究的结论为不管肩峰和喙肩韧带在撞击综合征的病理生理过程中扮演着何种角色，其在巨大、不可修复肩袖撕裂患者的治疗中极为重要。[32]

对巨大肩袖撕裂进行清理和肩峰下减压的效果不如肩袖修复，但是其在对功能要求较低的患者的治疗中仍有一定地位，对这些患者而言，缓解疼痛是首要的，患者对功能的要求不高。但是，清理和肩峰下减压的效果会随着时间的推移而下降。如果患者术前后方肩袖完整，表现为三角肌完整且外旋有力，通常很有可能获得令人满意的治疗效果。

部分修复与边缘重叠

"边缘重叠"这一术语指的是对巨大、U 形肩袖撕裂进行边对边缝合。大部分巨大肩袖撕裂并没有出现肌腱回缩，是由内向外纵向的 L 形撕裂，由于肌肉 - 肌腱单元的弹性而表现为 U 形撕裂。[33] 从 20 世纪 40 年代开始，研究者们推荐使用边对边、肌腱对肌腱的缝合以及肌腱末端到骨的缝合。对撕裂进行松解会导致修复失败，因为应力在撕裂的顶点超负荷，但是边对边缝合根据边缘重叠的生物力学原则更具力学优势。边缘重叠修复时，随着边对边缝合的进行，大的游离缘逐渐向大结节汇聚（图 16-3）。随着边缘的汇聚，游离缘的张力显著降低，最终覆盖在肱骨头上的游离缘在修复时几乎无张力。边对边缝合 2/3 的 U 形撕裂可以将肩袖游离缘的张力降低至缝合前的 1/6。该修复方式降低了通过缝合锚或骨通道将游离缘固定到骨的失败风险。不应将巨大、U 形撕裂的内侧缘从关节盂和肩胛颈上充分游离然后牵拉覆盖在肱骨骨床上，这种方式会在已修复的肩袖边缘中央产生非常大的张力，容易导致修复失败。

修复巨大肩袖撕裂时必须遵守边缘重叠和力偶的原理。在进行边缘重叠缝合后，如果肩袖的上部仍有缺损，且至少一半的冈下肌可以缝合至骨质，那么部分修复仍然有效。部分修复推荐用于无法完全修复缺损，而局部肩袖肌腱转移又无法实施时。对于真正无法移动的撕裂，间隔滑移有时可以使冈上肌获得 1~2 cm 的额外侧方移动，从而更多地完成部分修复。[34] 但是，该技术的效果报道不一。

一项对 48 只切断冈上肌和冈下肌 4 周以后的大鼠的研究比较了部分修复、不修复、仅修复

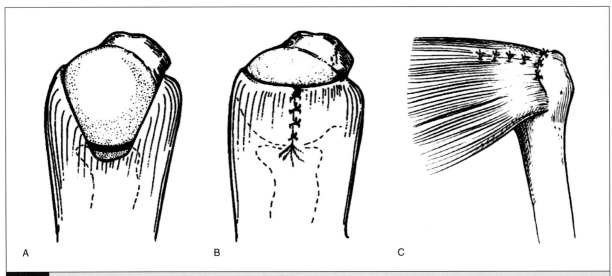

图 16-3　示意图分别显示了 U 形肩袖撕裂（A）、部分边对边缝合（B）和边对边缝合联合缝合锚以及将肩袖游离缘固定至骨质（C）。在修复过程中，大结节的边缘重叠缝合增加了横截面积，缩短了撕裂的长度，从而降低了张力。经允许引自 Burkhart SS: Arthroscopic treatment of massive rotator cuff tears. *Clin Orthop Relat Res* 2001;390:107–118.

冈下肌和两根肌腱均修复的效果。[35] 定量活动测试（内外应力、停止、加速和步宽）在无修复和仅修复冈下肌的大鼠之间存在显著差异，但在仅修复冈下肌和两根肌腱均修复的大鼠之间无差别。仅将冈下肌修复至原止点而不修复冈上肌与同时修复冈上肌和冈下肌，在重建前后力偶方面，对肩关节功能的改善程度相当。

　　一项尸体标本研究对边缘重叠技术在巨大肩袖撕裂修复中的生物力学原理进行了研究。将 20 例肩关节标本的冈上肌肌肉–肌腱单元去除，制作大的回缩性肩袖撕裂模型，然后运用切开手术的方式进行边缘重叠修复，在关节盂缘内侧 5 mm 处开始向外侧进行简单缝合。每缝合一针测量一次残留间隙。研究发现每一针缝合都能明显减小残留间隙，第一针时残留间隙减小 50%，第二针时减小 60%，第三针时减小 67%，第四针时减小 75%（$P < 0.05$）。分别在肩袖完整时、切除冈上肌后、每一次边缘重叠缝合后，在不同的旋转和外展位测量每个标本冈下肌和肩胛下肌应力，发现缝合后冈下肌和肩胛下肌的应力减小，在 0° 外展位旋转不同角度时应力减小 58%（$P <$

0.05）。外展 60° 时，在不同旋转位置上的绝对应力值均降低，但是除第 4 次边缘重叠后的冈下肌应力有统计学差异外（$P < 0.05$），其他情况下的变化均无统计学差异。在尝试打结和闭合间隙的过程中，同时测量盂肱关节移位和肩袖自身的张力。尽管在肌腱拉向一起时，冈下肌和肩胛下肌的应力会轻度增高，但是尝试打结时肩袖的张力和压力极低。第一针边缘重叠缝合所增加的肩袖内在张力最大，后续的缝合也有类似效应，但增加的幅度减小。4 针边缘重叠缝合后，肱骨头平均前移 4.97 mm。[36] 这些研究结果表明，边缘重叠可以降低撕裂间隙和应力，打结时盂肱关节的移位极小，肌腱内在应力的变化也很小。

肌腱转移

　　无法修复的撕裂可以定义为不能直接进行肌腱至骨的修复并愈合的撕裂。肌腱转移作为此类撕裂的治疗方法已经被学者们接受。局部肌腱转位、远处肌腱转移和三角肌瓣转位是目前提出的重建肩袖的方法。使用部分肩胛下肌和小圆肌覆盖上方肩袖缺损的效果有限，而且后续报道无法复制这种效果。[37] 可以重复并获得长期疗效的是远处肌腱转移，可以使用背阔肌转移修复巨大后上撕裂，或使用胸大肌转移修复相对少见的前上撕裂。

背阔肌转移

背阔肌转移于 1988 年被提出，用于重建冈上肌和冈下肌完全缺失的撕裂。[38] 将大圆肌和背阔肌转变为外旋肌最早被用于治疗儿童的臂丛神经产伤麻痹，将之用于重建巨大肩袖撕裂被认为是与该手术类似的成人手术。[39] 背阔肌可以提供大且有血供的肌腱覆盖肩袖缺损，肌腱从其在肱骨干的止点转移至肱骨头外上方。背阔肌肌腱近乎垂直的走行，可以起到下压肱骨头的效果，通过其止点与肱骨头的相对位置关系，发挥外旋作用。该技术曾被用于治疗 14 例巨大肩袖撕裂患者，其中 9 例患者有严重功能障碍，10 例患者需要背阔肌覆盖肩袖缺损。前 11 例患者的术后肌电图证实，患者肩胛上神经和胸背神经功能正常；1 例患者肩关节屈曲时有支配背阔肌的神经活动，3 例患者在外旋时有支配背阔肌的神经活动。肌电图研究表明，背阔肌主要通过肌腱固定作用发挥外旋功能。这些患者对术后第 1 年随访时的效果满意，前屈、外展和外展时的外旋控制能力均有改善，在腰部和肩关节之间活动上臂时的易疲劳性也降低。大圆肌并没有随背阔肌一起转移，因为大圆肌通常太粗大，无法穿过三角肌，而且大圆肌的伸缩范围和长度不足。

一项研究报道了 69 例使用背阔肌转移治疗巨大、不可修复肩袖撕裂的病例，结果表明其具有确切的长期疗效。在平均 53 个月的随访中，主观肩关节评分由术前的平均 28 分增加至平均 66 分。年龄和性别校正的 Constant-Murley 评分由平均 55 分增加至平均 73 分（$P < 0.0001$）；满分为 15 分的疼痛评分由 6 分改善为 12 分（$P < 0.0001$）；最大屈曲角度由 104° 增加至 123°，最大外展角度由 101° 增加至 119°，最大外旋角度由 22° 增加至 29°（$P < 0.05$）；肌力由 0.9 kg 增加至 1.8 kg（$P < 0.0001$）。13 例患者术前有肩胛下肌功能缺陷，表

现为抬离试验阳性。与肩胛下肌完整的患者不同，这些患者无明显功能改善和疼痛缓解。该研究的结论是背阔肌转移用于不可修复肩袖撕裂的治疗可以长期地缓解患者的慢性疼痛和改善肩关节功能障碍，尤其是对于肩胛下肌功能完整的患者。如果患者有肩胛下肌功能缺陷，该手术的效果不确定，很有可能不应进行背阔肌转移。[40]

术前肩关节的功能和力量会影响背阔肌转移的效果。[41] 对 14 例进行了背阔肌转移的巨大肩袖撕裂患者的研究发现，术前肩关节功能差的女性患者通常治疗效果不佳。该研究发现，影响预后的最重要预测因素是术前主动前屈和外旋的活动范围及力量。假性瘫痪不能进行背阔肌转移，为背阔肌转移的禁忌证。

一项研究对比了翻修手术组（16 例肩袖修复失败后使用背阔肌转移作为补救手术的患者）与初次手术组（6 例初次进行背阔肌转移的巨大、不可修复肩袖撕裂的患者）的效果，术者有 7 年的手术经验。[42] 在 16 例翻修患者中，3 例在此前进行了不只 1 次肩袖修复，7 例进行了锁骨远端切除。两组患者术前改良 Constant 肩关节评分无差异（初次手术组平均 37 分，翻修手术组平均 36 分）。在平均 25 个月的随访中，初次手术组前屈改善 60°（范围为 30°~90°），翻修手术组改善 43°（范围为 15°~75°）。翻修手术组中，6 例患者的主动前屈小于 90°，而初次手术组所有患者都在 100° 以上，这 6 例患者中有 5 例术中发现有三角肌止点剥离。初次手术组 6 例患者的改良 Constant 肩关节评分的改善超过 30%，而翻修手术组仅有 1 例患者有如此大的改善。肌腱质量差、严重脂肪退变和三角肌止点剥离是导致预后不良的因素。肌腱质量差和严重脂肪退变在两组患者中均较普遍，而三角肌止点剥离仅发生在翻修手术组患者（16 例患者中有 7 例）。三角肌损伤患者和三角肌完整患者的术后功能差别有统计学意义，在翻修手术组内比较和翻修手术组与初次手术组之间比较的结果均如此。在初次手术

组的 6 例患者中，1 例发生转移的背阔肌撕裂，在翻修手术组的 16 例患者中，有 7 例发生撕裂，发生时间为平均术后第 19 个月（3~38 个月）。总体撕裂率为 36%，初次手术组为 17%，翻修手术组为 44%。初次手术组患者的效果与其他初次背阔肌转移的报道相似，但是其作为肩袖修复失败的补救手术，主观和客观功能改善均有限。[40] 翻修手术组中，近 20% 的患者功能较差。该研究的作者认为，三角肌功能缺陷会明显影响翻修手术的临床效果，所有三角肌功能缺陷的患者早期肩袖修复均不成功。采取背阔肌转移作为补救性措施时，患者的选择非常重要，因为合并的肩关节病变及功能障碍会导致预后不良。肩袖撕裂的类型不影响手术效果。完整的三角肌是恢复肩关节功能所必需的。[42] 另一项研究也发现，在肩袖撕裂修复失败后行背阔肌转移的患者中，三角肌功能与功能改善的程度相关。[43]

近年来，又有对背阔肌转移技术进行改良的报道。例如，切取带一小片骨质的肌腱进行转移，使转移的肌腱实现直接骨与骨的愈合；还有单一切口技术，以及微创入路的单一切口技术，仅显露肌腱的肱骨侧止点及需要转移的部位。[44-47] 尽管这些改良技术具有理论上的优势，但是其效果与原始的手术相比并无优势。背阔肌转移可以改善肩关节功能，但是并无研究表明其可以延缓肩袖撕裂性疾病的进展。

胸大肌转移

胸大肌转移也是前上方巨大肩袖撕裂的一种治疗选择。慢性肩胛下肌撕裂的修复极具挑战性且治疗效果不满意。早期的研究报道了 Bristow 手术失败后采用胸小肌转移的 4 例患者和采用胸大肌转移的 1 例患者，均取得了良好的结果。[48] 由于胸大肌和（或）胸小肌转移在早期肩胛下肌部分撕裂患者中取得了好的效果，学者们开始将其用于肩胛下肌完全撕裂患者。[49] 在 1980—1994 年，通过胸大肌和（或）胸小肌转移治疗了 13 例

不可修复肩胛下肌撕裂（定义为肩胛下肌完全缺失）的患者，患者同时合并盂肱关节前方不稳定。在平均 5 年的随访中，按照 Neer 和 Foster 分级，10 例患者获得了满意的效果，其余 3 例效果不佳。3 例效果不佳的患者之前均接受了至少 2 次重建手术。这些患者存在持续的肩关节疼痛、力量差及肌腱转移后前方松弛的症状。1 例肌腱转移失败的患者还经历了一次新的外伤。10 例获得了满意效果的患者，其转移的肌腱均有主动收缩，盂肱关节几乎无前方移位。这些患者日常活动或工作时无疼痛，或仅有轻度疼痛。[49]

12 例（平均年龄 65 岁）不可修复肩胛下肌撕裂患者接受了喙突下胸大肌转移。[50] 上方 1/2~2/3 的胸大肌被转移以替代肩胛下肌腱。转移的胸大肌从联合腱（喙肱肌和肱二头肌短头）的后方穿过，止于小结节，使胸大肌的方向与肩胛下肌相适应（图 16-4）。在平均 28 个月的随访中，5 例患者的

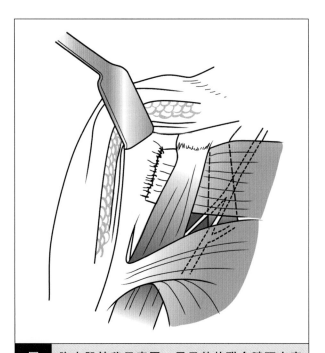

图 16-4　胸大肌转移示意图，显示其从联合腱下方穿过。经允许引自 Resch H, Povacz P, Ritter E, et al: Transfer of the pectoralis major muscle for the treatment of irreparable rupture of the subscapularis tendon. *J Bone Joint Surg Am* 2000;82（3）:372-382.

效果为优，4 例为良，3 例为一般。Constant 肩关节评分由平均 26.9 分增加至平均 67.1 分，所有患者的超声检查证实转移肌腱愈合。

一项研究将 30 例患者分为 3 组：Ⅰ组，11 例患者（平均年龄为 37 岁），不稳定手术失败；Ⅱ组，8 例患者（平均年龄为 55 岁），半肩关节或全肩关节置换后肩胛下肌撕裂；Ⅲ组，11 例患者（平均年龄为 58 岁），存在累及肩胛下肌腱的巨大肩袖撕裂。[51] 所有患者均接受了胸大肌转移，胸大肌胸骨头从胸大肌锁骨头下方穿过。该技术转移的胸大肌胸骨头在收缩时可以将胸大肌锁骨头作为支点，而且该技术可使胸大肌胸骨头拉力的方向与肩胛下肌更加一致。与拉力方向位于胸壁后方的肩胛下肌不同，转移的胸大肌的拉力方向仍位于胸壁前方。转移的胸大肌及肩胛下肌的拉力方向与胸壁关系的差异存在于所有的胸大肌转移技术（直接转移、通过联合腱后方至喙突下转移和胸大肌锁骨头后方转移）。在最短 2 年的随访中，Ⅰ组的 11 例患者中有 7 例疼痛缓解，Ⅲ组的 11 例患者中有 7 例疼痛缓解，但Ⅱ组的 8 例患者中仅有 1 例疼痛缓解；而且功能改善最少的也是关节置换术后肩胛下肌撕裂的患者（Ⅱ组）。Ⅱ组的 8 例患者中有 6 例肌腱转移失败，相比而言，Ⅰ组的 11 例患者中有 3 例手术失败，Ⅲ组的 11 例患者中有 4 例手术失败。该研究的作者认为，关节置换术后出现不可修复肩胛下肌撕裂的患者，行胸大肌转移的失败风险很高，尤其是肱骨头前方半脱位的患者。仅存在肩胛下肌功能不全且盂肱关节对合良好的稳定性手术失败的患者，很有希望获得疼痛缓解和功能改善。如果肩关节存在半脱位或对合关系不佳，胸大肌转移很可能失败，应考虑采用其他手术作为补救性手段，如骨性阻挡、转移至喙突及使用异体或自体肌腱进行关节囊重建等。

转移的胸大肌从联合腱后方通过比从联合腱前方通过更有生物力学优势，但是临床上并没

有证据表明后者的效果更差，胸大肌从联合腱前方转移对技术的要求更低 [52-53]（图 16-5）。在一项包含 30 例行胸大肌经联合腱前方转移患者（平均年龄 53 岁）的研究中，平均相对 Constant 肩关节评分在第 32 个月随访时由术前的 47 分改善至 70 分。[53] 仅存在单纯肩胛下肌撕裂，或肩胛下肌撕裂同时合并可修复的冈上肌撕裂的患者，术后相对 Constant 肩关节评分为 79 分。肩胛下肌撕裂同时合并不可修复冈上肌（和冈下肌）撕裂的患者临床效果明显更差，末次随访时相对 Constant 肩关节评分仅为 49 分。总体而言，经联合腱前方转移的效果与经联合腱后方转移相似。[53]

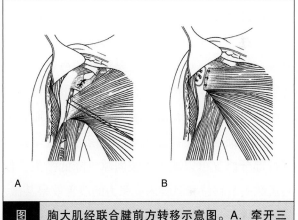

图 16-5　胸大肌经联合腱前方转移示意图。A. 牵开三角肌，分离肩胛下肌，尝试将残余肌腱、瘢痕和筋膜组织缝合到小结节。然后完全松解胸大肌止点，准备大结节的内侧区域作为胸大肌的转移位置。B. 将胸大肌肌腱经联合腱前方转移至大结节内侧。经允许引自 Jost B, Puskas GJ, Lustenberger A, Gerber C: Outcome of pectoralis major transfer for the treatment of irreparable subscapularis tears. *J Bone Joint Surg Am* 2003;85（10）:1944–1951.

三角肌瓣重建

欧洲的外科医师报道了三角肌瓣重建技术治疗后上方撕裂，结果各异。该技术在缓解疼痛和改善肩关节功能方面有满意的中期效果，但长期效果不佳。在平均 13.9 年的随访中，50% 的患者三角肌瓣撕裂，70% 的患者肩关节出现 1 期或 2 期关节炎。[54] 研究没有发现导致三角肌瓣撕

裂的预测因素。另一项研究报道患者功能改善很少，但疼痛改善和患者满意度尚可。[55]超声检查显示，中期随访时仅 16.5% 的三角肌瓣保持完整，长期随访只有 12.5% 保持完整。两项研究的作者均不推荐再使用该技术。

总结

巨大、不可修复肩袖撕裂在临床治疗上仍极具挑战性。仔细地询问病史和进行体格检查对于准确诊断和了解患者现状至关重要。可以使用多种影像学检查手段帮助判断病变的范围和严重程度，最常用的包括普通 X 线检查、CT 关节造影和 MRI 检查。该病的自然病程尚不清楚，部分患者经过物理治疗和疼痛控制等非手术治疗后症状缓解。不过，大部分患者疼痛和功能障碍加重并需要进一步治疗。对于对功能要求低的患者，单纯清理手术可以缓解疼痛，有时还可获得其他的功能改善。撕裂越大，清理手术效果越差，而且随着时间的推移，症状会加重。使用边缘重叠技术进行部分修复可以减小撕裂间隙、降低张力，但对盂肱关节移位和肌腱内在张力的改善效果甚微。如果巨大、不可修复肩袖撕裂患者的三角肌功能完好，且肩关节无力并非由假性瘫痪导致，那么肌腱转移的治疗效果良好。肌腱转移无法逆转肩袖撕裂关节病变的进展。对于巨大、不可修复肩袖撕裂治疗方式的选择必须结合患者的需求、期望及患者完成高强度康复训练的能力来确定。

参考文献

[1] Bedi A, Dines J, Warren RF, Dines DM: Massive tears of the rotator cuff. *J Bone Joint Surg Am* 2010;92(9):1894-1908.

A comprehensive review of massive rotator cuff tears included workup and treatment options.

[2] Cofield RH, Parvizi J, Hoffmeyer PJ, Lanzer WL, Ilstrup DM, Rowland CM: Surgical repair of chronic rotator cuff tears: A prospective long-term study. *J Bone Joint Surg Am* 2001;83-A(1):71-77.

[3] Zingg PO, Jost B, Sukthankar A, Buhler M, Pfirrmann CW, Gerber C: Clinical and structural outcomes of nonoperative management of massive rotator cuff tears. *J Bone Joint Surg Am* 2007;89(9):1928-1934.

A retrospective review of 19 patients with a nonsurgically managed massive rotator cuff tear found satisfactory shoulder function despite progression of degenerative structural joint changes and the risk of a repairable tear progressing to an irreparable tear during the 4-year study period. Level of evidence: IV.

[4] Harryman DT II, Hettrich CM, Smith KL, Campbell B, Sidles JA, Matsen FA III: A prospective multipractice investigation of patients with full-thickness rotator cuff tears: The importance of comorbidities, practice, and other covariables on self-assessed shoulder function and health status. *J Bone Joint Surg Am* 2003;85-A(4):690-696.

[5] Su W-R, Budoff JE, Luo Z-P: The effect of anterosuperior rotator cuff tears on glenohumeral translation. *Arthroscopy* 2009;25(3):282-289.

A biomechanical study evaluated the effect of an anterosuperior rotator cuff tear in cadaver shoulders. Tears of the superior subscapularis altered mechanics at low loads, and tears of the entire subscapularis altered mechanics at all loads.

[6] Burkhart SS: Fluoroscopic comparison of kinematic patterns in massive rotator cuff tears: A suspension bridge model. *Clin Orthop Relat Res* 1992;284:144-152.

[7] Parsons IM, Apreleva M, Fu FH, Woo SL: The effect of rotator cuff tears on reaction forces at the glenohumeral joint. *J Orthop Res* 2002;20(3):439-446.

[8] Oh JH, Jun BJ, McGarry MH, Lee TQ: Does a critical rotator cuff tear stage exist? A biomechanical study of rotator cuff tear progression in human cadaver shoulders. *J Bone Joint Surg Am* 2011;93(22):2100-2109.

A biomechanical study of cadaver shoulders evaluated the stage at which rotator cuff tears alter kinematics. A tear of the entire supraspinatus tendon was the stage of increasing rotational range of motion and decreasing abduction capability, and progression to the infraspinatus muscle was the critical stage for changes in humeral head kinematics.

[9] Gerber C, Wirth SH, Farshad M: Treatment options for massive rotator cuff tears. *J Shoulder Elbow Surg* 2011;20(2, suppl):S20-S29.

A review of massive rotator cuff tears included nonsurgical treatment, repair, transfers, and arthroplasty.

[10] Werner CM, Steinmann PA, Gilbart M, Gerber C:

Treatment of painful pseudoparesis due to irreparable rotator cuff dysfunction with the Delta III reverse-ball-and-socket total shoulder prosthesis. *J Bone Joint Surg Am* 2005;87(7):1476-1486.

[11] Zumstein MA, Jost B, Hempel J, Hodler J, Gerber C: The clinical and structural long-term results of open repair of massive tears of the rotator cuff. *J Bone Joint Surg Am* 2008;90(11):2423-2431.

At 10-year follow-up of 23 patients who underwent open repair of a massive rotator cuff tear, 22 patients were satisfied with the outcome, and the retearing rate was associated with preoperative fatty infiltration. Level of evidence: IV.

[12] Goutallier D, Postel J-M, Gleyze P, Leguilloux P, Van Driessche S: Influence of cuff muscle fatty degeneration on anatomic and functional outcomes after simple suture of full-thickness tears. *J Shoulder Elbow Surg* 2003;12(6):550-554.

[13] Nové-Josserand L, Costa P, Liotard J-P, Safar J-F, Walch G, Zilber S: Results of latissimus dorsi tendon transfer for irreparable cuff tears. *Orthop Traumatol Surg Res* 2009;95(2):108-113.

A retrospective review of 26 patients after latissimus dorsi transfer found a high satisfaction rate but a variable increase in active external rotation at a mean 34-month follow-up. Level of evidence: IV.

[14] Nové-Josserand L, Edwards TB, O'Connor DP, Walch G: The acromiohumeral and coracohumeral in-tervals are abnormal in rotator cuff tears with muscu- lar fatty degeneration. *Clin Orthop Relat Res* 2005;433:90-96.

[15] Hamada K, Fukuda H, Mikasa M, Kobayashi Y: Roentgenographic findings in massive rotator cuff tears: A long-term observation. *Clin Orthop Relat Res* 1990;254:92-96.

[16] Walch G, Edwards TB, Boulahia A, Nové-Josserand L, Neyton L, Szabo I: Arthroscopic tenotomy of the long head of the biceps in the treatment of rotator cuff tears: Clinical and radiographic results of 307 cases. *J Shoulder Elbow Surg* 2005;14(3):238-246.

[17] Hamada K, Yamanaka K, Uchiyama Y, Mikasa T, Mikasa M: A radiographic classification of massive rotator cuff tear arthritis. *Clin Orthop Relat Res* 2011;469(9):2452-2460.

A retrospective review of 75 patients, 41 of whom were surgically treated, found that those with more acromiohumeral interval narrowing had more muscle fatty degeneration and a higher rate of retearing. Level of evidence: III.

[18] Goutallier D, Postel JM, Bernageau J, Lavau L, Voisin MC: Fatty muscle degeneration in cuff ruptures: Pre- and postoperative evaluation by CT scan. *Clin Orthop Relat Res* 1994;304:78-83.

[19] Fuchs B, Weishaupt D, Zanetti M, Hodler J, Gerber C: Fatty degeneration of the muscles of the rotator cuff: Assessment by computed tomography versus magnetic resonance imaging. *J Shoulder Elbow Surg* 1999;8(6):599-605.

[20] Lippe J, Spang JT, Leger RR, Arciero RA, Mazzocca AD, Shea KP: Inter-rater agreement of the Goutallier, Patte, and Warner classification scores using preoperative magnetic resonance imaging in patients with rotator cuff tears. *Arthroscopy* 2012;28(2):154-159.

An MRI review by three board-certified orthopaedic surgeons evaluated the interobserver reliability of three classification schemes. None of the classifications had high interobserver reliability. Level of evidence: III.

[21] Burkhart SS, Barth JR, Richards DP, Zlatkin MB, Larsen M: Arthroscopic repair of massive rotator cuff tears with stage 3 and 4 fatty degeneration. *Arthroscopy* 2007;23(4):347-354.

In a retrospective review of 22 patients with grade 3 or 4 fatty infiltration who underwent repair of a massive rotator cuff tear, all 17 patients with grade 3 infiltration had clinical improvement at a mean 39.3-month follow-up, and 2 of the 5 with grade 4 infiltration had improvement. Level of evidence: IV.

[22] Mellado JM, Calmet J, Olona M, et al: Surgically repaired massive rotator cuff tears: MRI of tendon integrity, muscle fatty degeneration, and muscle atrophy correlated with intraoperative and clinical findings. *AJR Am J Roentgenol* 2005;184(5):1456-1463.

[23] Yoo JC, Ahn JH, Yang JH, Koh KH, Choi SH, Yoon YC: Correlation of arthroscopic repairability of large to massive rotator cuff tears with preoperative magnetic resonance imaging scans. *Arthroscopy* 2009;25(6):573-582.

In 51 consecutive patients who underwent arthroscopic repair of a large or a massive tear, those with grade 2 or 3 fatty infiltration had a greater risk of incomplete repair. Level of evidence: II.

[24] Meyer DC, Farshad M, Amacker NA, Gerber C, Wieser K: Quantitative analysis of muscle and tendon retraction in chronic rotator cuff tears. *Am J Sports Med* 2012;40(3):606-610.

In an MRI study of 130 shoulders with an intact or a torn supraspinatus (20 or 110 shoulders, respectively), fatty infiltration was graded and retraction of the tendon stump and the musculotendinous junction was measured. In advanced fatty infiltration, a component of shortening arises from the tendon. Level of evidence: III.

［25］ Iannotti JP, Ciccone J, Buss DD, et al: Accuracy of office-based ultrasonography of the shoulder for the diagnosis of rotator cuff tears. *J Bone Joint Surg Am* 2005;87(6):1305-1311.

［26］ Al-Shawi A, Badge R, Bunker T: The detection of full thickness rotator cuff tears using ultrasound. *J Bone Joint Surg Br* 2008;90(7):889-892.

An evaluation of the accuracy of portable ultrasonography for detecting rotator cuff tears found that experienced operators were able to most accurately detect large and massive tears.

［27］ Levy O, Mullett H, Roberts S, Copeland S: The role of anterior deltoid reeducation in patients with massive irreparable degenerative rotator cuff tears. *J Shoulder Elbow Surg* 2008;17(6):863-870.

A prospective assessment of 17 patients with a massive rotator cuff tear treated with an anterior deltoid rehabilitation program found significant clinical improvement at a minimum 9-month follow-up after treatment. Level of evidence: III.

［28］ Liem D, Lengers N, Dedy N, Poetzl W, Steinbeck J, Marquardt B: Arthroscopic debridement of massive irreparable rotator cuff tears. *Arthroscopy* 2008;24(7):743-748.

A retrospective review of 31 patients with a massive rotator cuff tear who underwent arthroscopic débridement with or without biceps tenotomy found improvement in clinical scores and no decrease in biceps strength for those with low demands at a mean 47-month follow-up. Level of evidence: IV.

［29］ Gartsman GM: Arthroscopic acromioplasty for lesions of the rotator cuff. *J Bone Joint Surg Am* 1990;72(2):169-180.

［30］ Fagelman M, Sartori M, Freedman KB, Patwardhan AG, Carandang G, Marra G: Biomechanics of coracoacromial arch modification. *J Shoulder Elbow Surg* 2007;16(1):101-106.

A biomechanical study evaluated several coracoacromial arch alterations and found that reconstruction best resisted anterosuperior migration.

［31］ Flatow EL, Weinstein XA, Duralde CA, et al: Coracoacromial ligament preservation in rotator cuff surgery. *J Shoulder Elbow Surg* 1994;3:573.

［32］ Fenlin JM Jr, Chase JM, Rushton SA, Frieman BG: Tuberoplasty: Creation of an acromiohumeral articulation—a treatment option for massive, irreparable rotator cuff tears. *J Shoulder Elbow Surg* 2002;11(2):136-142.

［33］ Burkhart SS: Arthroscopic treatment of massive rotator cuff tears. *Clin Orthop Relat Res* 2001;390:107-118.

［34］ Tauro JC: Arthroscopic "interval slide" in the repair of large rotator cuff tears. *Arthroscopy* 1999;15(5):527-530.

［35］ Hsu JE, Reuther KE, Sarver JJ, et al : Restoration of anterior-posterior rotator cuff force balance improves shoulder function in a rat model of chronic massive tears. *J Orthop Res* 2011;29(7):1028-1033.

In an in vivo study of rats, creation of a two-tendon tear of the supraspinatus and the infraspinatus was followed by no repair, infraspinatus-only repair, or two-tendon repair. Isolated infraspinatus repair and two-tendon repair restored similar function.

［36］ Mazzocca AD, Bollier M, Fehsenfeld D, et al: Biomechanical evaluation of margin convergence. *Arthroscopy* 2011;27(3):330-338.

A biomechanical study of 20 shoulders evaluated the effect of margin convergence on retracted rotator cuff tears. There was a significant decrease in rotator cuff strain and gap size after margin convergence in a large retracted tear.

［37］ Warner JJ: Management of massive irreparable rotator cuff tears: The role of tendon transfer. *Instr Course Lect* 2001;50:63-71.

［38］ Gerber C, Vinh TS, Hertel R, Hess CW: Latissimus dorsi transfer for the treatment of massive tears of the rotator cuff: A preliminary report. *Clin Orthop Relat Res* 1988;232:51-61.

［39］ L'Episcopo JB: Tendon transposition in obstetrical paralysis. *Am J Surg* 1934;25:122-125.

［40］ Gerber C, Maquieira G, Espinosa N: Latissimus dorsi transfer for the treatment of irreparable rotator cuff tears. *J Bone Joint Surg Am* 2006;88(1):113-120.

［41］ Iannotti JP, Hennigan S, Herzog R, et al: Latissimus dorsi tendon transfer for irreparable posterosuperior rotator cuff tears: Factors affecting outcome. *J Bone Joint Surg Am* 2006;88(2):342-348.

［42］ Warner JJ, Parsons IM IV: Latissimus dorsi tendon transfer: A comparative analysis of primary and salvage reconstruction of massive, irreparable rotator cuff tears. *J Shoulder Elbow Surg* 2001;10(6):514-521.

［43］ Birmingham PM, Neviaser RJ: Outcome of latissimus

dorsi transfer as a salvage procedure for failed rotator cuff repair with loss of elevation. *J Shoulder Elbow Surg* 2008;17(6):871-874.

Retrospective review of 18 patients who underwent latissimus dorsi transfer for a massive rotator cuff tear found improved clinical scores and motion at an average 25-month follow-up. Level of evidence: IV.

[44] Moursy M, Forstner R, Koller H, Resch H, Tauber M: Latissimus dorsi tendon transfer for irreparable rotator cuff tears: A modified technique to improve tendon transfer integrity. *J Bone Joint Surg Am* 2009;91(8):1924-1931.

Two latissimus dorsi harvesting techniques were compared: the standard tendon technique and a modification with removal of some bone. At a mean 47-month follow-up, the modified tendon technique led to better clinical scores. Level of evidence: III.

[45] Habermeyer P, Magosch P, Rudolph T, Lichtenberg S, Liem D: Transfer of the tendon of latissimus dorsi for the treatment of massive tears of the rotator cuff: A new single-incision technique. *J Bone Joint Surg Br* 2006;88(2):208-212.

[46] Gerhardt C, Lehmann L, Lichtenberg S, Magosch P, Habermeyer P: Modified L'Episcopo tendon transfers for irreparable rotator cuff tears: 5-year follow-up. *Clin Orthop Relat Res* 2010;468(6):1572-1577.

A retrospective review of 20 patients who underwent a modified L'Episcopo tendon transfer for a massive rotator cuff tear found an increase in shoulder function but some progression of rotator cuff arthropathy at 5-year follow-up. Level of evidence: IV.

[47] Lehmann LJ, Mauerman E, Strube T, Laibacher K, Scharf HP: Modified minimally invasive latissimus dorsi transfer in the treatment of massive rotator cuff tears: A two-year follow-up of 26 consecutive patients. *Int Orthop* 2010;34(3):377-383.

A retrospective review of 26 patients who underwent a modified minimally invasive latissimus dorsi transfer for a massive rotator cuff tear found improved clinical scores at a mean 24-month follow-up. Level of evidence: IV.

[48] Young DC, Rockwood CA Jr: Complications of a failed Bristow procedure and their management. *J Bone Joint Surg Am* 1991;73(7):969-981.

[49] Wirth MA, Rockwood CA Jr: Operative treatment of irreparable rupture of the subscapularis. *J Bone Joint Surg Am* 1997;79(5):722-731.

[50] Resch H, Povacz P, Ritter E, Matschi W: Transfer of the pectoralis major muscle for the treatment of irreparable rupture of the subscapularis tendon. *J Bone Joint Surg Am* 2000;82(3):372-382.

[51] Elhassan B, Ozbaydar M, Massimini D, Diller D, Higgins L, Warner JJ: Transfer of pectoralis major for the treatment of irreparable tears of subscapularis: Does it work? *J Bone Joint Surg Br* 2008;90(8):1059-1065.

The outcomes of pectoralis major transfer were evaluated in the setting of an unsuccessful procedure for instability of the shoulder, an unsuccessful shoulder replacement, or a massive rotator cuff tear. Patients who underwent the transfer after an unsuccessful shoulder replacement had the worst outcomes. Level of evidence: III.

[52] Resch H, Povacz P, Ritter E, Aschauer E: Pectoralis major muscle transfer for irreparable rupture of the subscapularis and supraspinatus tendon. *Tech Shoulder Elbow Surg* 2002;3:167-173.

[53] Jost B, Puskas GJ, Lustenberger A, Gerber C: Outcome of pectoralis major transfer for the treatment of irreparable subscapularis tears. *J Bone Joint Surg Am* 2003;85(10):1944-1951.

[54] Lu XW, Verborgt O, Gazielly DF: Long-term outcomes after deltoid muscular flap transfer for irreparable rotator cuff tears. *J Shoulder Elbow Surg* 2008;17(5):732-737.

A retrospective review of long-term outcomes of deltoid muscular flap transfer for a massive rotator cuff tear found satisfactory short- and mid-term results but poor long-term (13.9-year) results. The authors recommended against the procedure. Level of evidence: IV.

[55] Glanzmann MC, Goldhahn J, Flury M, Schwyzer HK, Simmen BR: Deltoid flap reconstruction for massive rotator cuff tears: Mid- and long-term functional and structural results. *J Shoulder Elbow Surg* 2010;19(3):439-445.

A retrospective review of 31 deltoid flap transfers found that ultrasound-confirmed deltoid flap survival was 16.5% at 53-month follow-up and 12.5% at 175-month follow-up. Deltoid flap survival was correlated with better clinical outcome. The authors did not recommend this procedure. Level of evidence: IV.

第十七章　肩袖愈合的生物增强

Kyle A. Caswell, DO; Todd C. Moen, MD; Wayne Z. Burkhead Jr, MD

引言

肩袖修复可以有效缓解有症状肩袖撕裂患者的疼痛，但对功能改善的效果不明确。如果要获得功能改善，修复的肌腱与骨之间必须愈合。研究发现，肌腱愈合失败的风险极高，大或巨大肩袖撕裂患者术后的再撕裂率为11%~94%。[1-2]过高的愈合失败风险促使学者们开始研究术中生物增强技术以提高肌腱愈合率。对切开和关节镜下肩袖修复的生物增强技术均有研究，目前被报道的体内和体外生物增强剂包括同种异体肌腱、细胞外基质（ECM）、富血小板血浆（PRP）、生长因子、干细胞和基因治疗。

术前评估

术前评估从仔细地询问病史和进行体格检查开始，判断患者是否可能从生物增强中获益。患者的病史对于发现肩袖修复失败的危险因素非常重要，危险因素包括糖尿病、高脂血症、吸烟史、

Dr. Burkhead or an immediate family member has received royalties from Tornier; is a member of a speakers' bureau or has made paid presentations on behalf of Tornier; serves as a paid consultant to or is an employee of Tornier, Wright Medical Technology, Stryker, and Bio2tech I-Flow; and serves as a board member, owner, officer, or committee member of the International Board of Shoulder and Elbow Surgery. Neither of the following authors nor any immediate family member has received anything of value from or owns stock in a commercial company or institution related directly or indirectly to the subject of this chapter: Dr. Caswell and Dr. Moen.

严重肌肉脂肪退变和高龄。[3-5]视诊观察是否存在冈上肌和冈下肌窝萎缩、肱二头肌腱断裂和巨大肩袖撕裂失代偿时的肱骨头固定或动态性前上方脱位。患者可能出现迟滞征，表明存在巨大肩袖撕裂。[6-8]肩袖萎缩且存在严重主动活动（尤其是外旋）受限的患者可能存在肩胛上神经病变，手术前应进行肌电图检查。[9]普通X线检查应至少包括无旋转时的正位片、腋位片和冈上肌出口位片。诊断巨大肩袖撕裂的更准确的手段包括普通（或增强）MRI和关节内增强CT。

适应证和禁忌证

肩袖修复生物增强技术的适应证仍存在争议，仅有少量循证医学证据的支持。目前生物增强技术的最佳适应证是切开或关节镜下修复巨大肩袖撕裂时患者存在影响愈合的合并症。生物增强技术还可用于修复失败后的翻修手术。巨大肩袖撕裂是指前后径大于5 cm或有两条及以上肌腱受累的撕裂。[10-11]根据Goutallier的描述，该类撕裂的可修复概率与肩袖肌腱纤维脂肪退变的程度有关。Goutallier分级为2级或以下表明肌肉成分多于脂肪成分。[12-14]在决定使用生物增强技术进行肩袖修复之前，必须考虑撕裂的大小、撕裂的慢性程度、肌肉萎缩的范围及纤维脂肪化程度。活动性感染和明显的盂肱关节炎是使用组织增强技术的禁忌证。

生物增强剂的类型和效果

目前临床上使用的生物增强剂主要是 ECM 和 PRP。ECM 有 3 种类型：同种异体 ECM、异种异体 ECM 和合成 ECM。[15] PRP 富含多种生长因子。一些因子由血小板演化而来，包括血小板衍生生长因子、血管内皮生长因子、转化生长因子 –β1、成纤维生长因子和表皮生长因子；其他因子由血浆演化而来，包括肝细胞生长因子和胰岛素样生长因子 –1。[16] 肩袖修复时使用生物增强技术在切开手术和关节镜手术中均有报道[17–20]（图 17–1，17–2）。

猪小肠黏膜下组织异种移植物

多项关于猪小肠黏膜下组织异种移植物的研究都没有得到良好结果。在一项前瞻性随机对照研究中，30 例肩袖存在两根肌腱慢性撕裂的患者接受了切开完全修复手术，其中 15 例患者同时接受了猪小肠黏膜下组织加强（加强组），另外 15 例患者未接受（非加强组）。[21] 修复 1 年后的关节内增强 MRI 显示，加强组有 4 例愈合，而非加强组有 9 例愈合。移植物加强不仅没能促进愈合，反而使术后的中期功能评分明显更低。加强组和非增强组的中期肩关节和患者满意度评分无显著差别。基于以上结果，学者们不推荐使用猪小肠黏膜下组织进行巨大、慢性肩袖撕裂后的加强修复。[21]

另一项随机对照研究将进行传统修复的患者按照是否接受了猪小肠黏膜下组织碎片增强分为加强组和对照组。[22] 研究最终在术后 2~4 周放弃，因为加强组的 19 例患者中有 4 例出现了严重局部术后反应，需进行手术清创、灌洗及移植物碎片移除。同时，研究发现加强组的再撕裂率与对照组类似，因此研究者反对使用该异种移植物。[22]

一项采用猪小肠黏膜下组织异种移植物加强修复巨大肩袖撕裂的前瞻性研究也取得了很差的结果。[23] 实验组的平均 UCLA 肩关节评分和平均 ASES 肩关节疼痛和功能障碍评分均优于对照组。但是，术后 MRA 证实仅 44% 的撕裂部分（或完全）愈合。3 例患者出现并发症，包括 1 例感染和 2 例皮肤反应。由于存在皮肤反应风险且 MRA 结果较差，研究者反对将猪小肠黏膜下组织作为移植物。[23]

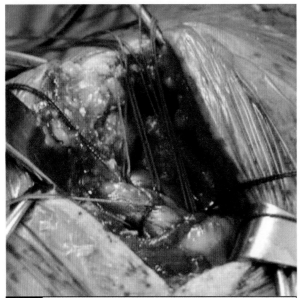

图 17-1　切开肩袖修复手术，在使用生物增强剂前，将缝合锚置于被修复的肩袖周围。经允许引自 Burkhead WZ, Schiffern SC, Krishnan SG: Use of GraftJacket as an augmentation for massive rotator cuff tears. *Semin Arthroplasty* 2007; 18（1）:11–18.

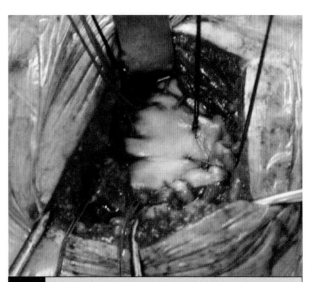

图 17-2　将生物增强剂牢固地缝合在被修复的肩袖上，形成密闭修复。经允许引自 Burkhead WZ, Schiffern SC, Krishnan SG: Use of GraftJacket as an augmentation for massive rotator cuff tears. *Semin Arthroplasty* 2007; 18（1）:11–18.

一项回顾性研究分析了 11 例进行切开肩袖修复的大或巨大肩袖撕裂患者，患者同时接受了猪小肠黏膜下组织加强修复，研究发现移植物加强并未提高临床效果，也没能实现强化愈合。在术后第 6 个月随访时，MRI 证实 10 例患者出现大的、回缩性再撕裂。5 例患者术后临床功能评分下降，但是患者术前和术后肩关节评分无显著差异。因此，研究者不推荐在治疗大或巨大肩袖撕裂时使用猪小肠黏膜下组织移植物。[24]

猪真皮胶原异种移植物

猪真皮胶原异种移植物的使用可以提高临床和影像学结果，但是一项研究的结论提示该移植物不能用于填补肩袖缺损。[25-26] 10 例巨大肩袖撕裂患者在修复肌腱时使用了猪真皮胶原增强移植物，在术后第 1 年随访时，患者的平均 Constant 肩关节评分，平均疼痛评分，外展力量以及内旋、外旋、外展活动范围均明显改善。所有患者均可进行日常活动。除 1 例患者不满意外，其余患者对结果均满意。在平均第 4.5 年随访时，MRI 和超声证实 8 例（80%）患者移植物完整，2 例患者移植物撕裂。术中和术后无并发症发生。研究者得出的结论为使用猪真皮胶原异种移植物作为生物增强剂修复巨大肩袖撕裂是安全的，而且有助于提高临床效果。[25]

一项对 20 例患者的研究得到了不同结果，该研究中有 4 例患者采用猪真皮胶原移植物桥接了巨大肩袖撕裂修复后的肩袖缺损。[26] 术后第 3~6 个月随访时，接受移植物桥接的患者出现了肩袖撕裂复发的症状和体征，体格检查和 MRI 均提示患者有炎症表现及残留移植材料连续性中断。4 例患者中有 2 例后来接受了反肩关节置换术，对术中标本进行了组织学检查，在慢性炎症背景下可见坏死性纤维蛋白材料，无感染表现。其余 16 例使用移植物进行肩袖修复增强的患者在术后第 2 年随访时无类似并发症或早期修复失败的表现。研究者认为该移植物在增强肩袖修复方面可能具有优势，但不推荐其用于桥接巨大肩袖撕裂。[26]

人尸体真皮胶原同种移植物

17 例患者在进行切开肩袖修复时接受了人真皮胶原同种移植物增强修复。[27] 其中，11 例患者的诊断为原发性巨大肩袖撕裂，6 例为复发性巨大肩袖撕裂。术后患者的疼痛评分、功能状态及 UCLA 肩关节评分明显改善。7 例患者进行了术后 MRI 检查，2 例患者发现有小的再撕裂。无其他并发症（如感染和无菌性炎症反应）发生。研究者的结论为，人真皮胶原同种移植物增强在初次或翻修巨大肩袖撕裂修复手术中可能安全、有效。[17]

人尸体真皮胶原同种移植物在关节镜手术研究中也同样取得了值得肯定的效果。一项前瞻性随机对照研究报道了 44 例双肌腱肩袖撕裂且撕裂大于 3 cm 的患者，所有患者都接受了关节镜下修复手术，其中 22 例接受了人真皮胶原基质增强（增强组，其余为对照组）。[27] 术后第 24 个月随访时，加强组患者的 ASES 肩关节疼痛和功能障碍评分及 Constant 肩关节评分明显优于对照组，差别有统计学意义。平均第 14.4 个月随访时，钆增强 MRI 证实，在接受随访的 35 例患者中，85% 的加强组患者（20 例患者中的 17 例）和 40% 的对照组患者（15 例患者中的 6 例）肩袖保持完整。研究者得出的结论为，使用人真皮胶原基质同种移植物加强修复双肌腱肩袖撕裂是有效的，可以增加肌腱完全愈合的概率。

45 例巨大、不可修复肩袖撕裂患者接受了关节镜下修复，并使用无细胞人真皮基质同种移植物进行了桥接。[19] 研究使用了 3 项临床效果评分（UCLA 肩关节评分、WORC 评分和 ASES 肩关节疼痛和功能障碍评分）评价临床疗效。在至少 24 个月的随访中，患者的所有临床评分均改善，其中 UCLA 肩关节评分的改善有统计学差异。研究者得出的结论为该技术安全且患者满意度高，能够避免肌腱转移或关节置换手术的并发症。[19]

1 例 62 岁行肩袖修复的患者进行了无细胞人真皮基质加强。[28] 3 个月后，患者存在轻度疼痛，肩关节可上举。MRI 显示移植物的前外侧缘未与骨附着。随后患者进行了关节镜检查和修复，并在移植部位取了活检组织。病理检查证实无细胞人真皮基质已与周围组织融合，有胶原纤维、大量新生血管、新生宿主细胞排列，几乎无炎症反应。研究者认为该移植物适用于初次修复的加强，可以作为组织重塑的支架。[28]

PRP

多项研究观察了 PRP 用于肩袖修复的效果。一项前瞻性研究将 53 例小至巨大肩袖撕裂患者随机分为单纯关节镜下单排肩袖修复组（27 例）和修复联合 PRP 加强组（26 例）。[29] 术后第 2 年随访时，MRI 证实两组巨大肩袖撕裂患者的再撕裂率相似（使用了 PRP 的巨大撕裂患者的再撕裂率为 40%，未使用 PRP 的患者为 52%）。第 3 个月随访时，接受 PRP 治疗的患者疼痛缓解，肩关节功能和力量（肩关节简明测试、UCLA 肩关节评分和 Constant 肩关节评分）以及外旋力量改善。后续随访时，两组无差别。2 年随访时，MRI 证实两组的愈合率无差别。[15,29]

一项前瞻性随机双盲对照研究将 88 例小至中等肩袖撕裂患者分为单纯关节镜修复组和修复联合自体富血小板纤维蛋白基质加强组。[30] 在术后第 16 个月随访时，两组的临床效果和 MRI 表现无统计学差异。

在一项包含 79 例行肩袖修复患者的随机对照研究中，患者分为单纯修复组和修复联合富血小板纤维蛋白基质增强组，术后第 6 周和第 12 周的超声检查证实两组在愈合方面无明显差异。[15,31] 2/3 的接受富血小板纤维蛋白基质治疗的患者实现了完全愈合，80% 的单纯修复组患者完全愈合。在临床效果评分和力量测量方面，两组相似。[15,31]

生物增强技术未来的研究方向

间充质干细胞

骨髓来源的间充质干细胞（MSC）或许也可用于生物增强。[32] MSC 在修复中可能可以促进肩袖肌腱 - 骨的修复，因为其具有向多种结缔组织结构分化的能力，包括肌肉、骨、韧带、肌腱和软骨。一项家兔模型研究发现 MSC 可以促进跟骨骨通道中踇长肌腱与骨之间的愈合。[16,33] 一项比较了分别使用 MSC（MSC 组）和纤维蛋白胶载体（纤维蛋白胶载体组）进行的前交叉韧带重建的家兔模型研究表明，MSC 组在术后第 2 周时，肌腱 - 骨界面有大片区域存在不成熟的纤维软骨细胞，第 8 周时在正常前交叉韧带止点处有类似软骨的物质填充，并出现纤维软骨连接骨和肌腱的成熟区域。[34] 术后第 8 周时的生物力学测试发现，与纤维蛋白胶载体组相比，MSC 组的前交叉韧带移植物具有更高的破坏负荷和强度。[16,34]

在一项大鼠模型研究中，MSC 被用于肩袖修复中促进骨 - 肌腱止点的愈合。[35] 研究者将大鼠分为三组，第一组在肌腱 - 骨修复处使用添加了 10^6 骨髓来源 MSC 的纤维蛋白黏合剂载体；第二组仅使用纤维蛋白黏合剂载体；第三组为对照组，仅进行修复。术后第 2 周和第 4 周的组织学检查和生物力学测试发现，这三组在胶原纤维构成、纤维软骨形成和失效负荷方面无差别。研究者得出的结论为，单纯使用 MSC 不能促进肩袖模型中肌腱 - 骨愈合，因为修复部位缺少分子或细胞信号诱导 MSC 进行合适的分化。[35] 在人体中，在关节镜下修复肩袖时从肱骨近端获取的结缔组织祖细胞可以作为成骨分化的介质。[36] 这些细胞可以作为自体移植物置于肌腱 - 骨界面，具有促进愈合的潜能。

生长因子

生长因子是细胞因子的一个亚类，具有促进细胞分裂、成熟和分化的功能，主要包括成纤维细胞生长因子、软骨韧带基质蛋白、结缔组织生长因子、血小板衍生生长因子、转化生长因子 -β、胰岛素样生长因子 -1 以及骨形态发生蛋白 12、13 和 14。[37] 目前研究主要聚焦于在肩袖修复模型中使用生长因子促进肌腱－骨界面的愈合。生长因子的种类、使用时机和使用方式正在研究中。

基因治疗

基因治疗也是生物增强研究的一个方面。胚胎发育研究已经发现了肌腱和韧带的特异性标志物。在鸡胚、鼠胚和小鼠肢体韧带发育中，scleraxis 是一种在发育早期肌腱内表达的螺旋－祥－螺旋转录因子。在鸡胚肌腱细胞的发育中，tenomodulin 受 scleraxis 调控。敲除 Tenomodulin 基因后小鼠的肌腱细胞强度下降、分化能力下降、肌腱超微结构发生改变。[5,38]

纳米纤维技术

纳米纤维工程也是一个研究的热点，纳米纤维的生物仿真属性使其成为了一个理想的肌腱组织－工程平台。目前，已经设计出一种聚乳酸－聚羟基乙酸纳米纤维支架用于肩袖肌腱组织工程，人肩袖成纤维细胞的附着、排列、基因表达和基质的加工可以在平行或非平行聚乳酸－聚羟基乙酸纳米纤维支架上评估。[39]成纤维细胞在平行纤维支架上可以比在非平行支架上生长得更长，更呈现纵向生长。Ⅰ型胶原纤维在平行支架上的生长方向更有规律。在所有时间点上，平行支架的抗张强度均优于非平行支架。这一研究结果表明，纳米纤维的结构对于细胞反应和支架的属性至关重要。未来的研究需要确定该类型支架是否有助于促进肩袖修复时肌腱－骨界面的恢复。[39]

总结

肩袖修复的生物增强技术仍存在争议，但在不断发展。生物增强技术可能适用于初次或翻修的巨大、可修复的、具有愈合潜能的肩袖撕裂。目前，临床上使用的生物增强技术主要是 ECM 技术和 PRP 技术。为了实现肩袖修复后的最佳愈合，未来的生物增强技术实验研究将集中在 MSC、生长因子、基因治疗和纳米技术的使用上。

参考文献

[1] Lafosse L, Brozska R, Toussaint B, Gobezie R: The outcome and structural integrity of arthroscopic rotator cuff repair with use of the double-row suture anchor technique. *J Bone Joint Surg Am* 2007;89(7):1533-1541. The functional and anatomic results of arthroscopic double-row suture anchor rotator cuff repair were studied using CT or MRA. Level of evidence: IV.

[2] Galatz LM, Ball CM, Teefey SA, Middleton WD, Yamaguchi K: The outcome and repair integrity of completely arthroscopically repaired large and massive rotator cuff tears. *J Bone Joint Surg Am* 2004;86(2):219-224.

[3] Nho SJ, Delos D, Yadav H, et al: Biomechanical and biologic augmentation for the treatment of massive rotator cuff tears. *Am J Sports Med* 2010;38(3):619-629. The clinical treatment of repair of a massive rotator cuff tear was reviewed, and methods for augmenting the healing of a degenerative rotator cuff tendon were explored.

[4] Abboud JA, Kim JS: The effect of hypercholesterolemia on rotator cuff disease. *Clin Orthop Relat Res* 2010;468(6):1493-1497. Patients with a rotator cuff tear were more likely to have hypercholesterolemia than control subjects. Level of evidence: II.

[5] Kovacevic D, Rodeo SA: Biological augmentation of rotator cuff tendon repair. *Clin Orthop Relat Res* 2008;466(3):622-633. This is a review of two studies of rotator cuff repair in sheep using a mixture of osteoinductive factors and bone morphogenetic protein–12, with a detailed review of the current understanding of biologic augmentation of rotator cuff repair healing. Level of evi- dence:V.

[6] Gerber C, Hersche O, Farron A: Isolated rupture of the subscapularis tendon. *J Bone Joint Surg Am* 1996;78(7):1015-1023.

[7] Gerber C, Krushell RJ: Isolated rupture of the tendon of the subscapularis muscle: Clinical features in cases. *J Bone Joint Surg Br* 1991;73(3):389-394.

[8] Hertel R, Ballmer FT, Lombert SM, Gerber C: Lag signs in the diagnosis of rotator cuff rupture. *J Shoulder Elbow Surg* 1996;5(4):307-313.

[9] Mallon WJ, Wilson RJ, Basamania CJ: The association of suprascapular neuropathy with massive rotator cuff tears: A preliminary report. *J Shoulder Elbow Surg* 2006;15(4):395-398.

［10］DeOrio JK, Cofield RH: Results of a second attempt at surgical repair of a failed initial rotator-cuff repair. *J Bone Joint Surg Am* 1984;66(4):563-567.

［11］Neer CS II, Craig EV, Fukuda H: Cuff-tear arthropa- thy. *J Bone Joint Surg Am* 1983;65(9):1232-1244.

［12］Goutallier D, Postel JM, Bernageau J, Lavau L, Voisin MC: Fatty muscle degeneration in cuff ruptures: Pre- and postoperative evaluation by CT scan. *Clin Orthop Relat Res* 1994;304:78-83.

［13］Fuchs B, Weishaupt D, Zanetti M, Hodler J, Gerber C: Fatty degeneration of the muscles of the rotator cuff: Assessment by computed tomography versus magnetic resonance imaging. *J Shoulder Elbow Surg* 1999;8(6):599-605.

［14］Goutallier D, Postel JM, Gleyze P, Leguilloux P, Van Driessche S: Influence of cuff muscle fatty degenera- tion on anatomic and functional outcomes after simple suture of full-thickness tears. *J Shoulder Elbow Surg* 2003;12(6):550-554.

［15］Montgomery SR, Petrigliano FA, Gamradt SC: Bio- logic augmentation of rotator cuff repair. *Curr Rev Musculoskelet Med* 2011;4(4):221-230.
Current research was reviewed pertaining to biologic augmentation of rotator cuff repair using allograft, ECMs, PRP, growth factors, stem cells, and gene ther- apy. Level of evidence: V.

［16］Edwards SL, Lynch TS, Saltzman MD, Terry MA, Nu- ber GW: Biologic and pharmacologic augmentation of rotator cuff repairs. *J Am Acad Orthop Surg* 2011; 19(10):583-589.
The basic science of rotator cuff healing was discussed, with a broad overview of current and future biologic and pharmacologic augmentation techniques for rota- tor cuff repair. Level of evidence: V.

［17］Burkhead WZ, Schiffern SC, Krishnan SG: Use of GraftJacket as an augmentation for massive rotator cuff tears. *Semin Arthroplasty* 2007;18(1):11-18.
A surgical technique for open rotator cuff repair with GraftJacket (Wright Medical Technology) allograft augmentation was reported, with early results. Level of evidence: IV.

［18］Labbé MR: Arthroscopic technique for patch augmentation of rotator cuff repairs. *Arthroscopy* 2006;22(10):e1-e6.

［19］Wong I, Burns J, Snyder S: Arthroscopic GraftJacket repair of rotator cuff tears. *J Shoulder Elbow Surg* 2010;19(2, suppl):104-109.
A surgical technique was presented for arthroscopic rotator cuff reconstruction using the GraftJacket al- lograft acellular human dermal matrix, with an update of earlier data. Level of evidence: IV.

［20］Seldes RM, Abramchayev I: Arthroscopic insertion of a biologic rotator cuff tissue augmentation after rotator cuff repair. *Arthroscopy* 2006;22(1):113-116.

［21］Iannotti JP, Codsi MJ, Kwon YW, Derwin K, Ciccone J, Brems JJ: Porcine small intestine submucosa aug- mentation of surgical repair of chronic two-tendon ro- tator cuff tears: A randomized, controlled trial. *J Bone Joint Surg Am* 2006;88(6):1238-1244.

［22］Walton JR, Bowman NK, Khatib Y, Linklater J, Mur- rell GA: Restore orthobiologic implant: Not recom- mended for augmentation of rotator cuff repairs. *J Bone Joint Surg Am* 2007;89(4):786-791.
The results of patients who underwent an open rotator cuff repair with xenograft allograft reconstruction were described. Level of evidence: III.

［23］Phipatanakul WP, Petersen SA: Porcine small intestine submucosa xenograft augmentation in repair of mas- sive rotator cuff tears. *Am J Orthop (Belle Mead NJ)*2009;38(11):572-575.
The results of using porcine small intestine submucosa xenograft to augment the repair of massive rotator cuff tears were described. Level of evidence: IV.

［24］Sclamberg SG, Tibone JE, Itamura JM, Kasraeian S: Six-month magnetic resonance imaging follow-up of large and massive rotator cuff repairs reinforced with porcine small intestinal submucosa. *J Shoulder Elbow Surg* 2004;13(5):538-541.

［25］Badhe SP, Lawrence TM, Smith FD, Lunn PG: An as- sessment of porcine dermal xenograft as an augmenta- tion graft in the treatment of extensive rotator cuff tears. *J Shoulder Elbow Surg* 2008;17(1, suppl):35S-39S.
Clinical, ultrasound, and MRI outcomes of massive rotator cuff repairs using porcine dermal collagen ten- don augmentation grafting were analyzed. Level of ev- idence: IV.

［26］Soler JA, Gidwani S, Curtis MJ: Early complications from the use of porcine dermal collagen implants (Per- macol) as bridging constructs in the repair of massive rotator cuff tears: A report of 4 cases. *Acta Orthop Belg* 2007;73(4):432-436.
The clinical, radiographic, and histologic results of re- pair of a massive rotator cuff tear using a porcine der- mal collagen implant in a bridging fashion were de- scribed in four patients. Level of evidence: IV.

［27］Barber FA, Burns JP, Deutsch A, Labbé MR, Litchfield

RB: A prospective, randomized evaluation of acellular human dermal matrix augmentation for arthroscopic rotator cuff repair. *Arthroscopy* 2012;28(1):8-15.

This study evaluated the safety and effectiveness of arthroscopic acellular human dermal matrix augmentation of large rotator cuff tear repairs. Level of evidence: II.

[28] Snyder SJ, Arnoczky SP, Bond JL, Dopirak R: Histologic evaluation of a biopsy specimen obtained 3 months after rotator cuff augmentation with Graft-Jacket Matrix. *Arthroscopy* 2009;25(3):329-333.

A biopsy specimen taken from a single rotator cuff augmented 3 months earlier with an acellular human dermal matrix graft was histologically evaluated. Level of evidence: IV.

[29] Randelli P, Arrigoni P, Ragone V, Aliprandi A, Cabitza P: Platelet rich plasma in arthroscopic rotator cuff repair: A prospective RCT study, 2-year follow-up. *J Shoulder Elbow Surg* 2011;20(4):518-528.

A prospective randomized controlled double-blind study reported the results of using autologous PRP in patients undergoing arthroscopic rotator cuff repair. Level of evidence: I.

[30] Castricini R, Longo UG, De Benedetto M, et al: Platelet-rich plasma augmentation for arthroscopic rotator cuff repair: A randomized controlled trial. *Am J Sports Med* 2011;39(2):258-265.

A randomized controlled study investigated the results of autologous platelet-rich fibrin matrix for augmentation of a double-row repair of small- or medium-size rotator cuff tears.

[31] Rodeo SA, Delos D, Williams RJ, Adler RS, Pearle A, Warren RF: The effect of platelet-rich fibrin matrix on rotator cuff tendon healing: A prospective, randomized clinical study. *Am J Sports Med* 2012;40(6):1234-1241.

This randomized controlled trial showed platelet-rich fibrin matrix had no effect on tendon healing, tendon vascularity, manual muscle strength, and clinical rating scales. Level of evidence: II.

[32] Caplan AI: Mesenchymal stem cells and gene therapy. *Clin Orthop Relat Res* 2000;379(suppl):S67-S70.

[33] Ouyang HW, Goh JC, Lee EH: Use of bone marrow stromal cells for tendon graft-to-bone healing: Histological and immunohistochemical studies in a rabbit model. *Am J Sports Med* 2004;32(2):321-327.

[34] Lim JK, Hui J, Li L, Thambyah A, Goh J, Lee EH: Enhancement of tendon graft osteointegration using mesenchymal stem cells in a rabbit model of anterior cruciate ligament reconstruction. *Arthroscopy* 2004;20(9):899-910.

[35] Gulotta LV, Kovacevic D, Packer JD, Deng XH, Rodeo SA: Bone marrow-derived mesenchymal stem cells transduced with scleraxis improve rotator cuff healing in a rat model. *Am J Sports Med* 2011;39(6):1282-1289.

Bone marrow–derived MSCs were transduced with scleraxis to augment rotator cuff healing at early time points in a rat model. Level of evidence: I.

[36] Mazzocca AD, McCarthy MB, Chowaniec DM, Cote MP, Arciero RA, Drissi H: Rapid isolation of human stem cells (connective tissue progenitor cells) from the proximal humerus during arthroscopic rotator cuff surgery. *Am J Sports Med* 2010;38(7):1438-1447.

A technique was described for arthroscopically obtaining bone marrow aspirate from the proximal humerus and then purifying and concentrating the connective tissue progenitor cells in the operating room. Level of evidence: III.

[37] Würgler-Hauri CC, Dourte LM, Baradet TC, Williams GR, Soslowsky LJ: Temporal expression of 8 growth factors in tendon-to-bone healing in a rat supraspinatus model. *J Shoulder Elbow Surg* 2007;16(5, suppl): S198-S203.

The temporal expression of eight different growth factors for tendon-to-bone healing was evaluated in a rat model. Level of evidence: II.

[38] Asou Y, Nifuji A, Tsuji K, et al: Coordinated expression of scleraxis and Sox9 genes during embryonic development of tendons and cartilage. *J Orthop Res* 2002;20(4):827-833.

[39] Moffat KL, Kwei AS, Spalazzi JP, Doty SB, Levine WN, Lu HH: Novel nanofiber-based scaffold for rotator cuff repair and augmentation. *Tissue Eng Part A* 2009;15(1):115-126.

Bench work efforts were aimed at creating a novel nanofiber-based scaffold for rotator cuff tendon tissue engineering and evaluating the attachment, alignment, gene expression, and matrix elaboration over time of human rotator cuff fibroblasts on aligned and unaligned polylactide-coglycolide nanofiber scaffolds. Level of evidence: II.

第十八章 肩袖手术预后的影响因素

Michael E. Angeline, MD; Joshua S. Dines, MD

引言

肩袖撕裂常常导致残疾和疼痛，美国每年约进行 75000 例肩袖修复手术。全关节镜肩袖修复术的预后良好，术后 5 年功能恢复满意。[1]尽管肩袖修复手术在临床上取得了成功，但修复部位常在肌腱 - 骨附丽点形成纤维血管瘢痕。应当注意，肩袖修复术并不能再生胚胎发育过程中形成的天然肌腱 - 骨附丽点。这种结构在机械力学上比正常的肌腱薄弱，更容易发生断裂。[2]最新的研究提出，术后肩袖完全愈合的患者往往具有更好的功能预后。[3]影响肩袖手术预后的危险因素及如何更好地提高治愈率为当前的研究热点。

天然的肩袖肌腱 - 骨附丽点的作用是使集中在肌腱和骨之间的应力最小化。该结构由 4 个不同的过渡区域组成：肌腱、纤维软骨、矿化的纤维软骨和骨（图 18-1）。胶原纤维含量因组织类型而异。[4]肌腱区域主要由 I 型和Ⅲ型胶原纤维组成，纤维软骨区域由 I 型、Ⅱ型和Ⅲ型胶原纤维组成。矿化的纤维软骨区域含有 I 型、Ⅱ型和 X 型胶原纤维。骨区域由 I 型胶原纤维组成。[5-6]

Dr. Dines or an immediate family member has received royalties from Biomet; serves as a paid consultant to Biomimetic and Tornier; and has received research or institutional support from Biomimetic. Neither Dr. Angeline nor any immediate family member has received anything of value from or has stock or stock options held in a commercial company or institution related directly or indirectly to the subject of this chapter.

生物学因素

肩袖撕裂的发病率为 5%~39%。[7]目前已知的危险因素包括外伤史、优势手损伤和年龄增长。一项中期随访显示，39%~49% 肩袖损伤后未经手术治疗的患者撕裂程度增加，且疼痛程度与撕裂程度增加及撕裂进展加快有关。[8-9]随着肩袖撕裂的发展和症状加剧，是否需要进行手术治疗要基于多种因素考虑。可能影响肩袖手术预后的生物学因素包括患者的年龄、遗传因素、并发症和肌腱完整性。

患者年龄

随着年龄的增长，骨质减少，肌腱细胞化、血管化都会对肩袖愈合产生不利影响。最近的一些案例研究回顾了 65 岁以上患者肩袖修复的结果。[10-12]与自身或其他年轻患者相比，有 10~12 名老年患者在行关节镜下肩袖修复术后疼痛程度、活动范围和功能状态均有所改善。这些研究表明，单独的年龄因素与老年患者的不良功能预后无关。但是，大多数相关研究处于Ⅳ级，仅对年龄和功能预后进行了单变量分析。其他混杂变量可能对结果产生影响，例如，年轻患者较高的功能需求可能影响了他们对手术预后的认识。

最近的一项多因素分析发现，在肌腱愈合过程中，即使采用双排修复使修复部位的生物力学强度最大化，高龄也是修复部位的主要生物学限制因素。[13]随着年龄的增长，冈下肌脂肪变性和肌腱撕裂后断端回缩加重，这会对手术预后产生负面影响。总体而言，老年患者在肩袖修复术后

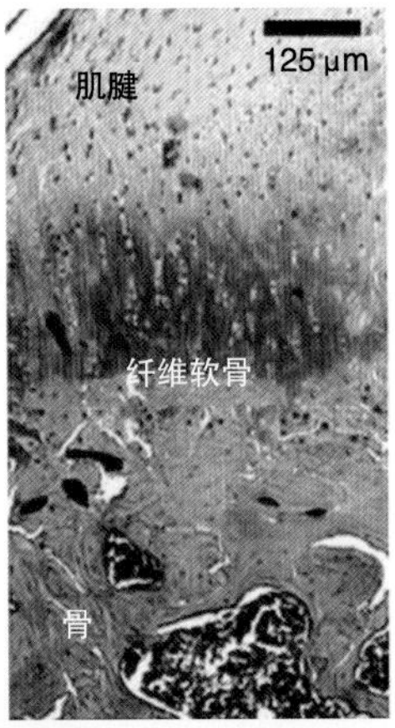

组织区域	细胞类型	基质主要成分
肌腱	成纤维细胞	Ⅰ型和Ⅲ型胶原纤维（直径 40~400 nm）
纤维软骨	纤维软骨细胞	Ⅰ型、Ⅱ型及Ⅲ型胶原纤维
矿化纤维软骨	肥大纤维软骨细胞	Ⅰ型、Ⅱ型及Ⅹ型胶原纤维
骨	成骨细胞 骨细胞 破骨细胞	Ⅰ型胶原纤维（直径 34.5~39.5 nm）

图 18-1 肌腱－骨附丽点的结构和组成。经允许引自 Zhang X, Bogdanowicz D, Eriksen C, et al. Biomimetic scaffold design for functional and integrative tendon repair. *J Shoulder Elbow Surg* 2012;21（2）：266-277.

的功能预后指标有所改善，但是修复部位的愈合能力随着年龄的增长而降低。

遗传因素

尽管没有与肩袖损伤直接相关的单个基因，但肩袖撕裂和肌腱病患者的基因途径发生了改变。这种改变表现在胶原纤维的组成、脉管系统、细胞内信号传导机制以及修复后原生结构的再生能力等方面，这些改变影响了肩袖肌腱的结构。在愈合的肌腱中，胶原纤维基因表达改变导致Ⅲ型胶原纤维增加和Ⅰ型胶原纤维减少，这和瘢痕愈合途径一致。调节Ⅰ型胶原纤维和Ⅲ型胶原纤维的比例可增强愈合肌腱的强度。

转化生长因子－β（TGF-β1、TGF-β2 和 TGF-β3）的表达水平为当前的研究热点之一，有研究表明其会影响愈合肌腱内细胞的增殖、分化和基质合成。在成年人的肌腱愈合过程中，TGF-β1 和 TGF-β2 的水平升高，导致瘢痕形成和 TGF-β3 低水平表达。而婴儿伤口愈合具有较高水平的 TGF-β3 表达，后续不会有瘢痕形成。[14]

在大鼠冈上肌修复模型中发现，局部注射 TGF-β3 可改善术后第 4 周的修复部位的强度并增加 Ⅰ型胶原纤维的表达，从而促进愈合。[15] 这些研究结果证实了这种治疗的可能性，但是需要进一步研究以确定最佳的 TGF-β3 剂量。

研究者发现改变基质金属蛋白酶（MMPs）的动态表达模式可调节肩袖撕裂中细胞外基质的重塑，因此最近进行了一些关于 MMPs 及其组织抑制剂的研究。MMPs 及其组织抑制剂之间的平衡失调会导致 MMPs 活性增加，可能通过影响肌腱降解进而影响肌腱愈合。[16] 在大鼠冈上肌修复模型中，局部注射 MMPs 组织抑制剂会导致胶原组织显著增加，胶原降解减少。[17] 这些结果表明，在肩袖修复后调节 MMPs 活性可增强修复部位肌腱－骨附丽点的愈合。

多西环素（一种抗生素）可通过与其抗菌功效无关的途径发挥抑制 MMPs 的作用。一项大鼠模型的相关研究评估了多西环素对肌腱愈合的影响。[16] 肩袖修复术后，多西环素介导的 MMPs 活性抑制可以改善肌腱－骨附丽点的生物力学和组织学愈合指标。需要进一步的研究来明确通过抑制 MMPs 改善肌腱愈合的确切机制，但是多西环素治疗可能成为改善肩袖手术预后的一种疗法。

最近的研究还评估了肩袖撕裂的遗传风险。[18-19] 这些研究证实了肩袖损伤具有很强的遗传易感性，患者的一级和二级亲属发病风险增加，研究者们认为具有遗传易感性的个体更容易受到年龄相关肌腱变性的影响。但现在还没有研究证实遗传因素对术后肌腱 – 骨附丽点愈合的作用。需要通过进一步研究充分筛查相关易感基因，并了解肩袖损伤相关基因的确切机制。

合并症

患者的合并症会严重影响肌腱的愈合。肥胖是与糖尿病、血管疾病和高胆固醇血症风险相关的全球性健康问题。这些疾病状态导致局部血管减少，可能影响肌腱 – 骨附丽点的愈合。近期的两项回顾性病例对照研究评估了肥胖与关节镜下肩袖修复术预后的相关性。[20-21]两项研究的结果相互矛盾，一项研究发现，肥胖与术后功能不良、住院时间延长和手术时间延长之间存在统计学上的显着相关性。[20]另一项研究控制了混杂变量之后发现，身体质量指数及肥胖与关节镜下肩袖修复术预后无关。[21]不同的研究基于不同的预后指标、随访时间及外科医师的技术，研究者很难直接对肥胖与肩袖修复的预后进行评估。因此，目前仍不清楚二者之间的关系。

糖尿病会影响肌腱的愈合。已有研究证实，与对照组大鼠相比，糖尿病组大鼠的肩袖在修复后生物力学性能较差，纤维软骨较少，肌腱 – 骨附丽点的胶原纤维减少。[22]这些研究证明持续的高血糖会损害肩袖肌腱 – 骨附丽点愈合。最近的一项回顾性研究根据是否患有糖尿病，对接受了关节镜下肩袖修复术的患者进行了比较。[23]两组患者术后的功能评分均得到改善，但非糖尿病患者的改善更明显，他们的前屈功能、外旋功能恢复得更好，日常活动和力量评分更高。糖尿病患者的前屈功能和外旋功能相对较差，感染发生率略高。不能将有关糖尿病对肌腱愈合的影响的基础和临床研究结果理解为糖尿病患者不适宜行关节镜下肩袖修复术，尽管糖尿病患者的预期结果可能不如非糖尿病患者，但在术后，他们的疼痛和功能依然能够得到改善。

肌腱完整性

虽然肩袖撕裂的时间和程度很重要，但就肌肉萎缩和脂肪浸润的程度而言，肩袖肌肉组织的质量可能对术后的解剖学和功能预后存在更大的影响。一项对绵羊慢性肩袖损伤模型的研究表明，引起冈下肌脂肪浸润的关键因素是羽状角（羽状肌纤维插入肌腱的角度）的改变。[24]随着羽状角角度的增加，肌纤维缩短，脂肪浸润加重。一些临床研究证实，羽状角角度增加可导致肌腱 – 骨附丽点愈合处的生物力学性能较差，肌腱机械性能降低。术前相对较严重的肌肉萎缩和脂肪浸润可能会引起手术失败率增加、肌肉功能丧失及其他不良预后。[25-27]肌肉质量和脂肪浸润程度对冈下肌预后的影响比对冈上肌更明显。一些研究者认为冈下肌功能较差可能损害盂肱关节的生物力学并导致患者预后较差。[25]

肩袖撕裂的自然病史和肌肉的脂肪浸润程度可能与撕裂大小、部位、发作时间和患者年龄相关。[28-29]例如，一名老年患者肩袖严重撕裂，肌腱断裂病程过长会导致更严重的脂肪浸润。在所有撕裂类型中，出现症状后平均 4 年，冈上肌出现 Goutallier 2 级脂肪浸润[30]（表 18-1）。如果是创伤导致的肩袖损伤或累及多根肌腱，则病程进展更快，症状发作后平均 2.5 年，在冈下肌中发生 Goutallier 2 级脂肪浸润。[28]无论冈下肌腱是否断裂，都会发生脂肪浸润。

表 18-1

Goutallier 脂肪浸润分级

分级	描述
0 级	肌肉组织完全正常，没有脂肪浸润
1 级	肌肉中可见脂肪组织
2 级	肌肉多于脂肪
3 级	肌肉与脂肪一样多
4 级	脂肪多于肌肉

理解了肩袖损伤的病程进展和影响因素后，外科医师应在术前了解肌肉萎缩和脂肪浸润的程度，并进行适当干预（图 18-2）。应尽量在出现 Goutallier 2 级脂肪浸润之前尝试进行外科手

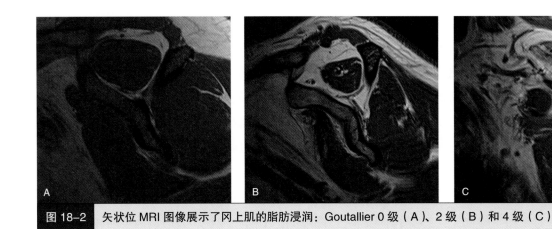

图18-2 矢状位 MRI 图像展示了冈上肌的脂肪浸润：Goutallier 0 级（A）、2 级（B）和 4 级（C）

术修复，以避免出现不良的解剖学和功能性结局。[25,27] 此外，尚无临床研究发现 Goutallier 2 级脂肪浸润及其相关结构改变在术后可逆。[23]

社会因素

社会因素，包括吸烟和工伤赔偿诉求，可能对肩袖手术的结果起着重要作用，这应引起外科医师的重视。有研究发现，在肩袖撕裂患者中，吸烟者的比例高于一般人群，对于体力劳动者，肩袖损伤引起的疼痛仅次于背痛，是体力劳动者最常见的上肢症状。[31-32] 此外，研究发现尼古丁会对手术切口部位的胶原纤维沉积和愈合产生负面影响，因为尼古丁的血管收缩作用会减少组织氧供。[31] 在大鼠肩袖损伤模型中，植入渗透泵输送尼古丁可延缓瘢痕的降解和重塑，从而影响肌腱 - 骨愈合。[33] 最近还有研究探究了吸烟对肩袖疾病的影响。[31,34] 一项对接受超声检查的单侧非创伤性肩关节疼痛患者的问卷调查显示，吸烟与肩袖疾病之间有很强的关联性，并且可能是因果关系。[31] 一项研究的结果显示，肩袖撕裂的程度与患者年龄无关，与吸烟的剂量和时间有关。吸烟剂量较大的患者，肩袖撕裂程度较严重，撕裂范围较大。[34]

一些研究发现，有工伤赔偿诉求的患者在行肩袖修复术后，预后相对较差。[32,35-36] 最近的两项研究使用多因素分析和病例对照研究，发现工伤赔偿诉求和肩袖手术预后呈负相关。[32,36] 肩袖修

复术后一年，这些患者的肩关节功能较其他患者差，且工伤赔偿诉求对康复有负面影响。尽管这些发现很有意义，但工伤赔偿诉求并不影响患者接受肩袖手术，这些患者也可从手术中受益。[32]

最近的一项横断面研究探究了导致工伤患者肩袖修复术后再损伤的潜在因素。[35] 在研究中，半数的手术失败的患者肩袖持续损伤的原因是解剖学异常（未治疗盂肱神经损伤或固定失败）或手术本身（复杂的局部疼痛综合征或开放手术三角肌复位失败）。外科医师应及时发现工伤患者手术失败的原因。

医师相关因素

手术时机

外科医师可以通过选择手术时机、手术方法和术后康复手段来影响肩袖手术的预后。慢性肩袖撕裂行手术治疗应充分考虑肌肉萎缩和脂肪浸润程度。应在患者进展至 Goutallier 2 级脂肪浸润之前进行手术。有研究发现，冈下肌脂肪变性与慢性退行性冈上肌腱撕裂有关。[37] 因为肌肉质量和冈下肌脂肪浸润的程度会影响手术预后，所以术前需要考虑冈上肌腱的情况。外科医师还应合理选择急性肩袖撕裂的手术时机。以前普遍认为，受伤 3 周内修复急性肩袖撕裂可以获得更好的功能预后。[38] 最近的两项回顾性研究发现，在受伤后 3~4 个月内进行手术的患者，其功能预后与早期进行开放手术的患者

的功能预后相似。[38]一般而言，急性肩袖撕裂患者在受伤后 3 周内接受手术，不会影响功能预后。

手术方法

手术方法的选择可能会影响肩袖手术的预后。由于研究者对解剖学上的愈合效果和（或）术后的再次撕裂的担心，最佳手术方案（特别是单排修复、双排修复或经骨无锚修复术）仍无定论。当前的双排和骨间修复技术增强了修复部位的生物力学强度，并增加了修复肌腱的表面积，但对于它们能否提供优良的功能预后仍存在争议（图 18-3）。

最近的一些前瞻性研究和系统评价比较了单排修复和双排修复的效果。[39-42]3 项前瞻性研究发现，在 1~2 年的随访中，单排修复和双排修复之间无明显的临床或解剖学差异。[39-41]最近的一项研究发现，两种修复之间没有明显的功能差异。[43]但是，对于大于 3 cm 的撕裂，双排修复术后肩关节肌肉力量更强。[41]此外，与单排修复相比，双排修复大于 1 cm 的撕裂，再撕裂率显著降低。[42]这些研究表明，对于较小的肩袖撕裂，单排修复和双排修复的预后几乎没有区别，而撕裂范围较大的患者可能更适合双排修复。在决定手术方案之前，外科医师应充分权衡利弊。患者的体型、功能需求和撕裂特征都需要纳入考虑范围。

术后康复

肩袖撕裂会导致手术前后肩关节僵硬。在肩袖损伤模型中，术后长时间制动可改善修复后肌腱插入部位的生物力学特性。[44]但是，长时间制动会导致肩关节僵硬。全层撕裂或急性外伤撕裂患者的术前肩关节僵硬程度明显更高。[45]在大鼠肩袖模型中，术后制动导致的关节僵硬很短暂，从长期预后来看，与未制动患者无明显差异。[46]此外，与持续制动相比，早期的肩关节被动活动可能不利于术后康复，进而导致冈上肌腱修复后活动范围丧失。[44]这些发现强调了术后制动对肌腱愈合的潜在有益作用。最近的一项回顾性临床研究支持这一观点，该研究发现，在行关节镜下肩袖修复后制动 6 周不会影响术后第 1 年随访时的肩关节僵硬率或功能预后。[47]此外，采用这种保守的术后康复方案，再撕裂率有降低的趋势。需要进一步进行前瞻性研究，以充分了解术后长期制动与关节僵硬和肌腱修复部位愈合的关系。

生物制剂

肩袖手术中的难点是如何刺激再生而非修复方法。患者自身或医师的治疗均无法使肌腱像天然形成的肌腱 - 骨界面一样愈合。因此，许多研

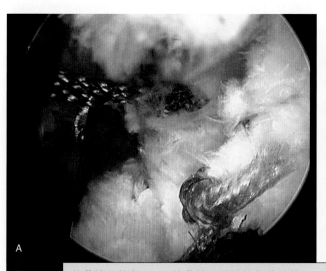
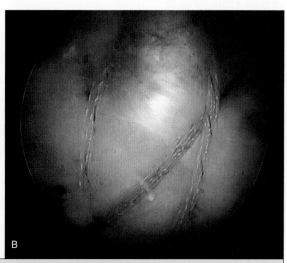

图 18-3　关节镜下修复。A. 关节镜下单排修复的照片。B. 关节镜下双排修复的照片

究者正在研究使用生物制剂和细胞疗法来增强修复效果，改善肌腱愈合。

血小板衍生生长因子

在肌腱愈合的早期炎症阶段，血小板衍生生长因子（PDGF）有助于促进细胞趋化、增殖、分化和基质合成。[4] PDGF蛋白家族由两个亚基（A链和B链）组成，这些亚基来自血小板和其他类型的细胞，如平滑肌细胞等。肩袖愈合会导致反应性瘢痕形成，而不是组织学上正常的附丽结构，未来可能通过添加PDGF来增强修复部位的生物学特性。

重组人PDGF-BB（rhPDGF-BB）是在肩袖修复的临床研究中测试的第一个外源性生长因子。使用绵羊肩袖模型来检查rhPDGF-BB对肩袖愈合的影响。[48] 发现与标准缝线相比，用生长因子包被的缝线在肩袖修复后可增强组织学特性，但不能改善生物力学特性。研究者还使用绵羊肩袖修复模型研究了由rhPDGF-BB和Ⅰ型胶原蛋白基质组成的移植物的作用。[49] 修复后第12周，与对照组或高剂量组相比，使用了低剂量和中剂量rhPDGF-BB的移植物显示出生物力学强度和解剖学外观改善。这些研究突出了生长因子的剂量、给药时间和给药方法的重要性。PDGF有望增强肌腱-骨愈合，目前正在使用rhPDGF-BB进行肩袖修复的Ⅰ期临床研究。

PRP

在肌腱-骨植入物自然愈合的过程中，许多生长因子（细胞因子）上调。提高这些因子的浓度具有增强肌腱细胞、干细胞和内皮细胞在愈合界面处募集和增殖的能力。PRP治疗已成为增强肌腱愈合的常用方法，因为其血小板和生长因子（包括PDGF、血管内皮生长因子、TGF-β、成纤维细胞生长因子-2和胰岛素样生长因子-1）的浓度为自体浓度。最近的一些研究评估了在肩袖修复部位使用PRP的临床效果。[50-53] 在两项队列研究中，与对照组患者相比，在关节镜下行肩袖修复时应用PRP未能改善功能预后指标。[52-53] 另一项Ⅰ级随访研究在术后第6、12和24个月的时间点得到了相似的结论。[54] 然而，与对照组相比，应用了PRP的患者在术后第1个月的疼痛评分较低，并且术后第3个月的临床结果有所改善。这些结果说明PRP可能对早期肌腱愈合产生积极影响。

关于PRP是否对肩袖修复术后愈合具有改善作用依然存在争议。对跟腱断裂的动物研究和临床研究发现，应用PRP可以增强愈合和功能恢复。[55-56] PRP的作用可能取决于愈合肌腱的机械负荷特性。最近的一项研究还发现了3种市售PRP分离系统中生长因子浓度的差异。[57] 需要进一步研究以充分了解PRP改善肌腱愈合的机制及不同生长因子浓度的重要性。

间充质干细胞

随着对再生肌腱愈合研究的进展，仅基于细胞生长因子的疗法可能不足以改善组织的物质特性。将这些因素与未分化的细胞结合可能会增强组织的愈合。间充质干细胞（MSC）具有自我更新和分化成其他细胞系（脂肪细胞、肌腱细胞和软骨细胞）的能力。目前，MSC仅能通过从骨髓中分离自体基质细胞获得，其他获取方法仍在研究中。细胞疗法可通过直接的局部旁分泌作用或抗炎作用影响修复过程。在大鼠肩袖模型中，仅添加骨髓来源的MSC并不会增强肌腱附着部位的生物力学或组织学特性。[58] MSC和其他因子的结合可能有助于增强修复部位。若要探究细胞和因子的最佳组合，应加深对肌腱自然形成机制和信号通路的认识。

一些使用MSC和转录因子scleraxis的研究突出了联合疗法的潜在益处。人们发现scleraxis通常在肌腱形成中具有重要作用，并且还存在于肌腱固有层及肌腱-骨插入位点。最佳的一项研究在大鼠肩袖模型中使用经腺病毒介导的scleraxis诱导的骨髓间充质干细胞，与对照组相比，实验组术后的生物力学性能明显更好。[59] 此外，实验组大鼠产生了纤维软骨，这与天然肌腱－骨附丽点非常相似。需要进行进一步的研究，以充分了解再生肌腱－骨附丽点所必需的复杂信号机制，以及可增加生物力学性能的最佳组合、给药剂量和输送载体。

仿生支架

研究者利用组织工程研究了仿生支架，该支架具有与宿主环境实现有机的整合的潜能。理想的支架能够恢复天然肌腱－骨界面的组织学和力学性能。当前的研究集中在由聚丙交酯乙交酯纳米纤维和一种复合物（由 PLGA 纳米纤维与羟基磷灰石纳米颗粒构成）组成的双相支架。[6] 这种双相设计的目的是促进天然的非矿化和矿化的纤维软骨结合区在修复后再生。在大鼠肩袖修复模型中发现，双相支架可刺激钙化和非钙化的基质形成，而不刺激对照组中纤维血管瘢痕形成。

尽管仿生支架有望增强和促进再生愈合，但仍需要进一步研究以深入了解天然结构中形成梯度结构的信号传导机制。[6] 对肌腱－骨附丽点的发育生物学的深入了解将直接影响未来的支架设计。后续可在支架中植入生长因子和其他信号分子。

总结

患者和医师相关的因素都会影响肩袖手术的结果。患者因素包括年龄、遗传因素、合并症、肌腱完整性和社会因素。患者年龄本身可能不会影响肩袖手术的功能预后，但年龄会对解剖学预后产生负面影响。肩袖疾病可能有遗传易感性，控制 MMPs 活性或将 TGF-β3 输送至修复部位可促进肌腱愈合。众所周知，糖尿病会对肌腱的愈合和肩袖手术的预后产生负面影响，但肥胖与肩袖病变之间的真实相关性尚不清楚。肩袖修复术后，肩袖肌肉萎缩和脂肪浸润的程度对解剖学预后和功能预后有重要影响。应在 Goutallier 2 级脂肪浸润发生之前进行手术。研究者发现，吸烟和工伤赔偿诉求会对肩袖修复的手术预后产生负面影响。

与医师相关的影响肩袖手术预后的因素包括

手术时机、手术方法和术后康复。急性肩袖撕裂在受伤后 3~4 个月内行手术治疗均相对安全。对于慢性肩袖撕裂，应评估肌肉萎缩和脂肪浸润程度，并在 Goutallier 2 级脂肪浸润之前进行修复。对于较大范围的撕裂，单排修复和双排修复的效果存在显著差异。大鼠模型的基础研究表明，长时间的制动可以提高修复部位的强度，但容易引起短暂的肩关节僵硬。早期的被动运动可能会对肩关节力学产生负面影响。

保守的术后固定康复治疗方案（固定期为 6 周）对手术修复 1 年后的活动范围或功能结局没有影响。但 MRI 检查可观察到这种方法有降低再撕裂率的趋势。

未来针对改善肩袖手术预后的研究方向包括使用 PDGF、PRP、MSC 和仿生支架。单独应用 PDGF 可改善肩袖术后的生物力学强度和解剖结构。而单独使用 PRP 或 MSC 可能不会显著增强修复部位的生物力学或组织学特性。进一步的研究应关注这些生长因子（细胞因子）的最佳组合、最佳剂量和输送方法。未来有希望使用仿生支架来增强肌腱的再生愈合能力，但仍需进一步研究证实。

参考文献

[1] Gulotta LV, Nho SJ, Dodson CC, Adler RS, Altchek DW, MacGillivray JD; HSS Arthroscopic Rotator Cuff Registry: Prospective evaluation of arthroscopic rotator cuff repairs at 5 years: Part I—functional outcomes and radiographic healing rates. *J Shoulder Elbow Surg* 2011;20(6):934-940.
At 5-year follow-up after arthroscopic rotator cuff repair in 106 patients, functional results remained constant. Healing rates on ultrasound improved over time. Level of evidence: II.

[2] Galatz LM, Sandell LJ, Rothermich SY, et al: Characteristics of the rat supraspinatus tendon during tendon-to-bone healing after acute injury. *J Orthop Res* 2006;24(3):541-550.

[3] Slabaugh MA, Nho SJ, Grumet RC, et al: Does the literature confirm superior clinical results in radiographically healed rotator cuffs after rotator cuff repair? *Ar-*

throscopy 2010;26(3):393-403.

A systematic review examined the correlation between the structural integrity of the rotator cuff after repair and the clinical outcome. Important differences were noted between patients with a healed or an unhealed rotator cuff repair. Level of evidence: IV.

[4] Bedi A, Maak T, Walsh C, et al: Cytokines in rotator cuff degeneration and repair. *J Shoulder Elbow Surg* 2012;21(2):218-227.

The use of cytokines during the healing process after rotator cuff repair is discussed.

[5] Galatz L, Rothermich S, VanderPloeg K, Petersen B, Sandell L, Thomopoulos S: Development of the supraspinatus tendon-to-bone insertion: Localized expression of extracellular matrix and growth factor genes. *J Orthop Res* 2007;25(12):1621-1628.

Using a murine model, the development of the rotator cuff tendon-to-bone insertion site was examined. The rotator cuff was morphologically distinct at 13.5 days postconception, and a shift from TGF-β3 to TGF-β1 expression occurred 2 days later.

[6] Zhang X, Bogdanowicz D, Erisken C, Lee NM, Lu HH: Biomimetic scaffold design for functional and integrative tendon repair. *J Shoulder Elbow Surg* 2012;21(2):266-277.

A review article examining the current approaches to functional and integrative tendon repair using biomimetic design principles. Level of evidence: Review article.

[7] Yamamoto A, Takagishi K, Osawa T, et al: Prevalence and risk factors of a rotator cuff tear in the general population. *J Shoulder Elbow Surg* 2010;19(1):116-120.

The epidemiology of rotator cuff tears was examined in 683 people (1,366 shoulders). A 20.7% prevalence of full-thickness rotator cuff tears was found. The risk factors involved a history of trauma, the dominant arm, and age. Level of evidence: III.

[8] Safran O, Schroeder J, Bloom R, Weil Y, Milgrom C: Natural history of nonoperatively treated symptomatic rotator cuff tears in patients 60 years old or younger. *Am J Sports Med* 2011;39(4):710-714.

Size change was examined in 61 nonsurgically treated full-thickness rotator cuff tears. At an average 29-month follow-up, half of the tears had increased in size. No correlation was found between tear size and patient age or initial tear size.

[9] Mall NA, Kim HM, Keener JD, et al: Symptomatic progression of asymptomatic rotator cuff tears: A prospective study of clinical and sonographic variables. *J*

Bone Joint Surg Am 2010;92(16):2623-2633.

A prospective study of 195 patients with asymptomatic rotator cuff tears found that pain development was associated with an increase in tear size, and larger tears were more likely to develop pain. Level of evidence: III.

[10] Verma NN, Bhatia S, Baker CL III, et al: Outcomes of arthroscopic rotator cuff repair in patients aged years or older. *Arthroscopy* 2010;26(10):1273-1280.

Thirty-nine patients age 70 years or older were evaluated after arthroscopic rotator cuff repair. At an average 36.1-month follow-up, American Shoulder and Elbow Surgeons Shoulder Index, Simple Shoulder Test, and visual analog pain scores had significantly improved. Level of evidence: IV.

[11] Charousset C, Bellaïche L, Kalra K, Petrover D: Arthroscopic repair of full-thickness rotator cuff tears: Is there tendon healing in patients aged 65 years or older? *Arthroscopy* 2010;26(3):302-309.

Eighty-eight patients age 65 years or older were evaluated after arthroscopic rotator cuff repair. At an average age 41-month follow-up, Constant and Simple Shoulder Test scores had significantly improved. The retear rate was 42% based on a CT arthrogram.

[12] Osti L, Papalia R, Del Buono A, Denaro V, Maffulli N: Comparison of arthroscopic rotator cuff repair in healthy patients over and under 65 years of age. *Knee Surg Sports Traumatol Arthrosc* 2010;18(12):1700-1706.

The outcomes of 28 pairs of matched patients older and younger than 65 years were compared after arthroscopic rotator cuff repair. At an average 27-month follow-up, there were no significant differences in motion or scores on the UCLA Scale or Medical Outcomes Study 36-Item Short Form.

[13] Tashjian RZ, Hollins AM, Kim HM, et al: Factors affecting healing rates after arthroscopic double-row rotator cuff repair. *Am J Sports Med* 2010;38(12):2435-2442.

Forty-eight patients were evaluated at a mean 16-month follow-up after double-row rotator cuff repair. Multivariate regression analysis showed that age was the most important factor influencing tendon healing at the repair site, even with a double-row con- struct. Level of evidence: IV.

[14] Manning CN, Kim HM, Sakiyama-Elbert S, Galatz LM, Havlioglu N, Thomopoulos S: Sustained delivery of transforming growth factor beta three enhances tendon-to-bone healing in a rat model. *J Orthop Res* 2011;29(7):1099-1105.

In a rat rotator cuff repair model, TGF-β3 was delivered to the repair site using a heparin-fibrin–based delivery system. Sustained delivery of TGF-β3 to the healing tendon-bone insertion led to significant improvement in structural properties at 28 days and material properties at 56 days, compared with controls.

[15] Kovacevic D, Fox AJ, Bedi A, et al: Calcium- phosphate matrix with or without TGF-β3 improves tendon-bone healing after rotator cuff repair. *Am J Sports Med* 2011;39(4):811-819.

In a rat rotator cuff repair model, delivery of TGF-β3 with an injectable calcium-phosphate matrix significantly improved the strength of the repair site at 4 weeks. TGF-β3 delivery also resulted in greater type I rather than type III collagen expression at the healing enthesis.

[16] Bedi A, Fox AJ, Kovacevic D, Deng XH, Warren RF, Rodeo SA: Doxycycline-mediated inhibition of matrix metalloproteinases improves healing after rotator cuff repair. *Am J Sports Med* 2010;38(2):308-317.

Modulation of MMP-13 activity was significantly reduced after oral administration of doxycycline in a rat rotator cuff repair model. The healing enthesis had an increased load to failure at 2 weeks compared with controls.

[17] Bedi A, Kovacevic D, Hettrich C, et al: The effect of matrix metalloproteinase inhibition on tendon-to-bone healing in a rotator cuff repair model. *J Shoulder Elbow Surg* 2010;19(3):384-391.

Local delivery of an MMP inhibitor resulted in reduced collagen degradation at the healing enthesis in a rat rotator cuff repair model. Biomechanical testing revealed no significant differences in stiffness or ultimate load to failure compared with controls.

[18] Gwilym SE, Watkins B, Cooper CD, et al: Genetic influences in the progression of tears of the rotator cuff. *J Bone Joint Surg Br* 2009;91(7):915-917.

The relative risk of full-thickness rotator cuff tears in siblings of patients with a tear was 2.85, compared with control subjects. Full-thickness tears in siblings were significantly more likely to progress over 5 years.

[19] Tashjian RZ, Farnham JM, Albright FS, Teerlink CC, Cannon-Albright LA: Evidence for an inherited predisposition contributing to the risk for rotator cuff disease. *J Bone Joint Surg Am* 2009;91(5):1136-1142.

Patients with diagnosed rotator cuff disease and a known genealogy were analyzed to describe the familial clustering of affected individuals. Significant excess relatedness of patients and elevated risks to both close and distant relatives of patients with rotator cuff disease were observed. Level of evidence: III.

[20] Warrender WJ, Brown OL, Abboud JA: Outcomes of arthroscopic rotator cuff repairs in obese patients. *J Shoulder Elbow Surg* 2011;20(6):961-967.

Retrospective review of 149 patients at 16.3-month follow-up after arthroscopic rotator cuff repair found a significant correlation between obesity and poor functional outcomes, longer surgical times, and longer hospital stay. Level of evidence: III.

[21] Namdari S, Baldwin K, Glaser D, Green A: Does obesity affect early outcome of rotator cuff repair? *J Shoulder Elbow Surg* 2010;19(8):1250-1255.

A retrospective review of 154 patients at a mean 54.8-week follow-up after rotator cuff repair compared preoperative and postoperative scores on the Disabilities of the Arm, Shoulder and Hand questionnaire; the Simple Shoulder Test; and the visual analog scale for pain, function, and quality of life. Obesity and body mass index did not influence early functional outcomes. Level of evidence: III.

[22] Bedi A, Fox AJ, Harris PE, et al: Diabetes mellitus impairs tendon-bone healing after rotator cuff repair. *J Shoulder Elbow Surg* 2010;19(7):978-988.

Diabetes was induced preoperatively in a rat rotator cuff repair model. The sustained hyperglycemia was found to impair both the biomechanical and histomorphometric properties of the healing tendon.

[23] Clement ND, Hallett A, MacDonald D, Howie C, McBirnie J: Does diabetes affect outcome after arthroscopic repair of the rotator cuff? *J Bone Joint Surg Br* 2010;92(8):1112-1117.

The outcomes of arthroscopic rotator cuff repair in patients with diabetes were compared with those of matched control subjects. Patients with diabetes had improvement in pain and function in the short term that was less than that of their counterparts without diabetes.

[24] Gerber C, Meyer DC, Frey E, et al: Neer Award 2007: Reversion of structural muscle changes caused by chronic rotator cuff tears using continuous musculotendinous traction. An experimental study in sheep. *J Shoulder Elbow Surg* 2009;18(2):163-171.

A sheep chronic rotator cuff tear model was used to demonstrate that continuous elongation of the infraspinatus muscle can lead to restoration of normal muscle architecture, partial reversal of muscle atrophy, and arrest of the progression of fatty infiltration.

[25] Gladstone JN, Bishop JY, Lo IK, Flatow EL: Fatty in-

filtration and atrophy of the rotator cuff do not improve after rotator cuff repair and correlate with poor functional outcome. *Am J Sports Med* 2007;35(5):719-728.

A prospective study of 38 patients found that muscle atrophy and fatty infiltration significantly affected the functional outcome after rotator cuff repair. Tear size significantly influenced repair integrity. Level of evidence: II.

[26] Oh JH, Kim SH, Ji HM, Jo KH, Bin SW, Gong HS: Prognostic factors affecting anatomic outcome of rotator cuff repair and correlation with functional outcome. *Arthroscopy* 2009;25(1):30-39.

Anatomic and functional outcomes after rotator cuff repair were evaluated in 177 patients at an average 29-month follow-up. Multivariate regression analysis showed that tear retraction and fatty degeneration of the infraspinatus were independent determinants of anatomic or functional outcome, but age was not. Level of evidence: IV.

[27] Liem D, Lichtenberg S, Magosch P, Habermeyer P: Magnetic resonance imaging of arthroscopic supraspinatus tendon repair. *J Bone Joint Surg Am* 2007;89(8):1770-1776.

The clinical and structural results of isolated supraspinatus arthroscopic repairs were evaluated in 53 patients at an average 26.4-month follow-up. Relatively great muscular atrophy and fatty infiltration preoperatively were associated with repair failure and an inferior clinical result. Level of evidence: IV.

[28] Melis B, Nemoz C, Walch G: Muscle fatty infiltration in rotator cuff tears: Descriptive analysis of 1688 cases. *Orthop Traumatol Surg Res* 2009;95(5):319-324.

The natural history of fatty infiltration was evaluated in 1,688 patients who underwent surgery for a rotator cuff tear. The mean time to severe fatty infiltration was 4, or 3 years in the supraspinatus, the infraspinatus, or the subscapularis, respectively. Level of evidence: IV.

[29] Kim HM, Dahiya N, Teefey SA, Keener JD, Galatz LM, Yamaguchi K: Relationship of tear size and location to fatty degeneration of the rotator cuff. *J Bone Joint Surg Am* 2010;92(4):829-839.

Shoulder ultrasound was performed bilaterally in patients to assess the type of rotator cuff tear and fatty degeneration in the supraspinatus and infraspinatus muscles. Fatty degeneration was found to be closely associated with tear size and location, especially in anterior supraspinatus tendon tears.

[30] Goutallier DB, Patte D: L'e´valuation par le scanner de la trophicite´ des muscles de la coiffe ayant une rupture tendineuse. *Rev Chir Orthop Reparatrice Appar Mot* 1989;75:126-127.

[31] Baumgarten KM, Gerlach D, Galatz LM, et al: Cigarette smoking increases the risk for rotator cuff tears. *Clin Orthop Relat Res* 2010;468(6):1534-1541.

A history of cigarette smoking was obtained in 584 patients who underwent diagnostic shoulder ultrasound for unilateral atraumatic shoulder pain. There was a strong association between smoking and rotator cuff disease, which was both dosage and time dependent. Level of evidence: III.

[32] Holtby R, Razmjou H: Impact of work-related compensation claims on surgical outcome of patients with rotator cuff related pathologies: A matched case- control study. *J Shoulder Elbow Surg* 2010;19(3):452-460.

In 110 patients with a workers' compensation–related injury, there was a significantly higher level of disability before and after rotator cuff surgery in comparison with a historical control group at 1-year follow-up. Level of evidence: III.

[33] Galatz LM, Silva MJ, Rothermich SY, Zaegel MA, Havlioglu N, Thomopoulos S: Nicotine delays tendon-to-bone healing in a rat shoulder model. *J Bone Joint Surg Am* 2006;88(9):2027-2034.

[34] Carbone S, Gumina S, Arceri V, Campagna V, Fagnani C, Postacchini F: The impact of preoperative smoking habit on rotator cuff tear: Cigarette smoking influences rotator cuff tear sizes. *J Shoulder Elbow Surg* 2012;21(1):56-60.

A correlation was found among cigarette smoking, rotator cuff tears, and tear size by analyzing 408 patients who underwent arthroscopic rotator cuff repair. Tear severity increased with increases in the average number of cigarettes and total lifetime cigarettes smoked.

[35] Razmjou H, Lincoln S, Axelrod T, Holtby R: Factors contributing to failure of rotator cuff surgery in persons with work-related injuries. *Physiother Can* 2008;60(2):125-133.

A cross-sectional study found that of 19 patients with continued impairment after surgical treatment of work-related shoulder injuries, 50% had at least one reason to explain their ongoing symptoms, emotional difficulties, and functional limitations.

[36] Henn RF III, Kang L, Tashjian RZ, Green A: Patients with workers' compensation claims have worse outcomes after rotator cuff repair. *J Bone Joint Surg Am* 2008;90(10):2105-2113.

After controlling for confounding factors, 39 patients

with a workers' compensation claim were found to have worse outcomes than comparable patients on outcome measures and visual analog shoulder pain, shoulder function, and quality-of-life scales 1 year after repair of a chronic rotator cuff tear. Level of evidence: I.

[37] Kim HM, Dahiya N, Teefey SA, et al: Location and initiation of degenerative rotator cuff tears: An analysis of three hundred and sixty shoulders. *J Bone Joint Surg Am* 2010;92(5):1088-1096.

Ultrasound of 360 shoulders showed that degenerative rotator cuff tears most commonly involve a posterior location near the junction of the supraspinatus and infraspinatus. These tears may originate in a region to 17 mm posterior to the biceps tendon.

[38] Petersen SA, Murphy TP: The timing of rotator cuff repair for the restoration of function. *J Shoulder Elbow Surg* 2011;20(1):62-68.

Acute, traumatic full-thickness rotator cuff tears in 36 patients were repaired as late as 4 months after injury, with no functional compromise according to American Shoulder and Elbow Surgeons and UCLA scores. Level of evidence: III.

[39] Burks RT, Crim J, Brown N, Fink B, Greis PE: A prospective randomized clinical trial comparing arthroscopic single- and double-row rotator cuff repair: Magnetic resonance imaging and early clinical evaluation. *Am J Sports Med* 2009;37(4):674-682.

One year after single-row or double-row rotator cuff repair, there were no differences in measures of postoperative motion or strength. MRI measurements of footprint coverage and the tendon thickness of patients in the two repair groups showed no differences. Level of evidence: I.

[40] Grasso A, Milano G, Salvatore M, Falcone G, Deriu L, Fabbriciani C: Single-row versus double-row arthroscopic rotator cuff repair: A prospective randomized clinical study. *Arthroscopy* 2009;25(1):4-12.

The clinical outcomes of arthroscopic rotator cuff repair were compared after single-row or double-row repair. At an average 24.8-month follow-up, no significant between-group clinical differences were noted. Level of evidence: I.

[41] Ma HL, Chiang ER, Wu HT, et al: Clinical outcome and imaging of arthroscopic single-row and double-row rotator cuff repair: A prospective randomized trial. *Arthroscopy* 2012;28(1):16-24.

A randomized study of patients with a rotator cuff tear larger than 3 cm found that double-row fixation resulted in significantly better muscle strength than single-row

fixation. There were no between-group differences in cuff integrity at 6-month and 2-year follow-up. Level of evidence: II.

[42] Duquin TR, Buyea C, Bisson LJ: Which method of rotator cuff repair leads to the highest rate of structural healing? A systematic review. *Am J Sports Med* 2010;38(4):835-841.

A systematic review found that double-row repair leads to significantly lower retearing rates in tears larger than 1 cm compared with single-row methods.

[43] Dines JS, Bedi A, ElAttrache NS, Dines DM: Single-row versus double-row rotator cuff repair: Techniques and outcomes. *J Am Acad Orthop Surg* 2010;18(2):83-93.

Although a double-row repair provides an improved mechanical environment for the healing enthesis, no clinical difference is noted between either repair technique. Level of evidence: Review article.

[44] Peltz CD, Dourte LM, Kuntz AF, et al: The effect of postoperative passive motion on rotator cuff healing in a rat model. *J Bone Joint Surg Am* 2009;91(10):2421-2429.

Early controlled passive motion had a detrimental effect on shoulder mechanics after surgery in a rat rotator cuff model.

[45] Seo SS, Choi JS, An KC, Kim JH, Kim SB: The factors affecting stiffness occurring with rotator cuff tear. *J Shoulder Elbow Surg* 2012;21(3):304-309.

The type and the direction of the rotator cuff tear and the presence of trauma were found to increase limitation of preoperative joint motion in 119 patients undergoing arthroscopic rotator cuff repair. Level of evidence: IV.

[46] Sarver JJ, Peltz CD, Dourte L, Reddy S, Williams GR, Soslowsky LJ: After rotator cuff repair, stiffness—but not the loss in range of motion—increased transiently for immobilized shoulders in a rat model. *J Shoulder Elbow Surg* 2008;17(1, suppl):108S-113S.

The increase in joint stiffness caused by immobilizing an injured and repaired rat rotator cuff was found to be transient.

[47] Parsons BO, Gruson KI, Chen DD, Harrison AK, Gladstone J, Flatow EL: Does slower rehabilitation after arthroscopic rotator cuff repair lead to long-term stiffness? *J Shoulder Elbow Surg* 2010;19(7):1034-1039.

Sling immobilization for 6 weeks after arthroscopic rotator cuff repair did not result in increased long-term stiffness at 1-year follow-up. MRI showed that conservative rehabilitation after repair may improve the rate of tendon healing. Level of evidence: IV.

[48] Uggen C, Dines J, McGarry M, Grande D, Lee T,

Limpisvasti O: The effect of recombinant human platelet-derived growth factor BB-coated sutures on rotator cuff healing in a sheep model. *Arthroscopy* 2010;26(11):1456-1462.

rhPDGF-BB coated sutures produced a more histologically normal tendon insertion site after a repair in a sheep model, but no biomechanical difference was noted compared to controls.

[49] Hee CK, Dines JS, Dines DM, et al: Augmentation of a rotator cuff suture repair using rhPDGF-BB and a type I bovine collagen matrix in an ovine model. *Am J Sports Med* 2011;39(8):1630-1639.

Recombinant human PDGF-BB combined with a type I collagen matrix improved the biomechanical strength and the anatomic appearance of the rotator cuff repair site in an ovine model.

[50] Jo CH, Kim JE, Yoon KS, et al: Does platelet-rich plasma accelerate recovery after rotator cuff repair? A prospective cohort study. *Am J Sports Med* 2011;39(10):2082-2090.

PRP application in 19 patients during arthroscopic rotator cuff repair did not accelerate recovery clinically or anatomically compared with patients in the control group. This study may have been underpowered, however. Level of evidence: II.

[51] Bergeson AG, Tashjian RZ, Greis PE, Crim J, Stoddard GJ, Burks RT: Effects of platelet-rich fibrin matrix on repair integrity of atrisk rotator cuff tears. *Am J Sports Med* 2012;40(2):286-293.

No difference was found in retearing rates and functional outcomes between 16 patients who had platelet-rich fibrin matrix augmentation of their rotator cuff repair and historical control subjects. Level of evidence: III.

[52] Barber FA, Hrnack SA, Snyder SJ, Hapa O: Rotator cuff repair healing influenced by platelet-rich plasma construct augmentation. *Arthroscopy* 2011;27(8):1029-1035.

Two matched groups of patients with or without PRP augmentation of their rotator cuff repair were compared at a mean 31-month follow-up. Patients in the PRP group had a lower retearing rate on MRI, but there was no between-group clinical difference aside from Rowe scores. Level of evidence: III.

[53] Castricini R, Longo UG, De Benedetto M, et al: Platelet-rich plasma augmentation for arthroscopic rotator cuff repair: A randomized controlled trial. *Am J Sports Med* 2011;39(2):258-265.

A comparison study found that autologous platelet-rich fibrin matrix augmentation of rotator cuff repairs did not improve functional outcomes at 16-month follow-up. There was no between-group difference in repair integrity based on MRI analysis. Level of evidence: I.

[54] Randelli P, Arrigoni P, Ragone V, Aliprandi A, Cabitza P: Platelet rich plasma in arthroscopic rotator cuff repair: A prospective RCT study, 2-year follow-up. *J Shoulder Elbow Surg* 2011;20(4):518-528.

During the first month after rotator cuff repair, autologous PRP augmentation was found to reduce pain. At 3 months after surgery, functional outcomes were significantly higher after PRP augmentation. No difference was noted at 6, 12, or 24 months. Level of evidence: I.

[55] Aspenberg P, Virchenko O: Platelet concentrate injection improves Achilles tendon repair in rats. *Acta Orthop Scand* 2004;75(1):93-99.

[56] Lyras DN, Kazakos K, Verettas D, et al: The influence of platelet-rich plasma on angiogenesis during the early phase of tendon healing. *Foot Ankle Int* 2009;30(11):1101-1106.

PRP enhanced neovascularization in a rabbit Achilles tendon model during the first 2 weeks of the healing process. The number of newly formed vessels in the PRP-treated rats at 4 weeks was less than that of control rats, and this fact suggests that the healing process was shortened.

[57] Castillo TN, Pouliot MA, Kim HJ, Dragoo JL: Comparison of growth factor and platelet concentration from commercial platelet-rich plasma separation systems. *Am J Sports Med* 2011;39(2):266-271.

The three different PRP concentration systems produced differing concentrations of growth factors and white blood cells.

[58] Gulotta LV, Kovacevic D, Ehteshami JR, Dagher E, Packer JD, Rodeo SA: Application of bone marrow-derived mesenchymal stem cells in a rotator cuff repair model. *Am J Sports Med* 2009;37(11):2126-2133.

The addition of MSCs to the healing rotator cuff insertion site in a rat model did not improve the structure, composition, or strength of the healing tendon attachment site.

[59] Gulotta LV, Kovacevic D, Packer JD, Deng XH, Rodeo SA: Bone marrow-derived mesenchymal stem cells transduced with scleraxis improve rotator cuff healing in a rat model. *Am J Sports Med* 2011;39(6):1282-1289.

MSCs genetically modified with scleraxis were used to augment rotator cuff healing in a rat rotator cuff model. At 4 weeks, fibrocartilage was increased and biomechanical properties were improved at the repair site.

第四部分

关节镜技术

栏目编委：
Augustus D. Mazzocca, MS, MD;
Marc Safran, MD

第十九章　关节镜治疗肩峰下及肩锁关节病变

Daniel Aaron, MD; Bradford Parsons, MD; Evan Flatow, MD

引言

　　肩峰下间隙和肩锁关节（AC 关节）的病变非常常见，其症状会严重影响患者的生活质量。非手术治疗可以发挥一定作用，但一般情况下需要行手术治疗。随着技术的发展，关节镜手术已成为许多此类疾病的标准治疗方法。本章讨论了影响肩峰下间隙和 AC 关节的最常见疾病的病因、评估和治疗，重点介绍了关节镜手术。

肩峰下病变

解剖学与病因学

　　外部压迫或撞击是导致肩袖疾病和撕裂的重要外在因素。内在因素也起着关键作用。然而，对于引起症状及肌腱病变的机械压迫程度，现仍存在争议。

　　笔者对肩峰下间隙的解剖进行了研究，其与肩袖疾病密切相关，比如肩峰下滑囊炎、撞击综

Dr. Parsons or an immediate family member is a member of a speakers' bureau or has made paid presentations on behalf of Zimmer and Arthrex; serves as a paid consultant to or is an employee of Zimmer and Arthrex; and has received research or institutional support from Wyeth. Dr. Flatow or an immediate family member has received royalties from Innomed and Zimmer; is a member of a speakers' bureau or has made paid presentations on behalf of Zimmer; and serves as an unpaid consultant to Zimmer. Neither Dr. Aaron nor any immediate family member has received anything of value from or has stock or stock options held in a commercial company or institution related directly or indirectly to the subject of this chapter.

合征、肩袖肌腱部分 / 完全撕裂等。目前关于肩峰下间隙的解剖学特征及其与肩袖病变和症状的关系已有许多定论。

　　Neer 首先提出前肩峰为肩袖和肱二头肌长头腱撞击的主要部位。[1] Neer 注意到前肩峰下表面上有一个尖状的隆起带，在部分尸体标本的前 1/3 发生了退变。这些解剖发现与术中观察到的冈上肌、冈下肌前部和肱二头肌最常发生肩袖损伤相关，当手臂处于中立位时，这些结构都位于肩锁关节前。Neer 的结论是，手臂在内旋或外旋时抬高，使这些结构位于前肩峰之下，它们在那里容易受到挤压、撞击，最终发生机械性病变。[1] 后来的解剖学研究表明，肩峰前缘的喙肩韧带在大结节于其下方通过时被拉伸，在屈曲和内旋时，结节和冈上肌撞击喙肩韧带和前肩峰。[2] 除此以外，肱二头肌也会撞击喙肩韧带。另一项尸体研究发现，肩肱间隙在手臂抬高 60°~120° 时减小，接触集中在冈上肌附丽处，前钩状肩锁关节的接触显著增加。[3] 肩锁关节前 1/3 的扁平结构对减少肩锁关节的撞击是必要的，这一发现支持了前钩状肩锁关节和喙肩韧带（CA 韧带）的解剖结构与肩袖撞击的相关性。[4]

　　目前，肩峰下减压术联合肩袖修补术的使用存在争议，并且有证据表明，如果没有明显刺痛，在常规肌腱修补时不需要行肩峰成形术。[5]

患者评估

　　肩峰下撞击的评估依赖于详细的病史、体格

检查以及影像学检查。撞击的典型症状是肩前外侧和（或）手臂疼痛。[6]患者常描述特定的位置和活动加剧了疼痛。疼痛可能会导致抬肩活动（例如，伸手拿高架子上的物体）或需要向内大幅旋转的活动（如穿上外套或系上胸衣）困难。而伸展手臂举起物体也经常引起症状。

体格检查

与任何肩部体格检查一样，临床医师应先对皮肤进行视诊，再通过与健侧对比，检查患侧肩关节和肩胛骨轮廓，辨别是否存在萎缩或畸形。应测量被动运动范围、主动运动范围和肩袖强度。肩峰下撞击可以通过激发动作来评估，其中最常用的是 Neer 试验和 Hawkins 试验。试验的原理是减少肩峰下间隙，增加肩袖与骨和韧带边界的接触。MRI 分析发现，肩袖在外展和内旋时与前下肩峰非常接近（Hawkins 试验阳性），而不是在完全外展时（Neer 试验阳性）。[7]一项关节镜检查发现，Neer 试验阳性更可能与肩袖和关节盂接触有关，而不是与肩峰接触，[8]另一项 MRI 研究发现，这两项检查都减少了冈上肌附丽点与肩峰下间隙骨缘之间的距离，但 Hawkins 试验的肩峰下间隙减少和肩袖接触更严重。[9]一项尸体研究也发现肩袖在这两项检查中都有接触。Neer 试验造成肩袖与内侧肩峰接触，Hawkins 试验造成肩袖与 CA 韧带接触，总之，这两种测试都造成了肩袖关节侧和前上关节盂之间接触。[10]在临床实践中，这两种测试的敏感性较高、特异性一般。[11]

影像学检查

除了病史和体格检查外，还应进行影像学评估。典型的肩位系列片包括标准 AP 位片、肩胛平面 AP 位片以及腋窝侧位和出口或肩胛骨 Y 位片。标准 AP 位可以看到 AC 关节周围的骨赘生物，肩胛平面 AP 位（真正的 AP 位）最能清楚地显示盂肱关节，也能显示大结节的囊性改变。腋位最适合显示肩峰，出口位最适合显示肩峰形态。在 AP 位片和冠状面 MRI 图片中可观察到撞击与肩肱距离之间存在相关性。[12]影像学检查结果可能支持撞击的诊断，但必须与临床症状和体征相结合。[13]

非手术治疗

肩峰撞击综合征确诊后必须制订治疗方案。明确是否存在相关的病理变化，特别是肩袖撕裂，这对任何治疗方案都至关重要。如果患者的肩袖没有全层撕裂，治疗手段通常倾向非手术治疗。

非甾体抗炎药

非甾体抗炎药（NSAIDs）常被推荐用于治疗肩峰下囊的炎症。这类药物在临床上是有效的。其作用的分子基础是减少肩胛下囊中的炎症细胞因子和介导受体。[14]NSAIDs 的全身和局部副作用使其使用存在争议。非选择性 NSAIDs（COX 抑制剂）增加了上消化道并发症（如溃疡和出血）的发生风险。COX-2 抑制剂减少了胃肠道不良反应，但可能存在心血管风险。[15]NSAIDs 在动物模型中显示出抑制肌腱 - 骨愈合的作用，这一发现使研究者对肩袖修复术后患者 NSAIDs 的使用产生了争议。[16]

物理治疗

物理治疗是一种常用的治疗方法。与接受非特异性物理治疗的肩峰下撞击患者相比，接受特殊康复方案（包括伸展、偏心肩袖加强和向心 - 偏心肩胛稳定运动）后需要手术治疗的患者比例显著降低。[17]

肩峰下注射

肩峰下注射通常用于肩峰下撞击综合征。类固醇激素是最常用的注射药物。类固醇激素也可以减少肩胛下囊的炎症细胞因子。[14]一项荟萃分析发现，在治疗肩袖疾病时，注射类固醇激素的患者受益不大。[18]某些患者由于血糖升高的风险而被禁止使用类固醇激素，接受多次类固醇激素注射的患者则被禁止进一步使用皮质类固醇。在动物模型中，注射甲泼尼龙后，肩袖肌腱的强度降低并发生组织学改变。[19]类固醇激素注射对大多数患者来说是一种低风险的干预措施，可能有助于进行物理治疗。目前，研究者正在研究新的药物，这些药物可能在临床上有效，但没有NSAIDs或皮质类固醇的不良反应。早期研究取得了较为满意的结果。[20]

目前美国骨科医师学会的实践指南建议使用物理疗法和NSAIDs初步治疗肩峰下撞击综合征，既不支持也不反对使用皮质类固醇注射、脉冲电磁场、离子导入、声透疗法、经皮电神经刺激、冷敷、热敷、按摩和活动调整。[5]

外科治疗

如果非手术治疗无效，可能需要手术治疗。在肩袖撕裂不超过50%的情况下，单纯肩峰下减压术是有效的。这个手术通常包括肩峰下囊切除、肩峰前成形术和CA韧带切除。削平肩锁关节前1/3足以消除外源性肩袖压迫。标准的减压方法是关节镜下减压术。

手术操作

关节镜下肩峰下减压（ASD）通常包括两个入路。标准的后侧入路在肩峰后外侧角内侧约2 cm，远端约2 cm。建议触诊盂肱关节后线的软点以确定入路的位置，但对于三角肌较大或脂肪层较厚的患者这一步骤可能较困难。用11号刀片切开皮肤。将套管针组件推至肩峰下空隙，可以沿着肩峰和CA韧带的下表面进行钝性分离以创建观察空间。手臂的纵向牵引可以增加肩肱距离，有助于手术操作。取出套管针，固定套管。将关节镜插入套管时，镜头对准上方，这样可以观察到肩峰。然后建立一个标准的外侧入路。将腰穿针放置在这个入路，使前肩峰和CA韧带接近。入路通常位于距肩峰外侧边缘3~4 cm、前缘1/3处。必须记住，腋神经穿过距肩峰外侧缘5~7 cm的区域。在确定了入路位置后，使用11号刀片制造一个5 mm的皮肤切口，创建一个横向入口。将一个透明的塑料套管置入间隙，以便简单地插入和移除仪器。先插入刨刀，去除滑囊组织，

扩大可视区域。立即烧灼出血部位。然后对肩袖的滑囊表面进行检查，并用探针排除肌腱撕裂。使用电刀去除肩峰下表面的所有附着软组织。在这一过程中应先创造一个低张力的切口，通过三角肌筋膜从套管入口直接进入肩峰边缘内侧；目的是促进器械进入肩峰前缘和CA韧带。肩峰外侧缘的定义是切开三角肌筋膜直到看到肌肉纤维，前缘的定义是剥离CA韧带直到没有纤维附着。如果肩袖有大的撕裂，韧带就不能完全松解，因为必须保持韧带弓的被动稳定作用。[5]随后，肩锁关节下表面的其余部分可以暴露。前肩峰成形术是用磨钻进行的。这一步的目的是磨平肩峰前缘。在确定需要切除多少骨性结构后，术者在前外侧角进行切除。阶梯切割技术为更内侧的切除创造了条件。当从外侧切除到内侧时，移动关节镜至外侧入路，以便在一个正交的切割平面上观察肩峰。磨钻从后侧入路进入，将肩峰磨至平滑的阶梯状。在整个手术过程中，必须注意充分界定骨边缘，避免切割三角肌。建议使用电刀进行仔细止血，在冲洗液中加入肾上腺素（1∶300 000）以尽量减少出血，并建议使用低泵压（35 mmHg）以避免肿胀。

结果

ASD能有效缓解撞击综合征的症状，其结果优于开放减压。1998年的一项回顾性研究得出结论：开放手术和ASD的成功率（分别为90.0%和89.3%）都很高，差异不显著，但是，由于三角肌没有分离，接受ASD的患者可以更早地进行康复训练。[21]而且关节镜技术相对较长的学习曲线已在很大程度上减短，因此它已经得到了更广泛的应用。最近的一项荟萃分析发现，这两种技术的临床效果相当，但是，接受ASD的患者恢复工作能力的速度比接受开放手术减压的患者更快且前者住院天数更少。[22]在行未修复肌腱的ASD后，小的全层冈上肌撕裂没有出现进展。[23]也有证据表明ASD可以降低肩峰下撞击患者未来肩袖撕

裂的风险；18% 的患者在 ASD 15 年后出现肩袖撕裂（4% 为全层撕裂），而按年龄匹配的对照组患者肩袖撕裂率约为 40%。[24]

肩袖修复术

ASD 是否可与关节镜下全层肩袖撕裂修复同时进行仍存在争议。在一项对全层肩袖撕裂患者进行的研究中，研究人员确定临床结果与几个变量相关，包括患者年龄、撕裂类型、肌腱质量、萎缩程度及修复方式，与修复的同时是否进行 ASD 无相关性。[25] 在一项前瞻性随机研究中，研究者对肩袖全层单肌腱撕裂患者进行了研究，根据患者（不包括肩峰骨刺患者）行肩袖修复术时是否进行 ASD 进行了分组，随访 1 年，没有发现明显的功能差异。[26] 另一项研究发现进行肩袖修复的患者无论是否进行 ASD，临床结果没有显著差异，但是接受 ASD 的患者再手术率较低。[27] 然而，最近的荟萃分析发现，再手术率或功能结果没有差异。[28] 在关节镜下观察到明显的撞击或患者感觉到明显的刺痛时，ASD 通常作为全层肩袖撕裂修复的辅助手段。

肩锁关节病变

病因学

AC 关节可能受到退行性疾病（如骨关节炎）或创伤性疾病（如脱位或分离）的影响。尽管与胸锁关节相比，AC 关节几乎没有运动，但 AC 关节炎较常见。这种情况可能由炎性或结晶性关节病、创伤及关节脓毒症发展而来。[29] AC 关节炎可以单独存在或与肩部其他病变伴发。锁骨远端的骨溶解也会导致 AC 关节疼痛和压痛，这一情况被认为是由软骨下小骨折后的血管增生和骨吸收引起的。AC 分离通常是由外伤造成的。

解剖学

AC 关节是肩峰和锁骨远端之间的关节，是上肢和轴向骨骼之间唯一的连接。它是一个双关节，包含一个纤维软骨盘。关节间隙的宽度通常为 1~3 mm。[30] 该关节由一组复杂的韧带和肌肉约束来保持稳定。前后移位主要受 AC 韧带，特别是上韧带的限制。下移位主要受两条喙锁（CC）韧带的限制，其中锥状韧带的强度最大。三角肌筋膜也可能有助于稳定，但其确切作用尚未得到很好的描述。医师应充分了解韧带的附着点，如果术中损伤附着点会导致医源性不稳定，而按照原始解剖结构重建韧带可能更有效。

一项对干骨标本和新鲜尸体标本锁骨和喙突的解剖研究发现，从锁骨远端到梯形结节中心的平均距离，男性为（25.4±3.7）mm，女性为（22.9±3.7）mm；到喙突内侧边缘的距离男性为（47.2±4.6）mm，女性为（42.8±5.6）mm。[31] 这些距离与锁骨总长度的比值在两性之间是一致的。具体来说，锁骨远端到梯形中心的距离与锁骨全长的比值为 0.17，到圆锥结节内侧缘的距离与锁骨全长的比值为 0.31。在新鲜尸体标本中，锁骨远端到梯形中心的距离与锁骨长度的比值为 0.17，到圆锥结节内侧缘的距离与锁骨全长的比值为 0.24。[31]

患者评估

有 AC 关节病变的患者经常在关节和颈部前外侧、斜方肌冈上区和前外侧三角肌处感到疼痛。[6] AC 关节的体格检查从视诊开始，注意检查锁骨远端的突出部分是否分离。如果怀疑分离，应检查关节前后平面和上下平面的稳定性。如果 AC 关节分离明显，应在肱骨远端上施加一个向上的力来评估其可复性。如果怀疑是慢性病变而未分离，应该触诊关节并注意压痛。据报道，直接压痛作为 AC 关节体格检查的敏感性为 96%~97%。[32-33] 交叉内收试验也较常应用，其中 AC 关节的疼痛是由手臂与肩膀在 90° 仰角最大内收引起的。根据报道，这一动作的敏感度为 67%。[33] O'Brien 试验也较常用，方法为手臂内收 15°，肩部内旋，患者主动抬起手臂抵抗阻力。这个过程中患者感觉到疼痛，且肩部处于外旋状态时疼痛减轻为试验阳性。O'Brien 试验报告的敏感性高达

83%，特异性为 90%。在交叉内收和 O'Brien 混合试验中，肩部抬高至 90°，手臂靠近躯干最大内收，患者在肩关节内旋时，主动地提高抵抗力。[33]患者在这个动作中感到疼痛而在外旋情况下只有轻微疼痛为试验阳性。据报道，交叉内收试验的敏感性为 98%。[33]也应检查 AC 关节是否有压痛、畸形和不稳定。

AC 关节的 X 线检查包括数个 AP 位检查：X 线向头侧、尾侧偏 15°；肱骨内旋外旋；手臂最大外展，X 线向头侧偏 30°~35°。在 AP 位影像中

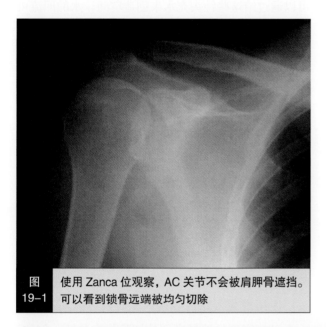

图 19-1 使用 Zanca 位观察，AC 关节不会被肩胛骨遮挡。可以看到锁骨远端被均匀切除

最常用的是 Zanca 位影像（图 19-1），X 线向头侧偏 15°。一般情况下可使用标准 AP 位片（图 19-2），但 Zanca 位可以可靠地避免肩胛骨遮挡 AC 关节，并且能观察到关节炎患者关节的侵蚀性变化、骨赘形成、关节间隙变窄以及创伤患者的关节间隙变宽和移位。[30,34]

MRI 检查非创伤性 AC 关节疼痛的敏感性为 85%，并且可以观察到 AC 分离患者的韧带结构。[32]核素骨扫描也有很高的准确性（76%）。[32]超声已经被用于检测 AC 关节炎，在一项研究中，65% 的无症状个体有阳性发现。[35]关节内注射麻醉剂是诊断非创伤性 AC 关节疾病的金标准，尽管确保麻醉剂真正进入关节的难度较大。[32]

肩锁关节炎及锁骨远端骨溶解的治疗

非手术治疗

对于影响 AC 关节的慢性疾病（如退行性关节病和骨溶解），首先尝试非手术治疗，例如，使用 NSAIDs 和物理疗法。如果这些方法无效，可向关节内注射皮质类固醇。最近的研究表明，虽然激素疗法短期内的效果一般，但如果疼痛能够缓解，则这种效果能够持续较久。[36]在该研究中，58 例患者中只有 16 例（28%）在注射皮质类固醇 1 个月后 AC 关节疼痛得到充分缓解，在平

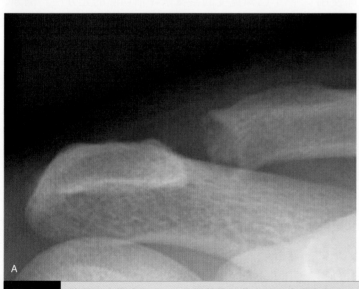
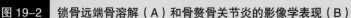
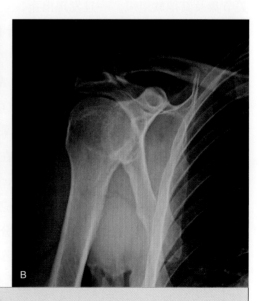

图 19-2 锁骨远端骨溶解（A）和骨赘骨关节炎的影像学表现（B）

均 42 个月的随访中，这 16 例患者中有 15 例有足够的缓解，避免了手术。尚未有皮质类固醇注射并发症的报道。[36] 注射皮质类固醇加局部麻醉药不仅可以协助疾病诊断，也是一种相对安全、有效的治疗方法。

外科治疗

锁骨远端切除术（DCR）是治疗 AC 关节炎或骨溶解的主要手术方法。锁骨远端切除术可以选择在开放手术或关节镜下进行，但标准疗法为关节镜下治疗。不管采用何种入路，手术的成功都取决于切除足够大小的锁骨远端，同时避免由于支撑韧带及其骨插入物的破坏而导致的关节稳定性降低。

关节镜下 DCR 手术的方法取决于 AC 关节病变是否与肩峰下撞击、肩袖撕裂等情况相关。当存在伴随性病变时，采用进行 ASD 的滑囊入路。在肩胛下间隙减压时，于后入路进镜，并在 AC 关节的前部建立一个额外的入路。从关节表面触诊，引入一根腰穿针，针头应准确地放置在前关节线的中线上，这样的器械角度才可为后续切除提供通道。当确定了入路的位置后，用 11 号刀片来制造一个 5 mm 的入路，并完全暴露关节。手术入路用钝套管针扩张，插入刨刀，切除下囊、关节盘及其他软组织。一旦发现出血，立即使用电刀灼烧。要特别注意，应完全暴露锁骨关节面，以便准确地测量骨切除术的均匀度。术中需显露锁骨远端的上半部分，同时避免切断上 AC 韧带以防止前后不稳定。当所有的软组织被切除时，用一个磨钻进行骨切除。与 ASD 一样，采用阶梯切割技术以确保切除的均匀性。用磨钻在锁骨前缘切除适量的骨，然后将磨钻向后推进，并将锁骨切除至阶梯状切割平面的水平。术者应仔细检查骨的轮廓，特别注意后面和上面的部分，这些部分通常不需要完全切除。任何需要切除的骨都用磨钻去除。然后重新插入刨刀，清除所有碎屑。有时很难从后方入口看到 AC 关节，如有必要，

可将肩峰小关节的后方部分切除。移除的骨不应超过确保关节充分可见所需的数量。

在患有孤立性 AC 关节病的患者中，直接入路在技术上比滑囊入路要求更高，但不会侵犯滑囊，从而最大限度地减少肿胀和出血。[37] 此外，由于根据 AC 关节解剖特点设计切口，该入路可以适应 AC 关节方向的解剖变异。在直接入路中，通过标准的前后入路，诊断性的盂肱关节镜可以排除关节内的伴随病变。AC 关节的准确位置和方向是通过使用 2 个或 3 个 22 号针头成功进入关节来确定的。可以通过给这些针头充水来创造空间，水的回流可以确定针尖已经位于关节腔内。在后关节线上制造一个 0.5 cm 的入口，并插入一个 2.7 mm 的关节镜（图 19-3）。AC 关节内的针头带有可视化装置。腰穿针用于引导前 AC 关节入路的操作，其方式与滑囊入路相同。建立一个 5.0 mm 的入口，插入一个 2.0 mm 的刨刀，取出软组织，明确 AC 关节的边缘，并用 2.0 mm 的磨钻以阶梯切割的方式开始骨切除。在创造出足够的空间后，可以使用标准的关节镜和较大的磨钻来完成重建。与滑囊入路一样，手术切除的深度、关节轮廓的均匀性和上 AC 韧带的保留也是非常重要的。

使用滑囊入路或直接入路时，可以通过插入一个已知宽度的器械来评估切除的充分性。例如，插入一把锉刀，还可以磨平剩余的粗糙边缘。解剖学研究发现，男性和女性的阶梯形切缘距离锁骨外侧缘分别 25.4 mm 和 22.4 mm，但临床研究发现，即使是完整的 CC 韧带和上、后 AC 韧带，切除 10 mm 也可以显著增加前移。[31,38] AC 关节囊的完全切开明显增加了不稳定性。因此，建议锁骨远端切除不超过 8 mm，并保留上方囊韧带结构。

与开放式 DCR 相比，关节镜下 DCR 有良好的疗效。一些研究发现，接受开放式或关节镜下 DCR 治疗 AC 关节炎的患者具有可预见的良好的疼痛缓解和较低的并发症发生率或再手术率。[39-41] 一项

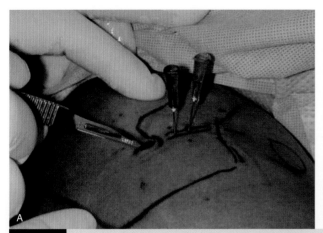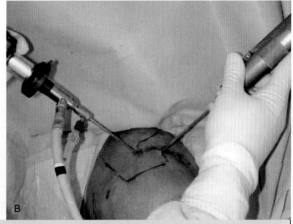

图 19-3　图片显示了用针头定位 AC 关节的方法和后 AC 入路的建立（A）；插入器械进行直接入路下锁骨远端切除（B）

比较研究发现，关节镜下 DCR 治疗的患者疼痛明显轻于开放式 DCR 治疗的患者。两组患者在手术量、手术时间、功能评分等方面无差异。[40] 关节镜下 DCR（尤其是采用直接入路）的患者术后恢复更快，[41] 但术后再手术率高，不过再手术率无统计学意义。[39] DCR 对治疗骨溶解有效；92.6% 的关节镜下 DCR 治疗锁骨远端骨溶解有良好的效果，但其对外伤性关节病的治疗效果不佳。[42] 关节镜下 DCR 通常与肩袖修复术联合应用于症状性 AC 关节炎患者。除了肩袖修复术外，肩袖修复时的 DCR 也可用于无症状 AC 关节炎伴下方骨赘生物，行 DCR 联合肩袖修复术的患者在术后第 2 年随访时的疗效更好，再手术率更低。[43]

肩锁关节损伤

损伤机制

关节脱位或分离通常是由直接冲击造成的（图 19-4）。冲击力的方向和大小决定了关节移位的方向和严重程度。最常见的损伤机制是肩膀的上部受到撞击，使肩峰受到向下的力。如果肩膀撞到地面，受伤的可能性更大，而且可能更严重。

分类

AC 分离最初根据肩锁关节相对于锁骨向下的移位距离分为 3 个等级。[44] 随后又增加了 3 个等级，这 3 个等级都是外科治疗的指征。[45] MRI 的出现使 X 线片分类与解剖学相联系，但这种关系可能并不一致。[46]

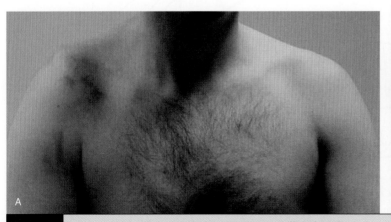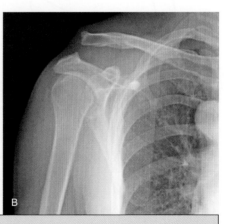

图 19-4　照片（A）和 Zanca 位片（B）显示 AC 关节完全分离

喙锁韧带的解剖学重建

大多数 AC 分离可采用非手术治疗，但当有手术治疗指征时，大多对喙锁韧带（CC 韧带）进行解剖学重建。生物力学研究发现，对两条 CC 韧带进行解剖学重建优于单一韧带重建的旧技术。在测试新鲜尸体标本中的天然 CC 韧带复合体时，移除失效后残余的韧带组织，并用半腱肌移植物进行解剖学重建。移植物从锁骨内侧（或外侧）骨道穿入并穿过喙突骨道，再从锁骨外侧（或内侧）骨道穿出。移植物在喙突骨道中的位置重塑了标本的原始方向。手术重建后进行的与手术重建前相同的生物力学测试显示，周期负载后没有显著的移植物永久性伸长，表明移植物能够承受早期康复锻炼。[47] 在尸体标本中比较解剖学重建与改良 Weaver-Dunn 手术的生物力学参数，解剖学重建是通过半腱肌移植物穿过锁骨远端的骨道实现的。[48] 锥状韧带的骨道位于锁骨后半轴远端内侧约 45 mm 处。斜方韧带的骨道更靠前，位于锁骨轴的中心，锥状韧带的骨道外侧约 15 mm 处（图 19-5）。在改善松弛和前后平移方面，解剖学重建优于改良 Weaver-Dunn 手术。因此，研究者得出结论，解剖学重建是生物力学重塑的最优方式，也有助于早期康复。解剖学重建的生物力学强度取决于移植物的强度。最近的一项分析发现，用掌长肌进行解剖学重建是不够的，用桡侧腕屈肌进行解剖学重建的效果优于改良 Weaver-Dunn 手术。[49]

关节镜下喙锁关节重建

早期的关节镜下 CC 关节重建技术涉及关节镜引导的在喙突基部经皮放置缝合锚和在锁骨经皮创建两个骨道。缝合穿通器用于将缝合线穿过锁骨骨道，并将之绑在钛板上（图 19-6）。在一项纳入 13 例患者的研究中，术后有 10 例患者保持解剖复位，2 例患者半脱位，1 例患者再次脱位。[50] 另一种关节镜手术方法使用钛缆（Arthrex）在喙突和锁骨之间进行非刚性固定。在一项纳入 12 例患者的研究中，有 2 例（16.7%）发生固定失败，但 12 例患者中有 11 例对结果满意。[51] 对尸体模型的研究显示，与天然配体相比，使用双钛缆在垂直平面和前方进行解剖重建，生物力学强度明显提

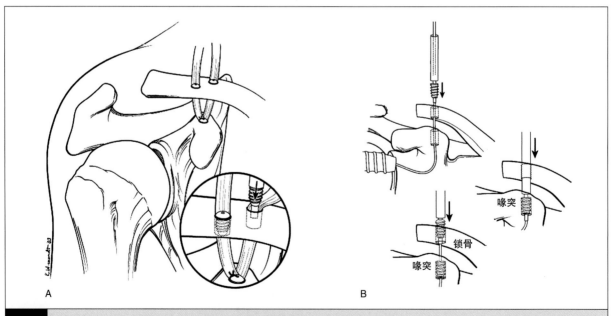

图 19-5　CC 韧带的解剖学重建（A）和关节镜下重建（B）的示意图。经允许引自 Mazzocca AD, Santangelo SA, Johnson ST, Rios CG, Dumonski ML, Arciero RA: A biomechanical evaluation of an anatomic coracoclavicular ligament reconstruction. *Am J Sports Med* 2006;34（2）:236–246.

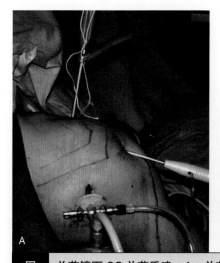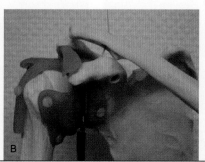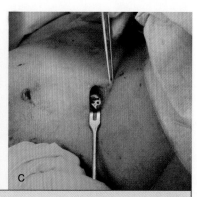

图 19-6　关节镜下 CC 关节重建。A. 关节镜设置，摄像头位于后侧入路，附加器械位于外侧入路和前侧入路。B. 模型示意缝合通道。C. 在锁骨钛板上打结。经允许引自 Chernchujit B, Tischer T, Imhoff AB: Ar throscopic reconstruction of the acromioclavicular joint disruption: Surgical technique and preliminary results. *Arch Orthop Trauma Surg* 2006;126（9）:575–581.

高[52]（图 19-7，19-8）。双钛缆结构也被临床用于关节镜下解剖学重建。[53]在平均 30 个月的随访中，23 例患者中有 8 例影像学检查发现骨缺损，但无明显临床表现。在一项对 10 例患者的研究中，全关节镜下（Weaver-Dunn 手术的 Chuinard

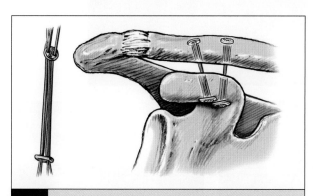

图 19-7　使用两个钛缆的 CC 关节解剖学重建示意图。经允许引自 Walz L, Salzmann GM, Fabbro T, Eichhorn S, Imhoff AB: The anatomic reconstruction of acromioclavicular joint dislocations using 2 Tight Rope devices: A biome chanical study. *Am J Sports Med* 2008;36（12）:2398–2406.

改良）包括 DCR 联合将前肩峰及 CA 韧带骨块转移到切除表面的手术，重建 4 股 CC 韧带，并将其缝合锚定在喙突和锁骨表面进行增强[54]（图 19-9）。该技术的基本原理是转移骨块愈合后通过移植物维持复位，进而形成动态重建。在该研究中，8 例患者骨块完全愈合，2 例患者部分愈合。由于没有发现缺损的影响，所有患者对结果都较满意。在最后一次随访中，只有 1 例患者在术后第 3 个月时没有恢复工作能力或达到受伤前的运动水平。[54]虽然这种重建方法不是解剖学重建，但两束钛缆在一定程度上模仿了 CC 韧带的走向和生物学性质。目前尚未发表关节镜下自体肌腱解剖学重建的临床研究。

一些外科医师在 CC 韧带重建时切除远端锁骨，发现原位 CC 移植物负荷随着 AC 关节的切除而增加，但 DCR 不会引起负荷的进一步增加。移植物增加的负荷远低于使其失效的负荷，并且没有明显的临床意义。[55]

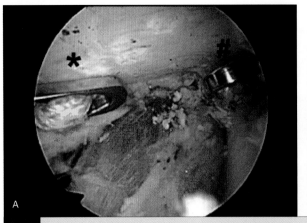
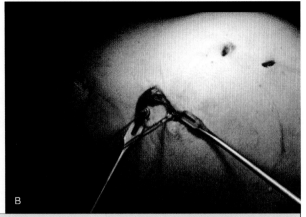

图 19-8 关节镜下使用两根钛缆辅助 CC 关节重建。A. 关节镜下前外侧入路的视图。B. 放置两枚锁骨侧纽扣后 AC 关节复位和固定。*= 后内侧入路可见锥状韧带；#= 前外侧入路可见斜方韧带。经允许引自 Salzmann GM, Walz L, Buchmann S, Glabgly P, Venjakob A, Imhoff AB: Arthroscopically assisted 2-bundle anatomic reduction of acute acromioclavicular joint separations. *Am J Sports Med* 2010;38（6）:1179-1187.

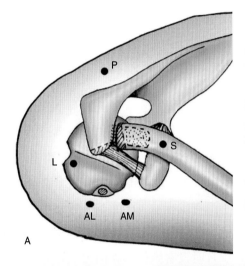
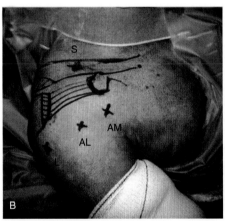
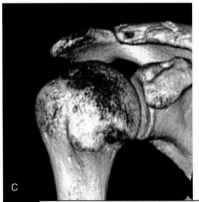
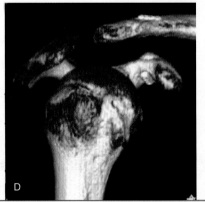
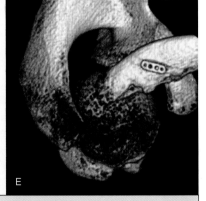

图 19-9 全关节镜下 Weaver-Dunn-Chuinard 改良修复。入路的示意图（A）和照片（B）。在冠状面（C）、矢状面（D）和轴向平面（E）上的三维 CT 重建显示锁骨外侧和喙突下方的纽扣放置。AL= 前外侧；AM= 前内侧；L= 外侧；P= 后部；S= 上部。经允许引自 Boileau P, Old J, Gastaud O, Brassart N, Roussanne Y: All-arthroscopic Weaver-Dunn-Chuinard procedure with double-button fixation for chronic acromioclavicular joint dislocation. *Arthroscopy* 2010;26（2）:149-160.

肩峰小骨

肩峰小骨由肩胛骨肩峰骨化中心未融合而产生。肩峰小骨通常在放射学检查中被偶然发现，它有可能导致疼痛和肩袖撞击。肩峰小骨的发病率约为 8%，最常见于男性和非洲人后裔。[56]

肩峰由肩峰基底、后部、中部和前部组成（图 19-10）。大约在 25 岁时整个肩峰融合在一起。后三角肌纤维、中三角肌纤维和前三角肌纤维分别附着于后肩峰、中肩峰和前肩峰。前肩峰也是 CA 韧带的锚定处。

诊断

肩峰小骨下撞击的任何症状都是肩峰下撞击的典型特征，包括抬高活动引起的疼痛。体格检查可发现冲击试验阳性、肩袖无力、骨不连处有触痛感。在 X 线检查、CT、MRI 和骨扫描中常可看到肩峰小骨（图 19-11）。

治疗

肩峰小骨引起的症状的初始治疗包括 NSAIDs 治疗、物理治疗和皮质类固醇注射。[56]如果非手术治疗不成功，可以选择几种手术方式。开放手术切除远端骨块可造成多种结果，其中三角肌损伤往往导致最差的预后。开放切除仅适用于小的前肩峰碎片。[57]关节镜切除可能具有较低的三角肌损伤率且可以去除较大的碎片，但尚未有对比

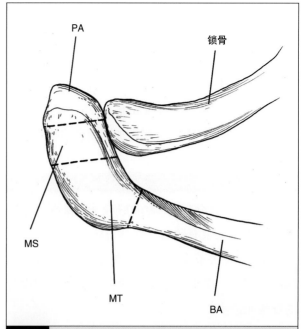

图 19-10　肩峰骨化中心的示意图。BA= 肩峰基部；MT= 肩峰后部；MS= 肩峰中部；PA= 肩峰前部。经允许引自 Kurtz CA, Humble BJ, Rodosky MW, Sekiya JK: Symptomatic os acromiale. *J Am Acad Orthop Surg* 2006;14（1）:12-19.

性研究文献。[58]已有成功的开放复位、空心螺钉内固定和张力带重建的报道，但不愈合的发生率很高，通常需要去除固定物。[58-59]

肩峰小骨下撞击通常采用简单的肩峰成形术治疗，只留下一个薄的皮质壳，并继续压缩到不愈合部位。应特别注意，不要侵犯三角肌附件，以

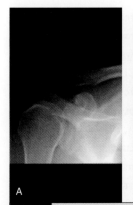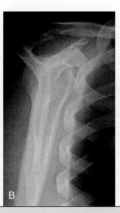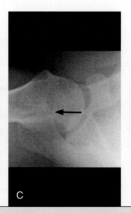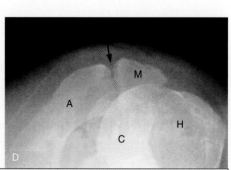

图 19-11　右肩的 AP 位（A）、出口位（B）、腋外侧位（C）和肩峰侧位（D）片显示在后肩峰和中肩峰之间的间隙（箭头）。A= 肩峰；C= 锁骨；H= 肱骨头；M= 肩峰中部。经允许引自 Kurtz CA, Humble BJ, Rodosky MW, Sekiya JK: Symptomatic os acromiale. *J Am Acad Orthop Surg* 2006;14（1）:12-19.

避免产生不稳定碎片。DCR 往往可避免这种情况，但通常无须进行，因为通过积极的肩峰成形术即可实现 AC 关节减压。[57] 在 13 例出现肩峰小骨不稳定症状的患者中，有 11 例在 ASD 后取得了较为满意的预后。[60] 然而，肩峰成形术难以治愈动态撞击，并且可能因碎片不稳定而加剧撞击症状。[59]

总结

关节镜治疗对许多影响肩峰下间隙和 AC 关节的疾病是安全有效的，包括肩峰下撞击、肩袖综合征、AC 关节炎、锁骨远端骨溶解、AC 分离和肩峰肥大。关节镜手术可能会随着技术和设备的发展而进步。

参考文献

[1] Neer CS II: Anterior acromioplasty for the chronic impingement syndrome in the shoulder: A preliminary report. *J Bone Joint Surg Am* 1972;54(1):41-50.

[2] Burns WC II, Whipple TL: Anatomic relationships in the shoulder impingement syndrome. *Clin Orthop Relat Res* 1993;294:96-102.

[3] Flatow EL, Soslowsky LJ, Ticker JB, et al: Excursion of the rotator cuff under the acromion: Patterns of subacromial contact. *Am J Sports Med* 1994;22(6):779-788.

[4] Flatow EL, Colman WW, Kelkar R, et al: The effect of anterior acromioplasty on rotator cuff contact: An experimental and computer simulation. *J Shoulder Elbow Surg* 1995;4:S53-S54 7856802

[5] Pedowitz RA, Yamaguchi K, Ahmad CS, et al: American Academy of Orthopaedic Surgeons Clinical Practice Guideline on: Optimizing the management of rotator cuff problems. *J Bone Joint Surg Am* 2012;94(2):163-167.
The authors discuss issues related to the Clinical Practice Guideline on management of the rotator cuff.

[6] Gerber C, Galantay RV, Hersche O: The pattern of pain produced by irritation of the acromioclavicular joint and the subacromial space. *J Shoulder Elbow Surg* 1998;7(4):352-355.

[7] Roberts CS, Davila JN, Hushek SG, Tillett ED, Corrigan TM: Magnetic resonance imaging analysis of the subacromial space in the impingement sign positions. *J Shoulder Elbow Surg* 2002;11(6):595-599.

[8] Jia X, Ji JH, Pannirselvam V, Petersen SA, McFarland EG: Does a positive Neer impingement sign reflect rotator cuff contact with the acromion? *Clin Orthop Relat Res* 2011;469(3):813-818.
The high correlation between arthroscopic evaluation of the arm position at which the rotator cuff contacts the superior glenoid and the position of pain in patients with a positive Neer impingement sign suggests that rotator cuff–glenoid contact, not rotator cuff–acromion contact, may be the immediate cause of impingement symptoms.

[9] Pappas GP, Blemker SS, Beaulieu CF, McAdams TR, Whalen ST, Gold GE: In vivo anatomy of the Neer and Hawkins sign positions for shoulder impingement. *J Shoulder Elbow Surg* 2006;15(1):40-49.

[10] Valadie AL III, Jobe CM, Pink MM, Ekman EF, Jobe FW: Anatomy of provocative tests for impingement syndrome of the shoulder. *J Shoulder Elbow Surg* 2000;9(1):36-46.

[11] Park HB, Yokota A, Gill HS, El Rassi G, McFarland EG: Diagnostic accuracy of clinical tests for the different degrees of subacromial impingement syndrome. *J Bone Joint Surg Am* 2005;87(7):1446-1455.

[12] Mayerhoefer ME, Breitenseher MJ, Wurnig C, Roposch A: Shoulder impingement: Relationship of clinical symptoms and imaging criteria. *Clin J Sport Med* 2009;19(2):83-89.
A cross-sectional study of the anatomic relationships and symptoms of impingement syndrome found that the Constant score was correlated with acromiohumeral distance but not with acromial morphology.

[13] Harrison AK, Flatow EL: Subacromial impingement syndrome. *J Am Acad Orthop Surg* 2011;19(11):701-708.
The pathophysiology and treatment of subacromial impingement syndrome were reviewed.

[14] Kim YS, Bigliani LU, Fujisawa M, et al: Stromal cell-derived factor 1 (SDF-1, CXCL12) is increased in subacromial bursitis and downregulated by steroid and nonsteroidal anti-inflammatory agents. *J Orthop Res* 2006;24(8):1756-1764.

[15] Labianca R, Sarzi-Puttini P, Zuccaro SM, Cherubino P, Vellucci R, Fornasari D: Adverse effects associated with non-opioid and opioid treatment in patients with chronic pain. *Clin Drug Investig* 2012;32(suppl 1):53-63.
The benefits and adverse effect profiles of opioid and nonopioid pain medications were described.

[16] Cohen DB, Kawamura S, Ehteshami JR, Rodeo SA: In-

domethacin and celecoxib impair rotator cuff tendon- to-bone healing. *Am J Sports Med* 2006;34(3):362-369.

[17] Holmgren T, Björnsson Hallgren H, Öberg B, Adolfsson L, Johansson K: Effect of specific exercise strategy on need for surgery in patients with subacromial impingement syndrome: Randomised controlled study. *BMJ* 2012;344:e787.

Compared with nonspecific physical rehabilitation, a 12-week course of manual mobilization, eccentric rotator cuff strengthening, and concentric-eccentric strengthening of scapular stabilizers led to decreases in pain and the need for surgery in patients with subacromial impingement after unsuccessful nonsurgical measures. Level of evidence: I.

[18] Buchbinder R, Green S, Youd JM: Corticosteroid injections for shoulder pain. *Cochrane Database Syst Rev* 2003;1:CD004016.

[19] Mikolyzk DK, Wei AS, Tonino P, et al: Effect of corticosteroids on the biomechanical strength of rat rotator cuff tendon. *J Bone Joint Surg Am* 2009;91(5):1172-1180.

In rats, a 50%-thickness infraspinatus tear was created. The rats receiving a single injection of methylprednisolone had a transient decrease in biomechanical strength and an increase in fat cells and collagen attenuation.

[20] Aaron DL, Bruce BG, Cote M, et al: Abstract: Novel anti-inflammatory agent and CXCR4 inhibitor (AMD3100)does not impede rotator cuff tendon healing in an animal model. *Annual Meeting Proceedings.* Rosemont, IL, American Academy of Orthopaedic Surgeons, presentation 074. http://www.aaos.org/ education/ education.asp. Accessed January 2, 2013.

In a biomechanical comparison of injured rat infraspinatus tendons, no weakening was noted with the administration of an inhibitor of SDF-1α–mediated subacromial bursal inflammation (AMD 3100).

[21] Checroun AJ, Dennis MG, Zuckerman JD: Open versus arthroscopic decompression for subacromial impingement: A comprehensive review of the literature from the last 25 years. *Bull Hosp Jt Dis* 1998;57(3):145-151.

[22] Davis AD, Kakar S, Moros C, Kaye EK, Schepsis AA, Voloshin I: Arthroscopic versus open acromioplasty: A meta-analysis. *Am J Sports Med* 2010;38(3):613-618.

A meta-analysis of studies of open and arthroscopic acromioplasty outcomes found that arthroscopic technique led to faster return to work and fewer inpatient hospital days. No other significant differences were found. Level of evidence: III.

[23] Norlin R, Adolfsson L: Small full-thickness tears do well ten to thirteen years after arthroscopic subacromial decompression. *J Shoulder Elbow Surg* 2008;17(1, suppl):12S-16S.

In a study of 181 patients who underwent arthroscopic subacromial decompression, those with a small, full-thickness supraspinatus tear had the best results at to 13-year follow-up. The authors concluded that repair of a small, full-thickness supraspinatus tear may be unnecessary and that subacromial decompression may be adequate.

[24] Björnsson H, Norlin R, Knutsson A, Adolfsson L: Fewer rotator cuff tears fifteen years after arthroscopic subacromial decompression. *J Shoulder Elbow Surg* 2010;19(1):111-115.

Rotator cuff integrity was determined by ultrasound in patients who had undergone subacromial decompression 15 years earlier. The prevalence of partial tears was 14% and full tears was 4%, compared with a 40%prevalence of degenerative tears in agematched historical control subjects. Level of evidence: III.

[25] Milano G, Grasso A, Salvatore M, Zarelli D, Deriu L, Fabbriciani C: Arthroscopic rotator cuff repair with and without subacromial decompression: A prospective randomized study. *Arthroscopy* 2007;23(1):81-88.

A prospective comparison of functional outcomes in patients undergoing rotator cuff repair with or without concurrent subacromial decompression found no significant differences at 2-year follow-up. Level of evidence: I.

[26] Gartsman GM, O'Connor DP: Arthroscopic rotator cuff repair with and without arthroscopic subacromial decompression: A prospective, randomized study of one-year outcomes. *J Shoulder Elbow Surg* 2004;13(4):424-426.

[27] MacDonald P, McRae S, Leiter J, Mascarenhas R, Lapner P: Arthroscopic rotator cuff repair with and without acromioplasty in the treatment of full- thickness rotator cuff tears: A multicenter, randomized controlled trial. *J Bone Joint Surg Am* 2011;93(21):1953-1960.

A comparison of outcomes after isolated rotator cuff repair or rotator cuff repair with acromioplasty found no differences in outcome scores, but patients who underwent isolated repair had a higher reoperation rate. Level of evidence: I.

[28] Chahal J, Mall N, MacDonald PB, et al: The role of

subcromial decompression in patients undergoing arthroscopic repair of full-thickness tears of the rotator cuff: A systematic review and meta-analysis. *Arthroscopy* 2012;28(5):720-727.

A meta-analysis of four level I studies found no differences in outcome after rotator cuff repair alone and with acromioplasty. Level of evidence: I.

［29］Noh KC, Chung KJ, Yu HS, Koh SH, Yoo JH: Arthroscopic treatment of septic arthritis of acromioclavicular joint. *Clin Orthop Surg* 2010;2(3):186-190.

Septic arthritis of the AC joint was successfully treated with arthroscopic débridement and distal clavicle resection in a case report.

［30］Zanca P: Shoulder pain: Involvement of the acromioclavicular joint: (Analysis of 1,000 cases). *Am J Roentgenol Radium Ther Nucl Med* 1971;112(3):493-506.

［31］Rios CG, Arciero RA, Mazzocca AD: Anatomy of the clavicle and coracoid process for reconstruction of the coracoclavicular ligaments. *Am J Sports Med* 2007;35(5):811-817.

In an anatomic description of the distance between the distal clavicle end and the insertion points of the CC ligaments in fresh-frozen cadaver and dry osteologic specimens, the ratios of clavicle length to the distance between the clavicle end and insertion points were found to be consistent in men and women and may serve as a guide to the creation of bone tunnels for an- atomic CC reconstruction.

［32］Walton J, Mahajan S, Paxinos A, et al: Diagnostic values of tests for acromioclavicular joint pain. *J Bone Joint Surg Am* 2004;86(4):807-812.

［33］van Riet RP, Bell SN: Clinical evaluation of acromioclavicular joint pathology: Sensitivity of a new test. *J Shoulder Elbow Surg* 2011;20(1):73-76.

A new test for AC pathology, consisting of cross-body adduction with elevation against resistance in internal rotation, had a sensitivity of 98%, which was higher than that of four other tests.

［34］Mazzocca AD, Spang JT, Rodriguez RR, et al: Biomechanical and radiographic analysis of partial coracoclavicular ligament injuries. *Am J Sports Med* 2008;36(7):1397-1402.

The authors studied whether injury to the conoid or trapezoid ligament would result in acromioclavicular joint instability following complete acromioclavicular joint injury.

［35］Girish G, Lobo LG, Jacobson JA, Morag Y, Miller B, Jamadar DA: Ultrasound of the shoulder: Asymptomatic findings in men. *AJR Am J Roentgenol* 2011;197(4):W713-719.

Ultrasound examination of the shoulder found abnormalities in 96% of the asymptomatic subjects, the most common of which were thickening of the subacromial and subdeltoid bursae, AC joint arthritis, and supraspinatus tendinosis.

［36］van Riet RP, Goehre T, Bell SN: The long term effect of an intra-articular injection of corticosteroids in the acromioclavicular joint. *J Shoulder Elbow Surg* 2012;21(3):376-379.

A prospective study of the efficacy of corticosteroid–local anesthetic injection into the AC joint found that the immediate diagnostic value was high; 28% of the patients had pain relief at 1-month follow-up that endured to the final average 42-month follow-up.

［37］Flatow EL, Cordasco FA, Bigliani LU: Arthroscopic resection of the outer end of the clavicle from a superior approach: A critical, quantitative, radiographic assessment of bone removal. *Arthroscopy* 1992;8(1):55-64.

［38］Beitzel K, Sablan N, Chowaniec DM, et al: Sequential resection of the distal clavicle and its effects on horizontal acromioclavicular joint translation. *Am J Sports Med* 2012;40(3):681-685.

A cadaver biomechanical study of AC joint stability after CC reconstruction and sequential resection of the distal clavicle found significantly greater instability after 10 mm of clavicle resection.

［39］Elhassan B, Ozbaydar M, Diller D, Massimini D, Higgins LD, Warner JJ: Open versus arthroscopic acromioclavicular joint resection: A retrospective comparison study. *Arthroscopy* 2009;25(11):1224-1232.

A retrospective comparison of open and arthroscopic distal clavicle resection found no statistically significant difference. Level of evidence: IV.

［40］Robertson WJ, Griffith MH, Carroll K, O'Donnell T, Gill TJ: Arthroscopic versus open distal clavicle excision: A comparative assessment at intermediate-term follow-up. *Am J Sports Med* 2011;39(11):2415-2420.

A review of functional and subjective outcomes of open and arthroscopic distal clavicle resection found similar functional scores. Patients who underwent arthroscopic resection had less pain at intermediate-term follow-up. Level of evidence: III.

［41］Pensak M, Grumet RC, Slabaugh MA, Bach BR Jr: Open versus arthroscopic distal clavicle resection. *Ar-*

throscopy 2010;26(5):697-704.

A review of outcome studies of open and arthroscopic distal clavicle resection found better subjective outcomes with arthroscopic procedures, with the direct approach permitting earlier return to athletics. Outcomes were worse in patients with posttraumatic arthrosis than in those with osteoarthritis or osteolysis. Level of evidence: III.

[42] Zawadsky M, Marra G, Wiater JM, et al: Osteolysis of the distal clavicle: Long-term results of arthroscopic resection. *Arthroscopy* 2000;16(6):600-605.

[43] Kim J, Chung J, Ok H: Asymptomatic acromioclavicular joint arthritis in arthroscopic rotator cuff tendon repair: A prospective randomized comparison study. *Arch Orthop Trauma Surg* 2011;131(3):363-369.

In a randomized prospective comparison of patients with a full-thickness rotator cuff tear and asymptomatic AC joint arthritis with inferior osteophytes, as diagnosed by radiographs, one group underwent isolated rotator cuff repair and the other group underwent rotator cuff repair with distal clavicle resection. Pain and functional scores were lower after distal clavicle resection at 6 and 12 weeks but were higher at 2 years.

[44] Tossy JD, Mead NC, Sigmond HM: Acromioclavicular separations: Useful and practical classification for treatment. *Clin Orthop Relat Res* 1963;28:111-119.

[45] Rockwood CA, Williams GR, Young DC: *Rockwood and Green's Fractures in Adults*, ed 3. Philadelphia, PA, JB Lippincott, 1991, pp 1181-1239.

[46] Barnes CJ, Higgins LD, Major NM, Basamania CJ: Magnetic resonance imaging of the coracoclavicular ligaments: Its role in defining pathoanatomy at the acromioclavicular joint. *J Surg Orthop Adv* 2004;13(2):69-75.

[47] Costic RS, Labriola JE, Rodosky MW, Debski RE: Biomechanical rationale for development of anatomical reconstructions of coracoclavicular ligaments after complete acromioclavicular joint dislocations. *Am J Sports Med* 2004;32(8):1929-1936.

[48] Mazzocca AD, Santangelo SA, Johnson ST, Rios CG, Dumonski ML, Arciero RA: A biomechanical evaluation of an anatomical coracoclavicular ligament reconstruction. *Am J Sports Med* 2006;34(2):236-246.

[49] Grutter PW, Petersen SA: Anatomical acromioclavicular ligament reconstruction: A biomechanical comparison of reconstructive techniques of the acromioclavicular joint. *Am J Sports Med* 2005;33(11):1723-1728.

[50] Chernchujit B, Tischer T, Imhoff AB: Arthroscopic reconstruction of the acromioclavicular joint disruption: Surgical technique and preliminary results. *Arch Orthop Trauma Surg* 2006;126(9):575-581.

[51] Thiel E, Mutnal A, Gilot GJ: Surgical outcome following arthroscopic fixation of acromioclavicular joint disruption with the TightRope device. *Orthopedics* 2011;34(7):e267-e274.

A cohort study of high-grade AC separations and one distal clavicle fracture treated with the TightRope device found a 16.67% rate of fixation failure. Patient satisfaction and functional scores were high.

[52] Walz L, Salzmann GM, Fabbro T, Eichhorn S, Imhoff AB: The anatomic reconstruction of acromioclavicular joint dislocations using 2 TightRope devices: A biomechanical study. *Am J Sports Med* 2008;36(12):2398-2406.

A biomechanical cadaver study of anatomic reconstruction of CC ligaments with two TightRope devices found a higher load to failure compared with native ligaments.

[53] Salzmann GM, Walz L, Buchmann S, Glabgly P, Venjakob A, Imhoff AB: Arthroscopically assisted 2-bundle anatomical reduction of acute acromioclavicular joint separations. *Am J Sports Med* 2010;38(6):1179-1187.

Arthroscopically assisted AC joint reduction with two flip-button devices to anatomically reconstruct the CC ligaments found improved pain and functional scores postoperatively, even in patients with radiographic loss of reduction (8 of 23 patients). Level of evidence: IV.

[54] Boileau P, Old J, Gastaud O, Brassart N, Roussanne Y: All-arthroscopic Weaver-Dunn-Chuinard procedure with double-button fixation for chronic acromioclavicular joint dislocation. *Arthroscopy* 2010;26(2):149-160.

Chronic, severe AC separations were treated with an all-arthroscopic Weaver-Dunn-Chuinard procedure augmented with a four-strand suture reconstruction of the CC ligaments. No loss of reduction was seen, all symptoms resolved, and functional outcome scores were high. Level of evidence:IV.

[55] Kowalsky MS, Kremenic IJ, Orishimo KF, McHugh MP, Nicholas SJ, Lee SJ: The effect of distal clavicle excision on in situ graft forces in coracoclavicular ligament reconstruction. *Am J Sports Med* 2010;38(11):2313-2319.

A biomechanical cadaver study assessed in situ graft forces in CC reconstruction, with or without sectioning of the AC ligaments and distal clavicle resection. Higher forces were seen with AC ligament sectioning, but distal clavicle resection did not substantially exacerbate this effect. Although the results were statistically significant, clinical significance could not be established because the increased forces on the graft after AC ligament sectioning and distal clavicle resection remained much lower than load to failure.

[56] Kurtz CA, Humble BJ, Rodosky MW, Sekiya JK: Symptomatic os acromiale. *J Am Acad Orthop Surg* 2006;14(1):12-19.

[57] Ortiguera CJ, Buss DD: Surgical management of the symptomatic os acromiale. *J Shoulder Elbow Surg* 2002;11(5):521-528.

[58] Harris JD, Griesser MJ, Jones GL: Systematic review of the surgical treatment for symptomatic os acromiale. *Int J Shoulder Surg* 2011;5(1):9-16.

A review of level I through IV evidence of surgical treatment of symptomatic os acromiale found that all evaluated techniques improved outcomes.

[59] Warner JJ, Beim GM, Higgins L: The treatment of symptomatic os acromiale. *J Bone Joint Surg Am* 1998;80(9):1320-1326.

[60] Wright RW, Heller MA, Quick DC, Buss DD: Arthroscopic decompression for impingement syndrome secondary to an unstable os acromiale. *Arthroscopy* 2000;16(6):595-599.

第二十章 关节镜下肩袖修复术

Charles M. Jobin, MD; Jay D. Keener, MD; Ken Yamaguchi, MD

引言

与开放手术相比，关节镜下肩袖修复术的预后良好，并发症发生率低，因而被广泛使用。肩袖修复的目标是减轻疼痛症状，获得肌腱－骨愈合，最大限度地恢复功能并尽可能改变肩袖疾病的自然病史。术后需要几个月的时间才能恢复功能，并且结构的愈合因患者及与撕裂相关的许多因素的不同而差别很大。相比再次撕裂后手术，初次手术的功能预后通常更好。最近的研究认为患者年龄、撕裂大小和慢性撕裂是影响修复完整性的最重要因素。结构修复的失败可能导致持续的肩关节无力，但是患者的满意度和临床结局不一定受肌腱愈合的影响。没有强有力的临床证据支持哪一种结构更优，最佳的修复固定结构仍是一个备受关注的研究课题。更好地了解肩袖撕裂的自然病史、年龄对肩袖疾病发生率和修复潜力的强烈影响，以及修复策略的优化，将有助于外科医师改良手术干预的适应证，并针对特定的患者和撕裂特征选择最佳的修复结构。

流行病学

年龄相关的退行性撕裂比创伤性撕裂更常见，尽管许多退行性撕裂是因剧烈伸展而出现症状的。[1]退行性肩袖撕裂的发病机制仍然存在争议，它可能是外在的机械撞击因素和内在的生物学因素共同作用的结果。[2]一项纳入 588 例单侧肩痛患者的自然病史研究发现，撕裂的发生率与患者年龄密切相关。[3]退行性肩袖撕裂通常发生在肩袖新月区内的冈上肌止点和冈下肌止点的交界处附近，此处是一个血运相对较差的区域，受周围的肩袖组织保护（图 20-1）。

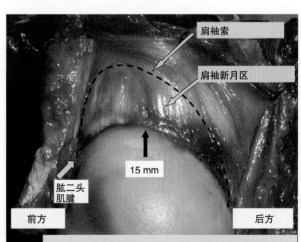

肩袖索

肩袖新月区

15 mm

肱二头肌腱

前方　　　　后方

图 20-1　照片显示了肩袖新月区，此处是肩袖撕裂的常见部位。肩袖新月区由肩袖索的悬吊结构支撑。经允许引自 Kim HM, Dahiya N, Teefey SA, et al: Location and initiation of degenerative rotator cuff tears: An analysis of three hundred and sixty shoulders. *J Bone Joint Surg Am* 2010;92（5）:1088–1096.

Dr. Yamaguchi or an immediate family member has received royalties from Tornier. Neither of the following authors nor any immediate family member has received anything of value from or has stock or stock options held in a commercial company or institution related directly or indirectly to the subject of this chapter: Dr. Jobin and Dr. Keener.

自然病史

肩袖疾病通常是进行性发展的，而且撕裂发生后肌腱自然愈合的能力很弱。自然病史研究发现，伴有疼痛的撕裂在2.5~5年内在撕裂大小方面的进展速度约为50%，而无症状撕裂的进展速度较慢，为30%。[4-5]年龄可能是撕裂进展的重要危险因素，60岁以上的患者撕裂进展率为54%，而较年轻的患者为17%。[6]有症状撕裂与冈上肌萎缩和Goutallier 2级及以上的脂肪浸润有关。[7]吸烟也与肩袖撕裂的进展有关，撕裂大小与之呈剂量和时间相关性。[8-9]

外源性因素与内源性因素

撞击是肩袖疾病中被描述最广泛的潜在外在因素。冈上肌出口处的肩袖反复机械磨损可能会导致撕裂。肩峰形态学分型的观察者间信度较差，并且很难与肩袖疾病相关联。肩峰骨刺因喙肩韧带内骨化而形成，可能提示存在慢性固有性肩袖病。肩峰骨刺的存在与年龄增长及囊侧和全层肩袖撕裂的发生有关。[10-11]在压力接触研究中，当处于诱发位时，未发现肩峰撞击。[12]3项随机对照研究和1项荟萃分析显示，在肩袖修复期间常规行肩峰成形术并未改善疼痛或预后评分。[13-16]应用肩峰成形术和清创术治疗的肩袖部分撕裂不能阻止撕裂随时间进展。[17]一项研究发现，肩峰横向指数，即肩峰相对于肱骨的横向投影的量度，与肩袖疾病和全层肩袖撕裂相关，然而其他研究没有发现这种关联。[10,18]肩袖疾病与年龄、双侧肩袖撕裂的频繁出现、与年龄相关的肩袖组织学变化，以及创伤与疼痛发作之间并不密切的联系密切相关，提示大多数退行性肩袖撕裂有一个主要的固有病因或生物学病因。

解剖学进展

肌腱止点的重建或许可以改善愈合效果和肩袖的解剖学功能。近期对肩袖止点的解剖学研究表明，冈上肌腱末端和冈下肌腱末端有重要的融合，冈上肌止点更小，冈下肌止点边缘更靠前方（图20-2）。较早期的研究将这些肌腱的止点分为两个不同的区域，这两个区域在大结节上的宽度几乎相等。在此之后，又发现一个冈上肌的更靠前的止点，它包裹了部分小结节。[19]冈下肌在大结节侧面止于结节间沟后2 mm处（图20-3）。这一发现或许可以解释之前认为是孤立存在的在冈上肌撕裂中见到的冈下肌脂肪变化。

累及前方肩袖索的冈上肌前方撕裂已逐渐被认为是冈上肌和冈下肌脂肪变化进展的危险因素。[20]前方的肩袖索撕裂紧邻肱二头肌腱，并牵涉肱二头肌侧方吊带。这些撕裂会破坏肩袖索的悬吊效果，从而使较薄的新月区产生更大的张力。一项研究发现，撕裂口与肱二头肌腱的接近程度与冈

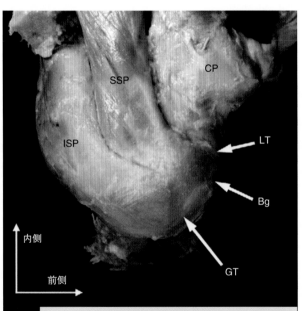

图 20-2 　照片显示了终末肩袖肌腱的附丽点，包括冈上肌（SSP）终末肌腱和冈下肌（ISP）终末肌腱的融合、冈下肌腱末端的前矢量以及跨越至小结节（LT）前方的冈上肌腱。CP = 喙突；Bg = 结节间沟；GT = 大结节。经允许引自 Mochizuki T, Sugaya H, Uomizu M, et al: Humeral insertion of the supraspinatus and infraspinatus: New anatomical findings regarding the footprint of the rotator cuff. *J Bone Joint Surg Am* 2008;90（5）:962-969.

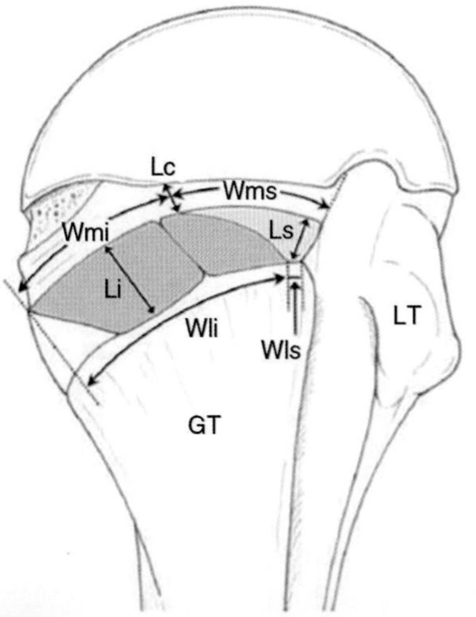

	平均值 ± 标准差（mm）
冈上肌	
最大内外径	6.9 ± 1.4
内侧缘前后宽度	12.6 ± 2.0
外侧缘前后宽度	1.3 ± 1.4
冈下肌	
最大内外径	10.2 ± 1.6
内侧缘前后宽度	20.2 ± 6.2
外侧缘前后宽度	32.7 ± 3.4
前方关节囊	
冈上肌止点后缘内侧长度	4.5 ± 0.5

图 20-3 肩袖止点的解剖尺寸示意及这些尺寸的平均值。冈上肌止点内外侧长度较此前研究小。冈上肌止点延伸至小结节，与关节囊融合，共用很长一段长度。GT= 大结节；Lc= 关节囊长度；Li= 冈下肌止点长度；Ls= 冈上肌止点长度；LT= 小结节；Wli= 冈下肌外侧止点宽度；Wls= 冈上肌外侧止点宽度；Wmi= 冈下肌内侧止点宽度；Wms= 冈上肌内侧止点宽度。经允许引自 Mochizuki T, Sugaya H, Uomizu M, et al:Humeral insertion of the supraspinatus and infraspinatus: New anatomical findings regarding the footprint of therotator cuff. *J Bone Joint Surg Am* 2008;90（5）:962-969.

上肌退行性改变密切相关。[21]超声检查发现，在冈上肌前侧肌腱完好无损的撕裂中，仅有11%发展为冈上肌退行性变。

肩袖肌肉的脂肪变性

肌肉脂肪变化和肌肉萎缩的发展与全层肩袖撕裂有关，这是一个具有时间依赖性的过程。肌肉脂肪变性通常被认为是不可逆的。Goutallier描述了脂肪浸润与撕裂大小和慢性撕裂的相关性。[22]脂肪变化的分级对外科医师确定最佳的手术适应证至关重要。在出现高等级脂肪变性之前，应尝试修复肌腱，这样能提高肌腱的愈合能力和手术的临床效果。此阈值可能是Goutallier 2级（脂肪量和肌肉量相等），研究发现，当处于这个等级或更高等级时，肌腱愈合能力降低，肩关节的力量和预后评分更低。[23-24]

对脂肪变性的自然病史研究表明，重要的肌肉变化在疼痛发作2.5年后发生。冈上肌在症状

发生后平均3年，出现中度的脂肪变化，到平均5年时出现严重的脂肪变化和肌肉萎缩。[25]急性冈上肌断裂后的6个月内就可发现进一步的变化。一项冈下肌脂肪变化的重点研究发现，发展为中度脂肪变化的时间为2.5年，发展为重度脂肪变化的时间为4年。[26]关于脂肪变性的回顾性报告有一些固有的局限性，因为撕裂的持续时间是未知的，特别是在退行性肩袖疾病中，可能从无症状撕裂开始。冈下肌脂肪变性的发生率高于冈上肌，并且可能在推测为仅冈上肌撕裂时发生。[27]冈下肌退行性改变尚未被完全了解，但可能与肩袖止点插入的异常解剖结构、冈下肌羽状角的改变、继发于肌腱回缩的肩胛上神经运动支牵拉以及失用性萎缩等有关。

修复伴有脂肪改变的肩袖后，可观察到持续性无力和功能评分降低。[22-23]撕裂修复后的肩袖肌腱可能会限制或减慢脂肪浸润的进程，但不能逆转。[23]在完整修复平均2年后，Goutallier等级

平均提高了 0.5 级。[24] 引起脂肪变化的生物学原因仍存在争议，脂肪变化进展导致的肌肉功能丧失是一个临床上的困境。一项动物模型研究发现，慢性肩袖撕裂会导致力量损失 50%、活动行为减少 68%、肌腱偏移减少 35%。[28] 应用电刺激的人体研究发现，肩袖肌张力与 Goutallier 等级具有很强的相关性。Goutallier 3 级时最大肌张力降低了 70%。[29] 即使肌腱成功愈合，不可逆的肌肉变化也可能影响功能预后和力量。

修复结构的生物力学

肩袖修复结构的生物力学已经在尸体模型中被广泛研究。虽然对最佳拔出强度、肌腱-骨加压和肌腱-骨间隙的理解逐渐深入，但是对这些研究进展的临床转化尚不清楚。修复的最终目标是在力学失效前将肌腱-骨界面进行生物学上的修复。肌腱-骨界面的微小运动、肌腱-骨界面的适当加压（或并置）以及最重要的良好的生物学条件，都可能促进生物学上的修复。

抓取组织的缝线结构，例如，改良的 Mason-Allen 针，能提供最佳的肌腱固定，但很难在关节镜下操作。经骨修复失败通常涉及拔出穿过骨的缝线。缝线锚定结构通常在缝线-肌腱界面处破裂，而且缝线会穿过肌腱。无论缝线结构最终拉力载荷和循环载荷的刚度如何，双排修复在生物力学上似乎都优于大多数单排修复。[30-31] 在肱骨旋转改变过程中，缝线承受循环载荷，相比于单排修复或经骨修复，双排修复具有更好的固定强度。[32]

经骨等效缝线桥技术将肌腱压到骨骼，其加压区域比单排固定宽（图 20-4）。[33] 传统的经骨修复与单排修复相比能恢复更大的止点，而双排锚定修复可以连续地重建大多数原始止点。从生物力学上来说，经骨等效修复具有更大的极限载荷强度，但在循环载荷下与传统的双排修复具有相似的刚度。[34] 与双排修复相比，经骨等效修复

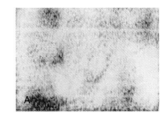
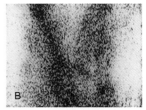
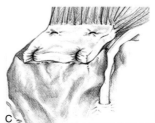
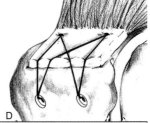

图 20-4 经骨等效缝线桥技术对肌腱到骨的加压比双排锚定的点固定修复更好。可以从内侧到外侧或从前方到后方创建缝线桥。压敏胶片（A 和 B）和示意图（C 和 D）显示了双排缝线锚定技术（A 和 C）和经骨等效缝线桥技术（B 和 D）的肌腱-骨加压情况。经允许引自 Park MC, ElAttrache NS, Tibone JE, Ahmad CS, Jun BJ, Lee TQ: Part I: Footprint contact characteristics for a transosseous-equivalent rotator cuff repair technique compared with a double-row repair technique. *J Shoulder Elbow Surg* 2007; 16（4）: 461-468.

还可以提供更大的肌腱-骨加压接触面积。[33] 结节性骨质减少或囊性变性可能影响锚定质量，因此应用缝线桥技术及选择更坚固的外侧皮质骨的策略被提倡使用。近期，防水修补再次被讨论，该技术在修补部位除去了滑液中的降解酶并保留了愈合因子。经骨等效结构在尸体模型中关节液外渗最少。[35]

多普勒超声发现，愈合部位的主要血供来自大结节锚定位点和肩袖浅表囊周层。[36] 肩袖修复增大的力量和压力可能会导致意想不到的后果，例如，内侧肌腱再撕裂概率增加及肌腱末端血供减少。一项对双排缝线桥结构的研究发现，60% 的再撕裂是由内行缝线周围断裂引起的，伴有到肌腱末端的连续性丧失。[37] 这些内侧的再撕裂（图 20-5）引起了研究者的担忧，因为缺乏肌腱末端可能会影响翻修肩袖的修复。目前，尚不

清楚导致这些再撕裂的原因，但一些证据表明，双排修复可能损害肌腱末端的血供。一项研究发现双排修复后肌腱末端的血流量直接减少了45%，这引起了研究者们对过度加压的修复结构的生物愈合潜力的担忧。[38] 然而，另一项超声研究发现，在肩袖修复后的最初几个月内，肌腱灌注增加，这表明尽管修复时进行了加压，但血管分布仍可恢复。[39]

影响修复完整性的因素

许多因素影响修复完整性，定义它们将有助于将研究重点放在影响患者预后的最重要因素上。影响修复完整性的最重要因素可能是年龄及其对修复后愈合能力的影响，而不是修复结构本身。[40-46] 一项关于孤立性冈上肌修复的研究发现，65岁以上患者的治愈率为45%，而年轻患者的治愈率为86%。[40] 另一项针对65岁以上患者的研究发现，

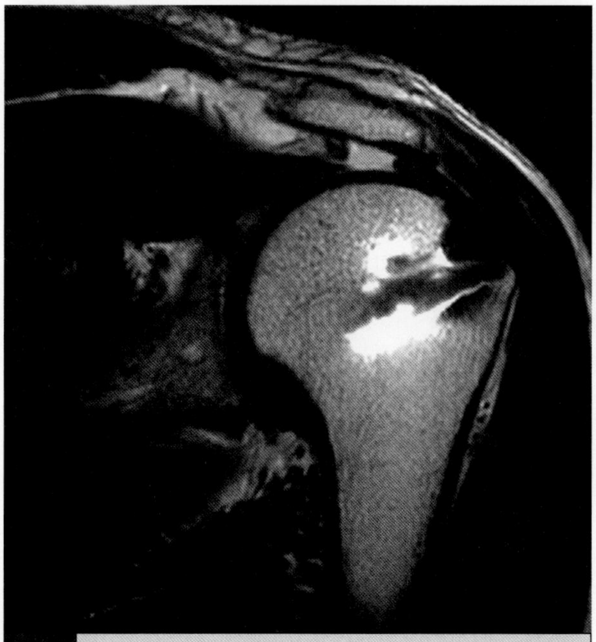

图 20-5　MRI 显示双排修复后再次撕裂。缺乏肌腱可能会阻碍肩袖修复。经允许引自 Koh KH, Kang KC, Lim TK, Shon MS, Yoo JC: Prospective randomized clinical trial of single- versus double-row suture anchor repair in 2- to 4-cm rotator cuff tears: Clinical and magnetic resonance imaging results. *Arthroscopy* 2011;27（4）:453-462.

术后第6个月的CT检查证实，部分再撕裂或全部再撕裂分别占25%和42%。[45] 术后第1年和第2年的超声检查发现，愈合的患者的平均年龄为58岁，而复发性撕裂的患者的平均年龄为64岁。此项研究发现，年龄因素可能被撕裂大小和慢性化等因素所掩盖了。

撕裂大小、慢性撕裂和Goutallier分级与修复失败密切相关。即使采用双排结构，较大的撕裂的愈合速度依然很慢。一项研究发现，双腱撕裂的愈合率为36%，而单腱撕裂的愈合率为67%。[43] 一项对23项研究中的1252例修复进行的系统评价发现，撕裂大小与修复后再撕裂之间存在很强的相关性。[29] 小于1 cm的撕裂的再撕裂率是7%~17%，而大于5 cm的撕裂的再撕裂率为41%~69%。肌肉变化也会影响修复的结果。一项研究发现，Goutallier 2级脂肪浸润患者的冈上肌再撕裂率高达40%，而Goutallier 0级或1级患者则为14%~18%。[24] 愈合受年龄、症状持续时间和肩袖肌肉萎缩的影响。

修复结构被认为是肌腱愈合的重要影响因素。一些对单排修复的研究发现，其术后再撕裂的发生率非常高。大和巨大（大于3 cm）肩袖撕裂行单排修复后的再撕裂率为76%~94%。[47] 平均大小为2.6 cm的撕裂在磁共振造影（MRA）上的缺陷率为88%。[48] 然而，这些研究没有足够的对照组来进行充分的比较。

大多数更高级别的研究还未发现双排修复可以大幅提高修复的完整性。一项对单排修复和双排修复进行比较的 I 级随机对照研究发现，如MRI所示，二者的全层或部分再撕裂率无统计学差异。[49] 另一项 I 级随机对照研究发现，单排和双排修复结构的再撕裂率均为10%，双排修复治疗的患者肌腱重度变薄的发生率为10%。[50] 第三个 I 级随机对照研究发现，单排修复和双排修复2年后，通过MRA检查得到的全层再撕裂率非常低，二者的差异无统计学意义（分别为8%和

4%）。[51] 一些证据水平较低的研究发现，双排修复结构具有更好的结构完整性，但这些研究存在设计缺陷，应谨慎参考。一项Ⅱ级队列研究发现，CT关节造影时双排修复在解剖学上获得了比单排修复更高的愈合率（分别为 61% 和 40%），但 Constant 肩关节评分无临床差异。[52] 一项Ⅲ级回顾性队列研究发现，单排修复后的再撕裂率为 25%，而双排修复后仅为 10%。[53] 一些研究者建议，具有更高的肩袖强度的年轻患者可能会受益于更坚固的双排结构。

人们对大量关于单排和双排修复的比较研究加以综合的尝试，得出了对临床预后和结构预后的系统综述。一篇对 6 项研究（3 项为Ⅰ级随机对照研究）的系统综述发现，对大于 3 cm 的撕裂采用双排修复似乎结构的愈合更好，患者有功能获益的可能性，但得到的证据是不确定的。[54] 一项对 23 项研究（包括 21 项Ⅳ级案例研究）的系统综述得出的结论是，撕裂大于 1 cm 的患者双排修复后的再撕裂率较低。[55] 这些系统综述的结论很难解释，因为从设计上讲，它们包含易于偏倚的研究。控制了年龄、撕裂大小和肌肉变化情况的研究应该能更好地确定双排修复的适应证。

手术治疗

适应证和禁忌证

传统上手术修复的适应证是在使用 NSAIDs、物理疗法和类固醇或局部止痛注射等非手术治疗失败后 3~6 个月的有症状的全层或较大的部分肩袖撕裂。相对于患者较年轻的创伤性撕裂，急性撕裂或慢性撕裂并发明确的急性延展伴功能下降是更加紧急的外科手术修复适应证。急性肩袖撕裂在受伤 3 周内被成功修复的可能性最大。[56]

文献中对肩袖手术干预的适应证没有明确定义。最常见的修复适应证是非手术治疗失败（52%）、日常生活活动受限（31%）、非手术治疗持续时间过长（26%）和夜间疼痛（16%）。[57] 在对肩袖撕裂的自然病史有了更好的了解后，手术干预的适应证也在不断完善。出现全层肩袖撕裂并不是手术干预的绝对适应证，非手术治疗可能会缓解疼痛，有些此类撕裂无明显症状。[3,58] 越来越多的数据表明，随着时间的延长，肩袖撕裂的大小逐渐进展，肩袖开始出现症状，并出现不可逆的肌肉变化。这些考量为在 65 岁以下的患者出现实质性肌肉变性之前早期修复小型（或中型）全层撕裂或累及前冈上肌的撕裂提供了依据。不建议手术治疗无症状撕裂，但建议进行连续评估以监测症状发展和撕裂的进展。

肩袖修复的禁忌证包括充分的非手术治疗和患者无能力遵循术后限制或无法进行术后康复锻炼。相对禁忌证包括 65 岁以上患者的慢性退行性撕裂、影像学发现肱骨头向近端移动以及脂肪浸润高于 Goutallier 2 级，尤其是当脂肪浸润涉及多个肩袖肌肉时。撕裂回缩并非禁忌证，但是如果肩袖修复时张力过大，则可能导致结构失效。尽管结构失效的可能性很高，尝试修复仍可能是合理的，因为即使肌腱再次断裂，患者仍有良好的或优异的临床预后。[48] 此外，对较大的或回缩的撕裂进行部分修复可得到良好的临床效果，理论上有使冈下肌 - 冈上肌力偶复原的益处。

术前评估

术前评估包括评估肩关节运动、肩胛控制、肩袖强度、减弱征以及任何可能影响肩关节的疾病，例如，颈椎病、肩锁关节炎和肱二头肌刺激征。应进行标准 X 线检查，包括肩关节正位（AP 位）、肩胛骨正位（真正 AP 位）、腋位和肩胛骨 Y 位检查，来评估盂肱关节炎、钙化肌腱炎、肱骨近端移位和肩胛下肌撕裂（提示前方半脱位）。肱骨近端移位在临床上很重要，它意味着正常运动学被破坏，这通常与冈下肌腱撕裂有关。肩峰间隔小于或等于 7 mm 提示慢性肩袖撕裂较大，并可能意味着不可修复。[59] 应使用 MRI 或超声检查以确认肩袖撕裂的存在。MRI 和超声检查均能预测关节镜检查的结果，二者能以几乎相等的准确度显示出全层撕裂和部分撕裂，能定量回缩、撕裂大小和脂肪浸润。[60] MRI 的优点是可以显示软骨、骨骼和盂唇，因此可以排除其他病理情况。超声检查便宜快捷，患者的耐受性更好，但是需要具有肩部超声检查经验的技术人员。

手术决策

影响肩袖手术成功率的因素主要有 3 类：生物学因素、手术技术因素和环境因素。三者在一定程度上都可以被外科医师控制。生物学因素通常由患者特征决定，包括患者年龄、撕裂大小、肌肉和肌腱质量、骨骼质量，以及遗传因素。患者的选择和手术适应证是外科医师控制生物学因素的最佳手段。65 岁以下的患者相比 65 岁以上的患者更容易愈合。[40-46] 使用生物制剂来促进肌腱愈合是一个令人非常感兴趣的领域，但是很少有证据支持生物制剂的临床使用。[61] 大量研究表明，双排修复结构在力学上优于单排修复结构，但二者的临床预后相似。[31-32,50-51,58,62-63] 环境因素，如术后康复方案、患者依从性、患者吸烟状况以及 NSAIDs 的应用情况，都可能是受外科医师影响的重要变量。

尽管仅有有限的临床证据表明双排修复或其等效修复后患者的临床预后更好，但这些修复在生物力学上更具优势，可以更好地重建止点的解剖结构，并且在特定情况下患者可以获得更高的肌腱愈合率。必须权衡双排修复的优缺点，其缺点主要与成本和手术时间有关。如果患者肩袖的愈合潜力不佳，许多外科医师会选择进行双排修复，希望通过使用更强的力学结构克服生物学上的局限性。这个策略可能效果有限。大多数发生部分撕裂、中小型全层撕裂和急性撕裂的 62~65 岁的患者具有良好的固有生物学因素，可以进行单排修复或双排修复。双排修复通常在肌腱质量差、撕裂较大或肌肉退行性改变进展的情况下才考虑使用，这些情况通常发生在年龄较大且愈合能力

有限的患者中。在这些患者中，牢固的修复结构可能获益有限。需要进一步研究以完善根据患者年龄和撕裂特征所使用的特定修复结构的适应证。

手术技术

肩袖修复常规使用局部麻醉，可根据需要采用气管内全身麻醉作为补充。在患者采用沙滩椅位时使用全身麻醉而非局部麻醉，可能会增加脑氧合下降的风险。[64] 尽管沙滩椅位最常用，但根据医师的经验，也可采用侧卧位。应用下肢连续加压装置以在围手术期机械预防深静脉血栓形成。铰接臂定位器用于在手术过程中控制患者四肢。肩峰下注射丁哌卡因与肾上腺素可能有助于止血。麻醉下检查可帮助确定伴随的关节僵硬或不稳定。

后视口可以位于标准位置，即距后外侧肩峰远端 2 cm，内侧 1 cm 处。而正对后外侧肩峰远端的更偏外侧的后视口可更好地观察肩峰下间隙。在肩袖间隔内建立前视口后，手术从对盂肱关节的诊断性关节镜检查开始。仔细评估肩胛下肌、关节盂、关节软骨、肱二头肌腱、吊索和锚定点。在肩峰下间隙内，根据撕裂大小建立一个或两个外侧口。非常重要的是，要将所有的入口设计在足够靠近远端的位置，使器械在肩部逐渐肿胀的情况下仍能够进入肩峰下间隙。如果在肌腱运动和修复过程中使用了一个外侧口用于观察，则建议设计一个额外的外侧工作口和一个前肩峰下间隙口用于处理缝线。

全关节囊切除术后能观察到撕裂的肌腱。若有以喙肩韧带下表面磨损为特征的肩峰骨赘形成或机械撞击的证据，则可能需要行前外侧肩峰成形术。确定肩袖边界后，清除其边缘直至显露健康的肌腱组织。用剃刀去除软组织，修整出大结节上的止点，并轻轻地去除大结节的皮质，以利于血运。如果需要锚定，应避免完全去除皮质，因为这样做可能影响固定效果。

撕裂模式识别和肩袖活动范围评估对于恢复肌腱止点至关重要。从外侧口观察有助于识别撕

裂模式并评估肌腱分层情况。确定撕裂的前缘和后缘以避免张力不平衡或复位不良是非常重要的。在有些时候撕裂比较复杂，不同层之间会出现分层和不同程度的回缩。新月形或 C 形撕裂通常可以在张力不会过大的前提下移动到解剖止点上。L形、反 L 形或 U 形撕裂可能需要使用边缘汇聚技术进行内侧闭合。

为获得足够的活动范围，可能需要将撕裂肌腱的全关节盂和肩峰侧松解。设置牵张缝线来辅助肌腱松解，以评估肌腱活动范围并确定进一步粘连的部位。对于可回缩的冈上肌撕裂，可通过切除从肱二头肌悬吊装置至喙突根部的组织来松解前肩袖间隙。在更靠内侧的区域，附着在前冈上肌腱的喙肱附着物也应被松解。肩袖间隙滑动是对间隙松解的修正，可保留外侧肩袖间隙组织为复位肩袖解剖位置提供参考。上关节盂和肩袖下表面之间的上关节囊松解通常是有效果的。很少需要在冈上肌腱和冈下肌腱之间进行后方的松解。

通过改善缝线到骨和缝线到肌腱的固定、最小化缝线的磨损、提高缝线的强度、确保结和环的安全性以及恢复肌腱止点，可以优化修复体的初始生物力学强度。由于肩袖固定设备的技术进步，现在缝线 – 肌腱界面是修复结构中最薄弱的环节。肩袖修复失败的患者通常存在缝线撕裂肌腱的情况。经骨修复经常因缝线穿骨而失败，缝线锚钉改善了骨固定部位，尤其是在循环载荷下。机械固定最终会在循环载荷下失效，因此必须进行生物学上的肌腱 – 骨愈合。

修复结构包括经骨缝合、单排、双排、经骨等效缝线桥、张力带、张力带与缝线桥相结合以及其他缝线桥结构，具有多样性（图 20-6）。所有结构都试图在张力不过大的前提下模仿解剖结构以减少肌腱并将其固定到肌腱止点上。如果使用内排锚钉，则将其放置在关节边缘附近。必须注意不要使内侧缝合太靠近内侧，因为这样做可能使肌腱外侧化并在修复过程中造成过大的张力。

可以使用内排结，若计划使用缝线桥结构，则将缝线尾部从结节上方的外侧引出并固定以将肌腱末端压到止点处。距离止点外缘远端 1~2 cm 处的大结节外侧面是坚硬的骨皮质，非常适合应用外排缝线桥技术。

在一些手术中，例如，在伴有结节骨丢失、大结节囊肿或骨质疏松的肩袖翻修手术中，结节可能不适合缝线锚钉固定。结合外侧骨皮质的经骨修复可能是唯一具有可靠强度固定点的修复技术。还有一种可行的技术是张力带技术，当肩关节内收时，它可以将肩袖的张力转变为将肌腱压至其止点的压力。[40,65] 张力带技术获得了早期的临床成功，其修复孤立的冈上肌撕裂有 70% 的修复完整性。

对复杂撕裂模式的纵向面的边缘汇聚或边到边修复有助于修复原本几乎无法修复的肩袖撕裂。关键是要识别出撕裂模式，并了解冈下肌常沿后内侧方向回缩，造成前内侧纵向撕裂。这些撕裂通常呈 U 形、L 形或反 L 形。在肌腱 – 骨修复之前，应从内侧到外侧进行边缘汇聚修复，使肌腱止点的位置推向更外侧，从而减少最终肌腱 – 骨修复结构的张力。

对于不能完全修复的撕裂应该考虑进行部分修复。较大的撕裂在部分修复后，即使修复结构失效，也可改善症状。[66] 一项针对大撕裂的Ⅲ级队列研究将 45 例完全修复与 41 例部分修复进行了比较，随访 2 年后发现患者的 UCLA 肩关节评分无明显差别。[67] 在一项纳入 27 例患者的病例研究中，1 例患者存在无法修复的 4.2 cm 撕裂，经部分修复和边缘汇聚后残留缺损为 1.2 cm，其预后良好。[68] 患侧肩关节的肩关节简明测试、Constant 肩关节评分和 UCLA 肩关节评分的得分显著提高，但力量显著弱于对侧肩关节。部分修复可使患者获益的原理尚不清楚。部分修复可能通过重新分配载荷来重新创建平衡的受力偶，并保护剩余的未受损肩袖免受过大的张力，或者其益处可能来自滑囊切除术、清创术或其他相关过程。

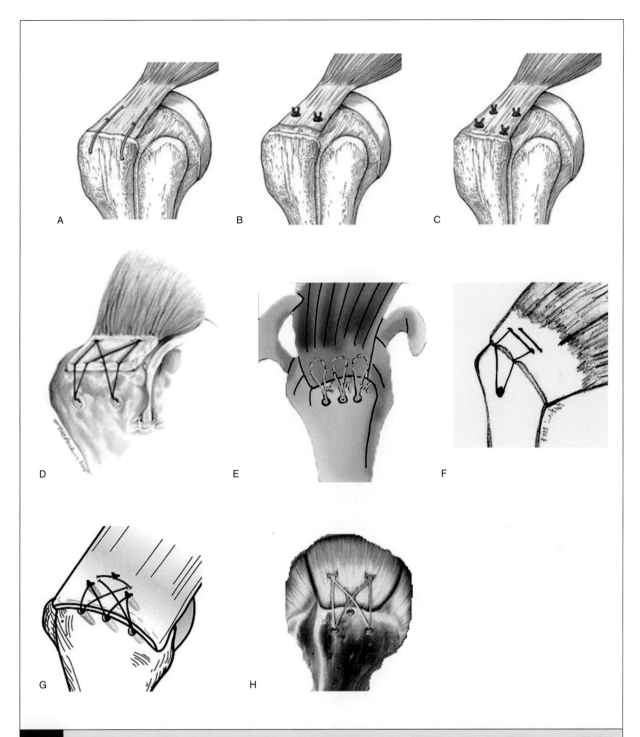

图
20-6　肩袖修复结构示意图。修复结构的多样性，共同的原则是点固定、缝线桥加压和张力带压迫。A. 经骨缝线结构。B. 单排结构。C. 双排结构。D. 经骨等效缝线桥（2 个内排锚钉和外侧缝线桥）。E. 张力带（水平垫倒置，缝线从侧面固定）。F. 罗马桥结构（2 个内排锚钉，带有 2 个前后缝线桥和 1 个外侧缝线桥的双内排、双载荷锚钉）。G. 菱纹缝线桥（2 个内排锚钉，带有 1 个前后缝线桥和 1 个外侧缝线桥的 3 个锚钉的双内排、双载荷锚钉缝线桥）。H. 三排结构（中央张力带修复和经骨等效缝合桥）

术后康复

尽管尚无高等级的证据支持，但术后康复对成功恢复至关重要。[69]一项设计巧妙的研究发现，在进行肩袖修复后，受监督的物理治疗的效果并未优于居家锻炼的效果。[70]肩袖修复后的康复方案反映出关于固定与早期运动的自相矛盾的观点。固定可以使肌腱修复免于过度拉伸，并有利于改善修复部位的结构特性，但早期会出现僵硬。早期运动可以预防僵硬并减轻疼痛，但会增加修复部位的压力。延后运动的康复方案通常为固定联合有限的被动运动6周，之后进行主动辅助运动，术后第3个月时开始主动运动，第4个月时进行抗阻力锻炼。早期运动方案为术后2周内进行被动运动，通常在6周内开始进行主动辅助运动。

肩袖修复后愈合时间较长是推迟术后早期运动的一种论据。修复结构在术后的前3个月内有撕裂或失效的可能性，这表明这段时间对于肌腱愈合至关重要。在一项对大于3 cm的撕裂的修复术后2天~2年的随访中，应用系列超声研究发现，再撕裂大多发生在术后的前3个月（78%），少数发生在术后3~6个月（22%）。[71]一项针对修复中型至大型肩袖撕裂的系列MRI研究发现，修复结构的状态在术后6~19个月未发现变化。[72]还有一项系列超声研究发现，在术后第1年随访中所有完整的修复结构在第2年随访中仍保持完整。[42]

肌腱愈合的生物力学影响康复方案。肩袖张力随盂肱关节的运动增加，例如，张力随向前抬高和外旋而增加。动物研究发现，与早期运动相比，固定可通过改善机械特性来促进肌腱-骨愈合，并改善组织学特性。[73]大鼠模型中，完全去除负荷对肌腱愈合不利。[74]

肩袖修复后的僵硬度与开放手术及三角肌下粘连的进展有关。一篇关节镜下肩袖修复的综述发现，必要时关节镜下松解后，成功恢复运动的患者的僵硬率为0~4%。[75]僵硬可能是肌腱愈合的指标。术后6周内肩关节僵硬的患者的再撕裂率低于肩关节活动范围较大的患者（两者的再撕裂率分别为30%和64%）。[76]

为了有足够的时间进行肌腱的早期愈合，建议大多数患者进行延后运动的物理治疗。肩关节使用吊带固定6周，在进行完好无损的结构修复后允许进行钟摆运动。在术后第6周时取下吊带，并开始进行被动运动。在术后第8~10周时，允许进行主动辅助运动。主动运动被推迟到术后第12周，4个月后才可以进行强化运动。

临床预后

在大多数患者中，肩袖修复的预后为良好到优秀。精心设计的研究通常发现预后得分、肩关节运动和疼痛程度均有改善。典型的手臂、肩膀和手部残疾（DASH）问卷的评分为10~20分，Constant肩关节评分为75~100分，ASES肩关节疼痛和功能障碍评分为85~95分，UCLA肩关节评分为28~35分，视觉模拟疼痛评分为1~3分，前举力量强度约6 kg。[54-55,63,77]肩袖修复的成功与否，不取决于修复的完整性，即使出现修复结构失效，疼痛、功能和预后评分得到改善的情况仍很常见。在一项研究中，有94%的患者发生了再撕裂，但是其中72%的患者的ASES肩关节疼痛和功能障碍评分高于90分。[66]患者满意度及临床成功与修复的完整性没有直接关系。[78]一篇包含13项关于修复完整性对临床预后影响的研究的系统评价发现，修复的完整性与强度的改善在统计学上和临床上都有相关性，但大多数预后指标未反映出这种改善。[79]该综述发现，基于最小的临床重要差异（超过5 kg或Constant肩关节评分的20%），前举强度在统计学上有改善。使用最小的临床重要差异标准进行评估，预后得分很少具有统计学显著性，并且没有临床意义上的显著差异。总之，这个系统评价支持以下观点：患者满意度和功能评分不取决于修复的完整性，但是完整愈合的修复可能会使力量提高。

肩袖修复后的长期临床预后令人满意，尽管

尚不清楚修复结构的长期完整性。一项对全层修复的为期 10 年的随访研究发现，临床预后并没有随着时间的推移而变差，患者残疾等级的提升可能由患者年龄的增长、活动量下降和肩关节需求下降所致。[80]一项对 33 例单排修复病例进行的术后平均 12.5 年的随访研究发现，88% 的患者的 UCLA 肩关节评分显示他们具有优异或良好的预后，并且没有运动障碍。[81]

单排修复与双排修复

无论采用单排修复还是双排修复，患者的预后一样好。一项 I 级随机对照研究对 62 例中型至大型撕裂（2~4 cm）的患者进行了 17 个月的随访，使用包含 MRI、视觉模拟量表或 ASES 肩关节疼痛和功能障碍评分、Constant 肩关节评分或 UCLA 肩关节评分进行了评估，发现其再撕裂率无差异，但双排修复的手术时间更长。[49]另一项 I 级随机对照研究对 80 名单排修复和双排修复患者随访 2 年后进行比较，发现他们的力量、DASH 评分及 Constant 肩关节评分无差异，但患者的年龄、性别和术前力量与预后相关。[63]一项 I 级研究使用连续 MRI 对 40 名平均撕裂大小为 1.8 cm 的单排和双排的修复患者进行了比较，发现他们的结构完整性、强度或运动情况、UCLA 肩关节评分、ASES 肩关节疼痛和功能障碍评分、Constant 肩关节评分、WOSI 评分和 SANE 评分等无差异。[50]一项 II 级队列研究对患者（平均年龄 56 岁）进行了 2 年以上的随访，发现双排修复和单排修复在 ASES 肩关节疼痛和功能障碍评分和 Constant 肩关节评分方面没有差异，但在对大到巨大撕裂（大于 3 cm）患者的亚组的分析中发现，双排修复的评分更高。[82]一项回顾性研究对单排修复或双排修复后的巨大撕裂病例进行了比较，发现在长期随访（超过 5 年）中双排修复的临床效果更好。[83]双排修复预后良好或优异的可能性是单排的 5 倍。双排修复还能提高 UCLA 肩关节评分，患者也感到肩膀接近正常的可能性更高。

有 4 篇系统综述没有提供重要的证据来支持双排修复在临床上优于单排修复，且均未发现二者的临床预后有显著差异。[54-55,77,84]其中，一篇系统综述基于一项 II 级研究说明大于 3 cm 的撕裂应用双排固定后可能有更好的 ASES 肩关节疼痛和功能障碍评分和 Constant 肩关节评分。[54]一篇系统综述发现，大于 1 cm 的撕裂可能从双排修复中获益，但是该综述仅包含一项 IV 级病例研究，并且经骨修复和单排修复被分在同一组。[55]还有一篇系统综述发现双排修复有功能优势的倾向。[84]

并发症

除再撕裂外，关节镜下肩袖修复很少出现并发症。一项纳入近 3000 例修复病例的回顾性研究发现，短暂性僵硬占 4%，内固定物相关问题占 0.5%，神经血管损伤占 0.2%，深层感染占 0.1%，血栓栓塞事件占 0.1%。[85]另一项研究发现，术后僵硬发生率仅为 10%，仅 3% 需要关节囊松解以恢复完全运动。[75]肩部功能的延迟恢复在肩袖修复后经常发生，尚未得到很好的描述。一项研究发现，只有 70% 的患者在术后 6 个月内恢复，延迟恢复的危险因素包括患者年龄、术前僵硬和撕裂大小。[86]

费用分析

与其他外科和内科治疗相比，肩袖修复是一种经济有效的治疗方法。肩袖修复的成本效益比约为每质量调整寿命年 3000~13 000 美元（约合人民币 20 000~85 000 元），具体取决于所使用的效用度量。与全髋关节置换术、冠状动脉搭桥术和高血压治疗相比，肩袖修复的成本效益比具有优势。[87]由于关节镜手术的器械和植入物的成本较高，所以开放式肩袖修复术比关节镜修复术的成本效益比更高。双排锚定修复的成本比单排修复更高，因为植入物成本更高且手术时间更长。[50-53,63,82]

循证策略

美国骨科医师学会最近发布了一篇治疗肩袖疾病的循证临床实践指南。[69]但遗憾的是，其中最重要的观点缺乏证据支持。该指南仅得出了少量结论：除全层撕裂外，应通过运动和使用非甾体抗炎药治疗肩袖疾病；肩袖修复时不需要常规行肩峰成形术；肩袖修复时不应使用猪肠补片；工伤赔偿诉求与肩袖修复的结果相对较差有关。

总结

如行关节镜下肩袖修复，需要对肌腱愈合的生物学潜力、环境因素和手术技术进行风险收益分析。影响肌腱愈合的最重要因素包括患者年龄、撕裂大小和慢性撕裂。如果进行外科手术修复，固定结构的选择可能对年轻患者的中小型撕裂不如对大撕裂或老年患者的撕裂重要，后者可能会从双排固定中受益。即使肌腱没有完整愈合，大多数患者也可从关节镜下肩袖修复中受益。与生物力学相比，肩袖修复受生物学的影响更大，必须加深对肌腱－骨愈合过程的理解以获得最佳预后。

参考文献

［1］ Mall NA, Kim HM, Keener JD, et al: Symptomatic progression of asymptomatic rotator cuff tears: A prospective study of clinical and sonographic variables. *J Bone Joint Surg Am* 2010;92(16):2623-2633.
The development of shoulder pain was associated with an increase in rotator cuff tear size in a prospective study of 195 patients who were asymptomatic. Level of evidence:III.

［2］ Papadonikolakis A, McKenna M, Warme W, Martin BI, Matsen FA III: Published evidence relevant to the diagnosis of impingement syndrome of the shoulder. *J Bone Joint Surg Am* 2011;93(19):1827-1832.
A systematic review tested the existence of impingement syndrome in terms of diagnosis, anatomy, pathophysiology, and surgical success and found little highlevel evidence. Level of evidence: II.

［3］ Yamaguchi K, Ditsios K, Middleton WD, Hildebolt CF, Galatz LM, Teefey SA: The demographic and morphological features of rotator cuff disease: A comparison of asymptomatic and symptomatic shoulders. *J Bone Joint Surg Am* 2006;88(8):1699-1704.

［4］ Yamaguchi K, Tetro AM, Blam O, Evanoff BA, Teefey SA, Middleton WD: Natural history of asymptomatic rotator cuff tears: A longitudinal analysis of asymptomatic tears detected sonographically. *J Shoulder Elbow Surg* 2001;10(3):199-203.

［5］ Safran O, Schroeder J, Bloom R, Weil Y, Milgrom C: Natural history of nonoperatively treated symptomatic rotator cuff tears in patients 60 years old or younger. *Am J Sports Med* 2011;39(4):710-714.
A longitudinal ultrasound study of 61 nonsurgically treated full-thickness cuff tears in patents younger than 60 years found an almost-50% progression of tear size at 2.5 years. Level of evidence: IV.

［6］ Maman E, Harris C, White L, Tomlinson G, Shashank M, Boynton E: Outcome of nonoperative treatment of symptomatic rotator cuff tears monitored by magnetic resonance imaging. *J Bone Joint Surg Am* 2009;91(8):1898-1906.
Age older than 60 years, a full-thickness tear, and fatty infiltration were the factors associated with progression of a rotator cuff tear on MRI. Level of evidence: IV.

［7］ Moosmayer S, Tariq R, Stiris MG, Smith HJ: MRI of symptomatic and asymptomatic full-thickness rotator cuff tears: A comparison of findings in 100 subjects. *Acta Orthop* 2010;81(3):361-366.
A retrospective case-control study found associations between symptoms and rotator cuff tear size greater than 3 cm, significant atrophy, and fatty degeneration of Goutallier grade 2 or higher. The causal relationships are unclear. Level of evidence: III.

［8］ Baumgarten KM, Gerlach D, Galatz LM, et al: Cigarette smoking increases the risk for rotator cuff tears. *Clin Orthop Relat Res* 2010;468(6):1534-1541.
A prospective cohort study found that the duration and dosage of cigarette smoking were correlated with an increased risk for rotator cuff tearing. Level of evidence: III.

［9］ Carbone S, Gumina S, Arceri V, Campagna V, Fagnani C, Postacchini F: The impact of preoperative smoking habit on rotator cuff tear: Cigarette smoking influences rotator cuff tear sizes. *J Shoulder Elbow Surg* 2012;21(1):56-60.
A cross-sectional survey of rotator cuff repairs found larger tears during arthroscopy among patients who were tobacco smokers compared with those who were not. A dosage and temporal relationship with tobacco use and rotator cuff tear size was seen. Level of evidence: IV.

［10］ Hamid N, Omid R, Yamaguchi K, Steger-May K, Stobbs G, Keener JD: Relationship of radiographic acromial characteristics and rotator cuff disease: A prospective investigation of clinical, radiographic, and sonographic findings. *J Shoulder Elbow Surg* 2012; 21(10):1289-1298.

The presence of an acromial spur was highly associated with rotator cuff tears in symptomatic and asymptomatic shoulders, but the acromial index had no association with rotator cuff tears. Level of evidence: III.

[11] Ogawa K, Yoshida A, Inokuchi W, Naniwa T: Acromial spur: Relationship to aging and morphologic changes in the rotator cuff. *J Shoulder Elbow Surg* 2005;14(6):591-598.

[12] Lee SB, Itoi E, O'Driscoll SW, An KN: Contact geometry at the undersurface of the acromion with and without a rotator cuff tear. *Arthroscopy* 2001;17(4): 365-372.

[13] Chahal J, Mall N, MacDonald PB, et al: The role of subacromial decompression in patients undergoing arthroscopic repair of full-thickness tears of the rotator cuff: A systematic review and meta-analysis. *Arthroscopy* 2012;28(5):720-727.

A systematic review of four level I studies found no statistically significant difference in subjective outcomes after arthroscopic rotator cuff repair with or without acromioplasty at intermediate follow-up. Level of evidence: I.

[14] Gartsman GM, O'Connor DP: Arthroscopic rotator cuff repair with and without arthroscopic subacromial decompression: A prospective, randomized study of one-year outcomes. *J Shoulder Elbow Surg* 2004; 13(4):424-426.

[15] Milano G, Grasso A, Salvatore M, Zarelli D, Deriu L, Fabbriciani C: Arthroscopic rotator cuff repair with and without subacromial decompression: A prospective randomized study. *Arthroscopy* 2007;23(1):81-88.

A randomized controlled study of 80 rotator cuff repairs with or without acromioplasty found no benefit in Constant, DASH, or work-DASH scores at shortterm follow-up. Level of evidence: I.

[16] MacDonald P, McRae S, Leiter J, Mascarenhas R, Lapner P: Arthroscopic rotator cuff repair with and without acromioplasty in the treatment of fullthickness rotator cuff tears: A multicenter, randomized controlled trial. *J Bone Joint Surg Am* 2011;93(21): 1953-1960.

A randomized controlled study of 86 rotator cuff repairs with or without acromioplasty found no difference in function and quality of life at 2-year follow-up, except a higher reoperation rate without acromioplasty.

There was no structural evaluation of healing. Level of evidence: I.

[17] Kartus J, Kartus C, Rostgård-Christensen L, Sernert N, Read J, Perko M: Long-term clinical and ultrasound evaluation after arthroscopic acromioplasty in patients with partial rotator cuff tears. *Arthroscopy* 2006; 22(1):44-49.

[18] Torrens C, López JM, Puente I, Cáceres E: The influence of the acromial coverage index in rotator cuff tears. *J Shoulder Elbow Surg* 2007;16(3):347-351.

A case control study found an increased acromial coverage index among patients with rotator cuff tears compared with normal control subjects. Level of evidence: III.

[19] Mochizuki T, Sugaya H, Uomizu M, et al: Humeral insertion of the supraspinatus and infraspinatus: New anatomical findings regarding the footprint of the rotator cuff. *J Bone Joint Surg Am* 2008;90(5):962-969.

A cadaver anatomic study of 113 shoulders found the supraspinatus tendon footprint to be much smaller than previously believed, and the greater tuberosity was occupied by a substantial amount of the infraspinatus.

[20] Kim HM, Dahiya N, Teefey SA, Keener JD, Galatz LM, Yamaguchi K: Relationship of tear size and location to fatty degeneration of the rotator cuff. *J Bone Joint Surg Am* 2010;92(4):829-839.

A prospective cohort of 262 tears evaluated by ultrasound found that fatty degeneration was closely associated with tear size and loss of integrity of the anterior supraspinatus tendon. Level of evidence: III.

[21] Kim HM, Dahiya N, Teefey SA, et al: Location and initiation of degenerative rotator cuff tears: An analysis of three hundred and sixty shoulders. *J Bone Joint Surg Am* 2010;92(5):1088-1096.

An ultrasound study of 360 rotator cuff tears found that degenerative tears most often involve the junction of the supraspinatus and infraspinatus tendons and may begin 13 to 17 mm posterior to the biceps tendon.

[22] Goutallier D, Postel JM, Gleyze P, Leguilloux P, Van Driessche S: Influence of cuff muscle fatty degeneration on anatomic and functional outcomes after simple suture of full-thickness tears. *J Shoulder Elbow Surg* 2003;12(6):550-554.

[23] Gladstone JN, Bishop JY, Lo IK, Flatow EL: Fatty infiltration and atrophy of the rotator cuff do not improve after rotator cuff repair and correlate with poor functional outcome. *Am J Sports Med* 2007;35(5): 719-728.

A MRI cohort study of rotator cuff repairs found that muscle fatty infiltration affected functional outcome, tear size affected repair integrity, and successful repair did not improve muscle degeneration. Muscle degeneration progressed after unsuccessful repair. Level of evidence: II.

[24] Liem D, Lichtenberg S, Magosch P, Habermeyer P: Magnetic resonance imaging of arthroscopic supraspinatus tendon repair. *J Bone Joint Surg Am* 2007;89(8): 1770-1776.

A cohort study found that fatty infiltration could not be reversed by successful rotator cuff repair. Severe preoperative fatty infiltration was associated with tear recurrence, progression of fatty infiltration, and inferior clinical results. Level of evidence: II.

[25] Melis B, DeFranco MJ, Chuinard C, Walch G: Natural history of fatty infiltration and atrophy of the supraspinatus muscle in rotator cuff tears. *Clin Orthop Relat Res* 2010;468(6):1498-1505.

A retrospective case study of 1,688 rotator cuff tears found that moderate supraspinatus fatty infiltration appeared 3 years after the onset of symptoms, and severe infiltration appeared at 5 years. Level of evidence: IV.

[26] Melis B, Wall B, Walch G: Natural history of infraspinatus fatty infiltration in rotator cuff tears. *J Shoulder Elbow Surg* 2010;19(5):757-763.

A retrospective case study of 1,688 rotator cuff tears found that relatively large tears, long duration, and older age were associated with more severe fatty infiltration of the infraspinatus. Grade 2 changes occurred 2.5 years after symptom onset. Level of evidence: IV.

[27] Cheung S, Dillon E, Tham SC, et al: The presence of fatty infiltration in the infraspinatus: Its relation with the condition of the supraspinatus tendon. *Arthroscopy* 2011;27(4):463-470.

This restrospective case series measured rotator cuff tears and MRI Goutallier changes of the supraspinatus and infraspinatus muscles. Increased infraspinatus fatty infiltration was correlated with severity of infraspinatus and supraspinatus tears. Significant infraspinatus fatty infiltration was seen in 18% of those shoulders without and infraspinatus tear. Level of evidence: IV.

[28] Meyer DC, Gerber C, Von Rechenberg B, Wirth SH, Farshad M: Amplitude and strength of muscle contraction are reduced in experimental tears of the rotator cuff. *Am J Sports Med* 2011;39(7):1456-1461.

An animal study created chronic rotator cuff tears in sheep and found loss of muscular strength and contractile amplitude in addition to retraction, fatty infiltration, and atrophy.

[29] Gerber C, Schneeberger AG, Hoppeler H, Meyer DC: Correlation of atrophy and fatty infiltration on strength and integrity of rotator cuff repairs: A study in thirteen patients. *J Shoulder Elbow Surg* 2007; 16(6):691-696.

A case series found that maximal tension of electrically stimulated supraspinatus muscles was strongly correlated with cross-sectional area and inversely with fatty infiltration. One year after successful tendon repair, fatty infiltration had not improved. Level of evidence: IV.

[30] Lorbach O, Bachelier F, Vees J, Kohn D, Pape D: Cyclic loading of rotator cuff reconstructions: Single-row repair with modified suture configurations versus double-row repair. *Am J Sports Med* 2008;36(8):1504- 1510.

A biomechanical study found that double-row anchor repairs with modified suture configurations offered the highest failure load and smallest gap formation.

[31] Kim DH, Elattrache NS, Tibone JE, et al: Biomechanical comparison of a single-row versus double-row suture anchor technique for rotator cuff repair. *Am J Sports Med* 2006;34(3):407-414.

[32] Ahmad CS, Kleweno C, Jacir AM, et al: Biomechanical performance of rotator cuff repairs with humeral rotation: A new rotator cuff repair failure model. *Am J Sports Med* 2008;36(5):888-892.

A cadaver study found that double-row repairs had better fixation strength than single-row repairs when exposed to cyclic loading and changes in humeral rotation.

[33] Park MC, ElAttrache NS, Tibone JE, Ahmad CS, Jun BJ, Lee TQ: Part I: Footprint contact characteristics for a transosseous-equivalent rotator cuff repair technique compared with a double-row repair technique. *J Shoulder Elbow Surg* 2007;16(4):461-468.

A cadaver rotator cuff repair study found better pressurized contact area and mean pressure with transosseous-equivalent suture-bridge repair when compared with double-row repair.

[34] Park MC, Tibone JE, ElAttrache NS, Ahmad CS, Jun BJ, Lee TQ: Part II: Biomechanical assessment for a footprint-restoring transosseous-equivalent rotator cuff repair technique compared with a double-row repair technique. *J Shoulder Elbow Surg* 2007;16(4): 469-476.

A cadaver biomechanical study found that a transosseous-equivalent suture-bridge repair improved failure loads and restored the footprint better than a double-row repair.

[35] Ahmad CS, Vorys GC, Covey A, Levine WN, Gardner TR, Bigliani LU: Rotator cuff repair fluid extravasation characteristics are influenced by repair technique. *J Shoulder Elbow Surg* 2009;18(6):976-981.

A cadaver study found better fluid extravasation characteristics with double-row suture-bridge repair than with single-row repair.

[36] Cadet ER, Adler RS, Gallo RA, et al: Contrastenhanced ultrasound characterization of the vascularity of the repaired rotator cuff tendon: Short-term and intermediate-term follow-up. *J Shoulder Elbow Surg* 2012;21(5):597-603.

A Doppler ultrasound study found that peribursal and bone anchor sites were the main conduits of blood flow for the rotator cuff tendon after arthroscopic repair and that flow increased with exercise.

[37] Cho NS, Lee BG, Rhee YG: Arthroscopic rotator cuff repair using a suture bridge technique: Is the repair integrity actually maintained? *Am J Sports Med* 2011; 39(10):2108-2116.

A case study of suture-bridge rotator cuff repairs found a 33% retear rate, with 66% of the retears at the musculotendinous junction. Retearing did not affect the subjective outcomes. Factors affecting healing were age, tear size, and fatty degeneration. Level of evidence:IV.

[38] Christoforetti JJ, Krupp RJ, Singleton SB, Kissenberth MJ, Cook C, Hawkins RJ: Arthroscopic suture bridge transosseous equivalent fixation of rotator cuff tendon preserves intratendinous blood flow at the time of initial fixation. *J Shoulder Elbow Surg* 2012;21(4): 523-530.

An immediate 45% reduction in terminal tendon blood flow was found by intraoperative laser Doppler flowmetry after the lateral row of a transosseousequivalent repair was tied down.

[39] Funakoshi T, Iwasaki N, Kamishima T, et al: In vivo vascularity alterations in repaired rotator cuffs determined by contrast-enhanced ultrasound. *Am J Sports Med* 2011;39(12):2640-2646.

A study measured tendon blood flow before and after rotator cuff repair and found increased flow at 1 and 2 months after surgery that decreased at 3 months, with more flow on the bursal side than on the articular tendon side.

[40] Boileau P, Brassart N, Watkinson DJ, Carles M, Hatzidakis AM, Krishnan SG: Arthroscopic repair of fullthickness tears of the supraspinatus: Does the tendon really heal? *J Bone Joint Surg Am* 2005;87(6):1229-1240.

[41] Keener JD, Wei AS, Kim HM, et al: Revision arthroscopic rotator cuff repair: Repair integrity and clinical outcome. *J Bone Joint Surg Am* 2010;92(3): 590-598.

A retrospective review found reliable outcomes after revision rotator cuff repair. Age and tear size were related to repair integrity, with only 27% of multitendon tears remaining healed. Repair integrity affected abduction strength and the Constant score. Level of evidence: IV.

[42] Nho SJ, Adler RS, Tomlinson DP, et al: Arthroscopic rotator cuff repair: Prospective evaluation with sequential ultrasonography. *Am J Sports Med* 2009; 37(10):1938-1945.

A sequential ultrasound study found the integrity of the repair was consistent at 1 and 2 years for 92.5% of patients. Level of evidence: III.

[43] Tashjian RZ, Hollins AM, Kim HM, et al: Factors affecting healing rates after arthroscopic double-row rotator cuff repair. *Am J Sports Med* 2010;38(12):2435-2442.

A case study found that older age and longer follow-up were associated with lower healing rates after double-row rotator cuff repair. Level of evidence: IV.

[44] Papadopoulos P, Karataglis D, Boutsiadis A, Fotiadou A, Christoforidis J, Christodoulou A: Functional outcome and structural integrity following mini-open repair of large and massive rotator cuff tears: A 3-5 year follow-up study. *J Shoulder Elbow Surg* 2011;20(1): 131-137.

A case study found that patient age, tear size, and retear size affected the final clinical outcomes. Level of evidence: IV.

[45] Charousset C, Bellaïche L, Kalra K, Petrover D: Arthroscopic repair of full-thickness rotator cuff tears: Is there tendon healing in patients aged 65 years or older? *Arthroscopy* 2010;26(3):302-309.

A case study of rotator cuff repairs in patients older than 65 years found a 42% retear rate despite improved function. These repairs were considered successful. Level of evidence: IV.

[46] Kamath G, Galatz LM, Keener JD, Teefey S, Middleton W, Yamaguchi K: Tendon integrity and functional outcome after arthroscopic repair of high-grade partial-thickness supraspinatus tears. *J Bone Joint Surg Am* 2009;91(5):1055-1062.

A case study found that arthroscopic repair of highgrade partial-thickness rotator cuff tears resulted in a high rate of tendon healing, and patient age was an important factor in tendon healing. Level of evidence: IV.

[47] Bishop J, Klepps S, Lo IK, Bird J, Gladstone JN, Flatow EL: Cuff integrity after arthroscopic versus open rotator cuff repair: A prospective study. *J Shoulder Elbow Surg* 2006;15(3):290-299.

[48] Meyer M, Klouche S, Rousselin B, Boru B, Bauer T, Hardy P: Does arthroscopic rotator cuff repair actually heal? Anatomic evaluation with magnetic resonance arthrography at minimum 2 years follow-up. *J Shoulder Elbow Surg* 2012;21(4):531-536.

A retrospective midterm study found good to excellent clinical outcomes after rotator cuff repair but an 88% rate of small or large defects on MRA. There was no correlation between clinical and anatomic outcomes. Level of evidence: IV.

[49] Koh KH, Kang KC, Lim TK, Shon MS, Yoo JC: Prospective randomized clinical trial of single- versus double-row suture anchor repair in 2- to 4-cm rotator cuff tears: Clinical and magnetic resonance imaging results. *Arthroscopy* 2011;27(4):453-462.

A randomized controlled study of 71 patients found similar clinical results and retear rates between doublerow and single-row repairs in medium-size to large rotator cuff tears. Level of evidence: I.

[50] Burks RT, Crim J, Brown N, Fink B, Greis PE: A prospective randomized clinical trial comparing arthroscopic single- and double-row rotator cuff repair: Magnetic resonance imaging and early clinical evaluation. *Am J Sports Med* 2009;37(4):674-682.

A randomized controlled study of 40 medium-size tears found no differences in clinical or MRI structural integrity between double- and single-row repairs as late as 1 year after surgery. Level of evidence: I.

[51] Franceschi F, Ruzzini L, Longo UG, et al: Equivalent clinical results of arthroscopic single-row and doublerow suture anchor repair for rotator cuff tears: A randomized controlled trial. *Am J Sports Med* 2007;35(8): 1254-1260.

A randomized controlled study of 60 patients found no clinical difference between single- and double-row repairs at 2-year follow-up, but there was a trend toward better structural healing in double-row repairs. Level of evidence: I.

[52] Charousset C, Grimberg J, Duranthon LD, Bellaiche L, Petrover D: Can a double-row anchorage technique improve tendon healing in arthroscopic rotator cuff repair? A prospective, nonrandomized, comparative study of double-row and single-row anchorage techniques with computed tomographic arthrography tendon healing assessment. *Am J Sports Med* 2007;35(8): 1247-1253.

A cohort study of 66 patients found no clinical difference between double- and single-row repairs, but there was better tendon healing on CT arthrography after double-row repair at 6-month follow-up. Level of evidence: II.

[53] Sugaya H, Maeda K, Matsuki K, Moriishi J: Functional and structural outcome after arthroscopic fullthickness rotator cuff repair: Single-row versus dualrow fixation. *Arthroscopy* 2005;21(11):1307-1316.

[54] Saridakis P, Jones G: Outcomes of single-row and double-row arthroscopic rotator cuff repair: A systematic review. *J Bone Joint Surg Am* 2010;92(3):732-742.

A systematic review of double- and single-row repairs found a trend toward improved structural healing with double-row fixation in large or massive rotator cuff tears.

[55] Duquin TR, Buyea C, Bisson LJ: Which method of rotator cuff repair leads to the highest rate of structural healing? A systematic review. *Am J Sports Med* 2010; 38(4):835-841.

A systematic review of 122 repairs from 23 studies, most of which contained level IV evidence, found that double-row repairs led to lower retear rates in tears larger than 1 cm. Level of evidence: IV.

[56] Lähteenmäki HE, Virolainen P, Hiltunen A, Heikkilä J, Nelimarkka OI: Results of early operative treatment of rotator cuff tears with acute symptoms. *J Shoulder Elbow Surg* 2006;15(2):148-153.

[57] Marx RG, Koulouvaris P, Chu SK, Levy BA: Indications for surgery in clinical outcome studies of rotator cuff repair. *Clin Orthop Relat Res* 2009;467(2): 450-456.

Patient characteristics and indications for surgery were found not to be described in most clinical outcome studies of rotator cuff repair. Level of evidence: III.

[58] Dunn W, Kuhn J: Effectiveness of physical therapy in treating atraumatic full thickness rotator cuff tears. *2011 Annual Meeting Proceedings*. Rosemont, IL, American Academy of Orthopaedic Surgeons, 2011, p 703.

This prospective cohort study of atraumatic full thickness rotator cuff tears found more than 90% of the patients elected for nonsurgical treatment after 3 months of physical therapy had significant improvement of ASES, Western Ontario Rotator Cuff, and Single Assessment Numeric Evaluation scores. This low rate of surgical care persisted at 2 years' follow-up, and data collection is ongoing. Level of evidence: II.

［59］Nové-Josserand L, Edwards TB, O'Connor DP, Walch G: The acromiohumeral and coracohumeral intervals are abnormal in rotator cuff tears with muscular fatty degeneration. *Clin Orthop Relat Res* 2005;433:90-96.

［60］Teefey SA, Rubin DA, Middleton WD, Hildebolt CF, Leibold RA, Yamaguchi K: Detection and quantification of rotator cuff tears: Comparison of ultrasonographic, magnetic resonance imaging, and arthroscopic findings in seventy-one consecutive cases. *J Bone Joint Surg Am* 2004;86(4):708-716.

［61］Isaac C, Gharaibeh B, Witt M, Wright VJ, Huard J: Biologic approaches to enhance rotator cuff healing after injury. *J Shoulder Elbow Surg* 2012;21(2):181-190.

A systematic review found a paucity of clinical research into the use of growth factors, stem cell therapy, and tissue-engineering augmentation for rotator cuff healing.

［62］Smith CD, Alexander S, Hill AM, et al: A biomechanical comparison of single and double-row fixation in arthroscopic rotator cuff repair. *J Bone Joint Surg Am* 2006;88(11):2425-2431.

［63］Grasso A, Milano G, Salvatore M, Falcone G, Deriu L, Fabbriciani C: Single-row versus double-row arthroscopic rotator cuff repair: A prospective randomized clinical study. Arthroscopy 2009;25(1):4-12.

A randomized controlled study of 80 patients found no difference between single- and double-row repairs clinically and structurally. Analysis showed that patient age, sex, and baseline strength influenced outcome. Level of evidence: I.

［64］Koh J, Levin S, Murphy G: Cerebral oxygenation in the beach chair position: The effect of general anesthesia compared to regional anesthesia. *2012 Annual Meeting* Proceedings. Rosemont, IL, American Academy of Orthopaedic Surgeons, 2012, p 911.

In a prospective study, 60 patients undergoing shoulder surgery in the beach chair position were tested for cerebral desaturation events to avoid neurologic injury. Patients with regional anesthesia and sedation had almost no cerebral desaturation events, unlike patients who had general anesthesia. Level of evidence: II.

［65］Millar NL, Wu X, Tantau R, Silverstone E, Murrell GA: Open versus two forms of arthroscopic rotator cuff repair. *Clin Orthop Relat Res* 2009;467(4):966- 978.

Arthroscopic knotless repairs had better healing rates compared with knotted or open repairs. The study was not controlled for tear size. Level of evidence: III.

［66］Galatz LM, Ball CM, Teefey SA, Middleton WD, Yamaguchi K: The outcome and repair integrity of completely arthroscopically repaired large and massive rotator cuff tears. *J Bone Joint Surg Am* 2004;86(2):219-224.

［67］Iagulli ND, Field LD, Hobgood ER, Ramsey JR, Savoie FH III: Comparison of partial versus complete arthroscopic repair of massive rotator cuff tears. *Am J Sports Med* 2012;40(5):1022-1026.

Retrospective review of 86 patients compared complete and partial repairs of massive rotator cuff tears, which had similarly good outcomes. Level of evidence: III.

［68］Kim SJ, Lee IS, Kim SH, Lee WY, Chun YM: Arthroscopic partial repair of irreparable large to massive rotator cuff tears. *Arthroscopy* 2012;28(6):761-768.

A case study of partial repairs of massive rotator cuff tears found satisfactory short-term outcomes. Level of evidence: IV.

［69］Pedowitz RA, Yamaguchi K, Ahmad CS, et al; American Academy of Orthopaedic Surgeons: Optimizing the management of rotator cuff problems. *J Am Acad Orthop Surg* 2011;19(6):368-379.

An AAOS workgroup found a lack of definitive evidence on most rotator cuff issues and made only four moderate-grade recommendations.

［70］Büker N, Kitis, A, Akkaya S, Akkaya N: [Comparison of the results of supervised physiotherapy program and home-based exercise program in patients treated with arthroscopic-assisted mini-open rotator cuff repair]. *Eklem Hastalik Cerrahisi* 2011;22(3):134-139.

No differences except cost were found between a home exercise program and supervised physical therapy in patients' pain, functional status, quality of life, and depression status.

［71］Miller BS, Downie BK, Kohen RB, et al: When do rotator cuff repairs fail? Serial ultrasound examination after arthroscopic repair of large and massive rotator cuff tears. *Am J Sports Med* 2011;39(10):2064-2070.

A serial ultrasound cohort study found that most retears occurred within the first 3 months and were associated with inferior clinical outcomes. Level of evidence: III.

［72］Koh KH, Laddha MS, Lim TK, Park JH, Yoo JC: Serial structural and functional assessments of rotator cuff repairs: Do they differ at 6 and 19 months postoperatively? *J Shoulder Elbow Surg* 2012;21(7):859-866.

A study found that the structural status of a rotator cuff repair could be assessed 6 months after surgery because the integrity of the rotator cuff did not change for as long as 2 years after surgery.

[73] Gimbel JA, Van Kleunen JP, Williams GR, Thomopoulos S, Soslowsky LJ: Long durations of immobilization in the rat result in enhanced mechanical properties of the healing supraspinatus tendon insertion site. *J Biomech Eng* 2007;129(3):400-404.

An animal study found that immobilizing the shoulder improves tendon-to-bone healing by increasing the organization of the collagen and subsequently increasing the mechanical properties.

[74] Galatz LM, Charlton N, Das R, Kim HM, Havlioglu N, Thomopoulos S: Complete removal of load is detrimental to rotator cuff healing. *J Shoulder Elbow Surg* 2009;18(5):669-675.

An animal study found that complete removal of load with pharmacologic paralysis was detrimental to rotator cuff healing, especially when combined with immobilization.

[75] Denard PJ, Lädermann A, Burkhart SS: Prevention and management of stiffness after arthroscopic rotator cuff repair: Systematic review and implications for rotator cuff healing. *Arthroscopy* 2011;27(6):842-848.

A systematic review found that postoperative stiffness resistant to nonsurgical management was uncommon, and arthroscopic capsular release could restore range of motion, if needed. Level of evidence: IV.

[76] Parsons BO, Gruson KI, Chen DD, Harrison AK, Gladstone J, Flatow EL: Does slower rehabilitation after arthroscopic rotator cuff repair lead to long-term stiffness? *J Shoulder Elbow Surg* 2010;19(7):1034-1039.

A retrospective case study found that sling immobilization for 6 weeks after arthroscopic rotator cuff repair did not result in increased long-term stiffness and could improve the rate of tendon healing.

[77] Nho SJ, Slabaugh MA, Seroyer ST, et al: Does the literature support double-row suture anchor fixation for arthroscopic rotator cuff repair? A systematic review comparing double-row and single-row suture anchor configuration. *Arthroscopy* 2009;25(11):1319-1328.

A systematic review found no clinical differences between single- and double-row repairs, but some studies reported that double-row repair might improve tendon healing. Level of evidence: III.

[78] Voigt C, Bosse C, Vosshenrich R, Schulz AP, Lill H: Arthroscopic supraspinatus tendon repair with suturebridging technique: Functional outcome and magnetic resonance imaging. *Am J Sports Med* 2010;38(5): 983-991.

A case study found similar functional outcomes with a suture-bridge technique compared with a double-row repair. Structural failure of the repair was not correlated with clinical failure. Age older than 60 years influenced tendon healing. Level of evidence: IV.

[79] Slabaugh MA, Nho SJ, Grumet RC, et al: Does the literature confirm superior clinical results in radiographically healed rotator cuffs after rotator cuff repair? *Arthroscopy* 2010;26(3):393-403.

A systematic review found increased strength in forward elevation in five of eight studies and improved Constant scores with an intact repair in six of nine studies. These results suggested that repair integrity may improve strength. Level of evidence: IV.

[80] Galatz LM, Griggs S, Cameron BD, Iannotti JP: Prospective longitudinal analysis of postoperative shoulder function: A ten-year follow-up study of fullthickness rotator cuff tears. *J Bone Joint Surg Am* 2001;83(7):1052-1056.

[81] Marrero LG, Nelman KR, Nottage WM: Long-term follow-up of arthroscopic rotator cuff repair. *Arthroscopy* 2011;27(7):885-888.

Retrospective review found that patients maintained good outcomes 10 years after rotator cuff repair. Level of evidence: IV.

[82] Park JY, Lhee SH, Choi JH, Park HK, Yu JW, Seo JB: Comparison of the clinical outcomes of single- and double-row repairs in rotator cuff tears. *Am J Sports Med* 2008;36(7):1310-1316.

A cohort study comparing double- and single-row repairs found better ASES scores, Constant scores, and strength in patients with a tear larger than 3 cm who were treated with a double-row technique. Level of evidence: II.

[83] Denard PJ, Jiwani AZ, Lädermann A, Burkhart SS: Long-term outcome of arthroscopic massive rotator cuff repair: The importance of double-row fixation. *Arthroscopy* 2012;28(7):909-915.

A retrospective comparative study found double-row repairs of massive rotator cuff tears to have 4.9 times more good or excellent outcomes than single-row repairs at a 5-year minimum follow-up. Level of evidence: III.

[84] DeHaan AM, Axelrad TW, Kaye E, Silvestri L, Puskas B, Foster TE: Does double-row rotator cuff repair improve functional outcome of patients compared with single-row technique? A systematic review. *Am J Sports*

Med 2012;40(5):1176-1185.

A systematic review found trends toward higher functional outcomes and a lower retear rate after a doublerow repair compared with a single-row repair.

[85] Randelli P, Spennacchio P, Ragone V, Arrigoni P, Casella A, Cabitza P: Complications associated with arthroscopic rotator cuff repair: A literature review. *Musculoskelet Surg* 2012;96(1):9-16.

Rotator cuff repair was found to be a low-risk surgical procedure. Failure of the repair was the most common complication.

[86] Manaka T, Ito Y, Matsumoto I, Takaoka K, Nakamura H: Functional recovery period after arthroscopic rotator cuff repair: Is it predictable before surgery? *Clin Orthop Relat Res* 2011;469(6):1660-1666.

Retrospective review found delayed recovery (more than 6 months) in 28% of patients after rotator cuff repair. Age, shoulder stiffness, and rotator cuff tear size influenced functional recovery time.

[87] Vitale MA, Vitale MG, Zivin JG, Braman JP, Bigliani LU, Flatow EL: Rotator cuff repair: An analysis of utility scores and cost-effectiveness. *J Shoulder Elbow Surg* 2007;16(2):181-187.

A cost-effectiveness study found that rotator cuff repairs compared favorably with other common healthcare interventions.

第二十一章　肱二头肌近端肌腱的镜下及切开治疗

Augustus D. Mazzocca, MS, MD; Mark P. Cote, PT, DPT, MSCTR; Knut Beitzel, MA, MD

引言

肱二头肌起自近端两个肌腱：肱二头肌长头腱（LHBT）及肱二头肌短头腱。LHBT 尤为重要，因其在肩胛盂关节中附着于盂上结节区域。[1] LHBT 起自上方盂唇的多条纤维，多数纤维起自上方盂唇的后方。[2] 关节内部分位于滑囊外，平均长度为 34.5 mm（±4.2 mm）。在进入结节间沟前，肌腱沿肱二头肌滑车结构走行。滑轮结构由前方的盂肱上韧带（SGHL）及肩胛下肌腱与后方的喙肱韧带及冈上肌腱前束组成[3]（图 21-1）。肱二头肌短头腱起自肩胛骨的喙突。与 LHBT 相反，肱二头肌短头腱起自关节外。

肱二头肌连接肩关节及肘关节。肱二头肌远端在肘关节主要参与前臂旋前，也参与肘关节屈曲。目前对肱二头肌在肩关节的作用尚有争论。[1,4] 以前认为 LHBT 存在下压肱骨头的作用，但近期的研究认为这一作用并不存在，因为 LHBT 在前方与盂肱关节相关。肱二头肌在肩关节的功能尚待讨论，但外科医师大多认为 LHBT 具有疼痛感受器的作用。[1,4]

Dr. Mazzocca or an immediate family member serves as a paid consultant to or is an employee of Arthrex and has received research or institutional support from Arthrex and Arthrosurface. Neither of the following authors nor any immediate family member has received anything of value from or has stock or stock options held in a commercial company or institution related directly or indirectly to the subject of this chapter: Dr. Cote and Dr. Beitzel.

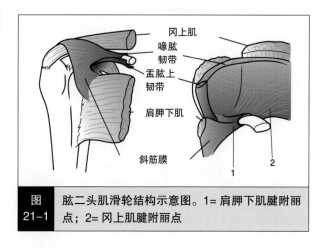

图 21-1　肱二头肌滑轮结构示意图。1= 肩胛下肌腱附丽点；2= 冈上肌腱附丽点

LHBT 的病理表现包括肌腱炎及撕裂。文献中类似的记录很多，但并没有被完全解释。由于 LHBT 独特的解剖特点，其关节内部分承受了压力、剪切力及摩擦力，其关节外部分主要承受张力。LHBT 的血管解剖在其病理过程中同样起着重要作用。LHBT 的关节内部分的长度为 3 cm，其血供比较特殊，为显著乏血管区。[5] 这一乏血管区与机械张力升高部位交叉。LHBT 的关节内退变可能源于多向力和节段性血供的协同作用。

病因学

多种关节内损伤可能继发 LHBT 撕裂，如滑囊炎、肩袖撕裂、SLAP 损伤及肩锁关节损伤。此外，也可见到原发的 LHBT 肌腱炎及撕裂。撕裂常见于附丽点或结节间沟近端附近。如撕裂位于附丽点远端，则肌腱残端可能于关节内嵌顿。LHBT 肌腱炎见于 50 岁以上人群，但既可单独引起肩关节疼痛，又可与其他一种或多种疾病共同引发肩关节疼痛。沙漏形肱二头肌也被认为是一种病变，LHBT 的关节内部分肥大，以致举臂时 LHBT 无法滑动，造成肌腱嵌顿。[6]

临床检查

如果肌腱完全撕裂，体格检查可能显示为 Popeye 畸形：近端及外侧凹陷。肌腱撕裂前患者常主诉肩关节前方疼痛，撕裂后疼痛缓解。如果肌腱没有撕裂，症状主要为活动时疼痛，特别是在对抗屈肘及前臂旋前时疼痛明显。肌腹上部触诊可有压痛。

胸肌下的肱二头肌肌腱炎检查对于发现肱二头肌病变有帮助。可通过上臂内收及外旋位时收缩辨认胸肌肌腱。检查者在腋部胸肌肌腱下缘触及肱二头肌，若触发疼痛则为阳性，提示肱二头肌病变，有时此处可见瘀斑。相关的肩袖病变检查很重要。评估肩关节活动范围，以发现肩胛盂关节内可能存在的残端嵌顿（沙漏形肱二头肌）。O'Brien 试验可检查 SLAP 损伤。Yergason 试验及 Speed 试验可评估相对远端（结节间沟内）的肌腱病变。由于单个试验的特异性有限，临床检查常需要整体考虑。

通常通过临床检查确定诊断，但影像学检查也有补充意义。超声检查价格低廉，可以发现结节间沟及附丽点处的 LHBT 缺如。MRI 不是做出诊断所必需的检查，但 MRI 关节造影是唯一可靠的区分 SLAP 损伤和滑轮损伤的方式。肌腱的劈裂，作为 IV 型 SLAP 损伤的一种，也可以通过这种方式诊断。

关节镜下检查是证实肌腱不稳的唯一客观方式。在进行任何外科操作前，应在关节镜下全程观察 LHBT 的关节内部分。建立前入路后，应以探针检查肌腱起始部及上盂唇，评估肌腱附着部情况，判断是否存在 SLAP 损伤。将肌腱从结节间沟中推出，并测试滑轮结构前后方向的稳定性。

分型

目前存在多种 LHBT 损伤的分型方法，尚未达成一致。分型主要聚焦于继发的肩关节疾病合并 LHBT 不稳定。LHBT 损伤可大致分为 3 型：单纯肌腱炎、肌腱炎合并 SLAP 损伤或不稳定，以及不稳定合并高级别肱二头肌滑轮结构损伤或肩袖损伤。

Habermeyer 分型将 LHBT 的滑轮结构损伤分为 4 型：I 型为 SGHL 损伤导致的 LHBT 前方不稳定；II 型为 SGHL 损伤合并冈上肌腱前部部分撕裂；III 型为 SGHL 损伤合并肩胛下肌腱部分撕裂；IV 型为冈上肌腱前部损伤合并肩胛下肌腱部分损伤，导致前后方向不稳定。[7]

Lafosse 镜下分型的依据是 LHBT 不稳定的方向和范围：LHBT 肉眼可见的损伤，并伴有肩胛下肌腱和（或）冈上肌腱的损伤。[8]

治疗

非手术治疗及手术治疗均已被详细表述过，但缺乏详细的数据证实哪种治疗更佳。[4,9] 非手术治疗尤其适用于自发性肌腱断裂。选择非手术治疗可能遗留一些畸形并在剧烈运动时出现痉挛。在结束运动后，痉挛通常会消失，但在一些患者中会持续存在。患者在康复治疗后，通常恢复较好，很少出现僵硬。为评价是否出现嵌顿，应鼓励患者进行关节全范围活动，包括过顶活动。

对于活动要求高或特别需要旋后力量的患者，一些医师建议手术治疗。体力劳动者的主力肢体受伤，通常选择手术治疗。患者经常在运动后出现疼痛和痉挛。年轻的患者、运动要求高的患者和不接受肱二头肌腱缺损的中年患者也应选择手术治疗。伤后 3 个月内手术效果更佳。

文献报道了数种固定 LHBT 的方法。近端方式通常为关节镜下进行 LHBT 的关节内部分固定，为肩袖修补的一部分。也可在关节外固定，固定位置通常位于关节面上方，结节间沟内。胸大肌上固定通常将 LHBT 固定于结节间沟下方，胸肌肌腱上缘以上。[10] 胸大肌下肌腱固定使用切开方式，经腋窝切口将 LHBT 固定在胸肌肌腱下方。

关节镜治疗

肌腱固定目前使用关节镜进行。[1] 在关节镜下于标准入路中用剪刀或射频刀将肌腱从肱二头肌附着处分离（图 21-2）。应避免关节盂唇损伤以保留功能。处理肌腱后，术者应检查确保肌腱滑入结节间沟中。对于老年患者的 SLAP 损伤，可予以清理。辨明解剖区域后，将肌腱残端固定，以完成 LHBT 固定术。

近端肌腱固定通常在关节镜下完成。肌腱残端可通过缝线、缝合锚或肌腱固定螺钉固定。[11-12] 一项固定技术的生物力学对比研究发现，锁孔缝合的肌腱固定方法优于传统的挤压螺钉固定，但不优于生物可吸收螺钉固定。锁孔缝合可能因肌腱断裂或滑脱而失败，而挤压螺钉固定失败则完全因为肌腱滑脱。[13] 研究者比较了以下 4 种固定方式的生物力学：胸肌下骨道固定（于骨道内缝合固定）、关节镜下挤压螺钉固定、胸肌下挤压螺钉固定，以及关节镜下缝合锚固定。骨道固定的移位显著多于其他 3 种方法，4 种方法都有显著的失效载荷特性。[14]

这些技术的优势在于保留了肌腱的长度，并能够在不增加切口的情况下实现肌腱的再固定。通常近端肌腱固定在其他手术（如肩袖修补）前进行。标准后方通道用于关节和 LHBT 的评估。使用探针将肌腱拉向关节侧以检查肌腱的结节间部分。使用穿刺针定位缝合钩部位，使用不可吸收缝线缝合钩经肌腱缝合。在这一部位，可以使用多种固定方式。经软组织固定可将肌腱与肩袖缝合。肌腱固定也可通过缝合锚实现，例如，带有两根 2 号缝合线的 5.5 mm 螺纹生物可吸收锚钉（Arthrex）（图 21-3）；也可使用生物肌腱固定螺钉，例如，4.5 mm 可吸收 SwiveLock 锚钉。在这些技术中，锚钉经去皮质化后，被放置于结节间沟入口处。缝合锚固定无须将肌腱拉出前缘。使用肌腱固定螺钉时，肌腱断端需拉出前缘，并承受螺钉的压力。在缝合部位近端，接近于起点处进行肌腱切断术（图 21-4）。

在关节镜下使用肌腱固定螺钉在胸大肌上固定肌腱断端于结节间沟中。经肌腱行缝合后，在肌腱上固定一根牵引线，在肌腱起点附近切断肌腱，并避免损伤上盂唇复合体。关节镜通过外侧入口移至肩峰下间隙。可以见到胸大肌肌腱镰状韧带，肱二头肌腱在其下方。使用腰穿针在肩袖间隙中确定辅助的前入路位置。需要切除肌腱近端的 20 mm，以清除病变的肌腱，并重建解剖关系。残端的最近

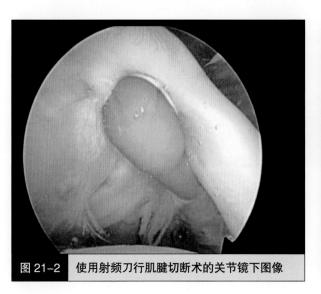

图 21-2　使用射频刀行肌腱切断术的关节镜下图像

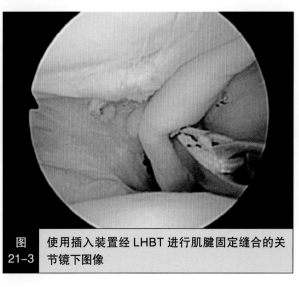

图 21-3　使用插入装置经 LHBT 进行肌腱固定缝合的关节镜下图像

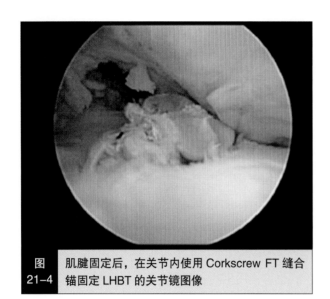

图
21-4 肌腱固定后，在关节内使用 Corkscrew FT 缝合锚固定 LHBT 的关节镜图像

端 15 mm 使用锁边缝合（或使用 Krakow 缝合法）。定位结节间沟，插入 2 mm 导针，使用 1 个直径为 7 mm 或 8 mm 的空心钻钻入 30 mm。将肌腱由前方辅助入口拉出，将 1 根缝线穿入肌腱固定螺钉并拉紧。最后，将螺钉拧入骨道，于关节镜下使用推结器在螺钉顶端打结。使用分叉的肌腱固定螺钉可以将肌腱穿入孔中（图 21-5）。

切开手术治疗

早期的肌腱固定技术将肌腱移位至喙突。由

于这项技术需要大范围切开，因此锁孔肌腱固定技术成为替代方法。通过胸大肌 – 三角肌入路暴露结节间沟，打出一个直径小于 1 cm 的尽可能窄的锁孔用于容纳肌腱。将肱二头肌腱打结，并固定于锁孔中。使用这种方法的肱二头肌撕裂患者，术后外旋力量及外观均有提高。[15]

另一种可以选择的方法是胸大肌下肌腱固定，使用挤压螺钉。胸大肌下入路的位置靠近肱二头肌肌腹部分。[16] 即使发生断裂，肌腱收缩也很少超过固定位置。在肌腱固定前，先行关节镜探查，观察有无合并损伤，行肌腱切断并做断端清理。上肢外展内旋，可触及胸大肌肌腱下缘。切口位于胸大肌肌腱下缘 3 cm 以内，上肢内侧（图 21-6A）。先切开至皮下组织，使用电刀止血，使用自动拉钩暴露视野。再清除脂肪组织，显露胸大肌、喙肱肌及肱二头肌表面筋膜。如未发现这些解剖标志，则可能是切口过于偏外。如果在三角肌与胸大肌之间找到头静脉，则切口可能过于靠近近端并偏外。找到胸大肌肌腱下缘，由近端向远端切开筋膜（图 21-6B）。将 Hohmann 拉钩放在胸大肌下及近端肱骨间，将肌肉拉向近端及外

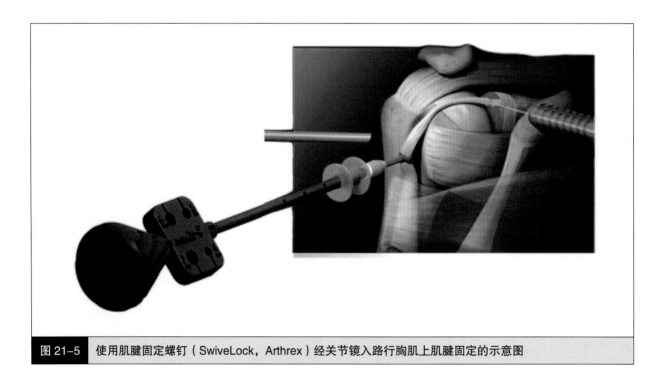

图 21-5 使用肌腱固定螺钉（SwiveLock，Arthrex）经关节镜入路行胸肌上肌腱固定的示意图

侧。钝的 Chandler 拉钩用于拉开喙肱肌及肱二头肌短头腱。内侧应避免暴力，以保护肌皮神经。辨别 LHBT 的腱腹交界处。确定 LHBT 张力合适，切除肌腱近端，保留腱腹交界处近端 20~25 mm 的肌腱。于胸大肌肌腱近端 1 cm 处显露骨膜。使用 2 号不可吸收缝线（如 FiberWire）缝合肌腱，固定 12 mm 的肌腱，以确保固定有效，并保证肱二头肌腱腹交界处位于胸大肌肌腱下方。这一步对于维持腱腹交界处张力及外观非常重要。

对大多数患者来说，8 mm 空心钻可以打出直径合适的骨道，使用直径 8 mm 的挤压螺钉固定。

钻孔深度不可超过 30 mm。（图 21-6C）钻透肱骨后方骨皮质会增加并发症风险，且毫无必要。

通过导向器穿入线环。一端由导向器穿过螺钉，术者持另一端，放松。穿过导向器的一端拉紧，直到肌腱末端被固定在导向器顶端。将导向器顶端置于骨道口上方，并插入，直到肌腱到达骨道底部。置入可吸收挤压螺钉，直到螺钉头部低于骨皮质表面（图 21-6D）。

手术治疗的临床效果

对肌腱切除术及肌腱固定的比较研究得出了

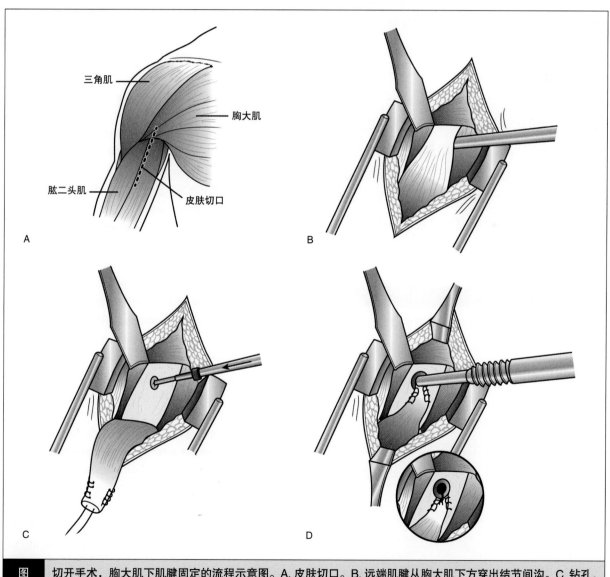

图 21-6　切开手术，胸大肌下肌腱固定的流程示意图。A. 皮肤切口。B. 远端肌腱从胸大肌下方穿出结节间沟。C. 钻孔，在胸肌下使用肌腱固定螺钉直接将回缩的肌腱固定。D. 拧入可吸收挤压螺钉，完成胸肌下肌腱固定

许多结论，但并没有一项技术显示出明显的临床优势。[4,9]因此，必须根据患者情况做出个体化选择。

关节镜治疗

对 LHBT 损伤的治疗究竟应该切除还是固定并未取得共识，两种方式均有较好的临床结果。[9]肌腱切除术后，疼痛明显减轻，功能改善，并发症的发生率为 13.3%。[17]近期的系统综述显示，肌腱切除术的结果与肌腱固定的结果相似。唯一的区别是肌腱切除术后的外观不满意率更高。[9]有一项研究显示，肌腱切除术后 30% 的患者对外观不满意。[18]也有肌腱切除术后剧烈活动时肌肉痉挛和肌力弱的报道。[1]肌腱切除术是解决 LHBT 损伤相关疼痛的有效方式。是老年患者或有严重合并症及存在腱固定术禁忌证患者的首选治疗方法。

切开手术治疗

文献报道切开行肌腱固定的结果满意。[4,19-20]肌腱近端固定可能引起肌腱滑囊炎及疼痛。[21]胸大肌下肌腱固定能够降低这一并发症的发生风险。[19,22]目前尚无一项技术被证明优于其他的技术，仍需更多的临床研究为决定 LHBT 手术方式提供证据。

总结

关于 LHBT 的肌腱炎和撕裂的文献很多，但目前尚未完全研究透彻。目前存在多种用于解决 LHBT 损伤相关疼痛的手术方式。肌腱切除术与肌腱固定结果相似，且尚无一种手术方式具有明显优势。关节镜技术包括单纯肌腱切除术及关节内或胸大肌上肌腱固定。肌腱断端可通过缝合锚或肌腱固定螺钉固定。切开手术方式首选胸大肌下肌腱固定。

参考文献

[1] Barber A, Field LD, Ryu R: Biceps tendon and superior labrum injuries: Decision-making. *J Bone Joint Surg Am* 2007;89(8):1844-1855.

Options for the surgical treatment of pathologic biceps conditions include decompression, débridement, tenotomy, and tenodesis. Factors to be considered include patient age, activity and cosmetic expectations, compliance, and associated pathologic entities that can be treated with a tenodesis.

[2] Vangsness CT Jr, Jorgenson SS, Watson T, Johnson DL: The origin of the long head of the biceps from the scapula and glenoid labrum: An anatomical study of 100 shoulders. *J Bone Joint Surg Br* 1994;76(6):951-954.

[3] Werner A, Mueller T, Boehm D, Gohlke F: The stabilizing sling for the long head of the biceps tendon in the rotator cuff interval: A histoanatomic study. *Am J Sports Med* 2000;28(1):28-31.

[4] Elser F, Braun S, Dewing CB, Giphart JE, Millett PJ: Anatomy, function, injuries, and treatment of the long head of the biceps brachii tendon. *Arthroscopy* 2011;27(4):581-592.

Biceps tenotomy and tenodesis were found to be effective for isolated LHBT pathology and combined lesions of the rotator cuff and biceps-labral complex. The function of the LHBT and its role in glenohumeral kinematics are only partially understood because of the difficulty of cadaver and in vivo biomechanical studies.

[5] Cheng NM, Pan WR, Vally F, Le Roux CM, Richardson MD: The arterial supply of the long head of biceps tendon: Anatomical study with implications for tendon rupture. *Clin Anat* 2010;23(6):683-692.

The LHBT was consistently supplied through its osseotendinous and musculotendinous junctions by branches of the thoracoacromial and brachial arteries, respectively, which divided the LHBT into two or three vascular territories, depending on the presence of the mesotenon-derived vascular supply.

[6] Ahrens PM, Boileau P: The long head of biceps and associated tendinopathy. *J Bone Joint Surg Br* 2007;89(8):1001-1009.

Current views on LHBT lesion pathology, diagnosis, and management were described. Surgical management was classified, with details of techniques.

[7] Habermeyer P, Magosch P, Pritsch M, Scheibel MT, Lichtenberg S: Anterosuperior impingement of the shoulder as a result of pulley lesions: A prospective arthroscopic study. *J Shoulder Elbow Surg* 2004;13(1):5-12.

[8] Lafosse L, Reiland Y, Baier GP, Toussaint B, Jost B: Anterior and posterior instability of the long head of

the biceps tendon in rotator cuff tears: A new classification based on arthroscopic observations. *Arthroscopy* 2007;23(1):73-80.

The authors assessed 200 patients with rotator cuff tears and reported that the direction of LHBT instability could be arthroscopically observed in 45% of the patients (posterior instability, 19%; anterior instability, 16%; and anteroposterior instability; 10%). The grade of the LHBT lesion became more significant with the increasing size of the tear. The authors used their findings to create a new arthroscopic classification for disorders of the LHBT. Level of evidence: IV.

[9] Slenker NR, Lawson K, Ciccotti MG, Dodson CC, Cohen SB: Biceps tenotomy versus tenodesis: Clinical outcomes. *Arthroscopy* 2012;28(4):576-582.

Tenotomy and tenodesis have comparably favorable results. The only major difference is a higher incidence of cosmetic deformity with biceps tenotomy.

[10] Lutton DM, Gruson KI, Harrison AK, Gladstone JN, Flatow EL: Where to tenodese the biceps: Proximal or distal? *Clin Orthop Relat Res* 2011;469(4):1050-1055.

Arthroscopic suprapectoral biceps tenodesis was described as a new technique for distal tenodesis. A more distal tenodesis location may decrease the incidence of persistent postoperative pain at the bicipital groove, but additional research is needed.

[11] Gartsman GM, Hammerman SM: Arthroscopic biceps tenodesis: Operative technique. *Arthroscopy* 2000;16(5):550-552.

[12] Geaney LE, Mazzocca AD: Biceps brachii tendon ruptures: A review of diagnosis and treatment of proximal and distal biceps tendon ruptures. *Phys Sportsmed* 2010;38(2):117-125.

Surgical repair of distal biceps ruptures was indicated to restore supination strength and endurance. Data suggest increased strength with the cortical button repair, although the best technique has not been determined. Proximal and distal biceps brachii ruptures were reviewed, with a treatment algorithm.

[13] Jayamoorthy T, Field JR, Costi JJ, Martin DK, Stanley RM, Hearn TC: Biceps tenodesis: A biomechanical study of fixation methods. *J Shoulder Elbow Surg* 2004;13(2):160-164.

[14] Mazzocca AD, Bicos J, Santangelo S, Romeo AA, Arciero RA: The biomechanical evaluation of four fixation techniques for proximal biceps tenodesis. *Arthroscopy* 2005;21(11):1296-1306.

[15] Froimson AI, Oh I: Keyhole tenodesis of biceps origin at the shoulder. *Clin Orthop Relat Res* 1975;112:245-249.

[16] Mazzocca AD, Rios CG, Romeo AA, Arciero RA: Subpectoral biceps tenodesis with interference screw fixation. *Arthroscopy* 2005;21(7):896.

[17] Gill TJ, McIrvin E, Mair SD, Hawkins RJ: Results of biceps tenotomy for treatment of pathology of the long head of the biceps brachii. *J Shoulder Elbow Surg* 2001;10(3):247-249.

[18] Osbahr DC, Diamond AB, Speer KP: The cosmetic appearance of the biceps muscle after long-head tenotomy versus tenodesis. *Arthroscopy* 2002;18(5):483-487.

[19] Mazzocca AD, Cote MP, Arciero CL, Romeo AA, Arciero RA: Clinical outcomes after subpectoral biceps tenodesis with an interference screw. *Am J Sports Med* 2008;36(10):1922-1929.

At a minimum 1-year follow-up, subpectoral biceps tenodesis with an interference screw was found to be a viable option for patients with symptomatic biceps tendinosis. Anterior shoulder pain and biceps symptoms were resolved, but patients with a coexistent rotator cuff lesion had less favorable outcomes.

[20] Millett PJ, Sanders B, Gobezie R, Braun S, Warner JJ: Interference screw vs. suture anchor fixation for open subpectoral biceps tenodesis: Does it matter? *BMC Musculoskelet Disord* 2008;9:121.

Retrospective review after open subpectoral biceps tenodesis with interference screw fixation or suture anchor fixation found reliable pain relief and improved function at an average 13-month follow-up. There was no statistically significant difference in outcomes. Residual pain may be an issue when suture anchors are used.

[21] Friedman DJ, Dunn JC, Higgins LD, Warner JJ: Proximal biceps tendon: Injuries and management. *Sports Med Arthrosc* 2008;16(3):162-169.

The LHBT is a known pain generator. Numerous pathologic entities may affect this tendon, including tendinitis, partial tearing, and subluxation, and often are associated with rotator cuff tears, especially those involving the subscapularis.

[22] Nho SJ, Reiff SN, Verma NN, Slabaugh MA, Mazzocca AD, Romeo AA: Complications associated with subpectoral biceps tenodesis: Low rates of incidence following surgery. *J Shoulder Elbow Surg* 2010;19(5):764-768.

In 353 patients treated with an open biceps tenodesis with bioabsorbable interference screw fixation, the 3-year incidence of complications was 2.0%.

第二十二章　肩胛下肌撕裂和喙突下撞击

Richard E. Duey, MD; Stephen S. Burkhart, MD

解剖学和功能

肩胛下肌对盂肱关节的稳定和运动至关重要，它是肩袖中最大且力量最强的肌肉，约提供肩袖总力量的 50%。[1]除了作为肩关节前方动态稳定肌，肩胛下肌还是内旋肌。近期的一项尸体研究发现，当上臂做外展和前屈运动时，肩胛下肌是盂肱关节中力量最强的内旋肌。[2]

肩胛下肌的主要作用之一是在冠状面和横断面上维持力偶（图 22-1）[3-4]。一项尸体研究发现，当肩袖前上撕裂累及肩胛下肌上部时，盂肱关节的生物力学在高负荷下会发生显著改变。[5]高负荷可以出现于巨大肩袖撕裂，由三角肌的生理性力量传输引起。[6]肩关节生物力学的改变可能由肩袖索从其附着点分离引起，肩袖索的前方附着点位于肩胛下肌上缘和冈上肌前缘[7]（图 22-2）。相反，当冈上肌完全撕裂而肩胛下肌保持完整时，肩关节的生物力学并不发生改变。[5]当冈上肌撕裂时，肩胛下肌必须产生更大的力来维持盂肱关节的生物力学稳定。[6]当冈上肌和冈下肌撕裂的前后径小于 7 cm 时，肩胛下肌尚可在生理范围内通过增加肌肉力量

Dr. Duey or an immediate family member serves as a paid consultant to or is an employee of Arthrex. Dr. Burkhart or an immediate family member serves as a board member, owner, officer, or committee member of the Arthroscopy Association of North America; has received royalties from Arthrex; serves as a paid consultant to or is an employee of Arthrex; and has received research or institutional support from Arthrex.

来代偿。上述发现证实了肩胛下肌在维持肩关节力偶平衡中的重要作用，尤其是当肩袖上部撕裂时，其作用更加显著。

治疗肩胛下肌撕裂必须掌握肩胛下肌腱止点的解剖。肩胛下肌腱的附着区比其他肩袖肌腱的更大。[8]肩胛下肌腱的附着区呈梯形，上部最宽，向下逐渐缩窄。[9-10]附着区从上到下长度约为 25 mm，上部宽度平均约为 17 mm，下部宽度平均约为 3 mm。在肌腱止点远端的肱骨颈处，有肩胛下肌肌肉附着区，其全长大约为 40 mm。[10]大约 60% 的肌腱止于肩胛下肌附着区的上 1/3，该区域被证实是肩胛下肌最牢固的附着点，同时还是最大的应力负荷受力点。[11]男性肩胛下肌附着区的面积明显大于女性的，附着区由上至下的长度和肱骨头的直径具有显著相关性。[10]

发病率和病理学

关节镜技术增强了外科医师辨识肩胛下肌病变的能力。对肩胛下肌撕裂的描述通常包括以下几部分：受累肌腱的位置、数量，撕裂的程度（部分撕裂或全层撕裂），以及病因（退行性或创伤性）。大多数肩胛下肌撕裂累及肩胛下肌附着点上部，且常位于关节侧，通常为部分撕裂及退行性改变。[12-13]这种撕裂模式多数是由喙突下间隙变窄和撞击（滚轴–挤压效应）导致的。[14]当肩胛下肌收缩并跨过喙突时，关节侧肌腱拉力增强导致张力侧纤维损伤（TUFF）的进展（图

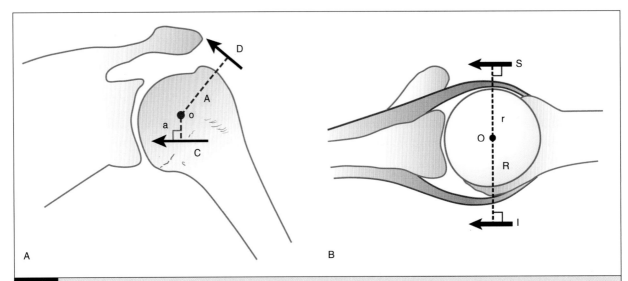

图 22-1　维持正常盂肱关系所需要的平衡力偶示意图。A. 在冠状面，肩袖下方的作用力（C）与三角肌（D）的作用力保持平衡。A = 三角肌的力臂；a = 肩袖下方的力臂；o = 旋转中心。B. 在水平轴面上，肩胛下肌的作用力（S）与冈下肌和小圆肌的作用合力保持平衡（I）。O = 旋转中心；R = 冈下肌和小圆肌的力臂；r = 肩胛下肌的力臂。经允许引自 Burkhart SS, Lo IKY, Brady PC, Denard PJ: Large and massive rotator cuff tears, in Burkhart SB: The Cowboy's Companion: A Trail Guide for the Arthroscopic Shoulder Surgeon. Philadelphia, PA, Lippincott Williams & Wilkins, 2012, pp 129–164.

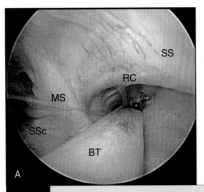
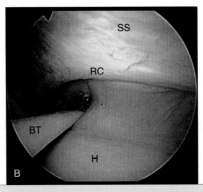
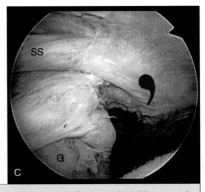

图 22-2　后方视角下的右肩关节镜照片，显示肩胛下肌（SSc）和冈上肌（SS）通过内侧吊索（MS）连接。A. 肩袖索（RC）与内侧吊索的前部融合。当内侧吊索在肩胛下肌处撕裂脱离时，可以根据逗号征定位肩胛下肌腱的上外侧角。B. 肩袖索（RC）的侧面观进一步显示了这种恒定的关系。C. 在巨大肩袖撕裂中，肩胛下肌和冈上肌之间的关系仍存在，逗号征（蓝色逗号）可用于识别上外侧的肩胛下肌腱。BT = 肱二头肌腱；G = 肩胛盂；H = 肱骨。经允许引自 Burkhart SS, Lo IKY, Brady PC, Denard PJ: Subscapularis tendon tears, in Burkhart SB: The Cowboy's Companion: A Trail Guide for the Arthroscopic Shoulder Surgeon. Philadelphia, PA, Lippincott Williams & Wilkins, 2012, pp 101–128.

22-3），喙突下撞击也会在肌腱深面引起纵向撕裂（图 22-4）。

最近的研究报道，27%~49% 的肩袖撕裂累及肩胛下肌，与冈下肌撕裂的发生率一致。[13,15-18] 几乎所有存在肩胛下肌撕裂的巨大肩袖撕裂，都会累及至少两块肩袖肌肉。[16-19] 然而，近期的两项研究发现，单纯性肩胛下肌腱撕裂大多数为创伤所致，损伤机制包括暴力外展外旋、上肢伸直位跌倒、强力牵拉、直接的暴力撞击、搬运重物。[16,20] 一项研究报道，单纯的肩胛下肌腱撕裂多为全层撕裂，且至少累及肌腱附着区的上 1/3。[16]

几项研究发现，肩胛下肌腱撕裂与肱二头肌

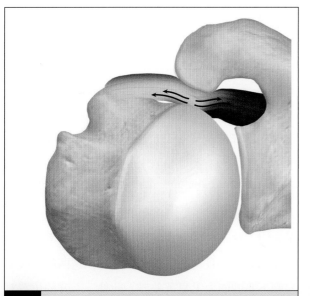

图
22-3

滚轴－挤压效应的示意图。在喙突下撞击患者中，突出的喙突使肩胛下肌腱表面受压，肩胛下肌腱在凸关节面产生张力（箭头所指），有时导致肩胛下肌纤维损伤（张力侧纤维损伤）。经允许引自 Burkhart SS, Lo IKY, Brady PC, Denard PJ: Subscapularis tendon tears, in Burkhart SS: *The Cowboy's Companion: A Trail Guide for the Arthroscopic Shoulder Surgeon*. Philadelphia, PA, Lippincott Williams & Wilkins, 2012, pp 101–128.

图
22-4

喙突下撞击的示意图。肩胛下肌腱纤维束被喙突尖端从前后方反复撞击，导致肌腱纤维向上下方扩张 (A)，从而导致肩胛下肌腱纤维束纵向断裂 (B)。C = 喙突；G = 肩胛盂。经允许引自 Burkhart SS, Lo IKY, Brady PC, Denard PJ: Subscapularis tendon tears, in Burkhart SS: *The Cowboy's Companion: A Trail Guide for the Arthroscopic Shoulder Surgeon*. Philadelphia, PA, Lippincott Williams & Wilkins, 2012, pp 101–128.

长头腱（LHBT）的病变有明显的相关性。[13,16-22] 与肩胛下肌撕裂相关的 LHBT 病变的发生率为 63%~85%。[16,18-20,22] 肩胛下肌撕裂几乎总伴有 LHBT 前方不稳定[13,17,21]（图 22-5）。当肩胛下肌全层撕裂，尤其是累及附着区的上 1/3 时，LHBT 脱位的发生率显著增高。[13,21]

　　肩胛下肌撕裂与 LHBT 半脱位或脱位显著相关，可能是由于肩胛下肌影响 LHBT 的稳定性。肩胛下肌上方止点可能是约束 LHBT 使其处于正常位置的最重要的结构。[23] 解剖学和组织学分析表明，肩胛下肌形成一个支点支撑着 LHBT，从结节间沟处向外急转后进入关节。[13,23] 肩胛下肌附着区最上方的宽阔部分形成独立的腱样条索并延伸至肱骨头凹，在 LHBT 转向肱骨头顶部时发挥作用，并维持 LHBT 的稳定性，该腱样条索还可作为盂肱韧带和喙肱韧带的内侧头的第二个附

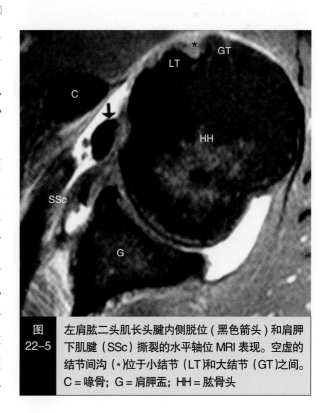

图
22-5

左肩肱二头肌长头腱内侧脱位（黑色箭头）和肩胛下肌腱（SSc）撕裂的水平轴位 MRI 表现。空虚的结节间沟（*）位于小结节（LT）和大结节（GT）之间。C = 喙骨；G = 肩胛盂；HH = 肱骨头

着点（除了骨附着位点外），后两者旋转并形成肱二头肌的内侧吊索，从而稳定 LHBT。

临床检查

可以通过临床检查来评估肩胛下肌的完整性和功能。研究者在关节镜下用 4 种常用的检查方法对 50 例可能存在肩胛下肌撕裂的患者进行了检查[24]。排除标准：钙化性肌腱炎、僵硬、不稳定、骨关节炎和既往手术史。所有患者术前均行 lift-off 试验、lag 征检查、压腹试验及 belly-off 征检查，并在关节镜下对肩胛下肌撕裂进行了评估和分级。结果显示，压腹试验和 belly-off 征检查的敏感性最高（分别为 88% 和 87%），belly-off 征检查的特异性最高（91%），其次是 lift-off 试验（79%）。belly-off 征检查的准确率是 90%，压腹试验的准确率是 74%。对于累及肩胛下肌上 1/4 的撕裂和全层撕裂，belly-off 征检查和压腹试验是最有效的体格检查。当累及范围超过 50% 时，lift-off 试验和 lag 征检查更准确。在通过外科手术确诊的肌腱撕裂病例中，体格检查的漏诊率为 15%。上述研究发现了更好的检测肩胛下肌撕裂的方式。然而，在临床诊疗过程中，患者经常合并肩关节病变，可能对上述临床检查方法的应用产生影响。

在另一项研究中，对 17 例接受关节镜治疗的单纯性肩胛下肌撕裂患者进行了改良的 lift-off 试验和压腹试验。[16]随后，将关节镜下发现与术前体格检查结果进行比较。在改良的 lift-off 试验中，患者被要求对检查者的手施加推力，检查者对其力量进行测量分级。5 例（29%）患者因疼痛或僵硬而无法进行测试。在能够进行该试验的患者中，lift-off 的敏感性为 92%。在改良的压腹试验中，检查者对患者的肘部施加压力，并对其应力进行测量分级，该试验的敏感性为 71%。在 17 例肩胛下肌腱撕裂患者中，采用这两种体格检查能检测出 16 例患者。然而，这些患者大部分是全层撕裂，至少累及肩胛下肌腱附着区的 30%。[16]

肌电图已被应用于临床检查，评估肩胛下肌上下部分的收缩能力。最近的一项研究记录了 lift-off 试验、压腹试验及熊抱试验过程中的各种肌电图数据。[25]在研究中，被检查者的手臂处于各种不同的位置，其中包括最佳位置（这些试验中手部本应在的标准位置），以此来判断手臂的位置对肌电图结果是否有影响。此外，研究者记录了 28 名健康志愿者的肩胛下肌上下部、冈上肌、冈下肌、大圆肌、背阔肌、肱三头肌和胸大肌的肌电图。结果表明，这三种试验均可评估肩胛下肌上下两部分的收缩能力，且与手臂的位置无关；这两部分收缩肩胛下肌的能力无显著差异。此外，手臂的位置对于肩胛下肌上、下两部分的收缩没有差异。[25]

另一项研究也比较了 lift-off 试验、压腹试验及熊抱试验过程中的肌电图数据。分别在肩关节前屈 0°、45° 和 90° 的位置进行熊抱试验，并监测胸大肌、背阔肌、肩胛下肌上下部的肌电图数据。肩关节前屈 45° 时，熊抱试验和压腹试验对肩胛下肌上下部的刺激比对胸大肌和背阔肌更强。lift-off 试验对肩胛下肌上下部和背阔肌的刺激无明显差异。相较于胸大肌和背阔肌，肩关节前屈 45° 时，熊抱试验可以更加特异性地刺激肩胛下肌，同时其对于肩胛下肌上部的刺激强度比对肩胛下肌下部高 20%，但这一结果没有统计学差异。肩关节前屈 90° 时，熊抱试验对肩胛下肌下部的刺激明显强于肩胛下肌上部、胸大肌和背阔肌。lift-off 试验对肩胛下肌的刺激效果仍有争议，肌电图数据表明压腹试验和熊抱试验都可以明显地刺激肩胛下肌。此外，根据肩关节位置的不同，熊抱试验可以选择性地偏向刺激肩胛下肌上部或下部。[26]

影像学检查

对于疑似肩袖撕裂的患者，首先选择 X 线检查。虽然肩胛下肌撕裂在 X 线片上无特殊征象，但 X 线片可以显示出伴随的病理改变，包括喙肱间隙变窄、盂肱关节炎和骨折。此外，在部分患者的 X 线片中还可以发现肱骨头上移，这可能是由长期的巨大肩袖撕裂或肩胛下肌的急性损伤所致，最终导致了肩关节冠状面和水平面的力偶失衡。

目前，MRI、磁共振关节造影、CT 关节造影（CTA）和超声检查已经用于评价肩胛下肌。超声检查既经济又有效，在临床上可用于对肩胛下肌的动态评估，但是它的实用性取决于超声医师是否具有丰富的专业知识。MRI、磁共振关节造影和 CTA 均能够检测到唇缘损伤、脂肪浸润和肌肉萎缩，但是超声检查却不具备这种能力。

最近的一项研究通过对比超声检查与关节镜检查对肩胛下肌撕裂的诊断结果，评价超声诊断的准确性。[15] 研究中的 96 例肩袖损伤患者先由一位经验丰富的超声医师进行超声检查，随后由一位外科医师进行肩关节镜检查。结果发现超声检查诊断肩胛下肌撕裂的敏感性为 30%，特异性为 100%，阳性预测值为 100%，阴性预测值为 78%。虽然超声检查的假阴性率较高，但是，在 19 例假阴性结果中，18 例存在肩胛下肌腱部分撕裂。超声检查肩胛下肌全层撕裂的敏感性为 86%。超声检查所明确的肩胛下肌全层撕裂均可在关节镜检查中得到证实。[15]

在一项探究关节镜下肩胛下肌修复效果的小样本前瞻性研究中，17 例单纯性肩胛下肌撕裂患者接受了 CTA 检查。[16] 结果显示，CTA 诊断肩胛下肌撕裂的敏感性为 94%。其中，15 例为累及 30% 以上肩胛下肌附着区的全层撕裂。

有研究评估了 MRI 在诊断肩胛下肌撕裂时的准确性。[18] 将肩关节的术前 MRI 检查结果与关节镜手术中的发现相对比，发现 MRI 的敏感性较低 (36%)，但特异性高 (100%)。MRI 总体准确率为 69%，较小的肩胛下肌撕裂常常被忽略，累及 50% 以上肩胛下肌附着区的撕裂更容易被发现，其敏感性为 56%，准确率为 86%。[18]

最近有研究调查了受过专业培训的骨科医师通过 MRI 准确发现肩胛下肌撕裂的能力。[17] 5 名骨科医师对 202 例患者的 4 个 MRI 特异性征象进行了前瞻性分析，包括：在轴位图像上，肩胛下肌腱从小结节上撕脱；在轴位图像上，肱二头肌长头腱的内侧半脱位 - 脱位（图 22-5）；在矢状面图像上，肩胛下肌在小结节处撕裂；在矢状面图像上，肩胛下肌萎缩。在 MRI 上观察到至少两个征象即可确定肩胛下肌撕裂。在检查患者或阅读放射科医师的报告之前，外科医师先自己评估患者的 MRI 结果。最终，在关节镜下明确肩胛下肌是否撕裂，该研究将肌腱附着区撕裂超过 10% 定义为肩胛下肌撕裂。该方法在诊断肩胛下肌撕裂方面的敏感性为 73%，特异性为 94%，阳性预测值为 90%，阴性预测值为 84%，准确率为 86%。MRI 诊断的整体准确性与 MRI 磁场强度及是否应用关节内造影剂无关。超过肌腱附着区 50% 的撕裂更容易被发现，检出率高于 97%。以上结果表明，上述 4 个 MRI 特异性征象的应用可以提高外科医师术前通过 MRI 诊断肩胛下肌撕裂的能力。[17] 这些研究表明，先进的影像学检查可以更有效地诊断较大的肩胛下肌全层撕裂，但对较小的部分撕裂的诊断价值不大。因此，如果临床表现符合肩胛下肌撕裂，就应该高度怀疑肩胛下肌撕裂的存在。

治疗

肩胛下肌撕裂的手术治疗与非手术治疗的指征尚存争议。急性创伤性撕裂通常需要通过手术修复，而较小的退行性撕裂可首先考虑非手术治疗，尤其是年龄超过 65 岁的对功能需求不高的老年患者。然而也有专家认为，鉴于肩胛下肌在肩关节功能中的重要作用，大部分肩胛下肌撕裂最终会导致肩关节功能障碍，故应予以修复。[27-28]，即使是在有大量脂肪浸润的情况下，一些研究者认为肩胛下肌也应该被修复，因为这样可以稳定肩关节，为肩关节的生物力学提供一个稳定的支点。[28-29]

当肩袖的前上部分撕裂时，研究者们提出了肩胛下肌修复的生物力学原则。[30] 冈上肌前部和肩胛下肌上部被逗号形状的弧形组织所连接，被称为"逗号征"。这处弧形组织由盂肱上韧带和喙肱韧带的内侧部分组成，它们在此处与肩胛下肌附着区的上外侧部分相互交错，形成了肱二头肌长头腱内侧悬吊的一部分。当前上肩袖撕裂长期存在时，弧形组织的止点沿着肩胛下肌上部发生骨性撕脱，"逗号征"成为识别肩胛下肌上外侧部分的主要标志（图22-2）。术者通过对弧形组织和肩胛下肌的修复，可使冈上肌前部恢复到解剖学位置。[30] 冈上肌肌肉－肌腱连接处的张力降低，使得随后对冈上肌的修复变得更加容易。此外，肩胛下肌和冈上肌前部的修复也恢复了肩袖索的前部连接。

虽然，在关节镜下治疗肩胛下肌撕裂及其并发症很有挑战性，但是不断发展的技术和器械给医师们带来了更多的便利。关节镜下修复肩胛下肌腱时，患者的体位可以是沙滩椅位或侧卧位。对于多条肌腱撕裂的情况，建议先修复肩胛下肌腱，以免肿胀进一步缩小本已变窄的喙突下间隙。前上外侧入路和前入路是标准的工作入路，后入路或侧方入路是用来观察的。通常使用30°关节镜从后入路观察肩胛下肌撕裂，70°关节镜可以显著改善关节镜下肩胛下肌附着区的视野。一些研究者认为30°关节镜从侧方入路观察肩胛下肌附着区的视野最佳，也有研究者认为70°关节镜从后入路观察的视野最佳。[16,27-28]

70°关节镜从后入路可以观察到结节间沟以下2 cm的部位，建立这种入路在关节镜下检查结节间沟内侧壁时是非常必要的。此外，这条入路还可以显露侧壁结构的断裂，包括肱二头肌的薄弱处和肩胛下肌腱的撕裂。这种撕裂可能被内侧悬吊的近端部分所遮挡（如果它是完整的），用70°关节镜向下仔细检查结节间沟是发现这种撕裂的唯一方法（图22-6）。

适当地调整患者手臂位置也有助于观察肩胛下肌。前屈和内旋手臂有助于检查肌腱附着点的情况。当患者处于侧卧位时，应用后杠杆推压不仅可增加前方的操作空间，还可改善肩胛下肌附着区的视野。[19,28] 这个动作是通过稳定患者的肘关节，一边用一只手稍微内旋手臂，一边用另一只手在肱骨近端施加向后的力来完成的。后杠杆推压被证实可以改善后方通道的视野，尤其是在应用70°关节镜时。相比之下，在沙滩椅位进行类似的操作对于改善肩胛下肌附着区视野的效果较差。

喙肱间隙狭窄与肩胛下肌病变有着显著相关性，因此，喙突下间隙必须与肩胛下肌撕裂同时处理。[32-33] 随着肩关节前后移动，内、外旋肩关节时可以从关节镜下观察到喙突尖端（看起来像肩胛下肌表面上一个滚动的凸轮）是否压迫和撞击肩胛下肌腱，也能观察到喙肱间隙是否明显变窄。将关节镜的尖端穿过在肩袖间隙制造的窗口放置在喙突和喙突下间隙处，可以判断它们的变化。同时，要注意保护弧形组织（图22-7）。用30°关节镜观察喙突尖端，因为70°关节镜开口偏下且容易在镜下迷失方向。许多外科医师在肩胛下肌修复时，仍以喙肱间隙小于或等于6 mm作为喙突成形术的手术指征。通过电凝和刨削可以将滑囊和其他软组织从喙突下间隙切除。[22,28,34] 切除联合腱和肩胛下肌所对应的喙突后外侧尖的毛糙缘，目的是将喙肱间隙扩大到7~10 mm（图22-8）。[19,28] 根据外科医师的习惯，喙突成形术也可以经肩峰下入路完成。熟悉解剖结构在喙突成形术中是很重要的，由于所有的主要神经血管结构距喙突尖端至少有28 mm，所以喙突尖端后外侧入路相对比较安全。[35]

为明确关节镜下喙突成形术的效果，一项研究切除了5例肩关节尸体标本中5~10 mm的喙突尖端。对每一个标本，在喙突尖端切除的前后均进行CT检查，并记录测量喙突重叠部分、喙突指数和喙肱间隙等指标。术后发现喙突下狭窄明显减轻，喙肩韧带和联合腱出现部分断裂。根据患者喙突的大小决定喙突切除范围，将切除范围控制在10 mm以内，可以预防术后并发软组织损伤。[36]

LHBT病变与肩胛下肌撕裂有明显相关性，通

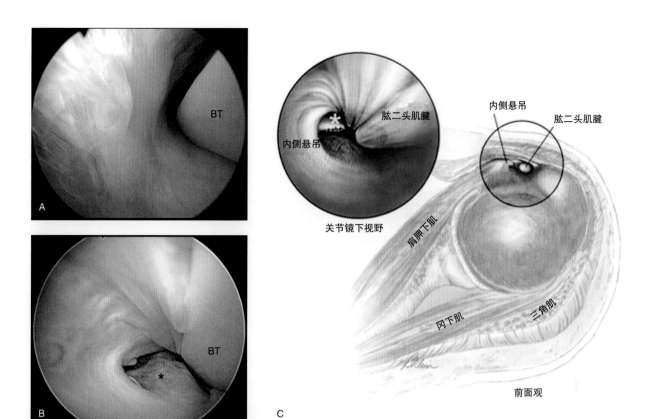

图 22-6　A. 使用 70° 关节镜从后入路观察到的正常肩关节，可见约 2 cm 长的结节间沟底部和侧壁。B. 结节间沟内侧壁破裂及远端小结暴露的肩关节镜照片。C. 图 22-6B 所示肩关节的示意图，显示了中远端肩胛下肌撕裂。*= 内侧壁断裂，BT= 肱二头肌腱。经允许引自 Burkhart SS, Lo IKY, Brady PC, Denard PJ: Subscapularis tendon tears, in Burkhart SS: *The Cowboy's Companion*: *A Trail Guide for the Arthroscopic Shoulder Surgeon*. Philadelphia, PA, Lippincott Williams & Wilkins, 2012, pp 101–128.

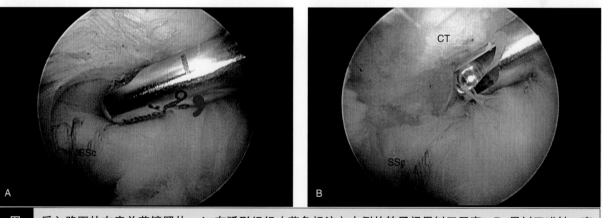

图 22-7　后入路下的右肩关节镜照片。A. 在弧形组织（蓝色标注）内侧的转子间用刨刀开窗。B. 用刨刀碰触，定位喙突尖端。CT= 喙突尖端；SSc= 肩胛下肌腱。经允许引自 Burkhart SS, Lo IKY, Brady PC, Denard PJ: Subscapularis tendon tears, in Burkhart SS: *The Cowboy's Companion*: *A Trail Guide for the Arthroscopic Shoulder Surgeon*. Philadelphia, PA, Lippincott Williams & Wilkins, 2012, pp 101–128.

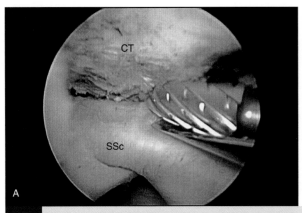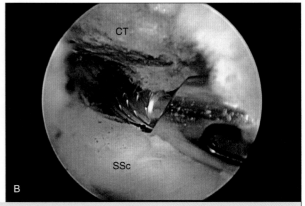

图 22-8　使用 70° 关节镜从盂肱关节后入路观察到的右肩关节，可以用来评估喙肱间隙。A. 喙肱间隙的宽度可以通过与已知的器械宽度相比较来评估；本图中喙肱间隙的宽度小于 5 mm 锉的宽度。B. 喙突成形术创造了至少 7 mm 宽的喙肱间隙。CT= 喙突尖端；SSc= 肩胛下肌腱。经允许引自 Burkhart SS, Lo IKY, Brady PC, Denard PJ: Subscapularis tendon tears, in Burkhart SS: *The Cowboy's Companion: A Trail Guide for the Arthroscopic Shoulder Surgeon*. Philadelphia, PA, Lippincott Williams & Wilkins, 2012, pp 101–128.

常，LHBT 病变的治疗必须与肩胛下肌的治疗同时进行。[13,16-22] 许多外科医师对肱二头肌的治疗主要依据关节镜检查的结果。[16,20,22] 除了年龄小于 35 岁者和投掷运动员外，多数患者在进行肩胛下肌修复时行 LHBT 的肌腱切断术或固定术。[28] 决定行肌腱切断术或固定术的主要依据是患者因素，包括年龄、活动水平、美观和个人偏好。解剖学研究强调了肩胛下肌上部对于 LHBT 的稳定作用。[13,23] 因此，通常肱二头肌的治疗目的是保护肩胛下肌。无论手术中 LHBT 的外观如何，对 LHBT 行肌腱切断术或固定术具有明显改善肩胛下肌的临床效果。[37] 两项研究发现，虽然手术过程中肱二头肌外观完整，患者在关节镜下修复后肩胛下肌愈合但是对临床疗效并不满意，这与 LHBT 的病变有明显相关性。[16,22] 关节镜下重建结节间沟区 LHBT 有良好的短期疗效，LHBT 的不稳定可能复发，导致肩胛下肌修复失败。[38] 因此，大多数专家更倾向于当存在肩胛下肌撕裂时，使用肌腱切断术或固定术来治疗 LHBT。[16,20,22,28,37]

附着区的准备是肩胛下肌修复成功的重要因素。使用电刀、刨刀和环形刮匙从骨床上小心地刮除所有软组织，形成一个均匀的出血骨面，以促进肩胛下肌愈合并形成有力的附着。在完全的慢性撕裂中，减少肌腱偏移可导致肌腱与原始附着区的不完全重合。如果需要，5~7 mm 的附着区可以在增大肌腱与原始附着区接触面的同时降低肌腱的张力。最近的一项研究对比了关节镜下修复 100% 全层肩胛下肌撕裂的患者，一组患者修复了原始附着区，另一组患者则将附着区内移了 7 mm。在至少 2 年的随访中，两组患者在功能评分、患者满意度和恢复活动方面没有显著差异。[39]

慢性撕裂可造成肩胛下肌严重收缩和邻近结构出现瘢痕。直接辨认肌腱边缘可能非常困难，但是通过识别弧形组织及其肩胛下肌腱止点上外侧角则非常方便。在牵引缝合下定位肩胛下肌，然后小心地进行肌腱的松解（图 22-2）。可见喙突后外侧骨化，肩胛下肌、联合腱和三角肌内侧筋膜之间的粘连，必须注意避免偏离肌腱下方或内侧太远（图 22-2）。[31] 通常，肩胛下肌与喙突下颈部和基底部之间有粘连，30° 骨膜剥离子在松解粘连方面非常有用。肩胛下神经止点距离喙突基部内侧约 11 mm。因此，在松解过程中避免向喙突内侧偏移是非常重要的。从关节盂颈前向后松解时也应如此。这个区域是相对无血管区。15° 骨膜剥离子有助于该部分的松解。保留弧形组织，从喙突基底部松解喙肱韧带可以大大改善肌腱的偏移。[40] 这部分释放被称为连续的前间隔滑动。肩胛下神经与腋神经和臂丛之间的粘连松解已被描述[16,41]。然而，这一步骤是非常危险的，许多外科医师发现，在修复前没有必要获得足够的肌腱偏移。[20,22,28]

缝合锚通常沿骨床从下到上植入。一般情况下，肌腱线性撕裂每1 cm（上下尺寸）使用1个锚。缝线可以顺行或逆行通过前入路或前上外侧入路，这取决于外科医师的习惯。下部缝线的打结可以早于上部缝线。上部缝线可以带到肌腱上缘的弧形组织的内侧并打结，从而使用弧形组织作为缝合切口的止裂点。

大多数肩胛下肌撕裂采用单排修复，并且有良好的短期和长期疗效。[16,19-20,22,42-43]而有些外科医师倾向于使用双排修复。[16,28,34,42-44]一些研究报道，使用双排修复能促进肌腱撕裂的愈合。[45]生物机制研究发现，使用双排缝线桥技术较使用单排修复能更明显地改善僵硬和最终负荷问题。[44]事实上，双排修复后，强度显著超过日常活动的预期负荷。在修复肩胛下肌的过程中，使用两个前辅助入路可以很方便地通过侧方入路应用缝线桥技术连接肌腱。[34]在该项技术中，低位前外侧入路可以作为工作入路和侧方锚钉的定位点。撑开器放置在低位前内侧入路，方便收缩联合腱和三角肌以便增大前方工作空间。

肩胛下肌撕裂通常累及止点的上部[12-13]。应用双排修复技术修复肩胛下肌上部被称为双反向垫修复。[46]该项技术较单排修复技术更能改善肌腱和骨床之间的压力。使用FiberTape缝合的无结技术是修复肩胛下肌撕裂的一种方式。[47]FiberTape是一种2.0 mm的尼龙材料非可吸收缝线带，与FiberWire（Arthrex）相似，但比FiberWire宽，在退变性肌腱病变的治疗中强度更高。将FiberTape放置于肩胛下肌腱的外上角，使整个上肢被拉向弧形组织内侧，并使用无线锚钉将FiberTape固定于外上角的附着区（图22-9）。宽的缝线带给肌腱和附着区带来了更大的压力，其较骨道有更强的抵抗能力。当固定牢固时，线尾能够将前部组织拉向弧形组织，侧方的固定使用肱二头肌腱固定结构或第二枚无线锚钉。[43]该技术应用双排结构固定肩胛下肌上部撕裂，是一种直接和有效的方式。

术后需要外展吊带固定患肢，可以进行肘关节的主动活动。上肢在侧方的被动外旋不能超过0°。吊带使用6周，然后逐步开始辅助下的主动活动。依据撕裂情况，术后第12~16周开始进行肌肉力量训练，恢复到正常的生活状态需要至少6个月。

结果

在过去的几年中，有多项研究的最终结果表

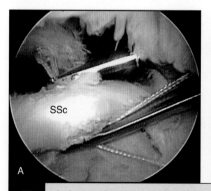
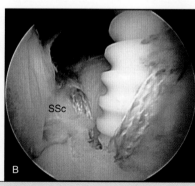
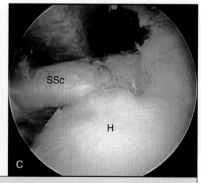

图22-9　右肩后入路下的关节镜照片显示上肩胛下肌腱撕裂的无结修复。A. 将FiberTape缝线带向前穿过上肩胛下肌腱。B. 缝线带用BioComposite SwiveLock C缝合锚（Arthrex)固定在骨床上。C. 使用无结修复技术修复止点。H= 肱骨；SSc =肩胛下肌腱。经允许引自Burkhart SS, Lo IKY, Brady PC, Denard PJ: Subscapularis tendon tears, in Burkhart SS: *The Cowboy's Companion: A Trail Guide for the Arthroscopic Shoulder Surgeon.* Philadelphia, PA, Lippincott Williams &Wilkins, 2012, pp 101–128.

明，关节镜下肩胛下肌修复术具有非常大的发展前景。在一项对 17 例孤立性肩胛下肌撕裂患者（平均手术年龄 47 岁）至少 2 年的随访研究中，13 例患者为创伤性撕裂，均通过关节镜手术修复，疼痛评分和 UCLA 肩关节评分明显改善，[16] 主动前屈、内旋和外旋显著改善，术后无肩关节僵硬表现，外展力量显著增强。在该研究中 9 例存在肱二头肌病变的患者应用了锚钉肌腱固定修复术，其中，2 例患者治疗失败。没有患者进行成形术治疗。术后应用 CTA 评估肩胛下肌的完整性，15 例患者获得完整的修复，2 例肩胛下肌上部撕裂患者复发。修复完整的患者总体功能恢复良好。术后患者未发现脂肪浸润。16 例（94%）患者对手术结果满意或非常满意。仅有 1 例患者对手术结果不满意，其虽然术前关节镜下肱二头肌外观完整，术后却出现肱二头肌不稳定。术后 CTA 检查确认诊断并显示肩胛下肌修复后愈合。[16]

在一项对 21 例孤立性肩胛下肌撕裂患者（平均年龄 43 岁）进行关节镜治疗的研究中，患者受伤时间和手术间隔的平均时间为 5.8 个月。[20] 由于其中 19 例患者均为创伤性撕裂，因此术者并未选择成形术。LHBT 的治疗依据术中表现：9 例患者采用肌腱固定、1 例采用肌腱切断术、2 例采用再中心化。1 例肌腱固定患者术后因为创伤性事件导致锚钉固定失败。随访 2 年以上后发现，患者的连续评分显著增高，19 例患者取得了很好或极好的疗效。1 例患者对于手术的疗效感到满意，1 例患者对术后疗效表示不满意。术后 MRI 检查提示，20 例患者的肩袖组织完整修复，但脂肪浸润程度加重；1 例肩胛下肌上部再撕裂患者出现显著的脂肪浸润表现。然而，患者对于临床结果表示满意，并不要求进行再手术治疗。4 例完整修复的患者出现肩胛下肌萎缩表现，患者表现出压腹试验阳性而 lift-off 试验阴性。手术治疗肩关会出现肩胛下肌横径和断面面积的减小。术后应用电子测力计测量患侧肌力和健侧肌力发现，患侧肌力明显降低。研究人员发现手术时

间越短肩关节的功能恢复越好、肌肉萎缩越少，但无显著统计学意义。[20]

一项研究报道了 23 例关节镜下治疗肩胛下肌撕裂的临床结果。[42] 61% 的患者接受了肱二头肌腱固定，没有患者接受成形术。在至少 2 年的随访中，患者的 Constant 肩关节评分、UCLA 肩关节评分和视觉模拟疼痛评分有显著改善。肩关节主观功能评分也有显著提高，85% 的患者有良好或非常好的临床效果。熊抱试验显示，经手术治疗的肩胛下肌力量显著降低。[42]

对 20 例关节镜下治疗的创伤性肩胛下肌撕裂患者（平均年龄 61.7 岁）进行前瞻性研究，其中 18 例（90%）疗效良好。[22] 所有的撕裂均累及肩胛下肌和冈上肌，其中 7 例还累及冈下肌。6 例患者需要行喙突成形术，MRI 检查显示，所有患者的喙肱间隙均小于 6 mm，并在关节镜下得到了证实。在至少 2 年的随访中，患者在 UCLA 肩关节评分和日本骨科协会临床量表的得分上有显著改善。术后用 MRI 评估修复完整性，7 例（35%）患者出现复发性撕裂，所有患者的临床评分均有所改善（6 例报告结果良好或优秀，1 例结果一般）。与未成功修复的患者相比，完整修复的患者在临床结果方面有更大的改善。高龄、严重肌腱收缩和复发性撕裂之间存在正相关关系。术后未见大量脂肪浸润，这一发现和良好的临床效果部分归因于受伤时间和手术的间隔时间短。1 例效果差的患者出现类似肱二头肌肌腱炎的表现。患者术中肱二头肌表现正常，第二次关节镜检查显示肩袖修复良好，但肱二头肌部分磨损。采用肱二头肌切断术后患者症状消失。[22]

一项研究对 40 例行关节镜下肩胛下肌撕裂修复术的患者进行了平均 5 年（3~7 年）的随访，包括所有接受原发性肩胛下肌修复的患者，无论是否伴有病理学改变。[19] 其中，19 例患者行肱二头肌腱止点或肌腱切断术，17 例（43%）患者的喙肱间隙小于 6 mm，在关节镜下行喙突成形术。患者的

视觉模拟疼痛评分、改良 UCLA 肩关节评分、改良 ASES 肩关节疼痛和功能障碍评分均明显改善，32 例（80%）患者的结果良好或优秀，33 例能恢复之前的活动水平，35 例（88%）对手术结果满意。[19]

一项研究回顾性分析了 79 例患者（平均手术年龄为 60.8 岁）在关节镜下治疗肩胛下肌撕裂后的远期功能结果。[41] 患者的撕裂是单独的或合并的类型，63% 是巨大的肩袖撕裂的一部分。39 例（49%）患者在手术时因喙肱间隙小于 6 mm，进行了喙突成形术。对 LHBT 的常规治疗方法是肌腱固定或肌腱切断术。在术后至少 7 年的随访中，患者的 UCLA 肩关节评分、ASES 肩关节疼痛和功能障碍评分和视觉模拟疼痛评分都有显著改善，83% 的患者结果良好或优秀。患者主观评价手术治疗的肩关节在最后随访时已达到正常功能的占 90%，92% 的患者能恢复正常活动，对手术结果满意。[41]

总结

肩胛下肌撕裂和喙突下撞击的诊断和治疗技术正在不断发展。关节镜下肩关节手术可以帮助医师更好地认识和理解这些临床实体，并进行微创治疗。对这些技术的短期和长期结果的评估都令人满意。需要进一步的工作以更好地描述肩胛下肌的腱索功能，以及喙突下撞击在肩胛下肌组织病理学中的特殊作用。双排修复技术在临床上可能有利于修复肩胛下肌撕裂，尽管在肌腱严重收缩的情况下，双排修复技术并不总是可行的。

参考文献

[1] Keating JF, Waterworth P, Shaw-Dunn J, Crossan J: The relative strengths of the rotator cuff muscles: A cadaver study. *J Bone Joint Surg Br* 1993;75(1):137-140.

[2] Ackland DC, Pandy MG: Moment arms of the shoulder muscles during axial rotation. *J Orthop Res* 2011;29(5):658-667.

A biomechanical cadaver study examined the moment arms of muscles that internally or externally rotate the humerus. The subscapularis was found to be the stron-gest internal rotator of the glenohumeral joint when the shoulder is in abduction or forward flexion.

[3] Burkhart SS: Fluoroscopic comparison of kinematic patterns in massive rotator cuff tears: A suspension bridge model. *Clin Orthop Relat Res* 1992;284:144-152.

[4] Burkhart SS, Lo IK: Arthroscopic rotator cuff repair. *J Am Acad Orthop Surg* 2006;14(6):333-346.

[5] Su WR, Budoff JE, Luo ZP: The effect of anterosuperior rotator cuff tears on glenohumeral translation. *Arthroscopy* 2009;25(3):282-289.

A cadaver model was used in finding that rotator cuff tears involving both the supraspinatus and the upper subscapularis substantially altered glenohumeral joint kinematics at physiologic loads. When the upper sub-scapularis tendon was left intact, no alteration in joint kinematics was noted.

[6] Hansen ML, Otis JC, Johnson JS, Cordasco FA, Craig EV, Warren RF: Biomechanics of massive rotator cuff tears: Implications for treatment. *J Bone Joint Surg Am* 2008;90(2):316-325.

When superior rotator cuff tears were created in a ca-daver model, increased force transmission was re-quired of the subscapularis for maintaining spheric glenohumeral joint kinematics. These force require-ments fell within the physiologic range for the sub-scapularis with tears as large as 7 cm in the anteropos-terior direction.

[7] Burkhart SS, Esch JC, Jolson RS: The rotator crescent and rotator cable: An anatomic description of the shoulder's "suspension bridge". *Arthroscopy* 1993;9(6):611-616.

[8] Curtis AS, Burbank KM, Tierney JJ, Scheller AD, Cur-ran AR: The insertional footprint of the rotator cuff: An anatomic study. *Arthroscopy* 2006;22(6):e1, e1.

[9] Richards DP, Burkhart SS, Tehrany AM, Wirth MA: The subscapularis footprint: An anatomic description of its insertion site. *Arthroscopy* 2007;23(3):251-254.

Nineteen cadaver shoulder specimens were used to in-vestigate the insertional anatomy of the subscapularis tendon. The upper 60% of the footprint formed a major attachment point for the tendon and probably plays an important role in load transmission.

[10] Ide J, Tokiyoshi A, Hirose J, Mizuta H: An anatomic study of the subscapularis insertion to the humerus: The subscapularis footprint. *Arthroscopy* 2008;24(7):749-753.

Forty cadaver shoulders were used to develop a de-tailed description of the anatomic footprint of the sub-scapularis tendon and the adjacent bare area. Certain dimensions were substantially larger in specimens from men than in those from women.

［11］Halder A, Zobitz ME, Schultz E, An KN: Structural properties of the subscapularis tendon. *J Orthop Res* 2000;18(5):829-834.

［12］Sakurai G, Ozaki J, Tomita Y, Kondo T, Tamai S: Incomplete tears of the subscapularis tendon associated with tears of the supraspinatus tendon: Cadaveric and clinical studies. *J Shoulder Elbow Surg* 1998;7(5):510-515.

［13］Arai R, Sugaya H, Mochizuki T, Nimura A, Moriishi J, Akita K: Subscapularis tendon tear: An anatomic and clinical investigation. *Arthroscopy* 2008;24(9):997-1004.

A clinical investigation established the prevalence of subscapularis tears and their association with biceps pathology. Anatomic dissection showed that the upper portion of the subscapularis insertion functions as an important stabilizer for the LHBT.

［14］Lo IK, Burkhart SS: The etiology and assessment of subscapularis tendon tears: A case for subcoracoid impingement, the roller-wringer effect, and TUFF lesions of the subscapularis. *Arthroscopy* 2003;19(10):1142-1150.

［15］Singisetti K, Hinsche A: Shoulder ultrasonography versus arthroscopy for the detection of rotator cuff tears: Analysis of errors. *J Orthop Surg (Hong Kong)* 2011;19(1):76-79.

The results of ultrasonography of 96 shoulders with rotator cuff symptoms were compared with arthroscopic surgical findings. Ultrasonography had a sensitivity of 30% and a specificity of 100% in the detection of subscapularis tears. Eighteen of the 19 false-negative results involved partial-thickness tears of the upper subscapularis.

［16］Lafosse L, Jost B, Reiland Y, Audebert S, Toussaint B, Gobezie R: Structural integrity and clinical outcomes after arthroscopic repair of isolated subscapularis tears. *J Bone Joint Surg Am* 2007;89(6):1184-1193.

Isolated subscapularis tears were arthroscopically repaired in 17 patients. Most of the tears were traumatic and full thickness. Significantly improved short-term clinical outcomes were reported. A retearing rate of 12% was observed on CTA. Sixteen patients were satisfied or very satisfied with the results of surgery. Level of evidence: IV.

［17］Adams CR, Brady PC, Koo SS, et al: A systematic approach for diagnosing subscapularis tendon tears with preoperative magnetic resonance imaging scans. *Arthroscopy* 2012;28(11):1592-1600.

Five orthopaedic surgeons systematically reviewed MRIs for 202 patients, using four specific criteria to determine whether a subscapularis tear was present. This approach led to improved accuracy in recognizing subscapularis tears, compared with previous studies. Level of evidence: III.

［18］Adams CR, Schoolfield JD, Burkhart SS: Accuracy of preoperative magnetic resonance imaging in predicting a subscapularis tendon tear based on arthroscopy. *Arthroscopy* 2010;26(11):1427-1433.

Preoperative shoulder MRI (as interpreted by radiologists) was compared with arthroscopic intraoperative findings. MRI had a sensitivity of 36% and a specificity of 100% for detecting subscapularis lesions. Larger tears were more readily identified using MRI. Level of evidence: III.

［19］Adams CR, Schoolfield JD, Burkhart SS: The results of arthroscopic subscapularis tendon repairs. *Arthroscopy* 2008;24(12):1381-1389.

Retrospective review at a median 5-year follow-up of patients who underwent arthroscopic subscapularis repair found that 80% had a good or excellent clinical outcome and 88% were satisfied with the results of surgery. Level of evidence: IV.

［20］Bartl C, Salzmann GM, Seppel G, et al: Subscapularis function and structural integrity after arthroscopic repair of isolated subscapularis tears. *Am J Sports Med* 2011;39(6):1255-1262.

At a minimum 2-year follow-up of 21 patients who underwent arthroscopic repair of a traumatic isolated subscapularis tear, 19 patients had a good or excellent result. MRI revealed an intact repair in 20 patients. Subscapularis strength was significantly decreased in the surgically treated extremity. Level of evidence: IV.

［21］Lafosse L, Reiland Y, Baier GP, Toussaint B, Jost B: Anterior and posterior instability of the long head of the biceps tendon in rotator cuff tears: A new classification based on arthroscopic observations. *Arthroscopy* 2007;23(1):73-80.

Instability of the LHBT and its association with rotator cuff tearing were evaluated in 200 consecutive patients undergoing arthroscopic rotator cuff repair. Ninety-six percent of patients with anterior instability of the biceps had a concomitant subscapularis tear.

［22］Ide J, Tokiyoshi A, Hirose J, Mizuta H: Arthroscopic repair of traumatic combined rotator cuff tears involving the subscapularis tendon. *J Bone Joint Surg Am* 2007;89(11):2378-2388.

Traumatic combined rotator cuff tears that included

the subscapularis were arthroscopically repaired in 20 patients. At a minimum 2-year follow-up, 90% reported a good or excellent result. The tear recurrence rate was 35%, based on postoperative MRI. One poor outcome occurred in a patient in whom biceps pathology developed after surgery. Level of evidence: IV.

[23] Arai R, Mochizuki T, Yamaguchi K, et al: Functional anatomy of the superior glenohumeral and coracohumeral ligaments and the subscapularis tendon in view of stabilization of the long head of the biceps tendon. *J Shoulder Elbow Surg* 2010;19(1):58-64.

The importance of the upper subscapularis insertion, superior glenohumeral ligament, and coracohumeral ligament in stabilizing the LHBT was investigated by means of anatomic and histologic analysis. The superior insertion of the subscapularis was found to be the most important restraint preventing dislocation of the LHBT.

[24] Bartsch M, Greiner S, Haas NP, Scheibel M: Diagnostic values of clinical tests for subscapularis lesions. *Knee Surg Sports Traumatol Arthrosc* 2010;18(12):1712-1717.

Four clinical tests were compared for their ability to accurately detect subscapularis tears in 50 consecutive patients undergoing shoulder arthroscopy. The Napoleon test had the highest sensitivity (88%), and the belly-off sign had the highest specificity (91%). Strict exclusion criteria probably had a substantial effect on the reported outcomes.

[25] Pennock AT, Pennington WW, Torry MR, et al: The influence of arm and shoulder position on the bear- hug, belly-press, and lift-off tests: An electromyographic study. *Am J Sports Med* 2011;39(11):2338-2346.

Electromyographic data were used to analyze the ability of three different physical examination tests to isolate the subscapularis. All three tests were effective for this purpose, and no test appeared superior to the others. None of the tests was able to selectively isolate the upper subscapularis.

[26] Chao S, Thomas S, Yucha D, Kelly JD IV, Driban J, Swanik K: An electromyographic assessment of the "bear hug": An examination for the evaluation of the subscapularis muscle. *Arthroscopy* 2008;24(11):1265-1270.

Electromyographic analysis showed that the bear hug test performed at 45° of shoulder flexion effectively isolates the subscapularis. A 20% increase in activation of the upper subscapularis compared with the lower subscapularis was not significant. At 90°of shoulder flexion, the bear hug test significantly isolated the lower subscapularis compared with the upper subscapularis and other muscles.

[27] Koo SS, Burkhart SS: Subscapularis tendon tears: Identifying mid to distal footprint disruptions. *Arthroscopy* 2010;26(8):1130-1134.

An arthroscopic technique for identifying mid to distal subscapularis tendon tears is described. A 70° arthroscope was used to carefully examine the medial sidewall of the bicipital groove for evidence of occult disruptions of the subscapularis tendon, which can easily be missed.

[28] Denard PJ, Lädermann A, Burkhart SS: Arthroscopic management of subscapularis tears. *Sports Med Arthrosc* 2011;19(4):333-341.

A review of subscapularis anatomy and function is presented along with the means to effectively identify and arthroscopically manage subscapularis pathology. The results of arthroscopic treatment of subscapularis lesions are discussed.

[29] Burkhart SS, Tehrany AM: Arthroscopic subscapularis tendon repair: Technique and preliminary results. *Arthroscopy* 2002;18(5):454-463.

[30] Ticker JB, Burkhart SS: Why repair the subscapularis? A logical rationale. *Arthroscopy* 2011;27(8):1123-1128.

Reasons are presented for repairing the subscapularis if it is part of an anterosuperior rotator cuff tear. Maintaining the soft-tissue attachment to the supraspinatus and repairing the subscapularis help reduce the supraspinatus tear, restore the anterior rotator cable attachment, and provide added security to the overall repair.

[31] Lo IK, Burkhart SS: The comma sign: An arthroscopic guide to the torn subscapularis tendon. *Arthroscopy* 2003;19(3):334-337.

[32] Nové-Josserand L, Edwards TB, O'Connor DP, Walch G: The acromiohumeral and coracohumeral intervals are abnormal in rotator cuff tears with muscular fatty degeneration. *Clin Orthop Relat Res* 2005;433(433):90-96.

[33] Richards DP, Burkhart SS, Campbell SE: Relation between narrowed coracohumeral distance and subscapularis tears. *Arthroscopy* 2005;21(10):1223-1228.

[34] Park JY, Park JS, Jung JK, Kumar P, Oh KS: Suture-bridge subscapularis tendon repair technique using low anterior portals. *Knee Surg Sports Traumatol Arthrosc* 2011;19(2):303-306.

Two low-anterior accessory portals were used for the arthroscopic repair of subscapularis tears. The purpose was to facilitate the use of a double-row suture-bridge technique for restoring the anatomic footprint of the subscapularis.

[35] Lo IK, Burkhart SS, Parten PM: Surgery about the

coracoid: Neurovascular structures at risk. *Arthroscopy* 2004;20(6):591-595.

[36] Kleist KD, Freehill MQ, Hamilton L, Buss DD, Fritts H: Computed tomography analysis of the coracoid process and anatomic structures of the shoulder after arthroscopic coracoid decompression: A cadaveric study. *J Shoulder Elbow Surg* 2007;16(2):245-250.

Arthroscopic coracoplasty was performed on five cadaver specimens. Preoperative and postoperative CT showed substantial changes in the morphology of the coracoid and the subcoracoid space. Resection of 10 mm or less of the coracoid tip appears to prevent undue disruption of the adjacent soft-tissue structures.

[37] Edwards TB, Walch G, Sirveaux F, et al: Repair of tears of the subscapularis. *J Bone Joint Surg Am* 2005;87(4):725-730.

[38] Bennett WF: Arthroscopic bicipital sheath repair: Two- year follow-up with pulley lesions. *Arthroscopy* 2004;20(9):964-973.

[39] Denard PJ, Burkhart SS: Medialization of the subscapularis footprint does not affect functional outcome of arthroscopic repair. *Arthroscopy* 2012;28(11):1608-1614.

Subscapularis tears involving 100% of the tendinous insertion were retrospectively reviewed. Some patients underwent a repair to the anatomic footprint, and the others had the footprint medialized an average of 5 mm before repair. At a minimum 2-year follow-up, there was no substantial between-group difference in functional outcomes. Level of evidence: III.

[40] Lo IK, Burkhart SS: The interval slide in continuity: A method of mobilizing the anterosuperior rotator cuff without disrupting the tear margins. *Arthroscopy* 2004;20(4):435-441.

[41] Denard PJ, Jiwani AZ, Lädermann A, Burkhart SS: Long-term outcome of a consecutive series of subscapularis tendon tears repaired arthroscopically. *Arthroscopy* 2012;28(11):1587-1591.

At a minimum 7-year follow-up of 79 patients who underwent arthroscopic repair of a subscapularis tendon tear, 83% had a good or excellent clinical result, and 92% were satisfied. Both isolated and combined tears were included; 63% involved a massive rotator cuff tear. Level of evidence: IV.

[42] Lafosse L, Lanz U, Saintmard B, Campens C: Arthroscopic repair of subscapularis tear: Surgical technique and results. *Orthop Traumatol Surg Res* 2010;96(8, suppl):S99-S108.

Extensive subscapularis tears were arthroscopically re- paired in 23 patients. The surgical technique is described. Short-term follow-up revealed significant improvement in clinical measures. The failure rate was 9%. Level of evidence: IV.

[43] Denard PJ, Lädermann A, Burkhart SS: Double-row fixation of upper subscapularis tears with a single suture anchor. *Arthroscopy* 2011;27(8):1142-1149.

A simplified, efficient technique for double-row fixation of upper subscapularis tears was described. Knotless anchor fixation was used to repair lesions involving as much as 50% of the superior tendon attachment.

[44] Wellmann M, Wiebringhaus P, Lodde I, et al: Biomechanical evaluation of a single-row versus double-row repair for complete subscapularis tears. *Knee Surg Sports Traumatol Arthrosc* 2009;17(12):1477-1484,48,4.

A biomechanical cadaver study found that a double- row repair of a simulated subscapularis tear had a substantially higher stiffness and ultimate load to failure than a single-row technique. Tendon elongation before failure was substantially lower with a double-row repair.

[45] Charousset C, Grimberg J, Duranthon LD, Bellaiche L, Petrover D: Can a double-row anchorage technique improve tendon healing in arthroscopic rotator cuff repair? A prospective, nonrandomized, comparative study of double-row and single-row anchorage techniques with computed tomographic arthrography tendon healing assessment. *Am J Sports Med* 2007;35(8):1247-1253.

Two groups of patients underwent arthroscopic repair of a rotator cuff tear using a single-row or double-row technique. No significant difference was noted in short-term clinical outcomes. CTA revealed significantly better tendon healing in those with a double- row repair. Level of evidence: II.

[46] Yoo JC, Kim JH, Lee YS, Park JH, Kang HJ: Arthroscopic double mattress repair in incomplete subscapularis tears. *Orthopedics* 2008;31(9):851-854.

A technique for the arthroscopic repair of upper subscapularis tendon tears was described. A double- loaded suture anchor was used in a double, inverted horizontal mattress repair of the torn tendon to its bone footprint.

[47] Denard PJ, Burkhart SS: A new method for knotless fixation of an upper subscapularis tear. *Arthroscopy* 2011;27(6):861-866.

A novel technique uses knotless fixation for the repair of subscapularis tears involving as much as 50% of the upper tendinous insertion. This efficient, straightforward technique can be used for most subscapularis tears.

第二十三章 运用关节镜技术对关节盂前下方骨缺损的评价和治疗

Frank Martetschläger, MD; Daniel Rios, MD; Robert E. Boykin, MD; Peter J. Millett, MD, MSc

引言

关节盂前下方骨缺损可能导致复发性盂肱关节不稳定。[1]导致这种骨缺损的主要原因包括急性肩关节脱位后骨折或慢性肩关节不稳定后骨侵蚀。急性肩关节脱位后 Bankart 损伤的发生率为4%~70%。男性比女性更容易出现 Bankart 损伤。[2]

Bankart 损伤通常发生在 2~4 点位置（右肩），根据骨缺损的百分比分为 3 种类型。Ⅰ型为移位性撕脱骨折，Ⅱ型为关节盂前下缘撕脱骨折畸形对合，Ⅲ型根据关节盂骨缺损的百分比来定义，ⅢA 型表示骨缺损小于 25%，ⅢB 型表示骨缺损大于 25%。

众所周知，关节盂骨缺损与关节镜下软组织修复失败的风险增加有关。因此，对于关节盂前下方骨缺损超过 20% 的患者，建议进行骨重建。[3]以往一般通过开放手术进行骨重建，近年来开放

手术逐渐被先进的关节镜手术所取代。[4-7]

生物力学

软组织修复术后会出现复发性不稳定，大量生物力学研究量化了骨缺损量。一项尸体研究表明，当关节盂宽长比小于 21% 时，关节的稳定性将显著降低。[8]另一项研究报道，当骨缺损宽长比大于 20% 时，关节前方稳定性显著降低。[9]另一项尸体研究发现，关节盂宽度减少 50% 可以使肩关节脱位的力降低 30%。[10]

肱骨头凸面与关节盂凹面的对应关系，以及肩袖的动态拉力阐明了关节盂凹面压缩对盂肱关节活动的影响。[11]关节盂骨缺损会导致压力升高进而产生疼痛和骨磨损。关节盂宽度减少 20% 会使其前下 1/4 象限压力增加 1 倍，峰值压力也随之增加。[12]因此，基于最新的生物力学研究数据，关节盂骨缺损宽长比下降 20%~25% 的患者建议进行修复，以防止因持续骨磨损和静态稳定性降低而出现反复性肩关节不稳定。

评估

病史和体格检查

详细的病史询问和体格检查有助于诊断盂肱关节不稳定。既往脱位次数、引起恐惧的动作及外伤或手术史都具有重要意义。

在与健侧做比较后，进行恐惧试验、再移位试验、负荷试验、前后抽屉试验，可以发现肩关节

Dr. Martetschläger or an immediate family member has received nonincome support (such as equipment or services), commercially derived honoraria, or other non–research-related funding (such as paid travel) from Arthrex and Steadman Philippon Research Institute. Dr. Millett or an immediate family member has received royalties from Arthrex; serves as a paid consultant to Arthrex; has stock or stock options held in Game Ready and VuMedi; and has received research or institutional support from Arthrex, OrthoRehab, Össur Americas, Siemens Medical Solutions USA, Smith & Nephew, and ConMed Linvatec. Neither of the following authors nor any immediate family member has received anything of value from or owns stock in a commercial company or institution related directly or indirectly to the subject of this article: Dr. Rios and Dr. Boykin.

前方和（或）后方不稳定。有研究表明，进行特定动作时患者出现恐惧比出现疼痛更容易诊断不稳定。[13]对全身性、症状性韧带松弛和凹陷征（0°和90°）的检查有助于诊断多向肩关节不稳定。

在麻醉下消除患者的不适和肌张力后，负荷试验、再移位试验和前后抽屉试验的结果更具参考价值。[13]在手术时，应在麻醉下评估患侧肱骨较健侧的移动量和有无提示骨缺损的骨擦感。[14]遗传性韧带松弛应与病理性韧带松弛相区别。

影像学检查

所有患者的初次影像学评估应包括正位（内旋位和外旋位）、腋位、肩胛骨冈上肌出口位、尖斜位。[15]此外，西点位可能有助于评估关节盂骨缺损，而喙突轴位可发现合并的 Hill-Sachs 损伤。骨缺损适合用轴位和矢状位 CT 序列图像进行评估，三维重建对于评估复杂骨缺损有一定帮助，其能准确测量骨缺损量及判断是否需要植骨[16-17]（图 23-1）。

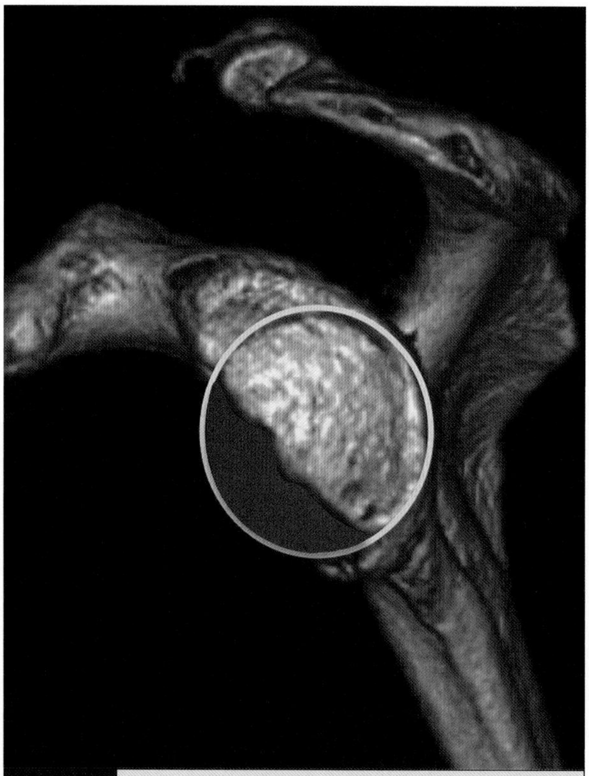

关节镜诊断

关节镜检查是诊断关节盂骨缺损的金标准。通过肩袖间隙可以观察到关节盂骨缺损的比例。在大多数急性损伤患者中，被周围韧带复合体隔开的骨片也可能受到损伤。[18]

2002 年，有学者提出一种关节镜下获取关节盂骨缺损量的方法，这种方法以关节盂裸点为参考点及下关节盂几何中心[1]（图 23-2）。因为以该点为中心的最佳区域直径大约为 24 mm，所以将从裸点到骨缺损处的测量值除以 24 来表示关节盂剩余部分的比例。例如，关节盂剩余 80% 表示有 20%的骨缺损。这项数据可用于指导手术决策。

关节盂骨缺损的关节镜治疗

手术适应证和决策

对于关节盂骨缺损后肩关节不稳定的患者，建议手术治疗。[13]基于临床和生物力学研究，如

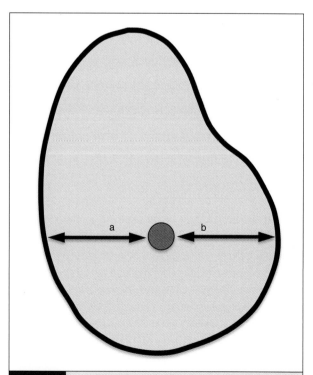

图 23-1　左肩三维重建 CT 图像显示前下方骨缺损。正常的关节盂应填满图中圆形。前方红色区域代表骨缺损量

图 23-2　示意图显示从关节盂裸点（中心圆圈）到关节盂后缘和前缘的距离，可用校正的探针测量。如果从中心到关节盂前缘的距离（b）小于中心到关节盂后缘的距离（a）的 50%，骨缺损量至少是关节盂下直径的 25%

果骨缺损超过关节盂直径的 20%~25%，建议进行骨重建。[3,8-9,12] 对于复发性肩关节不稳定风险较高的患者，如运动员，建议慎重考虑是否进行手术。

重建关节盂可以通过固定骨折块来实现。如果无法进行直接固定，可以使用自体骨或异体骨恢复稳定性。对于存在骨磨损的患者，可以考虑进行骨移植。[19]

生物力学研究发现，关节盂骨缺损为 20% 的患者可以通过软组织修复来恢复稳定性。[9] 因此，对于关节盂骨缺损小于 20% 的患者，建议进行软组织修复（Bankart 修补）。对于合并 Hill-Sachs 损伤的患者，Remplissage 术（2008 年被首次提出）可提高其肩关节生物力学稳定性。[20-21]

对于有条件进行骨折块固定的患者，可在关节镜下使用缝合锚或螺钉固定。[2,4-5,21-23] Bony Bankart Bridge 术（关节镜锚钉修补术）最早在 2009 年被提出，该手术使用锚钉将骨折块固定在关节盂边缘。[5] 对于无法修复的碎块或者磨损至缺损超过 25% 的患者，可以使用关节镜下 Bristow 术、Latarjet 手术和自体软骨（或异体骨）移植。[21-28]

关节镜下 Remplissage 术修复

当关节镜下发现关节盂骨缺损小于其直径 20% 时应进行标准的关节镜下 Bankart 修补。除了常规入路，可以在后侧的上方入路穿过锚钉。可以先固定锚钉，然后穿过肩胛骨盂唇组织对前方和前下方进行修补。缝合时不要打结，以便锚钉穿进肱骨。[20-28]

修复 Hill-Sachs 损伤部分时，先使用刨刀或环切器处理表面，造成轻度出血而不去皮质化。为了方便观察，关节镜从前上外侧入口进入。经典做法是将锚钉固定在骨缺损处，在冈下肌外侧穿出套管，从肩峰下间隙取出滑囊以方便缝合。将缝线从入口处同时穿过冈下肌腱和后囊的近端和远端以及肌肉肌腱连接处的外侧。患者手臂处于中立位时，先将下方缝线打结。最后，将冈下肌固定在肱骨缺损处，如此便完成了标准的 Bankart 修补。换言之，

Remplissage 术可在 Bankart 修补前进行，并在最后将缝线打结以调整前后方平衡。

Bony Bankart Bridge 术

Bony Bankart Bridge 术使用两点固定将骨折块压回原处。[5] 使用前上方高位入路和前下方辅助入路，关节镜放在 70° 的位置来观察骨折位置内侧的关节盂颈部。附着在骨折块上的盂唇和盂肱下韧带（IGHL）复合体应该被保留。器械通过前方两个入路进入使骨折块和 IGHL 位于 6 点位置。为了促进骨间愈合，应使用刨刀对关节盂颈部和骨折块接触面进行处理。通过前上方入路将骨折块抬高后，把第一个锚钉固定在关节盂颈部。这个锚钉为桥的内侧固定点。如果骨折块较小，一枚锚钉足以将骨折块固定在关节盂颈部内侧。如果骨折块较大，则在内侧放置两枚螺钉，缝线先穿过骨折块内侧的软组织，再穿过前下方套管。在关节盂边缘的骨折块下方放置一枚缝合锚，以固定盂唇和 IGHL 复合体。内侧缝线穿过 IGHL 复合体，将其向内上方牵拉，从而拉紧腋窝囊。移位大小通过前上方入路的抓取器来控制。缝线使用带滑锁的 Weston 结固定，背侧有两个交替的半结。如果骨折块较大，可以使用两枚锚钉。通过评估骨折复位后的张力来找到锚钉的最佳固定位置。在关节盂软骨骨折边缘钻孔。把内侧缝合锚的缝线放入 3.5 mm 无结锚后将锚钉放入钻孔。在此过程中，骨折块被压回原处以完成骨性愈合。用一个探头来测试其牢固性，剪除外侧锚钉的多余缝线。关节囊、盂唇、盂肱中韧带也可通过这种方法得到修复。建议固定撕裂的盂唇，以提供旋转稳定性。根据骨折块的大小，可采用一种或多种桥接技术来固定骨折块（图 23-3）。

关节镜下植骨修复

关节镜下植骨最早使用肩袖的前下方入路和肱二头肌后面的前上方入路。[26] 通过前上方入路观察可建立肩胛下肌前下方入路。从前下方入路和前下方深部入路插入 2 根 8.25 mm 套管针，从

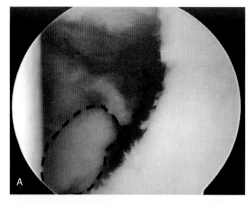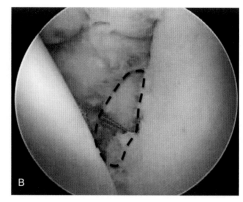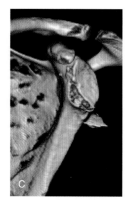

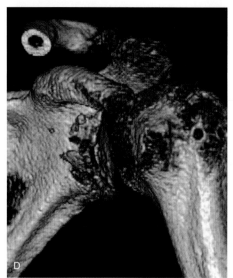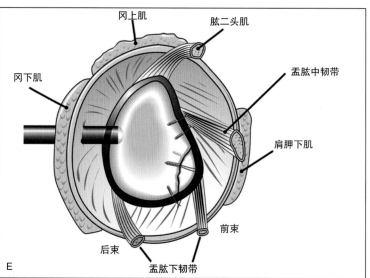

冈上肌　肱二头肌　盂肱中韧带　肩胛下肌　前束　后束　盂肱下韧带　冈下肌

图 23-3　左肩后入路关节镜照片显示采用 Bony Bankart bridge 技术再固定前方（A）和后方（B）的大块骨性 Bankart 损伤（虚线圈出）。左肩三维重建 CT 显示 Bony Bankart bridge 技术修复前方（C）和后方（D）的大块骨性 Bankart 损伤。E. 示意图显示 Bony Bankart bridge 技术修复后的情况，复位后的骨性 Bankart 损伤骨块，修复后的盂唇和移位的关节囊与 IGHL 复合体。经允许引自 Panel E adapted with permission from Millett PJ, Braun S: The "bony Bankart bridge" procedure: A new arthroscopic technique for reduction and internal fixation of a bony Bankart lesion. *Arthroscopy* 2009;25（1）:102–105.

后方入口插入 1 根 6 mm 套管针。从髂骨取一骨块，用摆锯修成合适形状。[29] 通过前下方入路，松解 6 点位置的盂唇关节囊复合体，使用骨钻或刨刀处理关节盂骨面使其出血后放置移植物。从前上方入路取出套管后，可用夹钳将移植物置入。当移植物放好后，可以用探针检查其与关节的对应关系，然后用克氏针临时固定。3 枚克氏针从前下方入路和前下方深部入路进入，经皮穿过肩胛下肌腱的上 1/3。用克氏针扩孔后，用 2 枚 2.7~3.7 mm 空心加压螺钉固定骨块。必要时，将骨块打磨至合适形状。最后在上方和下方用 2 枚锚钉重建关节囊韧带组织（图 23-4）。

关节镜下喙突转移术

2007 年关节镜下 Latarjet 手术被分为显露喙突、处理喙突、喙突钻孔截骨、转移喙突和植骨固定 5 个步骤。[25] 第 1 步，为了充分显露喙突，需切开关节囊，在喙肱韧带和肩胛下肌之间打开肩袖间隙。在右肩 2 点和 5 点位置切除盂唇前缘和盂肱中韧带，保留 IGHL 附着点。紧贴喙突切除喙肱韧带，并松解喙突深面的联合腱。在关节盂前下方（2~6 点位置）使用刨刀处理骨面。

第 2 步是在关节镜下通过前方和侧方入路暴

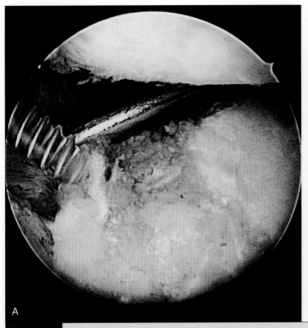
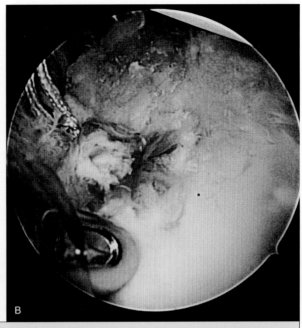

图 23-4　关节镜照片显示用两枚 2.7~3.7 mm 的加压螺钉进行骨移植物（A）和关节囊韧带复合体（B）的重建。将装有 FiberWire(Arthrex) 的 FasTak 缝合锚固定于移植物的上方和下方，采用水平褥式缝合固定。经允许引自 Scheibel M, Kraus N, Diederichs G, Haas NP: Arthroscopic reconstruction of chronic anteroinferior glenoid defect using an autologous tricortical iliac crest bone grafting technique. *Arch Orthop Trauma Surg* 2008;128（11）:1295-1300.

露喙突和腋神经（位于肩胛下肌前缘）。在胸小肌内外侧找到联合腱的边界，暴露臂丛神经，在喙突的基底部和尖端建立喙突入口。关节镜经前方入路进入，切除胸小肌时应尽量贴近喙突以避免损伤后方的臂丛神经。显露臂丛神经和腋神经血管束后，使用 2.9 mm 钻头在喙突下 8 mm 处钻 2 个孔。缝线穿过两孔后经喙突入口穿出，在距喙突尖端水平和垂直 2~2.5 cm 交界处进行截骨。切除喙突下方和内侧的联合腱，显露肩胛下肌前部。

第 3 步是将关节镜置于外侧入路。水平劈开肩胛下肌腱建立前下方入路。通过后方入路抬高肩胛下肌的上 1/3 使移植物通过。通过套管在钻孔中置入导针，以便通过缝线来控制移植物的位置。将移植物放在关节盂前缘 2~6 点位置。将关节镜从前方入路置入，经前下方入路在其中 1 枚螺钉中钻入 1 枚克氏针。在放入后一枚螺钉前应将前一枚螺钉完全置入以避免移植物移位。取出导针，使用 3.5 mm 钻头钻孔，置入 4.5 mm 螺钉。使用类似方法置入

第 2 枚螺钉，两枚螺钉应在视野下拧紧。处理关节盂移植物交界处可能存在的台阶。图 23-5 显示了手术完成时的关节镜下表现。

术后康复

应为患者制订个性化的康复方案。应该充分考虑修复的稳定性、骨缺损的大小、其他相关的操作和患者的整体身体条件及治疗目标。康复的进展和运动的恢复也应该考虑上述因素。

并发症

多篇文献报道，关节镜下治疗关节盂骨缺损的术后并发症发生率相对较低。[19,22,24,30-32] 然而，患者仍可发生感染、出血、神经血管损伤和麻醉意外。由于骨块较薄，可发生松动、尺寸过长刺激周围组织和移植物吸收等并发症。[33]

关节镜下骨移植由于操作邻近神经血管结构，可能造成神经血管的损伤。一项尸体研究表明，

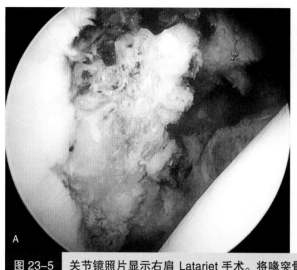
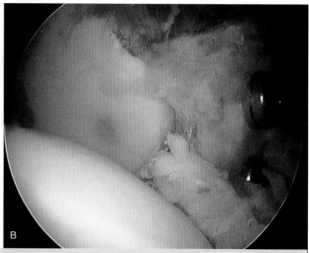

图 23-5　关节镜照片显示右肩 Latarjet 手术。将喙突骨移植物用两枚空心钉固定于关节盂的前缘。从后入路（A）和前入路（B）确认移植物的位置。经允许引自 Agneskirchner JD, Haag M, Lafosse M: Arthroskopischer Korakoidtransfer. *Der Orthopade* 2011;40:41-51.

关节镜辅助操作可以优化移植物的位置并可使医师更充分地处理关节盂骨面。[34] 这些优势可以降低开放手术的早期骨不连和晚期关节炎的风险。

结论

一些专家不建议骨缺损较大的患者进行关节镜下软组织增强术，因其失败率较高。[3, 8, 35] 然而，在三维 CT 评估中关节盂骨缺损超过 25% 的患者也可以在关节镜下成功进行 Bankart 修补。[18] 在一项进行了 34 个月随访的研究中，21 例骨缺损为 20%~30% 的患者接受了关节镜下治疗。其中 2 例（9.5%）出现反复半脱位，1 例（4.8%）出现反复脱位需要翻修。与骨磨损的患者相比，有骨折块存在的患者预后更好。在关节镜 Latarjet 手术后 26 个月的随访中，91% 的患者评价优秀，9% 的患者评价良好。[32] 然而 100 例患者中只有 35 例在第 26 个月时接受了复查。需要对严重骨缺损不稳定的患者进行更长期的研究，以评价手术的情况和患者的满意度。

开放手术

关节镜技术的进步使外科医师可以完成几乎所有的治疗肩关节不稳定的手术操作，尽管术后短期恢复效果很好，但是长期效果还没有得到验证。[19,22,32,36-37] 其中许多手术操作需要医师掌握先进的关节镜技术。需要注意的是，通过前入路进行开放手术确实可以有效缓解症状[38-40]。因此，当缺乏与关节镜修复相关的设备、经验或技术时，开放手术仍是一项重要的治疗选择。在翻修手术、软组织不足或显露困难时可能需要转为开放手术。随着关节镜技术的不断发展，外科医师应根据自身的技术水平及患者的盂肱关节不稳定类型来考虑手术适应证。[41]

总结

肩关节镜技术、内固定物和移植物等方面的改进，使因骨缺损导致肩关节不稳定的患者可以接受微创治疗。这些新兴技术必须通过更长期的研究来论证。相比之下，开放手术可以提供更可靠的治疗结果。因此，术者应熟练掌握开放手术技术，特别是复杂的关节镜手术有时可能需要转为开放手术。详细的手术计划是治疗由骨缺损导致的肩关节不稳定患者的关键。选择手术方式应该充分考虑外科医师的经验水平、最常见的病理类型及患者术中和术后的舒适度。

参考文献

[1] Burkhart SS, Debeer JF, Tehrany AM, Parten PM:

Quantifying glenoid bone loss arthroscopically in shoulder instability. *Arthroscopy* 2002;18(5):488-491.

［2］ Porcellini G, Paladini P, Campi F, Paganelli M: Long-term outcome of acute versus chronic bony Bankart lesions managed arthroscopically. *Am J Sports Med* 2007;35(12):2067-2072.

A modified Bankart technique was used to repair the capsulolabral complex and fix the avulsed bone fragment with suture anchors in 65 patients. One of the 41 patients with acute injury and 1 of the 24 with chronic injury had a traumatic redislocation. The mean Rowe score increased from 59 to 92 and from 43.5 to 61, respectively (*P* < 0.001).

［3］ Burkhart SS, De Beer JF: Traumatic glenohumeral bone defects and their relationship to failure of arthroscopic Bankart repairs: Significance of the invertedpear glenoid and the humeral engaging Hill-Sachs lesion. *Arthroscopy* 2000;16(7):677-694.

［4］ Kim KC, Rhee KJ, Shin HD: Arthroscopic three-point double-row repair for acute bony Bankart lesions. *Knee Surg Sports Traumatol Arthrosc* 2009;17(1):102-106.

An arthroscopic technique for bony Bankart repair was reported to confer effective, firm three-point fixation of the bony Bankart lesion without the suture material crossing the glenoid cavity.

［5］ Millett PJ, Braun S: The "bony Bankart bridge" procedure: A new arthroscopic technique for reduction and internal fixation of a bony Bankart lesion. *Arthroscopy* 2009;25(1):102-105.

An easy, reproducible technique for arthroscopic reduction and suture anchor fixation of bony Bankart fragments created a nontilting two-point fixation that compresses the fragment into its bed.

［6］ Mochizuki Y, Hachisuka H, Kashiwagi K, Oomae H, Yokoya S, Ochi M: Arthroscopic autologous bone graft with arthroscopic Bankart repair for a large bony defect lesion caused by recurrent shoulder dislocation. *Arthroscopy* 2007;23(6):e1-e4.

An arthroscopic autologous bone graft repair was used for a patient with recurrent dislocation of the shoulder joint and a large bony Bankart lesion. Two bones were harvested from the lateral side of the acromion and transplanted to the large bony defect of the glenoid.

［7］ Porcellini G, Campi F, Paladini P: Arthroscopic approach to acute bony Bankart lesion. *Arthroscopy* 2002;18(7):764-769.

［8］ Itoi E, Lee SB, Berglund LJ, Berge LL, An KN: The effect of a glenoid defect on anteroinferior stability of the shoulder after Bankart repair: A cadaveric study. *J Bone Joint Surg Am* 2000;82(1):35-46.

［9］ Yamamoto N, Itoi E, Abe H, et al: Effect of an anterior glenoid defect on anterior shoulder stability: A cadaveric study. *Am J Sports Med* 2009;37(5):949-954.

In eight cadaver shoulders, an osseous defect was created stepwise with a 2-mm increment of the defect width. The stability ratio was used to evaluate joint stability. An osseous defect of at least 20% of the glenoid length significantly decreased anterior stability.

［10］ Gerber C, Nyffeler RW: Classification of glenohumeral joint instability. *Clin Orthop Relat Res* 2002;400:65-76.

［11］ Lippitt S, Matsen F: Mechanisms of glenohumeral joint stability. *Clin Orthop Relat Res* 1993;291:20-28.

［12］ Greis PE, Scuderi MG, Mohr A, Bachus KN, Burks RT: Glenohumeral articular contact areas and pressures following labral and osseous injury to the antero-inferior quadrant of the glenoid. *J Shoulder Elbow Surg* 2002;11(5):442-451.

［13］ Bushnell BD, Creighton RA, Herring MM: Bony instability of the shoulder. *Arthroscopy* 2008;24(9):1061-1073.

Unrecognized large bony lesions have been identified as a primary cause of recurrent instability or failure of arthroscopic reconstruction for instability, and the diagnosis is difficult. Developments in the diagnosis and treatment of bony instability were reviewed.

［14］ Matsen FA III, Chebli C, Lippitt S: American Academy of Orthopaedic Surgeons: Principles for the evaluation and management of shoulder instability. *J Bone Joint Surg Am* 2006;88(3):648-659.

［15］ Bushnell BD, Creighton RA, Herring MM: Hybrid treatment of engaging Hill-Sachs lesions: Arthroscopic capsulolabral repair and limited posterior approach for bone-grafting. *Tech Shoulder Elbow Surg* 2007;8:194-203.

A hybrid technique is described in which an engaging Hill-Sachs lesion was treated through arthroscopic capsulolabral repair coupled with an open posterior approach to the humeral head, which involved splitting the posterior deltoid and the infraspinatus muscles.

［16］ Chuang TY, Adams CR, Burkhart SS: Use of preoperative three-dimensional computed tomography to quantify glenoid bone loss in shoulder instability. *Arthroscopy* 2008;24(4):376-382.

The glenoid index, which is calculated from three-dimensional CT, accurately predicted the need for bone grafting in 24 of 25 patients (96%). Three- dimensional

CT can be used for preoperative planning and patient counseling.

[17] Nofsinger C, Browning B, Burkhart SS, Pedowitz RA: Objective preoperative measurement of anterior glenoid bone loss: A pilot study of a computer-based method using unilateral 3-dimensional computed to- mography. *Arthroscopy* 2011;27(3):322-329.

A CT-based study confirmed that the normal inferior glenoid surface is a nearly perfect circle with remark- ably low variability. A simple, reliable method was de- scribed for determining the anatomic glenoid index, used to create an anatomic preoperative description of bone loss.

[18] Sugaya H, Moriishi J, Kanisawa I, Tsuchiya A: Arthro- scopic osseous Bankart repair for chronic recurrent traumatic anterior glenohumeral instability. *J Bone Joint Surg Am* 2005;87(8):1752-1760.

[19] Mologne TS, Provencher MT, Menzel KA, Vachon TA, Dewing CB: Arthroscopic stabilization in patients with an inverted pear glenoid: Results in patients with bone loss of the anterior glenoid. *Am J Sports Med* 2007;35(8):1276-1283.

Twenty-one of 23 patients undergoing arthroscopic stabilization surgery were found to have a bony defi- ciency of 20% to 30% at a mean 34-month follow- up. The procedure can yield a stable shoulder, but out- comes were less predictable with attritional bone loss.

[20] Koo SS, Burkhart SS, Ochoa E: Arthroscopic double- pulley remplissage technique for engaging Hill-Sachs lesions in anterior shoulder instability repairs. *Arthros- copy* 2009;25(11):1343-1348.

A new technique for arthroscopic remplissage was de- scribed, in which the eyelets of the two suture anchors were used as pulleys and a double-mattress suture was created.

[21] Purchase RJ, Wolf EM, Hobgood ER, Pollock ME, Smalley CC: Hill-Sachs "remplissage": An arthro- scopic solution for the engaging Hill-Sachs lesion. *Ar- throscopy* 2008;24(6):723-726.

An arthroscopic technique was described for the treat- ment of traumatic shoulder instability in patients with glenoid bone loss and a large Hill-Sachs lesion. Capsu- lotenodesis of the posterior capsule and infraspinatus tendon was used to fill the Hill-Sachs lesion.

[22] Sugaya H, Moriishi J, Kanisawa I, Tsuchiya A: Arthro- scopic osseous Bankart repair for chronic recurrent traumatic anterior glenohumeral instability: Surgical technique. *J Bone Joint Surg Am* 2006;88(suppl 1 pt 2:)159-169.

[23] Zhang J, Jiang C: A new "double-pulley" dual- row technique for arthroscopic fixation of bony Bankart lesion. *Knee Surg Sports Traumatol Arthrosc* 2011;19(9):1558-1562.

[24] Boileau P, Bicknell RT, El Fegoun AB, Chuinard C: Ar- throscopic Bristow procedure for anterior instability in shoulders with a stretched or deficient capsule: The "belt-and-suspenders" operative technique and prelim- inary results. *Arthroscopy* 2007;23(6):593-601.

A combined arthroscopic Bankart repair was used with a transfer of the coracobiceps tendon to reinforce the deficient anterior capsule in 36 patients. At a min- imum 1-year follow-up, 28 patients (78%) were very satisfied, 5 (14%) were satisfied, and 3 (8%) were disappointed.

[25] Lafosse L, Lejeune E, Bouchard A, Kakuda C, Gobezie R, Kochhar T: The arthroscopic Latarjet procedure for the treatment of anterior shoulder instability. *Arthros- copy* 2007;23(11):e1-e5.

The outcomes of 100 patients were reported at 26- month follow-up after an arthroscopic Latarjet proce- dure. Patient-reported outcome scores were 91% ex- cellent and 9% good. The all-arthroscopic Latarjet technique had excellent results through midterm follow-up, with minimal complications and good graft positioning.

[26] Scheibel M, Kraus N, Diederichs G, Haas NP: Arthro- scopic reconstruction of chronic anteroinferior glenoid defect using an autologous tricortical iliac crest bone grafting technique. *Arch Orthop Trauma Surg* 2008;128(11):1295-1300.

An all-arthroscopic reconstruction technique for the anteroinferior glenoid included autologous iliac crest bone grafting using Bio-Compression screws and a capsulolabral repair using suture anchors.

[27] Taverna E, Golanò P, Pascale V, Battistella F: An ar- throscopic bone graft procedure for treating anterior- inferior glenohumeral instability. *Knee Surg Sports Traumatol Arthrosc* 2008;16(9):872-875.

An arthroscopic method for treating anteroinferior glenohumeral instability was investigated in a cadaver model. There were six good, two fair, and two poor re- sults.

[28] Skendzel JG, Sekiya JK: Arthroscopic glenoid osteo- chondral allograft reconstruction without subscapularis takedown: Technique and literature review. *Arthroscopy* 2011;27(1):129-135.

The literature on the surgical treatment of glenoid bone

deficiency was reviewed. A novel technique of arthroscopic anteroinferior glenoid reconstruction used glenoid osteochondral allograft without subscapularis takedown.

[29] Warner JJ, Gill TJ, O'hollerhan JD, Pathare N, Millett PJ: Anatomical glenoid reconstruction for recurrent anterior glenohumeral instability with glenoid deficiency using an autogenous tricortical iliac crest bone graft. *Am J Sports Med* 2006;34(2):205-212.

[30] Lafosse L, Boyle S, Gutierrez-Aramberri M, Shah A, Meller R: Arthroscopic latarjet procedure. *Orthop Clin North Am* 2010;41(3):393-405.

The value of the arthroscopic Latarjet procedure was described for the treatment of complex shoulder instability. Results were excellent at short- to mid-term follow-up, with minimal complications.

[31] Sugaya H, Kon Y, Tsuchiya A: Arthroscopic repair of glenoid fractures using suture anchors. *Arthroscopy* 2005;21(5):635.

[32] Lafosse L, Boyle S: Arthroscopic Latarjet procedure. *J Shoulder Elbow Surg* 2010;19(2, suppl):2-12.

The arthroscopic Latarjet procedure is a valuable tool in the treatment of complex shoulder instability. Introduction of the procedure into practice was described. The procedure was recommended for surgeons with good anatomic knowledge and advanced arthroscopic skills.

[33] Tauber M, Resch H, Forstner R, Raffl M, Schauer J: Reasons for failure after surgical repair of anterior shoulder instability. *J Shoulder Elbow Surg* 2004;13(3):279-285.

[34] Nourissat G, Nedellec G, O'Sullivan NA, et al: Mini- open arthroscopically assisted Bristow-Latarjet procedure for the treatment of patients with anterior shoulder instability: A cadaver study. *Arthroscopy* 2006;22(10):1113-1118.

[35] Kim SH, Ha KI, Cho YB, Ryu BD, Oh I: Arthroscopic anterior stabilization of the shoulder: Two to six-year follow-up. *J Bone Joint Surg Am* 2003;85-A(8):1511-1518.

[36] Agneskirchner JD, Haag M, Lafosse L: [Arthroscopic coracoid transfer: Indications, technique and initial results]. *Orthopade* 2011;40(1):41-51.

The indications, surgical technique, and early results of coracoid transfer related to a completely arthroscopic technique were reviewed.

[37] Park MJ, Tjoumakaris FP, Garcia G, Patel A, Kelly JD IV: Arthroscopic remplissage with Bankart repair for the treatment of glenohumeral instability with Hill- Sachs defects. *Arthroscopy* 2011;27(9):1187-1194.

Twenty patients underwent arthroscopic Bankart repair with remplissage for the treatment of recurrent anterior glenohumeral instability and a large Hill- Sachs defect. At a mean 29-month follow-up, function was restored, pain was diminished, and 85% of the patients were satisfied.

[38] Auffarth A, Schauer J, Matis N, Kofler B, Hitzl W, Resch H: The J-bone graft for anatomical glenoid reconstruction in recurrent posttraumatic anterior shoulder dislocation. *Am J Sports Med* 2008;36(4):638-647.

Long-term results were reported for 47 patients after stabilization with a J-bone graft, which was found to be capable of creating a stable shoulder joint without causing extensive loss of motion. The patients had traumatic glenoid rim fracture after shoulder dislocation. Despite anatomic glenoid reconstruction, some patients had mild to moderate arthropathy.

[39] Hovelius L, Sandström B, Olofsson A, Svensson O, Rahme H: The effect of capsular repair, bone block healing, and position on the results of the Bristow-Latarjet procedure (study III): Long-term follow-up in shoulders. *J Shoulder Elbow Surg* 2012;21(5): 647-660.

At long-term follow-up of 319 patients after an open Bristow-Latarjet procedure, 837 had a good and consistent result. The rate of recurrence decreased and subjective results improved when a horizontal capsular shift was added to the coracoid transfer.

[40] Hovelius L, Vikerfors O, Olofsson A, Svensson O, Rahme H: Bristow-Latarjet and Bankart: A comparative study of shoulder stabilization in 185 shoulders during a seventeen-year follow-up. *J Shoulder Elbow Surg* 2011;20(7):1095-1101.

Eighty-eight consecutive shoulders underwent Bankart repair, and 97 consecutive shoulders underwent Bristow-Latarjet repair for traumatic anterior recurrent instability. At a mean 17-year follow-up, patients with the Bristow-Latarjet repair had better results than those with Bankart repair done with anchors, in terms of stability and subjective evaluation.

[41] Millett PJ, Clavert P, Warner JJ: Open operative treatment for anterior shoulder instability: When and why? *J Bone Joint Surg Am* 2005;87(2):419-432.

第二十四章　关节镜治疗多向不稳定

Brett McCoy, MD; Waqas Munawar Hussain, MD; Michael J. Griesser, MD; Anthony Miniaci, MD

引言

虽然基础医学、临床研究和影像学领域的发展改善了研究者们对肩关节不稳定的认识，但是多向不稳定（MDI）的临床诊断依然很困难。Neer 和 Foster 在 1980 年首次描述了这种复杂的肩关节不稳定类型，此后便在该领域开展了广泛的研究。[1]MDI 被定义为在两个或多个方向下、前和后（上）的盂肱关节的症状性、无意识的不稳定。[2]AMBRI（非创伤性、多向、双侧、康复、肩胛下移位）被用于描述 MDI。[3]但是，由于 MDI 的特征和描述存在许多不一致的地方，因此很难明确其发病率并比较相应的研究结果。[4]

尽管已发表的研究结果表明，包括物理疗法在内的非手术治疗对超过 80% 的患者有良好或优异的疗效，但并非所有患者都可以通过非手术治疗获得改善。[5]少数患者可能需要进行开放或关节镜手术来加强稳定性。[6]最初，开放手术的治疗重点在通过关节囊的再次拉紧减小关节容积（特别是在下部区域），从而降低关节囊松弛度。[7]改进的关节镜技术和仪器及对病理解剖学的更深理解带来了治疗这种复杂疾病的微创手术方法的发展。[8-10]

病理解剖学

盂肱关节使肩部具有很好的活动范围。稳定性和灵活性之间的微妙平衡被破坏可能导致 MDI。重要的是要理解，松弛度与不稳定性不直接相关，并且动态和静态约束都可以在一定程度上弥补结构上的缺陷。松弛确实起着重要的作用，但是当代偿机制失效时，它可能会表现出症状。[11]与创伤性不稳定患者不同，伴有松弛的患者可能具有孤立的盂唇 – 关节囊松弛，而并不伴有明确的盂唇撕裂。尽管该病原本是非创伤性的，但是由 MDI 引起慢性不稳定的患者仍可能有继发性的盂唇病变，如盂唇撕裂。[9,12]

肩部的静态稳定结构包括骨骼和韧带结构。关节凹与盂唇共同作用，为肩部稳定性提供了较小但关键的作用，研究人员观察到，与正常对照组相比，MDI 患者的关节凹表面相对平坦。[11,13]

Dr. Miniaci or an immediate family member serves as a board member, owner, officer, or committee member of the International Society of Arthroscopy, Knee Surgery, and Orthopaedic Sports Medicine; the American Shoulder and Elbow Surgeons; the Arthroscopy Association of North America; and the American Society for Sports Medicine; has received royalties from Arthrosurface and Zimmer; is a member of a speakers' bureau or has made paid presentations on behalf of Arthrosurface; serves as a paid consultant to or is an employee of Arthrosurface, Smith & Nephew, Stryker, and Zimmer; has stock or stock options held in DePuy, Medtronic, Zimmer, Stryker, and Arthrosurface; and has received nonincome support (such as equipment or services), commercially derived honoraria, or other non–research-related funding (such as paid travel) from Stryker and Arthrosurface. None of the following authors or any immediate family member has received anything of value from or has stock or stock options held in a commercial company or institution related directly or indirectly to the subject of this chapter: Dr. McCoy, Dr. Hussain, and Dr. Griesser.

盂唇过小可导致关节盂的总体有效深度下降。肩胛盂的扭转也有导致不稳定的倾向。[11] 目前，已明确了囊韧带（包括盂肱上韧带、盂肱中韧带、盂肱下韧带）的作用，即根据四肢的位置相互收紧或放松来抵抗关节的平移。这些结构中的任何一个缺失或存在缺陷都可能增加不稳定的倾向。同样，肩袖间隔中的缺陷也被认为会增加关节下移的量，并可能存在于 MDI 中。[2,14] 一项 MRA 评估发现，MDI 患者肩胛下肌和冈上肌之间的间隔（反映肩袖间隔的大小）并不大于其他类型肩关节不稳定患者的。[15]

动态稳定由在肩关节活动范围中最活跃的肌腱结构维持，而囊韧带结构并未参与。[2] 肩胸的肌肉系统会动态改变肩部的位置，以提供最合适的关节盂扭转角度和倾斜度，以保持稳定。[16] 斜方肌、菱形肌和前锯肌的异常或失衡会影响肩胛骨的旋转并最终影响肩部稳定。一项证实了 MDI 患者存在肩胛运动异常的研究强调了在康复过程中纳入定向稳定性练习的重要性。[17] 冈上肌、冈下肌和小圆肌通过关节凹的加压，增加了肱骨头与肩胛盂之间的接触力。[16] 肩袖的肌腹具有直接的加固或限制作用，以避免关节异常运动。[11] 活跃的神经肌肉控制和完整的本体感觉反馈机制对于维持盂肱关节的功能和动态稳定是必需的。有研究观察到了肩袖功能的差异，并比较了 MDI 患者与正常对照组患者在牵拉、向前出拳、抬高和过顶投掷运动中的肌电图结果。[18] MDI 肩部的不规则性可能削弱肩袖根据传入本体感觉的微小变化处理和调整其响应的能力。

与正常对照组患者相比，MDI 患者可能存在胶原和弹性蛋白的变化。在比较胶原的交联、胶原纤维的直径和密度，以及氨基酸和弹性蛋白的组成时发现，正常肩关节与存在 MDI 或单向不稳定的肩关节之间的组织之间具有组织化学差异。在 MDI 翻修手术的肩关节中获取的关节囊与在 MDI 初次手术干预时从肩关节中获取的关节囊组织不同。这些分析表明，该组 MDI 患者有潜在的结缔组织病变。[19]

除这些因素外，下方关节囊过大，以及随之而来的关节内负压丢失也可能导致 MDI。关节容积的增加被认为会导致关节内负压下降，从而使关节的稳定性下降。尸体研究评估了关节囊移位后、关节排气前后的关节内压力。尽管关节囊向下移位减少了关节容积并增加了关节内压力，以应对向下负荷，但是排气后，即使是在关节囊重叠加固后，所有标本的肱骨头均向下脱位。[20] MDI 患者的盂唇也不典型，而且盂唇-关节囊复合体在正常肩部的缓冲作用也未在 MDI 患者中发现。

临床评估

MDI 的诊断主要基于临床病史和体格检查。患者临床病史的特征可能是与活动有关的非特异性肩痛，通常在 30 岁之前开始。主要症状可能为疼痛、不稳定。运动表现和力量可能变差，四肢麻木或感觉异常程度较小。[11] 有关症状的发生频率、反复性和严重性，以及使症状加重或减轻的姿势或活动的信息，可以为判断不稳定的程度和方向提供重要依据。结缔组织疾病和相关的松弛在确诊为 MDI 的患者中并不少见，并且双肩均可受累。多向松弛在重复进行双上肢过顶运动的运动员中最为普遍，例如，游泳运动员、排球运动员和体操运动员。[11] 症状相对较重的患者可能在更细微的活动中表现出肩关节不稳定，例如，上肢举过头顶、将物体握持在身体侧面或睡觉时改变姿势。[2,21]

有症状的 MDI 通常是重复性微创伤导致关节囊松弛的结果。[7] 单次刺激性创伤或事件引发症状的情况不太常见。临床医师必须保持高度警惕，以确保诊断是合理的。与前方单向不稳定（通常表现为前下方盂唇-关节囊损伤）相反，MDI 可以表现为无解剖结构损伤的肩关节不稳定。在手术稳定肩关节后仍持续出现症状的 40 岁以下患者，医师应考虑 MDI 的可能。[11]

部分患者能够主动使肩关节脱位，他们可以选择性地控制肌肉的收缩和松弛，从而引起反复的不稳定。[2] 主动性肩关节脱位通常与情绪或精神疾病有关，这些患者在进行手术稳定后通常预后较差。[22] 重要的是，要把那些继发性肩关节脱位患者，与那些主动诱发肩关节脱位后小心避免刺激性动作或姿势的患者区别开来。继发性脱位患者通常会自我保护或自动调节位置性的不稳定，通常来说，他们进行手术稳定的效果良好。[11]

体格检查从视诊开始，仔细观察有无肌肉萎缩、双侧肩胛不对称或翼状肩胛。全身性松弛可包括掌指关节过伸、拇指到手腕的过伸、膝关节和肘关节过伸、髌骨不稳和扁平足（图 24-1）。患者可能表现出凹陷征，其特征是在向松弛内收的肩关节施加向下的应力时，肩峰的侧面边界下方有凹陷。当肢体远端外旋时（盂肱上韧带的张力增加）看到凹陷征，可证实与盂肱上韧带相关的更大程度的松弛。

尽管 MDI 的诊断主要基于临床病史和体格检查，但也应该获取影像学图像以排除解剖缺陷并评估可能伴随的肩部结构病变，例如，Hill-Sachs 损伤、反 Hill-Sachs 损伤和盂肱韧带撕裂。可以进行 MRI 检查以评估肩胛的解剖结构，如盂唇、肩袖和肱二头肌。[7] CT 对于评估骨质和骨缺损很有用。对于早期 MDI 手术未成功的患者，应将注意力集中在单个肩袖肌肉（肩胛下肌）的功能和强度上。肩胛下肌内旋强度的降低可能高达 30

%，从而导致动态稳定性下降。[21,23]

非手术治疗和手术治疗的注意事项

为 MDI 患者选择合适的治疗方法，需要对主观和客观评估结果进行仔细的评估。图 24-2 为临床医师进行决策的流程图。重要的是要注意，以疼痛为主要临床表现的患者，其病因可能与松弛无关。因此，需要对 MDI 患者的肩部疼痛进行广泛的鉴别诊断和彻底的检查。对于在体格检查中发现的任何不对称表现，除了 MDI 之外，还需要考虑解剖异常（例如，盂唇损伤、Bankart 损伤和 SLAP 损伤）。

非手术治疗

对于大多数 MDI 患者，非手术治疗被认为是一线治疗。康复治疗应治疗肩胸的运动障碍，包括本体感受训练和肩袖加强训练。一项对 MDI 非手术治疗的研究发现，在 39 例患者中，有 35 例结果良好或优异。随后的长期随访研究显示，年轻的运动员患者对非手术治疗的反应较差，非手术治疗的患者中有 49% 结果较差，需要手术的患者占 37%。[24] 单纯的物理治疗无法让肩部运动恢复正常，但是接受了物理治疗联合关节囊移位的患者在第 4 年的随访中充分恢复了正常运动。[25] 尽管有这些发现，但仍建议在进行任何外科手术之前至少进行 6 个月的物理治疗。[25]

手术治疗

进行了康复治疗但仍有持续的功能障碍的患者应保留手术干预的选择。手术的目的是治疗发

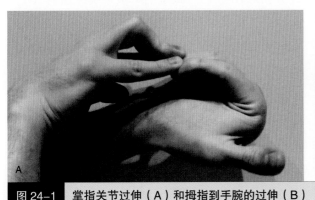

图 24-1　掌指关节过伸（A）和拇指到手腕的过伸（B）

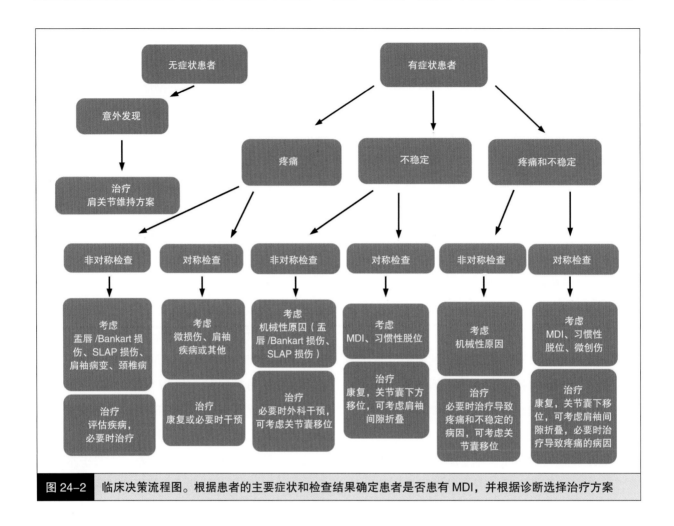

图 24-2 临床决策流程图。根据患者的主要症状和检查结果确定患者是否患有 MDI，并根据诊断选择治疗方案

生病变的结构，重点是使用关节囊－韧带技术减少关节囊的容积。诊疗全身性松弛症患者时，区分出真正的肩关节 MDI 与创伤性不稳定是很重要的。在 Neer 最初的关于下方关节囊移位的描述中，有超过一半的患者因严重创伤而出现不稳定。[1] 已发现 Bankart 修复中存在的弥漫性松弛会增加治疗的失败率，但这与真正的 MDI 是不同的。[26] 外科医师应仔细考虑患者的病情是创伤性盂唇撕裂还是真正的 MDI。诊断时应参考文献中相关的患者群体数据。

关节镜治疗注意事项

开放手术已用于外科手术治疗 MDI，但实验室数据显示开放手术和关节镜手术可实现的体积减小的量是相当的。[27] 在尸体模型中，1 cm 的褶皱缝合可使关节囊的体积减小 10%，5 个褶皱缝合的体积减小量类似开放移位手术。[28] 一项采用 ASES 肩关节疼痛和功能障碍评分的临床研究发现，与开放手术相比，关节镜治疗的效果具有统计学上的优势。早期手术患者的 ASES 肩关节疼痛和功能障碍评分相对较低。[29] 最近的一项系统综述纳入了 7 个比较开放手术和关节镜治疗 MDI 的研究，发现在肩关节不稳定的复发率、运动的恢复、外旋的丧失及并发症的发生率方面，二者没有显著差异。经关节镜治疗后，恢复运动的倾向略有增大。[30] 该系统综述适当地排除了具有 Bankart 损伤的患者，但仅包含具有Ⅳ级证据的研究。由于疾病过程和特定治疗机制的内在差异，这些发现难以得到很好的解释。但是，文献表明，有经验的术者可使关节镜治疗达到与开放手术相同的结果。

MDI 的关节镜治疗涉及不同的技术，最常见的技术为关节囊皱缩术和（或）肩袖间隙闭合术。关节囊热挛缩术由于报道的失败率、软骨溶解和神经损伤的发生率较高，因而已不再推荐。[31-32]多项实验室研究评估了关节镜治疗的特定技术。其中一项研究发现，单独的关节囊皱缩术虽然可以减少关节的过度运动，但必须联合肩袖间隙闭合术以减少盂肱关节平移。[33]与上－下肩袖间隙闭合术相比，内－外肩袖间隙闭合术可以更有效地减少关节的后移。[34]对 3 种类型的褶皱缝合进行比较后发现，简单缝合的效果可与 8 字缝合及褥式缝合相媲美。[35]

目前关于关节镜治疗 MDI 的临床数据有限。大多数研究仅进行到中期随访，并且许多研究包括患有 Bankart 损伤的患者。一项回顾性研究对 40 例接受关节镜治疗的 MDI 患者进行了 2~5 年的随访，结果显示：91% 的患者活动范围令人满意，86% 的患者可以极少受限或没有限制地恢复运动，并且临床结局评分为良好。[8]在一项对 9 例从事需要进行过顶运动的年轻运动员 MDI 患者的研究中，患者接受了关节囊褶皱缝合和肩袖间隙闭合治疗，其中有 7 例治疗结果评分为良好或出色；7 例患者可继续从事该运动项目，但其中 3 例可进行的运动级别较低。[36]

关节镜技术

麻醉下的检查是手术的第一步。所有 MDI 患者均具有向下的肩关节不稳定，重要的是要确定主要不稳定的方向是向前还是向后。这些发现应与对侧肩关节进行比较。检查后，令患者采取沙滩椅位或侧卧位。

在相对外侧的位置建立后方操作入路对于后续的关节囊和盂唇操作是有利的。在肩袖间隙建立 1~2 个前方入路（图 24-3）。应当对肩关节进行彻底的诊断检查，并注意肩袖间隙正常时是扩展的，并评估盂唇 Bankart 损伤（图 24-4）。在 MDI 中，盂唇可能有一些细微变化，但应保持贴附。牵拉肱骨可导致通过试验阳性，即关节镜可以在没有来自盂肱关节的阻碍的情况下，从后上方穿至前下方（图 24-5）。

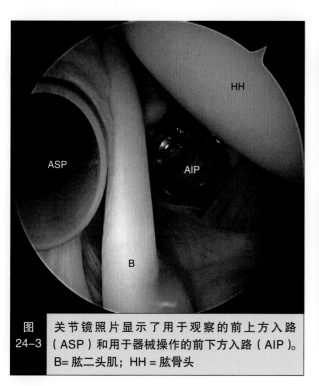

图 24-3　关节镜照片显示了用于观察的前上方入路（ASP）和用于器械操作的前下方入路（AIP）。B= 肱二头肌；HH = 肱骨头

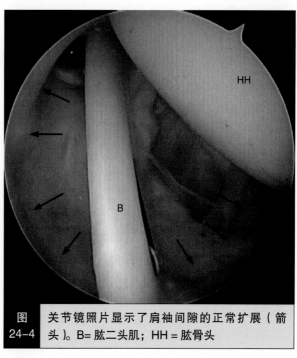

图 24-4　关节镜照片显示了肩袖间隙的正常扩展（箭头）。B= 肱二头肌；HH = 肱骨头

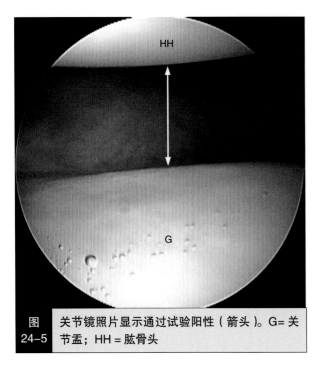

图 24-5　关节镜照片显示通过试验阳性（箭头）。G= 关节盂；HH = 肱骨头

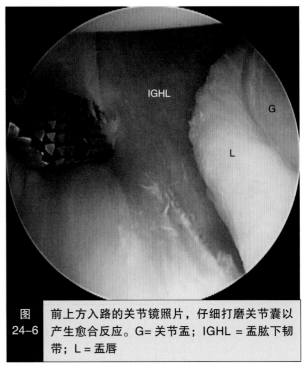

图 24-6　前上方入路的关节镜照片，仔细打磨关节囊以产生愈合反应。G= 关节盂；IGHL = 盂肱下韧带；L = 盂唇

对于关节囊皱缩术和肩袖间隙重叠术，目前存在着多种策略。在操作过程中，必须避免过紧或腋神经损伤。腋神经在关节盂的 6 点位置下方大约 12.4 mm 处走行，可以通过将手臂置于外展、外旋位并轻微牵引来保护腋神经。[37-38] 先进行关节囊的磨削，然后以连续的方式行关节囊皱缩术，通常从主要不稳定区域开始（前部或后部，图 24-6）。很重要的一点是从下到上逐步操作，因为每次皱缩都会减少关节的容积，从而限制操作的视野（图 24-7）。必须注意避免在内外方向上的组织移位，因为这样做会减小肩部的旋转运动范围。在处理了主要方向的不稳定后，将与主要不稳定方向相对的组织进行移位，以形成平衡稳定的肩关节（图 24-8）。缝合后，检查肱骨头中心在肩胛盂的位置，并检查肩关节的活动范围。缝线可能会断裂，如果运动受限，也可以将缝线拆下并重新拉紧。缝线可以穿过关节囊和盂唇或使用关节盂的缝合锚钉固定。目前尚未确定最佳的缝线数量、缝线构型和缝线材料。

研究者对肩袖间隙闭合的作用仍是有争议的。大多数支持肩袖间隙闭合的数据仅限于尸体研究，仅有很少的高级别临床证据。有一项研究表明，下方稳定性没有改善，但可以减小运动范围。[15] 避免缝合过紧和随后的外旋丢失是很重要的；可以通过在修复过程中将手臂放置在外展 20° ~30° 位置来防止这种情况的发生。该技术包含了内外和上下的闭合。

制动和康复

术后制动可以保持中立位，也可以基于原发不稳定的方向。例如，后下方不稳定的患者可以固定在外旋位。由于 MDI 术后僵硬的发生率远不如术后残余松弛的那么高，因此建议逐渐推进康复治疗。肩关节吊带固定 6 周（如果关节未出现僵硬，则吊带可佩戴更长的时间）。6 个月内，逐渐恢复运动。

总结

MDI 的诊断和治疗是一个临床难题。重要的是认识到真正的 MDI 本质上是非创伤性的。一线治疗是康复治疗，但是一些研究数据表明某些

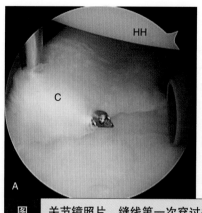
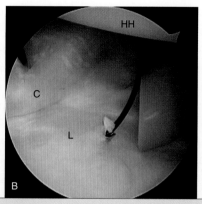
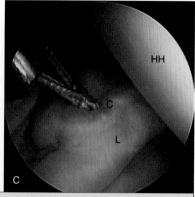

图
24-7　关节镜照片，缝线第一次穿过关节囊组织，在缝合盂唇之前使其上移（A）。缝合钩穿过盂唇，使可吸收的缝线穿过（B）。在组织的关节囊侧打结（C）。C= 关节囊组织；HH= 肱骨头；L= 盂唇

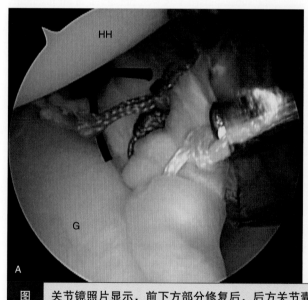
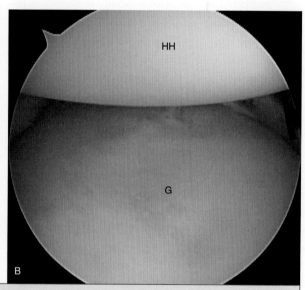

图
24-8　关节镜照片显示，前下方部分修复后，后方关节囊皱缩（A）。从前上方入路可以看到，经过多次褶皱缝合，肱骨头获得了平衡并位于关节盂关节面的中心位置（B）。G= 关节盂；HH= 肱骨头

患者对非手术治疗反应较差。目前，关于手术干预的证据有限，但多项研究表明，关节镜下治疗MDI可以达到与开放手术相同的效果。有必要继续研究以进一步明确关于手术技术的具体建议。

参考文献

[1]　Neer CS II, Foster CR: Inferior capsular shift for involuntary inferior and multidirectional instability of the shoulder: A preliminary report. *J Bone Joint Surg Am* 1980;62(6):897-908.

[2]　Bahu MJ, Trentacosta N, Vorys GC, Covey AS, Ah-mad CS: Multidirectional instability: Evaluation and treatment options. *Clin Sports Med* 2008;27(4):671-689. A general review of MDI and treatment options is provided. The initial treatment is with physical therapy, and surgical solutions are appropriate only after unsuccessful nonsurgical treatment.

[3]　Thomas SC, Matsen FA III: An approach to the repair of avulsion of the glenohumeral ligaments in the management of traumatic anterior glenohumeral instability. *J Bone Joint Surg Am* 1989;71(4):506-513.

[4]　McFarland EG, Kim TK, Park HB, Neira CA, Gutierrez MI: The effect of variation in definition on the diagnosis of multidirectional instability of the shoulder. *J*

Bone Joint Surg Am 2003;(11):2138-2144.

[5] Burkhead WZ Jr, Rockwood CA Jr: Treatment of instability of the shoulder with an exercise program. *J Bone Joint Surg Am* 1992;74(6):890-896.

[6] Caprise PA Jr, Sekiya JK: Open and arthroscopic treatment of multidirectional instability of the shoulder. *Arthroscopy* 2006;22(10):1126-1131.

[7] Cole B: *Surgical Techniques of the Shoulder, Elbow, and Knee in Sports Medicine.* Philadelphia, PA, WB Saunders, 2008.

A general review of surgical techniques in sports medicine is provided, including open surgical procedures for MDI.

[8] Baker CL III, Mascarenhas R, Kline AJ, Chhabra A, Pombo MW, Bradley JP: Arthroscopic treatment of multidirectional shoulder instability in athletes: A retrospective analysis of 2- to 5-year clinical outcomes. *Am J Sports Med* 2009;37(9):1712-1720.

The mean ASES score was 91.4 at 2- to 5-year follow-up of arthroscopic treatment of MDI in 43 shoulders in athletes age 14 to 39 years. Ninety-one percent of the patients had full or satisfactory range of motion, 98% had full or slightly decreased strength, and 86% had returned to sport with little or no limitation.

[9] Alpert JM, Verma N, Wysocki R, Yanke AB, Romeo AA: Arthroscopic treatment of multidirectional shoulder instability with minimum 270 degrees labral repair: Minimum 2-year follow-up. *Arthroscopy* 2008;24(6):704-711.

At a mean 56-month follow-up of 13 patients (mean age, 27.2 years) after arthroscopic stabilization for MDI and a labral tear of at least 270°, 85% had a good result on physical examination and measures including ASES.

[10] ElAttrache NS: *Surgical Techniques in Sports Medicine.* Philadelphia, PA, Lippincott, Williams & Wilkins, 2007.

Surgical techniques in sports medicine are reviewed, with a technique for arthroscopic surgical stabilization of MDI.

[11] Gaskill TR, Taylor DC, Millett PJ: Management of multidirectional instability of the shoulder. *J Am Acad Orthop Surg* 2011;19(12):758-767.

The definition, diagnosis, physical examination, physical therapy, and arthroscopic stabilization of MDI are reviewed.

[12] Werner AW, Lichtenberg S, Schmitz H, Nikolic A, Habermeyer P: Arthroscopic findings in atraumatic shoulder instability. *Arthroscopy* 2004;20(3):268-272.

[13] Kim SH, Noh KC, Park JS, Ryu BD, Oh I: Loss of chondrolabral containment of the glenohumeral joint in atraumatic posteroinferior multidirectional instability. *J Bone Joint Surg Am* 2005;87(1):92-98.

[14] Schenk TJ, Brems JJ: Multidirectional instability of the shoulder: Pathophysiology, diagnosis, and management. *J Am Acad Orthop Surg* 1998;6(1):65-72.

[15] Provencher MT, Dewing CB, Bell SJ, et al: An analysis of the rotator interval in patients with anterior, posterior, and multidirectional shoulder instability. *Arthroscopy* 2008;24(8):921-929.

The magnetic resonance arthrograms of patients with an anteriorly, posteriorly, or multidirectionally unstable shoulder were compared with those of control the subjects. The distance between the supraspinatus and the subscapularis was well preserved in all instability patterns. The long head of the biceps tendon assumes a more anterior position relative to the supraspinatus in posterior instability, compared with the anteriorly unstable or stable shoulder.

[16] Lippitt S, Matsen F: Mechanisms of glenohumeral joint stability. *Clin Orthop Relat Res* 1993;291:20-28.

[17] Ogston JB, Ludewig PM: Differences in 3-dimensional shoulder kinematics between persons with multidirectional instability and asymptomatic controls. *Am J Sports Med* 2007;35(8):1361-1370.

Patients with MDI had abnormal scapular kinematics in upward rotation, abduction, and internal rotation in comparison with control subjects. This finding highlights the importance of scapular stability and positioning exercises during MDI rehabilitation.

[18] Illyés A, Kiss RM: Electromyographic analysis in patients with multidirectional shoulder instability during pull, forward punch, elevation and overhead throw. *Knee Surg Sports Traumatol Arthrosc* 2007;15(5):624-631.

An electromyelography study compared patients with MDI and control subjects. Centralization of the glenohumeral joint is attempted by increasing rotator cuff musculature activation in patients with MDI, but there is an increased time difference in the peak activity of these muscle groups.

[19] Rodeo SA, Suzuki K, Yamauchi M, Bhargava M, Warren RF: Analysis of collagen and elastic fibers in shoulder capsule in patients with shoulder instability. *Am J Sports Med* 1998;26(5):634-643.

[20] Yamamoto N, Itoi E, Tuoheti Y, et al: The effect of the inferior capsular shift on shoulder intra-articular

pressure: A cadaveric study. *Am J Sports Med* 2006;34(6):939-944.

[21] Forsythe B, Ghodadra N, Romeo AA, Provencher MT: Management of the failed posterior/multidirectional instability patient. *Sports Med Arthrosc* 2010;18(3):149-161.

Presentation, physical examination findings, and radiographic analysis are described for patients after unsuccessful surgery for posterior instability or MDI, with options for a revision surgical solution.

[22] Rowe CR, Pierce DS, Clark JG: Voluntary dislocation of the shoulder: A preliminary report on a clinical, electromyographic, and psychiatric study of twenty-six patients. *J Bone Joint Surg Am* 1973;55(3):445-460.

[23] Warner JJ, Micheli LJ, Arslanian LE, Kennedy J, Kennedy R: Patterns of flexibility, laxity, and strength in normal shoulders and shoulders with instability and impingement. *Am J Sports Med* 1990;18(4):366-375.

[24] Misamore GW, Sallay PI, Didelot W: A longitudinal study of patients with multidirectional instability of the shoulder with seven- to ten-year follow-up. *J Shoulder Elbow Surg* 2005;14(5):466-470.

[25] Nyiri P, Illyés A, Kiss R, Kiss J: Intermediate biomechanical analysis of the effect of physiotherapy only compared with capsular shift and physiotherapy in multidirectional shoulder instability. *J Shoulder Elbow Surg* 2010;19(6):802-813.

A comparison of 32 patients with MDI treated only with physical therapy, 19 patients with MDI treated with capsular shift and physical therapy, and 50 healthy control subjects found that the alterations in kinematic parameters could be returned to normal with physical therapy alone but could be restored for at least 4 years with capsular shift and physical therapy.

[26] Chechik O, Maman E, Dolkart O, Khashan M, Shabtai L, Mozes G: Arthroscopic rotator interval closure in shoulder instability repair: A retrospective study. *J Shoulder Elbow Surg* 2010;19(7):1056-1062. In a retrospective review of patients with recurrent instability after arthroscopic Bankart repair, with or without arthroscopic rotator cuff interval closure, systemic joint hyperlaxity was associated with recurrent instability. Patients with arthroscopic rotator cuff interval closure had a more limited range of motion, with 75% having a good or an excellent functional result.

[27] Sekiya JK, Willobee JA, Miller MD, Hickman AJ, Willobee A: Arthroscopic multi-pleated capsular plication compared with open inferior capsular shift for reduc-

tion of shoulder volume in a cadaveric model. *Arthroscopy* 2007;23(11):1145-1151.

In seven fresh-frozen cadaver shoulders, arthroscopic plication resulted in a 58% mean volume decrease. Open inferior capsular shift resulted in a mean volume decrease of 45%. This study showed that the arthroscopic method could be as effective as the open method.

[28] Ponce BA, Rosenzweig SD, Thompson KJ, Tokish J: Sequential volume reduction with capsular plications: Relationship between cumulative size of plications and volumetric reduction for multidirectional instability of the shoulder. *Am J Sports Med* 2011;39(3):526-531.

In 12 fresh-frozen cadaver shoulders, a 1-cm plication stitch resulted in a 10% volume reduction. Five plication stitches resulted in a 49% to 52% reduction, which is similar to the result in an open lateral-based capsular shift.

[29] Yeargan SA III, Briggs KK, Horan MP, Black AK, Hawkins RJ: Determinants of patient satisfaction following surgery for multidirectional instability. *Orthopedics* 2008;31(7):647.

A review of 50 shoulders in 46 patients after stabilization surgery for MDI found that subjective variables, such as symptoms and motion, had the greatest correlation with patient satisfaction.

[30] Jacobson ME, Riggenbach M, Wooldridge AN, Bishop JY: Open capsular shift and arthroscopic capsular plication for treatment of multidirectional instability. *Arthroscopy* 2012;28(7):1010-1017.

A systematic review of seven studies with 197 patients found that arthroscopic capsular plication yielded results comparable to those of open capsular shift in terms of recurrent instability, return to sport, external rotation loss, and overall complications.

[31] D'Alessandro DF, Bradley JP, Fleischli JE, Connor PM: Prospective evaluation of thermal capsulorrhaphy for shoulder instability: Indications and results, two- to five-year follow-up. *Am J Sports Med* 2004;32(1):21-33.

[32] Hawkins RJ, Krishnan SG, Karas SG, Noonan TJ, Horan MP: Electrothermal arthroscopic shoulder capsulorrhaphy: A minimum 2-year follow-up. *Am J Sports Med* 2007;35(9):1484-1488.

At 2-year follow up, 37 of 85 thermal capsulorrhaphies had failed, and almost 60% had failed in patients with posterior, multidirectional, or anteroposterior instability. Augmenting these procedures with capsular plication and/or rotator cuff interval closure is recommended to improve results.

[33] Shafer BL, Mihata T, McGarry MH, Tibone JE, Lee TQ: Effects of capsular plication and rotator interval closure in simulated multidirectional shoulder instabil- ity. *J Bone Joint Surg Am* 2008;90(1):136-144.

Seven cadaver shoulders received anterior plication, posterior plication, and rotator cuff interval closure. Capsular plication alone resulted in reduced range of motion in the intact state, but reduction of glenohumeral translation required the addition of rotator cuff interval closure.

[34] Farber AJ, ElAttrache NS, Tibone JE, McGarry MH, Lee TQ: Biomechanical analysis comparing a traditional superior-inferior arthroscopic rotator interval closure with a novel medial-lateral technique in a cadaveric multidirectional instability model. *Am J Sports Med* 2009;37(6):1178-1185.

Eight match-paired cadaver shoulders underwent either superior-inferior or medial-lateral rotator cuff interval closure. Medial-lateral closure more closely restored range of motion to the intact state and significantly reduced posterior translation with the shoulder in an abducted, externally rotated position.

[35] Nho SJ, Frank RM, Van Thiel GS, et al: A biomechanical analysis of shoulder stabilization: Posteroinferior glenohumeral capsular plication. *Am J Sports Med* 2010;38(7):1413-1419.

Twenty-one fresh-frozen cadaver shoulders underwent capsulolabral plication with a simple stitch, a horizontal mattress, or a figure-of-8 configuration. All three configurations were effective in plication, but the simple stitch may be preferred because of technical ease.

[36] Voigt C, Schulz AP, Lill H: Arthroscopic treatment of multidirectional glenohumeral instability in young overhead athletes. *Open Orthop J* 2009;3:107-114.

Ten shoulders in nine young overhead athletes were treated with arthroscopic anteroposterior capsular plication and rotator cuff interval closure after unsuccessful nonsurgical treatment of MDI. Seven of the nine patients were able to return to their previous level of sport, but three returned at a lower level.

[37] Uno A, Bain GI, Mehta JA: Arthroscopic relationship of the axillary nerve to the shoulder joint capsule: An anatomic study. *J Shoulder Elbow Surg* 1999;8(3):226-230.

[38] Price MR, Tillett ED, Acland RD, Nettleton GS: Determining the relationship of the axillary nerve to the shoulder joint capsule from an arthroscopic perspective. *J Bone Joint Surg Am* 2004;(10):2135-2142.

第二十五章　肩关节上盂唇从前向后损伤

James R. Andrews, MD; Brett Shore, MD

引言

在肩关节镜技术出现之前，运动员的肩关节功能障碍主要被认为与肩峰撞击肩袖密切相关[1]，其主要治疗方法是切开式肩峰成形术，然而研究数据证实此种治疗方法的结果一般：失败率约为50%，只有约22%的患者恢复到伤前的运动水平。[2] 1985年，有学者首次报道了投掷运动员与肱二头肌长头相关的肩关节上盂唇损伤。[3] 其主要表现为盂唇的撕裂和分离，有时亦伴有肱二头肌腱的撕裂。与此同时，这些患者往往伴有肩袖损伤。针对这一系列的发现所提出的可能的损伤机制为肩袖和肱二头肌盂唇复合体反复张力过大导致磨损。1990年，肩关节SLAP损伤被用于描述这一损伤，其定义为从肱二头肌前缘至肱二头肌后缘广泛的损伤。[4] Snyder分型最初仅仅分为4型，后来分型范围逐步扩大到包括前盂唇所有

Dr. Andrews or an immediate family member has received royalties from Biomet Sports Medicine; serves as a paid consultant to or is an employee of Biomet Sports Medicine, Bauerfiend, Theralase, MiMedx, and Physiotherapy Associates; has stock or stock options held in Patient Connection and Connective Orthopaedics; and serves as a board member, owner, officer, or committee member of FastHealth, the American Orthopaedic Society for Sports Medicine, and Physiotherapy Associates. Neither Dr. Shore nor any immediate family member has received anything of value from or has stock or stock options held in a commercial company or institution related directly or indirectly to the subject of this chapter.

可识别的病理损伤。最新的研究重新探讨了SLAP损伤的发病机制、临床表现和治疗方法，从而提高了对这些损伤及其治疗的认识。

分型

尽管SLAP损伤已由最初的4型扩展至10型，但是使用最为广泛的分型还是4型[4-6]（图25-1）。已经有研究证实此分型的可靠性不佳。[7-8] I型病变是上盂唇内侧边缘的退行性磨损，但肱二头肌附着区完整。I型损伤为最常见的SLAP损伤，多

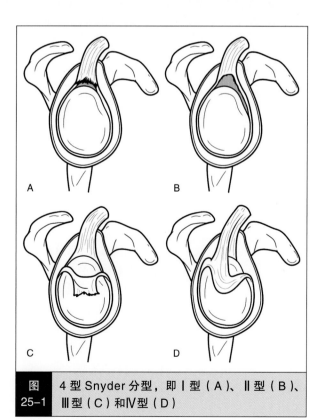

图 25-1　4型Snyder分型，即I型（A）、II型（B）、III型（C）和IV型（D）

不伴有明显的临床症状，往往在中年患者中被不经意地发现。Ⅱ型 SLAP 损伤往往表现为上盂唇与肱二头肌腱复合体从肩胛盂撕脱。这是临床最常见的、症状最明显的损伤。Ⅱ型 SLAP 损伤的撕裂可分为前方撕裂、后方撕裂或从前向后的撕裂（相对于肱二头肌起点）（图 25-2）。投掷运动员往往伴随着撕裂继续向后方延伸。Ⅲ型 SLAP 损伤

的特征是上盂唇的桶柄样撕裂，病变累及关节内，但盂唇与肱二头肌腱复合体仍旧附着于肩胛盂上。Ⅳ型 SLAP 损伤在桶柄样撕裂的基础上，延伸到肱二头肌长头腱，可能导致肌腱完全撕脱。其余的 Gartsman 和 Ryu 分型涉及相关的肩关节不稳定损伤，如 Bankart 损伤、后盂唇损伤、盂肱中韧带损伤或 360° 盂唇部损伤（表 25-1）。

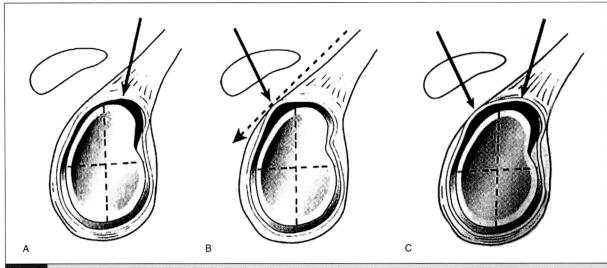

图 25-2　Snyder Ⅱ型 SLAP 损伤的前方撕裂（A）、后方撕裂（B）及从前向后撕裂（C）三种亚型。实线箭头所指为撕裂的原发位置（前部、后部或前后部均有），虚垂直线和虚水平线为关节盂象限的划分，虚线箭头为产生 SLAP 后方撕裂的力的方向（B）。经允许引自 Morgan CD, Burkhart SS, Palmeri M, Gillespie M. Type II SLAP lesions: Three subtypes and their relationships to superior instability and rotator cuff tears. *Arthroscopy* 1998;14（6）:553–565.

表 25-1

SLAP 损伤

分型	描述
Ⅰ型	上盂唇磨损
Ⅱ型	肱二头肌腱与上盂唇分离
Ⅲ型	上盂唇桶柄样撕裂，肱二头肌止点完整
Ⅳ型	上盂唇桶柄样撕裂延伸至肱二头肌腱
Ⅴ型	Bankart 损伤延伸并使肱二头肌腱止点分离
Ⅵ型	前方或后方盂唇瓣，伴Ⅱ型肱二头肌腱损伤
Ⅶ型	肱二头肌腱止点分离，延伸至盂肱中韧带
Ⅷ型	Ⅱ型合并后方盂唇延伸
Ⅸ型	Ⅱ型合并 360° 盂唇分离
Ⅹ型	Ⅱ型合并后下方盂唇分离

解剖学与生物力学

盂唇由一个纤维软骨环构成，外观呈新月形，从而加深肩关节盂。此外，盂唇亦作为盂肱韧带和肱二头肌腱的附着点。上盂唇外观呈黏液状，牢固地附着于关节盂周围，有时亦有部分附着于中央。

肱二头肌长头腱附着在盂唇后上方和盂上结节，肩胛盂内侧约 5 mm 处。40%~60% 的肱二头肌腱纤维附着于盂上结节，其余的则直接附着于盂唇。肱二头肌附着在盂唇上的主要部位不尽相同，在大多数人中，肱二头肌大部分或全部仅附着在盂唇后部，但也可以主要附着于前部。盂唇的血供主要通过关节及周边的动脉提供，主要包括肩胛上动脉、旋肱后动脉和旋肩胛动脉等。盂唇四周的血供最为丰富，中央部分相对欠缺，而上盂唇的血供最差。

肱二头肌腱可以视作肱骨头的一个压迫者，是在肩关节外展和外旋时限制其脱位的次要约束。[9] SLAP 损伤可降低肩关节在外展外旋时对外旋的抵抗。与之相关的 SLAP 损伤可增加旋前的移位，并增加肱骨下韧带复合体的张力。[10] 当盂肱关节功能下降时，肱二头肌在肩关节的稳定中起到了巨大的作用。[11]

剥离征是由投掷姿势对上盂唇和肱二头肌的影响所致[12]（图 25-3）。投掷姿势导致肩关节处于最大程度的外展外旋位，迫使肱二头肌腱处于相对靠后方且垂直的位置，从而在此过程中扭曲后盂唇。肱二头肌起点的完整性可有效地对抗这种移动，但是在存在 II 型 SLAP 损伤的情况下，盂唇可从关节盂上向内侧旋转并到达肩胛颈的后方。修复 II 型 SLAP 损伤可恢复上盂唇的稳定性，并消除剥离现象。

病理

现有的 SLAP 损伤的可能机制包括重复性投掷运动、牵引和压迫，这些均已在标本模型中得到证实。单一的创伤事件是导致缺如前一症状期的患者突然出现此类损伤的原因，而重复性的投掷活动是导致投掷运动员发病的主要原因。在标本研究中，特别是当手臂向前弯曲时，直接压迫或撞击会导致 SLAP 损伤。[13] 此外也有研究发现，对肩关节下方半脱位进行持续牵引可导致 SLAP 损伤。[14]

运动员的 II 型 SLAP 损伤的机制是复杂且具有争议的。其中一种说法是后方关节囊挛缩导致肱骨头内旋不足（GIRD）伴随着肱骨头后上移位、

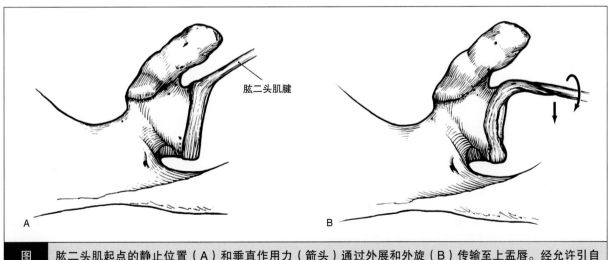

肱二头肌腱

A　　　　　　　　　　　B

图 25-3 肱二头肌起点的静止位置（A）和垂直作用力（箭头）通过外展和外旋（B）传输至上盂唇。经允许引自 Burkhart SS, Morgan CD. The peel-back mechanism: Its role in producing and extending posterior type II SLAP lesions and its effect on SLAP repair rehabilitation. *Arthroscopy* 1998;14（6）:637-640.

外展和外旋，然后在肱二头肌起点施加剪切力和扭力所致。[12,15]虽然在关节镜检查中发现了这种剥离机制的证据，但很少有直接证据表明伴有后关节囊挛缩的肱骨头内旋不足是发生 SLAP 损伤的主要原因。对运动员来说，剥离机制可能是常态，他们在投掷时肩关节的外旋增加，而内旋则减少（图 25-4）。可能是这种过度的外旋，使肱二头肌止点承受了异常压力，失去后关节囊的约束。在肩关节 90° 外展和 90° 外旋时，在肱骨大结节和肩胛盂后上盂唇之间会发生内侧撞击。[16]当这一过程在投掷的最后一个阶段，即肩关节上举的时候反复出现，则可以导致 SLAP 损伤。

尽管以上说法均适用于运动员 II 型 SLAP 损伤，但所谓的除草假说可能能够更加充分地解释大多数患者的 SLAP 损伤。[17]除草假说表明 SLAP 的撕裂是因为肩关节上举阶段反复交替作用力，这会在肱二头肌复合体上产生向后的作用力，而继之而来的减速则会产生向前的作用力。这一过程可导致投掷运动员的特征性 SLAP 损伤。

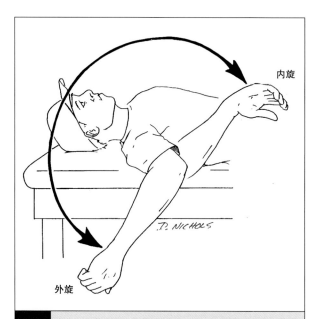

图
25-4
图示关节总活动弧的概念，其中外旋（ER）活动范围 + 内旋（IR）活动范围 = 总活动范围。经允许引自 Wilk KE, Meister K, Andrews JR. Current concepts in the rehabilitation of the overhead throwing athlete. *Am J Sports Med* 2002; 30（1）:136–151.

临床评估

有症状的 SLAP 损伤患者大致分为两类：一类是运动员，其中大多数是棒球投手（此外还包括游泳运动员、网球运动员、标枪运动员和排球运动员）；另一类是遭受了急性创伤，肩关节受到牵拉或者压缩的患者。此外，由于军事训练的严苛和重复，SLAP 损伤也常在军人中发生。在接受肩关节镜检查的军人中，约有 22% 的人存在 SLAP 损伤，而其中 69% 是 II 型。[18]

一份准确而完整的病史对于评估 SLAP 损伤至关重要。过顶运动运动员对其症状和发病时间的描述往往是含糊不清的，并且无法明确追溯到受伤原因。因此，对于此类患者最重要的是要了解其活动的特性，包括速度变化、机制、持续时间和是否伴有疼痛。肩关节撞击的症状通常类似于 SLAP 损伤，包括弥散的疼痛、上臂麻木综合征及肩关节活动范围的丧失。上臂麻木综合征被定义为由于疼痛和不适而无法以受伤前的速度和控制能力活动肩关节。[19]当肩关节旋转时，患者可能会出现机械症状，如交锁、卡住或弹出等。

当怀疑患者存在 SLAP 损伤时，体格检查应包括对肩关节功能障碍或病理性肩关节运动（如 GIRD 或摩擦音）的评估以及对肩关节病损的应力性检查。此外，应评估肌肉萎缩，冈下肌萎缩提示棘突处的囊肿，往往与 SLAP 损伤有关。在没有其他损伤的情况下，存在 SLAP 损伤的患者应具有正常的肩袖强度和肩关节主动活动范围（在投掷运动员中，定义为其优势手和非优势手之间的肩关节主动活动范围差距不超过 25°）。对肩关节不稳定的检查对于检测相关的盂唇损伤至关重要，应当包括针对前方不稳定的肩关节前脱位恐惧 – 再复位试验和针对后方不稳定的加载移位试验。此外还有 O'Brien（动态挤压）试验、肱二头肌负荷 II 试验、被动肩关节外展和肘关节屈曲、复位试验、曲柄试验和旋后外旋抵抗试验，这些试验均可用于发现 SLAP 损伤[20-25]（图 25-5）。

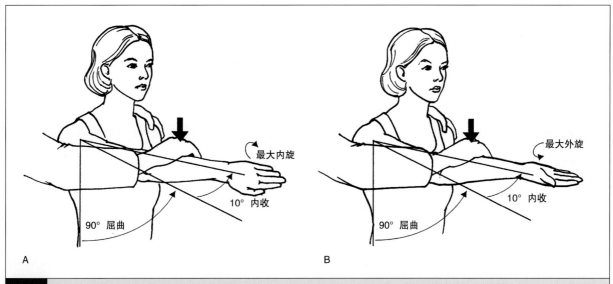

图
25-5
图示 O'Brien 试验。在肩关节屈曲内收时，内旋（A）或外旋（B）手臂抵抗向下的力。外旋时症状减轻是一个阳性结果。经允许引自 Parentis MA, Jobe CM, Pink MM, Jobe FW. An anatomic evaluation of the active compression test. *J Shoulder Elbow Surg* 2004;13（4）:410–416.

利用以上常用的新兴的查体方法进行充分的评估后，复位试验可能是最准确的试验，而复位实验结合 O'Brien 试验是检测 SLAP 损伤很有效的方式。[26] 一项最新的荟萃分析评估了针对 SLAP 损伤的各种体格检查的实用性，结果表明，主动加压试验、曲柄试验和肱二头肌张力试验具有非常高的敏感性和特异性，而前方滑动试验的准确性明显更低。[27] 一项病例对照研究发现，在仅有 SLAP 损伤的患者身上进行体格检查，肱二头肌负荷 II 试验最为准确，而 O'Brien 试验、复位试验、肱二头肌张力试验及盂唇张力试验不能准确辨别 SLAP 损伤。[28] 不过有部分研究者认为复位试验在此项研究中的实施可能存在问题。正确的方法是患者取仰卧位，肩关节离开检查床的一侧，使肩胛骨得到支撑，但肱骨没有活动。肩关节外展 90°，肘关节屈曲 90°。肩关节外旋至最大角度，肘关节后伸至最大角度，肩关节被动抬高，保持水平外展和外旋。阳性表现为当肩关节运动（通常 90°~120°）时，患者会出现疼痛，并听到弹响。

O'Brien 试验是在患者手臂向下加压的情况下进行的，此时肩关节前屈 90°，肘关节伸直，手臂轻微内收（10°~15°），手先最大内旋，然后旋后。如果在旋后过程中患者的疼痛减轻，则该试验结果为阳性。Speed 试验是在手臂向下施加压力的同时，肩关节前屈 60°，并且肘关节伸展。如果疼痛局限于结节间沟，则该试验结果为阳性。曲柄试验是在将肩关节抬高至 160°，并在肱骨内、外旋的同时施加轴向负荷的情况下进行的。如在外旋时患者出现疼痛，则为阳性，此外，亦可伴有弹响或交锁。肱二头肌负荷 II 试验是在患者仰卧，肩膀外展 120°，肘关节屈曲 90°，前臂旋后的情况下进行的。肩关节得以最大外旋，患者屈曲肘关节以抵抗阻力。若患者出现疼痛，则此试验为阳性。

尽管它们的整体准确性差异很大，但几种试验经常被结合使用。需要说明的是，阳性结果往往仅提示 SLAP 损伤而无法进行确诊。

影像学检查

最初的影像学检查仅仅是普通的 X 线片（肩关节前后位、肩胛骨前后位、肩关节腋位和出口位），这些 X 线片并不专门用于诊断 SLAP 损伤，但可以帮助分辨其他肩部的病变。MRI 是鉴定 SLAP 损伤及伴随的盂唇、软骨和肩袖损伤的首选检查方法。尽管 MRA 识别盂唇部分损伤的优势已被广泛认同，但仍值得一提的是，添加关节内造影剂对于鉴别盂唇的细微病变非常有用。在摄片时肩关节的外展和外旋可进一步显示上盂唇和前盂唇的损伤，并在研究上盂唇解剖变异时具有独特的优势。[29]肩关节的外旋可提高 MRA 识别 SLAP 损伤的敏感性和特异性。[30]与 SLAP 损伤相符的 MRA 表现包括 T2 加权成像上后上盂唇的信号增强，以及冠状位 MRA 上肩胛盂和上盂唇之间出现环状影（图 25-6）。在轴位 MRI 或 MRA 上发现前上方盂唇撕裂也提示 SLAP 损伤。MRI 有助于鉴别肩胛上囊肿和棘突囊肿，而这些囊肿往往与 SLAP 损伤有关。

MRI 对诊断 SLAP 损伤的准确性为 67%～98%，特异性为 63%～100%。[31-35]使用 3T 磁场进行 MRI 与 MRA 的敏感性并列比较的结果为 83%：98%，MRA 显然具有更高的敏感性。[36]CT 关节造影对 SLAP 损伤的诊断往往更为精确，

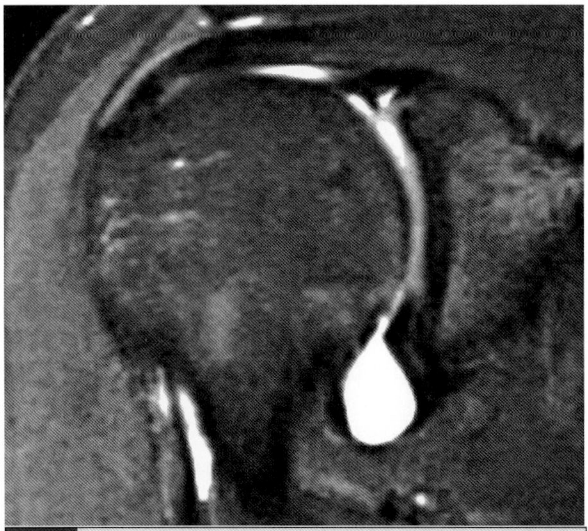

图 25-6　冠状位 T2 加权成像 MRA 显示盂唇和关节盂之间的造影剂。经允许引自 Keener JD, Brophy RH: Pathogenesis, evaluation and treatment. *J Am Acad Orthop Surg* 2009;17（10）:627–637.

相比于 MRA，其在观察者之间具有良好的一致性。[37-38]尽管肩关节的影像学应用时间较长，但 SLAP 损伤的准确诊断必须结合病史和体格检查结果。

治疗

非手术治疗

SLAP 损伤的非手术治疗包括：刺激性运动、镇痛消炎药、后方关节囊拉伸及肩袖和肩关节稳定性的增强。

四阶段恢复法适用于有肩部症状（如 SLAP 损伤、肩袖病变、肌腱炎或内撞击）的运动员的康复。[39]急性期，即第一阶段的目标是减轻疼痛、减少炎症、恢复正常运动（特别是内旋和水平内收），以及恢复肌肉力量和本体感觉。第二阶段的重点是逐渐增加力量，提高灵活性，并促进对肌肉的控制。第三阶段的内容是积极地增强力量和功能锻炼。第四阶段是重返投掷运动阶段，它包括一组间歇投掷运动或另一个类似的特定运动，该阶段持续至运动时疼痛消失。一项涉及 39 例患者的研究发现，其中 19 例（49%）患者在非手术治疗失败后需要进行手术治疗。[40]在决定进行手术前，运动员应首先尝试采用非手术治疗，并评估能否由此恢复正常活动，特别是内旋。

手术治疗

SLAP 损伤的手术治疗通常在肩关节镜下进行。其手术治疗方式多样，选择往往取决于损伤的类型、患者的活动水平，以及附加的损伤。手术治疗的适应证通常为 3 个月的非手术治疗效果不佳，但是对于高水平运动员，应考虑早期手术干预，尤其是在休赛期。而对于赛季中尚可以忍受疼痛并参加比赛的运动员，其手术治疗可以推迟至赛季结束。对于非高水平运动员的 SLAP 损伤，其治疗方法已经引起了广泛的争议，关于哪些患者可以从手术中获益，以及应该采用哪种手术方式的问题仍未得到解决。对于 SLAP 损伤，

当非手术治疗失败，患者的症状和体格检查结果提示与 SLAP 损伤有关，以及在关节镜下修复肱二头肌起点并不稳定时，常常建议行手术治疗。对于 40 岁以上有症状的 SLAP 损伤患者，肱二头肌固定往往比肱二头肌修复更为有利。

手术治疗的选择取决于 SLAP 损伤的类型，如使用最初的 4 型 Snyder 分型所确定的损伤类型。对于其他分型（特别是包括 SLAP 损伤伴肩关节不稳定）的患者，当病变没有延伸到上盂唇时，通常需要手术治疗以修复盂唇的连续性及肩关节的稳定性。Ⅰ型 SLAP 损伤可通过轻度病损清除术恢复肩关节的稳定性，但在没有症状的情况下可能并不需要手术治疗。Ⅱ型 SLAP 损伤由于累及肱二头肌腱起点，通常需要将肱二头肌盂唇复合体重新附着到上关节盂，但肱二头肌腱固定可以用于翻修术或 40 岁以上活动量较小的患者。对于Ⅲ型 SLAP 损伤，可采用病损清除术，以及对桶柄样撕裂进行固定并修复任何导致肩关节不稳定的盂唇损伤。另外，如果桶柄样撕裂累及盂肱中韧带，则应予以修复。Ⅳ型损伤的手术治疗方式的选择取决于肱二头肌损伤的严重程度。在肱二头肌受损极轻微的情况下，仅需要行肱二头肌病损清除术加盂唇修复，但在肱二头肌腱严重损伤的情况下，首选的治疗是切开或关节镜下肱二头肌腱固定。

手术技巧

在此之前已有多种 SLAP 损伤修复技术被广泛报道。本章作者偏好的手术技术将在后文具体阐述（图 25-7，25-8）。关节镜检查时患者可取沙滩椅位或侧卧位，且术者以标准方式建立后入路。如果还存在 Bankart 损伤，则建立一个更偏向内侧的入路（在关节盂附近）可能会更有帮助。入路越偏向内侧，对于向后侧延伸的 SLAP 损伤越有帮助。前入路在肩袖间隙内建立，并用于施行诊断性的关节镜检查以排除其他损伤。

根据 SLAP 损伤的程度，可考虑建立其他入路用于放置缝合锚，这些入路包括辅助外侧入路（距肩峰前外侧角约 1 cm）、Wilmington 入路（距肩峰后外侧角约 1 cm）和可用于过线的 Neviaser 入路。需要注意的是，术中往往并不需要建立所有的入路。套管不能穿过肩袖而仅能用于前入路。[41] 所有需要经过肩袖的入路均应使用 11 号刀片，沿肩袖纤维的走行切开从而建立入路，以最大限度地减少医源性损伤。

术中应充分探查 SLAP 损伤及其分型，从而选择合适的术式。确保肱二头肌腱的稳定性具有至关重要的作用。应从关节盂处游离盂唇，以完成彻底的撕裂，进而如所有的盂唇修复一样准备血供丰富的骨组织床以促进其愈合。这一步骤通常通

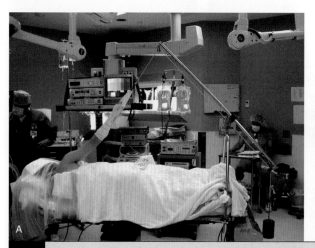
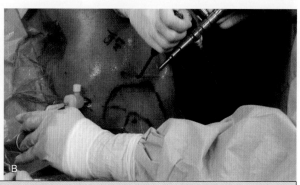

图 25-7　图示 SLAP 损伤的修复。A. 关节镜手术时首选侧卧位，但也可以使用沙滩椅位。B. 展示了前入路（绿色套管）、后入路和辅助入路（并非总是必要的）的位置

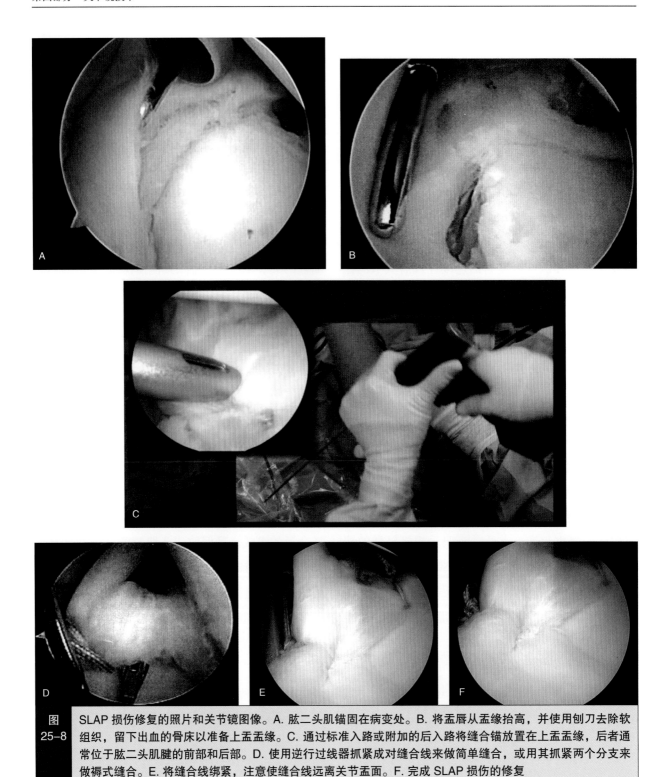

图 25-8　SLAP 损伤修复的照片和关节镜图像。A. 肱二头肌锚固在病变处。B. 将盂唇从盂缘抬高，并使用刨刀去除软组织，留下出血的骨床以准备上盂盂缘。C. 通过标准入路或附加的后入路将缝合锚放置在上盂盂缘，后者通常位于肱二头肌腱的前部和后部。D. 使用逆行过线器抓紧成对缝合线来做简单缝合，或用其抓紧两个分支来做褥式缝合。E. 将缝合线绑紧，注意使缝合线远离关节盂面。F. 完成 SLAP 损伤的修复

过前入路完成。良好地控制刨刀及熟悉反向设置的使用对于避免术中伤及关节面十分重要。接下来则需要将缝合锚放置在关节边缘。由于使用缝合钉可导致滑膜炎和关节损伤，现大部分医师已放弃使用此种技术。[42-43] 尽管无线结技术作为一种新兴技术已被广泛接受，但此处依旧推荐使用标准的 3.0 mm 生物复合缝合锚。[44] 一个缝合锚置入肱二头肌腱的前方，这时需要使用套管针以确定从辅助外侧入路（距关节盂中心 45°）进入的适当角度。该入路通常可用于将一个缝合锚放置在肱二头肌

的后方，但是如果 SLAP 损伤存在向后方延续的可能，则应当使用 Wilmington 入路。在术中切勿为了保护入路而导致缝合锚置入的位置或方向不佳。过线可以使用穿过套管针的缝合恢复装置、刚性逆行过线器、弯曲的缝合环或退线器来完成。缝合的形式可以是只穿过一次上盂的单结或穿过两次上盂的褥式缝合。生物力学数据表明，单结的滑脱率要高于褥式缝合，一个双负荷缝合锚相当于两个单负荷缝合锚，而两个后方的缝合锚则等于一个前方的缝合锚和一个后方的缝合锚（位于类似剥离机制的垂直向量上）。[45-47] 在关节镜下，可以同时进行盂唇旁囊肿的手术治疗。[48] 盂唇旁囊肿可以通过修复 SLAP 损伤而不直接减压解决，但如果发现肌肉萎缩严重，则建议直接减压。[49]

术后护理

SLAP 损伤修复后康复方案的选择取决于修复的程度（相对广泛的撕裂往往需要较长的时间），以及是否伴有其他术中发现的损伤。[50] 术后 6 周内专注于恢复肩关节活动范围和运动稳定性，接下来的 6 周致力于增强力量和恢复本体感觉。

简单的病损清除术后的恢复过程可能相当快，但修复 Ⅱ 型 SLAP 损伤需要一个更渐进、更结构化的方案。在术后前 4 周，允许的活动范围为上举不超过 90°，内旋活动范围可大于外旋活动范围。术后 8 周应充分恢复正常活动，术后 12 周可进行投掷运动。等长收缩活动应该于术后立即进行以加强活动时的动态稳定性，而负重运动及肱二头肌的锻炼则应在术后 7 周及 12 周后方可开始。

Ⅳ 型病变修复后的康复与 Ⅱ 型病变相似，但尚需注意肱二头肌腱的锻炼。如果对肱二头肌腱进行了松解，则建议肱二头肌主动运动从术后 6 周后开始。如果进行了成形，建议肱二头肌主动运动从术后 12 周后开始。

预后

关于 SLAP 损伤患者的预后研究大多数集中在 Ⅱ 型 SLAP 损伤上。在 1 年的随访中，78% 的

患者在接受了病损清除术后，取得了良好的预后；但在 2 年的随访中，只有 63% 的患者取得了良好的预后；44% 的患者重返赛场[51]。

SLAP 损伤修复的结果往往取决于其固定方式。使用可吸收材料常可导致预后不佳，包括夜间痛、术后活动范围不佳及无法重返赛场[41,52]。经关节镜修复 SLAP 损伤常可消除剥离征，优良率可达 97%。[53] 在一项对 53 例投手患者长达 1 年随访的研究结果中，其中有 44 例（87%）重新回到了赛场，但不幸的是，在那些伴有肩袖撕裂的患者中，都发现了一定程度的内旋活动范围的下降。一项纳入 23 名优秀投掷运动员的研究亦发现，伴有肩袖撕裂的患者重回赛场的比例较那些不伴有肩袖撕裂的患者低。[54] 在对于评估投掷运动员预后量表的选择上，一项平均 38 个月的随访中，有 22 例（96%）患者的美国肩肘指数评分等级可达良好的水平；然而，只有 12 例（52%）患者的 Kerlan-Jobe 评分可达良好水平，且仅有 13 例（57%）患者重返赛场。[55] 最近一项对 47 例患者平均 2.7 年的前瞻性研究发现，40 例（85%）患者在随访中显示出良好的预后；与非创伤性患者相比，因急性创伤性事件患病的患者具有更好的预后及更高的重返赛场的比例。[56] 在另一项平均 3.5 年的随访中，投掷运动员的总体满意度为 93%，恢复到伤前运动水平的比例为 84%，美国肩肘外科评分和 Kerlan-Jobe 评分量表的平均得分分别为 87.9 分和 73.6 分。[57] 这项研究结果提示 Kerlan-Jobe 评分可作为评估投掷运动员预后的一个较好的方法。

在一项对平均年龄为 39.7 岁的患者进行的研究中，总的优良率为 87%。[58] 工伤患者中仅有 65% 的患者认为其恢复良好，但这一比例在非工伤患者中可高达 95%，并且统计分析发现，40 岁以上的这两类患者中也有相似的趋势，但差异没有统计学意义。同样，另一项研究也发现，对年龄在 40 岁以下和 40 岁以上的患者进行 SLAP 损

伤修复后，其效果与非手术治疗没有显著性差异。[59]然而对老年患者（平均年龄为57岁）进行SLAP损伤修复和肩袖修补，可取得良好的效果。[60]一项针对45~60岁患者的研究发现，对于Ⅱ型SLAP损伤，病损清除术的效果优于SLAP损伤修复联合肩袖修补术。[61]关于SLAP修复翻修术的相关资料有限，但是在一项12例患者的小型研究中，修复翻修术的效果明显差于初次修复术，尤其是对于那些投掷运动员或工伤患者。[62]

最近，已有学者提出使用初次肱二头肌腱固定治疗SLAP损伤患者，特别是年龄较大或不参与投掷运动的患者。在关节镜下行该手术或SLAP修复术，发现前者的效果在术后评分、满意度及重返赛场的病例比例上明显优于后者。由于行前一种手术的患者的年龄明显高于行SLAP修复术的患者的年龄（平均年龄分别为52岁和37岁），因此将数据外推到年轻的患者是不合适的。[63]

并发症

SLAP损伤修复最常见的并发症是术后关节僵硬、活动范围下降，这两种并发症可通过适当的术后物理治疗将其发生率降至最低。此外，其他并发症还包括夜间痛、肩袖撕裂、滑膜炎和软骨损伤，这些可能与锚钉的松动有关。[52,64-66]也有少量文献宣称发现肩胛上神经损伤。[67-68]

总结

SLAP损伤通常是由两个截然相反的病因所导致的：特定的创伤事件或长期进行投掷运动。经典的Ⅱ型SLAP损伤多见于40岁以下的男性投掷运动员的优势臂。投掷运动员中SLAP损伤的发病机制尚存争议。仅对SLAP损伤进行临床评估尚不足以明确诊断，确诊往往依赖于高质量的影像学证据（3T MRA）或关节镜检查。非手术治疗有时是有效的，但外科干预则是投掷运动员的首选治疗方式。SLAP损伤的手术修复在缓解疼痛和提高肩关节功能方面可取得良好的效果，但对于能否恢复至伤前高水平的运动状态这一点尚无法确认。行修复术的术后并发症不常见。根据损伤的程度和性质行结构化康复对患者的预后至关重要。

参考文献

[1] Neer CS Ⅱ: Anterior acromioplasty for the chronic impingement syndrome in the shoulder: A preliminary report. *J Bone Joint Surg Am* 1972;54(1):41-50.

[2] Tibone JE, Jobe FW, Kerlan RK, et al: Shoulder impingement syndrome in athletes treated by an anterior acromioplasty. *Clin Orthop Relat Res* 1985;188:134-140.

[3] Andrews JR, Carson WG Jr, McLeod WD: Glenoid labrum tears related to the long head of the biceps. *Am J Sports Med* 1985;13(5):337-341.

[4] Snyder SJ, Karzel RP, Del Pizzo W, Ferkel RD, Friedman MJ: SLAP lesions of the shoulder. *Arthroscopy* 1990;6(4):274-279.

[5] Maffet MW, Gartsman GM, Moseley B: Superior labrum-biceps tendon complex lesions of the shoulder. *Am J Sports Med* 1995;23(1):93-98.

[6] Powell SE, Nord KD, Ryu RK: The diagnosis, classification and treatment of SLAP lesions. *Oper Tech Sports Med* 2004;12:99-110.

[7] Gobezie R, Zurakowski D, Lavery K, Millett PJ, Cole BJ, Warner JJ: Analysis of interobserver and intraobserver variability in the diagnosis and treatment of SLAP tears using the Snyder classification. *Am J Sports Med* 2008;36(7):1373-1379.

This is a cohort study in which 22 video vignettes of shoulder arthroscopy were sent to members of the Arthroscopy Association of North America, the American Shoulder and Elbow Surgeons, and the American Orthopaedic Society for Sports Medicine. They were asked to review the images, classify the SLAP lesions, and recommend treatment; a total of 73 members returned analyses. Surgeons had the most difficulty differentiating between type Ⅲ and type Ⅳ lesions and between type Ⅱ lesions and normal shoulders; additionally, the treatment of type Ⅲ lesions was most variable. Overall, moderate interobserver agreement was found with respect to the Snyder classification, which improved significantly when the diagnoses were analyzed based on treatment desision. Level of evidence: Ⅱ.

[8] Jia X, Yokota A, McCarty EC, et al: Reproducibility and reliability of the Snyder classification of superior labral

anterior posterior lesions among shoulder surgeons. *Am J Sports Med* 2011;39(5):986-991.

[9] Kumar VP, Satku K, Balasubramaniam P: The role of the long head of biceps brachii in the stabilization of the head of the humerus. *Clin Orthop Relat Res* 1989;244:172-175.

[10] Pagnani MJ, Deng XH, Warren RF, Torzilli PA, Altchek DW: Effect of lesions of the superior portion of the glenoid labrum on glenohumeral translation. *J Bone Joint Surg Am* 1995;77(7):1003-1010.

[11] Warner JJ, McMahon PJ: The role of the long head of the biceps brachii in superior stability of the glenohumeral joint. *J Bone Joint Surg Am* 1995;77(3):366-372.

[12] Burkhart SS, Morgan CD: The peel-back mechanism: Its role in producing and extending posterior type IISLAP lesions and its effect on SLAP repair rehabilita- tion. *Arthroscopy* 1998;14(6):637-640.

[13] Clavert P, Bonnomet F, Kempf JF, Boutemy P, Braun M, Kahn JL: Contribution to the study of the pathogenesis of type II superior labrum anterior-posterior lesions: A cadaveric model of a fall on the outstretched hand. *J Shoulder Elbow Surg* 2004;13(1):45-50.

[14] Bey MJ, Elders GJ, Huston LJ, Kuhn JE, Blasier RB, Soslowsky LJ: The mechanism of creation of superior labrum, anterior, and posterior lesions in a dynamic biomechanical model of the shoulder: The role of inferior subluxation. *J Shoulder Elbow Surg* 1998;7(4):397-401.

[15] Burkhart SS, Morgan CD, Kibler WB: The disabled throwing shoulder: Spectrum of pathology. Part I: Pathoanatomy and biomechanics. *Arthroscopy* 2003;19(4):404-420.

[16] Walch G, Boileau P, Noel E, Donell ST: Impingement of the deep surface of the supraspinatus tendon on the posterosuperior glenoid rim: An arthroscopic study. *J Shoulder Elbow Surg* 1992;1(5):238-245.

[17] Jazrawi LM, McCluskey GM III, Andrews JR: Superior labral anterior and posterior lesions and internal impingement in the overhead athlete. *Instr Course Lect* 2003;52:43-63.

[18] Kampa RJ, Clasper J: Incidence of SLAP lesions in a military population. *J R Army Med Corps* 2005;151(3):171-175.

[19] Burkhart SS, Morgan CD, Kibler WB: Shoulder injuries in overhead athletes: The "dead arm" revisited. *Clin Sports Med* 2000;19(1):125-158.

[20] O'Brien SJ, Pagnani MJ, Fealy S, McGlynn SR, Wilson JB: The active compression test: A new and effective test for diagnosing labral tears and acromioclavicular joint abnormality. *Am J Sports Med* 1998;26(5):610-613.

[21] Kim SH, Ha KI, Ahn JH, Kim SH, Choi HJ: Biceps load test II: A clinical test for SLAP lesions of the shoulder. *Arthroscopy* 2001;17(2):160-164.

[22] Nakagawa S, Yoneda M, Hayashida K, Obata M, Fukushima S, Miyazaki Y: Forced shoulder abduction and elbow flexion test: A new simple clinical test to detect superior labral injury in the throwing shoulder. *Arthroscopy* 2005;21(11):1290-1295.

[23] Liu SH, Henry MH, Nuccion SL: A prospective evaluation of a new physical examination in predicting glenoid labral tears. *Am J Sports Med* 1996;24(6):721-725.

[24] Myers TH, Zemanovic JR, Andrews JR: The resisted supination external rotation test: A new test for the diagnosis of superior labral anterior posterior lesions. *Am J Sports Med* 2005;33(9):1315-1320.

[25] Cheung EV, O'Driscoll SW: Abstract: The dynamic labral shear test for superior labral anterior posterior tears of the shoulder. *74th Annual Meeting Proceedings*. Rosemont, IL, American Academy of Orthopaedic Surgeons, 2007, p 574.
The authors assess the dynamic labral shear test in the diagnosis of SLAP tears in 105 shoulders.

[26] Ben Kibler W, Sciascia AD, Hester P, Dome D, Jacobs C: Clinical utility of traditional and new tests in the diagnosis of biceps tendon injuries and superior labrum anterior and posterior lesions in the shoulder. *Am J Sports Med* 2009;37(9):1840-1847.
In a cohort study of 325 consecutive patients who underwent six commonly described clinical tests and two new tests (uppercut and dynamic labral shear), clinical findings were correlated with findings at surgery. The uppercut test was the most accurate for biceps disease, and the dynamic labral shear test as the most accurate single test for SLAP lesions.

[27] Meserve BB, Cleland JA, Boucher TR: A meta-analysis examining clinical test utility for assessing superior labral anterior posterior lesions. *Am J Sports Med* 2009;37(11):2252-2258.
Six of 198 studies met the inclusion criteria for a meta-analysis of clinical tests for the diagnosis of SLAP lesions. The accuracy of the anterior slide test was poor. The recommendation was to use the active compression test first, the crank test second, and the Speed test third when a SLAP lesion is suspected.

[28] Cook C, Beaty S, Kissenberth MJ, Siffri P, Pill SG, Hawkins RJ: Diagnostic accuracy of five orthopedic clinical tests for diagnosis of superior labrum anterior

posterior (SLAP) lesions. *J Shoulder Elbow Surg* 2012;21(1):13-22.

A case control study of 87 patients with shoulder pathology evaluated the clinical accuracy and usefulness of five commonly described tests for the diagnosis of SLAP lesions. Only the biceps load II test had clinical usefulness for identifying isolated SLAP lesions, and none of the tests were accurate in isolation. Level of evidence: III.

[29] Borrero CG, Casagranda BU, Towers JD, Bradley JP: Magnetic resonance appearance of posterosuperior labral peel back during humeral abduction and exter- nal rotation. *Skeletal Radiol* 2010;39(1):19-26.

A retrospective review of patients younger than 40 years found MRI sensitivity of 73%, specificity of 100%, positive predictive value of 100%, and negative predictive value of 78% for the presence of a peel- back lesion.

[30] Jung JY, Ha DH, Lee SM, Blacksin MF, Kim KA, Kim JW: Displaceability of SLAP lesion on shoulder MR arthrography with external rotation position. *Skeletal Radiol* 2011;40(8):1047-1055.

MRA in neutral and external rotation of 210 patients who underwent shoulder arthroscopy found sensitivity improved from 64.4% (neutral) to 78.5% (external rotation), accuracy improved from 71% to 81.9%, and specificity constant at 93.6%.

[31] Connell DA, Potter HG, Wickiewicz TL, Altchek DW, Warren RF: Noncontrast magnetic resonance imaging of superior labral lesions: 102 cases confirmed at arthroscopic surgery. *Am J Sports Med* 1999;27(2):208-213.

[32] Bencardino JT, Beltran J, Rosenberg ZS, et al: Superior labrum anterior-posterior lesions: Diagnosis with MR arthrography of the shoulder. *Radiology* 2000;214(1):267-271.

[33] Jee WH, McCauley TR, Katz LD, Matheny JM, Ruwe PA, Daigneault JP: Superior labral anterior posterior (SLAP) lesions of the glenoid labrum: Reliability and accuracy of MR arthrography for diagnosis. *Radiology* 2001;218(1):127-132.

[34] Tung GA, Entzian D, Green A, Brody JM: High-field and low-field MR imaging of superior glenoid labral tears and associated tendon injuries. *AJR Am J Roentgenol* 2000;174(4):1107-1114.

[35] Pandya NK, Colton A, Webner D, Sennett B, Huffman GR: Physical examination and magnetic resonance imaging in the diagnosis of superior labrum anterior-posterior lesions of the shoulder: A sensitivity analysis. *Arthroscopy* 2008;24(3):311-317.

Fifty-one consecutive patients with a SLAP lesion confirmed arthroscopically and no shoulder instability were evaluated with MRI or MRA and physical examination. Test sensitivities were active compression, 90%; dynamic shear, 80%; and Jobe relocation, 76%. MRI sensitivity was 67% (surgeon) and 53% (radiologist); MRA sensitivity was 72% (surgeon) and 50% (radiologist). Level of evidence: II.

[36] Magee T: 3-T MRI of the shoulder: Is MR arthrography necessary? *AJR Am J Roentgenol* 2009;192(1):86-92.

In 150 consecutive patients younger than 50 years, MRA was more sensitive than MRI for detecting partial-thickness rotator cuff tears, SLAP lesions, and anterior labral tears.

[37] Kim YJ, Choi JA, Oh JH, Hwang SI, Hong SH, Kang HS: Superior labral anteroposterior tears: Accuracy and interobserver reliability of multidetector CT arthrography for diagnosis. *Radiology* 2011;260(1):207-215.

A review of 161 CT arthrograms for the detection of SLAP lesions found sensitivity of 94.3% to 97%, specificity of 72.6% to 76.7%, and accuracy of 86.3%, with good interobserver agreement ($\kappa = 0.72$).

[38] Oh JH, Kim JY, Choi JA, Kim WS: Effectiveness of multidetector computed tomography arthrography for the diagnosis of shoulder pathology: Comparison with magnetic resonance imaging with arthroscopic correlation. *J Shoulder Elbow Surg* 2010;19(1):14-20.

Similar sensitivity, specificity and interobserver agreement were found for CT arthrography and MRA in the diagnosis of labral pathology and full-thickness rotator cuff tears, but MRA was better at identifying partial-thickness rotator cuff tears. Level of evidence: I.

[39] Wilk KE, Obma P, Simpson CD, Cain EL, Dugas JR, Andrews JR: Shoulder injuries in the overhead athlete. *J Orthop Sports Phys Ther* 2009;39(2):38-54.

Shoulder anatomy, pathology, biomechanics, and rehabilitation of the overhead athlete were reviewed. Level of evidence: V.

[40] Edwards SL, Lee JA, Bell JE, et al: Nonoperative treatment of superior labrum anterior posterior tears: Improvements in pain, function, and quality of life. *Am J Sports Med* 2010;38(7):1456-1461.

Nineteen patients who were nonsurgically treated for a documented SLAP lesion had overall improvement on functional outcomes measures at a minimum 1-year follow-up, with 71% of the athletes returning to their earlier sports levels.

[41] O'Brien SJ, Allen AA, Coleman SH, Drakos MC: The

trans-rotator cuff approach to SLAP lesions: Technical aspects for repair and a clinical follow-up of 31 patients at a minimum of 2 years. *Arthroscopy* 2002;18(4):372-377.

[42] Freehill MQ, Harms DJ, Huber SM, Atlihan D, Buss DD: Poly-L-lactic acid tack synovitis after arthroscopic stabilization of the shoulder. *Am J Sports Med* 2003;31(5):643-647.

[43] Sassmannshausen G, Sukay M, Mair SD: Broken or dislodged poly-L-lactic acid bioabsorbable tacks in patients after SLAP lesion surgery. *Arthroscopy* 2006;22(6):615-619.

[44] Oh JH, Lee HK, Kim JY, Kim SH, Gong HS: Clinical and radiologic outcomes of arthroscopic glenoid labrum repair with the BioKnotless suture anchor. *Am J Sports Med* 2009;37(12):2340-2348.

A study of 97 patients with a labral tear repaired with the BioKnotless suture anchor found overall good results, with significant improvements in functional outcomes scores and a return to normal recreation and sport in 81.1% of the patients with anterior instability and 83.3% of those with a SLAP lesion. Level of evidence: IV.

[45] Domb BG, Ehteshami JR, Shindle MK, et al: Biomechanical comparison of 3 suture anchor configurations for repair of type II SLAP lesions. *Arthroscopy* 2007;23(2):135-140.

A biomechanical cadaver study evaluated the load to failure of three suture configurations used for SLAP repair. The single anchor with mattress suture through the biceps anchor was the strongest configuration, followed by two anchors with simple sutures anterior and posterior to the anchor. A simple suture anterior to the anchor was the weakest configuration.

[46] Baldini T, Snyder RL, Peacher G, Bach J, McCarty E: Strength of single- versus double-anchor repair of type II SLAP lesions: A cadaveric study. *Arthroscopy* 2009;25(11):1257-1260.

A biomechanical study found that using two single-loaded anchors is biomechanically equivalent to using a single double-loaded anchor with respect to mean load to failure in SLAP repair.

[47] Morgan RJ, Kuremsky MA, Peindl RD, Fleischli JE: A biomechanical comparison of two suture anchor configurations for the repair of type II SLAP lesions subjected to a peel-back mechanism of failure. *Arthroscopy* 2008;24(4):383-388.

A biomechanical study found an equivalent load to failure in two suture configurations for SLAP repair

(two anchors placed posterior to the biceps anchor, one anchor placed anterior and one placed posterior to the biceps anchor).

[48] Westerheide KJ, Dopirak RM, Karzel RP, Snyder SJ: Suprascapular nerve palsy secondary to spinoglenoid cysts: Results of arthroscopic treatment. *Arthroscopy* 2006;22(7):721-727.

[49] Youm T, Matthews PV, ElAttrache NS: Treatment of patients with spinoglenoid cysts associated with superior labral tears without cyst aspiration, debridement, or excision. *Arthroscopy* 2006;22(5):548-552.

[50] Wilk KE, Reinold MM, Dugas JR, Arrigo CA, Moser MW, Andrews JR: Current concepts in the recognition and treatment of superior labral (SLAP) lesions. *J Orthop Sports Phys Ther* 2005;35(5):273-291.

[51] Cordasco FA, Steinmann S, Flatow EL, Bigliani LU: Arthroscopic treatment of glenoid labral tears. *Am J Sports Med* 1993;21(3):425-430, discussion 430-431.

[52] Cohen DB, Coleman S, Drakos MC, et al: Outcomes of isolated type II SLAP lesions treated with arthroscopic fixation using a bioabsorbable tack. *Arthroscopy* 2006;22(2):136-142.

[53] Morgan CD, Burkhart SS, Palmeri M, Gillespie M: Type II SLAP lesions: Three subtypes and their rela- tionships to superior instability and rotator cuff tears. *Arthroscopy* 1998;14(6):553-565.

[54] Neri BR, ElAttrache NS, Owsley KC, Mohr K, Yocum LA: Outcome of type II superior labral anterior posterior repairs in elite overhead athletes: Effect of concomitant partial-thickness rotator cuff tears. *Am J Sports Med* 2011;39(1):114-120.

A cohort study evaluated the results of SLAP repair in overhead athletes using two outcomes measures. The Kerlan-Jobe score was more strongly correlated with return to play than the American Shoulder and Elbow Index score. Level of evidence: III.

[55] Alberta FG, ElAttrache NS, Bissell S, et al: The development and validation of a functional assessment tool for the upper extremity in the overhead athlete. *Am J Sports Med* 2010;38(5):903-911.

In a cross-sectional study, 282 competitive overhead athletes completing the new Kerlan-Jobe Orthopaedic Clinic questionnaire were self-stratified into three injury categories: playing without pain, playing with pain, or not playing as a result of pain. The new score correctly stratified patients by injury category and had excellent responsiveness after treatment of injury.

[56] Brockmeier SF, Voos JE, Williams RJ III, Altchek DW,

Cordasco FA, Allen AA; Hospital for Special Surgery Sports Medicine and Shoulder Service: Outcomes after arthroscopic repair of type-II SLAP lesions. *J Bone Joint Surg Am* 2009;91(7):1595-1603.

A prospective study of 47 patients who underwent repair of a type II SLAP lesion found good overall scores on outcomes measures and high patient satisfaction at a minimum 2-year follow-up. Patient satisfaction and return-to-play rates were higher in patients who had discrete trauma. Level of evidence: IV.

[57] Neuman BJ, Boisvert CB, Reiter B, Lawson K, Ciccotti MG, Cohen SB: Results of arthroscopic repair of type II superior labral anterior posterior lesions in overhead athletes: Assessment of return to preinjury playing level and satisfaction. *Am J Sports Med* 2011;39(9):1883-1888.

A review found overall good results and high patient satisfaction in 30 overhead athletes who underwent SLAP repair, at an average 3.5-year follow-up. Functional outcomes scores and overall satisfaction were relatively low. Level of evidence: IV.

[58] Denard PJ, Lädermann A, Burkhart SS: Long-term outcome after arthroscopic repair of type II SLAP lesions: Results according to age and workers' compensation status. *Arthroscopy* 2012;28(4):451-457.

A review of long-term outcomes of isolated type II SLAP repairs found a good to excellent result in 87%, with significantly poorer results in patients with a worker's compensation claim. Level of evidence: IV.

[59] Alpert JM, Wuerz TH, O'Donnell TF, Carroll KM, Brucker NN, Gill TJ: The effect of age on the outcomes of arthroscopic repair of type II superior labral anterior and posterior lesions. *Am J Sports Med* 2010;38(11):2299-2303.

A review of 52 patients at a minimum 2-year follow-up after type II SLAP repair found no significant difference in outcomes scores or patient satisfaction stratified by age (age 40 years or younger versus older than 40 years). Level of evidence: III.

[60] Forsythe B, Guss D, Anthony SG, Martin SD: Concomitant arthroscopic SLAP and rotator cuff repair. *J Bone Joint Surg Am* 2010;92(6):1362-1369.

A retrospective study compared the results of rotator cuff repair with or without concomitant SLAP repair in older patients. Functional outcomes scores were comparable. Level of evidence: III.

[61] Abbot AE, Li X, Busconi BD: Arthroscopic treatment of concomitant superior labral anterior posterior (SLAP) lesions and rotator cuff tears in patients over the age of 45 years. *Am J Sports Med* 2009;37(7):1358-1362.

In a cohort study of patients older than 45 years who had a rotator cuff tear and a type II SLAP lesion, all patients had a rotator cuff repair and were randomly assigned to débridement or SLAP lesion repair. The patients who underwent débridement had better outcomes scores, improved function, and better motion that those with SLAP repair. Level of evidence: II.

[62] Park S, Glousman RE: Outcomes of revision arthroscopic type II superior labral anterior posterior repairs. *Am J Sports Med* 2011;39(6):1290-1294.

At a mean follow-up of 50.5 months, 12 patients (mean age, 32.6 years) who underwent an isolated revision SLAP repair had overall worse results than with a primary repair. The worst results were in patients with a workers' compensation claim and overhead athletes. Level of evidence: IV.

[63] Boileau P, Parratte S, Chuinard C, Roussanne Y, Shia D, Bicknell R: Arthroscopic treatment of isolated type II SLAP lesions: Biceps tenodesis as an alternative to reinsertion. *Am J Sports Med* 2009;37(5):929-936.

Poorer results were found in 10 patients (mean age, 37 years) who had a SLAP repair than in 15 patients (mean age, 52 years) who had an arthroscopic biceps tenodesis. The significant age difference between the groups makes it difficult to draw any definitive conclusions. Level of evidence: III.

[64] Edwards DJ, Hoy G, Saies AD, Hayes MG: Adverse reactions to an absorbable shoulder fixation device. *J Shoulder Elbow Surg* 1994;3(4):230-233.

[65] Burkart A, Imhoff AB, Roscher E: Foreign-body reaction to the bioabsorbable Suretac device. *Arthroscopy* 2000;16(1):91-95.

[66] Kaar TK, Schenck RC Jr, Wirth MA, Rockwood CA Jr: Complications of metallic suture anchors in shoulder surgery: A report of 8 cases. *Arthroscopy* 2001;17(1):31-37.

[67] Yoo JC, Lee YS, Ahn JH, Park JH, Kang HJ, Koh KH: Isolated suprascapular nerve injury below the spinoglenoid notch after SLAP repair. *J Shoulder Elbow Surg* 2009;18(4):e27-e29.

An isolated suprascapular nerve injury occurred after arthroscopic SLAP repair.

[68] Kim SH, Koh YG, Sung CH, Moon HK, Park YS: Iatrogenic suprascapular nerve injury after repair of type II SLAP lesion. *Arthroscopy* 2010;26(7):1005-1008.

A suprascapular nerve injury at the spinoglenoid notch was caused by improper insertion of a suture anchor during a type II SLAP repair.

第二十六章　肩关节炎的关节镜治疗

Emilie V. Cheung, MD; Marc Safran, MD; John Costouros, MD

引言

对于有疼痛症状的年轻的或活动量大的肩关节炎患者，骨科医师常面临处理上的困境。至于如何定义年轻，必须根据在活动需求背景下的时间及生理年龄。治疗的首要目标是缓解疼痛和改善功能。非手术治疗可能无法提供令人满意的疼痛缓解效果，并且患者会因日常或娱乐活动时功能受限而感到沮丧。全肩关节置换术可以提供非常满意和确定的结果，但是对于年轻患者的长期疗效仍不可预测。主要的并发症包括肩胛盂侧部件的松动及肩胛盂溶解，这都需要手术翻修。对

Dr. Cheung or an immediate family member serves as a board member, owner, officer, or committee member of the American Academy of Orthopaedic Surgeons. Dr. Safran or an immediate family member has received royalties from Stryker; serves as a paid consultant to Cool Systems and Arthrocare; serves as an unpaid consultant to Cool Systems, Cradle Medical, Ferring Pharmaceuticals, Biomimedica, and Eleven Blade Solutions; has stock or stock options held in Cool Systems, Cradle Medical, Biomimedica, and Eleven Blade Solutions; has received research or institutional support from Ferring Pharmaceuticals and Smith & Nephew; and serves as a board member, owner, officer, or committee member of the American Orthopaedic Society for Sports Medicine; the International Society of Arthroscopy, Knee Surgery, and Orthopaedic Sports Medicine; and the International Society for Hip Arthroscopy. Neither Dr. Costouros nor any immediate family member has received anything of value from or has stock or stock options held in a commercial company or institution related directly or indirectly to the subject of this chapter.

于年轻的或活动量大的患者，选择肩关节置换术时这些都应考虑在内。

一项针对 78 例年龄在 50 岁及以下患者的半肩关节置换术或全肩关节置换术后至少 15 年的随访研究发现，在预估的 20 年关节存活率（未行翻修术）方面，全肩关节置换术是 84%，半肩关节置换术是 75%。[1]关节置换术后患者有显著的长期疼痛缓解和功能改善。然而使用 Neer 评分后，研究者发现几乎有一半的患者存在不满意的结果，通常是活动受限。因此，研究者认为对于年龄在 50 岁及以下的患者必须在治疗方式的选择上非常慎重，且需要在行关节置换术前考虑其他治疗方法。行全肩关节翻修术的原因包括感染、肩胛盂部松动和肩袖撕裂。行半肩关节翻修术的主要原因是肩胛盂溶解引起的疼痛。

另一项研究结果有相似的翻修率，共 1285 例行肩关节置换术的患者（半肩关节置换术 455 例，全肩关节置换术 830 例），分别诊断为原发性骨关节炎、类风湿关节炎或肱骨头坏死。[2]创伤患者被排除在外。两组在人口统计学和诊断方面都没有统计学差异。经过 42 个月的随访，翻修率有统计学差异，半肩关节置换术为 4.2%，全肩关节置换术是 1.9%。翻修的主要原因是肩胛盂磨损引起的症状和全肩关节置换术后肩胛盂侧假体松动。

这些研究的结果提示，针对年轻患者在行关节置换术前应积极考虑其他治疗方法。可选择的治疗方法包括关节镜下清理、去除游离体、软骨

成形术、关节囊松解及对引起疼痛的相关病理学因素的治疗。关节镜下重建手术相较于开放的重建手术有显著的优势，包括切口更小、手术时间短、出血量少、术后疼痛轻、感染率低、可安排门诊手术及康复更快。

Outerbridge 分型虽然最初是用来描述髌骨的软骨和骨软骨损伤的，但目前在临床上也广泛应用于描述其他关节（包括肩关节）的软骨和骨软骨损伤。Outerbridge I 级损伤是指关节面的软化，II 级损伤是关节面软骨的玻璃样裂隙，III 级损伤是软骨纤维样变，IV 级损伤是暴露了软骨下骨。[3] 对于伴有 III 级或 IV 级损伤的软骨软化，关节镜治疗时可清理关节面，制造一个光滑的负重面，去除可能引起机械性疼痛的松动软骨瓣。

临床评估

肩关节的影像学检查需包括纯正位片和格列希位（Grashey view）片。Grashey 位是垂直于肩胛骨的平面，而非身体的平面。通过 X 线向外侧成角大约 40° 投射，可以清晰地观察到盂肱关节的间隙。肩关节轴位像可用于评估关节盂偏心性的磨损情况及是否有盂肱关节的半脱位[4]（图 26-1）。骨关节炎的影像学改变包括关节间隙变小、肱骨下方骨赘形成、软骨下骨囊性变和软骨下骨硬化（图 26-2）。

Samilson-Prieto 影像学分类常用于描述肩关节病的严重程度。[5] 轻度关节病是指肱骨头下方和（或）关节盂骨赘高度 <3 mm。中度关节病是肱骨头下方和（或）关节盂骨赘高度为 3~7 mm，伴有轻度的盂肱关节不规则。重度关节病是肱骨头下方和（或）关节盂骨赘高度 >7 mm，伴有盂肱关节间隙变小和硬化。游离体也能在 X 线片上被发现。MRI 检查有助于判断肩袖损伤，盂唇或肱二头肌腱的病理改变，以及局灶性的软骨损伤。

关节炎通常不是单独存在的。与之并存的肩关节病理改变包括肩峰下撞击、肩袖撕裂、肩锁关节炎、肱二头肌长头腱肌腱炎、关节囊挛缩、盂唇撕裂和肩胛上神经病变。全面详细的物理检查可帮助医师分辨除严重的肩关节炎以外的可能

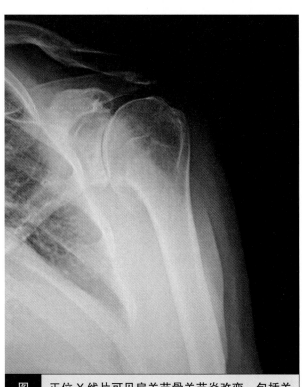

| 图 26-1 | 轴位 X 线片可见肱骨头变平和非对称性的关节盂后方磨损导致的 2 个凹陷（顶点位于关节盂的中心） |

| 图 26-2 | 正位 X 线片可见肩关节骨关节炎改变，包括关节间隙变小、肱骨下方骨赘形成、软骨下骨囊性变和软骨下骨硬化 |

潜在的疼痛原因。尽管存在骨关节炎，上述引起肩关节疼痛的病因仍可通过手术来治疗。

手术的禁忌证和指征

肩关节镜下清理的手术禁忌证包括存在活动性的感染及合并其他疾病而无法进行全身麻醉等。这与其他外科手术的禁忌证相似。无法进行全身麻醉是肩关节镜下清理的相对禁忌证，因为也可以在局部麻醉（肌间沟阻滞麻醉）下进行手术。

肩关节镜下清理的手术指征包括非手术治疗3个月症状无明显改善。非手术治疗包括维持活动范围的物理康复治疗，非甾体抗炎药治疗，以及关节内注射糖皮质激素。合并密尔沃基（Milwaukee）肩关节综合征的患者经过肩关节简单的闭合针刺灌洗及激素注射，可以达到其后6个月的疼痛缓解效果。[6]

关节镜下清理也可用于治疗年轻且活动量大的肩关节炎患者。这类患者通常不是关节置换术的候选者，而且不愿遵从术后的限制要求，这会增加假体早期失效的风险。手术的最佳候选者是生理年龄年轻（小于60岁），诊断为骨关节炎，存在中度活动范围丢失，以及有盂肱关节中心性磨损的患者。全肩关节置换术通常不推荐用于那些需要参加接触类运动项目的患者或需要参加重体力劳动或搬运重物的患者。这些患者可能更适合一种更微创的方法，如关节镜下清理。肩关节镜手术被证实是一种安全、低并发症发生率的技术。[7-8]然而，对于肩关节炎，关节镜治疗通常被认为是一种临时性的替代治疗方法，而非最终治疗方法。那些行关节镜下清理的患者，多年后通常需要行关节置换术。

手术技术

关节镜下清理的手术技术包括完整的盂肱关节和肩峰下间隙的诊断性关节镜探查（图26-3，26-4）。应用局部麻醉（肌间沟阻滞麻醉）有助于

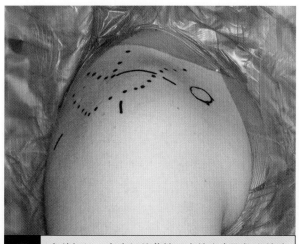

图 26-3　术前标记。右肩行关节镜手术的患者取标准的沙滩椅位。标注骨性标志，以虚线标注锁骨和肩胛冈，长实线标注肩锁关节，圆圈标注喙突。以短实线标注标准的后入路、外侧入路和前入路的位置

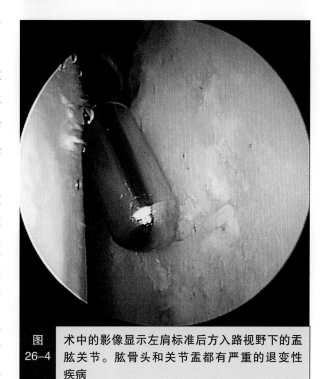

图 26-4　术中的影像显示左肩标准后方入路视野下的盂肱关节。肱骨头和关节盂都有严重的退变性疾病

在有挛缩的关节进行操作以及术后的疼痛控制。盂肱关节间隙会因进展性的骨关节炎和关节囊挛缩而变得极度狭小。一个技巧是在紧缩的肩关节进行关节镜操作以进入盂肱关节时，为避免穿刺针意外损伤软骨，可以向外牵引肱骨头。另外一个技巧是将穿刺点设置在比通常进入关节的位置

偏上方处，在关节线贴近肱骨头的上方。或者先将一个一次性塑料套管套在转换棒上并插入关节，再以金属套管替代塑料套管。使用由外向内的技术建立标准的前方工作通道以进入肩袖间隙。

术中需要处理可能引起肩关节疼痛的合并损伤。去除松动的骨软骨碎片，用电动刨刀刀头清理骨软骨损伤，使用刨刀刀头、刮勺或咬骨钳去除不稳定的软骨瓣膜直至见到稳定的基层。对Ⅲ级的关节软骨损伤，需要清理呈现光滑且逐渐变薄的边缘。

肱骨头下方大块的骨赘会引起机械症状，如交锁和磨擦音。术者可以使用电动毛锉从肱骨头上将骨赘刨削掉。使用前下方的工作入路及弯曲的设备可以更加容易地处理肱骨头下方。另外，调整肱骨头的旋转角度也有助于去除下方的骨赘。

虽然手术去除有潜在机械性阻挡的骨赘可改善活动范围，但从根本上改善活动范围的更重要的方法是关节囊松解。在清除腋窝处的骨赘时必须考虑到损伤臂丛神经的风险。[9]

对于中心性损伤，可使用微骨折（完整的软骨下骨钻孔）的方法。其目的是使多能干细胞内流至软骨下骨出血床，其进一步纤维软骨化，从而填充软骨的缺损。将软骨缺损部位处理至稳定的边缘后，使用刮勺在损伤的基底部去除钙化的软骨。微骨折的方法可用于肱骨头或关节盂全厚的软骨缺损，标准与膝关节的相似（如大小不超过 8 cm²）。使用微骨折的尖锥穿透软骨下骨2 mm，每隔 2 mm 做一次穿刺[10]（图 26–5）。肩关节微骨折的手术指征和疗效仍在观察中。

关节镜下的关节盂成形术及关节囊成形术对

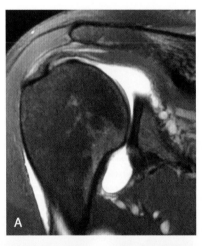
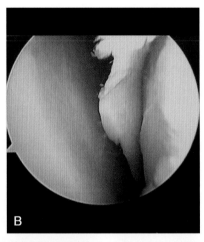
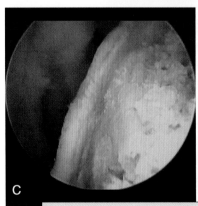
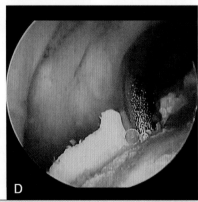
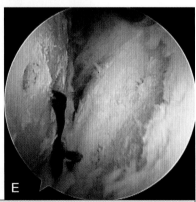

图 26–5　肱骨头的一处孤立的全厚软骨缺损。A. 术前 MRI。B. 术中影像显示关节软骨损伤，边缘游离形成瓣膜。C. 使用刮勺清理后的损伤情况。D. 微骨折的尖锥穿刺进入软骨下骨。E. 另外一例患者的术中影像，显示肱骨头微骨折后骨孔良好的渗血

于那些不适合行关节置换术的肩关节骨关节炎患者是行之有效的技术。[11]非中心性对称的盂肱关节可以通过纠正变形的关节盂轮廓来治疗，通常这类骨关节炎患者都有显著的后方磨损。手术的流程与开放手术做偏心的磨削相似。在关节镜下使用毛锉和锉刀将前方关节盂或将骨软骨的边缘修整光滑，磨削成 2 个凹陷的形状，再逐步修磨成中心性凹陷的形状，这样会显著缓解疼痛并改善关节活动范围。可能需要创建多个手术入路来清除围绕肱骨头的骨赘。如有指征，还需要进行关节镜下的滑膜清理和关节囊松解，以帮助恢复肱骨头的位置，甚至在理论上增加关节的接触面积。关节镜下的滑膜清理和关节囊松解从技术层面上来说是非常有挑战的操作，但是对于有经验的肩关节镜手术医师，这是必须掌握的技术。

大约 30% 行关节镜下清理的肩关节骨关节炎患者都合并有关节囊挛缩。[12-13]仅行关节镜下清理不能改善这些患者的活动范围。如果患者已有显著的活动受限，推荐进行关节囊松解，这也有助于重建中心匹配的关节。但即使进行了关节囊松解，扁平的肱骨头也无法转动，所以术前评估时要非常仔细地检查放射学影像，确保肱骨头仍是圆的且关节是匹配的。一些医师认为关节囊松解可减轻接触的压力，从而缓解疼痛。

关节囊松解可使用射频消融设备或手持咬钳进行。由外向内创建标准的前入路，进入肩袖间隙。用射频设备在关节盂外侧 1 cm 处切开肩袖间隙的关节囊和喙肱韧带。要完全松解肩袖间隙内致密的关节囊组织，也要松解中部的盂肱关节韧带（图 26-6）。在内收位，外旋手臂可便于显露肩袖间隙的组织。注意保护肩胛下肌腱和中段的肱二头肌悬吊结构，以防止肱二头肌腱不稳定。覆盖在肩胛下肌腱表面的致密关节囊需要完全松解至前下方的关节囊凹陷处。肩胛下肌腱和关节囊可通过其外观来区分：肩胛下肌腱纤维横向走行，而关节囊纤维走行不规则。

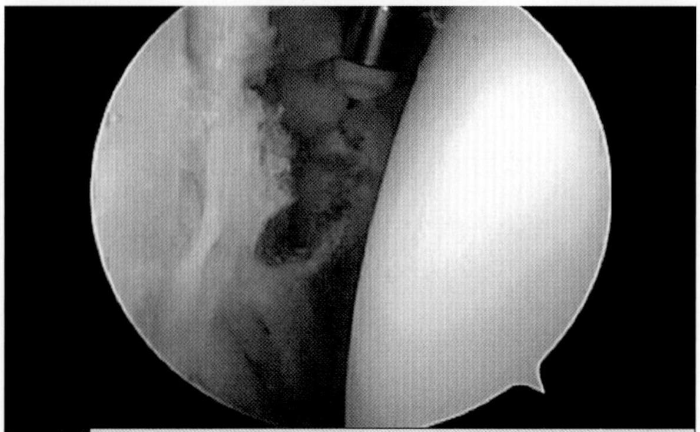

后方关节囊的松解可在前方通路或附属肩袖横向通路的视野下，自后方通路完成。[14]与前方关节囊组织相比，后方关节囊和相关的盂肱关节韧带通常没有那么致密。松解时内旋手臂有助于显露后方关节囊。

松解下方关节囊时需要上臂内收，放松紧挨着关节盂下方的臂丛神经，从而最大限度地降低损伤神经的风险。一些医师为了避免臂丛神经因射频或直接的机械外力损伤，而选择手法松解，即在稳定肩胛骨的同时最大限度地将手臂前上举。

关节镜可进入肩峰下间隙（图 26-7）并进行肩峰下减压，如果有临床指征，可切除锁骨远端。肩峰下滑囊切除是肩关节镜下清理盂肱关节骨关

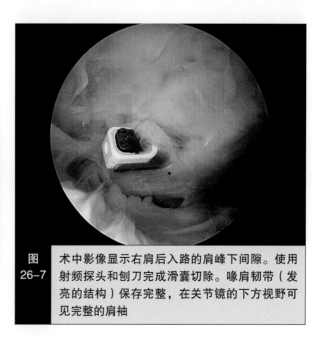

图 26-6　后方通路视野下的术中影像显示使用射频设备松解前方关节囊

图 26-7　术中影像显示右肩后入路的肩峰下间隙。使用射频探头和刨刀完成滑囊切除。喙肩韧带（发亮的结构）保存完整，在关节镜的下方视野可见完整的肩袖

节炎成功与否的极重要步骤。可使用射频设备消融肩峰下滑囊。应仔细保护喙肩韧带，特别是在合并有巨大肩袖撕裂的情况下，可减小肱骨头向前上脱位的风险，特别是那些最终需要行关节置换术的患者。

患者麻醉后，应以轻柔的手法活动肩关节。对于有骨质疏松以及手法活动可能导致医源性骨折的患者，更应特别小心。可用一只手稳定肩胛骨，另一只手尽可能地靠近腋窝处抓住肱骨干。这一方法可有效缩短手法操作时的杠杆力臂，减小骨折的风险。手法松解可使下方 6 点方向的关节囊纤维撕裂。手法松解肩关节时，需使手臂前屈、外展，在体侧做外旋和内旋运动，以及在外展位做外旋和内旋运动，并分别记录所能达到的角度。

术后康复

术后为了舒适可以使用吊带，并鼓励患者主动、被动活动手臂。术后应即刻开始物理康复治疗，进行积极的主动和被动活动练习，以防止发生粘连。教会患者以下动作：在肩胛骨平面上前屈、上举手臂，手臂在体侧时外旋，外展位时内旋和外旋。做功能锻炼时，患者仰卧以限制肩胛骨的活动，只锻炼盂肱关节。患者不仅要在指导下进行物理康复治疗，每天还应该进行居家练习。蜡疗有助于减轻术后的肿胀和疼痛。术后阶段使用抗炎药物也有一定的帮助。术后活动范围改善且疼痛减轻后，可加入力量练习。

结果

很多研究发现，在相对较短的随访期内，早期肩关节炎的关节镜处理是有效的。[15]其中一项研究包含 25 例早期关节炎患者（早期炎症定义为没有明显的影像学改变），对这些患者采用关节镜治疗，去除游离体和切除肩峰下滑膜。[16]在平均 34 个月的随访中，80% 的患者可获得良好的结果。最短的疼痛缓解期是 8 个月。上述研究的文章作者不建议对腋位影像上有盂肱关节间隙消失或关节不成对应性关系的患者进行关节镜治疗，但是研究数据并不能支持这一观点。

对于没有明显影像学改变的早期肩关节骨关节炎患者，手术操作对于同时存在的其他病理改变也有益处。例如，在一项研究中，合并 Outerbridge Ⅳ 级软骨损伤的 21 例患者在行关节镜下肩峰成形术后，疼痛得到了缓解，功能也得到了改善。[17]其他研究也报道了相似的可喜结果，这些研究的关节镜下清理方法包括滑囊切除、盂唇清理和部分致密肩袖组织的清理。[13,16,18]

在关节镜下处理单独的、中心性的盂肱关节 Ⅳ 级软骨损伤（不合并关节炎的影像学证据）被证实是有效的。[12]88% 的患者有至少 28 个月的显著疼痛缓解期。同时进行的手术操作如肩峰成形、锁骨远端切除、盂唇清理和盂唇修补都对功能恢复无负面影响。对于大于 2 cm^2 的骨软骨损伤，手术不会取得好的治疗效果，疼痛会很快再次出现。作者建议对肩关节有被动活动范围丢失的患者行关节镜下关节囊松解。

在一项前瞻性研究中，19 例患者合并有严重的退行性肩关节炎，对这些患者进行了关节镜下清理，去除了游离体并切除了肩峰下滑囊。[19]平均随访 24 个月（12~50 个月）。所有患者的关节间隙完全消失且合并有很大的骨赘。他们都被建议行全肩关节置换术。关节镜下没有行骨赘切除、关节盂成形、肩峰成形或其他操作，也没有行关节囊切开或关节囊松解。术后，16 例（84%）患者有良好的结果。术后 3 个月可获得最大程度的疼痛缓解，术后 6 个月获得最大程度的功能改善，患者满意度在术后 6 个月达到平台期。78% 的患者在其后 2~4 年的随访中都能维持满意的结果。一例患者 1 年后接受了关节置换术，另一例患者在术后第 3 年再次接受了关节镜下清理手术。

另一项纳入了 19 例患者的研究未在关节镜下行滑囊切除，长期（4 年）随访发现结果逐渐恶化。[20]13例（68%）患者对于疼痛缓解效果非常满意，虽然功能和活动范围相比术前水平没有变化。3例（16%）患者在随访期间接受了半肩关节置换术。

还有一项研究对19例年龄不大于55岁的患者，共20例肩关节进行了关节镜治疗，这些患者合并有Outerbridge Ⅱ~Ⅳ级软骨损伤。[21]除了关节镜下清理，9例患者行肩峰下减压，另4例患者行肩峰下滑囊切除（未行肩峰成形术），共13例患者行肩峰下滑囊切除。经过最少12个月的随访（平均20个月，12~33个月），关节存活率达85%，3例患者接受了肩关节置换术。Ⅱ级、Ⅲ级损伤患者的结果评分与Ⅳ级损伤患者的结果评分大体相似。合并单极损伤（关节盂侧或肱骨头侧）的患者的结果比两侧都有软骨缺损的患者的结果更好。这19例患者的平均ASES肩关节疼痛和功能障碍评分为75分，其中9例患者（5例为Ⅳ级软骨损伤）的评分大于80分。

只有一项研究特别调查了严重肩关节骨关节炎患者接受关节镜下清理及关节囊松解的效果。[22]8例患者接受了关节镜下清理及关节囊松解，短期随访显示其获得了良好的疼痛缓解和功能改善的评分。对于有中心性磨损的肩关节炎患者，关节囊松解可使患者获得活动范围的改善。而对于有后方磨损、关节盂呈双凹形态及肱骨头扁平合并骨赘的患者，不太可能通过松解关节囊来改善活动范围，关节囊松解反而可加重疼痛。虽然针对骨赘切除尚没有细致的研究，但是早期的文献报道认为这会改善关节镜下清理的预后。[9]

一项纳入14例合并严重肩关节炎、关节盂呈双凹形态的患者的研究提示，对这类患者建议行关节盂成形术及骨关节囊成形术。[11]术后3年的随访发现，采取上述治疗的这些患者获得了持续的疼痛缓解和撞击消除。在活动结束点出现撞击痛是术后最佳预后的指征，手术时可一并结构性处理大骨赘、关节盂后方磨损、肱骨头半脱位及大块的游离体。消极的预测因素是活动范围中段出现的疼痛，肱骨旋转时盂肱关节压紧导致的疼痛，以及同心圆匹配的盂肱关节。虽然这些操作步骤在技术上较为困难，但是对于严格挑选的患者，有经验的医师还是能够顺利完成的。

一项纳入了71例患者的研究报道，55例患者获得了平均随访期超过2年的疼痛缓解和肩关节功能康复。[23]其中20例患者接受了早期的手术。患者的Samilson-Prieto放射学评分为0~4分，都合并有Outerbridge Ⅱ~Ⅳ级的软骨损伤。基于患者的放射学疾病评分、年龄或活动量，以及不愿意行关节置换术的想法，这些患者并未被视为关节置换术的候选人。他们选择进行关节镜治疗。[23]手术由一个四人医师团队中的一人完成，包括不同的手术操作：关节囊松解（44例），肱二头肌腱固定或切断术（14例），微骨折（11例），游离体或骨赘切除（12例），以及肩峰下减压（28例）。由于没有对具体操作做进一步研究，因此并不清楚它们有何作用。16例（22%）患者在平均术后10个月接受了关节置换术。另外55例在平均27个月（12~90个月）的随访期内没有要求行关节置换术。接受全肩关节置换术的患者的平均关节间隙宽度为1.5 mm，平均Samilson-Prieto评分为2.4分。未接受全肩关节置换术的患者的平均关节间隙宽度为2.6 mm，平均Samilson-Prieto评分为1.9分。

通过微骨折方法治疗肱骨头或关节盂中心性软骨损伤仍是一个新兴的技术领域，该技术主要来源于膝关节的技术。一项研究应用微骨折方法治疗了30例合并全厚软骨损伤的患者，患者的平均年龄为43岁。[10]经过至少2年的随访，有19%的患者的治疗被认为是不成功的，这些患者在平均47个月的随访期内要求进行再一次的肩关节手术治疗。其余患者获得了疼痛的缓解及功能的改善。这一操作针对相对较小的损伤和只累及肱骨侧的缺损可能更加有效。

总结

针对年轻、活动量大的患者，关节镜下清理术及关节囊松解是肩关节骨关节炎的有效治疗方法。在手术时应同时处理伴随的肩关节病理改变，如肩袖疾病、撞击综合征、肱二头肌腱和盂唇的病理改变及肩锁关节炎。文献报道短期随访可获得令人满意的疼痛缓解和功能恢复效果，甚至对某些非常严重的盂肱关节炎也是如此。关节囊松解、骨赘切除和微骨折的益处仍待进一步研究。虽然关节镜下清理不能替代关节置换术，但其为一些患者提供了一种治疗的选择，并延后了行关节置换术的需求。

参考文献

[1] Sperling JW, Cofield RH, Rowland CM: Minimum fifteen-year follow-up of Neer hemiarthroplasty and total shoulder arthroplasty in patients aged fifty years or younger. *J Shoulder Elbow Surg* 2004;13(6):604-613.

[2] Yian EH, Navarro RA, Funahashi T, et al: Hemiarthroplasty and total shoulder arthroplasty (TSA) revision rates: Analysis of 1,311 elective shoulder replacements in a community setting. American Shoulder and Elbow Surgeons Specialty Day, February 2011. http://www.ases-assn.org. Accessed September 20, 2012.

[3] Outerbridge RE, Dunlop JA: The problem of chondromalacia patellae. *Clin Orthop Relat Res* 1975;110:177-196.

[4] Gerber C, Costouros JG, Sukthankar A, Fucentese SF: Static posterior humeral head subluxation and total shoulder arthroplasty. *J Shoulder Elbow Surg* 2009;18(4):505-510.

Static posterior subluxation of the humeral head often is associated with glenohumeral arthritis. This condition can be corrected in most shoulders undergoing total shoulder arthroplasty, but recentering is not correlated with glenoid version or its correction.

[5] Samilson RL, Prieto V: Dislocation arthropathy of the shoulder. *J Bone Joint Surg Am* 1983;65(4):456-460.

[6] Epis O, Caporali R, Scirè CA, Bruschi E, Bonacci E, Montecucco C: Efficacy of tidal irrigation in Milwaukee shoulder syndrome. *J Rheumatol* 2007;34(7):1545-1550.

Ten patients with Milwaukee shoulder syndrome underwent ultrasound examination, tidal irrigation, and instillation of methylprednisolone and tranexamic acid. This minimally invasive procedure led to a significant improvement in pain and active motion. Patients with recent-onset disease recovered completely.

[7] Bigliani LU, Flatow EL, Deliz ED: Complications of shoulder arthroscopy. *Orthop Rev* 1991;20(9):743-751.

[8] Small NC: Complications in arthroscopic surgery of the knee and shoulder. *Orthopedics* 1993;16(9):985-988.

[9] Millett PJ, Gaskill TR: Arthroscopic management of glenohumeral arthrosis: Humeral osteoplasty, capsular release, and arthroscopic axillary nerve release as a joint-preserving approach. *Arthroscopy* 2011;27(9):1296-1303.

A technique for arthroscopic management of glenohumeral arthrosis in young, high-demand patients combines traditional glenohumeral débridement and capsular release with inferior humeral osteoplasty and arthroscopic transcapsular axillary nerve decompression. Symptom relief may be greater than with débridement alone.

[10] Millett PJ, Huffard BH, Horan MP, Hawkins RJ, Steadman JR: Outcomes of full-thickness articular cartilage injuries of the shoulder treated with microfracture. *Arthroscopy* 2009;25(8):856-863.

In 30 patients, microfracture in glenohumeral joints with full-thickness chondral lesions led to significant improvement in ability to work, activities of daily living, and sports activity. The greatest improvement occurred with relatively small humeral lesions; the poorest was with bipolar lesions.

[11] Kelly EW, Steinmann SP, O'Driscoll SW: Arthroscopic glenoidplasty and osteocapsular arthroplasty for advanced glenohumeral osteoarthritis. *67th Annual Meeting Proceedings*. Rosemont, IL, American Academy of Orthopaedic Surgeons, 1999.

[12] Cameron BD, Galatz LM, Ramsey ML, Williams GR, Iannotti JP: Non-prosthetic management of grade IV osteochondral lesions of the glenohumeral joint. *J Shoulder Elbow Surg* 2002;11(1):25-32.

[13] Ogilvie-Harris DJ, Wiley AM: Arthroscopic surgery of the shoulder: A general appraisal. *J Bone Joint Surg Br* 1986;68(2):201-207.

[14] Costouros JG, Clavert P, Warner JJ: Trans-cuff portal for arthroscopic posterior capsulorrhaphy. *Arthroscopy*

2006;22(10):e1-e5.

[15] Elser F, Braun S, Dewing CB, Millett PJ: Glenohumeral joint preservation: Current options for managing articular cartilage lesions in young, active patients. *Arthroscopy* 2010;26(5):685-696.

Shoulder joint preservation techniques are reviewed, with a guide to surgical decision making and summaries of the current treatments for focal chondral defects and more massive structural osteochondral defects (microfracture, osteoarticular transplantation, autologous chondrocyte implantation, bulk allograft reconstruction, and biologic resurfacing).

[16] Weinstein DM, Bucchieri JS, Pollock RG, Flatow EL, Bigliani LU: Arthroscopic debridement of the shoulder for osteoarthritis. *Arthroscopy* 2000;16(5):471-476.

[17] Ellowitz AS, Rosas R, Rodosky MW, Buss DD: The benefit of arthroscopic decompression for impingement in patients found to have unsuspected glenohumeral osteoarthritis. *64th Annual Meeting Final Program.* Rosemont, IL, American Academy of Orthopaedic Surgeons, 1997, p 206.

[18] Ogilvie-Harris DJ: Arthroscopy and arthroscopic surgery of the shoulder. *Semin Orthop* 1987;2:246-258.

[19] Safran MR, Wolde-Tsadik G: Prospective outcome study of arthroscopic debridement for the treatment of grade IV glenohumeral arthritis. *Annual Meeting Proceedings.* Rosemont, IL, American Academy of Orthopaedic Surgeons, 2002, p 659.

[20] Feldmann DD, Orwin JF: Efficacy of arthroscopic debridement for treatment of glenohumeral arthritis. *Transactions of the 19th Open Meeting.* Rosemont, IL, American Shoulder and Elbow Surgeons, 2003, p. 30.

[21] Kerr BJ, McCarty EC: Outcome of arthroscopic débridement is worse for patients with glenohumeral arthritis of both sides of the joint. *Clin Orthop Relat Res* 2008;466(3):634-638.

Arthroscopic glenohumeral débridement in 19 patients (20 shoulders) younger than 55 years with Outer- bridge grade II to IV articular cartilage changes was found to be effective for managing symptoms and delaying the need for prosthetic replacement.

[22] Richards DP, Burkhart SS: Arthroscopic debridement and capsular release for glenohumeral osteoarthritis. *Arthroscopy* 2007;23(9):1019-1022.

Range of motion and pain were improved by using electrocautery to release the rotator cuff interval, the anterior capsule, the posterior capsule, and the axillary recess. A reduction in joint contact pressures is believed to be the primary mechanism for pain relief after capsular release.

[23] Van Thiel GS, Sheehan S, Frank RM, et al: Retrospective analysis of arthroscopic management of glenohumeral degenerative disease. *Arthroscopy* 2010;26(11):1451-1455.

A retrospective review of 71 shoulders after arthroscopic débridement for degenerative joint disease suggested that patients with residual joint space and an absence of large osteophytes can avoid arthroplasty at short-term follow-up and have increased function with decreased pain. Significant risk factors include the presence of grade IV bipolar disease, large osteophytes, and joint space of less than 2 mm.

第五部分

关节炎与关节成形术

栏目编委：
T. Bradley Edwards, MD

第二十七章　肱骨近端的解剖及假体的修复重建

Christopher R. Chuinard, MD, MPH

引言

　　最早记录的肱骨近端假体置换术是 1893 年法国医师 Jules Emile Pean 开展的一个两阶段的手术（切除肱骨头后二期再植入假体），患者被诊断为广泛的结核性骨髓炎。[1] 假体是牙科医师制作的，使用了铂金的柄，与非限制性假体相比，它的设计更像现代的反球关节。假体在一段很短的时间内表现良好，但最终还是会因为感染复发而失效。Pean 医师的灵感来自一个德国医师 Themistocles Gluck，后者设计了几个肱骨近端的替代物，包括一个模块化的象牙材质的肱骨头。[1] 这两位医师的思维方式相对超前，但并没有付诸实践。得益于当今世界发展的科学技术，现代的假体不再使用贵金属和象牙。目前，假体已经进化为一种近似天然肱骨解剖形态的设计和另一种完全不像肱骨天然形态的假体。

解剖学

　　肩关节首次非限制性关节置换术的目的是重

Dr. Chuinard or an immediate family member serves as a board member, owner, officer, or committee member of the ACESS and the American Academy of Orthopaedic Surgeons Upper Extremity Question Writing Committee; is a member of a speakers' bureau or has made paid presentations on behalf of Mitek, Tornier, Smith & Nephew, and Arthrex; serves as a paid consultant to or is an employee of Mitek and Tornier; has received research or institutional support from Tornier; and has stock or stock options held in Tornier.

建患者正常的、特有的肱骨解剖形态。为了可靠且可重复地实现这一目标，术者必须了解肱骨的正常解剖形态，肩胛盂的解剖，以及盂肱关节的运动学原理。对于全肩关节置换术，主要需要考虑的也是肱骨本身。理解关节面和运动轴的关系非常重要。这是因为在手术过程中，可能缺失肱骨头的标准形态，术者必须掌握肱骨头的大小、形态和旋转半径的关系，才能准确地重建正常的解剖关系。

肱骨头的大小和形态

　　虽然尸体研究提供了肱骨头的大小和形态的平均值，但是实际上，每个肱骨头的规格变异很大。肱骨头的关节面大概占整个球形面积的 1/3，在边缘略呈椭圆形，矢状面直径和冠状面直径相比平均少 2 mm。[2-6] 正因为这个关系，肱骨头的直径和厚度间存在一个相对固定的比例，这意味着每个不同的半径都对应着一个唯一的肱骨头高度。[2-8] 男性平均肱骨头旋转半径的厚度是 24 mm，女性是 19 mm。在两个维度上，男性肱骨头的平均直径都要比女性大 2 mm。[4,8-9] 研究显示在解剖颈水平，肱骨头的平均直径为 43.4 mm 或 44.5 mm。[2-4] 这些研究发现，肱骨头的半径和高度之间的占比为 70%~80%。各研究间的差异可能与研究方法有关[4-11]（图 27-1）。

　　使用大的肱骨头假体会限制外展的初始 20° 和最后 20°，导致肱骨向近端移位、外旋丢失及后移增加。使用小的肱骨头假体会导致下移。[10] 增

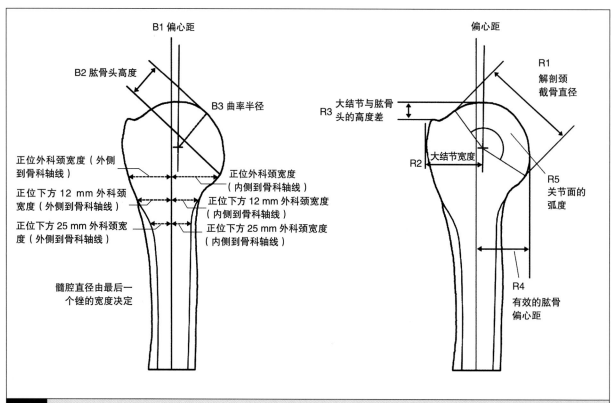

图 27-1　肱骨假体置换的关键解剖关系。B—生物力学参数，R—冗余参数。经允许引自 Wirth MA, Ondrla J, Southworth C, Kaar K, Anderson BC, Rockwood CA Ⅲ. Replicating proximal humeral articular geometry with a third-generation implant: A radiographic study in cadaveric shoulders. *J Shoulder Elbow Surg* 2007; 16（suppl 3）: S111-S116.

加肱骨头的高度超过正常值 5 mm 会使关节活动范围显著减小，高度减少 5 mm 也会使关节偏移减少 27°。[7] 移位 5 mm 对应着 20%的肱骨头半径，会改变 20%的肩袖杠杆力臂。[12]

肱骨颈干角

肱骨颈干角是指肱骨头中心线和肱骨干髓腔轴线的夹角（图 27-2）。研究报道的范围为 129.6°~137°，加权平均值为 134.4°。[2-5,13] 一项对 2058 具尸体的肱骨解剖研究发现，78%的颈干角范围为 130°~140°，135°是最常见的测量值，平均值为 134.7°（115°~148°）。[14] 其临床意义在于极度内翻或极度外翻的角度会给假体的重建带来极大的挑战，除非使用相应改良的假体。然而现在可通过变化的截骨技术使颈干角固定的假体被放置在与关节面相适应的重建位置。对于内翻的颈干角，肱骨截骨应从外上方开始；而对于外翻的颈干角，截骨应从内下方开始[14]（图 27-3）。由于假体植入时颈干角的不同会引起外展肌肉长度的变化，进而改变旋转中心，导致撞击或肩袖功能障碍，因此术者需使假体与肱骨头截骨线相匹配，恢复相适应的关节面弧度。[14-16]

肱骨头的偏心距

同时考虑横断面和冠状面这两个平面上肱骨头的旋转中心与肱骨干轴线之间的偏心距是非常重要的。由于肱骨头的旋转中心没有与肱骨干的轴线（也被称为骨科轴线）重合，很小的偏移就会导致盂肱关节运动学的改变。骨科轴线代表着肱骨中心锉孔的轴线；肱骨头实际的旋转中心位于后方平均 2.1 mm（范围为 2~4 mm，在矢状面上）、内侧 6.6 mm（范围为 6~9 mm，在冠状面上）处，因此造就了一个位于肱骨干髓腔轴线后内侧的旋转中心[2,5,8,13,16-19]（图 27-4）。

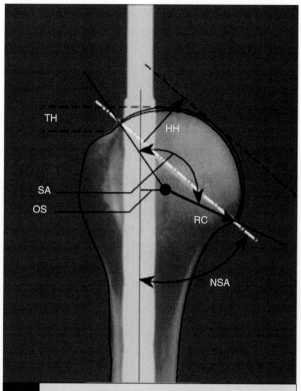

图
27-2
正位的 X 线片显示冠状面的肱骨近端解剖学参数。黑点—旋转中心，白色虚线—关节面的基底，竖直的黑线—扩髓后的髓腔中心线，HH—肱骨头的高度，NSA—颈干角，OS—内侧偏心距，RC—曲率半径，TH—大结节与肱骨头的高度差，SA—关节面的弧度。经允许引自 Pearl ML. Proximal humeral anatomy in shoulder arthroplasty: Implications for prosthetic design and surgical technique.*J Shoulder Elbow Surg* 2005;14（Suppl 1）:S99–S104.

肱骨头的后倾角

肱骨头的后倾角或后扭转角是指肱骨远端经髁上连线与肱骨头中心线之间的夹角。报道的范围为（17.9°±13.7°）至（21.4°±3.3°）。肱骨头的后倾角可能更易受到如患者的年龄、性别和种族等因素的影响，而且同一个体两侧的角度也可能不同。[2,20-23] 肱二头肌腱沟与肱骨头赤道存在一定的相关性；肱二头肌腱沟平均偏离赤道 8~9 mm，也被用作肱骨头后倾的标志。[5,20-22] 一项针对 120 具尸体的研究使用 CT 来测量后倾角，以经髁上连线为标准测量，平均后倾角为 17.6°，而以前臂轴线为标准测量则平均后倾角为 28.8°。[24] 通过

三维激光分析关节面，以关节几何学大致的质心，得出后倾角平均为 18.6°。[20] 另外一项研究发现：可以基于小结节的外侧边缘测量后倾角，平均为 48°，该方法较为可靠。[25] 研究人员使用特殊的夹具测量了 185 个干的骨骼标本，发现小结节是比肱二头肌腱沟和经髁上连线更加可靠的标志点。许多肱骨假体重建时是以前臂作为标志来确定后倾角度。当以前臂为标志使用截骨模板时，术者在截骨前应考虑到 10°~15° 的提携角所带来的天然性差异，以及肩袖止点的可视下操作[17]（图 27-5）。

肱骨干形态学

在过去 10 年中，人们开始越来越多地关注肱骨干近端和干骺端的形态学。现确认了 3 个肱骨近端的形态学模型：低偏心距型、标准型和高偏心距型[5]（图 27-6）。这些术语是根据肱骨头与干骺端骨干的偏心距相对值而定的。偏心距的减小可能使插入直柄假体更困难。正是基于理解了这一解剖特点现发展出了弧形柄假体（又称无翅柄假体）及几何形态简化型假体柄。由于更多注意力放在了创造各种适应性的假体上，因此一些压配设计方面的弊端逐步显现。部分压配型假体使旋转中心向上方和外侧分别移位 12 mm 和 8 mm，从而导致肩袖功能障碍。[26-27] 即使只抬高肱骨头假体 5 mm 也会减少肩袖肌肉的力臂，甚至当手臂内收时可以改变肌肉的矢量。[28-30] 大结节与肱骨头的平均高度差为 6 mm；如果肱骨过高，手臂外展时下方的关节囊会过紧，而内收时肩袖则会承担过分的张力[4,31]（图 27-1）。

假体设计的考虑因素

第一、第二和第三代肱骨假体

现代的肩关节置换术源自 Neer 在 1951 年的整体化设计。[32] 这一系统共有 5 个不同直径规格的柄和 1 个规格的肱骨头。假体柄与现代的骨折柄相似，多孔设计允许骨长入。Neer 使用这种假

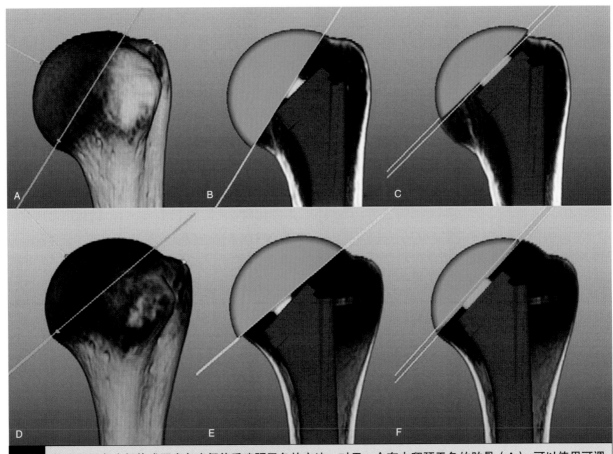

图 27-3 使用可调角度假体或固定角度假体重建颈干角的方法。对于一个有内翻颈干角的肱骨（A），可以使用可调角度假体在解剖颈截骨（B），或使用固定角度假体以 135° 从肱骨颈的外上点开始截骨（C）。对于一个有外翻颈干角的肱骨（D），可以使用可调角度假体可以在解剖颈截骨（E），或使用固定角度假体以 135° 从肱骨颈的内下点开始截骨（F）。绿线—解剖颈（确定了自然的颈干角），黄线—假体的颈部及颈干角。蓝色区域—固定角度假体的颈部，绿色区域—肱骨头假体，红色区域—假体柄，黄色区域—可调角度假体的颈部。经允许引自 Jeong J, Bryan J, Iannotti JP: Effect of a variable prosthetic neck–shaft angle and the surgical technique on replication of normal humeral anatomy. *J Bone Joint Surg Am* 2009;91（8）:1932–1941.

体获得了早期的成功，使得 1974 年引入了成功的髋关节假体设计，使用骨水泥柄、肱骨头（有 2 个规格）及聚乙烯的关节盂组件。第二代肩关节假体引入了模块化的肱骨头和假体柄设计，使得关节重建更接近解剖学重建。使用这一系统，更易解剖放置肱骨头（相对于肱骨结节和肩袖），提供了不同高度的肱骨头假体及可调的偏心距，使得软组织张力的调整更加容易。[33]然而许多第二代假体在肱骨头和假体柄的领之间存在一个间隙：更小的肱骨头假体和相应的关节面弧度减小会使肱骨的非关节面部分和关节盂不正常地接触。[26-27]假体柄的领和第二代肱骨头假体之间的

台阶使关节更易过度填充，或放置肱骨头时肱骨头相对于大结节的位置过高。[16]通常，通过软组织的张力可以判断肱骨头是否位于截骨平面上，但是由于台阶的存在，这一方法十分不确定。大部分第二代假体都有一个预设好的颈干角，需使用专门的截骨模板。使用骨水泥固定假体可以更好地恢复解剖形态，而以压配的方式固定假体是很难调整的。

现代的可适应性肩关节假体同样是基于解剖学的标准。[2-3]这些第三代假体柄有很多部分因考虑到颈干角的不同而做了相应调整，当然也包括肱骨头的大小和可变的偏心距。与第二代假体相比，解剖型假体能够更加准确地复原盂肱关节

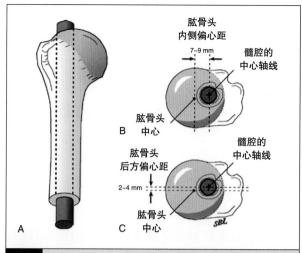

图 27-4 肱骨头的偏心距。A. 髓腔的中心轴线。B. 冠状面上肱骨头的偏心距（内侧距髓腔的中心轴线 7~9 mm）。C. 矢状面上肱骨头的偏心距（后方距髓腔的中心轴线 2~4 mm）。经允许引自 Iannotti JP, Lippitt SB, Williams GR Jr. Variation in neck-shaft angle: Influence in prosthetic design. *Am J Orthop (Belle Mead NJ)* 2007; 36（12, suppl 1）:9-14.

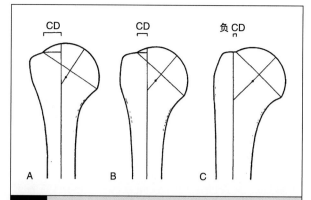

图 27-6 肱骨近端的形态和相对于干骺端关节面的偏心距模型。A. 高偏心距型。B. 标准型。C. 低偏心距型。CD—临界距离或大结节偏心距，指冈上肌腱止点内侧到肱骨干长轴的距离。如果 CD 值减少，插入直柄假体会更困难。斜线—肱骨头相对于骨干的倾斜角，黑点—旋转的几何中心，垂线—肱骨干的长轴。经允许引自 Hertel R, Knothe U, Ballmer FT. Geometry of the proximal humerus and implications for prosthetic design. *J Shoulder Elbow Surg* 2002;11（4）:331-338.

时旋转中心近似正常。[35] 通过使用第三代假体，医师可以进行肱骨头解剖截骨，并有充足的把握使假体复制解剖形态。假体可以适应患者，而不需患者适应假体。与第二代假体一样，第三代假体柄使用骨水泥固定，可提供额外的自由度。

长柄、短柄和无柄肱骨假体，以及肱骨表面置换

近些年，肱骨假体柄受到更多的关注。髋关节置换的理念也逐步渗透至肩关节假体。肱骨假体的许多原始理念源自股骨假体。肩关节的表面置换也是吸取了髋关节表面置换的经验，并且已经被应用了数年。表面置换只去除软骨和软骨下骨，能够轻松地恢复偏心距、旋转半径和肱骨头的高度及直径，在保留肱骨近端骨量的同时避免了假体柄相关的并发症。[36-38]

支持表面置换的学者认为这种能够保留骨量的手术方法与全肩关节置换术和带柄的半肩关节置换术相比，是年轻或活动量大的患者的首选治疗方式，而且后期很容易转换为带柄的假体置换或关节融合。[36-42] 在一项纳入 36 例年龄不超过

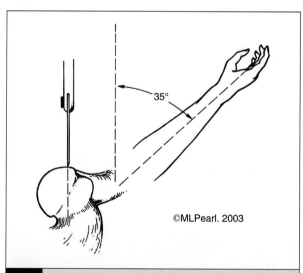

图 27-5 后倾角过大的肱骨截骨。以标准的 35° 后倾角截骨，很难解剖重建，而且有损伤肩袖的风险。经允许引自 Pearl ML. Proximal humeral anatomy in shoulder arthroplasty: Implications for prosthetic design and surgical technique. *J Shoulder Elbow Surg* 2005;14（1 suppl 1）:S99-S104.

的活动，并减小关节盂上的偏心负荷。此外，第二代假体可在关节盂的上部产生 8 倍的关节内反作用力。[34] 假体适应性的更多进化允许关节重建

55 岁的患者的研究中，使用表面置换，没有发现短期内假体松动或关节盂磨损，35 例患者具有非常高的满意度。[38] 如果没有使用假体柄，很容易重建旋转中心，这是因为关节面的位置与髓腔无关。然而在全肩关节置换术中，如果没有行肱骨截骨，则很难暴露关节盂（图 27-7A）。如果骨量不足、存在骨质疏松、骨坏死显著或肱骨近端存在畸形，需要谨慎进行表面置换。一些患者合并中心性的软骨缺损或骨坏死，可能需要进行局部病变区域的表面置换[43]（图 27-7B）。

目前，假体柄的设计重点集中在如何固定干骺端。这些压配的设计源自干骺端骨质的固定而非远端皮质骨的固定。目前欧洲正在开展关于无柄假体在截骨平面下固定的研究。无柄假体的设计不同于表面置换；医师需做肱骨头解剖型截骨，将假体放置在截骨面中心，可以不用考虑偏心距的问题，使术者重建原本的旋转中心而不受肱骨干轴线的影响。由于是固定在干骺端的，因此没有假体柄迫使假体处于内翻或不正确的角度的情况。近期的研究报道显示，短期的临床结果是令人满意的，即使是肱骨近端存在畸形，肱骨解剖重建后，使用保留骨量的假体经传统的关节盂入路进行关节盂置换的情况也是如此。[44-46] 无柄假体不适用于骨质疏松患者，后者通常是老年女性患者。[46-47]

长柄的设计的优势在于更大的骨长入界面可以分散应力，以及更大的接触面积可以用于抵抗旋转或扭转负荷，提供良好的长期稳定性。缺点包括与假体柄相关的并发症，如术中或术后出现的假体周围骨折、运动学的改变及翻修困难。无柄假体的优点包括保留了近端的骨量，便于后期的翻修或肩袖撕裂的修补。初次行关节置换术时都会切除肱骨头，以便显露关节盂。无柄假体的金属更少，因此关节僵硬的发生风险可能更小，会将更多的应力传导到骨质，因此会有更长期的存活率。[44]

如果有半肩关节置换术的手术指征，可能有必要行关节表面置换。相对年轻的患者或肱骨近端解剖结构异常（如存在骨折后遗症）的患者或者关节盂仍处于原始对称状态的患者都是表面置换的理想候选者，而非带柄的半肩关节置换术或传统的全肩关节置换术的候选者。[38] 通过对肱骨近端的磨削安装一个金属壳来恢复光滑的球形关节面，支持者认为，表面置换的过程能够很容易地重建肱骨的旋转中心。然而关节也易于被过分填充，因此术中需要特别注意导针是否垂直于解剖颈的平面。[39-40,43] 软组织松解与全肩关节置换术时是一样的，需在肱骨截骨前完成并保证手术部位充分显露，良好的长期满意度和假体存活率都是可实现的。[41-42,48]

短柄假体的设计代表着一种介于传统有柄假体和无柄假体或表面置换之间的妥协。更短的假体柄

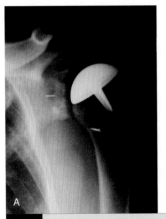
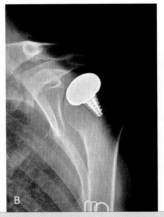
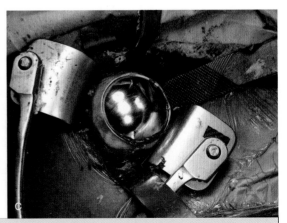

图 27-7　A. 肩关节 Grashey 位 X 线显示全肩表面置换。肩关节 Grashey 位 X 线片（B）和同一患者的术中照片（C）显示通过中心性表面置换治疗骨坏死

能提供旋转控制，具有与传统假体柄一样的优异稳定性，并可获得其肱骨近端干骺端压配的生物力学固定。长期随访发现短柄假体的应力遮挡更小，可伴有肱骨近端的骨溶解或吸收，这是因为应力集中在邻近肱骨头的部分，而非远侧的肱骨干。虽然短柄假体面临与长柄假体一样的长期效果问题，但是其短期数据仍是相对理想的。另外，柄更短的设计维持了骨保留手术的希望，对于翻修手术或未来病理改变的治疗（如肩袖疾病的治疗）是特别重要的。

骨性（解剖学）平衡或软组织的平衡

为了关节置换术后功能恢复，关节重建时必须恢复解剖学关系，对于肌肉的力量也必须予以恰当的平衡。通常，平衡软组织的常见方法是从关节前方松解过度紧张的组织，以维持正常的对线、稳定性和关节活动范围。不太常见的方法是将关节后方冗余的软组织折叠、短缩。在85%的人群中，肱骨头的大小有8个固定的组合；因此可选择合适的假体，使之提供理想的关节活动范围、稳定性及位移度。通过改变肱骨头假体的高度和厚度可调节软组织的相对张力。[4,18,49]

骨性平衡的概念意味着需要重建肱骨的解剖形态至必要的自然维度，或者至少根据肱骨头切除的量来决定。[3]假设肱骨头的厚度与解剖颈的直径或截骨平面相关，那么截骨量就决定了肱骨头的厚度。[2]因此，当完成去除骨赘、确认解剖颈及截骨这几个关键步骤后，剩下的问题就是如何填充截骨部分。

接下来恢复骨性解剖的步骤是恢复盂肱关节的运动学特性。如果截骨正确时假体柄内翻放置或假体放置正确而肱骨头截骨不足，则会出现过度填充的问题。[16,28-30]在任何一个病例中，肱骨头都应该被放置在干骺端的中心；如果使用现代适应性假体，那么放置肱骨头假体这一步骤可更容易地完成，这种假体可以最大限度地减小骨性平衡和软组织平衡间的差异。肱骨头的上缘应高于大结节的顶点5~10 mm。[4,7-8,31]带有偏心距的

肱骨干需要使用偏心的肱骨头，而非中心性肱骨头。[2-3,5]如果特定的系统缺少中心性肱骨头，术者应选择使肱骨头凸向恰当的方向；如果伴有小结节截骨，凸向前方的肱骨头与截骨重建区会很好地匹配。另外，可使用骨水泥型假体柄，欧洲比美国使用得更加普遍。使用骨水泥型假体柄允许医师在术中悬浮肱骨头假体，将其放置在理想的位置，以便重建关节的几何形态。

如果软组织出现对称性紧张，则提示肱骨头假体可能太大或截骨不足。[49]需要特别关注关节囊，确保软组织充分松解。为了纠正肱骨头过度后移，可使用更大型号的假体，但这样会牺牲关节活动范围（旋后运动）。此外，也可以增加后方的偏心距；或将后方关节囊折叠缝合，或经肱骨缝合（如同修复后方盂肱韧带撕脱）。[48-49]软组织重建后，手臂在内收位应该有40°外旋；肱骨头在向后应力的作用下会向后移位关节盂50%的宽度；手臂在外展位的内旋可达60°。[50]（这被称为40-50-60定律。）

骨水泥固定和非骨水泥固定

"固定"是一个相对的词语，因为骨骼是动态的、有活性的组织结构。术后即刻的骨–假体界面与2年后随访时的完全不同。当手术时的创伤被愈合的区域所替代，过渡区域越薄，应力就会越好地分散到周围的骨质。医师必须创造一个生态环境来支持从假体至骨的适当的应力传导，使假体不会随着时间的延长而松动，从而避免导致疼痛或假体失效。在材料科学成功地创造出一种可以复制自然组织硬度的假体之前，假体和骨骼之前仍然存在相对不匹配。这种硬度上的不匹配会导致微动和最终的假体松动。[51]假体的设计和界面应以紧压方式加载应力并尽可能均匀地分散应力，使微动小于70 μm。在最初的6~12周，最低程度的界面应力传导会促进愈合区域骨质的成熟，但是这不合实际。因此，非常重要的是尽可能地分散应力以减小剪切力并增加压力。为了获

得均匀的应力分布，假体必须与原关节盂或关节盂组件匹配放置，尽可能地恢复关节旋转功能，减少滚动或滑动。[52]

非骨水泥型假体的设计是为了通过假体表面和骨之间的主要连接获得初始固定。如果假体有髓腔塞存在，会出现剪切力，必须尽量减少剪切力或将其转化为骨 - 假体界面的压力。给假体施加压力会提高干骺端的吻合性，防止假体柄内翻。[53]理想状态下，应力从假体传导至骨，会使骨 - 假体界面产生最小的剪切力，并将负荷串联传递到骨，而不是以并联或负荷分担的方式。[54]下一阶段就是允许假体间隙处的骨长入或长出以将其锁定在原位。这是一个动态的过程，因为骨骼总是在不断地重建。[51]一些假体的设计明显优于其他假体，最近的放射学研究表明，带领的或远端压配型假体可能会在近端产生应力遮挡，导致内侧骨距的骨吸收。[55]肱骨近端的骨丢失会导致更多的微动，最终导致假体松动。[56]干骺端的压配比假体柄的远端压配更有效，在小型锥形柄的进化过程中这种设计趋势得以延续。[57]

与压配设计相关的实际问题和考虑因素与植入的相对容易程度有关，与初始压配的稳定性无关。假体上很长的翅可以使柄陷入内翻的位置，不能与截骨线平齐，或者可迫使柄倾斜或旋转。较小的圆柱体假体已经被更接近楔形体的假体所代替，以防止在骨内沉降；沿着内侧骨距打压植骨可以增强干骺端的紧密压配。[53,57]一个骨水泥型假体柄可以漂浮在水泥壳中，使手术医师能够将其精确地放置在截骨面上，以准确地重建截除的解剖结构和旋转中心。文献报道的非限制性肩关节置换术的松动率从骨性长入型的 0 或应用骨水泥的 1.5% 到有限长入整体柄的 10.0%。一些研究表明某些骨水泥型假体柄的设计可能优于非骨水泥型假体柄。[52,58-61]重要的是要认识到，假体柄会因对特定应用的适用性而有所变化。例如，如果设计用于骨水泥型的假体柄用作压配假体，则结果很差，反之亦然。一项纳入 1584 例初次行关节置换术患者的研究确定了肱骨侧假体失效的危险因素，相关危险因素包括男性、相对年轻的年龄、金属支持的关节盂和创伤后关节疾病。[58]使用近端骨水泥型假体柄的患者与使用压配型假体柄的患者相比，前者的旋转微动得到改善，完全的骨水泥固定型假体没有优势。[62]因此，对于没有骨折的患者，在植入前，最好只在假体柄的干骺端部分涂抹骨水泥。一项一级的研究比较了骨水泥型和非骨水泥型的特定假体柄，发现使用骨水泥型假体柄在关节的活动范围、力量和生活质量方面有更好的结果。[63]

软组织的考虑因素

肩胛下肌是肩关节置换术后功能恢复的关键。肩关节置换术中有 72% 的患者发现合并肩袖撕裂或肩胛下肌无力，而肩胛下肌无力预示着长期预后不良。[64-66]最近的经骨修复研究发现，肩胛下肌无力的发生率为 25%。[67]对于修复肩胛下肌完整性的关注导致了肌腱切开替代方法的发展。[68]替代方法包括骨膜袖套样剥离和几种不同方式的小结节截骨。这些方法中均是将肌腱和关节囊视为一个整体，从而保护血供（图 27-8）。在生物力学上，小结节截骨和双排修复失效需要超常的负荷，尽管最近的研究发现截骨术和肌腱切开术在修复强度上没有什么不同。[66,69-73]45 例患者在接受常规肌腱切开修复术后，41 例背后推离试验（lift-off test）结果均为阴性，45 例压腹试验（belly-press test）结果均为阴性。[74]小结节截骨术后骨与骨之间的愈合良好，临床结果良好；但仍有 44% 的患者有肌腹的脂肪浸润。[65-66]截骨术患者的肩胛下肌功能较以往同期肌腱切开术的患者更好。[75]归根结底，外科医师的偏好是肩胛下肌的入路和修复方式选择的决定性因素。

一份关于通过肩袖间隙保留肩胛下肌入路的报道指出了了在术中，肩关节活动不受限制的优势。这

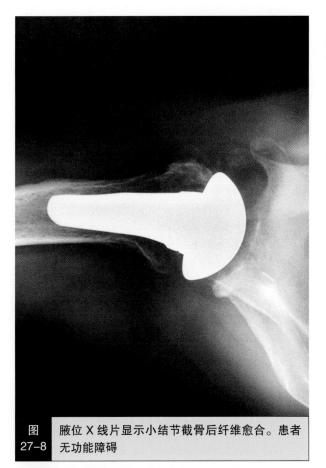

图 27-8 腋位 X 线片显示小结节截骨后纤维愈合。患者无功能障碍

未来的研究方向

人们仍然担心关节盂的磨损问题或关节盂植入假体的松动问题，而关于假体重建的研究仍在继续，假体重建可以提供与全肩关节置换术一样好的疼痛缓解效果，同时需要的手术时间更少、难度更小、费用更少。我们的愿望是找到一种硬度更低、耐磨性更好的肱骨假体材料。目前市面上还没有可用于肩关节置换术的关节假体，但正在为合适的应用进行研究。[77] 复合材料可能更适合肱骨，而陶瓷或金属并不适合。磁浮热解碳可能是肩关节假体的发展方向，因为它的弹性模量为 29.4 GPa，更接近皮质骨的弹性模量（23 GPa），对软骨有更好的磨损特性，因此对于半肩关节置换术是一个理想的选择。[78] 自 20 世纪 60 年代起，热解碳就被用于制作心脏的机械瓣膜，自 1979 年起用于小关节置换术；在欧洲，已经进行了数百次的热解碳肱骨置换术[79]（图 27-9）。

总结

现代非限制型肩关节置换术试图重建肱骨近端自然的解剖结构，从而减轻疼痛，恢复正常的肩关节运动学。假体设计的发展导致了模块化假体的出现，这种假体能够适应患者的解剖结构，

种方法的技术要求高，需要专门的器械，可能不适合肩关节僵硬、有大的下方骨赘或三角肌巨大的患者。[76] 在一项纳入 22 例患者的研究中，关注的问题是"6 例非自然形态的肱骨头截骨，8 例残余肱骨颈下方骨赘，5 例使用了过小的肱骨头假体。"[76]

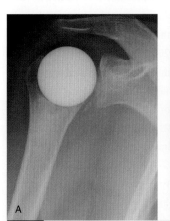
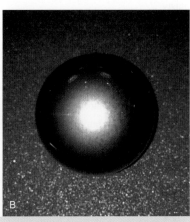
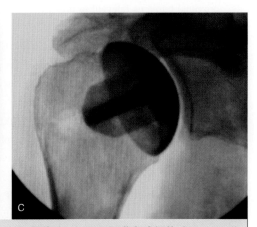

图 27-9 在欧洲市场上出售的两种热解碳假体。Grashey 位 X 线片（A）和照片（B）显示斯诺克球假体（Tornier 公司）；Grashey 位 X 线片（C）显示表面置换的假体（Integra 公司）（图 A 由 Gilles Walch 医学博士提供；图 C 由 Integra 公司提供）

同时最大限度地减少手术创伤，提高假体的长期存活率。[80]然而，改进的假体设计并不能取代严格的手术技术。软组织因素对于重建后提供长期的稳定和功能仍然至关重要。材料科学可以提供具有与宿主骨相似的生物力学特性的化合物，从而延长假体的寿命。

参考文献

[1] Bankes MJ, Emery RJ: Pioneers of shoulder replacement: Themistocles Gluck and Jules Emile Péan. *J Shoulder Elbow Surg* 1995;4(4):259-262.

[2] Boileau P, Walch G: The three-dimensional geometry of the proximal humerus: Implications for surgical technique and prosthetic design. *J Bone Joint Surg Br* 1997;79(5):857-865.

[3] Walch G, Boileau P: Prosthetic adaptability: A new concept for shoulder arthroplasty. *J Shoulder Elbow Surg* 1999;8(5):443-451.

[4] Iannotti JP, Gabriel JP, Schneck SL, Evans BG, Misra S: The normal glenohumeral relationships: An anatomical study of one hundred and forty shoulders. *J Bone Joint Surg Am* 1992;74(4):491-500.

[5] Hertel R, Knothe U, Ballmer FT: Geometry of the proximal humerus and implications for prosthetic design. *J Shoulder Elbow Surg* 2002;11(4):331-338.

[6] Pearl ML: Proximal humeral anatomy in shoulder arthroplasty: Implications for prosthetic design and surgical technique. *J Shoulder Elbow Surg* 2005;14 (1 Suppl S):99S-104S.

[7] Pearl ML, Volk AG: Coronal plane geometry of the proximal humerus relevant to prosthetic arthroplasty. *J Shoulder Elbow Surg* 1996;5(4):320-326.

[8] Robertson DD, Yuan J, Bigliani LU, Flatow EL, Yamaguchi K: Three-dimensional analysis of the proximal part of the humerus: Relevance to arthroplasty. *J Bone Joint Surg Am* 2000;82(11):1594-1602.

[9] Wataru S, Kazuomi S, Yoshikazu N, Hiroaki I, Takaharu Y, Hideki Y: Three-dimensional morphological analysis of humeral heads: A study in cadavers. *Acta Orthop* 2005;76(3):392-396.

[10] Vaesel MT, Olsen BS, Søjbjerg JO, Helmig P, Sneppen O: Humeral head size in shoulder arthroplasty: A kinematic study. *J Shoulder Elbow Surg* 1997;6(6):549-555.

[11] Wirth MA, Ondrla J, Southworth C, Kaar K, Anderson BC, Rockwood CA III: Replicating proximal humeral articular geometry with a third-generation implant: A radiographic study in cadaveric shoulders. *J Shoulder Elbow Surg* 2007;16(Suppl 3):S111-S116.

Radiographic measurements confirmed that a third-generation arthroplasty can accurately reproduce the native anatomy of the humerus.

[12] Fischer LP, Carret JP, Gonon GP, Dimnet J: Etude cinématique des mouvements de l'articulation scapulo-humérale (articulatio humeri). *Rev Chir Orthop Reparatrice Appar Mot* 1977;63(Suppl 2):108-115.

[13] Roche C, Angibaud L, Flurin PH, Wright T, Fulkerson E, Zuckerman J: Anatomic validation of an "anatomic" shoulder system. *Bull Hosp Jt Dis* 2006;63(3-4):93-97.

[14] Jeong J, Bryan J, Iannotti JP: Effect of a variable prosthetic neck-shaft angle and the surgical technique on replication of normal humeral anatomy. *J Bone Joint Surg Am* 2009;91(8):1932-1941.

Both fixed-angle and variable-angle prostheses have the ability to replicate native anatomy, but humeral head height may need to be adjusted when a fixed- angle device is used, and care must be taken not to alter the available surface arc.

[15] Takase K, Yamamoto K, Imakiire A, Burkhead WZ Jr: The radiographic study in the relationship of the glenohumeral joint. *J Orthop Res* 2004;22(2):298-305.

[16] Iannotti JP, Spencer EE, Winter U, Deffenbaugh D, Williams G: Prosthetic positioning in total shoulder arthroplasty. *J Shoulder Elbow Surg* 2005;14(1, Suppl S):111S-121S.

[17] Pearl ML, Volk AG: Retroversion of the proximal humerus in relationship to prosthetic replacement arthroplasty. *J Shoulder Elbow Surg* 1995;4(4):286-289.

[18] Pearl ML, Kurutz S, Postacchini R: Geometric variables in anatomic replacement of the proximal humerus: How much prosthetic geometry is necessary? *J Shoulder Elbow Surg* 2009;18(3):366-370.

A computer algorithm was used to conclude that increased geometric variability in a prosthesis allowed for closer approximation of normal anatomy.

[19] Iannotti JP, Lippitt SB, Williams GR Jr: Variation in neck-shaft angle: Influence in prosthetic design. *Am J Orthop (Belle Mead NJ)* 2007;36(12, Suppl 1):9-14.

Introducing variability in the neck-shaft angle of the prosthesis was thought to allow more accurate reproduction of the instant center of rotation.

[20] Harrold F, Wigderowitz C: A three-dimensional analysis of humeral head retroversion. *J Shoulder Elbow Surg* 2012;21(5):612-617.

The anterior cartilage–metaphyseal junction may not accurately reproduce true retroversion when used as the reference for humeral resection.

[21] Tillett E, Smith M, Fulcher M, Shanklin J: Anatomic determination of humeral head retroversion: The relationship of the central axis of the humeral head to the bicipital groove. *J Shoulder Elbow Surg* 1993;2(5):255-256.

[22] Doyle AJ, Burks RT: Comparison of humeral head retroversion with the humeral axis/biceps groove relationship: A study in live subjects and cadavers. *J Shoulder Elbow Surg* 1998;7(5):453-457.

[23] Edelson G: Variations in the retroversion of the humeral head. *J Shoulder Elbow Surg* 1999;8(2):142-145.

[24] Hernigou P, Duparc F, Hernigou A: Determining humeral retroversion with computed tomography. *J Bone Joint Surg Am* 2002;84(10):1753-1762.

[25] Hromádka R, Kubena AA, Pokorný D, Popelka S, Jahoda D, Sosna A: Lesser tuberosity is more reliable than bicipital groove when determining orientation of humeral head in primary shoulder arthroplasty. *Surg Radiol Anat* 2010;32(1):31-37.

Based on a study of 185 humeri, the lesser tuberosity was believed to be a more reliable landmark for retroversion because the bicipital groove is variable along its length.

[26] Pearl ML, Kurutz S: Geometric analysis of commonly used prosthetic systems for proximal humeral replacement. *J Bone Joint Surg Am* 1999;81(5):660-671.

[27] Pearl ML, Kurutz S, Robertson DD, Yamaguchi K: Geometric analysis of selected press fit prosthetic systems for proximal humeral replacement. *J Orthop Res* 2002;20(2):192-197.

[28] Nyffeler RW, Sheikh R, Jacob HA, Gerber C: Influence of humeral prosthesis height on biomechanics of glenohumeral abduction: An in vitro study. *J Bone Joint Surg Am* 2004;86(3):575-580.

[29] Favre P, Moor B, Snedeker JG, Gerber C: Influence of component positioning on impingement in conventional total shoulder arthroplasty. *Clin Biomech (Bristol, Avon)* 2008;23(2):175-183.

Component position had an effect on impingement through the arc of motion. One factor under the surgeon's control is the position of the implant along the resection line.

[30] Williams GR Jr, Wong KL, Pepe MD, et al: The effect of articular malposition after total shoulder arthroplasty on glenohumeral translations, range of motion, and subacromial impingement. *J Shoulder Elbow Surg* 2001;10(5):399-409.

[31] Takase K, Imakiire A, Burkhead WZ Jr: Radiographic study of the anatomic relationships of the greater tuberosity. *J Shoulder Elbow Surg* 2002;11(6):557-561.

[32] Neer CS II: Articular replacement for the humeral head. *J Bone Joint Surg Am* 1955;37-A(2):215-228.

[33] Fenlin JM Jr, Vaccaro A, Andreychik D, Lin S: Modular total shoulder: Early experience and impressions. *Semin Arthroplasty* 1990;1(2):102-111.

[34] Büchler P, Farron A: Benefits of an anatomical reconstruction of the humeral head during shoulder arthroplasty: A finite element analysis. *Clin Biomech (Bristol, Avon)* 2004;19(1):16-23.

[35] Irlenbusch U, End S, Kilic M: Differences in reconstruction of the anatomy with modern adjustable compared to second-generation shoulder prosthesis. *Int Orthop* 2011;35(5):705-711.

The variation in proximal humeral geometry supports the use of a prosthesis that can be adapted to patient anatomy. Modern prostheses more closely approximated the native humeral anatomy compared with second-generation implants.

[36] Hammond G, Tibone JE, McGarry MH, Jun BJ, Lee TQ: Biomechanical comparison of anatomic humeral head resurfacing and hemiarthroplasty in functional glenohumeral positions. *J Bone Joint Surg Am* 2012;94(1):68-76.

Humeral resurfacing may more accurately re-create the geometric center of rotation than hemiarthroplasty.

[37] Jensen KL: Humeral resurfacing arthroplasty: Rationale, indications, technique, and results. *Am J Orthop (Belle Mead NJ)* 2007;36(12, Suppl 1):4-8.

Guidelines for humeral resurfacing arthroplasty were provided in this report.

[38] Bailie DS, Llinas PJ, Ellenbecker TS: Cementless humeral resurfacing arthroplasty in active patients less than fifty-five years of age. *J Bone Joint Surg Am* 2008;90(1):110-117.

These data supported the use of resurfacing for arthritis in the young patient. Level of evidence: IV.

[39] Thomas SR, Sforza G, Levy O, Copeland SA: Geometrical analysis of Copeland surface replacement shoulder arthroplasty in relation to normal anatomy. *J Shoulder Elbow Surg* 2005;14(2):186-192.

[40] Thomas SR, Wilson AJ, Chambler A, Harding I, Thomas M: Outcome of Copeland surface replacement shoulder arthroplasty. *J Shoulder Elbow Surg* 2005;14(5):485-

491.

[41] Pritchett JW: Long-term results and patient satisfaction after shoulder resurfacing. *J Shoulder Elbow Surg* 2011;20(5):771-777.

The author reported that shoulder resurfacing had 96% survivorship and 95% patient satisfaction at 20- year follow-up.

[42] Burgess DL, McGrath MS, Bonutti PM, Marker DR, Delanois RE, Mont MA: Shoulder resurfacing. *J Bone Joint Surg Am* 2009;91(5):1228-1238.

The history, indications, technique, and advantages of resurfacing arthroplasty of the shoulder were thoroughly reviewed. Longer-term data will be necessary to determine whether resurfacing is preferable to total shoulder arthroplasty, but initial data are promising. This procedure may be the preferred option for younger patients.

[43] Scalise J, Miniaci A, Iannotti J: Resurfacing arthroplasty of the humerus: Indications, surgical technique, and clinical results. *Tech Shoulder Elbow Surg* 2007;8:152-160.

Techniques for shoulder resurfacing were reported, with particular attention given to surgical technique.

[44] Huguet D, DeClercq G, Rio B, Teissier J, Zipoli B; TESS Group: Results of a new stemless shoulder prosthesis: Radiologic proof of maintained fixation and stability after a minimum of three years' follow-up. *J Shoulder Elbow Surg* 2010;19(6):847-852.

In early results, the use of a stemless device was equivalent to that of stemmed implants.

[45] Collin P, McGourbey G, Boileau P, Walch G: Complications of the Simpliciti stemless prosthesis, in Walch G, Boileau P, Molé D, Favard L, Lévigne C, Sirveaux F, eds: *Shoulder Concepts 2012: Complications in Shoulder Arthroplasty*. Montpellier, France, Sauramps Medical, 2012, pp 57-61.

The combined experience from three shoulder centers in France was reported for 23 patients. The results were similar to those of standard arthroplasty, but caution may be needed in patients with poor bone quality.

[46] Tauber M, Habermeyer P, Magosch P: Is a stemless prosthesis better? in Walch G, Boileau P, Molé D, Favard L, Lévigne C, Sirveaux F, eds: *Shoulder Concepts Complications in Shoulder Arthroplasty*. Montpellier, France, Sauramps Medical, 2012, pp 49-56.

The results from a single institution and a multicenter study in France were reported at 3- to 5-year follow-up after the use of a stemless design. The results were similar to those of traditional third- and fourth-generation shoulder arthroplasty prosthesis. The complication rate was 9.8% to 12.1%.

[47] Barvencik F, Gebauer M, Beil FT, et al: Age- and sex-related changes of humeral head microarchitecture: Histomorphometric analysis of 60 human specimens. *J Orthop Res* 2010;28(1):18-26.

Regions of less dense bone in the proximal humerus were identified in humeri harvested at autopsy.

[48] Williams G, Iannotti J: Unconstrained prosthetic arthroplasty for glenohumeral arthritis with an intact or repairable rotator cuff: Indications, techniques, and results, in Iannotti J, Williams G, eds: *Disorders of the Shoulder*, ed 2. Philadelphia, PA, Lippincott, Williams, & Wilkins, 2007, pp 713-715.

The authors summarized the history, indications, results, and complications of shoulder arthroplasty.

[49] Harryman DT, Sidles JA, Harris SL, Lippitt SB, Matsen FA III: The effect of articular conformity and the size of the humeral head component on laxity and mo- tion after glenohumeral arthroplasty: A study in cadavera. *J Bone Joint Surg Am* 1995;77(4):555-563.

[50] Matsen F, Clinton J, Rockwood C, Wirth M, Lippitt S: *The Shoulder*, ed. 4. Philadelphia, PA, Saunders, 2009, pp 1093-1096.

The authors summarized the conventional theoretical and technical aspects of shoulder arthroplasty.

[51] Jobe CM, Phipatanakul WP, Bowsher JG: *Revision and Complex Shoulder Arthroplasty*. Philadelphia PA, Wolters Kluwer/Lippincott, Williams & Wilkins, 2010, pp 83-94.

The biomechanics of prosthetic fixation were clearly discussed, providing insight into possible modes of failure.

[52] Cofield R: Loosening of cemented and uncemented humeral stems, in Walch G, Boileau P, Molé D, Favard L, Lévigne C, Sirveaux F, eds: *Shoulder Concepts 2012: Complications in Shoulder Arthroplasty*. Montpellier, France, Sauramps Medical, 2012, pp 23-27.

The Mayo experience of cemented and cementless shoulder arthroplasty was concisely described. Cemented stems may have better survivability.

[53] Boorman RS, Hacker S, Lippitt SB, Matsen FA: A conservative broaching and impaction grafting technique for humeral component placement and fixation in shoulder arthroplasty: The procrustean method. *Tech Shoulder Elbow Surg* 2001;2:172-173.

[54] Orr TE, Carter DR: Stress analyses of joint arthroplasty

in the proximal humerus. *J Orthop Res* 1985;3(3):360-371.

[55] Edwards B: Can a short-stem avoid the potential complications of the longer stems? The Aequalis Ascend experience, in Walch G, Boileau P, Molé D, Favard L, Lévigne C, Sirveaux F, eds: *Shoulder Concepts 2012: Complications in Shoulder Arthroplasty.* Montpellier, France, Sauramps Medical, 2012, pp 147-149.
The author's experience with a short-stem humeral prosthesis was described. A near-term improvement in calcar resorption was reported.

[56] Cuff D, Levy JC, Gutiérrez S, Frankle MA: Torsional stability of modular and non-modular reverse shoulder humeral components in a proximal humeral bone loss model. *J Shoulder Elbow Surg* 2011;20(4):646-651.
Rotational stability with humeral stems in a reverse model was studied. Monoblock stems performed best, especially when the proximal humerus was intact.

[57] Matsen FA III, Iannotti JP, Rockwood CA Jr: Humeral fixation by press-fitting of a tapered metaphyseal stem: A prospective radiographic study. *J Bone Joint Surg Am* 2003;85(2):304-308.

[58] Cil A, Veillette CJ, Sanchez-Sotelo J, Sperling JW, Schleck CD, Cofield RH: Survivorship of the humeral component in shoulder arthroplasty. *J Shoulder Elbow Surg* 2010;19(1):143-150.
The least amount of radiolucency was seen around cemented components, but all maintained good survivability.

[59] Gonzalez JF, Alami GB, Baque F, Walch G, Boileau P: Complications of unconstrained shoulder prostheses. *J Shoulder Elbow Surg* 2011;20(4):666-682.
This meta-analysis of unconstrained shoulder arthroplasty reported excellent survivability, with a trend toward better results with cemented rather than cementless implants.

[60] Sperling JW, Cofield RH, O'Driscoll SW, Torchia ME, Rowland CM: Radiographic assessment of ingrowth total shoulder arthroplasty. *J Shoulder Elbow Surg* 2000;9(6):507-513.

[61] Throckmorton TW, Zarkadas PC, Sperling JW, Cofield RH: Radiographic stability of ingrowth humeral stems in total shoulder arthroplasty. *Clin Orthop Relat Res* 2010;468(8):2122-2128.
A press-fit design that included porous coating circumferentially around the metaphysis performed much better than earlier implants that had ingrowth surface only on the undersurface of the collar. No loosening was reported at short-term to midterm follow-up.

[62] Harris TE, Jobe CM, Dai QG: Fixation of proximal humeral prostheses and rotational micromotion. *J Shoulder Elbow Surg* 2000;9(3):205-210.

[63] Litchfield RB, McKee MD, Balyk R, et al: Cemented versus uncemented fixation of humeral components in total shoulder arthroplasty for osteoarthritis of the shoulder: A prospective, randomized, double-blind clinical trial—A JOINTs Canada Project. *J Shoulder Elbow Surg* 2011;20(4):529-536.
Cementation of a humeral arthroplasty implant had better results than cementless fixation. The stem originally was designed for cemented use. Level of evidence: I.

[64] Sperling JW, Potter HG, Craig EV, Flatow E, Warren RF: Magnetic resonance imaging of painful shoulder arthroplasty. *J Shoulder Elbow Surg* 2002;11(4):315-321.

[65] Gerber C, Yian EH, Pfirrmann CA, Zumstein MA, Werner CM: Subscapularis muscle function and structure after total shoulder replacement with lesser tuberosity osteotomy and repair. *J Bone Joint Surg Am* 2005;87(8):1739-1745.

[66] Gerber C, Pennington SD, Yian EH, Pfirrmann CA, Werner CM, Zumstein MA: Lesser tuberosity osteotomy for total shoulder arthroplasty: Surgical technique. *J Bone Joint Surg Am* 2006;88(Suppl 1, Pt 2):170-177.

[67] Liem D, Kleeschulte K, Dedy N, Schulte TL, Steinbeck J, Marquardt B: Subscapularis function after transosseous repair in shoulder arthroplasty: Transosseous subscapularis repair in shoulder arthroplasty. *J Shoulder Elbow Surg* 2012;21(10):1322-1327.
A 25% rate of subscapularis dysfunction was reported after a transosseous repair.

[68] Armstrong A, Lashgari C, Teefey S, Menendez J, Yamaguchi K, Galatz LM: Ultrasound evaluation and clinical correlation of subscapularis repair after total shoulder arthroplasty. *J Shoulder Elbow Surg* 2006;15(5):541-548.

[69] Krishnan SG, Stewart DG, Reineck JR, Lin KC, Buzzell JE, Burkhead WZ: Subscapularis repair after shoulder arthroplasty: Biomechanical and clinical validation of a novel technique. *J Shoulder Elbow Surg* 2009;18(2):184-192, discussion 197-198.
A sound reconstruction technique was described for lesser tuberosity osteotomy repair.

[70] Van Thiel GS, Wang VM, Wang FC, et al: Biomechanical similarities among subscapularis repairs after shoulder arthroplasty. *J Shoulder Elbow Surg*

2010;19(5):657-663.

No difference was found among multiple types of subscapularis repairs, including osteotomy.

[71] Van den Berghe GR, Nguyen B, Patil S, et al : A biomechanical evaluation of three surgical techniques for subscapularis repair. *J Shoulder Elbow Surg* 2008;17(1):156-161.

Tendon-to-bone repair was not as strong as bone-to-bone repair for an osteotomy or tendon-to-tendon repair.

[72] Giuseffi SA, Wongtriratanachai P, Omae H, et al: Biomechanical comparison of lesser tuberosity osteotomy versus subscapularis tenotomy in total shoulder arthroplasty. *J Shoulder Elbow Surg* 2012;21(8):1087-1095.

Little difference was found in a comparison of tendon-to-tendon and osteotomy repairs.

[73] Ahmad CS, Wing D, Gardner TR, Levine WN, Bigliani LU: Biomechanical evaluation of subscapularis repair used during shoulder arthroplasty. *J Shoulder Elbow Surg* 2007;16(Suppl 3):S59-S64.

Transosseous tunnels altered the anatomy and were less strong than tendon-to-tendon repairs or combined constructs.

[74] Caplan JL, Whitfield B, Neviaser RJ: Subscapularis function after primary tendon to tendon repair in patients after replacement arthroplasty of the shoulder. *J Shoulder Elbow Surg* 2009;18(2):193-197-198.

Excellent results were reported after traditional subscapularis tenotomy and repair.

[75] Qureshi S, Hsiao A, Klug RA, Lee E, Braman J, Flatow EL: Subscapularis function after total shoulder replacement: Results with lesser tuberosity osteotomy. *J Shoulder Elbow Surg* 2008;17(1):68-72.

Excellent results were reported after a lesser tuberosity osteotomy technique was used for total shoulder arthroplasty.

[76] Lafosse L, Schnaser E, Haag M, Gobezie R: Primary total shoulder arthroplasty performed entirely thru the rotator interval: Technique and minimum two-year outcomes. *J Shoulder Elbow Surg* 2009;18(6):864-873.

Good results were reported after the use of a subscapularis-sparing approach to the shoulder joint. The surgery is technically demanding.

[77] Williams GR Jr, Iannotti JP: Alternative bearing surfaces—do we need them? *Am J Orthop (Belle Mead NJ)* 2007;36(12, Suppl 1):15-17.

The risks and benefits of metal-on-metal, ceramic-on-ceramic, and ceramic-on-polyethylene bearings in the shoulder were described, as was cross-linking of the polyethylene.

[78] Cook SD, Thomas KA, Kester MA: Wear characteristics of the canine acetabulum against different femoral prostheses. *J Bone Joint Surg Br* 1989;71(2):189-197.

[79] Stanley J, Klawitter J, More R: Joint replacement technology, in Revell P, ed: *Joint Replacement Technologies.* Boca Raton, FL, CRC Press, 2008, pp 631-656.

The material properties, manufacturing, and clinical use of pyrolytic carbon for joint arthroplasty were described.

[80] Buzzell JE, Lutton DM, Shyr Y, Neviaser RJ, Lee DH: Reliability and accuracy of templating the proximal humeral component for shoulder arthroplasty. *J Shoulder Elbow Surg* 2009;18(5):728-733.

Preoperative templating was found to approximate surgical reconstruction with a modern prosthesis.

第二十八章 关节盂的解剖及假体的修复重建

Patric Raiss, MD; T. Bradley Edwards, MD; Gilles Walch, MD

引言

肱骨近端半肩关节置换术是治疗肩关节退行性病变的标准方法，可取得良好的效果。与半肩关节置换术相比，全肩关节置换术在疼痛缓解、功能恢复和患者满意度方面都有优势。[1]全肩关节置换术的主要问题是关节盂组件松动，这在中长期随访中经常观察到。[2-5]因此，一些医师避免使用关节盂组件，特别是在活动范围大、预期寿命长的相对年轻的患者中。[6]患者的结局因使用的固定理念（骨水泥固定或非骨水泥固定）和关节盂组件设计（龙脊型或短桩型，平背或凸背）的不同而不同。

Neither Dr. Raiss nor any immediate family member has received anything of value from or owns stock in a commercial company or institution related directly or indirectly to the subject of this article. Dr. Edwards or an immediate family member has received royalties from Tornier and Orthohelix; is a member of a speakers' bureau or has made paid presentations on behalf of Tornier; serves as a paid consultant to Kinamed and Tornier; serves as an unpaid consultant to Gulf Coast Surgical Services; has received research support from Tornier; has received nonincome support (such as equipment or services), commercially derived honoraria, or other non–research-related funding (such as paid travel) from Tornier; and serves as a board member, owner, officer, or committee member of the American Shoulder and Elbow Surgeons. Dr. Walch or an immediate family member has received royalties from Tornier, and has received nonincome support (such as equipment or services), commercially derived honoraria, or other non–research-related funding (such as paid travel) from Tornier.

解剖学

了解肩胛盂的解剖学知识对每一位肩关节外科医师来说都是至关重要的，尤其是在考虑行全肩关节置换术时。医师需要知道患者关节盂的角度、倾斜度、高度、宽度和形状。[7]可以利用这些信息制订手术计划。

关节盂的凹陷被软骨覆盖，最薄的部分在中心。软骨的厚度从中心向周围增加。软骨终止于盂唇，盂唇由强大的纤维软骨组成。关节盂面的形态可描述为梨形或倒置的逗号形。肱二头肌长头的止点（即盂上结节）是关节盂的最高点，肱三头肌长头的止点（即盂下结节）是关节盂的最低点。多项研究分析了无炎症的肩关节盂表面的平均尺寸，结果略有不同。[8-11]从上到下测得的关节盂的平均高度为35~39 mm，平均宽度为23~29 mm。[8-11]分析关节的表面积和关节盂凹陷的体积后发现，平均表面积为8.7 cm^2，平均体积为11.9 cm^3。[10]在CT上采用不同的方法常规测量关节盂的角度。[12]75%的被评估的肩关节有平均7.4°的后倾，另外25%的肩关节有2°~10°的前倾。[13]另一项研究发现344个肩胛骨的平均后倾角为1.2°。[8]

假体方面的考量因素

关节盂组件可以使用或不使用骨水泥固定。目前有几种不同的假体设计和固定理念。

非骨水泥固定的关节盂假体

使用非骨水泥固定的关节盂假体的手术翻修

率和并发症发生率高于使用骨水泥固定的关节盂假体。一项前瞻性、双盲随机研究比较了使用非骨水泥固定的后背金属骨长入型关节盂组件与使用骨水泥固定的平背龙脊型关节盂组件的结果（每组各 20 个肩关节）。[2] 使用骨水泥固定的关节盂组件周围的放射线透光率明显较高（85% ： 25%，P<0.01），但有 4 个（20%）由非骨水泥固定的关节盂组件出现松动，其中 3 个假体需要翻修（图 28-1）。使用骨水泥固定的关节盂假体未见松动。2005 年，有研究人员报道了 147 例连续进行的肩关节置换术的结果，平均随访期为 7.5 年。[14] 由于临床未见到效果，11% 的肩关节中后背金属型关节盂假体已经被移除；8% 的肩关节在 X 线片上有组件断裂的征象，但无临床症状。最近的多项调查证实，使用不同的后背金属

型关节盂假体设计，并发症发生率都很高。[15-17] 最常见的并发症显然是假体松动，其次是聚乙烯严重磨损或聚乙烯部分从假体的金属部分上分离。只有一项研究描述了良好的中长期结果。[18] 在这项研究中，1996—2005 年，35 例患者进行了 35 例人工肩关节置换术，使用后背金属型关节盂假体，该部件由涂有多孔钛和羟基磷灰石的钛合金外壳组成，并以两枚 6.5 mm 螺钉固定。这种关节盂假体的适应证尚不清楚。研究人员在平均 6 年的随访中没有发现松动或并发症。为了证实这些发现，有必要对这种新的非骨水泥型关节盂假体进行进一步的中长期研究。

使用骨水泥固定的关节盂假体

使用骨水泥固定的聚乙烯关节盂组件的结果有较多的文献报道。在使用骨水泥固定的关节盂假体周围，放射线透亮带很常见，报告率为 0~96%。[19] 尽管放射线透亮带通常在术后即刻的 X 线片上即可见，但它们的存在并不总是预示着假体松动或临床症状。

使用骨水泥固定的关节盂假体的两种主要类型是龙脊型和短桩型（图 28-2）。一项对 328 例全肩关节置换术后即刻放射学影像的分析发现，当使用龙脊型假体时，放射线透亮带的出现率显著升高。[19] 这些数据得到了两项前瞻性随机研究的支持，这两项前瞻性随机研究发现，在 2 年的随访中，龙脊型假体周围的放射线透亮带明显比短

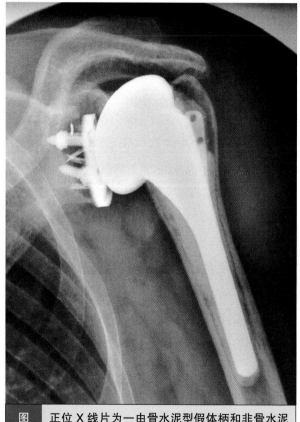

图 28-1　正位 X 线片为一由骨水泥型假体柄和非骨水泥型后背金属型关节盂假体组成的全肩关节置换术后第 14 年的影像。可以看到肱骨向近端移位，关节盂假体明显松动伴有一枚螺钉断裂及聚乙烯内衬磨损

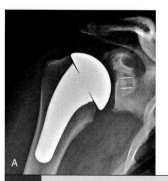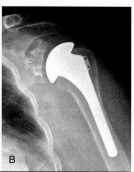

图 28-2　全肩关节置换术后即刻正位 X 线片。其中非骨水泥柄与骨水泥龙脊型关节盂组件（A）或骨水泥短桩型关节盂组件（B）相结合

桩型假体周围的放射线透亮带多。[20-21]一项生物力学研究发现，短桩型假体的最大张力缘的位移程度明显小于龙脊型假体。[22]然而，另一项研究经过平均 4 年的随访发现，50 例使用龙脊型假体的患者的放射线透亮带的出现率与 50 例使用短桩型假体的患者没有差异。[23]

使用骨水泥固定的龙脊型关节盂假体的长期结果有较多的文献报道。最近显示报道了 972 个使用全聚乙烯骨水泥型关节盂假体的存活率，并以翻修为终点。[24]10 年的总体存活率为 95%，15 年的总体存活率为 92%；15 年时，Cofield 1 型假体（施乐辉公司）的存活率为 87%，Neer 2 型假体（施乐辉公司）的存活率为 94%。Cofield 2 型假体（施乐辉公司）的存活率也很高，术后 5 年时为 99%，术后 10 年时为 94%。两个多中心研究的平背或凸背的关节盂假体的存活率显示有着相似的结果。[3-4]在没有肩袖撕裂或术前不稳定的 263 例骨关节炎患者中，使用骨水泥固定的平背龙脊型假体行全肩关节置换术，术后平均随访 10 年（5~20 年）。[3]以关节盂假体翻修为终点，假体的 10 年存活率为 94.5%，15 年存活率为 79.4%。以放射学影像上的假体松动为终点时，结果不太理想，10 年存活率为 80.3%，15 年存活率仅为 33.6%。相同的研究者分析了 333 例使用骨水泥固定的凸背关节盂假体行全肩关节置换术，以关节盂组件翻修为终点，5 年存活率为 99.7%，10 年存活率为 98.3%。以放射学影像上的假体松动为终点时，假体的 5 年存活率为 99.7%，10 年存活率仅为 51.5%。在这两项研究中，在患者的疼痛水平、活动水平和肩关节运动方面，放射学影像上的假体松动与临床恶化有显著的相关性。

最近一项研究纳入了 518 例使用凸背或平背龙脊型关节盂假体的全肩关节置换术患者，通过对其进行平均 8.6 年（5~18 年）的随访，研究分析了关节盂组件的松动模式。[25]失败的 3 个主要机制是内侧塌陷（7.9%）、上倾（10%）和后倾（6.4%）。关节盂假体的内陷与准备关节盂时过度磨削及软骨下骨完全切除有关（P<0.001）。导致上倾的危险因素有关节盂假体放置过低，术后即刻 X 线片显示关节盂假体面向上方放置，以及肱骨头向上移位（P<0.05）。导致后倾的危险因素有术前肱骨头向后半脱位、准备关节盂时过度磨削及软骨下骨完全切除（P<0.001）。放射学假体松动率约为 32%，故该文献作者认为保护软骨下骨对关节盂假体的长期存活十分重要。[25]

尽管在比较性研究中显示了良好的前景，但这种短桩型关节盂假体的中长期研究数据很少。已发表的最长随访期（平均 5 年）的研究报道显示，以翻修为终点时，短桩型全聚乙烯 Cofield 2 型假体的存活率与龙脊型假体相似。[24]这种假体不同于目前大多数的短桩型假体，它有 3 个线性排列的短桩，而不是 4 个或 5 个非线性排列的短桩。仍需要更长时间的随访以更好地阐明短桩型设计相对于龙脊型设计的优势。

使用部分骨水泥固定的全聚乙烯假体

在过去的 10 年中，假体的设计已经发展到包括组件的形态、固定短桩的数量和位置以及固定方法的变化。锚栓固定的关节盂假体（如锚栓式关节盂假体，DePuy 公司；Cortiloc 假体，Tornier 公司）是一种需要最小量骨水泥固定的全聚乙烯设计；在这种设计中，鳍样的中心短桩埋入中心钻孔中，无须骨水泥，而周边的小短桩则需常规骨水泥固定。虽然松质骨生长到中心短桩的机制尚不清楚，但已有其取得良好效果的文献报道。[26-28]使用这种类型的关节盂假体进行了超过 33 000 例的肩关节置换，但仅有 3 篇患者数量有限的研究报道。[28]在经过平均 43 个月的随访后，一项基于 CT 的研究发现在 35 例接受这种假体治疗的患者中，有 32 例（91%）假体的 6 个中心非骨水泥固定的短桩鳍里平均有 4.5 个在周围有骨长入，3 例（9%）假体中没有骨长入。[27]另一项研究在透视控制下使用放射线检测了 20 例患者的骨形成情况，并经过至少 5 年的随访，发现其中的 15 例患者的锚栓鳍周围有骨形成，[26] 其余 5 例患者的中心短桩周围发现有放射线透亮带或骨溶解。针对这类假体的另一项研究在 44 个肩部进行了平均 3 年的 X 线随访。[28] 当 Lazarus 等人设计的系统用于分析关节盂组件的骨水泥固定情况和假体位置情况时，86% 的假体被评为"骨水泥固定良好"和"假体位置良好"。[19] 在中心短桩周围骨溶解的发生率为 7%，68% 的假体在中心短桩鳍的周围有足够的骨生长。有一个假体出现了明显松动。

另一种混合型关节盂假体（综合肩关节系统，Biomet 公司）也有骨水泥固定的外周短钉和能够长入骨的使用非骨水泥固定的多孔钛涂层中心短桩设计。但使用结果尚未公布。

平背假体与凸背假体

关节盂假体的背面可以是平的或带弧度的。凸背假体试图使假体的背部形状与患者关节盂本身的凹面相匹配。半球形的铰刀通常可用于凸背假体系统中的关节盂制备，而平面的铰刀用于平背假体的骨准备。与凸背假体相比，平背假体的一个缺点是通常需要在磨削过程中切除更多的骨，因为原始的关节盂必须修锉平整以匹配假体背部的形状。从生物力学角度来看，凸背假体比平背假体更能抵抗微动。[22] 然而，临床研究并没有显示任何一种假体有优越性。

通过对 X 线片观察发现，使用平背假体在短期内会导致更多的放射线透亮带，但长期的随访发现这种差异会逐渐变小。[29-30] 一项对 66 例人工肩关节置换术的前瞻性研究发现，经过 2 年的随访，平背假体的平均放射线透亮带 Molé 评分（4.2 分）和凸背假体（3.2 分）有明显差异。[31-32] 同组患者经过 10 年随访，存活 56 例肩关节，但平背假体组的平均放射线透亮带 Molé 评分增加到 9.8 分，凸背假体组增加到 8.3 分。[33] 这 10 年的差异没有统计学意义，但作者发现在

这些经过 10 年随访的患者中，行关节置换术时年龄小于 60 岁的患者的放射线透亮带评分明显更高（P<0.03），如果手术侧肩关节是主力侧，则放射线透亮带更多（P<0.017），而且术后即刻 X 线片中放射线透亮带的存在情况可有效预测其进展程度（P<0.018）。这项研究是平背和凸背关节盂假体使用结果唯一可用的临床比较研究。

假体不匹配

假体不匹配是指关节盂和肱骨组件之间曲率半径的差异。盂肱关节骨性不匹配的半径为 8~9 mm，软骨不匹配的半径可以小至 0.1 mm。[34] 在全肩关节置换术中，不匹配的范围取决于假体，而假体最终由手术医师选择。肱骨和关节盂组件之间的完全一致性增加了组件的接触面积，从而降低了接触压力。[35] 然而，在一个协调的系统中，当肱骨头在关节盂上移动时，各组件之间的接触面积会明显减小，并且增加的力会传递到关节盂组件的边缘。[36] 这种边缘负荷会增加关节盂组件松动的风险。[37] 相反地，增加盂肱关节的不匹配度会减少肱骨头和关节盂组件之间的接触面积，从而导致接触压力增加，加速聚乙烯的磨损并增加盂肱关节的不稳定。[34-36] 大多数研究者建议组件应有一定的不匹配度，以避免关节盂组件边缘负荷过大。[34-35] 只有一项临床研究分析了假体不匹配度对使用骨水泥固定的关节盂组件周围放射线透亮带形成的影响。[34] 在 319 个肩关节中，采用 Aequalis 全肩关节置换系统（Tornier 公司）治疗，所有患者的诊断相同，均为盂肱关节原发性骨关节炎，并且都使用了骨水泥固定的龙脊型关节盂组件。[34] 将患者分为 4 组不同的匹配度：第 1 组，0~4 mm；第 2 组，4.5~5.5 mm；第 3 组，6~7 mm；第 4 组，大于 7 mm。经过平均 4.5 年的随访，第 3 组和第 4 组（分别为 3.8 分和 3.7 分）的平均放射线透亮带 Molé 评分要低于第 1 组和第 2 组（分别为 6.4 分和 5.8 分）。作者的结论是，6~10 mm 的盂肱关节不匹配最有利于控制放射线透亮带的进展。[34]

技术因素

关节盂的准备技术

在假体植入过程中，充分暴露关节盂表面是原关节盂准备的关键。许多关节盂暴露和准备的技术已被描述。这里只描述资深作者的首选技术。

在切断肩胛下肌腱后，将肱骨头牵开器插入关节内。松解内侧和下方的盂肱韧带，将肱骨头向后牵拉，显露关节盂的前缘。肩胛下肌腱置于肩胛骨前方的肩胛下隐窝内，以关节盂前缘的牵开器固定。将肱二头肌长头腱从其在肩胛上结节的止点处游离，并在胸大肌肌腱的上缘以不可吸收缝线缝合固定。盂唇和关节囊从喙突的前下方开始游离，在 5 点位（右肩）或 7 点位（左肩）终止。将下方的关节囊和肱三头肌腱的外侧部分游离至 8 点（右肩）或 4 点左右（左肩）。下方的松解是充分暴露关节盂和假体的关键步骤（图 28-3）。使肱骨头向后方脱位并切除。当肱骨侧准备完成后，向后牵拉肱骨近端，暴露关节盂。用刮匙从关节盂处刮除残余的软骨。可以看到骨赘，将其移除。用电刀标记关节盂表面的中心。如果使用空心钻系统，则可在中心插入导针；如果使用非空心钻系统，则可直接在中心钻孔。使用机动铰刀制备关节盂的表面。为了延长假体的寿命，需要保护软骨下骨，进行最小限度的磨削。[4,24]如果使用的是短桩型假体，则可以钻剩余的周围孔。如果使用龙脊型假体，则建议使用击打压配的方式准备关节盂。[31]此技术可最小限度地去除骨质，并使用龙脊冲头压缩关节盂骨质。研究表明，与传统的刮除技术相比，该技术可以显著改善龙脊型关节盂组件周围的放射线透亮带评分。[31]假体可以按照制造商的建议进行固定。

骨水泥技术

关节盂准备完成后，用脉冲枪冲洗龙脊槽或短桩孔，以清除松质骨中的血液和碎片。脉冲枪在髋关节置换术中的益处已得到充分证实，但在肩关节置换术中，类似的疗效尚未得到证实。关节盂的

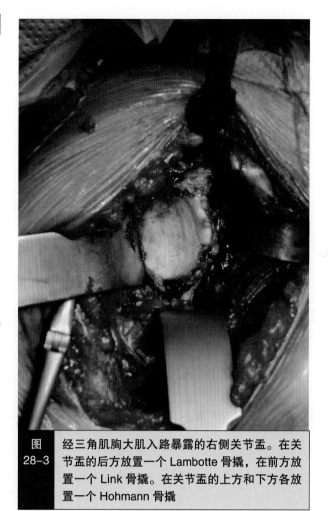

图 28-3　经三角肌胸大肌入路暴露的右侧关节盂。在关节盂的后方放置一个 Lambotte 骨撬，在前方放置一个 Link 骨撬。在关节盂的上方和下方各放置一个 Hohmann 骨撬

骨质应在冲洗后干燥。在用骨水泥固定龙脊型假体前，使用 3 种不同的保持关节盂干燥的方法（使用被凝血酶浸泡过的凝胶海绵，压缩气体冲洗或生理盐水冲洗，然后使用普通的海绵），比较其在术后即刻的影像学检查中关节盂周围的放射线透亮带情况，并没有发现有统计学上的显著差异。[38]另一种干燥关节盂凹陷的排水孔技术是在喙突上钻一个孔，使其与关节盂凹陷相通，在假体的骨水泥固定过程中，对这个孔持续进行抽吸。[39]一项临床研究发现，使用排水孔技术可显著改善骨水泥的覆盖，减少龙脊型或短桩型假体周围的放射线透亮带。[39]一项基于 CT 的体外研究发现，与标准技术相比，在使用排水孔技术时，关节盂凹陷内的骨水泥渗透明显更深。[40]该技术的一个潜在问题是，钻孔可能会削弱喙突，导致骨折。

有许多类型的骨水泥可供使用，包括慢固化或快固化骨水泥，高、中、低黏度骨水泥，含有抗生素的骨水泥。水泥可以在碗中手动搅拌，也可以使用真空离心机搅拌以降低孔隙率。没有数据可以用于比较不同类型的骨水泥应用于关节盂假体植入的效果。

已经有研究人员描述了多种直接或用注射器将骨水泥注入关节盂凹陷的技术。体外使用注射器注射的骨水泥渗透性比手动填充的更好，骨质疏松症患者的骨水泥渗透得更深。[41]这一发现在一项研究中得到证实，该研究发现关节盂凹陷局部的骨密度与骨水泥的渗透性呈强负相关性。[29]加压是一种行之有效的提高髋关节和膝关节置换术中骨水泥渗透性的方法。关于这项技术在全肩关节置换术中的应用，已经有一些已发表的研究结果。根据是否使用"徒手填塞技术"或"新设备加压技术"，有研究人员比较了全聚乙烯关节盂组件周围放射线透亮带的出现情况。[30]术后即刻影像学检查显示使用手动填充骨水泥的关节盂假体周围放射线透亮带的出现率和厚度值明显更高（P<0.05）。短桩型关节盂假体组的放射线透亮带明显少于龙脊型假体组（P<0.05）。当60 ml注射器与加压海绵一起用于短桩孔内的骨水泥填充时，69例肩关节中90%的肩关节在术后即刻的影像学检查中没有放射线透亮带。[42]该研究的研究者使用一个尺寸匹配的短桩部件使骨水泥加压，发现放射线透亮带的出现率低。目前，尚无较长期的后续数据。最近出现了一种硅胶的加压装置，该装置具有用于龙脊型假体的槽或短桩型假体的孔。[43]这个装置可以很容易地连接到骨水泥枪上。在一项体外研究中，与传统的骨水泥技术相比，使用该设备会使骨水泥更均匀和更深地渗入关节盂骨质中。在对骨水泥加压后，研究人员建议在骨水泥固化之前将假体保持在原位，并去除挤出的骨水泥，以避免关节中出现异物，从而预防异物引起的聚乙烯磨损。

未来的研究方向

关节盂假体的松动是全肩关节置换术的薄弱环节。关节盂假体松动与否对相对年轻的患者来说尤其重要，因为他们的预期寿命比大多数老年患者更长且有更高的活动水平。[6,44]为了避免传统的关节盂假体植入，现已引入了可替代的耐磨界面。

表面生物学重建

一种不用植入传统假体的关节盂表面重建的方法是使用软组织移植。其原理是创造一个光滑的生物性关节盂表面，从而减少肱骨和关节盂人工组件之间的机械摩擦。[45]可用的移植材料包括同种异体半月板、关节囊、自体阔筋膜、异体跟腱和细胞外基质产物等。[45-48]对36例存在不同肩关节疾病的患者使用生物方式进行关节盂表面重建联合肱骨头置换治疗。[48]7例肩关节使用前方关节囊，11例肩关节使用自体阔筋膜，18例肩关节使用同种异体跟腱。[48]随访2~15年，ASES肩关节疼痛和功能障碍评分的平均分由术前的39分提高到91分。根据Neer标准，50%的患者对手术结果非常满意，36%的患者满意，14%的患者不满意。所有患者的肩关节间隙均在术后有所减小，但5年后并无进展。在盂肱关节活动范围和影像学上的关节盂侵蚀度方面，使用同种异体移植物的患者的效果比使用自体移植物的患者的效果更好。4例患者后续进行了手术，1例是与伤口感染有关的清创术，3例转为全肩关节置换术。3例转为全肩关节置换术的患者都将前方关节囊用于关节盂表面重建。作者推荐将异体跟腱移植用于关节盂的生物表面修复。

另一项研究将半肩关节置换术与关节盂生物表面重建术相结合，取得了相反的结果。[49]在13例患者（平均年龄为34岁）中，11例使用同种异体跟腱，1例使用自体阔筋膜，1例使用自体前方关节囊。术后3年仅1例满意，其余12例接受了翻修手术。由于严重的肩痛和关节间隙狭小，

10 例患者需要行全肩关节置换术。2 例患者因为感染接受了清创术和最终的关节切除成形手术。作者的结论是，在这些患者中使用的移植物材料不耐用，应该谨慎使用关节盂生物重建技术。

在另一项研究中，30 例肩关节采用金属肱骨头置换和异体半月板移植以生物重建关节盂。[47] 虽然在所有临床结果测量方面都有显著改善，但仍有 17% 的肩关节在 1 年的随访中需要翻修。其中 2 例患者接受了全肩关节置换术，1 例患者接受了保留半肩关节假体的移植物移除术。1 例患者发生了感染，需要移除所有植入物。还有 1 例患者接受了关节镜下清理。

有研究分析了关节镜下仅使用补片来生物学重建关节盂而不置换肱骨的效果，75% 的患者经 3~6 年的随访，结果显示其获得了满意的结果。[50] Constant 肩关节评分和 ASES 肩关节疼痛和功能障碍评分都有很大的改善，但仍有 25% 的患者改为半肩关节置换术。这些不一致的结果导致了这样一个结论：生物学表面重建可能是年轻人肩关节退行性病变治疗的一个选择，但应谨慎使用。需要进行前瞻性研究，以比较生物学表面重建、半肩关节置换术和全肩关节置换术等技术的结果。

"锉完即用"的操作

虽然半肩关节置换术患者比全肩关节置换术患者有更差的功能结果和疼痛缓解效果，但它仍是治疗肩关节退行性病变的一个可行选择。[1] 特别是对于相对年轻的患者，关节盂假体松动是一个值得关注的问题。合并关节盂偏心磨损的肩关节与肱骨头位于关节盂中心的肩关节相比，前者行半肩关节置换术的效果较差。[51] 因此，出现了一种"锉完即用"的操作，作为在不使用关节盂假体的情况下纠正关节盂偏心磨损形成的双凹面的一种方法。[36,52] 在这个过程中，使用一个大直径的锉来磨锉关节盂，并选择一个比关节盂锉的曲率直径小 2 mm 的肱骨头假体。[36] 虽然已经有研究证实磨锉过的关节盂的内在稳定性可以恢复，

并且纤维软骨会重新覆盖表面，但是关于此类手术的临床和放射学结果的研究数据很少。[52-54] 一项研究中，经过平均 2.7 年的随访，35 例肩关节的功能显著改善，32 例肩关节术后疼痛减轻，只有 1 例肩关节的功能无变化，2 例肩关节的疼痛加重。[52] 1 例肩关节术后疼痛和僵硬的患者接受了翻修手术，术中重新磨锉了关节盂并进行了关节囊松解。11.4% 的肩关节有进行性内侧侵蚀，17.1% 的肩关节再次出现后方磨损。

嵌入式关节盂假体

与传统关节盂假体的套入技术相比，嵌入式关节盂假体技术是指将整个假体插入骨内。关节盂表面的磨锉深度应为 2~3 mm，从而制造一个环状皮质边缘来围绕假体。[55] 嵌入式假体用于关节盂严重偏心磨损的表面重建。在一项对 7 例患者的病例研究中，经过平均 4.3 年的随访发现，7 例患者有显著的功能改善和疼痛缓解，但没有发现组件松动的放射学征象。[55] 尽管力学测试和有限元分析表明，与传统假体相比，嵌入式假体具有良好的效果；但必须认识到，使用这种假体需要磨锉原本关节盂的皮质骨，而软骨下骨的保留对于骨水泥固定的龙脊型关节盂假体的寿命至关重要。[56]

总结

根据预期，全肩关节置换术后患者的功能会有明显改善，疼痛会有明显缓解。其结果似乎优于半肩关节置换术。然而，关节盂组件似乎是全肩关节置换术的薄弱环节。骨水泥固定的龙脊型假体有较高的松动率，而短桩型假体没有长期（超过 5 年）的研究数据。在过去，由于非骨水泥固定的关节盂假体有很高的失效率，许多已被废弃。需要进行进一步的研究，分析使用根据新理念设计的新的关节盂假体的长期结果，并确定关节盂侧的理想治疗方案。

参考文献

［1］ Radnay CS, Setter KJ, Chambers L, Levine WN, Bigliani LU, Ahmad CS: Total shoulder replacement compared with humeral head replacement for the treatment of primary glenohumeral osteoarthritis: A systematic review. *J Shoulder Elbow Surg* 2007;16(4):396-402.

　　The results of hemiarthroplasty and total shoulder arthroplasty are systematically reviewed.

［2］ Boileau P, Avidor C, Krishnan SG, Walch G, Kempf JF, Molé D: Cemented polyethylene versus uncemented metal-backed glenoid components in total shoulder arthroplasty: A prospective, double-blind, randomized study. *J Shoulder Elbow Surg* 2002;11(4):351-359.

［3］ Young A, Walch G, Boileau P, et al: A multicentre study of the long-term results of using a flat-back polyethylene glenoid component in shoulder replacement for primary osteoarthritis. *J Bone Joint Surg Br* 2011;93(2):210-216.

　　A multicenter study examined the long-term results of cemented glenoid implantation. Level of evidence: IV.

［4］ Walch G, Young AA, Melis B, Gazielly D, Loew M, Boileau P: Results of a convex-back cemented keeled glenoid component in primary osteoarthritis: Multicenter study with a follow-up greater than 5 years. *J Shoulder Elbow Surg* 2011;20(3):385-394.

　　A multicenter study examined the mid- and long-term results of cemented convex-back glenoid implantation. Level of evidence: IV.

［5］ Kasten P, Pape G, Raiss P, et al: Mid-term survivorship analysis of a shoulder replacement with a keeled glenoid and a modern cementing technique. *J Bone Joint Surg Br* 2010;92(3):387-392.

　　The midterm results of cemented keeled glenoid implantation are reported. Level of evidence: IV.

［6］ Burroughs PL, Gearen PF, Petty WR, Wright TW: Shoulder arthroplasty in the young patient. *J Arthroplasty* 2003;18(6):792-798.

［7］ Schrumpf M, Maak T, Hammoud S, Craig EV: The glenoid in total shoulder arthroplasty. *Curr Rev Musculoskelet Med* 2011;4(4):191-199.

　　The options for glenoid replacement are presented.

［8］ Churchill RS, Brems JJ, Kotschi H: Glenoid size, inclination, and version: An anatomic study. *J Shoulder Elbow Surg* 2001;10(4):327-332.

［9］ Mallon WJ, Brown HR, Vogler JB III, Martinez S: Radiographic and geometric anatomy of the scapula. *Clin Orthop Relat Res* 1992;277(277):142-154.

［10］ Kwon YW, Powell KA, Yum JK, Brems JJ, Iannotti JP: Use of three-dimensional computed tomography for the analysis of the glenoid anatomy. *J Shoulder Elbow Surg* 2005;14(1):85-90.

［11］ Iannotti JP, Gabriel JP, Schneck SL, Evans BG, Misra S: The normal glenohumeral relationships: An anatomical study of one hundred and forty shoulders. *J Bone Joint Surg Am* 1992;74(4):491-500.

［12］ Rouleau DM, Kidder JF, Pons-Villanueva J, Dynamidis S, Defranco M, Walch G: Glenoid version: How to measure it? Validity of different methods in two-dimensional computed tomography scans. *J Shoulder Elbow Surg* 2010;19(8):1230-1237.

　　The validity of two-dimensional CT for evaluating glenoid version is examined. Level of evidence: IV.

［13］ Saha AK: The classic: Mechanism of shoulder movements and a plea for the recognition of "zero position" of glenohumeral joint. *Clin Orthop Relat Res* 1983;173:3-10.

［14］ Martin SD, Zurakowski D, Thornhill TS: Uncemented glenoid component in total shoulder arthroplasty: Survivorship and outcomes. *J Bone Joint Surg Am* 2005;87(6):1284-1292.

［15］ Fucentese SF, Costouros JG, Kühnel SP, Gerber C: Total shoulder arthroplasty with an uncemented soft-metal-backed glenoid component. *J Shoulder Elbow Surg* 2010;19(4):624-631.

　　The use of a new uncemented glenoid component led to high failure rates. Level of evidence: IV.

［16］ Groh GI: Survival and radiographic analysis of a glenoid component with a cementless fluted central peg. *J Shoulder Elbow Surg* 2010;19(8):1265-1268.

　　The short-term results of using the anchor-peg glenoid implant are presented. Level of evidence: IV.

［17］ Taunton MJ, McIntosh AL, Sperling JW, Cofield RH: Total shoulder arthroplasty with a metal-backed, bone-ingrowth glenoid component: Medium to long-term results. *J Bone Joint Surg Am* 2008;90(10):2180-2188.

　　The mid- and long-term results of using uncemented glenoid components were found to be unsatisfactory. Level of evidence: IV.

［18］ Castagna A, Randelli M, Garofalo R, Maradei L, Giardella A, Borroni M: Mid-term results of a metal-backed glenoid component in total shoulder replacement. *J Bone Joint Surg Br* 2010;92(10):1410-1415.

　　The use of an uncemented glenoid component design led to excellent midterm results. Level of evidence: IV.

［19］ Lazarus MD, Jensen KL, Southworth C, Matsen FA

III: The radiographic evaluation of keeled and pegged glenoid component insertion. *J Bone Joint Surg Am* 2002;84(7):1174-1182.

[20] Gartsman GM, Elkousy HA, Warnock KM, Edwards TB, O'Connor DP: Radiographic comparison of pegged and keeled glenoid components. *J Shoulder Elbow Surg* 2005;14(3):252-257.

[21] Edwards TB, Labriola JE, Stanley RJ, O'Connor DP, Elkousy HA, Gartsman GM: Radiographic comparison of pegged and keeled glenoid components using modern cementing techniques: A prospective randomized study. *J Shoulder Elbow Surg* 2010;19(2):251-257.

The short-term results of using a cemented pegged glenoid component were superior to those of using a keeled glenoid component. Level of evidence: I.

[22] Anglin C, Wyss UP, Pichora DR: Mechanical testing of shoulder prostheses and recommendations for glenoid design. *J Shoulder Elbow Surg* 2000;9(4):323-331.

[23] Throckmorton TW, Zarkadas PC, Sperling JW, Cofield RH: Pegged versus keeled glenoid components in total shoulder arthroplasty. *J Shoulder Elbow Surg* 2010;19(5):726-733.

No difference was found in the development of radiolucent lines after a cemented pegged or keeled glenoid component was used. Level of evidence: IV.

[24] Fox TJ, Cil A, Sperling JW, Sanchez-Sotelo J, Schleck CD, Cofield RH: Survival of the glenoid component in shoulder arthroplasty. *J Shoulder Elbow Surg* 2009;18(6):859-863.

The survival of different glenoid components is compared. Level of evidence: IV.

[25] Walch G, Young AA, Boileau P, Loew M, Gazielly D, Molé D: Patterns of loosening of polyethylene keeled glenoid components after shoulder arthroplasty for primary osteoarthritis: Results of a multicenter study with more than five years of follow-up. *J Bone Joint Surg Am* 2012;94(2):145-150.

Patterns of loosening are described at mid- and long-term follow-up after implantation of cemented keeled glenoid components. Level of evidence: IV.

[26] Churchill RS, Zellmer C, Zimmers HJ, Ruggero R: Clinical and radiographic analysis of a partially cemented glenoid implant: Five-year minimum follow- up. *J Shoulder Elbow Surg* 2010;19(7):1091-1097.

The 5-year results of the use of anchor-pegged glenoid components is presented. Level of evidence: IV.

[27] Arnold RM, High RR, Grosshans KT, Walker CW, Fehringer EV: Bone presence between the central peg's radial fins of a partially cemented pegged all poly glenoid component suggest few radiolucencies. *J Shoulder Elbow Surg* 2011;20(2):315-321.

Anchor-pegged glenoid components are analyzed. Level of evidence: IV.

[28] Wirth MA, Loredo R, Garcia G, Rockwood CA Jr, Southworth C, Iannotti JP: Total shoulder arthroplasty with an all-polyethylene pegged bone-ingrowth glenoid component: A clinical and radiographic outcome study. *J Bone Joint Surg Am* 2012;94(3):260-267.

The short- and mid-term results of using anchorpegged glenoid components are presented. Level of evidence: IV.

[29] Raiss P, Pape G, Kleinschmidt K, et al: Bone cement penetration pattern and primary stability testing in keeled and pegged glenoid components. *J Shoulder Elbow Surg* 2011;20(5):723-731.

A CT examination of cement mantles and biomechanical testing of primary stability in cemented glenoid components is presented.

[30] Klepps S, Chiang AS, Miller S, Jiang CY, Hazrati Y, Flatow EL: Incidence of early radiolucent glenoid lines in patients having total shoulder replacements. *Clin Orthop Relat Res* 2005;435(435):118-125.

[31] Szabo I, Buscayret F, Edwards TB, et al: Radiographic comparison of two glenoid preparation techniques in total shoulder arthroplasty. *Clin Orthop Relat Res* 2005;431:104-110.

Glenoid preparation technique influences implant survival and the occurrence of radiolucent lines when a cemented keeled glenoid component is used. Level of evidence: IV.

[32] Molé D, Roche O, Riand N, Levigne C, Walch G: Results in osteoarthritis and rheumatoid arthritis, in Walch G, Boileau P, eds: *Shoulder Arthroplasty.* New York, NY, Springer, 1998.

[33] Collin P, Tay AK, Melis B, Boileau P, Walch G: A ten-year radiologic comparison of two-all polyethylene glenoid component designs: A prospective trial. *J Shoulder Elbow Surg* 2011;20(8):1217-1223.

Cemented keeled flat-back and convex-back glenoid components are prospectively compared. Level of evidence: II.

[34] Walch G, Edwards TB, Boulahia A, Boileau P, Molé D, Adeleine P: The influence of glenohumeral prosthetic mismatch on glenoid radiolucent lines: Results of a multicenter study. *J Bone Joint Surg Am* 2002;84(12):2186-2191.

［35］Terrier A, Büchler P, Farron A: Influence of glenohumeral conformity on glenoid stresses after total shoulder arthroplasty. *J Shoulder Elbow Surg* 2006;15(4):515-520.

［36］Matsen FA III, Bicknell RT, Lippitt SB: Shoulder arthroplasty: The socket perspective. *J Shoulder Elbow Surg* 2007;16(5, suppl):S241-S247.

An overview of hemiarthroplasty, total shoulder arthroplasty, and the ream-and-run procedure is presented.

［37］Collins D, Tencer A, Sidles J, Matsen F III: Edge displacement and deformation of glenoid components in response to eccentric loading: The effect of preparation of the glenoid bone. *J Bone Joint Surg Am* 1992;74(4):501-507.

［38］Edwards TB, Sabonghy EP, Elkousy H, et al: Glenoid component insertion in total shoulder arthroplasty: comparison of three techniques for drying the glenoid before cementation. *J Shoulder Elbow Surg* 2007;16(3, suppl):S107-S110.

Drying methods before cementation of glenoid components are compared. Level of evidence: I.

［39］Gross RM, High R, Apker K, Haggstrom J, Fehringer JA, Stephan J: Vacuum assist glenoid fixation: Does this technique lead to a more durable glenoid component? *J Shoulder Elbow Surg* 2011;20(7):1050-1060.

The results of using the weep-hole technique for cementation of glenoid components are presented. Level of evidence: IV.

［40］Hasan SA, Cox WK, Syed M, Suva LJ: Microcomputed tomography assessment of glenoid component cementation techniques in total shoulder arthroplasty. *J Orthop Res* 2010;28(5):559-564.

The standard and weep-hole techniques for cementation of glenoid components are compared.

［41］Nyffeler RW, Meyer D, Sheikh R, Koller BJ, Gerber C: The effect of cementing technique on structural fixation of pegged glenoid components in total shoulder arthroplasty. *J Shoulder Elbow Surg* 2006;15(1):106-111.

［42］Barwood S, Setter KJ, Blaine TA, Bigliani LU: The incidence of early radiolucencies about a pegged glenoid component using cement pressurization. *J Shoulder Elbow Surg* 2008;17(5):703-708.

Fewer radiolucent lines developed when cement pressurization of glenoid components was used. Level of evidence: IV.

［43］Raiss P, Sowa B, Bruckner T, et al: Pressurisation leads to better cement penetration into the glenoid bone: A cadaveric study. *J Bone Joint Surg Br* 2012;94(5):671-677.

Cement mantle thickness and homogeneity are analyzed after insertion of a cemented pegged or keeled glenoid component using the standard technique or a cement restrictor.

［44］Raiss P, Aldinger PR, Kasten P, Rickert M, Loew M: Total shoulder replacement in young and middle-aged patients with glenohumeral osteoarthritis. *J Bone Joint Surg Br* 2008;90(6):764-769.

The clinical results of young patients who underwent cemented total shoulder replacement are presented. Level of evidence: IV.

［45］Burkhead WZ Jr, Krishnan SG, Lin KC: Biologic resurfacing of the arthritic glenohumeral joint: Historical review and current applications. *J Shoulder Elbow Surg* 2007;16(5, suppl):S248-S253.

Options and outcomes of biologic resurfacing of the glenoid are reviewed.

［46］Creighton RA, Cole BJ, Nicholson GP, Romeo AA, Lorenz EP: Effect of lateral meniscus allograft on shoulder articular contact areas and pressures. *J Shoulder Elbow Surg* 2007;16(3):367-372.

Biomechanical testing of pressures and contacts after meniscus allograft on the glenoid are described.

［47］Nicholson GP, Goldstein JL, Romeo AA, et al: Lateral meniscus allograft biologic glenoid arthroplasty in total shoulder arthroplasty for young shoulders with degenerative joint disease. *J Shoulder Elbow Surg* 2007;16(5, suppl):S261-S266.

Clinical results are described after glenoid resurfacing using meniscal allografts. Level of evidence: IV.

［48］Krishnan SG, Nowinski RJ, Harrison D, Burkhead WZ: Humeral hemiarthroplasty with biologic resurfacing of the glenoid for glenohumeral arthritis: Two to fifteen-year outcomes. *J Bone Joint Surg Am* 2007;89(4):727-734.

Short- to long-term results are reported after biologic resurfacing of the glenoid. Level of evidence: IV.

［49］Elhassan B, Ozbaydar M, Diller D, Higgins LD, Warner JJ: Soft-tissue resurfacing of the glenoid in the treatment of glenohumeral arthritis in active patients less than fifty years old. *J Bone Joint Surg Am* 2009;91(2):419-424.

Results are reported for biologic resurfacing of the glenoid in young patients. Level of evidence: IV.

［50］Savoie FH III, Brislin KJ, Argo D: Arthroscopic glenoid resurfacing as a surgical treatment for glenohumeral arthritis in the young patient: Midterm results.

Arthroscopy 2009;25(8):864-871.

The midterm results are reported after arthroscopic resurfacing of the glenoid. Level of evidence: IV.

[51] Hettrich CM, Weldon E III, Boorman RS, Parsons IM IV, Matsen FA III: Preoperative factors associated with improvements in shoulder function after humeral hemiarthroplasty. *J Bone Joint Surg Am* 2004;86(7):1446-1451.

[52] Lynch JR, Franta AK, Montgomery WH Jr, Lenters TR, Mounce D, Matsen FA III: Self-assessed outcome at two to four years after shoulder hemiarthroplasty with concentric glenoid reaming. *J Bone Joint Surg Am* 2007;89(6):1284-1292.

The clinical outcomes of the ream-and-run procedure are reported. Level of evidence: IV.

[53] Matsen FA III, Clark JM, Titelman RM, et al: Healing of reamed glenoid bone articulating with a metal humeral hemiarthroplasty: A canine model. *J Orthop Res* 2005;23(1):18-26.

[54] Weldon EJ III, Boorman RS, Smith KL, Matsen FA III: Optimizing the glenoid contribution to the stability of a humeral hemiarthroplasty without a prosthetic glenoid. *J Bone Joint Surg Am* 2004;86(9):2022-2029.

[55] Gunther SB, Lynch TL: Total shoulder replacement surgery with custom glenoid implants for severe bone deficiency. *J Shoulder Elbow Surg* 2012;21(5):675-684.

The short-term results of a glenoid inset implant for bone deficiency are reported. Level of evidence: IV.

[56] Gunther SB, Lynch TL, O'Farrell D, Calyore C, Rodenhouse A: Finite element analysis and physiologic testing of a novel, inset glenoid fixation technique. *J Shoulder Elbow Surg* 2012;21(6):795-803.

Biomechanical testing and finite element analysis of inlay and onlay glenoid components are reported.

第二十九章　半肩关节置换和反肩关节置换治疗急性肱骨近端骨折

Pascal Boileau, MD; Daniel Grant Schwartz, MD; Tjarco D. Alta, MD

引言

肱骨近端骨折约占所有骨折的 5%。然而，在 70 岁以上的患者中，肱骨近端骨折是第三常见的骨折（发生率仅次于髋部骨折和桡骨远端骨折）。[1] 通常只有三部分和四部分移位的肱骨近端骨折采用关节置换术治疗。其余很少使用关节置换术，再加上手术医师治疗策略的组间和组内一致性评价较低，使得即使是最有经验的外科医师也难以处理肱骨近端骨折。[2] 手术成功需要清楚地了解适应证、治疗方案的选项、假体设计的基本原理以及与结节修复和假体放置相关的技术细节。

1953 年，Neer 首次描述了通过半肩关节置换治疗肱骨近端骨折，他的"满意但不完美"的结果包括：90% 的患者在用假体置换治疗三部分和四部分移位骨折时获得了满意或非常满意的结果。[3-4] 但没有后续的研究能够复制 Neer 的结果。[5-6] 在

Dr. Boileau or an immediate family member has received royalties from Tornier; serves as a paid consultant to or is an employee of Smith & Nephew and DePuy; and serves as a board member, owner, officer, or committee member of the European Society for Surgery of the Shoulder and the Elbow. Dr. Alta or an immediate family member has received nonincome support (such as equipment or services), commercially derived honoraria, or other non-research-related funding (such as paid travel) from Tornier. Neither Dr. Schwartz nor any immediate family member has received anything of value from or has stock or stock options held in a commercial company or institution related directly or indirectly to the subject of this chapter.

过去的几十年中，对材料科学的发展、制作解剖型肩关节假体能力的提升以及对结节修复和假体放置技术的发展提高了医师使用关节置换术恢复关节原本解剖形态的能力。

对 70 岁以上的肱骨近端骨折患者采用反肩关节置换术越来越普遍，但这一概念并不新颖。1989—1993 年，Grammont 医师为 22 例肱骨近端骨折或骨折后遗症患者施行了反肩关节置换术。[7] 多项研究显示，反肩关节置换术是骨科医师的重要技术手段。

骨折的分类

1934 年，Codman 根据解剖骨块的位置（位于大结节、小结节、外科颈还是肱骨头）对肱骨近端骨折进行分类。[8] Neer 发展了这个概念，提出解剖骨块必须移位至少 1 cm 或成角 45°，才能被认为是移位骨折的一部分。[9] 因此，四部分骨折会涉及肱骨头移位和（或）骨干成角、大结节与小结节移位和（或）成角。骨折的部分越多，就越可能危及肱骨头的血供。

AO-ASIF 骨折分类系统在临床实践中并不常用，但它是基于骨折的粉碎程度和肱骨头血供中断的可能性来分类的。[10] A 型骨折是完全关节外骨折，只有一条骨折线。B 型骨折也是完全关节外骨折，但有两条骨折线。C 型骨折为关节内骨折并包含亚型，按严重程度从轻到重分为 C1 型骨折（轻微移位）至 C3 型骨折（脱

位，肱骨头缺血风险最大）。基于 Hertel 二进制的分类法和 LEGO 分类法也未在临床实践中使用。[11]

手术适应证和禁忌证

典型的半肩关节置换术适用于严重的骨折类型，包括骨折脱位、某些三部分和四部分骨折、肱骨头劈裂骨折和累及 40% 以上关节面的骨折。[7,12-14] 外翻嵌插型的四部分骨折相对不太可能导致肱骨头坏死，因此与其他一些类型的骨折相比，部分医师的治疗方案更为保守。[15] 内侧软组织铰链完整、干骺端骨折片大于 8 mm 以及骨膜完整是外翻嵌插型四部分骨折骨坏死风险相对较低的原因。[11] 将患者的年龄作为半肩关节置换术的适应证存有争议，一些医师将半肩关节置换术的年龄下限定为 70 岁，但另一些医师则将年龄下限定为 55 岁，在某些情况下，更年轻的患者也可行半肩关节置换术。[2,14,16] 谨慎的医师应仔细考虑患者的生理年龄，包括任何并存的医疗状况，并在做出治疗决定之前与患者充分讨论所有风险和获益。

对于功能需求较低的 70 岁以上患者，反肩关节置换术可以替代半肩关节置换术。[17] 由于粉碎性骨折或骨质疏松，结节部骨量很少，会影响与骨干和假体的愈合，这也是选择反肩关节置换术的有利因素。既往存在的肩袖病变和巨大肩袖撕裂是反肩关节置换术的附加手术适应证。

半肩关节置换术和反肩关节置换术的禁忌证是患者有活动性感染或者临床上不稳定不能耐受手术。虽然半肩关节置换术或反肩关节置换术没有绝对的年龄下限，但较年轻的严重粉碎性骨折患者应首先尝试切开复位内固定。除非患者能够参与结构化康复计划，否则医师不应选择半肩关节置换术，因为物理治疗是获得良好效果的基础。对于有腋神经麻痹或关节盂骨缺损不足以支撑假体基座的患者，不应行反肩关节置换术。

肩袖外旋肌的作用

一般来说，外科医师应该把移位的肱骨近端三、四部分骨折看作是需要修复的巨大肩袖撕裂。骨折的结节被肩袖肌肉和肌腱牵引向内侧移位；大结节由冈上肌、冈下肌和小圆肌向后内侧牵引，小结节由肩胛下肌向前内侧牵引。结节必须与骨干愈合，才能发挥适当的肩袖功能。大结节的移位、畸形愈合或不愈合是半肩关节置换术治疗骨折后效果不佳的主要原因。[5] 大结节的位置正确和愈合良好是手术成功的关键。由于肩部处于一种不利平衡中，包括内旋肌（胸大肌、肩胛下肌、背阔肌和大圆肌）、大结节及其附丽肌肉（冈下肌和小圆肌）丢失会使肩部真正的外旋肌缺失。所以医师必须高度重视大结节的牢固固定；否则，当大结节畸形愈合或不愈合时，肩关节内旋的自然优势会变得更加强大。

大结节的固定和愈合在反肩关节置换术中是非常重要的。尽管反肩关节置换术可以恢复肩袖损伤的肩关节的主动前屈上举，但大结节移位或畸形愈合而导致的肩袖外旋肌肉缺失会使肩关节丧失主动外旋。主动外旋对于患者控制手臂在空间中的位置和进行日常生活活动（如刮胡子、刷牙、梳头、握手、开门和使用勺子）的能力至关重要。[18] 当大结节畸形愈合或不愈合时，外旋肌功能丧失，上臂在抬高或外展时没有肌肉可以负担前臂的重量，从而出现朝向躯体的上肢摆动。

部分医师在创伤后反肩关节置换术中常忽略结节的修复，这种疏漏会导致外旋肌丧失。最近的一项研究比较了反肩关节置换术和半肩关节置换术的结果，发现反肩关节置换术后的 Constant 肩关节评分、外展和前屈更好，而半肩关节置换术后的外旋更好。[19] 这个结果是可以预测的，因为只有 1 例行反肩关节置换术的患者再次植入了结节。为了最大限度地恢复包括外旋在内的日常生活活动能力，应尽可能为每例患者修复结节。外科医师必须明白，从功能角度来看，无论是半肩关节置换术还是反肩关节置换术，大结节的位置和愈合都是至关重要的。

假体设计的考量因素

第三代解剖型肩关节假体的发展有助于重建骨性关节炎患者肱骨近端的正常解剖结构。[6]传统的肱骨解剖型假体体积太大，阻碍了结节的解剖复位，且使结节和骨干之间仅有很小的接触面。由于假体颈部的金属体积大，骨愈合的可能性很低，结节移位和畸形愈合的风险很高（图 29-1）。

手术中结节的准确复位及其保持不移位的能力与临床结果的改善呈正相关。[5,20-21]最近开发出了可辅助这一过程的假体柄。低切迹的假体的金属体积相对较小，允许未经改变的结节解剖复位，并有更多的空间可容纳植骨，以进一步促进愈合（图 29-2）。低切迹的假体柄在干骺端有一个窗口，

可以放置额外的植骨，以促进大小结节骨块间的愈合。[16]另外一些假体干骺端周围的金属被粗糙化，通过骨长入粗糙的羟基磷灰石涂层表面或多孔钽微表面来增加骨性稳定。需要在假体的颈部放置环扎线，如果接触到粗糙的金属表面，这些缝线可能会断裂，而假体颈的内侧光滑，可以避免这个问题。[6]使用低切迹的骨折专用型假体，结节的移位和不愈合的发生率可减少 50%。[21]

骨折型的反肩关节假体柄也正在研发中。一种具有光滑干部的混合型假体允许使用骨水泥固定，其近端部分是粗糙的羟基磷灰石涂层（带有植骨窗口），可促进结节的愈合[7]（图 29-3）。建议在行半肩关节置换术和反肩关节置换术时使用低切迹假体，以允许植骨并最大限度地提高结节愈合的可能性（图 29-4）。

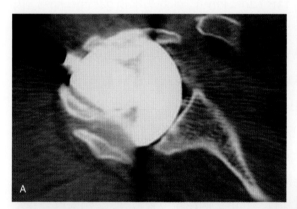
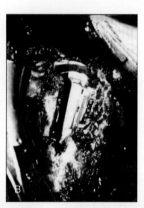

图 29-1　轴位 CT 图像（A）和翻修手术的照片（B）显示，传统解剖型半肩关节假体的设计不利于肱骨近端骨折的治疗。假体颈部金属过多，阻碍了大结节的复位和愈合（版权所有：法国尼斯的 Pascal Boileau 医师）

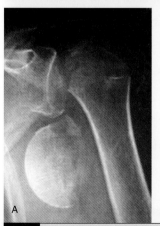
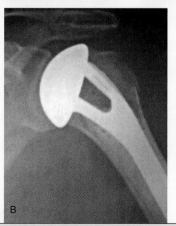
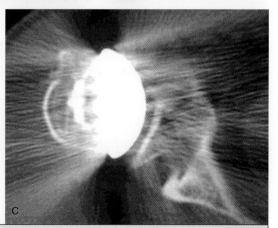

图 29-2　肱骨近端四部分骨折脱位重建术后的图像，使用了骨折型假体。A. 术前正位 X 线片显示肱骨头骨块位于腋窝处，与关节囊的所有联系中断，血供中断。B. 术后正位 X 线片显示使用骨折型假体柄，结节解剖重建在柄周围。C. 轴位 CT 图像显示结节准确复位，从肱骨头骨块中取出骨松质，植于假体柄的周围以促进结节愈合（版权所有：法国尼斯的 Pascal Boileau 医师）

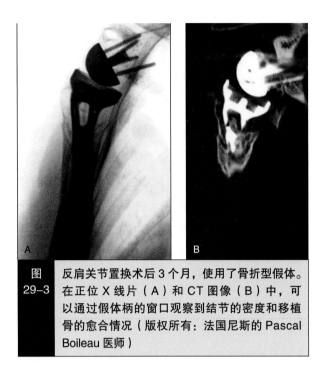

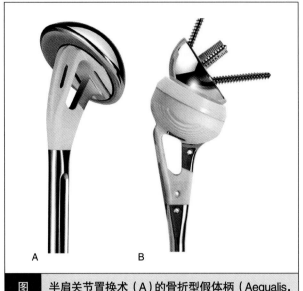

图 29-3　反肩关节置换术后 3 个月，使用了骨折型假体。在正位 X 线片（A）和 CT 图像（B）中，可以通过假体柄的窗口观察到结节的密度和移植骨的愈合情况（版权所有：法国尼斯的 Pascal Boileau 医师）

图 29-4　半肩关节置换术（A）的骨折型假体柄（Aequalis，Tornier 公司）和反肩关节置换术的假体（B）（版权所有：法国尼斯的 Pascal Boileau 医师）

骨折型假体

半肩关节置换术

在最近一项对 61 例患者的研究中，如果大结节在解剖位置愈合（P=0.0004），那么患者术后 Constant 肩关节评分显著改善，假体的类型影响了解剖和功能的恢复。经平均 45 个月的随访，在 30 例使用骨折型假体柄的患者中，26 例（87%）患者的大结节在解剖位置愈合；经平均 81 个月的随访，在 31 例使用传统假体柄的患者中，14 例（45%）患者的大结节愈合（$P<0.0001$）。骨折型假体柄的主动前屈上举角度、主动外旋角度和 Constant 肩关节评分（分别为 136°、34° 和 68 分）明显优于传统假体柄（分别为 113°、23° 和 58 分；$P<0.0001$）。无论使用何种类型的假体，女性患者和 75 岁以上的患者的功能结果都明显低于其他患者，结节的并发症发生率也更高（$P<0.0001$）。[22]

反肩关节置换术

在一项前瞻性多中心队列研究中，75 例肱骨近端移位骨折患者（76 个肩关节）使用骨折型反肩关节假体柄进行治疗。[23] 49 例患者（50 个肩关节）经至少 1 年的随访，主动前屈上举的角度为平均 131°（40°~170°），外旋为平均 24°（0°~50°），内旋为 5 分（0~10 分）。视觉模拟疼痛评分表（满分为 10 分）的平均得分为 1 分（0~5 分）。校正了年龄和性别后，平均 Constant 肩关节评分为 64 分（31~91 分）和 93%（45%~142%）。平均 SSV 评分为 70%（50%~90%）。未记录有并发症发生，没有患者需进一步手术。43 个（86%）肩关节的大结节的影像学检查显示完全愈合。5 例发生术后早期的结节移位，其中 2 例在新位置愈合，2 例未愈合并发生骨溶解，1 例部分愈合伴骨溶解。2 例出现迟发性的结节移位：1 例大结节不愈合伴骨溶解，1 例部分愈合伴骨溶解。未见关节盂或肱骨侧假体松动。

无论患者年龄大小，结节的愈合都可以通过在特定的反肩关节骨折型假体的周围重新附着和植骨来实现。骨折型假体为促进结节愈合创造了一个可靠的环境。

技术因素

结节的植骨和固定

结节的愈合对临床疗效的影响巨大，因此，其固定技术应便于解剖复位和牢固固定。[5,20-21,24-25]

理想的结构是使用6根缝线（4根水平环扎线和2根垂直张力带缝线）将大小结节、假体和肱骨干牢固地固定在一起，从而最大限度地提高骨块间的稳定性[26]（图29-5）。将2根缝线穿入小圆肌，2根缝线穿入冈下肌。在肱骨干上放置2根垂直的缝线，1根用于缝合肩胛下肌和冈上肌，另1根用于缝合冈上肌和冈下肌。2根环扎线从假体

颈内侧绕过固定大结节。用2根环扎线（分别来自冈下肌和小圆肌）固定小结节。反肩关节假体的结节修复也使用同样的技术。[17,26]

尼斯结（Nice结）是一个滑动结，可自我稳定（防滑）且牢固（因为它使用了双股缝合线），容易打结和收紧（图29-6）。在过去的7年中，这项新的技术已经成功地用于固定半肩关节假体或

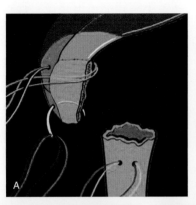
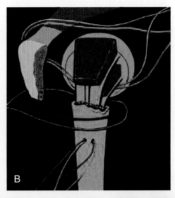
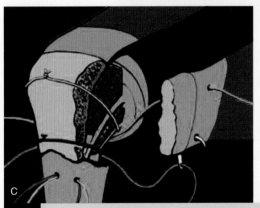
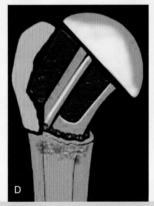
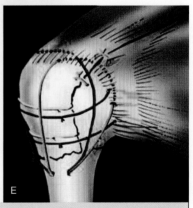

图29-5 结节的修复过程示意图。共使用6根缝线，包括4根水平环扎线和2根垂直张力带缝线。A. 6根缝线2根一组分别穿入小圆肌、冈下肌和肱骨干。B. 4根水平环扎线从假体颈的后方绕过。C. 先将2根水平环扎线绕过假体颈内侧固定大结节。然后，用另外2根水平环扎线固定小结节，最后用2根垂直张力带缝线调节整个结构。D. 植骨窗口内的骨折型假体。E. 使用水平环扎线和垂直张力带缝线捆扎后的最终结构（版权所有：法国尼斯的 Pascal Boileau 医师）

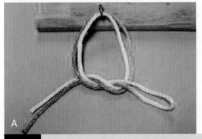
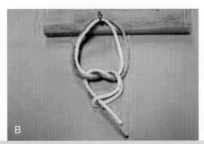
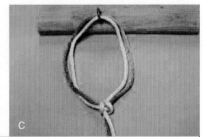

图29-6 用于环扎固定假体周围结节的双线尼斯结（Nice结）。先打一个方结（A），将2根游离线穿入环中（B），通过同时拉动2根游离线收紧该结（C）。另添加3个半挂结，最终锁定该结（版权所有：法国尼斯的 Pascal Boileau 医师）

反肩关节假体周围的结节。[27]

假体的定位

以人工肩关节置换术治疗骨折时恢复肱骨长度的必要性，已经被多种方法肯定。恢复原本解剖形态这一原则是不变的，无论方法是恢复肩胛骨外侧缘和肱骨内侧之间的哥特式弓，还是测量胸大肌上缘到肱骨头最高点的距离（平均为5.5 cm）。[28-30]带有比例尺的健侧和患侧手臂X线片有助于医师根据健侧的肱骨高度和肱骨头大小来评估患侧（图29-7）。借助骨折连接导向杆，可以很容易地确定有多少假体柄必须被保留在骨干外，以恢复肱骨的解剖长度，进而促进结节的修复（图29-8）。骨折连接导向杆（Tornier公司）也

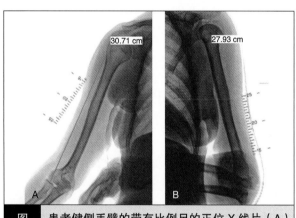

30.71 cm   27.93 cm

A   B

图 29-7 患者健侧手臂的带有比例尺的正位 X 线片（A）可用作评估患侧手臂（B）的肱骨高度模板（版权所有：法国尼斯的 Pascal Boileau 医师）

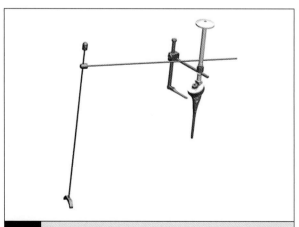

图 29-8 假体的骨折连接导向杆（Tornier 公司），可以在骨折重建时精确控制假体的角度和高度（版权所有：法国尼斯的 Pascal Boileau 医师）

有助于根据前臂的角度来调整假体的后倾。

结果

最近的研究证实了肩关节置换术对创伤性骨折的治疗有益，但仍然存在几十年前 Neer 所指出的令人满意但不完美的结果。[4,9]一项对移位的肱骨近端四部分骨折患者的随机对照研究发现，与非手术治疗的患者相比，行半肩关节置换术的患者生活质量显著提高，疼痛评分明显更低。[31]这项研究强调了手术治疗对某些患者的重要性。目前的一项研究正在进一步论证这一发现。[32]在已发表的文献中，患者常见术后疼痛减轻但活动范围不全。[33-39]在一项对 57 例患者的研究中，30例患者对治疗结果不满意，其中 11 例患者有中重度疼痛或需要翻修。[35]根据挪威关节置换登记记录，在术后的前 10 年内，半肩关节置换术的翻修率为 8%，相对年轻的患者翻修率更高。[40]一项非随机研究发现，骨折患者在内固定术后的功能结果与半肩关节置换术相似，尽管半肩关节置换术患者的平均年龄更大。[41]另一项研究发现，半肩关节置换术后的结果比切开复位内固定术后的结果差。[25]这些发现可能说明患者的选择和手术医师的经验在治疗结果方面具有重要作用。尽管结果并不完美，但经验丰富的骨科医师可使半肩关节置换术达到较为令人满意的疗效。

反肩关节置换术是一种较半肩关节置换更新的技术，但尚未被证实对骨折患者有明显更优的疗效。一项对 43 例三部分或四部分骨折接受反肩关节置换术治疗的患者的回顾性研究发现，反肩关节置换术的功能结果与半肩关节置换术相似。[42]另一项研究发现，除了较低的外旋评分外，反肩关节置换术后的效果略好于半肩关节置换术，但经常出现关节盂切迹。[19]70% 的反肩关节置换术后X 线片发现有关节盂切迹。[43]表 29-1 总结了反肩关节置换术治疗肱骨近端骨折的结果。[19,23,42-53]

表 29-1

反肩关节置换后功能结果的相关研究报道

研究发表（年份）	病例数	患者平均年龄（岁）	平均随访时间（月）	平均主动外旋角度
结节切除				
Cazeneuve 和 Cristofari[44]（2006）	30	75		
Cazeneuve 等[45]（2008）	25/36	75	72	
Cazeneuve 和 Cristofari[43]（2009），Cazeneuve 和 Cristofari[46]（2010），Cazeneuve 和 Cristofari[47]（2011）	30/41	75	78 (12~168)	
Gallinet 等[19]（2009）	16	74	12 (6~18)	98°
Klein 和 Juschka[48]（2008）	20	75	33 (24~52)	122°
结节保留				
Bufquin 等[42]（2007）	40	78	22 (6~58)	97°
Sirveaux 等[49]（2006）	20	79		107°
Levy 和 Badman[50]（2011）	7	86	14 (12~23)	117°
Reitman 和 Kerzhner[51]（2011）	13	70	28 (8~46)	125°
Lenarz 等[52]（2011）	30	77	23 (12~36)	138°
Tisher 等[53]（2008）	1	79	33	150°
骨折假体保留结节				
Alta 等[23]（2012）	50	80	18 (12~39)	131°

表 29-1

反肩关节置换后功能结果的相关研究报道（续）

平均主动外旋角度	平均 Constant 肩关节评分（范围）	年龄和性别校准后的平均 Constant 肩关节评分	并发症
	59		12 例（40%）：7 例肱骨近端骨溶解，2 例不稳定，1 例感染，1 例肩胛盂侧松动，1 例肱骨侧松动
	59		1 例不稳定，1 例感染，2 例急性呼吸窘迫综合征，1 例肩胛盂侧松动，6 例肱骨近端骨溶解
	53		4 例（13%）：2 例急性呼吸窘迫综合征，1 例感染，1 例脱位。18 例（60%）进行性透亮线、肩胛侧切迹和骨刺形成
9°	53 (34~76)		1 例深部感染，1 例浅表感染，1 例急性呼吸窘迫综合征，5 例肱骨侧透亮线但无松动
25°	67 (47~98)		1 例脱位和 2 例早期感染
8°	44 (16~69)	66%(25%~97%)	11 例（28%）：1 例肩胛盂骨折，1 例肩峰骨折，1 例脱位，1 例三角肌撕裂，5 例一过性神经麻痹，3 例急性呼吸窘迫综合征
10°	55 (31~73)	81%(45%~106%)	
19°			1 例结节不愈合和肩峰骨折，1 例非桥接性异位骨化形成
	67 (45~77)		2 例术后腋神经麻痹，1 例损伤后桡神经麻痹，1 例术后切口血肿形成
27°			1 例复杂区域疼痛综合征、深静脉血栓形成和结节吸收
0°	61	88%	
24°	64 (31~91)	93%(45%~142%)	1 例血肿形成，1 例肺栓塞

总结

关于肱骨近端骨折的最佳治疗方法仍存在争议。外科医师很难确定患者的最佳治疗方法是非手术治疗、切开复位内固定、半肩关节置换还是反肩关节置换。外科医师对适当处理的具体内容也没有一致意见。[2]正在进行的研究将有助于确定哪些骨折类型可能有不良的结果[54-55]，但需要临床研究来确定在何种情况下使用半肩关节置换和反肩关节置换。

参考文献

[1] Baron JA, Barrett JA, Karagas MR: The epidemiology of peripheral fractures. *Bone* 1996;18(3, suppl):209S-213S.

[2] Petit CJ, Millett PJ, Endres NK, Diller D, Harris MB, Warner JJ: Management of proximal humeral fractures: Surgeons don't agree. *J Shoulder Elbow Surg* 2010;19(3):446-451.
Interobserver and intraobserver reliability were evaluated in proximal humeral fracture treatment. The moderate interobserver reliability improved when fewer surgical choices were presented. Intraobserver reliability was low. Level of evidence: IV.

[3] Neer CS, Brown TH Jr, McLaughlin HL: Fracture of the neck of the humerus with dislocation of the head fragment. *Am J Surg* 1953;85(3):252-258.

[4] Neer CS II: Displaced proximal humeral fractures: II.Treatment of three-part and four-part displacement. *J Bone Joint Surg Am* 1970;52(6):1090-1103.

[5] Boileau P, Krishnan SG, Tinsi L, Walch G, Coste JS, Molé D: Tuberosity malposition and migration: Reasons for poor outcomes after hemiarthroplasty for displaced fractures of the proximal humerus. *J Shoulder Elbow Surg* 2002;11(5):401-412.

[6] Boileau P, Sinnerton RJ, Chuinard C, Walch G: Arthroplasty of the shoulder. *J Bone Joint Surg Br* 2006;88(5):562-575.

[7] Sirveaux F, Roche O, Molé D: Shoulder arthroplasty for acute proximal humerus fracture. *Orthop Traumatol Surg Res* 2010;96(6):683-694.
This is an excellent review of current concepts in arthroplasty for acute fractures, including hemiarthroplasty and reverse shoulder arthroplasty.

[8] Codman E: *The Shoulder: Rupture of the Supraspinatus Tendon and Other Lesions in or About the Subacromial Bursa*. Boston, MA, Thomas Todd, 1934.

[9] Neer CS II: Displaced proximal humeral fractures: I.Classification and evaluation. *J Bone Joint Surg Am* 1970;52(6):1077-1089.

[10] Müller ME: *Manual of Internal Fixation: Techniques Recommended by the AO-ASIF Group*, 3rd ed. Berlin, Germany, Springer, 1991, pp 118-125.

[11] Hertel R, Hempfing A, Stiehler M, Leunig M: Predictors of humeral head ischemia after intracapsular fracture of the proximal humerus. *J Shoulder Elbow Surg* 2004;13(4):427-433.

[12] Cadet ER, Ahmad CS: Hemiarthroplasty for three- and four-part proximal humerus fractures. *J Am Acad Orthop Surg* 2012;20(1):17-27.
Treatment algorithms, techniques, and results related to hemiarthroplasty are reviewed.

[13] Nho SJ, Brophy RH, Barker JU, Cornell CN, MacGillivray JD: Management of proximal humeral fractures based on current literature. *J Bone Joint Surg Am* 2007;89(suppl 3):44-58.
The management options for proximal humeral fractures are discussed based on a review of the current literature.

[14] Voos JE, Dines JS, Dines DM: Arthroplasty for fractures of the proximal part of the humerus. *J Bone Joint Surg Am* 2010;92(6):1560-1567.
The rationale, surgical technique, rehabilitation, and outcomes of arthroplasty for fractures of the proximal humerus are discussed.

[15] Iannotti JP, Ramsey ML, Williams GR Jr, Warner JJ: Nonprosthetic management of proximal humeral fractures. *Instr Course Lect* 2004;53:403-416.

[16] Boileau P, Pennington SD, Alami G: Proximal humeral fractures in younger patients: Fixation techniques and arthroplasty. *J Shoulder Elbow Surg* 2011;20(2, suppl):S47-S60.
This excellent review is focused on the difficulties of treating younger patients with a proximal humeral fracture, with surgical tips.

[17] Sirveaux F, Navez G, Roche O, Mole D, Williams MD: Reverse prosthesis for proximal humerus fracture: Technique and results. *Tech Shoulder Elbow Surg* 2008;9:15-22.
The indications, contraindications, and technique for a reverse shoulder arthroplasty are discussed with respect to a proximal humeral fracture.

[18] Boileau P, Rumian AP, Zumstein MA: Reversed shoul-

der arthroplasty with modified L'Episcopo for combined loss of active elevation and external rotation. *J Shoulder Elbow Surg* 2010;19(2, suppl):20-30.

The technique, outcomes, and rationale for latissimus dorsi and teres major transfer during reverse shoulder arthroplasty are described for patients with no active external rotation. The importance of external rotation in activities of daily living is highlighted. Level of evidence: IV.

[19] Gallinet D, Clappaz P, Garbuio P, Tropet Y, Obert L: Three or four parts complex proximal humerus fractures: Hemiarthroplasty versus reverse prosthesis. A comparative study of 40 cases. *Orthop Traumatol Surg Res* 2009;95(1):48-55.

The 16 patients who received a reverse prosthesis had higher postoperative Constant scores and better forward flexion and abduction than the 17 who under- went hemiarthroplasty. However, both internal and external rotation were poorer in those with a reverse prosthesis. Level of evidence: IV.

[20] Kralinger F, Schwaiger R, Wambacher M, et al: Outcome after primary hemiarthroplasty for fracture of the head of the humerus: A retrospective multicentre study of 167 patients. *J Bone Joint Surg Br* 2004;86(2):217-219.

[21] Loew M, Heitkemper S, Parsch D, Schneider S, Rickert M: Influence of the design of the prosthesis on the outcome after hemiarthroplasty of the shoulder in displaced fractures of the head of the humerus. *J Bone Joint Surg Br* 2006;88(3):345-350.

[22] Boileau P, Winter M, Cikes A, et al: Can surgeons predict what makes a good hemiarthroplasty for fracture? in Boileau P, ed: *Shoulder Concepts 2012: Arthroscopy, Arthroplasty, and Fractures.* Paris, France, Sauramps Medical, 2012, pp 329-344.

In a study of 61 patients, postoperative Constant scores significantly improved if the greater tuberosity healed in an anatomic position. The type of implant influenced both anatomic and functional outcomes. Regardless of the type of implant, women and patients older than 75 years had significantly lower functional results and higher rates of tuberosity complication.

[23] Alta T, Decroocq L, Moineau G, et al: Reverse shoulder arthroplasty for the treatment of proximal humeral fractures in the elderly: Results with a minimum one-year follow-up. Saint Genis Laval, France, *24th Congress Scientific Program.* European Society for Surgery of the Shoulder and the Elbow, 2012, paper OP16.

http://secec.com. Accessed September 10, 2012.

Seventy-five consecutive patients (76 shoulders) with a displaced proximal humeral fracture were treated using a fracture-specific reverse shoulder arthroplasty stem. At a minimum 1-year follow-up of 49 patients (50 shoulders), the mean active mobility measurements were 131° for anterior elevation and 24° for external rotation. The mean score on a 10-point visual analog scale for pain was 1, and the mean Constant score was Forty-three shoulders (86%) had complete radio- graphic greater tuberosity healing.

[24] Mighell MA, Kolm GP, Collinge CA, Frankle MA: Outcomes of hemiarthroplasty for fractures of the proximal humerus. *J Shoulder Elbow Surg* 2003;12(6):569-577.

[25] Solberg BD, Moon CN, Franco DP, Paiement GD: Surgical treatment of three and four-part proximal humeral fractures. *J Bone Joint Surg Am* 2009;91(7):1689-1697.

A retrospective study of 122 consecutive patients with proximal humeral fractures found that patients who received locked plating had higher postoperative Constant scores than those who had hemiarthroplasty. Level of evidence: III.

[26] Boileau P, Walch G, Krishnan SG: Tuberosity osteosynthesis and hemiarthroplasty for four-part fractures of the proximal humerus. *Tech Shoulder Elbow Surg* 2000;1:96-109.

[27] Boileau P, Rumian AP: A non-slipping and secure fixation of bone fragments and soft tissues usable in open and arthroscopic surgery, in Boileau P, ed: *Shoulder Concepts 2010: Arthroscopy and Arthroplasty.* Paris, France, Sauramps Medical, 2010, pp 245-251.

The technique for using a novel double-limbed suture was described for both soft-tissue and bony fixation in open or arthroscopic surgery.

[28] Krishnan SG, Bennion PW, Reineck JR, Burkhead WZ: Hemiarthroplasty for proximal humeral fracture: Restoration of the Gothic arch. *Orthop Clin North Am* 2008;39(4):441-450, vi.

A technique is described for establishing anatomic humeral length with hemiarthroplasty for proximal humeral fractures. The alignment of the lateral border of the scapula with the medial calcar of the humerus was found to be helpful.

[29] Murachovsky J, Ikemoto RY, Nascimento LG, Fujiki EN, Milani C, Warner JJ: Pectoralis major tendon reference (PMT): A new method for accurate restoration of humeral length with hemiarthroplasty for fracture. *J*

Shoulder Elbow Surg 2006;15(6):675-678.

[30] Torrens C, Corrales M, Melendo E, Solano A, Rodríguez-Baeza A, Cáceres E: The pectoralis major tendon as a reference for restoring humeral length and retroversion with hemiarthroplasty for fracture. *J Shoulder Elbow Surg* 2008;17(6):947-950.

CT was used to measure the distance between the superior border of the tendon and the apex of the humeral head.

[31] Olerud P, Ahrengart L, Ponzer S, Saving J, Tidermark J: Hemiarthroplasty versus nonoperative treatment of displaced 4-part proximal humeral fractures in elderly patients: A randomized controlled trial. *J Shoulder Elbow Surg* 2011;20(7):1025-1033.

A randomized controlled study compared health-related quality of life in patients with a four-part proximal humeral fracture treated nonsurgically or with hemiarthroplasty. Those treated with hemiarthroplasty had higher quality-of-life scores and less pain. Level of evidence: I.

[32] Den Hartog D, Van Lieshout EM, Tuinebreijer WE, et al: Primary hemiarthroplasty versus conservative treatment for comminuted fractures of the proximal humerus in the elderly (ProCon): A multicenter randomized controlled trial. *BMC Musculoskelet Disord* 2010;11:97.

This is the protocol for an ongoing level I randomized controlled study to detect differences between nonsurgical management and hemiarthroplasty.

[33] Kontakis G, Koutras C, Tosounidis T, Giannoudis P: Early management of proximal humeral fractures with hemiarthroplasty: A systematic review. *J Bone Joint Surg Br* 2008;90(11):1407-1413.

This systematic review examined the results and the complications of hemiarthroplasty for proximal humeral fractures. In 808 patients from 16 studies, the postoperative mean active anterior elevation was 105.7°, mean abduction was 92.4°, and the mean Constant score was 56.63.

[34] Grönhagen CM, Abbaszadegan H, Révay SA, Adolphson PY: Medium-term results after primary hemiarthroplasty for comminute proximal humerus fractures: A study of 46 patients followed up for an average of 4.4 years. *J Shoulder Elbow Surg* 2007;16(6):766-773.

A retrospective study evaluated the midterm functional and radiographic results of hemiarthroplasty for fracture. The mean Constant score was 42, with near-universal relief of pain. Radiographic examination found that 24 of the 46 prostheses had superiorly migrated. Level of evidence: IV.

[35] Antuña SA, Sperling JW, Cofield RH: Shoulder hemiarthroplasty for acute fractures of the proximal humerus: A minimum five-year follow-up. *J Shoulder Elbow Surg* 2008;17(2):202-209.

A retrospective study evaluated long-term outcomes of hemiarthroplasty for acute fractures. The average external rotation was 30°, and average forward elevation was 100°, with 16% of the patients reporting moderate to severe pain. Level of evidence: IV.

[36] Fallatah S, Dervin GF, Brunet JA, Conway AF, Hrushowy H: Functional outcome after proximal humeral fractures treated with hemiarthroplasty. *Can J Surg* 2008;51(5):361-365.

A retrospective study of 45 patients after hemiarthroplasty for proximal humeral fracture found that mean active elevation was 87°, mean abduction was 63°, 15% of the patients reported severe pain, and 25% were unable to sleep on the affected extremity.

[37] Greiner SH, Kääb MJ, Kröning I, Scheibel M, Perka C: Reconstruction of humeral length and centering of the prosthetic head in hemiarthroplasty for proximal humeral fractures. *J Shoulder Elbow Surg* 2008;17(5):709-714.

The study focused on whether using the pectoralis major tendon reference to determine the length of the humerus after hemiarthroplasty led to better results. The overall mean postoperative Constant score was 47.7, but it was higher in patients for whom the pectoralis major tendon was used to reference humeral height.

[38] Padua R, Bondì R, Ceccarelli E, Campi A, Padua L: Health-related quality of life and subjective outcome after shoulder replacement for proximal humeral fractures. *J Shoulder Elbow Surg* 2008;17(2):261-264.

Patient-relevant quality-of-life measures were assessed after hemiarthroplasty for proximal humeral fracture. Scores were lower in the patients compared with healthy control subjects.

[39] Pavlopoulos DA, Badras LS, Georgiou CS, Skretas EF, Malizos KN: Hemiarthroplasty for three- and four-part displaced fractures of the proximal humerus in patients over 65 years of age. *Acta Orthop Belg* 2007;73(3):306-314.

A prospective case study followed patients with three- or four-part fracture treated with hemiarthroplasty. No patients had complete recovery of strength and full range of motion. Of the 50 patients, 34 were able to resume all activities of daily living.

[40] Fevang BT, Lie SA, Havelin LI, Skredderstuen A, Furnes O: Risk factors for revision after shoulder arthroplasty: 1,825 shoulder arthroplasties from the Norwegian Arthroplasty Register. *Acta Orthop* 2009;80(1):83-91.

In a review of 1,825 arthroplasties performed in Norway during a 12-year period, Kaplan-Meier failure curves and a Cox regression revealed revision rates of approximately 8%, with higher rates for younger patients.

[41] Bastian JD, Hertel R: Osteosynthesis and hemiarthroplasty of fractures of the proximal humerus: Outcomes in a consecutive case series. *J Shoulder Elbow Surg* 2009;18(2):216-219.

A prospective nonrandomized comparison study found that osteosynthesis and hemiarthroplasty had similar functional results. The average Constant score was points for patients treated with osteosynthesis and points for those treated with hemiarthroplasty. Level of evidence: II.

[42] Bufquin T, Hersan A, Hubert L, Massin P: Reverse shoulder arthroplasty for the treatment of three- and four-part fractures of the proximal humerus in the elderly: A prospective review of 43 cases with a short-term follow-up. *J Bone Joint Surg Br* 2007;89(4):516-520.

A prospective review of 43 patients with three- or four-part fractures who were treated with reverse shoulder arthroplasty found a mean active anterior elevation of 97° and a mean active external rotation in abduction of 30°. The Constant score improved to a mean of 44.

[43] Cazeneuve JF, Cristofari DJ: Delta III reverse shoulder arthroplasty: Radiological outcome for acute complex fractures of the proximal humerus in elderly patients. *Orthop Traumatol Surg Res* 2009;95(5):325-329.

A retrospective review of radiographic results after reverse shoulder arthroplasty for fracture of the proximal humerus found unsatisfactory images, notching, radiolucent lines, or inferior spurring for 70% of the patients.

[44] Cazeneuve JF, Cristofari DJ: Grammont reversed prosthesis for acute complex fracture of the proximal humerus in an elderly population with 5 to 12 year follow-up. *Rev Chir Orthop Reparatrice Appar Mot* 2006;92(6):543-548.

[45] Cazeneuve JF, Hassan Y, Kermad F, Brunel A: Delta III reverse-ball-and-socket total shoulder prosthesis for acute complex fractures of the proximal humerus in elderly population. *Eur J Orthop Surg Traumatol* 2008;18:81-86.

A Grammont style prosthesis was used to treat 25 consecutive patients with three- or four-part fractures or fracture-dislocations. The results were good with respect to pain, activity, strength, anterior elevation, and abduction but poor for internal and external rotation.

[46] Cazeneuve JF, Cristofari DJ: The reverse shoulder prosthesis in the treatment of fractures of the proximal humerus in the elderly. *J Bone Joint Surg Br* 2010;92(4):535-539.

The clinical and radiologic outcomes of 36 patients with a proximal humeral fracture were reported at a mean 6.6-year follow-up. The mean Constant score was 53, in contrast to 58.5 at an earlier mean 6-year follow-up (range, 1 to 12 years). The reduction in Constant score and the further development of scapular notching was of concern.

[47] Cazeneuve JF, Cristofari DJ: Long term functional outcome following reverse shoulder arthroplasty in the elderly. *Orthop Traumatol Surg Res* 2011;97(6):583-589.

Thirty-five patients had improvement in function with limitations in rotation after receiving a reverse prosthesis for a complex proximal humerus fracture. Scapular notching was present in 20 patients, with associated decreased function and abnormal humeral radiographic images.

[48] Klein M, Juschka M, Hinkenjann B, Scherger B, Ostermann PA: Treatment of comminuted fractures of the proximal humerus in elderly patients with the Delta III reverse shoulder prosthesis. *J Orthop Trauma* 2008;22(10):698-704.

Twenty patients (mean age, 74.85 years) were followed for 33.3 months after receiving a reverse shoulder prosthesis. The average range of motion in abduction was 112.5°(± 38.2°) and in anterior elevation was 122.7°(± 32.84°). The mean Constant Score was 67.85° (± 13.56°). The good functional outcomes and the short intervention times, with no need for a sufficient rotator cuff for implementation purposes, suggested that the Delta III reverse shoulder prosthesis is a useful treatment option for older patients with a comminuted fracture of the proximal humerus.

[49] Sirveaux F, Navez G, Favard L, Boileau P, Walch G, Molé D: The multi-centre study, in Walch G, Boileau P, Molé D, eds: *Reverse Shoulder Arthroplasty: Clinical Results, Complications, Revision.* Montpellier, France,

Sauramps Medical, 2006, pp 73-80.

[50] Levy JC, Badman B: Reverse shoulder prosthesis for acute four-part fracture: Tuberosity fixation using a horseshoe graft. *J Orthop Trauma* 2011;25(5):318-324.

This technical article described the use of a horseshoe graft technique to increase the possibility of tuberosity repair in patients receiving a reverse prosthesis for fracture. Six of seven patients had healing with good functional results.

[51] Reitman RD, Kerzhner E: Reverse shoulder arthoplasty as treatment for comminuted proximal humeral fractures in elderly patients. *Am J Orthop (Belle Mead NJ)* 2011;40(9):458-461.

At short-term follow-up of 13 patients after reverse shoulder arthroplasty for a proximal humeral fracture, the mean Constant score was 67, and no recurrent instability occurred. Three nerve palsies were reported, but no revisions were required.

[52] Lenarz C, Shishani Y, McCrum C, Nowinski RJ, Edwards TB, Gobezie R: Is reverse shoulder arthroplasty appropriate for the treatment of fractures in the older patient? Early observations. *Clin Orthop Relat Res* 2011;469(12):3324-3331.

At short-term follow-up after the use of reverse shoulder arthroplasty for a proximal humeral fractures, functional scores had improved, and the complication rate compared favorably with those of other treatment alternatives.

[53] Tischer T, Rose T, Imhoff AB: The reverse shoulder prosthesis for primary and secondary treatment of proximal humeral fractures: A case report. *Arch Orthop Trauma Surg* 2008;128(9):973-978.

An older woman required bilateral reverse shoulder arthroplasty for bilateral proximal humerus fractures. Her functional and radiographic outcomes were reported.

[54] Lee CW, Shin SJ: Prognostic factors for unstable proximal humeral fractures treated with locking-plate fixation. *J Shoulder Elbow Surg* 2009;18(1):83-88.

Forty-five unstable proximal humeral fractures were analyzed to determine risk factors for loss of reduction. Lack of comorbidities and restoration of the medial metaphysis predicted a good result from osteosynthesis.

[55] Solberg BD, Moon CN, Franco DP, Paiement GD: Locked plating of 3- and 4-part proximal humerus fractures in older patients: The effect of initial fracture pattern on outcome. *J Orthop Trauma* 2009;23(2):113-119.

Worse clinical outcomes and radiographic results were found in 24 patients with initial varus displacement of the humeral head than in 46 patients with initial valgus displacement.

第三十章　肱骨近端骨折后遗症的关节置换

Armodios M. Hatzidakis, MD; Benjamin W. Sears, MD

引言

肱骨近端骨折相对常见，美国每年约有 185 000 例急诊病例。[1]虽然绝大多数病例可通过非手术方法成功治疗，但仍可见许多严重的功能障碍，主要是损伤引起的骨性畸形、不愈合、骨坏死和骨塌陷。[2-4]肱骨近端骨折的后期并发症轻者为单纯的大小结节畸形愈合（或不愈合），可通过关节镜手术或切开复位内固定来处理，重者为复杂的关节面不匹配，常导致关节面破坏和早期关节炎。[4-5]对于肱骨近端解剖严重畸形或关节面严重破坏的病例，假体置换可能是重建关节功能和减轻疼痛的唯一可靠方法。

由于损伤复杂、肩袖功能不全、骨量丢失、瘢痕形成和骨性解剖变异，肱骨近端骨折后遗症的假体置换难度很大。有症状的肱骨近端骨折后遗症患者通常相对年轻、活动量较大，做出关节置换的决定甚至更有挑战性。这类患者的手术难度比原发性骨关节炎患者的更大，结果更不可预测。[3,6]

骨折后遗症分型

肱骨近端骨折后遗症的 Boileau 分型基于 71 例非限制性（解剖型）关节置换患者的影像学评估。[2]骨折后期并发症分为 4 型（图 30-1）。Ⅰ 型指骨折后遗症伴肱骨头压缩、塌陷或坏死，Ⅱ 型指肱骨近端向前或向后的锁定脱位或骨折脱位。Ⅰ 型和 Ⅱ 型是关节内后遗症，采用非限制性关节置换预计可获得较满意的预后。Ⅲ 型是累及外科颈的骨折不愈合，Ⅳ 型是存在严重的结节畸形愈合或肱骨近端畸形。Ⅲ 型和 Ⅳ 型是关节外后遗症，解剖型假体关节置换术后的结果不可预测。这一分型系统的重要作用是在关节置换时评估是否需要大结节截骨或固定。大结节畸形愈合或需要大结节截骨时，通常非限制性肩关节置换术的结果很差。[2-4,7-8]

Boileau 分型对术前计划的制订十分有用。在关节内后遗症（Ⅰ 型和 Ⅱ 型）中，肱骨近端解剖结构的改变很轻微，结节和骨干连续性是完整的。无须进行结节截骨，非限制性关节置换可获得可预测的较好结果（图 30-2），这类患者无须进行截骨就可使大结节和肱骨头的关系恢复至接近解剖重建。使用组配型、可调的第三代肱骨假体有助于重建二者的关系。

关节外后遗症（Ⅲ 型和 Ⅳ 型）常伴有肱骨近端解剖的严重改变和（或）结节与骨干连续性中断。这类患者使用非限制性假体的长期结果不可预测，主要是因为很难获得大结节相对于肱骨头在解剖位置的愈合。因此，可考虑一期固定结合

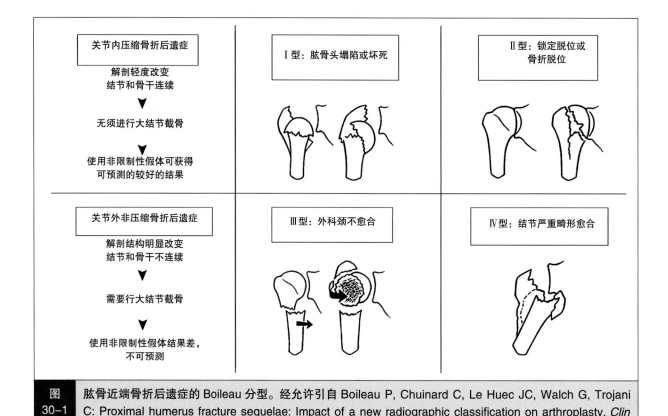

图 30-1 肱骨近端骨折后遗症的 Boileau 分型。经允许引自 Boileau P, Chuinard C, Le Huec JC, Walch G, Trojani C: Proximal humerus fracture sequelae: Impact of a new radiographic classification on arthroplasty. *Clin Orthop Relat Res* 2006;442:121–130.

植骨（Ⅲ型，不愈合）或半限制性（反肩关节）假体。

关节置换的适应证和禁忌证

患者存在有症状的骨折后遗症、疼痛和功能障碍时，可考虑行关节置换。关节置换的禁忌证包括急性感染、严重的神经损伤、禁忌手术的合并疾病和骨量极差假体无法有效固定。可选择使用非限制性肩关节假体置换技术（半肩关节置换、肱骨头表面置换和全肩关节置换）和半限制性假体置换技术（反肩关节置换）。

半肩关节置换、全肩关节置换和肱骨头表面置换

若骨折后遗症包括结节轻微畸形愈合或不愈合，则肱骨近端解剖畸形很小，如Ⅰ型、Ⅱ型和一部分Ⅲ型后遗症，半肩关节置换仍是主要的治疗选择。[3-4]假体设计的进步（如组配型和肱骨头偏心）使假体可更好地适应骨性结构的改变。

通常没有必要进行全肩关节置换，因为即使肱骨头有严重的退行性改变，患者的肩胛盂也很少有关节炎改变。但是最好在手术时检查肩胛盂是否有退行性改变，有时候肩胛盂的表面置换可明显减轻疼痛、恢复功能、避免翻修（图 30-2）。

解剖型假体包括带肱骨柄的假体和表面置换型假体。虽然过去更喜欢使用带肱骨柄的假体，但其适应性局限于髓内组件。表面置换假体无须与肱骨干相连，这种特点增加了其对严重畸形愈合的适应性，特别是对与颈干角相关的问题。近期文献报道，28 例行表面置换的Ⅰ型或Ⅱ型肱骨近端骨折后遗症患者的 Constant 肩关节评分结果良好，仅 1 例出现并发症。对于创伤后骨关节炎且骨量充足、肱骨头形态相对保存完好的患者（图 30-3），可行表面置换。[9]对于肱骨头塌陷或严重解剖异常的患者，肱骨头表面置换并不是一种理想的术式，因为假体必须牢固地固定在骨面上，可能无法充分适应骨性解剖。

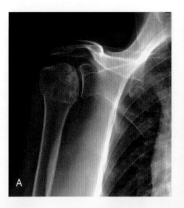
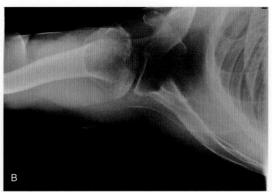
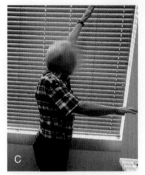
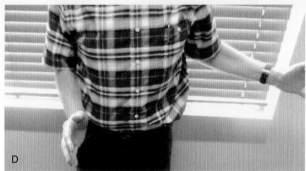
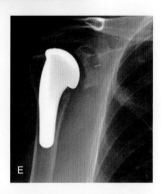
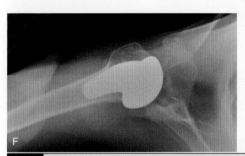
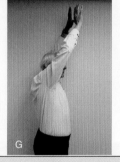
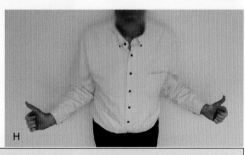

图 30-2　1例66岁的患者，肱骨近端囊内骨折愈合后出现肱骨头塌陷和骨坏死（Ⅰ型），手术时可见严重的肩胛盂关节面磨损，进行了肩胛盂表面置换。患者术后第1年随访时功能优，有轻微疼痛。术前正位片可见肱骨头塌陷和骨坏死（A）。术前腋位片可见关节面塌陷和结节轻微异常（B）。术前照片显示主动前屈（C）和主动外旋（D）。全肩关节置换术后1年的正位片（E）和腋位片（F）可见结节和肱骨头的关系接近解剖重建。全肩关节置换术后1年的照片显示主动前屈（G）和主动外旋（H）

反肩关节置换

对于70岁以上的骨折后遗症患者，以及伴有严重结节畸形愈合、不愈合和（或）肩袖缺损的患者，反肩关节置换是最常用的治疗方法。[10-11]反肩关节置换很大程度上降低了结节解剖位置或肩袖功能对盂肱关节活动和稳定性的影响，对于活动要求较低、结节严重畸形愈合、肱骨近端解剖异常（Ⅳ型）和伴有肩袖功能缺失的后遗症患者，是一种可选择的治疗方式。[3,10]对于70岁以上合并关节内后遗症（Ⅰ型或Ⅱ型）的患者，反肩关节置换可很好地减轻疼痛，改善术后上举。[4,12]反肩关节置换术也可作为一种半肩关节置换术失败后的挽救性手术，而对于肩袖质量差或肩袖不可修复的Ⅰ型后遗症患者，反肩关节置换应作为一期治疗选择（图30-4）。存在慢性前方不稳定的患者行反肩关节置换后可明显改善肩关节的稳定性。[10]有两项研究报道对于肱骨近端不愈合（Ⅲ型）患者，反肩关节置换可获得优良的结果。[13-14]

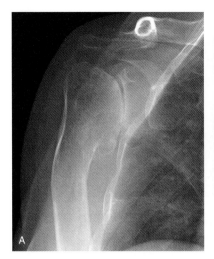
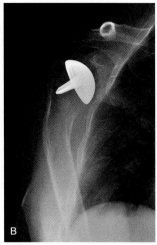

图 30-3　肱骨近端外科颈或肱骨近端骨干严重畸形愈合使肱骨假体柄无法插入，除非进行肱骨截骨。使用肱骨侧表面置换假体，例如，本例 72 岁男性患者，无论是否进行肩胛盂置换，可能都无须进行肱骨近端截骨。A. 术前正位片显示肱骨近端畸形愈合伴盂肱关节严重骨关节炎。B. 正位片显示使用肱骨侧表面置换假体进行全肩关节置换

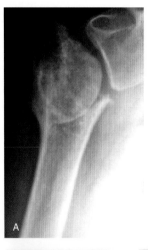
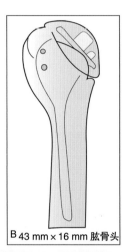

B 43 mm × 16 mm 肱骨头

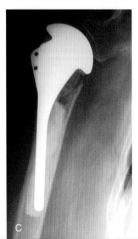
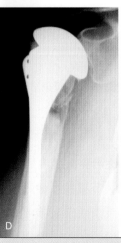
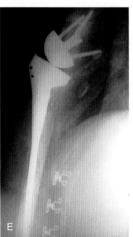
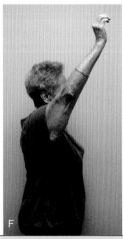

图 30-4　一例 67 岁女性患者，Ⅰ型肱骨近端骨折后遗症致肩关节疼痛、功能障碍。由于肩峰 - 肱骨头间隙正常，肩袖完整，因此采用了第三代半肩关节假体进行治疗。术中发现冈上肌腱变薄，需要修补。最初，肱骨头与肩胛盂匹配良好，但 1 年后，肱骨头向上和向后移位。患者出现慢性疼痛和功能障碍，且非手术治疗无效果。使用长柄反肩关节假体翻修后，舒适度和功能明显改善。A. 半肩关节置换前的肩关节正位片显示Ⅰ型肱骨近端骨折后遗症，大结节位置接近解剖重建。B. 术前模板可见大结节 - 肱骨头关节接近解剖重建。C. 半肩关节置换术后正位片可充分显示半肩关节置换的位置。D. 半肩关节置换术 1 年后的正位片显示肱骨头上移。E. 长柄反肩关节置换术后的正位片。F. 照片显示反肩关节置换术后的主动前屈

但是，与采用非限制性假体成功治疗的病例相比，接受反肩关节置换的病例通常伴有更广泛的永久性活动受限及肩关节主动旋转功能受限。

反肩关节置换的相对禁忌证包括患者的年龄和功能水平。对于小于 70 岁的患者无论是何种肱骨近端骨折后遗症，都应谨慎使用反肩关节置换。但是，对于许多严重结节不愈合或畸形愈合的患者，反肩关节置换是唯一能获得满意疗效的治疗方法。

结果

在近期的一项对 55 例肱骨近端骨折后遗症患者的研究中，研究者采用解剖型假体置换的方法治疗 Ⅰ 型和 Ⅱ 型后遗症患者，采用反肩关节置换的方法治疗 Ⅲ 型和 Ⅳ 型后遗症患者。对 36 例解剖型假体置换患者平均随访 24 个月，对 19 例反肩关节置换患者平均随访 19.3 个月后发现，两组患者术后在疼痛和功能方面均有明显改善，但并没有报道改善程度和后遗症类型的相关性。在平均 Constant 肩关节评分方面，接受解剖型假体置换的患者从 19 分提高到了 68 分，接受反肩关节置换的患者从 9 分提高到了 47.5 分。

一些研究专门报道了慢性脱位患者（Ⅱ 型）采用解剖型假体治疗的结果。其中一项回顾性研究报道了 11 例盂肱关节锁定前脱位患者在使用非限制性假体进行置换后，疼痛和功能评分明显改善。[15]但是，4 例（36%）患者术后出现前方不稳定，这 4 例患者中有 2 例在影像学检查中发现肩胛盂假体明显松动。还有一项对 12 例慢性盂肱关节后脱位患者的研究发现，采用非限制性肩关节置换后疼痛和功能明显改善，但 3 例（25%）患者因不稳定或假体松动须行翻修术。[16]总之，肩关节锁定脱位患者采用解剖型肩关节假体置换后可有效减轻疼痛，改善肩关节功能，但可能会残留不稳定和出现后期假体松动。总体来说，慢性盂肱关节后脱位假体置换的结果比前脱位行关节置换的结果更好一些。

反肩关节置换的适应证在过去的十几年中逐渐增多。最初，这一术式用于 70 岁以上对功能要求较低的患者，并用作骨折后遗症患者的挽救性手术，以处理既往无法处理的盂肱关节疾病。近期的一些研究报道了采用反肩关节置换治疗肱骨近端骨折后遗症的病例。一项研究对 18 例肱骨近端不愈合患者采用反肩关节置换，患者术后活动（如旋转）以及主观肩关节评分明显改善。[14]但是 5 例患者出现术后并发症，包括 2 例感染、1 例神经麻痹以及 2 例假体脱位（需使用更大直径的反球翻修）。研究者们认为虽然反肩关节置换有很高的并发症发生率，但可明显改善无法进行解剖型肩关节置换的有症状的肱骨近端不愈合患者的功能。在一项研究中，16 例肱骨近端骨折畸形愈合患者因严重疼痛或功能受限，采用反肩关节置换进行治疗，没有对畸形愈合的结节或残留的肱骨近端进行截骨。[17]术后第 2 年随访时，根据 ASES 肩关节疼痛和功能障碍评分、视觉模拟量表和肩关节简明测试，患者的疼痛和功能评分（包括旋转）明显改善，无明显并发症。研究者们认为使用反肩关节置换治疗肱骨近端骨折畸形愈合可获得满意的结果。

技术考虑

无须进行大结节截骨的肱骨侧假体插入

若肱骨近端假体插入时无须进行大结节截骨（如 Ⅰ 型和 Ⅱ 型后遗症时），可采用三角肌胸大肌入路显露盂肱关节。维持大结节愈合的位置十分重要，但可行小结节截骨进入关节，并处理肩胛下肌。[18]清理肩峰下间隙、三角肌下间隙和喙突下间隙中的瘢痕组织，活动肩关节，以最大限度显露盂肱关节。

显露肱骨头、肩袖和肩胛盂表面，肱骨头截骨需重建正常的盂肱关节解剖（假体上表面位于大结节上方 5 mm 处），同时保留大结节的完整性。一部分严重坏死的患者（Ⅰ 型），肱骨头可能塌陷以至于无须进行截骨。若选择带柄假体，假体柄必须较细，并用骨水泥固定，以适应增加的偏移。若颈干角严重畸形，可选择表面置换，此时无须插入肱骨侧假体柄。

大结节畸形愈合的截骨

虽然文献已报道大结节畸形愈合行关节置换时，大结节截骨的结果比不截骨的明显更差，但因为结节移位、患者年龄、功能水平或退变程度等因素，通常不能很好地维持结节的完整性。[3-4,7-8] 大结节截骨的相对适应证包括后移超过 1 cm，以及解剖结构改变导致无法充分插入假体。[19] 大结节畸形愈合相对更严重时进行解剖重建的患者，其肩关节功能的恢复情况可能更加不可预测（图 30-5）。

当必须进行大结节截骨时，可斜行截骨，尽

可能制造更大的接触面积以利于后期骨性愈合。应尽可能保护肩袖在大结节上的止点，同时松解肩袖以利于后期外展等动作。大结节远端骨膜应尽可能剥离而不切断，维持骨块上的软组织和血供。假体插入后，从肱骨头上取骨块置于假体近端和结节下表面之间，以促进愈合。最后用粗的不可吸收缝线将结节环扎固定于假体上。根据术中肩关节的活动范围，术后 6 周内可开始进行有限的肩关节被动活动，以减少僵硬的风险，同时促进大结节和肩胛下肌的愈合。

肱骨近端不愈合的关节置换

切开复位内固定及植骨（或不植骨），仍是不伴有严重退行性改变的Ⅲ型后遗症的第一治疗选择[3]（图 30-6）。对于严重关节炎或愈合能力较差

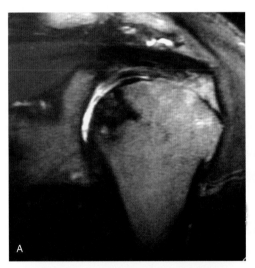
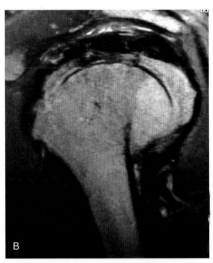
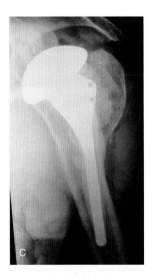
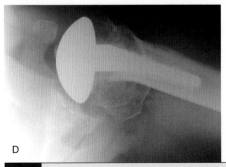
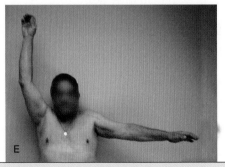
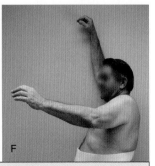

图 30-5　1 例 63 岁男性患者，肱骨近端大结节向后移位畸形愈合，选择解剖型肱骨假体以充分重建，没有进行大结节截骨。术后 1 年随访时，患者疼痛明显减轻，但仍然上举受限。A. 冠状面 MRI 图像显示肱骨近端骨折愈合，Ⅰ型后遗症。B. 斜矢状位 MRI 图像显示大结节后移并愈合。C. 全肩关节置换术后 1 年的正位片显示假体位置满意。D. 全肩关节置换术后 1 年的腋位片显示肱骨头相对于肩胛盂向前半脱位。E. 照片显示主动外展受限。F. 全肩关节置换术后 1 年的照片显示主动前屈上举受限

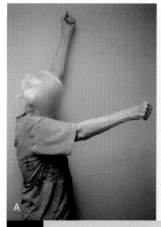
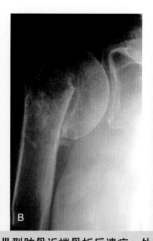
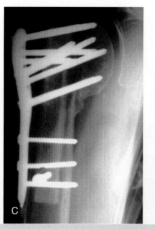
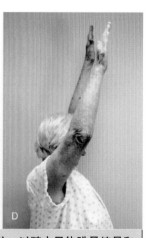

图 30-6　1例72岁女性患者，Ⅲ型肱骨近端骨折后遗症，外科颈不愈合，切开断端清理复位，以髓内异体腓骨植骨和锁定钢板螺钉内固定。术后第2年随访时，骨折愈合，主动活动明显改善。A. 术前照片显示主动前屈上举受限。B. 正位片显示Ⅲ型肱骨近端骨折后遗症（外科颈不愈合）。C. 术后1年正位片显示肱骨近端骨折锁定钢板固定后骨愈合。D. 照片显示前屈上举功能改善

（骨量差或肱骨头空化）的患者，解剖型肱骨头置换或反肩关节置换的结果最好。[13-14] 无论使用哪种类型的假体（解剖型或反肩关节假体），结节与肱骨侧假体的固定和愈合对于关节功能都十分重要，包括反肩关节置换术后的主动旋转。

通常采用三角肌胸大肌入路，以肱二头肌长头腱为标志找到肩袖间隙。尽可能保留小结节和大结节的连续性，将肩胛下肌剥离或切断，牵开以显露关节，肱骨头截骨时要注意保护大结节的活性。准备好肱骨干后，将最终的肱骨柄穿过环形的大小结节骨块，用骨水泥将骨块固定于肱骨干。在近端骨块与肱骨干和假体之间植骨，然后修复肩胛下肌。根据术中肩关节的活动范围，在术后6周内开始进行有限的肩关节被动活动。

陈旧性锁定脱位的处理

受伤超过6个月或肱骨关节面缺损超过40%的陈旧性盂肱关节锁定脱位（Ⅱ型后遗症）患者需行假体置换。[15-16] 陈旧性后方脱位时，可选择半肩关节置换或表面置换（图30-7）。若单纯重建肱骨头解剖形态后仍无法获得稳定性或后方关节囊过度松弛，可考虑行后方关节囊折叠紧缩术。

向前骨折脱位的患者比后方脱位的患者不稳定的风险更高。[15] 若肱骨不稳定或肩胛盂假体无

法有效固定，必须对肩胛盂缺损进行植骨。肩胛盂植骨的选择包括使用截除的肱骨头、使用自体髂骨嵴、喙突移位、或异体胫骨远端植骨。若需重建稳定性或肩袖无法修补，可考虑行反肩关节置换术。

将来的方向

采用解剖型肩关节置换或反肩关节置换治疗肱骨近端骨折后遗症的适应证和手术技术仍然在不断更新和进步，大结节的愈合对采用解剖型或反肩关节假体治疗急性骨折或骨折后遗症的患者的术后功能具有重要影响。新的解剖型和反肩关节假体的骨折假体柄设计可能提高急性骨折和骨折后遗症患者的大结节的愈合率。[20]

有许多文献详细讨论了肱骨近端畸形愈合行半肩关节置换时是否需要行大结节截骨。肱骨近端畸形愈合行反肩关节置换时可能也需要行大结节截骨。大结节通常相对于肱骨干向上、向外、向后移位，插入反肩关节肱骨侧假体柄，而不行大结节截骨，可能导致畸形愈合的大结节在外展时与肩峰发生撞击，在外旋时与肩峰和（或）肩胛盂发生撞击。这种撞击可能导致活动范围减小和不稳定（图30-8）。这种因素可能使行反肩关节置换的骨折后遗症患者的满意率低于肩袖病变行反肩关节置换的患者。

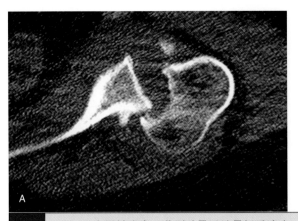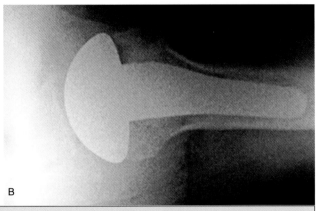

图
30-7
1例30岁男性患者，Ⅱ型肱骨近端骨折后遗症，锁定后方骨折脱位，肱骨头严重骨缺损。采用解剖型半肩关节置换重建肩关节解剖对位。A. 轴位CT图像显示锁定后方骨折脱位，伴有巨大的反 Hill-Sachs 损伤。B. 术后腋位片显示解剖型肱骨头置换，盂肱关节对位良好

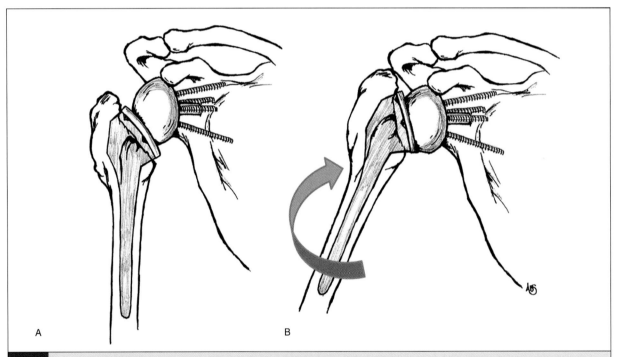

图
30-8
反肩关节置换时，大结节位置好（A）则无须行大结节截骨，外展外旋（B）时大结节和肩峰相撞击。大结节严重畸形愈合时，行反肩关节置换而不行大结节截骨可能导致肩峰撞击，从而影响手术结果，可能需要行大结节截骨以避免撞击

总结

肱骨近端骨折后遗症可导致严重的疼痛和功能障碍，通常需要行假体置换。骨折后遗症手术治疗的术前计划需仔细评估肱骨近端的解剖变异，判断是否需要行大结节截骨。总体来说，需要行大结节截骨的关节置换患者的功能结果比大结节

-肱骨头关系正常无须截骨的患者更差。肱骨头坏死或压缩（Ⅰ型），或慢性脱位（Ⅱ型）无须进行大结节截骨，可通过解剖型关节置换来治疗。肱骨近端不愈合（Ⅲ型）通常需要行内固定和植骨，虽然近期研究发现一部分患者反肩关节置换术后的结果优良。存在严重解剖异常和大结节畸

形愈合（Ⅳ型）或无法修补的肩袖缺损的患者，其行反肩关节置换术的效果更佳。

参考文献

［1］ Kim SH, Szabo RM, Marder RA: Epidemiology of humerus fractures in the United States: Nationwide emergency department sample, 2008. *Arthritis Care Res (Hoboken)* 2012;64(3):407-414.

An analysis of the 2008 Nationwide Emergency Department Sample revealed 370,000 US emergency room visits resulting from humeral fractures. More than 490,000 annual emergency room visits resulting from humeral fractures are projected to occur by 2030.Level of evidence: IV.

［2］ Boileau P, Trojani C, Walch G, Krishnan SG, Romeo A, Sinnerton R: Shoulder arthroplasty for the treatment of the sequelae of fractures of the proximal humerus. *J Shoulder Elbow Surg* 2001;10(4):299-308.

［3］ Boileau P, Chuinard C, Le Huec JC, Walch G, Trojani C: Proximal humerus fracture sequelae: Impact of a new radiographic classification on arthroplasty. *Clin Orthop Relat Res* 2006(442):121-130.

［4］ Cheung EV, Sperling JW: Management of proximal humeral nonunions and malunions. *Orthop Clin North Am* 2008;39(4):475-482, vii.

The results of corrective osteotomy, osteosynthesis with bone grafting, and arthroplasty are reviewed for patients with nonunion or malunion of the proximal humerus.

［5］ Martinez AA, Calvo A, Domingo J, Cuenca J, Herrera A: Arthroscopic treatment for malunions of the proximal humeral greater tuberosity. *Int Orthop* 2010;34(8):1207-1211.

Eight patients with malunion of the greater tuberosity were treated with arthroscopic acromioplasty, tuberoplasty of the greater tuberosity, and repair of the rotator cuff. One patient had an excellent result, six had a good result, and one had a poor result on the UCLA Shoulder Rating Scale.

［6］ Norris TR, Green A, McGuigan FX: Late prosthetic shoulder arthroplasty for displaced proximal humerus fractures. *J Shoulder Elbow Surg* 1995;4(4):271-280.

［7］ Antuña SA, Sperling JW, Sánchez-Sotelo J, Cofield RH: Shoulder arthroplasty for proximal humeral malunions: Long-term results. *J Shoulder Elbow Surg* 2002;11(2):122-129.

［8］ Mansat P, Guity MR, Bellumore Y, Mansat M: Shoulder arthroplasty for late sequelae of proximal humeral fractures. *J Shoulder Elbow Surg* 2004;13(3):305-312.

［9］ Pape G, Zeifang F, Bruckner T, Raiss P, Rickert M, Loew M: Humeral surface replacement for the sequelae of fractures of the proximal humerus. *J Bone Joint Surg Br* 2010;92(10):1403-1409.

Surface replacement arthroplasty in 28 shoulders resulted in good outcomes in shoulders with types I, II, and III proximal humeral fracture sequelae. The advantages of surface replacement include improved implant position, the preservation of bone stock, and the avoidance of periprosthetic fracture.

［10］ Neyton L, Garaud P, Boileau P: Results of reverse shoulder arthroplasty in proximal humerus fracture sequelae, in Walch G, Boileau P, Mole D, Favard L, Levigne C, Sirveaux F, eds: *Reverse Shoulder Arthroplasty*. Montpellier, France, Sauramps Medical, 2006.

［11］ Stechel A, Fuhrmann U, Irlenbusch L, Rott O, Irlenbusch U: Reversed shoulder arthroplasty in cuff tear arthritis, fracture sequelae, and revision arthroplasty. *Acta Orthop* 2010;81(3):367-372.

At a mean 4-year follow-up of 59 patients, reverse shoulder arthroplasty for severe arthropathy (rotator cuff tear, fracture sequelae, or revision) was suitable for restoring function and attaining pain relief, but reverse shoulder arthroplasty should be reserved for patients in whom conventional methods were unsuccessful.

［12］ Martin TG, Iannotti JP: Reverse total shoulder arthroplasty for acute fractures and failed management after proximal humeral fractures. *Orthop Clin North Am* 2008;39(4):451-457, vi.

Reverse shoulder arthroplasty was used for conditions involving insufficient rotator cuff function and proximal humeral malunion after unsuccessful hemiarthroplasty.

［13］ Kılıç M, Berth A, Blatter G, et al: Anatomic and reverse shoulder prostheses in fracture sequelae of the humeral head. *Acta Orthop Traumatol Turc* 2010;44(6):417-425.

In 55 patients with fracture sequelae who underwent anatomic total shoulder arthroplasty (for type I or II) or reverse total shoulder arthroplasty (for type III or IV), there was significant improvement in pain and function.

［14］ Martinez AA, Bejarano C, Carbonel I, Iglesias D, Gil-Alvaroba J, Herrera A: The treatment of proximal humerus nonunions in older patients with the reverse shoulder arthroplasty. *Injury* 2012.

Eighteen patients with proximal humeral atrophic nonunion were followed for 28 months after reverse shoulder arthroplasty. Two postoperative dislocations occurred, and one patient developed transient axillary neurapraxia. Average active motion including rotation significantly improved in all patients.

[15] Matsoukis J, Tabib W, Guiffault P, et al: Primary unconstrained shoulder arthroplasty in patients with a fixed anterior glenohumeral dislocation. *J Bone Joint Surg Am* 2006;88(3):547-552.

[16] Sperling JW, Pring M, Antuna SA, Cofield RH: Shoulder arthroplasty for locked posterior dislocation of the shoulder. *J Shoulder Elbow Surg* 2004;13(5):522-527.

[17] Willis M, Min W, Brooks JP, et al: Proximal humeral malunion treated with reverse shoulder arthroplasty. *J Shoulder Elbow Surg* 2012;21(4):507-513.

Sixteen patients underwent reverse shoulder arthroplasty for proximal humeral malunion. Active motion including rotation significantly improved, and no major complications were reported. Reverse shoulder arthroplasty was indicated for treating severe fracture sequelae.

[18] Scalise JJ, Ciccone J, Iannotti JP: Clinical, radiographic, and ultrasonographic comparison of subscapularis tenotomy and lesser tuberosity osteotomy for total shoulder arthroplasty. *J Bone Joint Surg Am* 2010;92(7):1627-1634.

Arthroplasty in 35 shoulders was performed with a standard subscapularis tenotomy or a lesser tuberosity osteotomy to release the subscapularis. The lesser tuberosity osteotomy resulted in higher outcome scores, a lower rate of tendon tears, and healing of the osteotomy. Level of evidence: III.

[19] Tauber M, Resch H: Prosthetic arthroplasty for delayed complications of proximal humerus fracture, in Cofield RH and Sperling JW, eds: *Revision and Complex Shoulder Arthroplasty*. Philadelphia, PA, Lippincott Williams & Wilkins, 2010.

[20] Krishnan SG, Reineck JR, Bennion PD, Feher L, Burkhead WZ Jr: Shoulder arthroplasty for fracture: Does a fracture-specific stem make a difference? *Clin Orthop Relat Res* 2011;469(12):3317-3323.

A retrospective review of 170 proximal humeral fractures treated with hemiarthroplasty found that the use of a fracture-specific stem resulted in better function and tuberosity healing than the use of a standard stem. Level of evidence: IV.

第三十一章　慢性肩关节病变的反肩关节置换

Randall J. Otto, MD; Phillip T. Nigro, MD; Mark A. Frankle, MD

引言

在过去的半个世纪，反肩关节置换（RSA）的出现是肩关节置换治疗终末期肩关节疾病的一个巨大进步。使用解剖型全肩关节置换（TSA）治疗软组织平衡良好的盂肱关节骨关节炎可获得长期的良好结果。但是，软组织不平衡的关节炎患者若采用全肩关节置换可能会因受力不均匀导致肩胛盂假体失败。反肩关节置换最早被设计用于改善肩袖缺损患者的功能。早期限制性假体的失败促使 Grammont 设计了一种非解剖型半限制性假体。[1]这种假体可改善功能，减轻疼痛。[2]随着时间的推移，这种设计不断被改良，发展成为现代的反肩关节假体。

Dr. Otto or an immediate family member is a member of a speakers' bureau or has made paid presentations on behalf of DJ Orthopaedics. Dr. Nigro or an immediate family member is a member of a speakers' bureau or has made paid presentations on behalf of DJ Orthopaedics. Dr. Frankle or an immediate family member has received royalties from DJ Orthopaedics; is a member of a speakers' bureau or has made paid presentations on behalf of DJ Orthopaedics; serves as a paid consultant to DJ Orthopaedics; serves as an unpaid consultant to DePuy; has received research or institutional support from DJ Orthopaedics, EBI, Eli Lilly, and Encore Medical; has received nonincome support (such as equipment or services), commercially derived honoraria, or other non–research-related funding (such as paid travel) from DJ Orthopaedics, EBI, Eli Lilly, and Encore Medical; and serves as a board member, owner, officer, or committee member of the American Shoulder and Elbow Surgeons, American Academy of Orthopaedic Surgeons, and Florida Medical Association.

设计原理

使用反肩关节假体的目的是提供一个稳定的盂肱关节支点。[1]反肩关节可阻挡肱骨上移，三角肌向上牵拉的力量可转化为旋转力臂。当重建盂肱关节后，残余的肩袖肌肉和肩胛周围肌肉通过三角肌的连接可重建肱骨和躯干之间的活动。

Grammont 设计的反肩关节假体包括极度外翻（155°）的肱骨侧假体和以肩胛盂骨性表面固定基座为中心的半球（图 31-1）。外翻的肱骨假体可通过延长力臂维持三角肌张力，提供肱骨侧假体和半球之间的压应力，因此可稳定关节对合。另外，半球旋转中心的内移可增强三角肌的收缩力量，因而可获得更有效的三角肌杠杆力臂。[3]假体的肱骨旋转中心尽可能贴近肩胛盂表面可降低基座的松动率。

尽管使用了 Grammont 型反肩关节假体的患者的临床结果明显改善，但也发现了许多机械性问题，包括盂肱关节无撞击活动范围的明显减小以及肱骨近端向外和向下偏移的明显改变。[4-5]这种与正常肩关节解剖结构的差异和相应的力学改变可能导致不可预见的并发症，包括假体止点改变引起的骨与软组织的改变以及肩关节功能改变引起的肩关节外形改变。许多临床和生物力学研究致力于改进反肩关节的假体设计和手术技术。

适应证和禁忌证

适应证

反肩关节置换的适应证不断增加，已被广泛

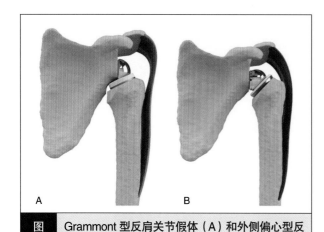

图 31-1 Grammont 型反肩关节假体（A）和外侧偏心型反肩关节假体（B）

用于治疗严重的肩关节病变患者。最初，反肩关节置换用于治疗肩袖缺损的盂肱关节炎患者。近些年也成功用于治疗严重肩袖缺损但没有盂肱关节炎、肩袖完整但盂肱关节不稳定的骨关节炎、类风湿关节炎、肱骨近端三部分或四部分骨折和骨折畸形愈合患者。此外，反肩关节置换也成功用于肿瘤切除后需行重建的患者、因骨折或肩袖损伤性关节病变行半肩关节置换失败的患者，以及全肩关节置换或早期反肩关节置换失败的患者。

若患者疼痛严重，10 分疼痛量表得分超过 5 分和（或）有严重的肩关节功能障碍时，可考虑行反肩关节置换术。由于缺乏稳定的止点，通常患者有临床和影像学上的肩关节假性麻痹，最常见的为前上方脱位。虽然不是必须如此，但是手术时修复残留的前方和后方肩袖有助于恢复反肩关节置换术后的旋转功能。反肩关节置换比较少见的一种适应证是肌肉骨骼肿瘤或肩关节深部感染。此时可选择一期或二期手术。[6] 将来需进一步研究来明确反肩关节置换的适应证。

禁忌证

反肩关节置换需有完整的三角肌功能以抬起上臂。因此，若患者存在因神经损伤、三角肌撕裂、肌肉间瘢痕形成或其他神经肌肉损伤等因素引起的三角肌功能障碍，是反肩关节置换的绝对禁忌证。若三角肌中央束肌腹损伤，反肩关节置换术后三角肌的功能可能受限。通过一期或分期手术，反肩关节置换可有效治疗感染病例，但急性感染时，应选择抗生素间隔物 Spacer。

过去，受限于假体的使用年限，通常不建议年龄低于 70 岁的患者行反肩关节置换。随着假体设计和手术技术的进步，这一因素变得不再那么重要。中期随访时发现，反肩关节置换较为持久耐用且有较好的结果。[7-9] 相对年轻的患者需考虑临床症状的严重程度、疼痛、肩关节功能障碍、损伤的程度，以及患者对假体可能没有那么经久耐用的接受度。患者的损伤相对较小时（如巨大肩袖损伤不合并关节炎），临床症状的严重程度对于预测满意度十分重要。若患者术前活动范围相对良好，则很难判断术后临床改善的程度。因此，综合考虑患者的症状和损伤严重程度对于决定治疗方式十分重要。

过去，肩胛盂缺损是反肩关节置换的绝对禁忌证。近期，很多研究发现了采用反肩关节置换成功治疗肩胛盂缺损的病例，并且反肩关节置换技术也在不断改进，被扩展用于治疗中度或重度肩胛盂缺损的病例。[10] 但是，十分严重的肩胛盂缺损会影响假体固定，仍是反肩关节置换的禁忌证。

关节置换的所有禁忌证也适用于反肩关节置换，包括严重的疾病、无法耐受手术、存在金属过敏和无法遵从术后活动限制的医嘱。另外，术者必须注意反肩关节置换治疗严重肩关节病变的学习曲线。跟其他所有新技术一样，术者的经验水平影响预后和并发症发生率。[11]

假体设计改进

Grammont 型反肩关节假体的临床局限性促使研究者们对假体设计不断改进，在保留反肩关节的同时，使肱骨的偏移最小化，并使肩关节的无撞击活动范围最大化。目前的设计尽可能减少了肩胛盂下撞击缺损、旋转功能缺乏、不稳定和肩胛盂侧失败等的发生率。设计上的改变包括使反肩半球相对于肩胛盂偏心化、肱骨侧假体相对于原始设计外翻减小。目前的假体设计使球体的旋转中心偏离肩胛盂表面，这种球体比原始设计的大，旋转中心相对于肩胛盂表面向外偏移 10 mm，向下偏移 4 mm。[12-13] 目前的许多设计也使颈干角更加接近解剖状态，在一些设计中，颈干角是 135°。

肩胛盂下撞击缺损

使肩关节无撞击活动范围最大化十分重要，这样做既有助于患者的功能，又有利于假体存活率、假体稳定性和减轻无法解释的疼痛。无撞击活动范围减小的一个后果是当患者尝试进行肩关节内收时，肩胛颈与肱骨聚乙烯衬垫的下表面发生撞击（图 31-2）。这种撞击会导致聚乙烯衬垫磨损和肩胛盂侧假体松动。内收受限在影像学上表现为肩胛盂下的撞击切迹，这种撞击切迹的出现和大小对功能评分有负面影响，会引起肩胛盂侧假体松动。[14-15] 无撞击活动范围的减小也增加了假体与骨或软组织撞击的可能性，导致疼痛和假体的杠杆性松动。

Grammont 型假体置换时，无法充分平衡软组织，无法提供足够的无撞击活动范围，因此无法最大限度地恢复肩关节功能。可通过改进手术技术来避免内收受限。使用虚拟电脑模型辅助研究造成肩胛下撞击的因素时，发现内翻型肱骨侧颈干角（130°）可很好地避免内收受限。[4-5] 使无撞击活动范围最大化的最重要因素是使用旋转中心相对于肩胛盂表面外移的反球。临床研究已经证实了这

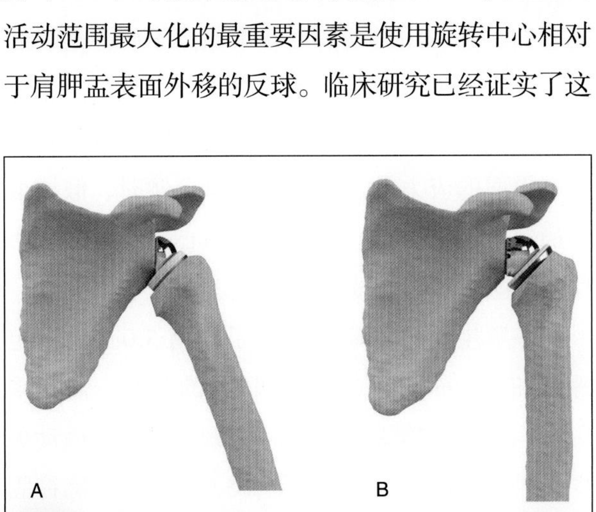

图 32-2 图示显示 Grammont 型假体（A）置换时，肱骨侧组件与肩胛颈撞击引起肩关节内收受限，外侧偏移假体（B）置换时，肱骨侧组件与肩胛颈无撞击

个结论，若使用偏心距外移的反球可避免肩胛下撞击的风险。[7,16-20] Grammont 型假体的一项改良是在肩胛盂和基座之间采用自体骨移植，以增加向外的偏心距。[13] 19% 的患者发现有肩胛下撞击，这一概率低于使用标准的中置型 RSA 假体。

外旋功能改善欠佳

Grammont 型假体已被证实有助于改善功能，减轻疼痛，但其对外旋功能的改善并不可靠。[21-24] Grammont 推测反肩关节置换时可通过三角肌后束收缩增加外旋角度，但没有生物力学数据支持这一观点。[25] 外旋力量丧失可能是因为肩袖损伤后的解剖改变，使残留的肩袖收缩力量减弱。另外，旋转中心内移使残留的肩袖松弛，无法有效收缩（图 31-3）。一些研究发现外旋没有改善的患者对他们的功能结果并不满意。[22]

旋转中心外移的反肩关节假体比 Grammont 型假体对外旋的改善效果更好。[12] 肩袖功能障碍的患者，其肱骨向近端移位可能会使完整的肩袖肌肉无法发挥正常功能。将肱骨置于相对更解剖的位置时，可重建关节稳定性，恢复残留肩袖的张力，使外旋功能改善。一些临床研究证实，重建肩关节向外的偏心距可改善不同病理状态患者的术后外旋功能。[7,16-20] 但是，术前就有小圆肌缺如或萎缩的患者无法恢复外旋功能，需行背阔肌转位来改善外旋功能。

肩关节不稳定

反肩关节置换术后的不稳定仍令人担忧。文献报道采用 Grammont 型假体置换后的肩关节脱位率高达 30%。导致肩关节不稳定的因素包括反球的直径、肱骨侧聚乙烯衬垫的约束力、软组织张力、撞击、假体型号错误和肱三头肌功能障碍等。

许多研究者建议通过重建肌肉张力从而增加肱骨侧的压应力来提高肩关节的稳定性。[7,16-20] 肱骨内移继发残留肩袖松弛，会影响肩关节稳定性。若肩胛盂有骨缺损，肱骨内移会将三角肌提供的力转为牵张力，增加脱位的可能性。[26] 提高肩关

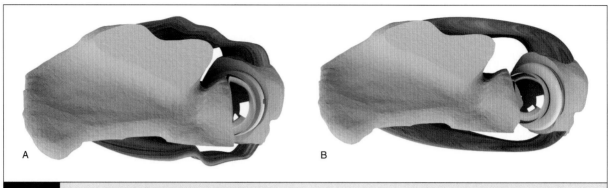

图 31-3 A. 偏心距内移的假体置换时，残留的外旋肩袖松弛。B. 偏心距外移的假体置换时，残留的外旋肩袖紧张

节稳定性的另一种方法是延长肱骨，同时使用外翻型肱骨侧衬垫。[21]但是这种方法增加了肩峰骨折、臂丛损伤、三角肌张力过大和活动障碍的风险。通过外移肱骨增加肩胛盂与大小结节的距离、增加通过肩关节的压应力是另一种提高稳定性的方法。

一些假体设计因素包括衬垫深度、反球大小和压应力被认为与肩关节不稳定相关。[27]改善稳定性的最重要方法是通过增加肱骨侧衬垫的厚度来提高经过肩关节的压应力。通过外移肱骨重建残留肩袖的张力，从而增加经过肩关节的压应力。研究发现外移肱骨可增加关节的反作用力。[27-28]

反肩关节置换术后脱位肩关节的早期处理为闭合复位并吊带制动一段时间。闭合复位失败或闭合复位后复发性不稳定，为切开翻修手术的指征。必须彻底松解假体周围组织，去除引起假体撞击和杠杆性松动的软组织。必须评估软组织张力，选择加厚的聚乙烯衬垫来增加外侧偏移和张力。可选择限制性更强的衬垫或更大的反球来增加稳定性。若这些方法都不成功，就得考虑可能是假体的型号不合适和位置不当引起的关节不稳定。

基座失效

许多研究报道了肩胛盂骨性结构与肩胛盂假体组件的连接失效。[2,12,20,29-33]1985 年以来所有的反肩关节假体设计都致力于促进肩胛盂侧的骨长入。若骨长入不佳，这种连接通常是纤维组织连接，并不持久稳定。造成骨长入失败的因素包括假体的设计

不佳、肩胛盂骨性缺损和假体位置不佳。Grammont的理论认为，将反球置于肩胛盂的固定基座中间可减小肩胛盂侧失效的风险，但这一理论并没有获得证实。在早期的研究中，高达 50% 的类风湿关节炎患者和出现肩胛盂下撞击的患者出现肩胛盂侧假体失效。[29-30]其他的假体也有很高的机械性失效率。

在对一种假体的早期研究中，研究者采用椭圆形的反球，同时将其旋转中心外移至距关节盂表面 10 mm 处，肩胛盂侧假体的失效率约为12%。[12]当反球旋转中心外移时，将反球下倾15°可使骨与基座界面承受均匀一致的压应力和最小的微动。[34]研究者们认为这可降低基座的失效率。这些研究者进行了另一项研究，证实了之前的研究，并采用早期的旋转中心位于肩胛盂表面的反球假体（Grammont 型假体）研究发现，相较于垂直于骨表面时，当基座有一定的下倾，骨与基座界面的应力最佳。[5]当基座上倾时，假体最不稳定（图 31-4）。选择向下偏心的反球时则相反，基座下倾时机械环境最不稳定。

一项生物力学研究对比了采用 5.0 mm 锁定螺钉和 3.5 mm 非锁定螺钉固定的基座，发现采用 5.0 mm 锁定螺钉固定基座的效果更好，微动更少。[35]后续的一项关于采用 5.0 mm 锁定螺钉固定有一定下倾的改良假体的临床研究发现，在最短 2 年的随访中，患者肩胛盂侧假体松动率降低至 0.4%。[19]

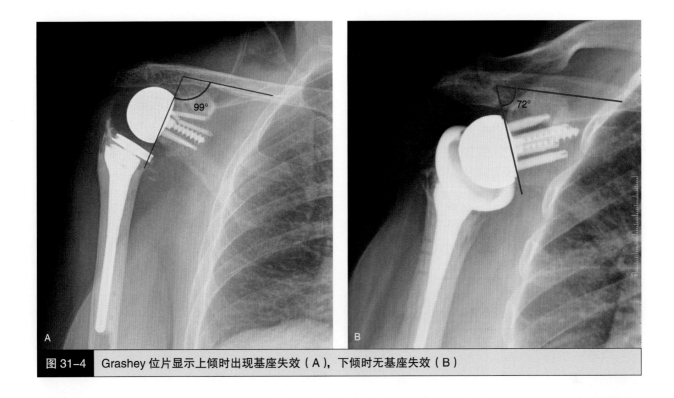

图 31-4　Grashey 位片显示上倾时出现基座失效（A），下倾时无基座失效（B）

当采用现在的假体置换技术，使用锁定螺钉固定的 Grammont 型假体也有相对很低的基座松动率，一期反肩关节置换患者的基座松动率为 0~5%[15,21,24]，而类风湿关节炎患者或翻修患者在反肩关节置换后的松动率为 0~8%[9,21,36]。现代的手术技术使 Grammont 型假体和外侧偏心型假体都可获得持久的肩胛盂侧假体固定。患者的自身疾病或早期关节置换造成肩胛盂骨量减少时，肩胛盂侧假体的固定仍是稳定的。

技术考虑

反球位置

研究者通过改进假体设计降低了肩胛下撞击的发生率。另外，研究者们还改良了手术技术，改变了反球的位置，以避免上臂贴近身体时引起肩胛颈下撞击。[37]一项生物力学研究评估了 4 种不同的肩胛盂假体位置对活动范围和机械性撞击的影响。[3]他们发现将反球放置在超过肩胛盂下缘处，并下倾 15°，可明显减少机械性撞击。反球下移以避免撞击的重要性也逐渐被临床所证实。[14]

另一项生物力学研究通过计算机模拟来探索减小内收受限和撞击风险的因素。[4]避免肩胛下撞击的第二重要因素是反球下移，最重要的因素是使用内翻型（130°）肱骨颈干角。

肩胛盂骨缺损

正常的肩关节中，肩胛盂中心线垂直于肩胛盂关节面，前倾约 10°。该中心线是骨性支柱，肱骨头在其下方，对合关系在整个盂肱关节和肩胛胸壁关节的活动范围内维持恒定。肩袖缺损时，肌肉力量不平衡，这一关系被破坏，引起力学改变和肩胛盂病理性磨损，其中高达 36% 的患者需行反肩关节置换。[38]根据损伤情况，磨损类型分为无磨损、上磨损、前磨损、后磨损和整体磨损。认识磨损类型对于制订术前计划十分重要。

最理想化的状态下，肩胛盂侧假体应沿着肩胛盂中心线置入，正常形态的肩胛骨在此处有 2.5~3.5 cm 的骨量用于固定。若肩胛盂有大块磨损或偏心磨损，在这一中心线插入假体并不总是可行的。有学者提出，使用一条改良的肩胛盂中心线，这条线在肩胛冈与肩胛体交界处的高密度骨处，与残余的肩胛盂表面重合。[38]沿着这条线将肩胛盂侧假体插入肩胛冈和肩胛体连接处，此处可提供充足的骨量用于固定。

一项回顾性研究纳入了9例采用Grammont型假体进行反肩关节置换的患者，患者术前严重骨缺损，行肩胛盂植骨，在最少2年的随访中，患者疼痛明显减轻，但功能结果评分低。其中6例患者影像学检查可见肩胛盂撞击切迹。[39]一项研究对比了使用外侧偏心型反肩关节假体置换的56例肩胛盂骨缺损患者和87例肩胛盂形态正常患

者。[10]在56例肩胛盂异常患者中，有22例进行了植骨，56例患者均使用改良的肩胛盂中心线进行肩胛盂侧假体固定（图31-5）。肩胛盂异常患者使用更大的反球，植骨患者采用带扩展边的反球加压植骨。文献报道肩胛盂异常患者和肩胛盂正常患者间无明显差异，两类患者的活动范围和功能结果均明显改善。其中1例患者对结果不满意，5例患者出现并发症（2例肩峰骨折、2例感染和1例假体周围骨折）。这些结果显示，在手术技术改进后，肩胛盂骨缺损并不是禁忌证。

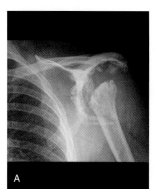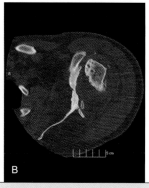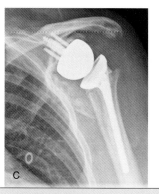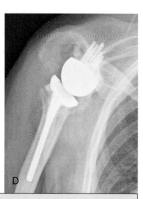

图 31-5 　Grashey位片（A）和腋位CT（B）显示严重的肩胛盂骨缺损。术后Grashey位片显示采用改良的肩胛盂中心线充分固定（C）和使用肩胛盂植骨及大的反球进行置换（D）

肱骨骨缺损

肱骨近端骨缺损时行反肩关节置换术可改善功能、减轻疼痛。[16]但是，肱骨近端骨缺损有较大可能引起肩关节不稳定、早期假体松动和旋转力弱。[16]肱骨近端严重骨缺损时，采用肱骨近端异体骨植骨结合反肩关节置换可改善功能结果（图31-6）。[16,18]异体骨植骨可提高肱骨柄假体的旋转稳定性。这对于组配型肱骨假体特别重要，肱骨近端骨缺损时，这种假体机械性失效的风险比非组配型肱骨假体高。[40]异体骨植骨可重建肱骨近端骨性外形，维持假体与骨结构的高度，防止肱骨假体下沉，从而有助于保持三角肌张力。异体骨植骨可外移三角肌牵拉的力线，作为支点增加三角肌的合力。

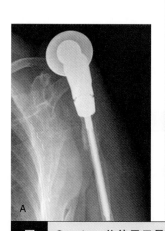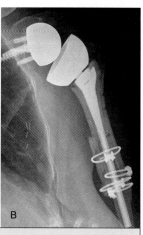

图 31-6 　Grashey位片显示骨缺损者半肩关节置换失败（A）以及肱骨近端骨缺损患者采用异体骨植骨结合假体置换（B）

背阔肌腱转位

若许多日常生活所需的主动外旋没有改善，

反肩关节置换患者会对结果不满意。[22,41] 将肱骨外移的假体改良设计是为了恢复肩关节外旋功能和力量，小圆肌缺如或萎缩意味着外旋不会改善。当侧抬上臂时，患者会出现吹号手征（the hornblower's sign）和外旋无力（an external rotation lag）。对于这些患者，建议采用改良的背阔肌－大圆肌肌腱转位结合反肩关节置换，以恢复主动上举和外旋，从而改善功能并提高满意度。[40-44]

对 17 例巨大肩袖损伤和小圆肌缺如的患者采用反肩关节置换和背阔肌－小圆肌转位进行治疗，其功能结果、活动范围和进行日常生活活动的能力均明显改善。[43] 对主动上举和外旋假性麻痹的 11 例患者（12 个肩关节）采用反肩关节置换和背阔肌转位进行治疗，患者的功能结果、活动范围和进行日常生活活动的能力均明显改善。[44]

只有在修复肩胛下肌腱后才能决定是否行背阔肌－大圆肌肌腱转位。若软组织将被动外旋限制在不超过 45° 的范围内，则手术获益可能无法抵消肌腱转移相关的并发症。

结果

在早期对使用反肩关节假体治疗肩袖缺损患者的报道中，患者均有较高的并发症发生率。然而，即使是使用早期的假体类型，反肩关节已被证实是一种可靠的治疗方法。假体设计的改进和手术技术的进步可能会在将来进一步提高假体的耐用性。表 31-1~31-4 列出了一些值得关注的研究及其结果。

并发症

反肩关节置换是治疗终末期肩关节病变的一个有效方法，但非解剖型的假体设计也会带来一些并发症。

感染

反肩关节置换术后感染发生率为 1%~12%。[12,29,45] 感染可能由手术期间直接接种、术后血肿播散、血行播散和多次肩部手术后惰性生物重新激活导致。反肩关节置换术后感染发生率比传统肩关节置换高，这可能是因为前者的肩峰下死腔更大、患者年龄更大，且反肩关节置换常用于翻修手术。血肿形成可能引起深部感染，特别是在持续引流时。

类风湿关节炎患者反肩关节置换术后和其他关节置换术后一样，感染风险相对较高。一项前瞻性研究发现，在 21 例类风湿关节炎患者中，术后感染的发生率为 9.5%。[46] 翻修手术也会增加反肩关节置换术后感染的发生率。文献报道半肩关节或传统全肩关节置换术后采用反肩关节置换进行翻修的患者感染发生率高达 6.7%。[9,15-17,21]

预防感染的措施包括细致的无菌技术和术前抗生素的使用。急性感染（少于 6 周）可通过清创、使用抗生素和更换聚乙烯衬垫等方法进行治疗。而慢性感染则需通过一期或二期翻修手术结合静脉注射抗生素进行治疗。要根据一期清创的程度来决定是否进行一期翻修。[6]

肩峰骨折和术中骨折

反肩关节置换术后肩峰骨折会严重影响结果（图 31-7）。术前患者可能有肩峰的髋臼化表现，使骨质变薄。反球下置引起三角肌张力增加，可能会导致反肩关节置换术后肩峰骨折。一项纳入了 527 例患者的回顾性研究发现，肩峰骨折的发生率为 3%。[47] 其他研究报道肩峰骨折的发生率为 0~4.4%。[46,48-50] 若患者疼痛没有缓解、术后早期疼痛和功能急性变化、康复进展缓慢，术者应怀疑存在肩峰骨折。X 线检查可能发现肩峰骨折，但通常 CT 检查更可靠。发现肩峰骨折后需早期制动。

在扩孔过程中可能发生肩胛盂骨折。[33,46,48] 应在扩孔器接触关节盂骨质之前小心地启动扩孔器，以避免导致扭矩过大。关节盂骨质下降也易导致骨折。在放置基座之前或穿过基座放置螺钉，可以实现稳定的骨折固定。在带有中心螺钉的假体中，将螺钉改变方向打入其他骨骼中可以实现稳定的固定。如果不能通过改变螺钉方向获得牢固固定，可

表 31-1

肩袖缺损行反肩关节置换的研究

研究发表（年份）	病例数	病因（病例数）	平均随访时间	术前/术后活动范围 前屈角度
旋转中心内移型假体				
Boulahia 等[2]（2002）	16	肩袖损伤型关节病	35 个月	70°/138°
Sirveaux 等[33]（2004）	77	肩袖损伤型关节病	44 个月	73°/138°
Vanhove 和 Beugnies[45]（2004）	24	肩袖损伤型关节病	31 个月	–
Seebauer 等[32]（2005）	57	肩袖损伤型关节病	18.2 个月	–/145°
Guery 等[15]（2006）	57	肩袖损伤（48）类风湿关节炎（6）骨折（2）翻修（1）	69.6 个月	–
Wall 等[23]（2007）	191	不同病因	39.9 个月	86°/137°
Gerber 等[44]（2007）	10	巨大肩袖损伤（曾行背阔肌转位）	18 个月	94°/139°
Simovitch 等[22]（2007）	77	肩袖损伤型关节病	44 个月	65°/115°
		无肩胛下撞击（43）	47 个月	–/127°
		肩胛下撞击（34）	42 个月	–/110°
Favard 等[8]（2011）	148	肩袖损伤型关节病	7.8 年	69°/129°
Melis 等[9]（2011）	68	非骨水泥型（34）	9.6 年	–/123°
		骨水泥型（34）	9.6 年	–/132°
旋转中心外移型假体				
Frankle 等[12]（2005）	60	肩袖损伤关节病	33 个月	55°/105.1°
Cuff 等[19]（2008）	96	肩袖缺损（70）关节置换术后肩袖缺损（23）肱骨近端不愈合（30）	27.5 个月	63.5°/118°
Mulieri 等[7]（2010）	60	无关节炎的肩袖损伤	52 个月	53°/134°
Klein 等[10]（2010）	143	肩袖缺损：肩胛盂正常（87）肩胛盂磨损（56）	30.9 个月	67°/140°

注：评价采用 Constant 肩关节评分或 ASES 肩关节疼痛和功能障碍评分。

表 31-1

肩袖缺损行反肩关节置换的研究（续）

术前/术后外展角度	术前/术后外旋角度	术前/术后功能评分	并发症（病例数）
–	6°/3°	31/85（Constant 肩关节评分）	创伤性肩胛盂侧松动（1），肩胛下撞击（10），脱位（1），术后静脉炎（1），术后血肿（1）
–	3.5°/11.2°	22.6/65.6（Constant 肩关节评分）	肩胛盂侧松动（5），肩胛盂侧假体组件分离（7），假体失效（3），肩胛下撞击（49），感染（1）
–	–	–/60（Constant 肩关节评分）	假体失效（1），肩胛下撞击（12）
–/140°	–	–/67（Constant 肩关节评分）	反球松动（1），聚乙烯衬垫磨损（1），深部感染（2），反射性交感神经营养不良（1），肩胛下撞击（13）
–	–	–/>30（Constant 肩关节评分）（72 个月时的假体存活率为 88%，120 个月时的假体存活率为 58%）	感染（3），脱位（3），肩胛盂侧松动（3）
–	8°/6°	23/60（Constant 肩关节评分）	脱位（15），感染（8），肩胛盂骨折（1），肱骨骨折（1），有症状的假体刺激（1），肌皮神经麻痹（1），桡神经麻痹（1），反球松动（1），肩胛盂基座松动（1）
87°/145°	12°/19°	34/70（Constant 肩关节评分）	感染（1），血肿（1）
63°/111°	–	38/78（Constant 肩关节评分）	没有报道
–/118°	15°/17°	–/83（Constant 肩关节评分）	–
–/102°	34°/31°	–/61（Constant 肩关节评分）	–
–	5°/11°	24/62（Constant 肩关节评分）	22% 的并发症发生率
–	–/7°	–/53（Constant 肩关节评分）	不稳定（4），肱骨骨折（2），肩峰骨折（1）
–	–/11°	–/60（Constant 肩关节评分）	
41.4°/101.8°	12°/41.1°	34.3/68.2（ASES 肩关节疼痛和功能障碍评分）	肩胛骨骨折（1），肩峰骨折（2），假体失效（1），感染（2），肱骨侧假体分离（1），基座失效（8）
61°/109.5°	13.4°/28.2°	30/77.6（ASES 肩关节疼痛和功能障碍评分）	脱位（2），创伤性脱位（2），创伤性肩峰骨折（1），感染（2），血肿（1），肩胛盂侧松动（1）
49°/125°	27°/51°	33/75（ASES 肩关节疼痛和功能障碍评分）	肱骨近端骨折（1），基座失效（4），中心螺钉断裂（1），深部感染（1），血肿（1），肩峰骨折（2），肩胛体骨折（1），脱位（1）
65°/126°	19.8°/49°	39.1/79.1（ASES 肩关节疼痛和功能障碍评分）	肩峰骨折（2），肱骨骨折（1），感染（2）

表 31-2

反肩关节置换治疗肱骨近端骨折的研究

研究发表（年份）	病例数	平均随访时间	术后活动范围 前屈角度
Bufquin 等[48]（2007）	43	22 个月	97°
Klein 等[53]（2008）	20	33 个月	122°
Gallinet 等[54]（2009）	16	12 个月	98°
Cazeneuve 和 Cristofari[55]（2010）	36	6.6 年	–
Lenarz 等[56]（2011）	30	23 个月	139°

注：评价采用 Constant 肩关节评分或 ASES 肩关节疼痛和功能障碍评分。

表 31-2

反肩关节置换治疗肱骨近端骨折的研究（续）

术后活动范围

外展角度	外旋	术后功能评分	并发症（病例数）
86°	30°	44（Constant 肩关节评分）	神经损伤（5），反射性交感神经营养不良（3），脱位（1），肩胛盂骨折（1），肩峰骨折（1），三角肌前间隙裂开（1）
113°	25°	68（ASES 肩关节疼痛和功能障碍评分）68（Constant 肩关节评分）	复发性脱位（1），感染（2）
–	9°	53（Constant 肩关节评分）	深部感染（1），表浅感染（1），反射性交感神经营养不良（1）
–	–	53（Constant 肩关节）	反射性交感神经营养不良（2），感染（1），脱位（4），基座松动（1）
–	27°	78（ASES 疼痛和功能障碍评分）	复杂性区域疼痛综合征、深静脉血栓形成和结节吸收（1）

注：评价采用 Constant 肩关节评分或 ASES 肩关节疼痛和功能障碍评分。

表 31-3

反肩关节置换治疗类风湿关节炎的研究

研究发表（年份）	病例数	平均随访时间	术前 / 术后活动范围 前屈角度
Rittmiester 等[29]（2001）	7	54 个月	–
Young 等[36]（2011）	18	3.8 年	78° /139°
Holcomb 等[46]（2010）	21	36 个月	52° /126°

注：评价采用 Constant 肩关节评分或 ASES 肩关节疼痛和功能障碍评分。

表 31-3

反肩关节置换治疗类风湿关节炎的研究（续）

术前 / 术后活动范围

外展角度	外旋角度	术前 / 术后功能评分	并发症（病例数）
–	–	17/63（Constant 肩关节评分）	翻修（3），肩胛盂侧假体松动（2），肩峰切开复位内固定失败（1）
–	17° /46°	22/64.9（Constant 肩关节评分）	肩峰骨折（1），肩胛冈骨折（1），喙突骨折（1），大结节撕脱（2），短暂性腋神经麻痹（1）
55° /116°	19° /33°	28/82（ASES 肩关节疼痛和功能障碍评分）	肩胛盂假体周围骨折（1），感染（2），肩胛冈骨折（1），术中肩胛盂骨折（1），影像学可见的基座松动（1）

注：评价采用 Constant 肩关节评分或 ASES 肩关节疼痛和功能障碍评分。

表 31-4

反肩关节置换翻修术的相关研究

研究发表（年份）	病例数	手术和（或）原发疾病（病例数）	平均随访时间	术前/术后活动范围 前屈角度
内侧旋转中心假体				
Werner 等[24]（2005）	58	原发性肩袖损伤关节置换（17） 关节置换翻修（41） 原发性肩袖损伤关节置换（17）	38 个月	42°/100°
Boileau 等[21]（2006）	45	半肩关节置换术后翻修（19） 骨折并发症翻修（7）	40 个月	55°/121°
Melis 等[57]（2012）	37	全肩关节置换转为反肩关节置换	47 个月	68°/121°
外侧旋转中心假体				
Levy 等[17]（2007）	19	半肩关节置换术后翻修	35 个月	49.7°/76.1°
Werner 等[24]（2005）	29	半肩关节置换术后翻修 肩袖缺如（70）	35 个月	38.1°/72.7°
Cuff 等[19]（2008）	96	关节置换后肩袖缺如（23） 肱骨近端不愈合（3）	27.5 个月	63.5°/118°
Holcomb 等[58]（2009）	14	反肩关节置换	33 个月	51°/118°
Chacon 等[18]（2009）	25	异体骨移植的半肩关节置换术后翻修	30 个月	33°/82°
Walker 等[50]（2012）	22	全肩关节置换失败后的翻修	40 个月	50°/130°

表 31-4

反肩关节置换翻修术的相关研究（续）

术前/术后活动范围 外展	外旋	术前/术后结果评分	并发症（病例数）
43°/90°	17°/12°	18/56（Constant 肩关节评分）	总发生率（50%），再手术率（33%） 血肿（12），脱位（5），感染（1），神经损伤（1），肩胛侧松动（3），肱骨柄松动（1），肩胛骨骨折（4），聚乙烯衬垫脱位（1）
	7°/11°	17/58（Constant 肩关节评分）	脱位（3），深部感染（3），无菌性肱骨侧松动（1），肱骨侧假体周围骨折（2），术中肩胛盂骨折（1），伤口血肿（1），肩峰骨折（2），腋神经麻痹（1）
		24/55（Constant 肩关节评分）	肩胛盂侧松动（3），不稳定（3），肱骨侧下沉（2），感染（2），血肿（1）
外侧旋转中心假体			
42.2°/77.2°		29.1/61.2（ASES 肩关节疼痛和功能障碍评分）	聚乙烯失效（2），肱骨侧假体周围骨折（1），肱骨侧松动（2），肩胛侧假体周围骨折（2），基座松动（2），感染（1），血肿（1）
34.1°/70.4°	11.2°/17.6°	22.3/52.1（ASES 肩关节疼痛和功能障碍评分）	假体周围骨折（1），聚乙烯断裂（4），聚乙烯脱位（1），脱位（4），感染（1），基座失效/螺钉断裂（1），肱骨柄松动（1），桡神经麻痹（1）
61°/109.5°	13.4°/28.2°	30/77.6（ASES 肩关节疼痛和功能障碍评分）	脱位（2），创伤性脱位（2），创伤性肩峰骨折（1），感染（2），血肿（1），肩胛盂侧松动（1）
38°/112°	8°/22°	23/70（ASES 肩关节疼痛和功能障碍评分）	肩胛盂侧失效（1），脱位（1），血肿（1）
40°/82°	10°/18°	32/69（ASES 肩关节疼痛和功能障碍评分）	复发性不稳定（1），肩峰骨折（1），异体骨骨折（1），异体骨和聚乙烯断裂（1）
45°/100°	12.5°/49.5°	38.5/67.5（ASES 肩关节疼痛和功能障碍评分）	肩胛骨骨折（1），肩峰骨折（1），脱位（1），肩胛盂侧松动（1），肩胛盂侧和肱骨侧松动（1）

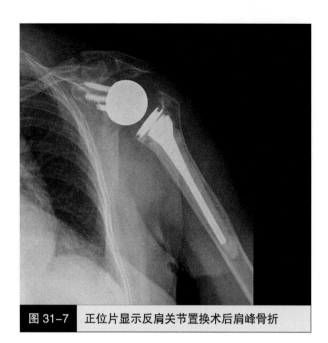

图31-7　正位片显示反肩关节置换术后肩峰骨折

能需要分期进行关节盂重建。

　　术中肱骨骨折可能由于对肱骨施加了过大的扭矩或使用了压配型假体所致。如果骨骼系统整体骨质下降，必须注意避免暴露期间肱骨过度旋转。由于骨折也可能发生在肱骨髓腔扩髓时，因此首选手动扩髓。骨折应在插入肱骨侧假体之前用钢丝环扎固定，用或不用钢板均可。也可以考虑使用长柄假体。

神经损伤

　　文献报道反肩关节置换术后有1%~4%的患者出现神经功能障碍，通常是暂时性的。术中对臂丛神经的牵拉，特别是在显露肩胛盂时以及延长上臂以维持三角肌张力时，都可能引起神经损伤。一篇文献报道，在191例反肩关节置换患者中，有1例肌皮神经损伤患者和1例桡神经麻痹患者。[23]一篇文献报道，在16例行反肩关节置换的类风湿关节炎患者中，有1例短暂性腋神经麻痹患者。[36]其他大量研究也报道了反肩关节置换术后神经损伤较罕见，但亚临床神经损伤的发生率可能相对较高。文献报道，采用解剖型肩关节置换和半肩关节置换时，术中神经损伤的发生率高达57%。[51]19例患者中有9例反肩关节置

换术后4周内出现肌电图改变。[52]反肩关节置换术后出现急性神经损伤的风险是全肩关节置换的10.9倍。绝大多数为腋神经损伤，9例肌电图改变的患者中有8例在6个月内完全恢复。

其他并发症

　　文献报道，反肩关节置换术后相对少见的并发症包括肱骨侧假体松动、假体周围骨折、反球分离、聚乙烯衬垫分离和聚乙烯衬垫碎裂等。

未来方向

　　反肩关节置换是一种相对较新的治疗由不同病因导致的肩袖损伤的方法。现有的随访数据仅限于中期结果。未来的研究需要确定现有反肩关节假体的长期耐用性，以及在相对年轻、活动量较大的患者中的耐用性。专注于改进假体设计和手术技术可能会扩大目前反肩关节置换的适应证范围。

参考文献

［1］Grammont PM, Baulot E: Delta shoulder prosthesis for rotator cuff rupture. *Orthopedics* 1993;16(1):65-68.

［2］Boulahia A, Edwards TB, Walch G, Baratta RV: Early results of a reverse design prosthesis in the treatment of arthritis of the shoulder in elderly patients with a large rotator cuff tear. *Orthopedics* 2002;25(2):129-133.

［3］Nyffeler RW, Werner CM, Gerber C: Biomechanical relevance of glenoid component positioning in the reverse Delta III total shoulder prosthesis. *J Shoulder Elbow Surg* 2005;14(5):524-528.

［4］Gutiérrez S, Comiskey CA IV, Luo Z-P, Pupello DR, Frankle MA: Range of impingement-free abduction and adduction deficit after reverse shoulder arthroplasty: Hierarchy of surgical and implant-design- related factors. *J Bone Joint Surg Am* 2008;90(12):2606-2615.
A virtual computer model of RSA was used to evaluate five surgical and implant-related factors and their effect on abduction-adduction. A lateral center of rotation resulted in the largest impingement-free abduction motion, followed by an inferior glenosphere placement, an inferior glenosphere tilt, a varus humeral neckshaft angle, and glenosphere size.

[5] Gutiérrez S, Levy JC, Lee WE III, Keller TS, Maitland ME: Center of rotation affects abduction range of motion of reverse shoulder arthroplasty. *Clin Orthop Relat Res* 2007;458:78-82.

The effects of glenosphere center of rotation on abduction motion in RSA were biomechanically evaluated using an electronic goniometer and digital video analysis of a model. There is a positive lineal correlation between glenosphere offset and abduction range of motion.

[6] Cuff DJ, Virani NA, Levy J, et al: The treatment of deep shoulder infection and glenohumeral instability with debridement, reverse shoulder arthroplasty and postoperative antibiotics. *J Bone Joint Surg Br* 2008;90(3):336-342.

Deep shoulder infection was treated in 21 patients (22 shoulders) using débridement, RSA, and antibiotics. At a mean 43-month follow-up, there was no evidence of recurrent infection, and patients had improvement in range of motion and in all measured outcomes. Outcomes of single-stage and two-stage procedures did not differ. Level of evidence: IV.

[7] Mulieri P, Dunning P, Klein S, Pupello D, Frankle M: Reverse shoulder arthroplasty for the treatment of irreparable rotator cuff tear without glenohumeral arthritis. *J Bone Joint Surg Am* 2010;92(15):2544-2556.

Irreparable cuff tear without arthritis was treated with RSA in 69 patients (72 shoulders). At a minimum 2-year follow-up, 60 shoulders had significant improvement in range of motion in all planes and im- proved pain and function scores. Level of evidence: IV.

[8] Favard L, Levigne C, Nerot C, Gerber C, De Wilde L, Mole D: Reverse prostheses in arthropathies with cuff tear: Are survivorship and function maintained over time? *Clin Orthop Relat Res* 2011;469(9):2469-2475. In 464 patients at a minimum 2-year follow-up after

RSA and 148 patients at a minimum 5-year follow-up, there were 107 complications. Survivorship at 10 years was 89% with revision as an end point and was 72% with a Constant score lower than 30 as the end point. Despite the low 10-year revision rate, radiographic and outcome deterioration occurred over time. Caution is warranted when RSA is considered for younger patients. Level of evidence: IV.

[9] Melis B, DeFranco M, Lädermann A, et al: An evaluation of the radiological changes around the Grammont reverse geometry shoulder arthroplasty after eight to 12 years. *J Bone Joint Surg Br* 2011;93(9):1240-1246.

A multicenter study with a mean 9.6-year follow-up evaluated radiographic changes in 68 RSAs. Scapular notching was observed in 88% of patients and was associated with a superolateral approach. Glenoid lucency was observed in 16% of patients. Stem subsidence was more common after cemented than uncemented RSA. Stress shielding and tuberosity resorption were more common in uncemented components.

[10] Klein SM, Dunning P, Mulieri P, Pupello D, Downes K, Frankle MA: Effects of acquired glenoid bone defects on surgical technique and clinical outcomes in reverse shoulder arthroplasty. *J Bone Joint Surg Am* 2010;92(5):1144-1154.

Acquired glenoid bone defects treated with RSA in 56 patients were compared with normal glenoids in 87 patients to detect any difference in clinical outcome. At 2-year follow-up, there were no graft failures or resorption; five complications and one unsatisfactory result occurred. Level of evidence: IV.

[11] Kempton LB, Ankerson E, Wiater JM: A complication-based learning curve from 200 reverse shoulder arthroplasties. *Clin Orthop Relat Res* 2011;469(9):2496-2504.

In 200 consecutive RSAs performed by one surgeon, shoulder-related complications occurred in 23.1% of the first 40 patients and 6.5% of the remaining 160 patients. After revision surgery, the local complication rate was 17.5%, compared with 7.9% after primary surgery. Level of evidence: IV.

[12] Frankle M, Siegal S, Pupello D, Saleem A, Mighell M, Vasey M: The Reverse Shoulder Prosthesis for glenohumeral arthritis associated with severe rotator cuff deficiency: A minimum two-year follow-up study of sixty patients. *J Bone Joint Surg Am* 2005;87(8):1697-1705.

[13] Boileau P, Moineau G, Roussanne Y, O'Shea K: Bony increased-offset reversed shoulder arthroplasty: Minimizing scapular impingement while maximizing glenoid fixation. *Clin Orthop Relat Res* 2011;469(9):2558-2567.

In a prospective study, 42 patients with rotator cuff deficiency were treated with bony increased-offset RSA to reduce notching and prosthetic instability. At a mean 28-month follow-up, the graft was completely incorporated in 98% of patients, with no graft resorption, glenoid failure, or prosthetic instability. Level of evidence: IV.

[14] Simovitch RW, Zumstein MA, Lohri E, Helmy N, Gerber C: Predictors of scapular notching in patients managed with the Delta III reverse total shoulder replacement. *J Bone Joint Surg Am* 2007;89(3):588-600.

In 76 patients (77 shoulders) treated with RSA, inferior notching occurred in 44%, posterior notching in 30%, and anterior notching in 8%. Inferior notching was associated with significantly poorer clinical outcome and can be avoided with optimal positioning of the glenosphere. Level of evidence: II.

[15] Guery J, Favard L, Sirveaux F, Oudet D, Mole D, Walch G: Reverse total shoulder arthroplasty: Survivorship analysis of eighty replacements followed for five to ten years. *J Bone Joint Surg Am* 2006;88(8):1742-1747.

[16] Levy J, Frankle M, Mighell M, Pupello D: The use of the reverse shoulder prosthesis for the treatment of failed hemiarthroplasty for proximal humeral fracture. *J Bone Joint Surg Am* 2007;89(2):292-300.

In 29 patients, revision to an RSA was required after unsuccessful hemiarthroplasty for proximal humeral fracture. Pain and function scores improved. Forward elevation improved from 38° to 73°, and abduction improved from 34° to 70°. The complication rate was 28%. Level of evidence: IV.

[17] Levy JC, Virani N, Pupello D, Frankle M: Use of the reverse shoulder prosthesis for the treatment of failed hemiarthroplasty in patients with glenohumeral arthritis and rotator cuff deficiency. *J Bone Joint Surg Br* 2007;89(2):189-195.

In 18 patients (19 shoulders) who underwent RSA after unsuccessful hemiarthroplasty with rotator cuff deficiency and joint arthritis, pain and functional outcomes significantly improved. Mean flexion improved by 26°, and abduction improved by 35°. The complication rate was 32%, mostly associated with severe glenoid or proximal humeral bone loss. Level of evidence: IV.

[18] Chacon A, Virani N, Shannon R, Levy JC, Pupello D, Frankle M: Revision arthroplasty with use of a reverse shoulder prosthesis-allograft composite. *J Bone Joint Surg Am* 2009;91(1):119-127.

In 25 patients with mean proximal humeral bone loss of 53.6 mm (range, 34.5 to 150.3 mm) who were treated using a revision prosthesis-allograft composite, pain and function scores were significantly improved at a minimum 2-year follow-up. Forward elevation, abduction, and internal rotation significantly improved. Nineteen patients had a good or excellent result, 5 had a satisfactory result, and 1 reported an unsatisfactory result. Level of evidence: IV.

[19] Cuff D, Pupello D, Virani N, Levy J, Frankle M: Reverse shoulder arthroplasty for the treatment of rotator cuff deficiency. *J Bone Joint Surg Am* 2008;90(6): 1244-1251.

In 112 patients (114 shoulders) treated with RSA for rotator cuff deficiency, pain and function scores had significantly improved at a minimum 2-year follow-up. Blinded range-of-motion analysis showed significantly improved motion in all planes, including external rotation. Fifty-five percent of patients had an excellent result, 27% had a good result, 12% had a satisfactory result, and 6% had an unsatisfactory result. Level of evidence: IV.

[20] Valenti P, Sauzières P, Katz D, Kalouche I, Kilinc AS: Do less medialized reverse shoulder prostheses increase motion and reduce notching? *Clin Orthop Relat Res* 2011;469(9):2550-2557.

In 76 patients treated with a lateral offset RSA for pseudoparalytic shoulder with rotator cuff deficiency, Constant scores had improved from 24 to 59 at a minimum 24-month follow-up. Active elevation improved by 61°, external rotation at the side improved by 15°, and external rotation with 90° of abduction improved by 30°. Level of evidence: IV.

[21] Boileau P, Watkinson D, Hatzidakis AM, Hovorka I: Neer Award 2005: The Grammont reverse shoulder prosthesis: Results in cuff tear arthritis, fracture sequelae, and revision arthroplasty. *J Shoulder Elbow Surg* 2006;15(5):527-540.

[22] Simovitch RW, Helmy N, Zumstein MA, Gerber C: Impact of fatty infiltration of the teres minor muscle on the outcome of reverse total shoulder arthroplasty. *J Bone Joint Surg Am* 2007;89(5):934-939.

In 42 patients treated with RSA for rotator cuff deficiency or cuff tear arthropathy, Goutallier stage 3 or 4 fatty infiltration led to significantly lower Constant scores and Subjective Shoulder Value (SSV) scores, as well as significantly less external rotation and a lower score for extremity positioning. Level of evidence: II.

[23] Wall B, Nové-Josserand L, O'Connor DP, Edwards TB, Walch G: Reverse total shoulder arthroplasty: A review of results according to etiology. *J Bone Joint Surg Am* 2007;89(7):1476-1485.

Outcome based on etiology was evaluated in 232 patients (240 shoulders) at a minimum 2-year follow-up after RSA. The results were good for several pathologies, but patients who underwent revision arthroplasty or had posttraumatic arthritis had less improvement and higher complication rates. Level of evidence: II.

[24] Werner CM, Steinmann PA, Gilbart M, Gerber C: Treatment of painful pseudoparesis due to irreparable rotator cuff dysfunction with the Delta III reverse-ball-and-socket total shoulder prosthesis. *J Bone Joint Surg Am* 2005;87(7):1476-1486.

[25] Boileau P, Watkinson DJ, Hatzidakis AM, Balg F: Grammont reverse prosthesis: Design, rationale, and biomechanics. *J Shoulder Elbow Surg* 2005;14(1, Suppl S):147S-161S.

[26] Norris TR, Kelly JD, Humphrey CS: Management of glenoid bone defects in revision shoulder arthroplasty: A new application of the reverse total shoulder prosthesis. *Tech Shoulder Elbow Surg* 2007;8:37-46.

A technique is described for a single-stage reconstruction for RSA using iliac crest bone graft for glenoid bone defects.

[27] Gutiérrez S, Keller TS, Levy JC, Lee WE III, Luo Z-P: Hierarchy of stability factors in reverse shoulder arthroplasty. *Clin Orthop Relat Res* 2008;466(3):670-676.

A biomechanical study assessed the hierarchy of stability factors by evaluating the force required to dislocate the humerosocket from the glenosphere in eight commercially available reverse shoulder prostheses. The most important factor was joint compressive force, followed by socket depth and glenosphere size.

[28] Terrier A, Reist A, Merlini F, Farron A: Simulated joint and muscle forces in reversed and anatomic shoulder prostheses. *J Bone Joint Surg Br* 2008;90(6):751-756.

A finite element model was used to compare joint forces in reversed and anatomic prostheses. With the reversed prosthesis, abduction was possible without rotator cuff muscles and required 20% less deltoid force to achieve. The mechanical advantage of RSA in cuff deficiency was thus confirmed.

[29] Rittmeister M, Kerschbaumer F: Grammont reverse total shoulder arthroplasty in patients with rheumatoid arthritis and nonreconstructible rotator cuff lesions. *J Shoulder Elbow Surg* 2001;10(1):17-22.

[30] Delloye C, Joris D, Colette A, Eudier A, Dubuc JE: [Mechanical complications of total shoulder inverted prosthesis]. *Rev Chir Orthop Reparatrice Appar Mot* 2002;88(4):410-414.

[31] Frankle MA, Siegal S, Pupello DR, Gutierrez S, Griewe M, Mighell M: Coronal plane tilt angle affects risk of catastrophic failure in patients treated with a reverse shoulder prosthesis. *J Shoulder Elbow Surg* 2007;16:e46.

Coronal tilt was evaluated in 262 patients treated with RSA to determine whether there was a correlation between tilt angle and baseplate fixation failure. Patients with a superior-tilted baseplate were at a greater risk of catastrophic mechanical failure.

[32] Seebauer L, Walter W, Keyl W: Reverse total shoulder arthroplasty for the treatment of defect arthropathy. *Oper Orthop Traumatol* 2005;17(1):1-24.

[33] Sirveaux F, Favard L, Oudet D, Huquet D, Walch G, Molé D: Grammont inverted total shoulder arthroplasty in the treatment of glenohumeral osteoarthritis with massive rupture of the cuff: Results of a multicentre study of 80 shoulders. *J Bone Joint Surg Br* 2004;86(3):388-395.

[34] Gutiérrez S, Walker M, Willis M, Pupello DR, Frankle MA: Effects of tilt and glenosphere eccentricity on baseplate/bone interface forces in a computational model, validated by a mechanical model, of reverse shoulder arthroplasty. *J Shoulder Elbow Surg* 2011;20(5):732-739.

The forces at the bone-baseplate interface in concentric and eccentric glenospheres, as well as the effect of tilt on these forces, were biomechanically evaluated. For lateralized and concentric glenospheres, inferior tilt provided the most even distribution of forces, and a superior tilt provided the most uneven distribution. For eccentric glenospheres, an inferior tilt provided a more uneven distribution of forces than a neutral tilt.

[35] Harman M, Frankle M, Vasey M, Banks S: Initial glenoid component fixation in "reverse" total shoulder arthroplasty: A biomechanical evaluation. *J Shoulder Elbow Surg* 2005;14(1, Suppl S):162S-167S.

[36] Young AA, Smith MM, Bacle G, Moraga C, Walch G: Early results of reverse shoulder arthroplasty in patients with rheumatoid arthritis. *J Bone Joint Surg Am* 2011;93(20):1915-1923.

Sixteen patients (18 shoulders) with rheumatoid arthritis and rotator cuff deficiency were treated with RSA and followed for a mean 3.8 years. Patients had significant improvement in functional outcome scores and range of motion. Scapular notching was observed in 10 of 18 shoulders. There was no component loosening or revision. Level of evidence: IV.

[37] Lévigne C, Boileau P, Favard L, et al: Scapular notching in reverse shoulder arthroplasty. *J Shoulder Elbow Surg* 2008;17(6):925-935.

At an average 47-month follow-up (range, 24 to 120 months), notching occurred in 62% of 326 consecutive patients (337 shoulders) treated with RSA and was more common with preoperative cuff tear arthropathy, grade 3 or 4 fatty infiltration of the infraspinatus, narrowed acromiohumeral distance, and superiorly oriented glenoids. Glenosphere placement influences notching; superior positioning and superior tilting should be avoided.

[38] Frankle MA, Teramoto A, Luo Z-P, Levy JC, Pupello D: Glenoid morphology in reverse shoulder arthroplasty: Classification and surgical implications. *J Shoulder Elbow Surg* 2009;18(6):874-885.

The morphology of 216 glenoids was evaluated with CT, and the effect on possible glenoid component fixation was determined. The subjects were graded on the presence of an abnormality, with subclassification based on location of erosions. The standard centerline was significantly shorter in abnormal glenoids, and the peripheral screw placement area was reduced by 42%.

[39] Neyton L, Boileau P, Nové-Josserand L, Edwards TB, Walch G: Glenoid bone grafting with a reverse design prosthesis. *J Shoulder Elbow Surg* 2007;16(3, Suppl): S71-S78.

Nine patients treated with RSA required glenoid bone grafting for bone loss. Most patients were satisfied and had pain relief despite low Constant scores. There was no glenoid component loosening or graft failure at a minimum 2-year follow-up, but six patients had inferior notching. Level of evidence: IV.

[40] Cuff D, Levy JC, Gutiérrez S, Frankle MA: Torsional stability of modular and nonmodular reverse shoulder humeral components in a proximal humeral bone loss model. *J Shoulder Elbow Surg* 2011;20(4):646-651.

Modular and nonmodular reverse humeral stem designs were evaluated biomechanically in the setting of proximal humeral bone loss compared with the intact humerus. The proximal bone loss constructs had significantly greater rotational micromotion. Two of 12 intact humerus constructs failed testing, and 5 of 12 bone loss constructs failed; all 7 were modular humeral designs.

[41] Boileau P, Chuinard C, Roussanne Y, Bicknell RT, Rochet N, Trojani C: Reverse shoulder arthroplasty combined with a modified latissimus dorsi and teres major tendon transfer for shoulder pseudoparalysis associated with dropping arm. *Clin Orthop Relat Res* 2008;466(3):584-593.

Eleven consecutive patients with combined loss of active elevation and external rotation were treated with RSA and latissimus dorsi–teres major tendon transfer. Mean active elevation improved from 70° to 148°, and external rotation improved from −18 to 18°. All patients had improvement in Constant scores, subjective assessment, and activities of daily living. Level of evidence: IV.

[42] Boileau P, Chuinard C, Roussanne Y, Neyton L, Trojani C: Modified latissimus dorsi and teres major transfer through a single delto-pectoral approach for external rotation deficit of the shoulder: As an isolated procedure or with a reverse arthroplasty. *J Shoulder Elbow Surg* 2007;16(6):671-682.

Fifteen consecutive patients underwent latissimus dorsi-teres major tendon transfer through a deltopectoral incision (eight were combined with RSA). The mean active elevation improved by 34.7°, and the mean active external rotation improved by 28°. Constant and SSV scores improved, with 14 of 15 patients satisfied or very satisfied with the result.

[43] Boileau P, Rumian AP, Zumstein MA: Reversed shoulder arthroplasty with modified L'Episcopo for combined loss of active elevation and external rotation. *J Shoulder Elbow Surg* 2010;19(2, Suppl): 20-30.

Seventeen consecutive patients underwent RSA combined with latissimus dorsi–teres major tendon transfer for loss of active elevation and external rotation. Mean elevation improved from 74° to 149°, and mean external rotation improved from −21° to 13°. Patient satisfaction, Constant scores, SSV scores, and activities of daily living all improved. Level of evidence: IV.

[44] Gerber C, Pennington SD, Lingenfelter EJ, Sukthankar A: Reverse Delta-III total shoulder replacement combined with latissimus dorsi transfer: A preliminary report. *J Bone Joint Surg Am* 2007;89(5):940-947.

Eleven patients (12 shoulders) underwent RSA combined with latissimus dorsi transfer for loss of active elevation and external rotation. Mean elevation improved from 94° to 139°. External rotation improved only from 12° to 19°, but functional external rotation improved on Constant scores. SSV scores and activities of daily living also significantly improved. Level of evidence: IV.

[45] Vanhove B, Beugnies A: Grammont's reverse shoulder prosthesis for rotator cuff arthropathy: A retrospective study of 32 cases. *Acta Orthop Belg* 2004;70(3):219-225.

[46] Holcomb JO, Hebert DJ, Mighell MA, et al: Reverse shoulder arthroplasty in patients with rheumatoid arthritis. *J Shoulder Elbow Surg* 2010;19(7):1076-1084.

RSA was performed in 21 patients with rheumatoid arthritis. Outcome scores, pain, and range of motion improved postoperatively. Severe glenoid erosion occurred in 10 shoulders, 5 of which required structural grafting. Reoperation was required for infection in 2 patients and periprosthetic fracture in 1 patient. Level of evidence: IV.

[47] Molé D, Favard L: [Excentered scapulohumeral osteoarthritis]. *Rev Chir Orthop Reparatrice Appar Mot* 2007;93(6, Suppl):37-94.

A fracture of the acromion occurred in 16 of 527 patients who underwent RSA (3%). The risk factors included a deltopectoral approach and high tension of the deltoid caused by excessive lateralization and hu- meral lengthening. Level of evidence: IV.

[48] Bufquin T, Hersan A, Hubert L, Massin P: Reverse shoulder arthroplasty for the treatment of three- and four-part fractures of the proximal humerus in the elderly: A prospective review of 43 cases with a short-term follow-up. *J Bone Joint Surg Br* 2007;89(4):516-520.

The 43 patients treated with RSA for proximal humerus fracture had good range of motion and functional scores despite tuberosity healing in only 58%. There was a 28% complication rate. Level of evidence: IV.

[49] Walch G, Mottier F, Wall B, Boileau P, Molé D, Favard L: Acromial insufficiency in reverse shoulder arthroplasties. *J Shoulder Elbow Surg* 2009;18(3):495-502.

Of 457 patients treated with RSA, 41 had preoperative acromial insufficiencies that were not found to contraindicate RSA. Patients with postoperative scapular spine fracture had a worse outcome. Level of evidence: III.

[50] Crosby LA, Hamilton A, Twiss T: Scapula fractures after reverse total shoulder arthroplasty: Classification and treatment. *Clin Orthop Relat Res* 2011;469(9):2544-2549.

Forty of 400 patients had acromial fracture after RSA. The authors proposed a classification and recommended treatment. Because a scapular spine fracture (type III) is likely to have a relatively poor result, open reduction and internal fixation is recommended. Level of evidence: II.

[51] Nagda SH, Rogers KJ, Sestokas AK, et al: Neer Award 2005:Peripheral nerve function during shoulder arthroplasty using intraoperative nerve monitoring. *J Shoulder Elbow Surg* 2007;16(3, Suppl):S2-S8.

Continuous intraoperative monitoring of the brachial plexus was done in 30 consecutive patients undergoing shoulder arthroplasty. Seventeen (57%) patients had episodes of nerve dysfunction during surgery. Of the 7 patients whose intraoperative nerve dysfunction did not return to normal with repositioning, 4 had electromyographic abnormalities at 4 weeks.

[52] Lädermann A, Lübbeke A, Mélis B, et al: Prevalence of neurologic lesions after total shoulder arthroplasty. *J Bone Joint Surg Am* 2011;93(14):1288-1293.

The correlation of neurologic injury with lengthening of the arm after RSA was evaluated in a comparison of patients treated with RSA with 23 patients treated with anatomic TSA. Postoperative electromyography showed evidence of neurologic lesions in 9 of 19 patients with RSA and 1 of 23 patients with TSA, although the lesions usually were transient. The mean lengthening of the arm in patients with RSA was 2.7 cm (± 1.8 cm).

[53] Klein M, Juschka M, Hinkenjann B, Scherger B, Ostermann PA: Treatment of comminuted fractures of the proximal humerus in elderly patients with the Delta III reverse shoulder prosthesis. *J Orthop Trauma* 2008;22(10):698-704.

Twenty patients treated with RSA for acute proximal humeral fracture were evaluated based on clinical and radiographic outcome. Good outcomes were attain- able at a mean 33-month follow-up. Level of evidence: IV.

[54] Gallinet D, Clappaz P, Garbuio P, Tropet Y, Obert L: Three or four parts complex proximal humerus fractures: Hemiarthroplasty versus reverse prosthesis. A comparative study of 40 cases. *Orthop Traumatol Surg Res* 2009;95(1):48-55.

Twenty-one patients treated with hemiarthroplasty for proximal humeral fracture were compared with 19 patients treated with RSA. Elevation and abduction range of motion and Constant scores were better after RSA, and internal and external rotation were better after hemiarthroplasty. There were 3 abnormal tuberosity fixations with hemiarthroplasty, and 15 of 19 patients had notching with RSA. Level of evidence: IV.

[55] Cazeneuve JF, Cristofari DJ: The reverse shoulder prosthesis in the treatment of fractures of the proximal humerus in the elderly. *J Bone Joint Surg Br* 2010;92(4):535-539.

In 36 patients with proximal humeral fracture treated with RSA and followed for a mean 6.6 years, Constant scores declined with longer follow-up, and 63% had radiographic evidence of notching, with development over time. One patient had aseptic loosening at 12- year follow-up. Level of evidence: IV.

[56] Lenarz C, Shishani Y, McCrum C, Nowinski RJ, Edwards TB, Gobezie R: Is reverse shoulder arthroplasty appropriate for the treatment of fractures in the older patient? Early observations. *Clin Orthop Relat Res* 2011;469(12):3324-3331.

In 30 patients treated with RSA for three- or four-part proximal humeral fracture (mean age, 77 years), there were significant improvements in pain and function scores and range of motion at a minimum 12-month follow-up. Three complications were noted. Level of evidence: IV.

[57] Melis B, Bonnevialle N, Neyton L, et al: Glenoid loosening and failure in anatomical total shoulder arthroplasty: Is revision with a reverse shoulder arthroplasty a reliable option? *J Shoulder Elbow Surg* 2012;21(3):342-349.

Thirty-seven patients underwent revision to RSA after unsuccessful TSA. Mean forward elevation improved from 68°to 120° Constant scores improved from 24 to 55. Three patients had postoperative glenoid baseplate loosening, and 3 had instability. Level of evidence: IV.

[58] Holcomb JO, Cuff D, Petersen SA, Pupello DR, Frankle MA: Revision reverse shoulder arthroplasty for glenoid baseplate failure after primary reverse shoulder arthroplasty. *J Shoulder Elbow Surg* 2009;18(5):717-723.

Revision RSA was performed in 14 patients for glenoid baseplate failure after primary RSA. Range-of-motion and American Shoulder and Elbow Surgeons Index scores improved postoperatively, and there were no differences between prefailure and postrevision outcome data. Revision RSA was found to restore pain relief and function to levels obtained after the index RSA. Two patients underwent a second revision RSA because of baseplate failure and dislocation. Level of evidence: IV.

[59] Walker M, Willis MP, Brooks JP, Pupello D, Mulieri PJ, Frankle MA: The use of the reverse shoulder arthroplasty for treatment of failed total shoulder arthroplasty. *J Shoulder Elbow Surg* 2012;21(4):514-522.

Twenty-two patients treated with RSA for unsuccessful TSA were followed for a minimum of 2 years. There were significant improvements in scores on the American Shoulder and Elbow Surgeons Index, Simple Shoulder Test, and visual analog scale as well as range of motion in all planes. Fourteen patients reported an excellent result, 3 a good result, 3 a satisfactory result, and 2 an unsatisfactory result. The overall complication rate was 22.7%. Level of evidence: IV.

第三十二章 反肩关节置换的并发症

Stephanie Muh, MD; Reuben Gobezie, MD

引言

研究者们推测，各种类型肩关节置换术的需求将持续增长。[1] 随着反肩关节置换的适应证范围的扩大，相关的并发症数量也在逐渐增加。文献报道反肩关节置换术后总的并发症发生率为11%~50%，[2-5] 高于传统的一期全肩关节置换术，更高于反肩关节翻修术。[4,6-7] 反肩关节相关的特异性并发症与假体的非解剖型设计、主要用于骨形态解剖异常的患者及术者的反肩关节置换经验水平等有关。若术者关节置换的经验相对较少，患者可能有更高的并发症发生率和死亡率。[8-9] 反肩关节置换相关的并发症包括术中的神经损伤、骨折，术后的感染、肩胛下撞击切迹、肩关节不稳定、肩胛盂基座失效和肩峰应力性骨折等。

术中并发症

神经损伤

文献报道反肩关节置换术后神经损伤的发生率为1%~10%，但通常能自行恢复。[2,10-13] 术中，旋转中心向内和向下移动，可以维持患侧上肢长

Dr. Gobezie or an immediate family member has received royalties from Arthrex; serves as a paid consultant to or is an employee of Arthrex and Tornier; and has received research or institutional support from Arthrex and Tornier. Neither Dr. Muh nor any immediate family member has received anything of value from or has stock or stock options held in a commercial company or institution related directly or indirectly to the subject of this chapter.

度，但也会牵拉臂丛神经。[14-15] 症状的严重程度从一过性的疼痛到永久性麻痹，可能造成肩关节功能严重障碍，特别是腋神经损伤时。

尸体研究发现，神经损伤与其紧张程度有关。[14] 8%的神经延长即可造成坐骨神经的血供减少，15%的牵拉延长可完全阻断血供。反肩关节置换术后臂丛神经承受很大的牵张应变（高达19.3%）。这一研究结果提示反肩关节置换引起的神经延长是导致一些患者臂丛神经损伤的因素之一。

术中牵引、肢体操作和假体的非解剖设计所需的手臂延长，这几个因素共同增高了神经损伤的风险。在一项前瞻性研究中，19例患者行一期反肩关节置换，9例出现亚临床的肌电图改变，主要为腋神经所支配的肌肉。[16] 与解剖型全肩关节置换相比，反肩关节置换术后神经损伤的风险增高了10.9倍。反肩关节置换术后患肢平均延长2.7 cm。但9例神经损伤的患者中有8例在6个月内自行恢复。一项关于肩关节置换术中神经损伤的前瞻性研究发现，56.7%的患者术中出现神经功能障碍或神经警报。[17] 这些神经警报中的大多数（76.7%）在手臂从处理肩胛盂时的极端外旋、过伸、外展或内收位置回到中立位置后，重新回到基线。研究人员得出结论，应尽量避免使手臂处于极端位置和牵开器的使用。

骨折

术中肩胛盂骨折是一种罕见但严重的并发症，与骨锉的使用和假体的植入固定有关。肩胛盂骨折

的常见原因包括在接触肩胛骨之前未启动骨锉，以及磨锉肩胛骨时超过软骨下骨，从而导致骨锉磨掉本应保留的软骨下骨。周围边缘的小骨折通常可以忽略，因为它们对反球基座的稳定固定没有影响。然而，延伸至中央孔的较大关节盂骨折则会造成不良后果。在插入反球之前，必须通过增强的基座固定或植骨来稳定地固定关节盂。如果采用中心螺钉基座设计，螺钉可以重新定位在关节盂内位置，以达到类似的效果。如果不能达到足够的稳定性，反肩关节置换可能需要转为半肩关节置换。

医源性肱骨骨折是最常见的肱骨侧并发症。患者常出现骨质降低，有骨折的危险。通过限制施加在肱骨上的扭矩和在准备过程中始终注意肱骨的位置，特别是当上臂在后伸、内收和外旋位置进行肱骨髓腔扩髓时，可以使风险最小化。治疗肱骨干骨折患者时，应在复位后插入一个长柄肱骨假体。用钢板和环扎钢丝复位固定骨折时，应显露桡神经。

术后并发症

感染

感染是反肩关节置换术后的一类严重并发症。诊断延迟可能引起慢性疼痛、不稳定、功能活动差、脓毒症等，或需要广泛的翻修手术。文献报道，传统全肩关节置换后感染率约为 0.7%，但反肩关节置换相关的感染率为 1%~15%。[3,5,11,18-21] 感染可能与无菌技术、术后血肿形成、手术时间过长和翻修手术等有关。当患者有合并症（如糖尿病、炎症性关节病和其他免疫抑制性疾病）时，感染风险增高。行翻修手术的患者感染风险也增高。

肩关节置换的感染诊断很困难。常见肩部病原体的惰性特征使大部分临床表现无特异性。疼痛常是第一主诉。痤疮丙酸杆菌、表皮葡萄球菌和金黄色葡萄球菌是肩部手术后感染的最常见病原体。[22] 痤疮丙酸杆菌是肩关节置换术后感染的常见病原体[23-24]，这种革兰阳性、耐氧、非芽孢形成的厌氧芽孢杆菌通常存在于健康皮肤和皮脂

腺的潮湿区域（如腋窝）。由于其毒性低，对痤疮丙酸杆菌感染的诊断和治疗很困难。痤疮丙酸杆菌感染患者可能有慢性非特异性主诉，实验室检查结果通常是正常的。标准实验室检查，如 C 反应蛋白（C-reactive protein，CRP）水平、红细胞沉降率（exchangeable sodium ratio，ESR）和白细胞计数，通常无法诊断假体周围感染。

在一项回顾性研究中，19 例肩关节置换患者经证实有假体周围感染，该研究发现最优 ESR 临界值（26 mm/h）检测肩关节置换术感染的敏感性为 32%，特异性为 93%。[25] 最优 CRP 临界值（7 mg/L）的敏感性为 63%，特异性为 73%。研究者认为 ESR 和 CRP 水平对肩关节假体感染的诊断敏感性较差。

新的生化标志物，包括白介素 -6、肿瘤坏死因子 α 和降钙素原 -C，正在作为诊断工具被研究。与传统的术中组织培养相比，超声技术诊断肩关节置换术后感染具有更高的敏感性和与之相似的特异性。[26] 此外，诊断的困难在于微生物需要相对较长的培养期，文献报道培养期平均为 13.3 天（4~21 天）[27]。

围手术期预防感染至关重要。应在建立切口 1 小时内预防性使用围手术期抗生素。使用氯己定消毒液是清除肩部凝固酶阴性葡萄球菌和丙酸杆菌最有效的方法。[28] 手术时长也是感染的一个危险因素。[24] 与无抗生素的骨水泥相比，抗生素骨水泥可降低一期反肩关节置换术后深部感染率。[29] 一些证据表明，与反肩关节置换相关的死腔内血肿形成是感染的一个危险因素。[30] 因此，通过术中细致的止血和术后放置引流管来避免术后血肿形成十分重要。

反肩关节置换术后感染的处理与其他全关节置换术后感染的处理相似。一些作者指出，早期使用微生物特异性抗生素对根除感染具有重要作用。[31] 目前的外科治疗方案包括冲洗和清创、抗生素抑制、一期或分期翻修手术、切除式关节置换术和关节融合术。[32-33] 急性感染（小于 6 周）

可以通过积极清创、静脉注射抗生素和更换聚乙烯衬垫或一期再置换成功治疗。[31,34-35] 对慢性感染（持续时间超过 3 个月）的最佳治疗方法存在争议。关于一期和分期翻修术根除慢性感染的疗效，研究证据是相互冲突的。[31,33-35] 大多数医师的经验是分期翻修，符合下肢关节置换文献的建议。通过分期翻修，包括积极清创、假体取出和放置聚甲基丙烯酸骨水泥间隔物，静脉使用抗生素 6 周后再次植入关节假体，可在功能结果和根除感染方面获得最可重复的结果。[32,36] 切除式关节置换术被用于那些无法手术再植入假体或其他治疗方法失败的患者。切除式关节置换术可较好地缓解疼痛，但限制了术后功能。

肩胛下撞击切迹

肩胛下撞击切迹（scapular notching），第一次被描述于 1997 年，是一个仅与反肩关节置换相关的放射学发现（图 32-1）。肱骨侧组件内侧缘撞击肩胛盂下缘导致肩胛下撞击切迹出现。肩胛下撞击切迹的发生率随假体的设计不同而变化。传统的 Grammont 型反肩关节假体的肩胛下撞击切迹发生率为 19%~96%。[3-5,11,13,37-39] 较新的旋转中心相对外移的反肩关节假体降低了肩胛下撞击切迹的发生率（0~16%）。[18,37,40] 其他因素，如手术入路、反球位置、自体肩胛骨解剖（肩胛颈长度、肩胛盂磨损和肩胛颈角）、假体颈角和患者活动水平，也会造成肩胛下撞击切迹。[39,41-42] 对引起肩胛下撞击的因素进行生物力学研究发现，肱骨组件颈干角相对内翻、反球相对下移和大的反球旋转中心外移是减少撞击的重要因素。[43]

通过肩关节的真实正位（Grashey 位）片来诊断肩胛下撞击切迹。切迹通常发生在术后 6 周至 14 个月。在 Sirveaux 分型中，Ⅰ 级切迹仅限于肩胛下柱，Ⅱ 级切迹与基座下方螺钉接触，Ⅲ 级切迹超过下方螺钉，Ⅳ 级切迹延伸至基座下方并接近中心柱[44]（图 32-2）。肩胛盂内下方骨赘通常伴随肩胛下撞击切迹同时出现（图 32-3）。

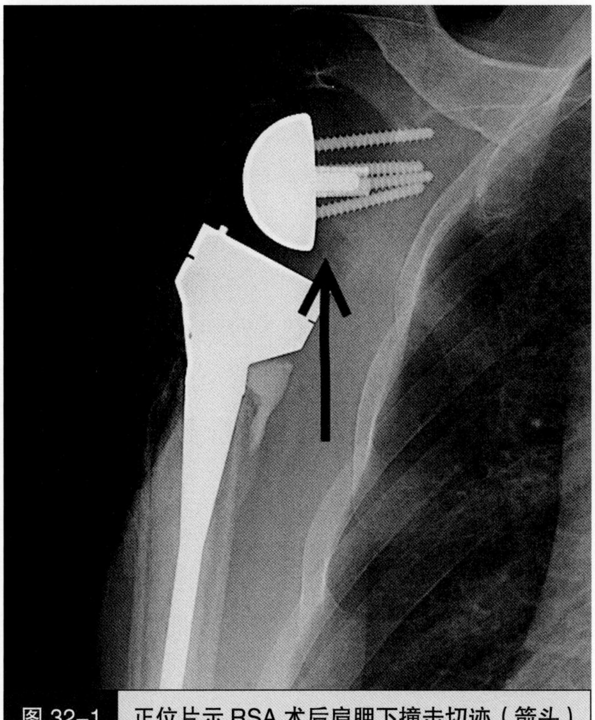

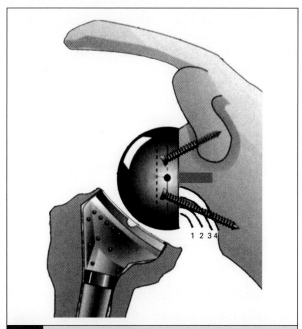

图 32-2　肩胛下撞击切迹的 Sirveaux 分型示意图。经允许引自 Sirveaux F, Favard L, Oudet D, Huquet D, Walch G, Molé D: Grammont inverted total shoulder arthroplasty in the treatment of glenohumeral osteoarthritis with massive rupture of the cuff: Results of a multicentre study of 80 shoulders. *J Bone Joint Surg Br* 2004;86（3）:388-395.

图 32-1　正位片示 RSA 术后肩胛下撞击切迹（箭头）

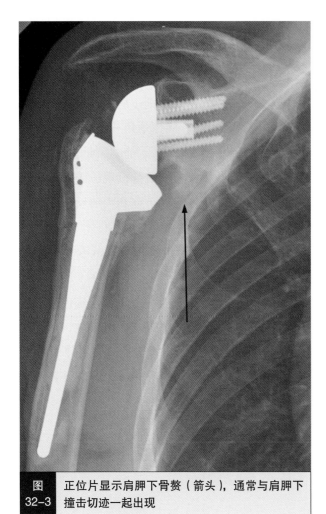

肩胛下撞击切迹的重要性和是否随着时间进展存在争议。肩胛下撞击切迹在术后平均 4.5 个月开始出现，在术后平均第 18 个月时稳定。[42]切迹进展的发生率在术后第 1 年为 48%，第 2 年为 60%，第 3 年为 68%，Ⅲ级和Ⅳ级切迹的发生率随着时间的推移而增高。[38]

肩胛下撞击切迹的影响也一直存在争议。多项研究发现肩胛下撞击切迹与 Constant-Murley 疼痛评分和主动前屈无关。[4-5,39,41]但有研究发现，肩胛下撞击切迹与 Constant-Murley 疼痛评分、主观肩关节值、主动前屈角度和外展角度呈负相关。[2,38,42,44]虽然肩胛下撞击切迹的长期影响还不清楚，但大多数专家认为，手术技术应该避免撞击切迹的出现，通常是将反球尽可能下移。目前已经有旋转中心更偏外的假体和新的肩胛侧假

体外移以避免撞击切迹出现的设计，如 BIO-RSA（Tornier）。新的 BIO-RSA 技术通过将患者肱骨头的自体骨移植到一个带有相对较长中心柱的基座上以实现旋转中心外移。当骨移植愈合后，旋转中心主要位于关节盂骨 - 假体界面。[10]

肩关节不稳定

脱位是反肩关节置换术后最常见的并发症之一，其发生率为 1%~31%[4-6,11,13,15,19-20]。造成不稳定的因素有很多，包括软组织张力、机械撞击、假体型号、近端骨量丢失、假体高度和腋神经功能障碍。反肩关节置换骨折后遗症患者不稳定的发生率比行反肩关节置换的原发性肩袖撕裂性关节病、巨大肩袖撕裂伴假性麻痹、急性骨折或不稳定性关节病患者高。[6]足够的软组织张力对稳定性十分重要。如果患者缺少功能正常的肩袖，必须适当延长三角肌，以增加经过假体的压应力，从而维持稳定性。如果三角肌没有合适的张力，脱位的风险就会增加。[15]通过手术技术，如减少肱骨切除、反球向下倾斜及反球偏心放置，可以使肱骨相对于肩胛骨的位置下移，从而增加三角肌张力，以获得稳定性。通过更大的头颈角外翻、更大的反球直径、外侧偏心和更厚的聚乙烯衬垫等假体设计也可以获得适当的软组织张力。肱骨侧组件与肩胛下方发生机械性撞击引起杠杆作用，是一个不太常见的肩关节不稳定原因，往往与肩胛侧假体位置过高有关。肩关节不稳定的另一个可能的危险因素与肩胛下肌腱的状态有关。最近的一些研究发现，与肩胛下肌腱可修复的患者相比，手术时肩胛下肌腱功能不全患者的不稳定率更高，但另一项研究发现肩胛下肌腱功能不全对脱位风险没有显著影响。[6,45-46]

大多数脱位发生在后伸、内收和内旋时，即手放在背后的位置时，脱位的方向是前脱位（图 32-4，32-5）。大多数患者的假体脱位可通过闭合复位来治疗。假体复位后，应在 X 线透视下检查肩关节，以确定机械性撞击是否是肩关节不稳定

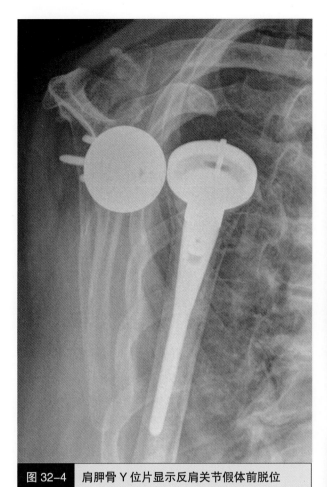

图 32-4　肩胛骨 Y 位片显示反肩关节假体前脱位

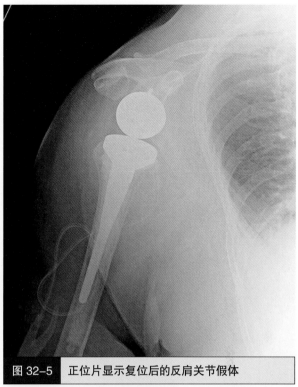

图 32-5　正位片显示复位后的反肩关节假体

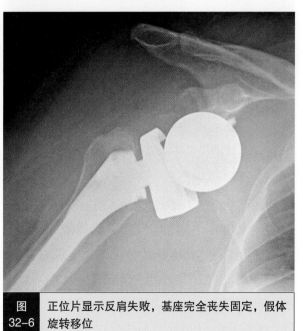

图 32-6　正位片显示反肩失败，基座完全丧失固定，假体旋转移位

的原因。如果不能闭合复位，则必须采取切开手术来复位肩关节。早期脱位（在手术的前 3 个月内）通常是由技术错误引起的，不能单独用闭合复位治疗。在翻修手术中，外科医师应评估合适的假体型号、软组织撞击和三角肌张力。如果这些变量中的任何一个导致了不稳定，都应该矫正。晚期脱位（术后 1 年以上）通常可采用闭合复位和固定一段时间来治疗。[47]

肩胛盂基座失效

肩胛盂基座或组件失效常发生在反肩关节置换术后早期[18,21]（图 32-6，32-7）。在早期反肩关节假体的设计中，旋转中心外侧偏移的反球在基座和肩胛盂的连接处产生了过大的扭矩和剪切力。假体设计的创新和改进降低了肩胛盂基座的失效率。[20-21] Grammont 型反肩关节假体使旋转中心居中，从而产生更大的向心力，降低了骨 – 假体连接

处的扭矩。这种设计可使肩胛盂基座稳定固定，据报道，术后第 10 年随访时，假体存活率为 84%。[48]

假体的骨长入最小孔径为 150 μm。[49] 基座缺乏骨长入与基座失效有关。无论选择什么类型的假体，假体下倾和使用锁定螺钉都能最大限度

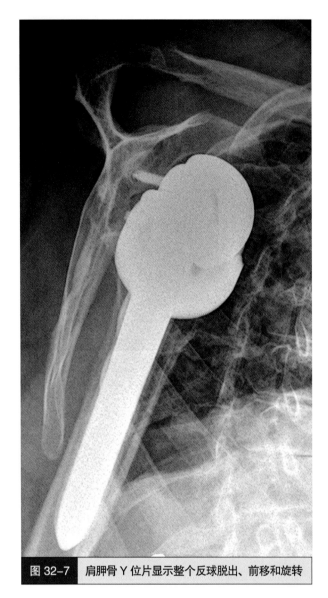

图 32-7 肩胛骨 Y 位片显示整个反球脱出、前移和旋转

发生率为 0.8%~6.9%。[3,5,15,18,20,37,51] 肩峰应力性骨折通常发生在术后 1 年内，可能与创伤事件无关[5,18,51]（图 32-8）。通常，患者术后恢复良好，但突然出现疼痛或功能丧失，无外伤史。在对 45 例患者的回顾性研究中，4.4% 的患者发生肩峰应力性骨折；研究者认为三角肌张力过大可能使严重骨质疏松症患者或肩峰骨磨损（如严重肩袖关节病）患者发生肩峰骨折。[21] 一项对 457 例患者的研究报道，肩峰应力性骨折的发生率为 0.8%。[51]

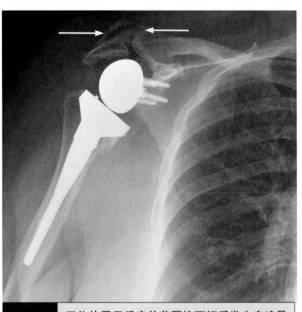

图 32-8 正位片显示反肩关节置换下倾后发生肩峰骨折（箭头）

地减小基座 - 骨界面处的应力，从而降低失败率。[50] 具有外侧偏心旋转中心的新型假体使用 5.0 mm 外周锁定螺钉，可降低基座机械性失效的风险。[20] 现代的反肩关节假体设计将锁定技术融入基座中，相关文献报道，应用此技术的肩胛盂松动率很低。医师应尽一切努力以最佳的方式将反球固定在肩胛盂下缘良好的骨质上。

肩峰应力性骨折

肩峰应力性骨折是另一种仅与反肩关节置换相关的并发症。这种骨折作为反肩关节置换的并发症很少引起注意，但最近引起了人们对它的关注。据报道，反肩关节置换术后肩峰骨折的

对肩峰应力性骨折的治疗存在争议。骨折移位较小时，通过一段时间制动的非手术治疗可获得满意的结果。[15,18,20] 在一项对 457 例反肩关节置换患者的研究中，4 例患者术后发生肩峰骨折，3 例骨折行非手术治疗，1 例采用张力带切开复位，最终失败，需要取出内固定。[51] 2 例出现永久性不愈合，2 例非手术治疗后骨愈合，但肩峰下倾至少 40°。与其他患者相比，4 例术后肩峰骨折患者在 Constant 肩关节评分、主动上举和主观满意度方面的结果较差。目前还不能确定最佳的治疗方法，但建议用外展支具固定非手术治疗 6 周，以减轻疼痛和肩峰倾斜。当反肩关节置换术后患

者康复进展缓慢、疼痛或在术后第 1 年内突然恶化时，建议高度怀疑肩峰应力性骨折。[51]

总结及未来方向

尽管与初次全肩关节置换相比，反肩关节置换并发症的发生率更高，但在适宜的患者中，反肩关节置换已被证明能恢复功能和缓解疼痛。为了减少反肩关节置换并发症的发生风险，术者必须熟悉肩关节的解剖、手术入路和与手术相关的并发症。随着术者手术经验的增加，并发症的发生率将持续降低。虽然反肩关节置换的中期结果十分乐观，但长期结果和并发症发生率仍然未知。长期结果将阐明肩胛下撞击切迹的临床后果。此外，反肩关节置换的长期存活率也值得关注；在反肩关节置换术后 6~8 年，患者的 Constant 肩关节评分、放射学结果和存活率都明显变差。[48] 反肩关节置换翻修手术需求的增高及其更高的并发症发生率也需要被进一步研究。

参考文献

［1］ Day JS, Lau E, Ong KL, Williams GR, Ramsey ML, Kurtz SM: Prevalence and projections of total shoulder and elbow arthroplasty in the United States to 2015. *J Shoulder Elbow Surg* 2010;19(8):1115-1120.
Trends and projections of procedure volume for shoulder and elbow arthroplasty in the United States were examined. The number of procedures is expected to increase 192% to 322% by 2015.

［2］ Cazeneuve JF, Cristofari DJ: The reverse shoulder prosthesis in the treatment of fractures of the proximal humerus in the elderly. *J Bone Joint Surg Br* 2010;92(4):535-539.
The clinical and radiographic outcomes of RSA were reported for 36 fractures at a mean 6.6-year follow- up. Mean Constant scores decreased with longer follow-up and progressive scapular notching.

［3］ Naveed MA, Kitson J, Bunker TD: The Delta III reverse shoulder replacement for cuff tear arthropathy: A single-centre study of 50 consecutive procedures. *J Bone Joint Surg Br* 2011;93(1):57-61.
Active forward elevation, American Shoulder and El- bow Surgeons Disability Index scores, and Oxford scores were improved at a mean 39-month follow-up after 50 RSAs for rotator cuff tear arthropathy.

［4］ Wall B, Nové-Josserand L, O'Connor DP, Edwards TB, Walch G: Reverse total shoulder arthroplasty: A review of results according to etiology. *J Bone Joint Surg Am* 2007;89(7):1476-1485.
A review of 91 RSAs by etiology found that patients with primary rotator cuff tear arthropathy, rotator cuff tear with primary arthritis, or a massive rotator cuff tear had best outcomes. Level of evidence: II.

［5］ Werner CM, Steinmann PA, Gilbart M, Gerber C: Treatment of painful pseudoparesis due to irreparable rotator cuff dysfunction with the Delta III reverse-ball-and-socket total shoulder prosthesis. *J Bone Joint Surg Am* 2005;87(7):1476-1486.

［6］ Trappey GJ IV, O'Connor DP, Edwards TB: What are the instability and infection rates after reverse shoulder arthroplasty? *Clin Orthop Relat Res* 2011;469(9):2505-2511.
A prospective review of 284 RSAs found a 5% insta-bility rate after primary RSA and an 8% rate after re-vision surgery. Patients with a repairable subscapularis tendon had a 1% rate of instability. Rates of infection were higher after revision than primary RSA. Level of evidence: III.

［7］ Zumstein MA, Pinedo M, Old J, Boileau P: Problems, complications, reoperations, and revisions in reverse total shoulder arthroplasty: A systematic review. *J Shoulder Elbow Surg* 2011;20(1):146-157.
A review of studies on postoperative complications af-ter RSA found global rates of 44%, 24%, 3.5%, and 10%, respectively, for notching, glenoid lucent lines, or hematoma formation without clinical significance; complications; reoperations; and revision procedures. Instability and infection were the most common causes of revision.

［8］ Walch G, Bacle G, Lädermann A, Nové-Josserand L, Smithers CJ: Do the indications, results, and complica- tions of reverse shoulder arthroplasty change with surgeon's experience? *J Shoulder Elbow Surg* 2012;21(11):1470-1477.
Two consecutive series of 240 RSAs were compared. The rates of revision surgery and complications were found to decrease with increased surgeon experience. Changes were noted in patient selection and clinical results but not in rates of notching. Level of evidence: IV.

[9] Lyman S, Jones EC, Bach PB, Peterson MG, Marx RG: The association between hospital volume and total shoulder arthroplasty outcomes. *Clin Orthop Relat Res* 2005;432:132-137.

[10] Boileau P, Moineau G, Roussanne Y, O'Shea K: Bony increased-offset reversed shoulder arthroplasty: Minimizing scapular impingement while maximizing glenoid fixation. *Clin Orthop Relat Res* 2011;469(9):2558-2567.

A prospective review of 42 patients who underwent RSA using an autologous humeral head graft found an early 98% rate of complete graft incorporation, improved clinical function, and a 19% incidence of scapular notching. Level of evidence: IV.

[11] Boileau P, Watkinson D, Hatzidakis AM, Hovorka I: The Grammont reverse shoulder prosthesis: Results in cuff tear arthritis, fracture sequelae, and revision arthroplasty. *J Shoulder Elbow Surg* 2006;15(5):527-540.

[12] Wierks C, Skolasky RL, Ji JH, McFarland EG: Reverse total shoulder replacement: Intraoperative and early postoperative complications. *Clin Orthop Relat Res* 2009;467(1):225-234.

Complications were compared after the first and second groups of 10 RSAs. Intraoperative complications were found to decrease after the first 10 procedures, but there was no significant difference in postoperative complications. Level of evidence: II.

[13] Valenti P, Sauzières P, Katz D, Kalouche I, Kilinc AS: Do less medialized reverse shoulder prostheses increase motion and reduce notching? *Clin Orthop Relat Res* 2011;469(9):2550-2557.

A retrospective review of 76 RSAs using a lateralized center-of-rotation glenosphere found a 0% incidence of scapular notching or glenoid loosening and improved forward flexion, external rotation, and Constant scores. Level of evidence: IV.

[14] Van Hoof T, Gomes GT, Audenaert E, Verstraete K, Kerckaert I, D'Herde K: 3D computerized model for measuring strain and displacement of the brachial plexus following placement of reverse shoulder prosthesis. *Anat Rec (Hoboken)* 2008;291(9):1173-1185.

Three-dimensional reconstruction of the cadaver brachial plexus and changes in strain and displacement after RSA showed 15% and 19% increases in strain in the lateral and medial roots of the median nerve, respectively, and a 10% decrease in the length of the axillary nerve.

[15] Lädermann A, Williams MD, Melis B, Hoffmeyer P, Walch G: Objective evaluation of lengthening in reverse shoulder arthroplasty. *J Shoulder Elbow Surg* 2009;18(4):588-595.

A radiographic review of 58 RSAs found an average 2 mm of humeral lengthening and 23 mm of arm lengthening. Humeral and arm lengthening occurred less often in patients with postoperative instability. Level of evidence: III.

[16] Lädermann A, Lübbeke A, Mélis B, et al: Prevalence of neurologic lesions after total shoulder arthroplasty. *J Bone Joint Surg Am* 2011;93(14):1288-1293.

A comparison of the incidence of neurologic lesions in 19 RSAs and 23 total shoulder arthroplasties found a 10.9 higher relative risk of acute postoperative nerve injury after RSA, with a mean lengthening of 2.7 cm. Nerve lesions usually were transient.

[17] Nagda SH, Rogers KJ, Sestokas AK, et al: Peripheral nerve function during shoulder arthroplasty using intraoperative nerve monitoring. *J Shoulder Elbow Surg* 2007;16(3, suppl):S2-S8.

A 56.7% incidence of nerve alerts during shoulder arthroplasty was reported; most returned to baseline after retractors were removed and the arm was repositioned to neutral. Extreme arm positions and retractors should be used for the minimal time necessary.

[18] Frankle M, Siegal S, Pupello D, Saleem A, Mighell M, Vasey M: The reverse shoulder prosthesis for glenohumeral arthritis associated with severe rotator cuff deficiency: A minimum two-year follow-up study of sixty patients. *J Bone Joint Surg Am* 2005;87(8):1697-1705.

[19] De Wilde L, Sys G, Julien Y, Van Ovost E, Poffyn B, Trouilloud P: The reversed Delta shoulder prosthesis in reconstruction of the proximal humerus after tumour resection. *Acta Orthop Belg* 2003;69(6):495-500.

[20] Cuff D, Pupello D, Virani N, Levy J, Frankle M: Reverse shoulder arthroplasty for the treatment of rotator cuff deficiency. *J Bone Joint Surg Am* 2008;90(6):1244-1251.

In 96 RSAs with a lateralized center of rotation, the overall complication rate was 6.25%, with improved postoperative abduction, forward flexion, and external rotation. There was no evidence of scapular notching at a mean 27.5-month follow-up. Level of evidence: IV.

[21] Boileau P, Watkinson DJ, Hatzidakis AM, Balg F: Grammont reverse prosthesis: Design, rationale, and biomechanics. *J Shoulder Elbow Surg* 2005;14(1, suppl):147S-161S.

［22］Topolski MS, Chin PY, Sperling JW, Cofield RH: Revision shoulder arthroplasty with positive intraoperative cultures: The value of preoperative studies and intraoperative histology. *J Shoulder Elbow Surg* 2006;15(4):402-406.

［23］Dodson CC, Craig EV, Cordasco FA, et al: *Propionibacterium acnes* infection after shoulder arthroplasty: A diagnostic challenge. *J Shoulder Elbow Surg* 2010;19(2):303-307.

Eleven patients were diagnosed with *P acnes* infection after shoulder arthroplasty. The diagnosis was difficult because of indolent clinical symptoms, resistance to broad-spectrum antibiotics, and the need to keep cultures at least 2 weeks. Level of evidence: IV.

［24］Kanafani ZA, Sexton DJ, Pien BC, Varkey J, Basmania C, Kaye KS: Postoperative joint infections due to Propionibacterium species: A case-control study. *Clin Infect Dis* 2009;49(7):1083-1085.

P acnes that occurred a mean 210 days after shoulder arthroplasty was diagnosed in 40 patients. Only 23% of cases occurred within 1 month of surgery. A history of earlier surgery and male sex were independent risk factors.

［25］Piper KE, Fernandez-Sampedro M, Steckelberg KE, et al: Creactive protein, erythrocyte sedimentation rate and orthopedic implant infection. *PLoS One* 2010;5(2):e9358.

CRP level and ESR were analyzed in patients who underwent hip, knee, or shoulder arthroplasty. CRP level and ESR were found to have poor sensitivity for the diagnosis of shoulder infection. Sensitivity and specificity for detecting shoulder infection were 23% and 93%, respectively.

［26］Piper KE, Jacobson MJ, Cofield RH, et al: Microbiologic diagnosis of prosthetic shoulder infection by use of implant sonication. *J Clin Microbiol* 2009;47(6):1878-1884.

The accuracy of sonicate fluid for detecting prosthetic shoulder infection in revision or resection shoulder arthroplasty was studied. Sonicate fluid was 66.7% sensitive and periprosthetic tissue culture was 54.5% sensitive for detecting prosthetic shoulder infection in revision or resection shoulder arthroplasty.

［27］Lutz MF, Berthelot P, Fresard A, et al: Arthroplastic and osteosynthetic infections due to Propionibacterium acnes: A retrospective study of 52 cases, 1995-2002. *Eur J Clin Microbiol Infect Dis* 2005;24(11):739-744.

［28］Saltzman MD, Nuber GW, Gryzlo SM, Marecek GS, Koh JL: Efficacy of surgical preparation solutions in shoulder surgery. *J Bone Joint Surg Am* 2009;91(8):1949-1953.

A prospective study comparing three surgical preparation solutions (ChloraPrep, DuraPrep, and povidone-iodine scrub) found ChloraPrep to be the most effective for eliminating bacteria before surgery. Level of evidence: I.

［29］Nowinski RJ, Gillespie RJ, Shishani Y, Cohen B, Walch G, Gobezie R: Antibiotic-loaded bone cement reduces deep infection rates for primary reverse total shoulder arthroplasty: A retrospective, cohort study of 501 shoulders. *J Shoulder Elbow Surg* 2012;21(3):324-328.

A retrospective study compared the incidence of deep infection after RSA in patients treated with antibiotic-loaded cement or plain cement. No deep infections developed in patients with antibiotic-loaded cement, compared with 3% in those with plain cement. Level of evidence: III.

［30］Cheung EV, Sperling JW, Cofield RH: Infection associated with hematoma formation after shoulder arthroplasty. *Clin Orthop Relat Res* 2008;466(6):1363-1367.

Hematoma formation required reoperation after 12 of 4,147 shoulder arthroplasties. Six of nine patients had positive cultures, and two eventually had a resection arthroplasty. Hematoma formation is often associated with a positive intraoperative culture. Level of evidence: IV.

［31］Weber P, Utzschneider S, Sadoghi P, Andress HJ, Jansson V, Müller PE: Management of the infected shoulder prosthesis: A retrospective analysis and review of the literature. *Int Orthop* 2011;35(3):365-373.

In a retrospective review of 10 patients treated for an infected shoulder prosthesis, a two-stage exchange yielded only slightly better results than resection arthroplasty. Level of evidence: IV.

［32］Sabesan VJ, Ho JC, Kovacevic D, Iannotti JP: Two-stage reimplantation for treating prosthetic shoulder infections. *Clin Orthop Relat Res* 2011;469(9):2538-2543.

A retrospective review found that two-stage reimplantation for prosthetic shoulder infection led to improved shoulder function and pain. There was a 35% incidence of complications, including five dislocations and one reinfection. Level of evidence: IV.

［33］Grosso MJ, Sabesan VJ, Ho JC, Ricchetti ET, Iannotti JP: Reinfection rates after 1-stage revision shoulder arthroplasty for patients with unexpected positive intraoperative cultures. *J Shoulder Elbow Surg* 2012;21(6):754-758.

Infection recurred in 5.9% of 17 patients who underwent a one-stage revision without prolonged antibiotic therapy after unsuccessful shoulder arthroplasty and a positive intraoperative culture. Infection recurred in 5.9%. Level of evidence: IV.

[34] Beekman PD, Katusic D, Berghs BM, Karelse A, De Wilde L: One-stage revision for patients with a chronically infected reverse total shoulder replacement. *J Bone Joint Surg Br* 2010;92(6):817-822.

Ten of 11 patients who underwent a one-stage revision of infected shoulder arthroplasty were considered free of infection at a median 24-month follow-up. The mean postoperative score gain on the Constant- Murley Scale was 10.

[35] Coste JS, Reig S, Trojani C, Berg M, Walch G, Boileau P: The management of infection in arthroplasty of the shoulder. *J Bone Joint Surg Br* 2004;86(1):65-69.

[36] Sperling JW, Kozak TK, Hanssen AD, Cofield RH: Infection after shoulder arthroplasty. *Clin Orthop Relat Res* 2001;382:206-216.

[37] Mulieri P, Dunning P, Klein S, Pupello D, Frankle M: Reverse shoulder arthroplasty for the treatment of irreparable rotator cuff tear without glenohumeral arthritis. *J Bone Joint Surg Am* 2010;92(15):2544-2556.

A retrospective review found that American Shoulder and Elbow Surgeons Disability Index scores, Simple Shoulder Test scores, visual analog scale scores, active forward flexion, abduction, internal rotation, and external rotation improved after RSA in 72 shoulders with an irreparable rotator cuff tear. Level of evidence: IV.

[38] Lévigne C, Garret J, Boileau P, Alami G, Favard L, Walch G: Scapular notching in reverse shoulder arthroplasty: Is it important to avoid it and how? *Clin Orthop Relat Res* 2011;469(9):2512-2520.

A retrospective review found that notching occurred in 68% of 448 patients after RSA and increased with longer follow-up time. Notching was associated with decreased strength and forward elevation but not with pain or the Constant-Murley score. Level of evidence: IV.

[39] Boileau P, Gonzalez JF, Chuinard C, Bicknell R, Walch G: Reverse total shoulder arthroplasty after failed rotator cuff surgery. *J Shoulder Elbow Surg* 2009;18(4): 600-606.

A retrospective review of RSA in 42 patients after unsuccessful rotator cuff surgery found that patients with poor preoperative motion were able to restore active elevation. Patients with maintained preoperative motion (more than 90°) risked loss of motion and lower satisfaction.

[40] Kempton LB, Balasubramaniam M, Ankerson E, Wiater JM: A radiographic analysis of the effects of prosthesis design on scapular notching following reverse total shoulder arthroplasty. *J Shoulder Elbow Surg* 2011;20(4):571-576.

A comparison of two prosthesis designs found that patients having the prosthesis with a lateralized center of rotation had a lower incidence of notching compared with those having the prosthesis with no center of rotation. Level of evidence: III.

[41] Lévigne C, Boileau P, Favard L, et al: Scapular notching in reverse shoulder arthroplasty. *J Shoulder Elbow Surg* 2008;17(6):925-935.

A retrospective review of 337 shoulders with a 62% incidence of notching after RSA found that the highest incidence of notching was in those with rotator cuff tear arthropathy. The rate was higher if an anterosuperior approach was used rather than a deltopectoral approach.

[42] Simovitch RW, Zumstein MA, Lohri E, Helmy N, Gerber C: Predictors of scapular notching in patients managed with the Delta III reverse total shoulder replacement. *J Bone Joint Surg Am* 2007;89(3):588-600.

The angle between the glenosphere and the scapular neck and the height of glenosphere implantation were highly correlated with the development of scapular notching. Patients with notching had a relatively poor clinical outcome. Level of evidence: II.

[43] Gutiérrez S, Levy JC, Frankle MA, et al: Evaluation of abduction range of motion and avoidance of inferior scapular impingement in a reverse shoulder model. *J Shoulder Elbow Surg* 2008;17(4):608-615.

A biomechanical study found that the glenosphere center of rotation offset had the greatest effect on range of motion. The neck-shaft angle had the greatest effect on scapular notching.

[44] Sirveaux F, Favard L, Oudet D, Huquet D, Walch G, Molé D: Grammont inverted total shoulder arthroplasty in the treatment of glenohumeral osteoarthritis with massive rupture of the cuff: Results of a multicentre study of 80 shoulders. *J Bone Joint Surg Br* 2004;86(3):388-395.

[45] Edwards TB, Williams MD, Labriola JE, Elkousy HA, Gartsman GM, O'Connor DP: Subscapularis insufficiency and the risk of shoulder dislocation after reverse shoulder arthroplasty. *J Shoulder Elbow Surg* 2009;18(6):892-896.

The incidence of dislocation was compared in patients with a repairable or irreparable subscapularis. An irreparable subscapularis tendon was found to be a significant risk factor for postoperative dislocation. Level of evidence: IV.

[46] Clark JC, Ritchie J, Song FS, et al: Complication rates, dislocation, pain, and postoperative range of motion after reverse shoulder arthroplasty in patients with and without repair of the subscapularis. *J Shoulder Elbow Surg* 2012;21(1):36-41.

No correlation was found between subscapularis repair and post-RSA complications, dislocation, pain, or motion. Level of evidence: III.

[47] Gerber C, Pennington SD, Nyffeler RW: Reverse total shoulder arthroplasty. *J Am Acad Orthop Surg* 2009;17(5):284-295.

The design rationale, indications, and the technique for RSA are reviewed, and clinical experience and common complications are discussed.

[48] Guery J, Favard L, Sirveaux F, Oudet D, Mole D, Walch G: Reverse total shoulder arthroplasty: Survivorship analysis of eighty replacements followed for five to ten years. *J Bone Joint Surg Am* 2006;88(8):1742-1747.

[49] Jasty M, Bragdon C, Burke D, O'Connor D, Lowenstein J, Harris WH: In vivo skeletal responses to porous-surfaced implants subjected to small induced motions. *J Bone Joint Surg Am* 1997;79(5):707-714.

[50] Gutiérrez S, Keller TS, Levy JC, Lee WE III, Luo ZP: Hierarchy of stability factors in reverse shoulder arthroplasty. *Clin Orthop Relat Res* 2008;466(3):670-676.

A biomechanical study concluded that compressive forces generated by muscles are the most important factor in maintaining stability after RSA.

[51] Walch G, Mottier F, Wall B, Boileau P, Molé D, Favard L: Acromial insufficiency in reverse shoulder arthroplasties. *J Shoulder Elbow Surg* 2009;18(3):495-502.

In 457 patients with RSA, preoperative acromial lesions had no effect on range of motion, Constant score, or subjective results. Those with postoperative acromial fracture had inferior functional and subjective results. Level of evidence: III.

第六部分

创伤与骨折

栏目编委：
Anand M. Murthi, MD

第三十三章　肱骨近端骨折

John-Erik Bell, MD, MS

引言

在年龄大于 65 岁的人群中，肱骨近端骨折是第三常见的肢体脆性骨折，仅次于髋部和桡骨远端骨折。虽然这些骨折最常发生于老年人的低能量创伤（如跌倒），但也可发生于较年轻患者的高能量创伤。大多数肱骨近端骨折无移位或只有轻度移位，通常可行非手术治疗。轻度移位骨折的非手术治疗可获得可预期的良好结果。移位骨折的处理方法包括非手术治疗、经皮穿针、切开复位内固定和一期关节置换。移位骨折的治疗较为复杂和困难，目前仍然存在争议。美国人口的老龄化使骨质疏松症的发生率增高，意味着与其他脆性骨折一样，肱骨近端骨折的发生率可能会增高。肱骨近端骨折很可能对医疗系统造成重大负担且该负担会日益加重。

解剖和分型

Codman 在 1934 年首次描述肱骨近端的骺线，他将肱骨近端分成 4 个解剖骨块：关节面骨块、大结节、小结节和肱骨干。[1]Neer 的四部分分型被广泛接受，他将 Codman 提出的 4 个骨块中任一骨块成角大于 45° 或移位大于 1 cm 定义为一部分。[2]任一部分的移位由其肌腱附着所决定。冈上肌和冈下肌将大结节拉向后上方。肩胛下肌向

Neither Dr. Bell nor any immediate family member has received anything of value from or has stock or stock options held in a commercial company or institution related directly or indirectly to the subject of this chapter.

前内侧牵拉小结节。胸大肌和三角肌将肱骨干向近端和内侧牵引，产生向前成角。

了解肱骨近端的血供十分重要，因为在某些骨折类型中骨坏死的风险很高，并且这种风险影响手术适应证和预后。最初认为前循环是肱骨头的主要供血来源。旋肱前动脉前外侧支在肱二头肌长头外侧缘向上走行，在结节间沟和大结节的交界处近端进入骨内，在骨内走行形成弓状动脉。[3]最近的研究强调了后循环的重要性。[4-5]旋肱后动脉的血供占关节面骨块血供的 64%，这一发现有助于解释为什么不是所有前循环完全断裂的骨折均会进展到骨坏死。

Neer 分型比较直接，相对容易应用，但没有考虑肱骨近端的血供，并且观察者间和观察者内可靠性一般。AO-ASIF 分型基于骨折的复杂性和肱骨头血供的破坏程度，将肱骨近端骨折分为 3 种基本类型共 27 个组和亚组。[6]该分类系统是综合性的，与预后和骨坏死相关，但它非常复杂，具有比 Neer 分型更差的观察者间和观察者内可靠性。

外展嵌插型骨折不包含在最初的 Neer 分型中，但它包含在 2002 年更新的 Neer 分型中。[7]在三部分或四部分骨折中，肱骨头相对于肱骨干外翻，并被压缩到肱骨干上（图 33-1）。大结节通常相对于头向上移位。认识这种骨折类型很重要，因为与大多数移位的三部分和四部分骨折不一样，其血供通常是保留的。四部分外展嵌插型骨折的骨坏死率低于移位的四部分骨折和骨折脱位的骨

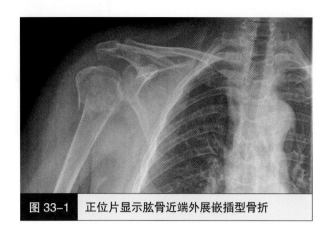

图 33-1　正位片显示肱骨近端外展嵌插型骨折

坏死率，可能是因为保留了内侧铰链的血供。[8-9]

肱骨近端神经和骨折结构之间密切的解剖关系导致这些骨折的神经损伤发生率较高。肌电图记录的腋神经异常率为 58%，肩胛上神经异常率高达 48%。[10] 腋动脉损伤被认为是肱骨近端骨折的并发症，最常见于骨折脱位。

评估和影像学检查

患者的病史应包括任何可能提示肩袖病变、关节炎或受伤前不稳定的肩关节症状。病史还应包括损伤机制、任何可能影响手术或麻醉安全的全身合并症及患者的社会状况。评估应包括彻底的神经血管检查、皮肤检查、相关损伤评估和恰当的影像学检查。神经血管检查应包括桡神经、正中神经、尺神经、肌皮神经（和前臂外侧皮肤感觉）、腋神经和肩胛上神经。对于腋神经，应确认三角肌收缩功能和完整的肩部外侧感觉。血管检查总是很重要的，在肩关节脱位时更为重要。如果怀疑有血管损伤，可以进行多普勒检查或血管造影成像。

标准肩关节创伤系列片包括真实正位片、肩胛骨 Y 位片和腋位片。其他用于评估特殊病变的 X 线片包括评估隐匿性外科颈或大结节骨折的内外旋位片，评估肩胛盂前缘骨折的西点腋位片，以及评估 Hill-Sachs 损伤的 Stryker 切迹位片。目前，这些特殊位片已被 CT 所取代，CT 通常可为手术决策和计划提供更详细的信息。

治疗决策和非手术治疗

在确定最佳治疗方案时，必须考虑患者的特点和骨折情况。患者的合并症、活动水平、优势手、年龄和遵守术后限制及指示的能力是重要的考虑因素。骨折特征包括骨质量、骨折类型和移位程度、肱骨头血管和神经系统状况也应作为考虑因素。

肱骨头坏死的风险随着骨折的复杂性的增高而增高。[11] 血供破坏和随后的骨坏死的预测因素包括干骺端延伸的长度（小于 8 mm）、骨折类型和内侧铰链的完整性。解剖颈骨折、四部分移位骨折和所有三部分骨折的骨坏死风险较高，除非结节之间没有骨折。干骺端延伸长度被认为与通过旋肱后动脉维持后内侧血供有关。[12]

对于无移位和轻度移位骨折普遍采用非手术治疗。这种治疗方法没有争议，作为治疗标准被广泛接受。大多数患者，即使是骨折稳定的患者，也需要 2~4 周的吊带制动。建议早期物理治疗，可改善稳定骨折的预后。通常轻柔的全范围运动练习是安全的，从钟摆运动和滑轮运动开始，并在几周后进行被动全范围运动练习。[13] 在术后第 6 周时，通常可以开始主动辅助和主动全范围运动练习，前提是 X 线片显示没有进一步的移位，并且有早期愈合的迹象。患者通常可获得较好的结果，文献报道患者有很高的影像学愈合率、良好的功能结果，以及很低的并发症发生率，伤侧和对侧的有效结果评分差异很小。[14-15]

一些患者的骨折脱位也可以进行闭合复位的非手术治疗。应仔细检查复位前的 X 线片，因为在复位操作过程中，隐匿的外科颈骨折可能会移位，继而可能将无须进行手术的骨折病例转变为困难的需要进行手术的病例（图 33-2）。骨折无移位的脱位可能需要在全身麻醉和 X 线透视下进行，以尽量减小所需的力和避免移位。

移位的三部分或四部分肱骨近端骨折的手术适应证更具争议性。最近有文献对这些骨折类型

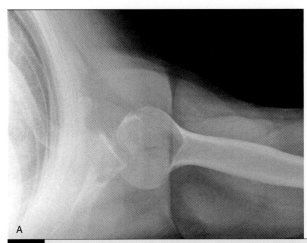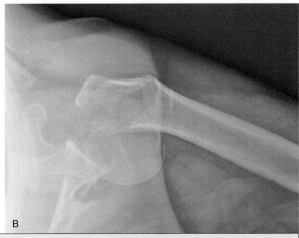

图 33-2　A. 腋位片显示后侧骨折脱位伴交锁的反 Hill-Sachs 损伤，一条无移位的裂缝延伸到外科颈。B. 尝试闭合复位后，骨折移位

进行了前瞻性随机研究，对比了接受切开复位锁定钢板内固定与接受非手术治疗的移位的三部分骨折，结果无统计学显著差异，但是，30% 接受切开复位内固定的患者需要再次手术。[16] 这些研究人员进行了另一项前瞻性随机对照研究，对比了移位的四部分骨折的半关节置换术和非手术治疗的效果，采用半关节置换术治疗的患者在疼痛缓解和生活质量方面有显著改善，但在活动范围方面两种治疗方法没有差异。[17] 2004 年发表的一篇系统综述发现，没有足够的证据确定四部分骨折的最佳治疗方法。[18]

对于移位的肱骨近端骨折，没有明确的证据支持手术或非手术的治疗策略，因此治疗往往取决于术者的经验和习惯。手术或非手术治疗的骨折比例存在明显的区域差异。[19-20]

手术治疗

肱骨近端骨折的手术治疗通常采用沙滩椅位或仰卧位，使用全身麻醉、局部麻醉或联合麻醉。透视机与手术台平行，可以在不需要明显移动手臂的情况下获得肩部的垂直 X 线片。标准的胸大肌三角肌入路和前外侧三角肌劈开入路是最常用的入路。对于骨折固定和关节置换胸大肌三角肌入路，具有可扩展性和实用性，虽然该入路很难显露肱骨近端的外侧和后方。前外侧三角肌劈开入路可为骨折固定提供良好的肱骨外侧和大结节的显露，但增加了腋神经损伤的风险，且无法扩展。[21]

经皮穿针是治疗外科颈骨折或内侧铰链完整的外展嵌插型骨折的一个好选择。内侧骨距严重粉碎是穿针固定的相对禁忌证。经皮穿针固定的优点包括保留骨折血肿，减少切开、软组织剥离和永久性内固定残留的需要，以及骨坏死风险相对较低；缺点包括技术难度较大，需要去除固定针，以及由于固定不牢固和针尾突出而无法开始早期的全范围运动练习。图 33-3 说明了经皮穿针的步骤。在胸大肌三角肌间隙线上做一个 1 cm 的小切口，插入止血钳或骨膜剥离子将肱骨头抬高到正确的位置。用 2.8 mm 的螺纹针将头部固定在肱骨干上。用止血钳经皮复位大结节，并用 1.25 mm 空心螺钉导针固定至肱骨头，扩孔后拧入 4.0 mm 空心螺钉。通常在 3~4 周时拔出针，然后可以开始运动练习。经皮穿针的结果通常较好。[22-25] 一项对 27 例二部分、三部分或四部分骨折患者的研究发现，在经皮穿针后平均第 35 个月随访时，10 分视觉模拟疼痛评分的平均评分为 1.4，ASES 肩关节疼痛和功能障碍评分为 83.4，Constant 肩关节评分为 73.9 分。[26]

自 10 年前采用锁定钢板技术以来，切开复位

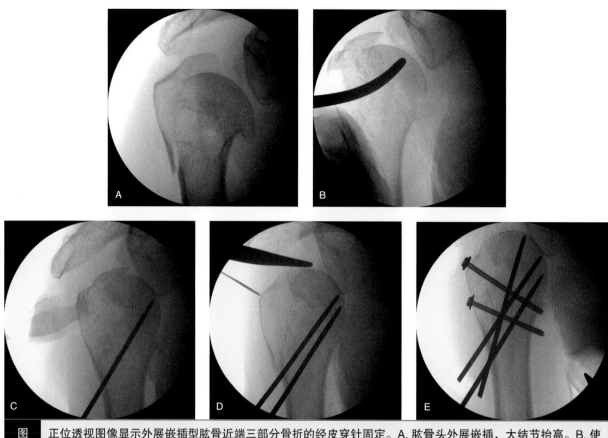

图 33-3　正位透视图像显示外展嵌插型肱骨近端三部分骨折的经皮穿针固定。A. 肱骨头外展嵌插，大结节抬高。B. 使用经皮放置的止血钳将头部抬起纠正外翻。C. 用 2.8 mm 的螺纹针将肱骨头固定至肱骨干上。D. 使用止血钳经皮复位大结节，使用 4.0 mm 空心螺钉导针进行临时固定。E. 经导针拧入带垫圈的空心螺钉进行牢固固定

内固定成了一种日益普遍的治疗方法。除锁定钢板外，还有许多其他的切开复位和内固定方法，包括缝合，使用钢丝、钢板、螺钉、空心螺钉的方法，以及髓内固定。最佳的固定结构取决于骨折类型和骨量。患者的骨量通常很差，尤其是肱骨头。通常，结节的最佳固定方法要避免完全依靠结节的骨性固定，还需结合肩袖止点的缝线固定。如果存在明显的干骺端粉碎，最好使用角度固定结构（角钢板或锁定钢板）或髓内固定，以防止失败，出现内翻。

最初显示锁定钢板在生物力学上优于现有的固定结构（包括 T 形钢板和支撑钢板）。肱骨近端锁定钢板的主要特征是螺钉朝向肱骨头，但锁定在不同的方向上，从而增加了整个结构的拔出强度。[27-29] 锁定钢板技术为骨质疏松患者的切开复位内固定提供了一种选择，在过去，关节置换术或非手术治疗是骨质疏松患者的唯一选择。锁定钢板技术也为骨量相对较好的年轻患者高度不稳定的高能量骨折和肱骨头劈裂骨折提供了一个理想的选择（图 33-4）。

虽然锁定钢板的使用已经变得很普遍，并且其使医师能够对以前不可能固定的骨折进行切开复位和内固定，但并发症发生率和再手术率很高。文献报道，大多数并发症与内固定物和技术有关，并强调即使是对经验丰富的外科医师来说，治疗这些骨折也十分困难。最近的许多研究都报道了很高的并发症发生率和再手术率[19,30-35]。一项纳入 187 例患者的大型多中心研究报道，使用肱骨近端锁定钢板的并发症发生率为 34%，其中 19% 的患者术后 12 个月内需要进行第二次非计划内的

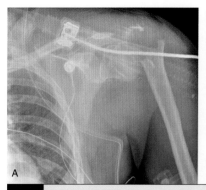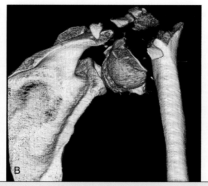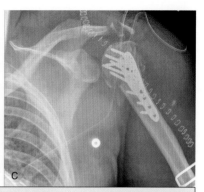

图 33-4　A. 正位片显示 28 岁男性患者在一次车祸后的高能量粉碎性四部分肱骨近端骨折。B. 三维 CT 重建显示肱骨头关节内劈裂。C. 术后 X 线片显示肱骨近端锁定钢板切开复位内固定

手术。[30] 并发症包括内固定物穿出、内固定失败引起的内翻塌陷、畸形愈合、骨不连、感染、神经损伤、粘连性关节囊炎、骨坏死，以及由肱骨头塌陷导致的后期内固定物穿出（图 33-5）。

注意以下几点可以减少发生内固定相关并发

症的风险。最常见的早期并发症是肱骨头螺钉穿出。应仔细测量每枚螺钉的长度并减去 5 mm，在离开手术室前检查所有螺钉的正侧位图像，可以很好地避免这种并发症的发生。辅以粗的缝线固定，缝线先穿过肩袖腱骨连接处，再通过钢板，

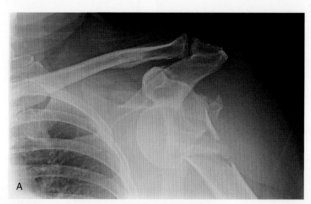

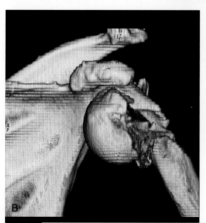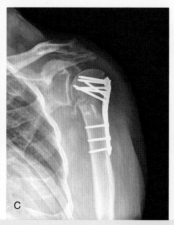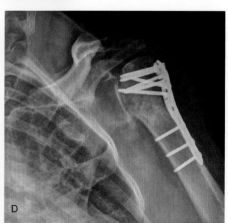

图 33-5　正位片（A）和三维 CT 重建图像（B）显示 45 岁男性患者的肱骨近端骨折脱位。术后正位片显示肱骨近端锁定钢板切开复位内固定（C）。术后 1 年的正位片（D）显示骨坏死，其可引起疼痛、弹响和肱骨头塌陷。因为螺钉是锁定的，所以当头部塌陷时螺钉并没有退后并保持固定，最终穿过软骨下骨进入了盂肱关节

有助于避免结节固定失败或内翻塌陷。大多数肱骨近端锁定钢板设计可通过近端进行缝线固定。治疗肱骨近端切开复位内固定失败的技术难度很高。治疗一些并发症（如骨坏死、慢性肩袖功能不全或结节骨不连）时，转为关节置换术可能是最好的选择。治疗由技术因素引起的固定失败时，改用角钢板固定是一个合理的选择，因为肱骨头通常有足够的残余骨量，可以成功翻修（图 33-6）。

结合髓内同种异体骨对内固定结构进行增强的技术在 2008 年被首次报道，近来颇受关注。[36] 临床结果和最近的生物力学数据证实，锁定钢板内固定结合髓内腓骨支撑加强，可以提高最大失效载荷和初始结构强度。[36-38] 这项技术在内翻成角和失去内侧支撑的骨折类型中最有用，并且已经被证实可以防止内翻塌陷（图 33-7）。

一期肩关节置换术是治疗三部分、四部分和肱骨头劈裂骨折的一种选择。是否行肩关节置换术或切开复位内固定，不仅取决于骨折类型，还取决于患者因素（如年龄、活动水平和期望值）（图 33-8）。传统的标准治疗方法是半肩关节

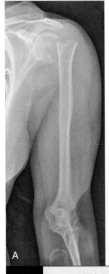
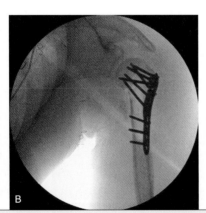
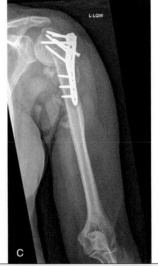
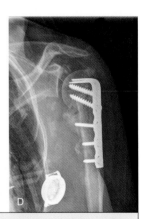

图 33-6 A. 正位片显示一例 60 岁女性患者的二部分肱骨近端移位骨折。B. 正位透视图像显示用肱骨近端锁定钢板进行治疗。C. 术后 6 周正位片显示内翻塌陷。D. 正位片显示用 90° 角钢板进行翻修，最终无痛骨愈合

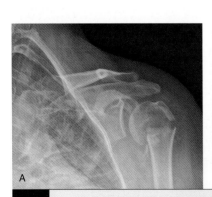
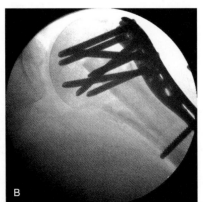
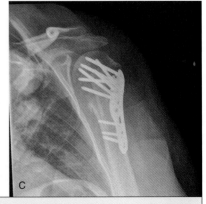

图 33-7 A. 60 岁类风湿关节炎患者肱骨近端二部分外科颈骨折后 4 周的正位片。最初采用非手术治疗，但患者在进行性内翻成角和骨折边缘吸收后选择切开复位内固定。正位透视图像（B）和正位片（C）显示采用标准肱骨近端锁定钢板结合髓内异体腓骨支撑以加强内侧支撑，从而避免内翻塌陷

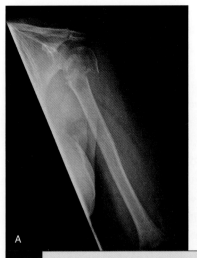
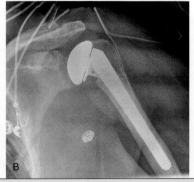
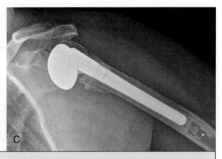

图 33-8　活动量较大的 62 岁女性肱骨近端四部分移位骨折患者行半关节置换术前（A）和术后（B）的正位片。术后，结节相对于肱骨头的位置合适。术后第 4 年随访时的正位片（C）显示结节愈合良好，患者主动抬高患肢 150° 无疼痛

置换术，但是反肩关节假体在治疗这些骨折方面越来越普及，特别是在对功能要求相对较低的 70 岁以上患者中。在肱骨近端骨折后，一期半肩关节置换术的疗效优于二期肩关节置换术。[39] 骨折行半肩关节置换术时影响结果的最重要的因素是结节是否位于合适的位置和是否愈合。[40-41] 结节位置不佳可导致术后力量和活动范围恢复不佳。[42] 结节修复的理想结构为水平和垂直方向的粗缝线直接穿过肩袖的腱骨连接处，如有可能还应穿过假体。内侧环扎缝合对修复结构的稳定性具有重要的生物力学意义。[43]

反肩关节置换术的适应证仍在不断完善，近年来，纳入了 70 岁以上功能要求相对较低患者的急性肱骨近端骨折。最近几项研究评价了反肩关节置换术作为肱骨近端骨折一期治疗的结果。在短期内，反肩关节置换术可以预见性地减轻疼痛并改善功能。[44-45] 与半肩关节置换术不同，即使结节没有很好地愈合，反肩关节置换术也可以缓解疼痛和改善功能。然而，为了重建最大外旋功能，反肩关节置换时仍建议进行结节重建。一项直接比较反肩关节置换术和半肩关节置换术结果的研究

发现，反肩关节置换术有更好的外展和过头上举，而半肩关节置换术有更好的内旋和外旋恢复。[46] 最近的研究显示，患者在中期随访时出现功能轻度恶化，肩胛盂假体周围出现透亮线。[47-48] 在第 1 年和平均第 6.6 年随访时，患者主诉疼痛加剧、力量丧失，Constant 肩关节评分恶化。只有 58% 的患者对治疗结果满意或非常满意。并发症发生率为 23%，再手术率为 17%。[48] 虽然早期的结果较好，但这项研究强调，在广泛推广对肱骨近端急性骨折行反肩关节置换术之前需要进行更长期的研究。

总结

肱骨近端骨折很常见，在美国，其发病率可能会根据人口统计学的变化而增加。理解肱骨近端的解剖和血供对骨折精确分型和制订适当的治疗计划十分必要。每一种治疗方案都有不同的适应证和并发症。目前，普遍认为无移位和轻度移位的骨折应行非手术治疗，但关于手术是否可显著改善移位骨折的结果以及特定骨折模式的最佳手术治疗方案尚无共识，需要更多的一级研究来提供相关证据。

参考文献

[1] Codman E: *The Shoulder: Rupture of the Supraspinatus Tendon and Other Lesions in or About the Subacromial Bursa*. Brooklyn, NY, G Miller, 1934.

[2] Neer CS II: Displaced proximal humeral fractures: Part I. Classification and evaluation. 1970. *Clin Orthop Relat Res* 2006;442:77-82.

[3] Laing PG: The arterial supply of the adult humerus. *J Bone Joint Surg Am* 1956;38-A(5):1105-1116.

[4] Hettrich CM, Boraiah S, Dyke JP, Neviaser A, Helfet DL, Lorich DG: Quantitative assessment of the vascularity of the proximal part of the humerus. *J Bone Joint Surg Am* 2010;92(4):943-948.

A cadaver study evaluated the vascularity of the humeral head using gadolinium and polymer injections. The posterior circumflex humeral artery was found to contribute 64% and the anterior humeral circumflex artery to contribute 36%.

[5] Brooks CH, Revell WJ, Heatley FW: Vascularity of the humeral head after proximal humeral fractures: An anatomical cadaver study. *J Bone Joint Surg Br* 1993;75(1):132-136.

[6] Marsh JL, Slongo TF, Agel J, et al: Fracture and dislocation classification compendium - 2007: Orthopaedic Trauma Association classification, database and outcomes committee. *J Orthop Trauma* 2007;21(10, suppl):S1-S133.

[7] Neer CS II: Four-segment classification of proximal humeral fractures: Purpose and reliable use. *J Shoulder Elbow Surg* 2002;11(4):389-400.

[8] Jakob RP, Miniaci A, Anson PS, Jaberg H, Osterwalder A, Ganz R: Four-part valgus impacted fractures of the proximal humerus. *J Bone Joint Surg Br* 1991;73(2):295-298.

[9] DeFranco MJ, Brems JJ, Williams GR Jr, Iannotti JP: Evaluation and management of valgus impacted four-part proximal humerus fractures. *Clin Orthop Relat Res* 2006;442:109-114.

[10] Visser CP, Coene LN, Brand R, Tavy DL: Nerve lesions in proximal humeral fractures. *J Shoulder Elbow Surg* 2001;10(5):421-427.

[11] Lee CK, Hansen HR: Post-traumatic avascular necrosis of the humeral head in displaced proximal humeral fractures. *J Trauma* 1981;21(9):788-791.

[12] Hertel R, Hempfing A, Stiehler M, Leunig M: Predictors of humeral head ischemia after intracapsular fracture of the proximal humerus. *J Shoulder Elbow Surg* 2004;13(4):427-433.

[13] Koval KJ, Gallagher MA, Marsicano JG, Cuomo F, McShinawy A, Zuckerman JD: Functional outcome after minimally displaced fractures of the proximal part of the humerus. *J Bone Joint Surg Am* 1997;79(2):203-207.

[14] Iyengar JJ, Devcic Z, Sproul RC, Feeley BT: Nonoperative treatment of proximal humerus fractures: A systematic review. *J Orthop Trauma* 2011;25(10):612-617.

A systematic review of nonsurgically treated proximal humeral fractures found a 98% rate of radiographic union and a predictably good Constant score averaging 74. The complication rate was 13%, with varus malunion the most common.

[15] Hanson B, Neidenbach P, de Boer P, Stengel D: Functional outcomes after nonoperative management of fractures of the proximal humerus. *J Shoulder Elbow Surg* 2009;18(4):612-621.

A prospective case study followed 124 patients for 1 year after a nonsurgically treated proximal humeral fracture. The difference between the injured and normal shoulders on the Constant and Disabilities of the Arm, Shoulder and Hand questionnaire scores was only 8.2 and 10.2, respectively.

[16] Olerud P, Ahrengart L, Ponzer S, Saving J, Tidermark J: Internal fixation versus nonoperative treatment of displaced 3-part proximal humeral fractures in elderly patients: A randomized controlled trial. *J Shoulder Elbow Surg* 2011;20(5):747-755.

A comparison of locking-plate and nonsurgical treatment of displaced three-part fractures found a trend toward better outcomes in patients treated with a locking plate, but there was no statistically significant between-group difference in pain or function. The surgically treated patients had a 30% reoperation rate. Level of evidence: I.

[17] Olerud P, Ahrengart L, Ponzer S, Saving J, Tidermark J: Hemiarthroplasty versus nonoperative treatment of displaced 4-part proximal humeral fractures in elderly patients: A randomized controlled trial. *J Shoulder Elbow Surg* 2011;20(7):1025-1033.

A comparison of hemiarthroplasty and nonsurgical treatment of displaced four-part proximal humeral fractures found that pain relief was significantly better in patients treated with hemiarthroplasty; there was no between-group difference in range of motion. Level of evidence: I.

[18] Bhandari M, Matthys G, McKee MD; Evidence-Based Orthopaedic Trauma Working Group: Four part

fractures of the proximal humerus. *J Orthop Trauma* 2004;18(2):126-127.

[19] Bell J-E, Leung BC, Spratt KF, et al: Trends and variation in incidence, surgical treatment, and repeat surgery of proximal humeral fractures in the elderly. *J Bone Joint Surg Am* 2011;93(2):121-131.

Using Medicare data, this study found a 25.6% increase in surgically managed proximal humeral fractures from 1999 to 2005, with significant regional variation in the proportion of fractures treated surgically and increasing rates of reoperation.

[20] Sporer SM, Weinstein JN, Koval KJ: The geographic incidence and treatment variation of common fractures of elderly patients. *J Am Acad Orthop Surg* 2006;14(4):246-255.

[21] Nicandri GT, Trumble TE, Warme WJ: Lessons learned from a case of proximal humeral locked plating gone awry. *J Orthop Trauma* 2009;23(8):607-611.

A case report documented entrapment of the axillary nerve between the plate and the humerus during open reduction and internal fixation using the direct lateral approach.

[22] Herscovici D Jr, Saunders DT, Johnson MP, Sanders R, DiPasquale T: Percutaneous fixation of proximal humeral fractures. *Clin Orthop Relat Res* 2000;375(375):97-104.

[23] Jaberg H, Warner JJ, Jakob RP: Percutaneous stabilization of unstable fractures of the humerus. *J Bone Joint Surg Am* 1992;74(4):508-515.

[24] Resch H, Povacz P, Fröhlich R, Wambacher M: Percutaneous fixation of three- and four-part fractures of the proximal humerus. *J Bone Joint Surg Br* 1997;79(2):295-300.

[25] Magovern B, Ramsey ML: Percutaneous fixation of proximal humerus fractures. *Orthop Clin North Am* 2008;39(4):405-416, v.

Indications, techniques, and outcomes are reviewed for percutaneous pinning of proximal humeral fractures.

[26] Keener JD, Parsons BO, Flatow EL, Rogers K, Williams GR, Galatz LM: Outcomes after percutaneous reduction and fixation of proximal humeral fractures. *J Shoulder Elbow Surg* 2007;16(3):330-338.

A case study reviewed proximal humeral fractures reduced and treated percutaneously in 35 patients. At an average 35-month follow-up, all fractures had healed and ASES and Constant scores were 83.4 and 73.9, respectively, with a mean visual analog pain score of only 1.4.

[27] Liew AS, Johnson JA, Patterson SD, King GJ, Chess DG: Effect of screw placement on fixation in the humeral head. *J Shoulder Elbow Surg* 2000;9(5):423-426.

[28] Weinstein DM, Bratton DR, Ciccone WJ II, Elias JJ: Locking plates improve torsional resistance in the stabilization of three-part proximal humeral fractures. *J Shoulder Elbow Surg* 2006;15(2):239-243.

[29] Hessmann MH, Hansen WS, Krummenauer F, Pol TF, Rommens PM: Locked plate fixation and intramedullary nailing for proximal humerus fractures: A biomechanical evaluation. *J Trauma* 2005;58(6):1194-1201.

[30] Südkamp N, Bayer J, Hepp P, et al: Open reduction and internal fixation of proximal humeral fractures with use of the locking proximal humerus plate: Results of a prospective, multicenter, observational study. *J Bone Joint Surg Am* 2009;91(6):1320-1328.

In a prospective observational study of 187 proximal humeral fractures treated with locking plates, the average Constant score was 85% of that of the contralateral shoulder at 1-year follow-up. There was a 34% complication rate with a 19% reoperation rate.

[31] Brunner F, Sommer C, Bahrs C, et al: Open reduction and internal fixation of proximal humerus fractures using a proximal humeral locked plate: A prospective multicenter analysis. *J Orthop Trauma* 2009;23(3):163-172.

At 1-year follow-up of 157 patients treated with a proximal humeral locking plate, good functional outcomes were reported. The average Constant score was 72 87% of the contralateral side score), but with a 35% complication rate.

[32] Ricchetti ET, Warrender WJ, Abboud JA: Use of locking plates in the treatment of proximal humerus fractures. *J Shoulder Elbow Surg* 2010;19(2, suppl):66-75.

In 54 patients with a proximal humeral fracture treated with a locking plate who were followed for a minimum of 6 months, overall good results were reflected in an average ASES score of 70.8, but with a 20.4% complication rate.

[33] Röderer G, Erhardt J, Kuster M, et al: Second generation locked plating of proximal humerus fractures: A prospective multicentre observational study. *Int Or- thop* 2011;35(3):425-432.

In a multicenter prospective study of 131 patients who underwent locked plating of proximal humeral frac- tures through a deltopectoral or direct lateral approach, the complications included screw perforation (15%) and displacement after open reduction and internal fixation (8%).

[34] Röderer G, Erhardt J, Graf M, Kinzl L, Gebhard F: Clinical results for minimally invasive locked plating of proximal humerus fractures. *J Orthop Trauma* 2010;24(7):400-406.

In a prospective study of 13 patients treated with a locking plate, three fractures had not healed at a minimum 6-month follow-up. The general complication rate was 21%, and the implant-related complication rate was 17%.

[35] Ong C, Bechtel C, Walsh M, Zuckerman JD, Egol KA: Three- and four-part fractures have poorer function than one-part proximal humerus fractures. *Clin Orthop Relat Res* 2011;469(12):3292-3299.

Outcomes were compared for patients with a two-part fracture treated nonsurgically and patients with a three- or four-part fracture treated with a locking plate. The patients with a locking plate had inferior outcomes, as shown by Medical Outcomes Study 36- Item Short Form and ASES scores, with more complications. Range of motion was similar between groups.

[36] Gardner MJ, Boraiah S, Helfet DL, Lorich DG: Indirect medial reduction and strut support of proximal humerus fractures using an endosteal implant. *J Orthop Trauma* 2008;22(3):195-200.

The steps were outlined for using a fibular allograft in the endosteal canal to support fixation of proximal humerus locking plate constructs.

[37] Osterhoff G, Baumgartner D, Favre P, et al: Medial support by fibula bone graft in angular stable plate fixation of proximal humeral fractures: An in vitro study with synthetic bone. *J Shoulder Elbow Surg* 2011;20(5):740-746.

A synthetic bone study compared the biomechanics of locking-plate fixation with those of locking plate fixation with intramedullary fibular allograft. Treatment with allograft was found to decrease migration and increase stiffness.

[38] Bae J-H, Oh J-K, Chon C-S, Oh CW, Hwang JH, Yoon YC: The biomechanical performance of locking plate fixation with intramedullary fibular strut graft augmentation in the treatment of unstable fractures of the proximal humerus. *J Bone Joint Surg Br* 2011;93(7):937-941.

A biomechanical study compared two-part surgical neck fractures in cadavers treated with a proximal humeral locking plate or a locking plate with intramedullary fibular strut graft. Maximum load to failure and stiffness were greater and displacement was less for those with

fibular strut graft combined with a locking plate.

[39] Bosch U, Skutek M, Fremerey RW, Tscherne H: Outcome after primary and secondary hemiarthroplasty in elderly patients with fractures of the proximal humerus. *J Shoulder Elbow Surg* 1998;7(5):479-484.

[40] Kralinger F, Schwaiger R, Wambacher M, et al: Outcome after primary hemiarthroplasty for fracture of the head of the humerus: A retrospective multicentre study of 167 patients. *J Bone Joint Surg Br* 2004;86(2):217-219.

[41] Boileau P, Krishnan SG, Tinsi L, Walch G, Coste JS, Molé D: Tuberosity malposition and migration: Reasons for poor outcomes after hemiarthroplasty for displaced fractures of the proximal humerus. *J Shoulder Elbow Surg* 2002;11(5):401-412.

[42] Frankle MA, Greenwald DP, Markee BA, Ondrovic LE, Lee WE III: Biomechanical effects of malposition of tuberosity fragments on the humeral prosthetic reconstruction for four-part proximal humerus fractures. *J Shoulder Elbow Surg* 2001;10(4):321-326.

[43] Frankle MA, Ondrovic LE, Markee BA, Harris ML, Lee WE III: Stability of tuberosity reattachment in proximal humeral hemiarthroplasty. *J Shoulder Elbow Surg* 2002;11(5):413-420.

[44] Lenarz C, Shishani Y, McCrum C, Nowinski RJ, Edwards TB, Gobezie R: Is reverse shoulder arthroplasty appropriate for the treatment of fractures in the older patient? Early observations. *Clin Orthop Relat Res* 2011;469(12):3324-3331.

At 12-month follow-up, 30 patients who underwent primary reverse shoulder arthroplasty for acute three- or four-part proximal humeral fracture had a mean ASES score of 78, a mean active forward elevation of 139°, and a visual analog scale pain score of only 1.1. The complication rate was 10%.

[45] Bufquin T, Hersan A, Hubert L, Massin P: Reverse shoulder arthroplasty for the treatment of three- and four-part fractures of the proximal humerus in the elderly: A prospective review of 43 cases with a short-term follow-up. *J Bone Joint Surg Br* 2007;89(4):516-520.

A case study of 43 patients who underwent reverse shoulder arthroplasty for proximal humeral fracture reported satisfactory clinical outcomes despite tuberosity migration at a mean 22-month follow-up.

[46] Gallinet D, Clappaz P, Garbuio P, Tropet Y, Obert L: Three or four parts complex proximal humerus fractures: Hemiarthroplasty versus reverse prosthesis. A

comparative study of 40 cases. *Orthop Traumatol Surg Res* 2009;95(1):48-55.

This study is the only direct comparison of reverse shoulder arthroplasty and hemiarthroplasty for three- and four-part proximal humeral fractures. Forty patients were studied. Patients treated with reverse shoulder arthroplasty had greater active forward elevation, and those treated with hemiarthroplasty had greater active external rotation. Their scores on the Disabilities of the Arm, Shoulder and Hand questionnaire scores were equivalent.

[47] Cazeneuve JF, Cristofari D-J: The reverse shoulder prosthesis in the treatment of fractures of the proximal humerus in the elderly. *J Bone Joint Surg Br* 2010;92(4):535-539.

A case study of reverse shoulder arthroplasty for proximal humerus fractures found radiographic glenoid loosening in 23 of 36 patients (63%) at a mean 6.6-year follow-up, with advancing scapular notching and decreasing Constant scores compared with short-term outcomes.

[48] Cazeneuve J-F, Cristofari D-J: Long term functional outcome following reverse shoulder arthroplasty in the elderly. *Orthop Traumatol Surg Res* 2011;97(6):583-589.

When 36 reverse shoulder arthroplasties were followed for a mean 6.6 years, a 63% incidence of radiographic glenoid loosening was found, with progressive notching and gradual deterioration of Constant scores over time.

第三十四章　新鲜严重肱骨近端骨折的治疗

Mark J. Jo, MD; Michael J. Gardner, MD

引言

绝大多数肱骨近端骨折移位小，骨折端稳定，非手术治疗效果好。目前尚未完全确定手术适应证。治疗的主要目标是恢复肩关节的良好功能，以及消除疼痛症状。在确定最佳治疗方案时，需要认真考虑患者的自身因素，尤其是要重点关注患者的生理年龄而不是实际年龄。以往，患者的实际年龄被当作判断适应证的明确指标。通常将年龄超过 65 岁的人群定义为老年人群，他们往往被认为平时久坐或肩关节活动范围相对较小。然而，患病人群的年龄分布正在发生迅速变化。目前，六七十岁人群对肩关节的功能需求比以往更高，实际年龄已经成为一个泛泛的变量。

治疗方案应该根据患者个人的实际需求和期望来制订。本身肩关节功能差或认知受限的患者可以耐受骨折不愈合但无疼痛的僵硬肩，而肩关节活动良好的年轻患者则希望骨折愈合并有较大的肩关节活动范围。大多数肱骨近端骨折患者的状况介于这两者之间、患者年龄相对较大、活动能力较低，可以接受骨折部分畸形愈合、活动范围减少、功能较差的情况。手术治疗的危险因素，如全身麻醉或局部麻醉风险、手术切口问题、内固定失效等，也应与患者的期望值、术前的活动范围以及精神状态等一起被衡量。另外，骨折是位于上肢的优势侧还是非优势侧也是需要考虑的因素。

流行病学和损伤机制

肱骨近端骨折占全身所有骨折的 5%，美国每年大约发生 8 万例肱骨近端骨折。[1] 随着骨质疏松患者的增多，肱骨近端脆性骨折的发生率也会增高。像大多数骨折一样，肱骨近端骨折在统计学上也是呈双模态分布，在相对年轻（20~30 岁）和老年（大于 65 岁）人群中的发病率较高。女性的发病率较男性高。绝大多数肱骨近端骨折发生在老年人群，多为站立位摔倒所致的低能量损伤。这类骨折应该被认为是真正的病理性骨折，并进行骨质疏松的检查。受伤时胳膊的体位（内收或外展、是否手掌伸展着地）决定了骨折的类型（内翻或外展）。而年轻患者的骨折多由高能量损伤引起，如摩托车事故或高处坠落。

临床检查

体格检查

体格检查应该包含全身检查，若是高能量损伤，应按高级创伤生命支持标准处理。老年人摔伤后也要进行中枢神经系统检查以排除颅内损伤。

Dr. Gardner or an immediate family member serves as a paid consultant to or is an employee of Synthes, DGIMed, Amgen, Stryker, and RTI Biologics; has received research or institutional support from Synthes and Amgen; and serves as a board member, owner, officer, or committee member of the Orthopaedic Trauma Association. Neither Dr. Jo nor any immediate family member has received anything of value from or has stock or stock options held in a commercial company or institution related directly or indirectly to the subject of this chapter.

应仔细检查肩关节周围皮肤，尤其要注意有无撕裂伤以排除开放性骨折。轻轻触诊检查疼痛程度及有无骨擦感以确定有无合并其他部位损伤，如锁骨、肩胛骨、肘关节和腕关节损伤等。另外，也要仔细全面地检查肢体末端的血运和神经状况。

肱骨近端骨折多累及外科颈，在骨折端的腋神经近侧段容易因为挫伤或嵌压受损。在急性损伤时准确评估腋神经的运动功能是比较困难的，但经常能发现三角肌的异常表现，尤其是三角肌前侧头不能主动上举。此外，也应该在肩关节的外侧仔细检查腋神经的感觉功能。

肱骨近端骨折合并脱位时会经常出现肩袖撕裂。年经患者往往肩袖撕裂范围较大，而老年患者则多表现为肩袖慢性磨损基础上的撕裂。最近的一项研究对 76 例非手术治疗的肱骨近端骨折患者行 MRI 检查后发现，存在 22 例肩袖撕裂，其中 4 例为全层撕裂。[2] 在肱骨近端骨折发生时评估肩袖的功能和完整性是非常困难的，在骨折愈合和康复锻炼至主动活动的过程中要注意评估。

影像学检查

合理且高质量的影像学检查对准确评估肱骨近端骨折和制订治疗计划至关重要。在真正的肩胛骨正位（前后位）中，肩胛骨与身体躯干大约成角 30°，真正的肩胛骨正位片可以清晰地显示盂肱关节。内旋正位可更好地显示大小结节，尤其适用于单独的结节骨折时，但在典型的肱骨近端干骺端骨折时则不是必需的。肩胛骨侧位（Y 型位）可显示矢状位的骨折脱位，尽管腋位片可以很好地显示盂肱关节脱位、外科颈骨折移位及小结节骨折移位，但是标准腋位片很难获得，因为需要患者外展上臂，在急性骨折时患者疼痛明显，而大多数患者能够耐受上臂 30° 外展，这足以满足腋位的要求。改良 Velpeau 腋位可以替代真正的腋位。

大多数肱骨近端骨折的评估不需要 CT 检查，但是对于高能量损伤导致的粉碎性骨折移位，CT检查还是有很大帮助的。如果 X 线片不能清晰地显示骨折移位情况，则需要行 CT 检查以更好地评估和制订治疗方案。尽管三维 CT 应用越来越多，但其检查费用较高，对治疗方案鲜有帮助。

肩袖对于肱骨近端骨折患者的功能恢复是非常重要的。术前可以行 MRI 检查来评估肩袖损伤情况，也可以在术中直视下探查。术后因内固定材料对 MRI 检查有影响，可以采用 B 超检查。有些专家应用 MRI 检查肱骨近端骨折合并肩袖损伤的情况，尤其是在大结节骨折移位超过 5 mm、三部分或四部分骨折、AO11B 型和 11C 型骨折中。[3-4]

非手术治疗

适应证

患者选择非手术治疗时需要考虑多种因素。应当分析不同类型骨折移位与骨折的两个主要并发症之间的关系，以及骨折不愈合的风险和畸形愈合对功能的影响。骨折不愈合对功能影响明显。如果骨折端间接触面积小，如外科颈骨折，骨折不愈合风险高。典型的骨折向前成角和肱骨干向前移位在腋位片上最容易评估（图 34-1）。根据患者的体位不同会有不同的 X 线片表现，因为仰卧位可使重力加重畸形。许多骨折因为发生在干骺端且血供丰富而容易愈合，但畸形愈合会导致关节功能受损。

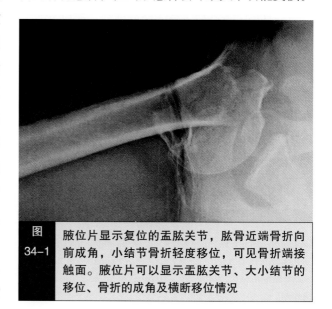

图 34-1　腋位片显示复位的盂肱关节，肱骨近端骨折向前成角，小结节骨折轻度移位，可见骨折端接触面。腋位片可以显示盂肱关节、大小结节的移位、骨折的成角及横断移位情况

大结节骨折畸形愈合会导致肩袖力臂缩短，以及肩袖在肩关节外展外旋时与肩峰撞击，从而使肩关节活动受限。同样的，内翻畸形愈合也会导致肩峰撞击和活动受限。尚不清楚会导致活动受限的具体骨折移位距离。不建议严格遵循 Neer 分型中的骨折移位大于 1 cm，成角大于 45° 的手术适应证，因为这个指标也不能准确地评估稳定性和功能。对于移位比较大的骨折，应同时对肩袖进行检查。

除了受伤后骨折原位愈合对关节功能有影响外，骨折的稳定性也必须受到重视。尽管难以预料非手术治疗时的骨折移位是否会加重，但某些特定骨折的移位可能进一步加重。发生在解剖颈或外科颈的骨折，尤其骨折端接触面较小时，骨折的不稳定性增高。内翻性骨折比外翻性骨折更不稳定。内侧柱（骨距区）粉碎性骨折移位可能会出现移位距离增大。

治疗

当根据骨折稳定性确定进行非手术治疗后，应尽早制动肩关节。[5] 选用合适的吊带制动肩关节几天足以控制疼痛，随后进行被动钟摆活动锻炼。无论如何，在康复师指导下的被动功能锻炼最晚在伤后 14 天开始进行，以尽可能减小肩关节局部粘连和僵硬。主动辅助功能锻炼在伤后 4~6 周内进行。针对三角肌和肩胛骨周围肌肉的力量练习在 X 线片显示骨折愈合后进行。

如果因为功能需求低或精神性疾病而对不稳定骨折患者采用非手术治疗，至少制动 2~4 周，以减小骨折移位距离增大和骨折不愈合的风险。

早期康复锻炼时难以评估骨折的稳定性或再移位的风险，需要考虑很多因素，如骨折类型和患者的能动性。被认为稳定的骨折也可能再移位，继而需要改变治疗方案。因此，非手术治疗患者早期需要多次随访和 X 线片复查。

一些患者可能受益于骨折闭合复位，闭合复位可以改善骨折对线和增加骨折端接触面积，从而促进骨折愈合和功能恢复。[6] 闭合复位可以在诊室进行，尤其适合有手术禁忌证和骨折移位严重而又不愿进行手术的患者。

手术治疗

手术治疗的目的是使骨折复位固定以确保骨折愈合和功能恢复。成功的治疗基于良好的骨量、肱骨头活力以及骨折愈合前复位不变的能力。骨量是患者的治疗基础，术前可以进行评估，在制订治疗计划前需要认真考虑。[7] 骨量较差时需要在生物力学上加强固定，如应用异体腓骨或带生物活性的人工骨。肱骨头的活力取决于其血供。X 线片或 CT 图像可以评估骨折的粉碎和移位程度。肱骨头血供可以通过骨折类型及累及内侧距的情况来判断。肱骨头与干骺端之间的距离小于 8 mm 或内侧软组织铰链断裂容易导致肱骨头缺血性坏死。[8] 肱骨头劈裂骨折往往会出现缺血，随着对骨折认识的深入和微骨折复位固定技术的发展，这类骨折可以行切开复位内固定，尤其是年轻患者的骨折。

肱骨近端骨折复位固定应用最多的是传统的胸大肌三角肌入路，也可以上下延伸切口探及盂肱关节和肱骨干。因为切口位于前方，所以可以很容易地探及肩胛下肌、肱二头肌长头腱、联合腱及小结节等结构。自胸大肌和三角肌间的神经界面间隙进入可以减小神经损伤的风险。尽管医师仔细操作，但仍有损伤肌皮神经和腋神经的风险，尤其是当过度牵拉联合腱和三角肌时。前入路会增高损伤头静脉和旋肱前动脉的风险，因为旋肱前动脉是供应肱骨头的主要血管，所以其损伤后会导致肱骨头缺血性坏死和骨折不愈合。[9] 为了到达骨折部位而过度分离软组织会剥离骨组织的血供。胸大肌三角肌入路的最大缺点是不能很好地探及大结节及肱骨头的外侧面，即大多数锁定钢板的近端标记点。内旋肱骨近端有利于显露近端外侧和缝合肩袖。

使用肩峰前外侧入路可以避免一些胸大肌三角肌入路的缺点。[10-11] 但该入路有损伤腋神经的风险。解剖研究发现，腋神经前束距肩峰约65 mm。术前应该测量和标记神经的位置。该入路为纵行切口，起自肩峰前角，向远端纵向延伸12~15 cm（图34-2）。沿肩关节皮肤张力线切开的手术切口更美观也更容易被接受。[12-15] 在三角肌

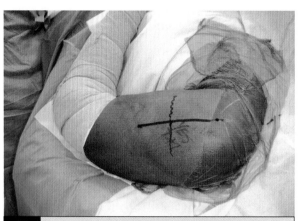

图34-2　肩峰前外侧入路的皮肤切口的体表标记，标记自肩峰前外侧角沿肱骨干轴线向远端延伸。腋神经大致标记于肩峰外远端 6.5 cm 处。经允许引自 Gardner MJ: Open reduction and internal fixation of fractures of the proximal humerus: The anterolateral acromial approach, in Levine WN, Cadet ER, Ahmad CS, eds: *Shoulder and Elbow Trauma*. London, England, JP Medical Publishers, 2012, pp 51–60.

前侧头和中间头之间深层钝性分离显露非血管间隙。触及并保护腋神经，在神经血管束的远端和近端分别建立两个窗以复位和固定骨折。

肩峰前外侧入路在直视下易探及大结节骨折块及确定钢板放置的位置。手术切口的平面也在钢板及螺钉固定的位置。该入路可以直达骨折线，有利于对骨折进行复位和固定。如果主要骨折线位于干骺端，则钢板可以间接起到复位的作用（图34-3）。该入路可以向上延伸到肩峰下间隙，探查冈上肌和冈下肌等肩袖肌肉的撕裂情况，并进行修复。该入路具有微创、软组织损伤小的特点。该入路的主要缺点是可能伤及腋神经，因此要仔细辨认并分离腋神经，在整个手术过程中都要小心保护腋神经。该入路也不能过度牵拉切口，除非牵张腋神经，否则不能探及肱骨前侧面。

胸大肌三角肌入路和肩峰前外侧入路都能很好地对肱骨近端骨折进行复位和固定。手术入路的选择需要根据骨折的特点、复位技术和医师的经验来决定。因为胸大肌三角肌入路前后牵拉范围更广，所以适用于关节置换、严重的骨折不愈合和畸形愈合。关节置换技术和手术器械多是根据前入路

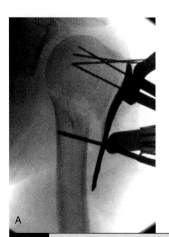
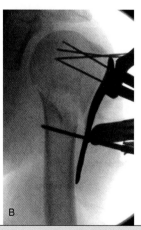
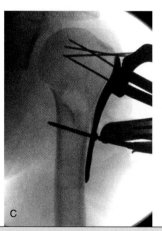
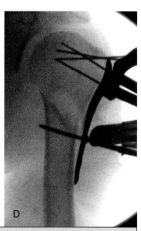

图34-3　透视图像显示通过肩峰前外侧入路利用钢板作为间接复位工具对肱骨近端骨折进行复位。A. 钢板位置放置合适，肱骨骨干骨折向内侧移位。B 和 C. 利用钢板进行复位，当把螺钉打入肱骨骨干并拧紧时，骨折远端骨干外移达到解剖复位。D. 骨折复位良好。复位螺钉尽量能长到足以帮助骨折端复位，最后通过钢板其他孔固定完毕后可以再更换短钉。经允许引自 Gardner MJ: Open reduction and internal fixation of fractures of the proximal humerus: The anterolateral acromial approach, in Levine WN, Cadet ER, Ahmad CS, eds: *Shoulder and Elbow Trauma*. London, England, JP Medical Publishers, 2012, pp 51–60.

来设计的，因此关节置换多采用前入路。胸大肌三角肌入路可以探及肱骨近端前侧面，尤其是当小结节在肩胛下肌牵拉下向内侧移位超过 1 cm 时。肩峰前外侧入路也可用于骨折不愈合或畸形愈合，但显露范围有限且不能过度牵拉以免损伤腋神经。如果医师对该入路非常熟悉，也可以用于关节置换。

胸大肌三角肌入路和肩峰前外侧入路都可在仰卧位或沙滩椅位进行。嘱患者取沙滩椅位时，可以在患者对侧进行前后位透视和从头侧进行腋位透视（图 34-4）。利用不遮挡肩后部的特殊手术床可以提高透视的清晰度。推荐使用仰卧位，患肢放于靠近手术床边缘的桌上。一定要确保手术床边缘可被 X 线穿透，不影响前后位透视。C 臂置于头侧，可以移动至肩关节前后位和腋位透视（图 34-5）。除了透视技术外，术前一定要确认影像屏及连接线等可正常使用以确保术中能够透视。

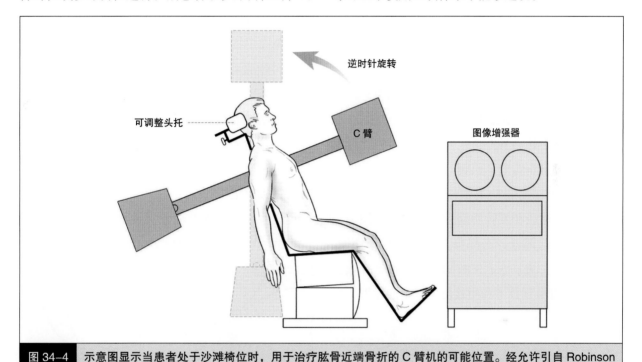

图 34-4　示意图显示当患者处于沙滩椅位时，用于治疗肱骨近端骨折的 C 臂机的可能位置。经允许引自 Robinson CM, Page RS: Severely impacted valgus proximal humeral fractures. *J Bone Joint Surg Am* 2004;86（suppl 1）:143–155.

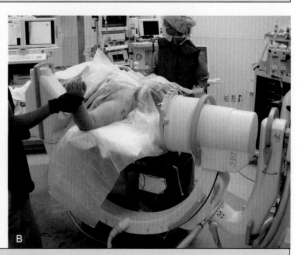

图 34-5　患者处于仰卧位（A），并用 X 线可透的桌子支撑手臂（B）以获取无阻挡的前后位和腋位透视片。经允许引自 Gardner MJ: Open reduction and internal fixation of fractures of the proximal humerus: The anterolateral acromial approach, in Levine WN, Cadet ER, Ahmad CS, eds: *Shoulder and Elbow Trauma*. London, England, JP Medical Publishers, 2012, pp 51–60.

闭合复位经皮穿针固定

闭合复位骨折要在透视下进行，可以徒手牵引或经皮肤小切口插入骨撬或其他器械进行骨折复位。复位成功后可以使用克氏针或经皮螺钉固定骨折。[16-19] 经皮固定技术的优点在于对软组织的剥离和破坏小。手术中对软组织剥离过大容易导致骨折不愈合和肱骨头坏死。[18] 在肱骨干外侧三角肌止点下方打入 1 枚或 2 枚克氏针：1 枚克氏针自前方皮质进入；如果需要的话，第 2 枚克氏针自大结节向内侧骨距打入。[16] 相关解剖学研究已经确定克氏针的最佳放置位置（图 34-6）。[19-20] 为了避免损伤腋神经前束，外侧针的入点应该在距离肱骨头高点远端至少两个肱骨头直径长度处。另外，也要注意前侧克氏针不要伤及头静脉和肱二头肌腱。自肱骨大结节处打向内侧骨距的克氏针距离肱骨头下缘至少 2 cm 以避免损伤腋神经和旋肱后动脉。经皮穿针固定技术已被用于二部分、三部分，甚至四部分骨折，应注意如果大结节固定失败则会导致临床疗效较差。[19] 随着微创技术和间接复位技术的发展，经皮固定技术越来越受到挑战，小切口复位和固定技术应该会引起更多的重视。

缝合固定

肱骨近端骨折的缝合固定技术可以消除或减小钢板固定和关节置换的相关手术风险。经骨缝合固定可以减少软组织损伤并有利于保护肱骨头血供。最初，缝合固定和克氏针固定技术被 Neer 介绍用于三部分骨折的治疗，但未被广泛应用。[21] 最近有几项研究报道了这项技术，一项应用缝合固定技术治疗 28 例两部分或三部分大结节或外科颈肱骨近端骨折的研究发现，78% 的病例结果优秀，11% 的病例结果良好。[22] 还有一项研究在应用经骨缝合技术治疗 165 例二部分、三部分、四部分骨折时发现，患侧改良后的 Constant 肩关节评分平均为健侧的 94%（图 34-7）。[23-24]

钢板固定

近些年，肱骨近端骨折手术治疗的适应证更

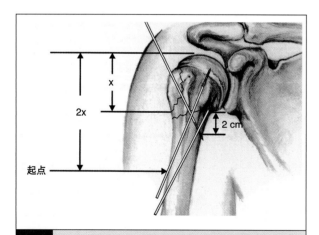

图 34-6 示意图显示了外侧和大结节固定针的位置。近端外侧针的起点应位于从肱骨头上方到肱骨头最下缘距离两倍处或更远端。大结节固定针应固定至与肱骨头最下端相距 20 mm 的肱骨外科颈皮质骨处。经允许引自 Rowles DJ, McGrory JE: Percutaneous pinning of the proximal part of the humerus: An anatomic study. *J Bone Joint Surg Am* 2001;83（11）:1695–1699.

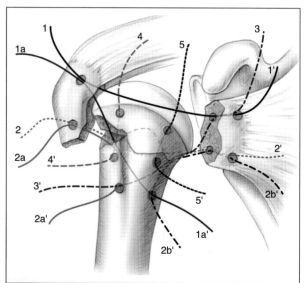

图 34-7 仅用缝合固定移位的四部分肱骨近端骨折的缝合技术。缝线以指定的编号顺序穿过指定的钻孔。1. 缝合固定大结节和肱骨干；1a 和 2. 缝合固定大小结节；2a. 缝合固定大结节和肱骨干；3. 缝合固定小结节和肱骨干；4 和 5. 缝合固定肱骨头和肱骨干。经允许引自 Dimakopoulos P, Panagopoulos A, Kasimatis G: Transosseous suture fixation of proximal humeral fractures: Surgical technique. *J Bone Joint Surg Am* 2009;91（suppl 2）:8–21.

加完善，内固定技术发展迅速。早期治疗的一些弊端是由螺钉在肱骨头内的把持力差引起的。许多肱骨近端骨折患者的肱骨近端及肱骨头骨质差，术后容易出现螺钉穿出和肱骨头塌陷。复杂肱骨近端骨折钢板内固定失效率高，所以建议对三部分、四部分骨折患者行人工肱骨头置换术。解剖锁定钢板及角度锁定螺钉技术的发展大大降低了内固定失效的风险。从不同角度方向打入较多的锁定螺钉可以更好地或最大程度地固定肱骨头。与其他固定方式相比，钢板螺钉固定提供了更加刚性的结构，但是需要充分地显露软组织以便更好地对骨折进行复位和固定。可以采用肩峰前外侧入路和微创设计的钢板内固定系统来减少软组织的损伤。[25-26]微创新技术尽管可以避免一些问题，但仍然存在螺钉切出肱骨头及内固定失效等并发症。

骨折的准确复位为骨折固定提供充分的力学稳定性、骨折愈合和肩关节功能的恢复很重要。[6,27-29]在肱骨近端内侧骨距复位合适后置入内下方骨距螺钉对于维持复位很重要。[29]对于内翻位骨折，过度复位至外翻位固定可以更好地增加骨接触面积和防止复位失效。钢板的放置位置决定了螺钉在肱骨头内的方向和轨迹。需要注意的是，尽管钢板是针对肱骨近端的解剖结构设计的，但是仍然存在个体差异。钢板位置应尽可能偏下以防止外展时撞击肩峰。需要检查肱骨头内螺钉及内下方骨距螺钉的位置和数目以确保固定作用的最大化和排除螺钉穿出肱骨头的风险。钢板必须放置于肱二头肌腱沟后侧以保护肱骨头内血供。结节骨折的复位和愈合会极大影响肩关节功能和手术效果。需要应用不可吸收缝线将结节骨折块相互缝合固定或缝合固定于钢板上。

加强固定

一些骨折可能需要进行结构性和（或）生物性的加强或支撑。尽管准确复位对于骨折的生物力学稳定性非常重要，但如果存在骨质疏松，尤其是肱骨近端及肱骨头内松质骨稀疏，会大减小骨折端的接触面积。许多骨折在损伤时就出现塌陷，骨折复位时需要撬起塌陷，从而导致骨缺损。自体骨、异体骨、骨水泥和骨替代物可以用于填充骨缺损，给骨折提供结构性或生物性支撑。[30-31]同种异体骨可被用于后内侧骨距粉碎性骨折、骨折不愈合及翻修手术等。同种异体腓骨或股骨头可以用于结构性支撑或增加螺钉对于骨质的把持力。[32]

髓内钉固定

髓内钉固定是肱骨近端骨折治疗的另一个选择。新式髓内钉的钉中钉设计能更好地进行角度固定。髓内钉的优点是软组织破坏小，可更好地保护血供。以前髓内钉入点位于大结节，容易损伤肩袖复合体，导致肩关节术后疼痛。新式髓内钉自大结节内侧软骨进入，可以避免损伤肩袖止点。[33-34]髓内钉的主要适应证是累及外科颈的肱骨近端二部分骨折，结合大小结节缝合固定也可适用于三部分和四部分骨折，其对于向干骺端或骨干延伸的肱骨近端骨折具有更大的优势。[35-40]

外固定

外固定也可以用于肱骨近端骨折的治疗，类似其他微创技术，外固定技术能够减少软组织损伤和血供破坏。[41-43]但是外固定也有缺点，例如，置钉时可能损伤重要解剖结构，外固定架螺钉容易松动和感染。外固定架笨重，在美观方面患者难以接受。外固定架可以用于多发创伤、难以耐受长时间手术和局部软组织损伤严重的患者。有研究报道，肱骨近端骨折应用外固定架可以取得较好的效果。[41-43]像之前介绍的经皮固定技术一样，需要采用间接复位技术，经皮小切口打入螺钉后，再连接外固定架螺栓及连接杆。

循证医学结果

来自美国医学中心的数据表明，65岁以上老年人群的肱骨近端骨折的发生率在1990—2005年没有发生太大的变化，但手术率增加了25%。[1]

美国不同州间的手术率不同，这表明对切开复位内固定手术适应证的认识仍存在差异。最近，一些高水平论文证据开始分析和解释这些差异。

治疗肱骨近端骨折时，选择内固定还是关节置换依赖很多因素，也一直未有定论，尤其是在锁定钢板问世以后。很少有研究对治疗方法进行直接比较，也没有相关随机对照研究。在最近一项对 55 岁以上的三部分、四部分肱骨近端骨折患者的回顾性研究中，38 例患者应用锁定钢板，48 例行半肩关节置换。[27] 对于三部分骨折，应用钢板的疗效比半肩关节置换好（Constant 肩关节评分为 60~72，P < 0.001），在四部分骨折患者中也得到类似结果（Constant 肩关节评分为 60~65，P=0.19）。研究结果显示，内翻型骨折的并发症，如复位丢失，发生率比其他类型骨折高，疗效也差。[26] 对于合并肩袖损伤的老年严重粉碎性骨折患者，应用反肩关节置换治疗越来越普遍。[44] 确认结节骨折的复位固定无论对于内固定还是肩关节置换都是非常重要的。

一项对 53 例应用锁定钢板治疗的 60 岁以上老年肱骨近端骨折患者的研究发现，并发症的发生率为 36%，其中螺钉切出肱骨头的发生率为 43%。[45] 但是，该项研究没有对应用锁定钢板起关键作用的骨折复位准确性进行评价。[30] 另外，也可应用多向锁定钢板治疗肱骨近端骨折，尽管理论上该治疗方法有很多优势，但最近一项随机对照研究发现，标准锁定钢板治疗肱骨近端骨折的疗效与多向锁定钢板没有差别。[46]

髓内钉也是治疗肱骨近端骨折的选择。最近一项针对 51 例二部分肱骨近端骨折的随机对照研究发现，无论是在术后第 1 年随访时还是在第 3 年随访时，肩关节功能都得到了很好的恢复，但在第 1 年随访时，钢板的疗效优于髓内钉，但并发症发生率更高。[36] 在第 3 年随访时，二者疗效差别不大。另外一项对 38 例二部分肱骨近端骨折应用多轴髓内钉的研究发现，骨折愈合及功能结果良好，肩关节疼痛副作用少。[35]

非手术治疗对一些患者仍然有效，尽管还不完全清楚其理想的适应证。一项对 70 例 60~85 岁患者使用非手术方法治疗移位和无移位的肱骨近端骨折的研究发现，移位骨折的效果差（Constant 肩关节评分为 59），无移位骨折的效果好（Constant 肩关节评分为 74），四部分骨折的效果最差（Constant 肩关节评分为 34）。[47] 一项研究报道，对 18 例生活要求低的三部分、四部分骨折患者采取非手术治疗，平均随访 39 个月，疗效欠佳（平均 Constant 肩关节评分为 61）。[48] 最近，一项随机对照研究比较了非手术治疗与手术治疗疗效，结果与上述研究结果不一致，研究对象为 50 例大于 60 岁的有移位的三部分和四部分骨折患者，非手术治疗组对骨折采取闭合复位，早期功能锻炼，随访 1 年后，功能恢复结果在组间无差异。[6]

总结

肱骨近端骨折的治疗具有一定挑战性，但是在详细了解患者的期望后审慎地选择现有的治疗方法往往可以取得较好的效果。肱骨近端骨折的理想治疗方案还没有完全定论。新技术、新方法的产生往往会使治疗方式产生重大转变，甚至有机会持续改善患者预后。既往的研究已经清楚地表明，肱骨近端骨折的非手术治疗有很好的效果。手术治疗应该用于对功能要求高或非手术治疗不愈合风险高的患者。患者的自身因素对决定是否行手术治疗是最重要的。随着人口的老龄化和寿命的延长，与以往相比，现在的患者在生命晚期的活动能力会越来越强，肱骨近端骨折后对预后的期望也越来越高。外科医师应根据骨折的类型和自己的经验选择手术方式。

参考文献

[1] Bell JE, Leung BC, Spratt KF, et al: Trends and variation in incidence, surgical treatment, and repeat sur-

gery of proximal humeral fractures in the elderly. *J Bone Joint Surg Am* 2011;93(2):121-131.

An analysis of Medicare data on treatment trends for proximal humeral fractures over 5 years found that the incidence of proximal humeral fractures was unchanged, but the rate of surgical treatment increased significantly.

[2] Fjalestad T, Hole MO, Blücher J, Hovden IA, Stiris MG, Strømsøe K: Rotator cuff tears in proximal humeral fractures: An MRI cohort study in 76 patients. *Arch Orthop Trauma Surg* 2010;130(5):575-581.

[3] Gallo RA, Sciulli R, Daffner RH, Altman DT, Altman GT: Defining the relationship between rotator cuff injury and proximal humerus fractures. *Clin Orthop Relat Res* 2007;458:70-77.

An analysis of radiographic and MRI characteristics of proximal humeral fractures revealed that greater severity of rotator cuff injury was correlated with a higher AO or Neer classification and with 5 mm or more displacement of the greater tuberosity. Level of evidence: II.

[4] Gallo RA, Altman DT, Altman GT: Assessment of rotator cuff tendons after proximal humerus fractures: Is preoperative imaging necessary? *J Trauma* 2009;66(3):951-953.

The usefulness of MRI for proximal humeral fractures was reviewed, and a treatment algorithm was proposed. One- and two-part fractures associated with less than 5 mm of greater tuberosity displacement were found not to warrant MRI. MRI may be useful for two-part fractures with more than 5 mm of greater tuberosity displacement as well as three- and four-part fractures.

[5] Lefevre-Colau MM, Babinet A, Fayad F, et al: Immediate mobilization compared with conventional immobilization for the impacted nonoperatively treated proximal humeral fracture: A randomized controlled trial. *J Bone Joint Surg Am* 2007;89(12):2582-2590.

Patients with a proximal humeral fracture were randomly assigned to mobilization earlier than a few days or at 3 weeks. Early mobilization led to improved outcomes and no complications. Level of evidence: I.

[6] Fjalestad T, Hole MO, Hovden IA, Blücher J, Strømsøe K: Surgical treatment with an angular stable plate for complex displaced proximal humeral fractures in elderly patients: A randomized controlled

trial. *J Orthop Trauma* 2012;26(2):98-106.

A comparison study of the surgical and nonsurgical treatment of older patients with a proximal humeral fracture found no difference in functional outcome at 1-year follow-up. Level of evidence: I.

[7] Tingart MJ, Apreleva M, von Stechow D, Zurakowski D, Warner JJ: The cortical thickness of the proximal humeral diaphysis predicts bone mineral density of the proximal humerus. *J Bone Joint Surg Br* 2003;85(4):611-617.

[8] Hertel R, Hempfing A, Stiehler M, Leunig M: Predictors of humeral head ischemia after intracapsular fracture of the proximal humerus. *J Shoulder Elbow Surg* 2004;13(4):427-433.

[9] Gardner MJ, Voos JE, Wanich T, Helfet DL, Lorich DG: Vascular implications of minimally invasive plating of proximal humerus fractures. *J Orthop Trauma* 2006;20(9):602-607.

[10] Gardner MJ, Griffith MH, Dines JS, Briggs SM, Weiland AJ, Lorich DG: The extended anterolateral acromial approach allows minimally invasive access to the proximal humerus. *Clin Orthop Relat Res* 2005;434:123-129.

[11] Gardner MJ, Boraiah S, Helfet DL, Lorich DG: The anterolateral acromial approach for fractures of the proximal humerus. *J Orthop Trauma* 2008;22(2):132-137.

Fifty-two patients with a proximal humeral fracture were treated using a minimally invasive anterolateral approach, which led to a good functional outcome and no axillary nerve injuries.

[12] Robinson CM, Murray IR: The extended deltoid-splitting approach to the proximal humerus: Variations and extensions. *J Bone Joint Surg Br* 2011;93(3):387-392.

Variations and extensions of the anterolateral surgical approach for the surgical treatment of proximal humeral fractures were presented, with a description of the indications and approaches used in 386 patients during a 12-year period.

[13] Robinson CM, Khan L, Akhtar A, Whittaker R: The extended deltoid-splitting approach to the proximal humerus. *J Orthop Trauma* 2007;21(9):657-662.

Experience with an extended deltoid-splitting approach for the treatment of proximal humeral frac- tures was presented. During a 9-year period, 226 patients underwent surgical fixation using this approach, with no major complications.

［14］ Robinson CM, Page RS: Severely impacted valgus proximal humeral fractures: Results of operative treatment. *J Bone Joint Surg Am* 2003;85-A(9):1647-1655.

［15］ Robinson CM, Page RS: Severely impacted valgus proximal humeral fractures. *J Bone Joint Surg Am* 2004;86-A(Suppl 1, Pt 2):143-155.

［16］ Jaberg H, Warner JJ, Jakob RP: Percutaneous stabilization of unstable fractures of the humerus. *J Bone Joint Surg Am* 1992;74(4):508-515.

［17］ Resch H, Povacz P, Fröhlich R, Wambacher M: Percutaneous fixation of three- and four-part fractures of the proximal humerus. *J Bone Joint Surg Br* 1997;79(2):295-300.

［18］ Keener JD, Parsons BO, Flatow EL, Rogers K, Williams GR, Galatz LM: Outcomes after percutaneous reduction and fixation of proximal humeral fractures. *J Shoulder Elbow Surg* 2007;16(3):330-338.

A cohort study revealed that in selected patients, percutaneous fixation led to reliable union and good clinical outcome.

［19］ Rowles DJ, McGrory JE: Percutaneous pinning of the proximal part of the humerus: An anatomic study. *J Bone Joint Surg Am* 2001;83(11):1695-1699.

［20］ Kamineni S, Ankem H, Sanghavi S: Anatomical considerations for percutaneous proximal humeral fracture fixation. *Injury* 2004;35(11):1133-1136.

［21］ Neer CS II: Displaced proximal humeral fractures: II. Treatment of three-part and four-part displacement. *J Bone Joint Surg Am* 1970;52(6):1090-1103.

［22］ Park MC, Murthi AM, Roth NS, Blaine TA, Levine WN, Bigliani LU: Two-part and three-part fractures of the proximal humerus treated with suture fixation. *J Orthop Trauma* 2003;17(5):319-325.

［23］ Dimakopoulos P, Panagopoulos A, Kasimatis G: Transosseous suture fixation of proximal humeral fractures. *J Bone Joint Surg Am* 2007;89(8):1700-1709.

In a large study of selected patients treated with a transosseous suture fixation technique, radiographic and clinical outcomes were favorable at 5-year follow-up.

［24］ Dimakopoulos P, Panagopoulos A, Kasimatis G: Transosseous suture fixation of proximal humeral fractures: Surgical technique. *J Bone Joint Surg Am* 2009;91(Suppl 2, Pt 1):8-21.

Experience with transosseous suture fixation in 165 patients over an 11-year period was presented. The mean Constant score was 94%. Level of evidence: IV.

［25］ Egol KA, Ong CC, Walsh M, Jazrawi LM, Tejwani NC, Zuckerman JD: Early complications in proximal humerus fractures (OTA Types 11) treated with locked plates. *J Orthop Trauma* 2008;22(3):159-164.

A retrospective analysis over a 3-year period revealed that locked plating of the proximal humerus had a very good union rate but a large number of complications, most of which were screw penetration of the humeral head.

［26］ Solberg BD, Moon CN, Franco DP, Paiement GD: Locked plating of 3- and 4-part proximal humerus fractures in older patients: The effect of initial fracture pattern on outcome. *J Orthop Trauma* 2009;23(2):113-119.

A retrospective analysis of older patients with a three- or a four-part fracture treated with locked plating revealed that varus angulation of the fracture was associated with relatively poor outcomes and an increased rate of complications. Valgus fractures with an intact metaphysis had the best outcomes.

［27］ Solberg BD, Moon CN, Franco DP, Paiement GD: Surgical treatment of three and four-part proximal humeral fractures. *J Bone Joint Surg Am* 2009;91(7):1689-1697.

A retrospective analysis of older patients with a three- or four-part fracture found that internal fixation led to better outcomes than hemiarthroplasty, especially in three-part fractures, but was associated with a higher complication rate.

［28］ Olerud P, Ahrengart L, Ponzer S, Saving J, Tidermark J: Internal fixation versus nonoperative treatment of displaced 3-part proximal humeral fractures in elderly patients: A randomized controlled trial. *J Shoulder Elbow Surg* 2011;20(5):747-755.

Older patients with a moderately displaced three-part fracture proximal humeral fracture were randomly assigned to be treated nonsurgically or with locking plate fixation. Surgery had a slight short-term benefit, but no significant long-term difference was reported between the two groups.

［29］ Gardner MJ, Weil Y, Barker JU, Kelly BT, Helfet DL, Lorich DG: The importance of medial support in locked plating of proximal humerus fractures. *J Orthop Trauma* 2007;21(3):185-191.

A retrospective study of proximal humeral fractures treated with locked plating revealed the importance of the inferomedial calcar region to the mechanical stability of the fracture reduction.

[30] Robinson CM, Wylie JR, Ray AG, et al: Proximal humeral fractures with a severe varus deformity treated by fixation with a locking plate. *J Bone Joint Surg Br* 2010;92(5):672-678.

Patients with varus displacement were successfully treated with anatomic reduction, locked plating, and structural allograft.

[31] Gerber C, Werner CM, Vienne P: Internal fixation of complex fractures of the proximal humerus. *J Bone Joint Surg Br* 2004;86(6):848-855.

[32] Gardner MJ, Boraiah S, Helfet DL, Lorich DG: Indirect medial reduction and strut support of proximal humerus fractures using an endosteal implant. *J Orthop Trauma* 2008;22(3):195-200.

Fibula strut allograft was used to improve the stability of a locking plate construct for a proximal humeral fracture.

[33] Mittlmeier TW, Stedtfeld HW, Ewert A, Beck M, Frosch B, Gradl G: Stabilization of proximal humeral fractures with an angular and sliding stable antegrade locking nail (Targon PH). *J Bone Joint Surg Am* 2003;85(suppl 4):136-146.

[34] Park JY, Pandher DS, Chun JY, Md ST: Antegrade humeral nailing through the rotator cuff interval: A new entry portal. *J Orthop Trauma* 2008;22(6):419-425.

An alternative starting portal for intramedullary nail fixation of proximal humeral fractures was used to avoid some of the complications associated with the classic starting point.

[35] Hatzidakis AM, Shevlin MJ, Fenton DL, Curran-Everett D, Nowinski RJ, Fehringer EV: Angular-stable locked intramedullary nailing of two-part surgical neck fractures of the proximal part of the humerus: A multicenter retrospective observational study. *J Bone Joint Surg Am* 2011;93(23):2172-2179.

Patients with a two-part surgical neck fracture were successfully treated using an articular starting portal. Patients had reliable healing and good functional outcomes with minimal postoperative shoulder pain.

[36] Zhu Y, Lu Y, Shen J, Zhang J, Jiang C: Locking intramedullary nails and locking plates in the treatment of two-part proximal humeral surgical neck fractures: A prospective randomized trial with a minimum of three years of follow-up. *J Bone Joint Surg Am* 2011;93(2):159-168.

Locked plating and intramedullary nail fixation were compared in randomly assigned patients with two-part surgical neck fractures. Between-group functional scores were similar at 3 years. Patients treated with in- tramedullary nailing had fewer complications. Those treated with plating had a better 1-year outcome. Level of evidence: I .

[37] Park JY, Kim JH, Lhee SH, Lee SJ: The importance of inferomedial support in the hot air balloon technique for treatment of 3-part proximal humeral fractures. *J Shoulder Elbow Surg* 2012;21(9):1152-1159.

A study of 43 patients over a 12-year period analyzed the importance of medial calcar support in three-part proximal humeral fractures treated with intramedullary nail and suture fixation. Reduction of the medial calcar and the use of an inferomedial screw improved stability and clinical outcomes.

[38] Konrad G, Audigé L, Lambert S, Hertel R, Südkamp NP: Similar outcomes for nail versus plate fixation of three-part proximal humeral fractures. *Clin Orthop Relat Res* 2012;470(2):602-609.

Intramedullary nail and locking plate fixation were compared in 211 patients treated for a three-part proximal humeral fracture. Outcome scores were similar at 1-year follow-up.

[39] Koike Y, Komatsuda T, Sato K: Internal fixation of proximal humeral fractures with a Polaris humeral nail. *J Orthop Traumatol* 2008;9(3):135-139.

Intramedullary nail fixation was used to treat 54 patients with a three-part proximal humeral fracture. No major complications were reported, and 79% of the patients had a satisfactory to excellent result.

[40] Adedapo AO, Ikpeme JO: The results of internal fixation of three- and four-part proximal humeral fractures with the Polaris nail. *Injury* 2001;32(2):115-121.

[41] Ebraheim NA, Patil V, Husain A: Mini-external fixation of two- and three-part proximal humerus fractures. *Acta Orthop Belg* 2007;73(4):437-442.

External fixation was used to treat two-part and three- part proximal humeral fractures, with good results. The minimally invasive procedure was suggested for patients with polytrauma.

[42] Martin C, Guillen M, Lopez G: Treatment of 2- and 3-part fractures of the proximal humerus using external fixation: A retrospective evaluation of 62 patients. *Acta Orthop* 2006;77(2):275-278.

[43] Zhang J, Ebraheim N, Lause GE: Surgical treatment of proximal humeral fracture with external fixator. *J Shoulder Elbow Surg* 2012;21(7):882-886.

External fixation was used to treat 32 patients with a proximal humeral fracture. The result was good to excellent in 81% of the patients. Level of evidence: IV.

[44] Cazeneuve JF, Cristofari DJ: The reverse shoulder prosthesis in the treatment of fractures of the proximal humerus in the elderly. *J Bone Joint Surg Br* 2010;92(4):535-539.

At 6-year follow-up of 36 proximal humeral fractures treated with reverse shoulder arthroplasty, a drop in Constant score was reported as well as increased evidence of glenoid component loosening and scapular notching compared with previously reported data.

[45] Owsley KC, Gorczyca JT: Fracture displacement and screw cutout after open reduction and locked plate fixation of proximal humeral fractures [corrected]. *J Bone Joint Surg Am* 2008;90(2):233-240.

A retrospective analysis revealed that locked plating led to a high rate of complications, most of which involved screw cutout, in older patients with a three- or four-part fracture.

[46] Voigt C, Geisler A, Hepp P, Schulz AP, Lill H: Are polyaxially locked screws advantageous in the plate osteosynthesis of proximal humeral fractures in the elderly? A prospective randomized clinical observational study. *J Orthop Trauma* 2011;25(10):596-602.

Polyaxial and nonpolyaxial locked screw-plate constructs were compared for treating proximal humeral fractures in older patients. No clinically significant difference was reported in functional outcomes.

[47] Torrens C, Corrales M, Vilà G, Santana F, Cáceres E: Functional and quality-of-life results of displaced and nondisplaced proximal humeral fractures treated conservatively. *J Orthop Trauma* 2011;25(10):581-587.

Nonsurgical treatment led to good pain relief but decreased function in older patients. Quality-of-life perception was unchanged.

[48] Yüksel HY, Yimaz S, Akşahin E, Celebi L, Muratli HH, Biçimoğlu A: The results of nonoperative treatment for three- and four-part fractures of the proximal humerus in low-demand patients. *J Orthop Trauma* 2011;25(10):588-595.

Eighteen patients older than 65 years were nonsurgically treated for a proximal humeral fracture. Functional outcomes were satisfactory and not well correlated with radiographic appearance.

第三十五章　肱骨近端骨折并发症

Robert Z. Tashjian, MD

引言

　　肱骨近端骨折约占所有骨折的5%，属于最常见的骨折之一。这类骨折大多数几乎没有移位，可以通过非手术治疗来达到完全愈合，肩关节活动范围恢复至接近正常，功能良好。[1]但是，仍有一些并发症（包括肱骨头坏死、畸形愈合、骨折不愈合、退行性关节炎和肩关节僵硬等）可能在肱骨近端骨折的非手术或手术治疗后发生。

肱骨头坏死

　　肱骨头坏死是由血供丧失导致骨细胞死亡所致。缺血区最初试图通过死骨的吸收和新骨的沉积进行自我修复，但是可能引起软骨下骨折，导致关节表面塌陷和盂肱关节炎。[2]肱骨头坏死的原因既可能是非创伤性的（例如，过量使用皮质类固醇激素、酗酒和患有镰状细胞病等），也可能是由肱骨近端骨折等外伤引起的。无论是非手术治疗还是手术治疗肱骨近端骨折，都可能发生创伤性骨坏死。骨折的严重程度决定了骨坏死风险的大小。[3]据报道，大组病例分析得出的总体骨坏死发生率在非手术治疗组为2%，在手术治疗组为8%。[1,4]对三部分和四部分骨折的研究发现，非手术治疗的骨坏死率为28%，手术治疗的骨坏

Neither Dr. Tashjian nor any immediate family member has received anything of value from or has stock or stock options held in a commercial company or institution related directly or indirectly to the subject of this chapter.

死率为35%。[3,5]这些研究表明，损伤越重，肱骨头坏死发生率越高。创伤后肱骨头坏死最常与临床残疾相关，尽管随着时间的推移，创伤后肱骨头坏死患者的残疾程度会比曾经预期的最坏结果有所降低。在一项对25例创伤后肱骨头部分或完全塌陷患者的研究中发现，临床结果取决于肱骨头塌陷的程度和骨折畸形愈合范围。[6]另一项研究也有类似的发现，在四部分骨折后创伤性肱骨头坏死中是否存在畸形愈合是影响预后的主要指标之一。[7]尽管许多没有实质性塌陷或畸形愈合的肱骨头坏死患者都有较好的临床结果，但如果出现严重的塌陷和畸形愈合，根据大结节的畸形愈合位置，通常需要进行半肩关节置换或反肩关节置换。[8]在没有实质性肱骨头塌陷或畸形愈合的情况下，治疗因肱骨头坏死而存在持续疼痛症状的患者时，可以考虑采用更加微创的手术方法，如关节镜清创术、切开或关节镜下核心减压术。[9-12]

评估和分类

　　肱骨头坏死的最初症状通常是存在于肩关节深部的广泛疼痛，与早期盂肱关节炎相似。疼痛经常放射到肘部，当过度使用肩关节时症状加剧。肱骨头坏死病灶的典型位置是内上部，当外展和前屈肩关节时，肱骨头的坏死部位会接触关节盂表面，可能引起症状。一些患者的症状相对不明显。

　　标准的肩部X线检查和MRI检查是主要的影像

学诊断方法。肩部 X 线片应包括肩关节内旋正位片、肩关节外旋正位片及腋位片。影像学改变通常发生在疾病的后期，但是可以在 MRI 上检测到早期改变。骨扫描结果不足以明确肩部肱骨头坏死的诊断。

肱骨头坏死分期非常重要，因为它决定了治疗方式及预后。最常用的分期是 Cruess 系统，是根据 Ficat-Arlet 髋关节股骨头坏死分期系统修改而来的[13]。该分期主要基于肱骨头塌陷的严重程度（图 35-1）。Ⅰ期，X 线片上看不到变化，在 MRI 上仅见水肿表现。Ⅱ期，在 X 线片上表现为局部硬化，MRI 能够更加明确地显示局部坏死病变。Ⅲ期，出现软骨下骨折伴肱骨头变扁，肱骨头球形丧失。Ⅳ期，肱骨头塌陷。Ⅴ期，在Ⅳ期

表现的基础上累及关节盂。[14]

最近描述的 Sakai 酒井分类系统，是基于病变大小和塌陷程度来分类的。[14] 肱骨头坏死的病变大小通过定义中斜冠状位和中斜矢状位 MRI 图像上的坏死角来评估。研究发现，在 46 个 Cruess Ⅰ期或Ⅱ期的肱骨头中，有 12 个肱骨头的坏死角超过 90°。其中 11 个肱骨头（占 92%）后期出现塌陷；4 个进展至 Cruess Ⅲ期，7 个进展至 Cruess Ⅳ期。坏死角小于 90° 的 34 个肱骨头没有一个进展为 Cruess Ⅲ期、Ⅳ期或Ⅴ期。

治疗

创伤后肱骨头坏死的治疗取决于 3 个因素：是否存在症状、坏死分期和畸形愈合的程度。如

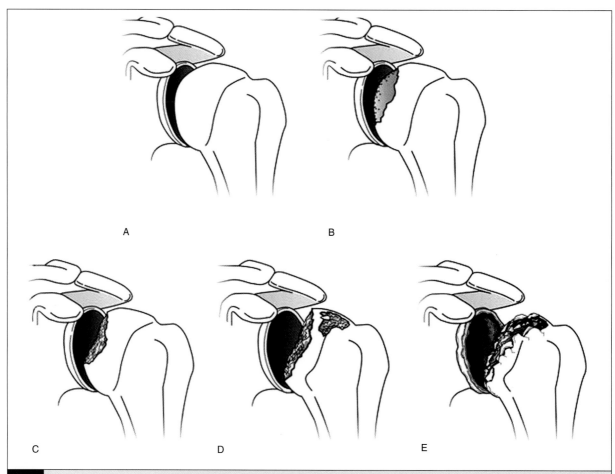

图 35-1　肱骨头坏死的 Cruess 系统示意图。A. Ⅰ期，没有影像学证据显示骨坏死，肱骨头看起来正常，保持球形并且没有硬化。B. Ⅱ期，出现斑驳的硬化迹象，但肱骨头的球形外观保持完整。C. Ⅲ期，发展为新月征，软骨下骨折伴肱骨头的球形丧失。D. Ⅳ期，累及软骨下骨并出现肱骨头塌陷。E. Ⅴ期，进展到早期关节盂的退行性改变。经允许引自 Harreld KL, Marker DR, Wiesler ER, Shafiz B, Mont MA: Osteonecrosis of the humeral head. *J Am Acad Orthop Surg* 2009;17:345–355.

果无症状，建议随访观察，通过影像学检查监测病变。如果有症状，则选取合理的治疗方法。非手术治疗方法包括物理康复疗法和使用消炎镇痛药物。非人工关节手术包括髓心减压术、行（或不行）髓心减压术的关节镜清理术、带血管蒂的骨移植等。通常对非手术治疗无效患者，有症状的Ⅰ期、Ⅱ期和Ⅲ期患者，以及肱骨头外形无畸变的患者，才会选择上述非人工关节手术。关节置换术适用于有症状的Ⅳ期和Ⅴ期病变及肱骨头畸变明显的Ⅲ期病变。

自然史和非手术治疗

肱骨头坏死病变的自然转归尚不清楚。目前仅有的研究是针对具有多种病因和相对较差的放射学分类的一小群患者。

最初，研究报道78%的类固醇性肱骨头坏死患者的长期预后良好。仅22%的患者需要手术治疗（行肩关节置换术），所有这些患者最初都为Cruess Ⅳ期或Ⅴ期。[13]一项对151例患者（200例肩关节）的研究发现，坏死分期越晚、坏死范围越大，则坏死进展越快、手术需求越高。[15]患者最初接受非手术治疗，平均随访8.6年，77%的患者轻度疼痛或无疼痛。但3年后需要行关节置换术的创伤性骨坏死患者为78%，非创伤性骨坏死患者为47%。一项对65例肱骨头坏死患者的研究发现，非手术治疗的长期预后较差。[16]在至少2年的随访中，有20%的患者接受了立即手术，在评估期间有34%的患者接受了手术，而非手术治疗后有23%的患者结果较差。所有接受手术或非手术治疗后结果较差的患者均存在Ⅲ期、Ⅳ期或Ⅴ期病变。存在Ⅰ期、Ⅱ期病变的患者长期预后良好，进展有限，不需要手术。还有一项研究报道，在中斜冠状位和中斜矢状位MRI图像上，坏死角小于90°的Ⅰ期和Ⅱ期肱骨头坏死病变没有进展。[14]

非手术治疗的主要目标是缓解肩关节疼痛和保持运动能力。建议进行物理康复治疗以预防粘连性滑囊炎。需要限制过顶活动。通常，大多数患者最初可以考虑采用非手术治疗。最初的非手术治疗很有效，最适合Ⅰ期或Ⅱ期病变的患者，尤其是病变较小的情况，也为获得满意的临床效果提供了很好的机会。非手术治疗也可能对相对较小的Ⅲ期病变有效，大多数Ⅲ期、Ⅳ期或Ⅴ期病变需要某种形式的手术干预。

非关节置换手术治疗

对于肱骨头坏死，不使用关节置换术的手术方式的选择有限，包括髓心减压、关节镜下清理术及髓心减压联合关节镜清理术。适应证包括对非手术治疗无效的Ⅰ期、Ⅱ期病变和塌陷有限的Ⅲ期病变。严重的Ⅲ期病变或Ⅳ期和Ⅴ期病变应通过部分或完全肩关节置换进行治疗。使用关节镜清理术治疗肱骨头坏死的数据有限，主要目标是延缓骨坏死进展并清理松动的软骨片或游离体。可以预期短期内的功能改善和疼痛缓解。一般认为，关节镜清理术可以不用联合髓心减压单独进行，即使是在治疗Ⅲ期或Ⅳ期病变时，对于减轻滑膜炎引起的疼痛和缓解松动软骨片或游离体的磨损症状最有用。

研究者对髓心减压治疗股骨头坏死的效果已进行了广泛的研究和应用。降低骨髓压力可以减轻疼痛并可能在坏死区域刺激新血管的重建和新生骨的积聚，从而达到较好的临床效果。但是，其成功率各不相同。尽管该方法存在一定争议，但对于股骨头Ⅰ期和Ⅱ期病变的患者似乎有效。

通常认为，对于非手术治疗无效的Ⅰ期和Ⅱ期肱骨头坏死，髓心减压具有长期的优良效果，影像学检查可见病变的进展有限，并且不需要行人工关节置换术。[12,18]目前尚不清楚Ⅰ期和Ⅱ期坏死影像学进展有限是由髓心减压所致还是自然转归。有研究报道髓心减压治疗Ⅲ期坏死取得了一些好的治疗效果，在平均5.6年的随访中，有70%的患者临床效果优良，其余30%的患者需要行关节置换术。[12]

有几种肱骨近端髓心减压技术已经被报道。在一项切开减压技术中，在胸大肌三角肌间隙下方、胸大肌止点正上方做一小切口钝性分离至肱二头肌长头腱沟外侧。[12]也可以使用较小的横向三角肌劈开方法，使用正侧位 X 线透视来定位坏死区，并使用 5 mm 取芯装置进行减压。根据病变的大小，也可以使用大的活检套管（6~10 mm）。[8]最近报道的经皮减压技术使用直径 3.2 mm 斯氏针，从常见的入点穿刺入坏死区 2~3 次。[18]一项研究报道，使用经皮减压技术成功治疗了 25 例 I 期或 II 期病变的肩关节（共 26 例，96％），平均随访 32 个月，通过 UCLA 评分系统评估，只有 1 例患者影像学检查有加重坏死表现。[17]报道的关节镜技术都强调了影像学实现可视化的优点，包括可以对坏死病变进行分期，行滑膜切除或清理术以减轻疼痛，使减压范围局限化，并避免取芯装置穿透关节软骨（图 35-2）。使用前十字韧带（ACL）导向器通过前口，然后使用来自侧门的导针，该导针能被 7 mm 空心钻扩孔。[9]也有类似的技术使用 ACL 导向器，先放置几个直径 3.2 mm 的斯氏针，然后再用直径

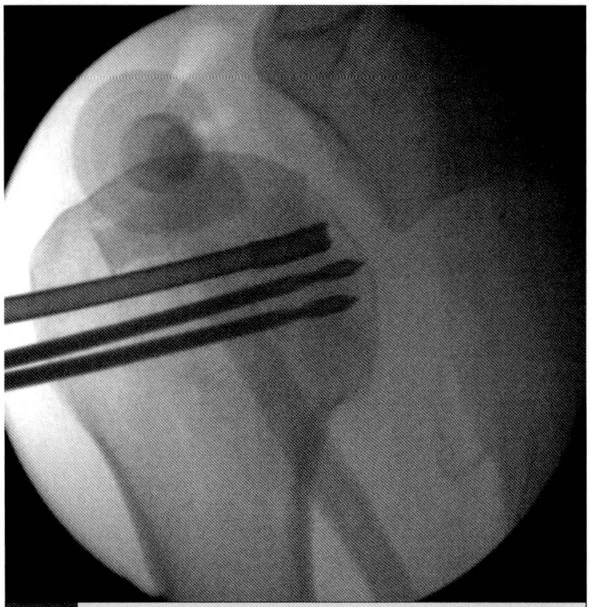

图 35-2　关节镜辅助髓心减压治疗 III 期肱骨头坏死的术中透视图像。（版权所有：Pat Greis, MD, Salt Lake City, UT）

4 mm 的取芯装置进行过度钻孔。[10]两项合并研究中的所有 4 例患者均恢复平稳并且疼痛立即减轻。通常认为关节镜和切开减压技术都可安全有效地治疗有症状的 I 期病变，II 期病变以及可能的 III 期坏死病变。

肱骨近端骨折畸形愈合

骨折畸形愈合的原因可能是术中复位不足、术后复位丢失以及移位骨折非手术治疗过程中未复位或移位距离增大。最近的一篇综述报道，在 650 例非手术治疗的肱骨近端骨折中，内翻畸形的发生率为 7％。[1]畸形愈合的患者通常会感到疼痛、活动受限及力量下降，其程度取决于骨折的类型及肱骨头塌陷或关节炎的情况。骨折端的肌肉牵拉决定了畸形愈合的最后位置。由于肩袖向后上牵拉导致大结节骨折畸形愈合于肱骨近端后上侧，从而造成肩峰下撞击和肩袖无力。非解剖位置生物力学导致疼痛和运动受限。由于胸大肌向内牵拉肱骨干而肩袖向上牵拉肱骨头，单纯外科颈骨折往往畸形愈合于屈曲内翻位，从而导致外展和屈曲功能丧失。

肱骨近端骨折愈合的临床评估应包括损伤机制和治疗史。骨质疏松症、过度锻炼或固定不足可能使骨折倾向于畸形愈合。影像学评估应包括普通 X 线照相（肩关节正位、肩胛骨正侧位、腋位）及三维重建 CT，可准确评估大小结节的位置和移位范围。如果怀疑早期肱骨头坏死或肩袖损伤，则应通过 MRI 检查来确定，根据结果可能需要调整外科治疗方案。

尽管有几种肱骨近端骨折畸形的分类系统，但均没有得到公认。使用区域分类法改良的 Neer 骨折分类系统相对简便，可能是最常用的方法。Beredjiklian 系统同时评估骨和软组织异常。[19]骨折畸形包括大小结节移位大于或等于 1 cm（I 型）、关节面台阶大于 5 mm（II 型）和肱骨近端成角超过 45°（III 型）。软组织异常包括僵硬、肩袖撕裂和撞击。Boileau 分型强调了治疗的适应证

和非限制性关节置换术的结果。[20] Ⅰ型肱骨近端骨折发展为肱骨头塌陷或坏死；Ⅱ型慢性脱位或骨折脱位；Ⅲ型外科颈骨折不愈合；Ⅳ型严重的结节畸形愈合，需要行大结节截骨术。

由于不需要行大结节截骨术，Ⅰ型和Ⅱ型在非限制性关节置换术后效果满意；而Ⅲ型和Ⅳ型需要行大结节截骨术，非限制性关节置换术后的效果较差。尽管肱骨近端骨折后会发生畸形愈合，但很少需要再次手术治疗。单独大结节或外科颈骨折畸形愈合但肩袖完整且无伴随关节炎的患者最适合手术治疗。这些损伤的非关节置换术包括单纯的关节镜清理术、关节镜清理联合结节截骨肩袖张力重建术。[19,21-27]

复杂的三部分或四部分骨折畸形愈合后合并关节炎、肱骨头塌陷、骨量不足或肩袖损伤时，可通过解剖型肩关节置换或反式全肩关节置换进行治疗。

大结节畸形愈合

单独的大结节畸形愈合最常见，固定大结节骨折的手术指征是移位超过 1 cm；但是，有些医师建议对移位超过 5 mm 的大结节骨折也进行手术固定。移位超过 1 cm 的被忽略的骨折、内固定后失效的骨折、移位小于 1 cm 非手术治疗失败的大结节骨折畸形愈合后往往会产生症状。[28-29] 大结节向后移位通常会阻碍外旋，向上移位则会导致外展、撞击和肩袖无力功能丧失。大结节畸形愈合的手术指征包括上移超过 5 mm 或后移超过 1 cm，并伴有疼痛、运动功能丧失和撞击。治疗大结节骨折畸形愈合的手术方式包括切开截骨术、关节镜清理术及关节镜下肩袖修复大结节成形术。在一项对 11 例单独大结节畸形愈合病例的研究中，有 2 例大结节后上移位 1~1.5 cm 采用关节镜下肩峰成形术治疗获得了满意的结果，其余 9 例大结节移位超过 1.5 cm 的病例接受了大结节截骨术、肩袖修复和关节囊松解术，恢复至偏离解剖位置 5 mm 以内。手术修复主要采用缝合固定。

最近一些报道介绍了关节镜下使用结节成形术及肩袖离断再修复术治疗单独向上移位的大结节骨折畸形愈合。对 4 例单独大结节畸形愈合进行了滑囊松解、肩峰下粘连松解、肩峰下减压、大结节成形术和肩袖离断再修复术，患者的 ASES 肩关节疼痛和功能障碍评分平均提高了 52 分，而视觉模拟评分法评分平均降低了 4.5 分。[23] 8 例大结节向后上移位 5~10 mm 的患者接受了相似的手术，其中 7 例患者的结果优良，毫无限制地重返以前的工作。[24] 对于有症状且大结节骨折移位超过 5 mm 的患者，建议行关节镜下大结节成形术和肩袖修复。[30] 建议在骨折后至少 6 个月，待畸形完全愈合后再行结节成形术和肩袖修复。

大结节向后移位较大（超过 1 cm）时，通常需要进行切开大结节截骨、滑囊和肩袖松解、缝合固定，若大结节骨折块足够大，可加用螺钉固定。

三维重建 CT 对于截骨术的术前计划很有帮助。常规使用胸大肌三角肌入路，但可能需要使用第二条后侧入路来发现和游离大结节骨折块。大结节向上移位 5~10 mm 且存在症状时，应采用关节镜下肩峰成形术，或者联合大结节截骨和肩袖重置术。

外科颈骨折畸形愈合

单独外科颈骨折畸形愈合相对不常见，而且相关手术治疗适应证和手术方法的报道有限。外科颈骨折畸形愈合通常由切开和闭合复位不良或非手术治疗时的复位失败导致。颈干角小于 120° 往往会减少肩关节主动活动范围并加重疼痛。[31] Neer 认为骨折成角大于 45° 是手术适应证，因为这将导致颈干角减小至 90°~100°。所有文献报道的颈干角均小于 110°，大多数为 90°~105°，这些文献可作为肱骨近端内翻畸形截骨矫正术前计划的参考。[21,25,27]

大多数外科医师建议采用简单的闭合外翻楔形截骨术，以恢复正常的颈干角角度（130°~140°）。[21,25,27] 尽管也普遍存在屈曲和旋转畸形，但恢复外翻至关重要。内固定可选 T 形钢板或肱骨近端锁定钢板，当前应用最多的是锁定钢板（图 35-3）。术前使用 X 线片和 CT 图像制作模板对于准确测量合适的楔形尺寸至关重要。行截骨术前要先进行关节囊松解以恢复肩关节被动活动范围。截下的楔形骨块可用于骨移植。应在畸形最大的干骺端区域进行截骨。[21,25] 截骨术后颈干角增加 20°，前屈会相应地增加 90°，上举会增加 56°。[27] 因此，外翻闭合楔形截骨术是治疗单独肱骨近端外科颈畸形愈合且颈干角小于约 110° 的合理选择，能够很好地缓解疼痛、扩大活动范围和改善肩关节功能。

肱骨外科颈骨折不愈合

肱骨近端骨折不愈合相对少见，但会导致严重的残疾，并且治疗难度极大。外科颈骨折不愈合占所有肱骨近端骨折的 1.1%，手术治疗可以成功地使连枷肩恢复到正常肩关节。[32] 外科颈骨折不愈合的治疗选择大致分为切开复位内固定（通常结合骨移植术）和关节置换术（解剖型假体置换术和反肩关节置换术）。[33] 外科颈骨折不愈合可分为肥大性不愈合（骨折端出现大量骨痂）和萎缩性不愈合（骨折端生物活性低）。影响外科颈骨折愈合的因素包括骨折移位大小、粉碎程度、肱二头肌等软组织嵌入情况、全身性疾病情况、骨质疏松症和过早康复锻炼等。[32-34] 外科颈骨折粉碎或横移超过骨干的 1/3 会使骨折不愈合的发生率增加 8%~10%。[32] 在 Boileau 分型中，肱骨近端骨折不愈合属于 III 型。[20] 根据此分类，通常需要大结节截骨，因此非限制性关节置换术治疗外科颈骨折不愈合的效果可能比较差。如果肱骨头完好，建议进行切开复位和内固定，如果肱骨头受损且患者年龄在 70 岁以上并需求较低，则建

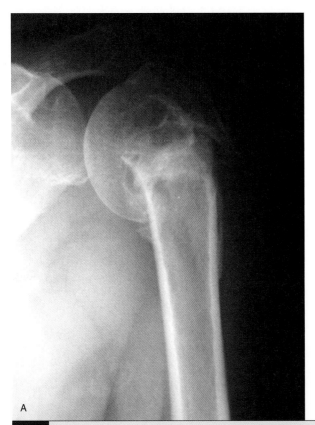

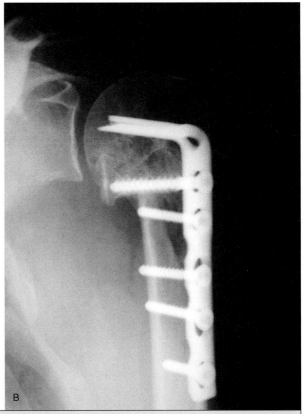

图 35-3 肩关节正位片。A. 术前，肱骨外科颈骨折内翻畸形愈合。B. 外翻闭合楔形截骨术后透视图，使用肱骨近端刀片钢板内固定。（版权所有：Andrew Green, MD, Providence, RI）

议进行反肩关节置换。外科颈骨折不愈合合并肱骨头坏死在相对年轻的患者中则很难处理，非限制性肩关节置换结合大结节截骨术通常是唯一的选择，但预后较差。[20]若不需要大结节截骨，非限制性肩关节置换结合内侧骨距植骨治疗外科颈骨折不愈合可能会取得较好的效果，尤其是在肩关节前屈上举方面。[35]

外科颈骨折不愈合的治疗选择受很多因素影响，包括患者年龄、骨量、有无肱骨头坏死、有无盂肱关节炎及肩袖损伤状况。外科颈骨折不愈合一般有 3 种治疗方法：切开复位内固定并植骨、解剖型肩关节置换（全肩关节置换术或肱骨头置换术）和反肩关节置换。

当无肱骨头坏死和盂肱关节炎时，切开复位钢板内固定是治疗外科颈骨折不愈合的最佳选择。有研究报道，结合切开复位 T 形钢板内固定和肩袖张力缝合固定及自体骨移植治疗 13 例外科颈骨折不愈合，其中 12 例完全骨性愈合；9 例恢复良好，无痛且功能活动恢复到伤前状态；4 例恢复差，存在轻到中度疼痛，功能难以恢复到伤前水平，不能继续伤前的工作。[34]一项研究报道，钢板固定结合自体骨移植治疗 25 例肱骨近端骨不连的患者，有 23 例（92%）骨折愈合良好，20 例（80%）临床结果优良。[36]最近有研究报道采用切开复位肱骨近端解剖锁定板加髓内同种异体植骨治疗 18 例有症状的肱骨近端骨折不愈合患者，随访 5.4 个月以上，17 例（94%）骨折愈合，平均主动前屈上举为 115°。[37]其中 4 例加用脱钙骨基质和同种异体松质骨打压植骨。之后，缝合固定大小结节于钢板上以加强固定。

目前有几种治疗外科颈骨折不愈合的方法，包括骨移植（自体骨移植或结构性同种异体骨移植）、体外冲击波、脉冲电磁场、低强度脉冲超声和骨形态发生蛋白（BMP）。自体骨移植是骨移植的金标准，因为自体骨具有骨传导性、骨诱导性和成骨活性。在所有外科颈骨折不愈合的治疗中应首选自体骨移植。髓内结构性同种异体骨移植可有效增强局部生物力学结构，也可以选择使用。[37]一些证据表明，低强度脉冲超声，脉冲电磁场和体外冲击波在治疗长骨骨不连方面具有积极作用，但尚无关于肱骨近端骨折不愈合使用这些治疗方法的具体资料。一些数据表明，低强度脉冲超声和体外冲击波的疗效要强于脉冲电磁场。[38-40]这些方法风险低又具有刺激骨折愈合的潜力，应被视为合理的辅助治疗方法。

BMP-7 被发现在 I 型胶原蛋白载体中可安全有效地治疗胫骨骨不连。BMP-7 治疗的临床和影像学检查结果与自体骨移植相当，但无移植供体部位损伤问题。[41]已证实 BMP-2 能降低新鲜胫骨干开放性骨折的骨不连和感染风险。[42]BMP-2 被 FDA 批准仅用于急性开放性胫骨骨折和前路腰椎椎间融合术；BMP-7 被 FDA 批准用于难治性长骨骨不连的治疗。但目前，BMP-7 已从市场上撤出仅用于临床研究，BMP-2 的标签外使用是唯一促进手术后外科颈骨不连愈合的治疗选项。

目前对于肩袖功能完好、无肱骨头坏死、无盂肱关节炎的外科颈骨折不愈合推荐进行切开复位钢板固定加自体或异体骨移植。如果早期内固定失效导致骨不连，应进行术前感染筛查，包括检查红细胞沉降率和 C 反应蛋白水平。胸大肌三角肌入路是经典的手术入路，可以向远侧延伸到肱骨干前外侧以增大肱骨干的显露。应对不愈合的骨折端进行彻底清理，并向远端髓内和近端肱骨头内钻孔，直到骨出血为止。如果由于早期内固定失效导致骨不连，则应取局部组织进行细菌培养和病理切片以检测局部有无急性感染迹象，并且应清除所有内固定和其他异物。修整同种异体腓骨形状以便植入髓腔[37]（图 35-4）。肱骨近端锁定板通常与加压装置一起使用，以帮助对骨不连部位进行加压固定。通常，将肩袖缝合于钢板上以加强固定，于自体骨上添加 BMP-2（标签外使用）并在骨不连部位周围压紧。

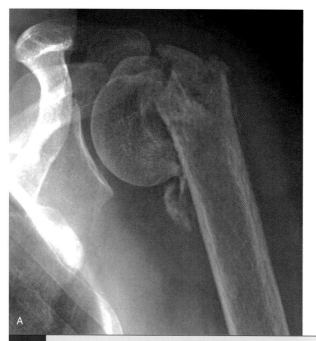
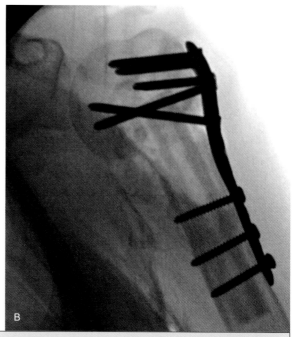

图 35-4　肩关节正位片。A. 术前，肱骨外科颈骨折不愈合，无肱骨头坏死，无盂肱关节炎。B. 术后，肱骨近端锁定钢板加同种异体腓骨髓内支撑和髂骨移植

应根据患者年龄及与肩相关的影响因素来选择治疗外科颈骨折不愈合的手术方式。如果患者年龄小于 70 岁且肩袖完整，无肱骨头坏死，无盂肱关节炎，则应考虑行切开复位植骨术。如果患者年龄超过 70 岁，外科颈骨不连并且存在肩袖损伤和肱骨头坏死，则应选择反式全肩关节置换术。如果患者年龄为 60~70 岁，自身需求相对较低，且存在肩袖损伤、肱骨头坏死及盂肱关节炎，那么也可以考虑行反式全肩关节置换术。若患者年龄为 60~70 岁，并且自身需求高，术中不需要大结节截骨和内侧骨距植骨，也可考虑行半肩关节置换术；若仅需要内侧骨距植骨而不需要大结节截骨，则可行非限制性肩关节置换术。若患者年龄小于 60 岁，且存在肩袖损伤、肱骨头坏死及盂肱关节炎，则与常规的半肩关节置换术相比，肩关节置换术后的主动被动活动功能较差。

盂肱关节炎

创伤后盂肱关节炎的治疗可能很困难，尤其对于不希望行关节置换术的相对年轻的患者。非

关节置换术的手术方法包括关节镜清理术（或联合关节囊松解）以及关节镜下关节盂表面重建术。治疗方案要考虑以下几个因素：患者的年龄、工作需求、是否存在运动受限或神经系统缺陷、关节间隙狭窄的程度、磨损的同心度、是否存在双相性（肱骨头和关节盂）疾病以及骨软骨病变的大小和分级。这些因素中的每一个都可能影响关节镜手术的效果，治疗创伤后盂肱关节炎，在选择行人工关节置换手术或非人工关节置换手术时也应考虑这些因素。

创伤后关节炎患者的病史应包括与早期手术治疗、患者的年龄和活动水平、患侧为优势侧、症状的严重程度、阻挡症状及患者将来对肩关节的需求（如体力劳动或运动）相关的信息。体格检查应特别注意对运动范围的评估，这可能影响手术治疗的选择及结果。应该进行全面的神经系统检查，包括腋神经检查和肩袖功能检查。影像学评估应包括肩胛骨正侧位片和腋位片。肩胛骨正位片用于评估关节间隙变窄以及残留骨折片的大小。腋位片用于评估关节盂形态及检测肩胛盂关节是否匹配，例

如，肩关节后半脱位和关节盂后侧磨损。只要没有植入金属固定物，MRI 即可用于检查肩袖形态。另外，可以使用超声和 CT 检查。MRI 和 CT 均可用于对关节盂形态的进一步分类。

创伤后骨关节炎的早期阶段通常可以通过减少活动、使用非甾体抗炎药、物理治疗和注射糖皮质激素等非手术方法治疗。AAOS 对这些治疗方法进行了评估，得出的结论是，目前的文献既不支持也不否定它们的有效性，因此可以合理应用这些方法。[43] 由于缺乏证据支持皮质类固醇注射的功效，因此除非有特殊情况，否则建议将单个关节的注射次数上限限制为 3 次。[44] AAOS 还确定，治疗盂肱关节骨关节炎患者时可以考虑补充透明质酸。[43] 研究发现，接受 hylan G-F 20（Synvisc；Genzyme）治疗的盂肱关节骨关节炎患者，在每周注射 3 次后，疼痛缓解，运动范围和生活质量改善长达 6 个月。[45] 一项研究发现与安慰剂治疗组相比，接受 3~5 次弥散性关节内透明质酸钠注射液治疗的盂肱关节炎患者的疼痛缓解明显，两组患者在统计学上存在显著差异。尽管这种改善具有统计学意义（在 100 mm 视觉模拟评分法为 7.8 mm），但其临床意义仍存异议。[46]

如果非手术治疗无效，则可考虑关节镜清理术（联合或不联合关节囊松解）、关节镜下关节盂表面重建术及人工关节置换术。由于缺乏高水平的证据，AAOS 没有对盂肱关节炎患者进行关节镜清理或生物学干预的建议。[43]

一项研究中，25 例早期盂肱关节炎患者接受了关节镜手术，进行了软骨盂唇清理、游离态清除、滑膜切除、灌洗和肩峰滑囊切除。[47] 在术后 3 年的随访中，优良率达到 80%。研究人员认为仅在关节间隙可见且关节炎局部累及的情况下才建议进行关节镜检查。另一项研究发现，在 IV 级骨软骨病变关节镜清理术后至少 2 年的随访中，有 88% 的患者疼痛缓解。[48] 如果患侧肩部的活动范围与对侧的差距在 15° 以内，则不进行关节囊松解。如果检查发现活动范围减少明显（与对侧相比，上举或外旋减少超过 15°），则行清理术及关节囊松解。关节囊松解术后患者肩关节前屈上举和外旋活动范围分别平均改善 23° 和 38°。研究人员建议，如果病变大于 2 cm[2]，则应避免手术，因为较大的病变范围似乎与疼痛的复发和治疗失效有关。另一项研究也有类似报道，关节囊松解后肩关节前屈上举活动范围和外旋活动范围有所改善（分别为 21° 和 17°）。[49] 关节囊松解后关节面接触压力的降低被认为是疼痛缓解的主要机制。一项对 36 例患者的研究发现，如果盂肱关节炎低于 Outerbridge 分型 IV 级，则结果明显更好。[50] 而对软骨病变范围的评估发现，单面 IV 级病变的表现与低级别病变相同。[51] 双面病变比单面病变具有更差的结果。同样，如果患者患有双面 IV 级病变，则关节镜清理术后失败的风险也很高。87% 的双面 IV 级病变患者后来需要行关节置换术。[52] 其他失败的危险因素包括关节间隙小于 2 mm 和较大的骨赘（Samilson-Prieto 2 级；3~7 mm，在肱骨头或关节盂）。

既往的研究表明，治疗局限性盂肱关节炎时，关节间隙在 2 mm 以上以及单面病变相对较小，病变不重于 IV 级及骨赘较小的患者，关节镜清理术是合理可行的。关节囊松解可以改善关节僵硬和关节炎患者的前屈上举和外旋活动范围。如果患者关节软骨广泛磨损、关节间隙小于 2 mm、肱骨头或关节盂上的骨赘较大（3~7 mm）或存在双面 IV 级病变，则关节镜清理术的效果可能较差，后期更可能需要行关节置换术。这类患者应避免单独行关节镜清理术。

关节镜下关节盂重建术最近被报道适用于单独行关节镜清理术无效的病变严重的患者。在关节镜清理术后，将关节面植入物缝合到关节盂表面（图 35-5）。一项研究报道，对 32 例患者行关节镜清理术并用无细胞真皮基质进行生物性关节盂重建，术后在疼痛缓解和功能预后方面效果明显，在平均第 3 年随访时成功率达 72%。[53] 在

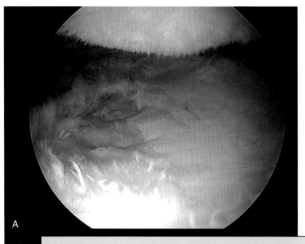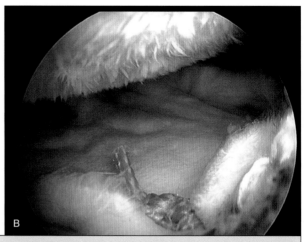

图 35-5 关节镜图像。A. 清理术前，肱骨头Ⅲ期病变，关节盂Ⅳ期骨软骨病变（双面关节病变）。B. 清理术后，生物性关节盂重建。（版权所有：Robert T. Burks, MD, Salt Lake City, UT）

这些患者中，94%的患者磨损广泛；59%的患者存在中度骨赘和关节间隙狭窄；41%的患者有大型骨赘、明显的关节间隙狭窄和严重的硬化症。患肢为优势侧同时合并糖尿病、类风湿关节炎或骨关节炎等全身性疾病时，预后较差，尽管影像学表现的分级不高。

一项对 20 例关节镜下利用猪小肠黏膜补片进行关节盂重建的研究发现，在 3~6 年的随访中，成功率为 75%。[54] 所有患者均为Ⅳ级双面病变，初次复查 X 线片显示 25% 的患者肩关节后半脱位，术后 1~5 年，有 25% 的患者需要行关节置换术。这些研究数据表明，对于有双面Ⅳ级骨软骨改变、磨损广泛、盂肱关节严重狭窄的年轻患者，关节镜清理术联合关节盂生物表面置换术可能是一种治疗选择。但是，必须注意，大约有 25% 的患者可能需要在手术后的 3~5 年内行关节置换术。

无关节炎的创伤后肩关节僵硬

肱骨近端骨折治疗后常见运动功能减弱，发生率约为 3%。[55] 活动范围减小通常较轻。有研究发现，移位较小的肱骨近端骨折，在平均随访 3.5 年后，前屈上举和外旋活动范围分别平均为对侧的 89% 和 87%，长久残留轻微的运动活动受限。[56] 这

种轻微的功能活动受限也常见于肱骨近端骨折内固定术后。肱骨近端骨折切开复位锁定钢板术后，前屈上举和外旋活动范围分别为平均 156° 和 46°。[57]

非手术治疗和手术治疗的治疗结果均可接受，但一小部分患者术后会出现病理性僵硬或粘连性滑膜炎。粘连性滑膜炎可以由关节外或关节内病因引起。关节内病因包括关节囊挛缩、关节炎、骨坏死和关节软骨畸形愈合等；关节外病因包括肩峰下粘连、撞击及大结节或外科颈骨折畸形愈合。需要了解病因以适当处理创伤后粘连性滑膜炎。

非手术骨折患者的病史资料应包括与固定时间相关的信息。尽管有些争议，但有证据表明，采取非手术治疗的轻微移位的肱骨近端骨折应立即进行早期功能锻炼，与悬吊固定 2~3 周后锻炼相比，前者功能恢复得更快，短期内疼痛缓解得更好，长期的肩关节活动范围更大。[56,58-59] 肩关节僵硬患者应接受全面的身体检查以评估早期的外科手术切口，并接受神经系统检查，尤其是腋神经检查和肩胛上神经检查。应当检查肩袖的功能状态以及主动和被动活动范围。患者通常活动受限并在达到活动范围上限时感到疼痛。创伤后肩关节僵硬常伴有与肩峰撞击相关的症状，尤其

是采用切开复位钢板内固定的患者。

影像学评估应包括肩关节正位片、肩胛骨正侧位片和腋位片，主要用于观察术后内固定位置，评估大小结节和外科颈骨折的畸形愈合状态，以及关节炎或骨坏死导致的关节软骨损伤。如果怀疑伴有肩袖损伤或早期骨坏死，尤其是患者出现阻挡症状或肩袖抗阻试验疼痛时，需要进行 MRI 检查。CT 检查只在怀疑骨折畸形愈合导致疼痛或运动受限时才有帮助。如果存在内固定材料，CT 关节造影可能有助于评估肩袖的完整性。

骨折后肩关节僵硬的治疗计划应考虑所有关节内或关节外病因。通常应在手术前先进行非手术治疗。物理康复治疗应着重于整体的被动和主动辅助牵拉锻炼。非甾体抗炎药可以减轻关节内炎症，从而减轻疼痛并改善运动功能。关节内皮质类固醇注射可使炎症局限并缓解早期疼痛。因为与安慰剂相比没有明显的益处，不推荐使用透明质酸钠关节腔内注射治疗单独存在的滑膜炎。[46] 非手术治疗应至少持续 2~3 个月。骨折后至少应经过 4~6 个月，才能考虑手术治疗。如果确诊存在骨坏死或关节炎，应考虑行关节置换术。如果仅有结节骨折或外科颈骨折畸形愈合而没有关节内软骨病变，应考虑矫正截骨和关节囊松解术。如果骨折愈合且力线

良好、没有关节内软骨病变，则仅行关节囊挛缩松解术即可。

关节镜下清理松解术治疗肩关节僵硬已被证明是一种有效的方法，可缓解疼痛，改善关节功能和活动范围。[60-62] 关节镜下松解的第一步是探查盂肱关节。最初关节镜位于标准的后入路，将前肩袖间隔入路作为工作入路。松解时首先要确定冈上肌前缘和肩胛下肌上缘。使用关节镜组织刨刀去除视窗中所有的瘢痕组织，直到喙肩韧带的下缘此处为松解的浅层标记。应注意避免损伤肱二头肌悬韧带，防止肱二头肌侧向不稳定。接下来，钝性分离肩胛下肌和盂肱骨中韧带间隙。松解盂肱韧带中部和下部并将关节囊松解至盂唇附近。松解至盂唇下方时应避免损伤邻近的腋神经。如果没有神经损伤麻痹，则可以使用神经刺激仪探测与神经之间的距离。看到肩胛下肌下缘，表明松解比较彻底，继续松解至 6 点位置以下。然后关节镜自前入路进入，并在进入后继续消融松解后下方关节囊（图 35-6）。去除并松解肩峰下粘连组织。任何用于内固定的螺钉都可以通过关节镜移除（图 35-7）。如果患者接受内固定术后至少 12 个月并且骨折已经愈合，那么在完成关节镜下清理松解术后，可以通过胸大肌三角肌入路去

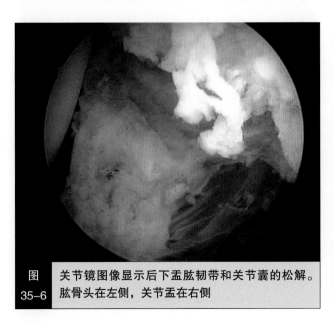

图 35-6　关节镜图像显示后下盂肱韧带和关节囊的松解。肱骨头在左侧，关节盂在右侧

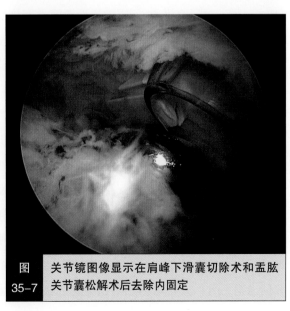

图 35-7　关节镜图像显示在肩峰下滑囊切除术和盂肱关节囊松解术后去除内固定

除钢板。麻醉下推拿松解可能在特发性滑囊炎的治疗中有作用，但不建议用于治疗创伤后粘连性滑囊炎，因为大多数患者具有关节内或关节外僵硬的病因。

手术后可立即开始物理康复治疗，重点是进行被动和主动的辅助拉伸。带导管的肌间沟神经阻滞通常可缓解疼痛 24~48 小时，并允许患者立即进行物理康复锻炼。在一项对 200 例患者的研究中，超声引导下使用留置导管的成功率为99%，短暂性神经功能损伤的发生率为 1%，患者无永久性损伤。[63] 也可以使用非甾体抗炎药、麻醉剂和普瑞巴林来控制疼痛。连续被动运动可以用作术后物理康复治疗的辅助手段，尤其适合缺少陪护帮助的患者。

有些研究报道了关节镜下清理对治疗创伤后僵硬关节的效果。一项回顾性研究对 21 例创伤后关节僵硬患者（包括 14 例肱骨近端骨折后的关节僵硬患者）在斜角肌间隙神经阻滞麻醉下进行了关节镜下关节囊挛缩及肩峰下粘连松解术，术后立即进行物理康复治疗。[61]该研究平均随访 33 个月（至少随访 12 个月），其中 95% 的患者对最终结果感到满意。与术后即刻活动能力相比，术后 6个月的活动能力减少了 48%，但在最后的随访中，活动能力逐渐增加，且最后的状态为术后即刻的110%。另一项研究将 50 例因粘连性滑膜炎而接受关节镜下松解的关节僵硬患者分为 3 类：术后僵硬患者（33 例）、骨折后僵硬患者（6 例，2 例关节盂骨折、2 例肱骨近端骨折、2 例肱骨近端骨折脱位）和特发性僵硬患者（11 例）。[60] 在平均 20 个月的随访中，所有患者活动范围增大的程度相似。骨折后僵硬患者前屈上举活动范围较术前增加 39°、外旋活动范围较术前增加 38°。与骨折后僵硬和特发性僵硬患者相比，术后僵硬患者的疼痛、满意度和功能活动评分更差。还有研究将 68 例肩关节僵硬患者分为特发性组、创伤后组、术后组、糖尿病组和撞击组 5 组。关节镜下松解后，组间的疼痛、运动和功能的改善无显著差异，但糖尿病组患者的结果明显比其他组患者差。[62]一般来说，关节镜下松解术对创伤后冻结肩的治疗有效，能预期疼痛缓解和运动改善（上举活动范围增加约 40° 和外旋活动范围增加约 40°），这与关节镜下松解术对特发性冻结肩治疗效果是相当的。术后最终恢复需要 1年多的时间。

总结

肱骨近端骨折的手术或非手术治疗均可导致多种并发症。肱骨头坏死进展风险有限，通常可以采取非手术治疗，非手术治疗在 I 期和 II 期病变中可取得良好的效果，但 III 期和 IV 期病变通常需要手术治疗。关节镜下清理术和髓心减压是出现持续症状的 I 期、II 期和 III 期病变的合理选择，在 I 期和 II 期病变中结果更佳。肱骨近端骨折畸形愈合少见。颈干角小于 110° 且有疼痛症状的外科颈骨折畸形愈合可以采用截骨矫正手术治疗。大结节骨折畸形愈合可通过截骨术（通常用于向后移位）或肩袖修复结节成形术（用于向上移位）进行治疗。如果患者年龄小于 70 岁，且无肱骨头坏死及盂肱关节炎外科颈骨折不愈合，则应考虑采用切开复位髓内异体骨植骨解剖锁定钢板。对于轻到中度的创伤后肩关节盂肱关节炎伴软骨磨损局限，关节间隙部分保留和骨赘较小或主要是单极骨赘的情况，可以通过关节镜下清理术和关节囊松解术有效地治疗。对于患有创伤后粘连性滑囊炎且骨畸形愈合或关节炎变化较小的患者，关节镜下松解是恢复其运动和功能的最佳选择，功能的恢复效果与特发性粘连性滑囊炎相似。

参考文献

[1] Iyengar JJ, Devcic Z, Sproul RC, Feeley BT: Nonoperative treatment of proximal humerus fractures: A systematic review. *J Orthop Trauma* 2011;25(10):612-617.

A systematic review of 12 studies with 650 patients

examined the results of nonsurgical treatment of proximal humeral fractures. The healing rate was 98%, and the complication rate was 13%, with varus malunion most common and osteonecrosis relatively rare (2%).

[2] Harreld KL, Marker DR, Wiesler ER, Shafiq B, Mont MA: Osteonecrosis of the humeral head. *J Am Acad Orthop Surg* 2009;17(6):345-355.

The etiology, diagnosis, evaluation, staging, natural history, and treatment of humeral head osteonecrosis were reviewed.

[3] Gerber C, Werner CM, Vienne P: Internal fixation of complex fractures of the proximal humerus. *J Bone Joint Surg Br* 2004;86(6):848-855.

[4] Thanasas C, Kontakis G, Angoules A, Limb D, Giannoudis P: Treatment of proximal humerus fractures with locking plates: A systematic review. *J Shoulder Elbow Surg* 2009;18(6):837-844.

A systematic review of 12 studies with 791 patients evaluated the efficacy and early results of using locking plates for proximal humeral fractures. Osteonecrosis occurred in 7.9% of the patients, and screw cutout occurred in 11.6%. Further surgery was needed in 13.7% of the patients.

[5] Yüksel HY, Ȳimaz S, Aks¸ahin E, Celebi L, Muratli HH, Biçimog lu A: The results of nonoperative treatment for three- and four-part fractures of the proximal humerus in low-demand patients. *J Orthop Trauma* 2011;25(10):588-595.

A retrospective review of 18 patients with a nonsurgically treated three- or four-part proximal humeral fracture found osteonecrosis in 28%. The results were satisfactory in patients older than 65 years, but the best results were found in younger patients who had a three-part fracture. Level of evidence: IV.

[6] Gerber C, Hersche O, Berberat C: The clinical relevance of posttraumatic avascular necrosis of the humeral head. *J Shoulder Elbow Surg* 1998;7(6):586-590.

[7] Lee CK, Hansen HR: Post-traumatic avascular necrosis of the humeral head in displaced proximal humeral fractures. *J Trauma* 1981;21(9):788-791.

[8] Boileau P, Chuinard C, Le Huec JC, Walch G, Trojani C: Proximal humerus fracture sequelae: Impact of a new radiographic classification on arthroplasty. *Clin Orthop Relat Res* 2006;442:121-130.

[9] Chapman C, Mattern C, Levine WN: Arthroscopically assisted core decompression of the proximal humerus for avascular necrosis. *Arthroscopy* 2004;20(9):1003-1006.

[10] Dines JS, Strauss EJ, Fealy S, Craig EV: Arthroscopic-assisted core decompression of the humeral head. *Arthroscopy* 2007;23(1):e1-e4.

An arthroscopic technique used an ACL drill guide to locate and drill humeral head osteonecrosis.

[11] Hardy P, Decrette E, Jeanrot C, Colom A, Lortat- Jacob A, Benoit J: Arthroscopic treatment of bilateral humeral head osteonecrosis. *Arthroscopy* 2000; 16(3):332-335.

[12] Mont MA, Maar DC, Urquhart MW, Lennox D, Hungerford DS: Avascular necrosis of the humeral head treated by core decompression: A retrospective review. *J Bone Joint Surg Br* 1993;75(5):785-788.

[13] Cruess RL: Experience with steroid-induced avascular necrosis of the shoulder and etiologic considerations regarding osteonecrosis of the hip. *Clin Orthop Relat Res* 1978;130(130):86-93.

[14] Sakai T, Sugano N, Nishii T, Hananouchi T, Yoshikawa H: Extent of osteonecrosis on MRI predicts humeral head collapse. *Clin Orthop Relat Res* 2008;466(5):1074-1080.

MRI was used to evaluate the necrotic angle (the extent of the necrotic lesion on midoblique-coronal and midoblique-sagittal studies) in 46 patients with humeral head osteonecrosis. No lesions collapsed if the necrotic angle was less than 90° , but 92% of the lesions collapsed if the angle was greater than 90° .

[15] Hattrup SJ, Cofield RH: Osteonecrosis of the humeral head: Relationship of disease stage, extent, and cause to natural history. *J Shoulder Elbow Surg* 1999;8(6):559-564.

[16] L'Insalata JC, Pagnani MJ, Warren RF, Dines DM: Humeral head osteonecrosis: Clinical course and radiographic predictors of outcome. *J Shoulder Elbow Surg* 1996;5(5):355-361.

[17] Harreld KL, Marulanda GA, Ulrich SD, Marker DR, Seyler TM, Mont MA: Small-diameter percutaneous decompression for osteonecrosis of the shoulder. *Am J Orthop (Belle Mead NJ)* 2009;38(7):348-354.

Twenty-six shoulders underwent decompression with a surgical technique that used small-diameter (3-mm) percutaneous perforations. The radiographic progression rate was 4% compared with a 48% rate in nonsurgically treated shoulders.

[18] LaPorte DM, Mont MA, Mohan V, Pierre-Jacques H, Jones LC, Hungerford DS: Osteonecrosis of the humeral head treated by core decompression. *Clin Orthop Relat Res* 1998;355:254-260.

[19] Beredjiklian PK, Iannotti JP, Norris TR, Williams GR:

Operative treatment of malunion of a fracture of the proximal aspect of the humerus. *J Bone Joint Surg Am* 1998;80(10):1484-1497.

[20] Boileau P, Trojani C, Walch G, Krishnan SG, Romeo A, Sinnerton R: Shoulder arthroplasty for the treatment of the sequelae of fractures of the proximal humerus. *J Shoulder Elbow Surg* 2001;10(4):299-308.

[21] Benegas E, Zoppi Filho A, Ferreira Filho AA, et al: Surgical treatment of varus malunion of the proximal humerus with valgus osteotomy. *J Shoulder Elbow Surg* 2007;16(1):55-59.

Five patients with a proximal humeral surgical neck varus malunion underwent a valgus wedge osteotomy of the proximal humerus with plate and screws. All patients had union at 6 weeks and were satisfied.

[22] Calvo E, Merino-Gutierrez I, Lagunes I: Arthroscopic tuberoplasty for subacromial impingement secondary to proximal humeral malunion. *Knee Surg Sports Traumatol Arthrosc* 2010;18(7):988-991.

An arthroscopic tuberoplasty technique for isolated greater tuberosity malunion with severe upward displacement included intra-articular and extra-articular transtendinous abrasion of the greater tuberosity with rotator cuff insertion preservation.

[23] Lädermann A, Denard PJ, Burkhart SS: Arthroscopic management of proximal humerus malunion with tuberoplasty and rotator cuff retensioning. *Arthroscopy* 2012;28(9):1220-1229.

Nine patients underwent arthroscopic tuberoplasty and rotator cuff advancement for malunion of a proximal humeral fracture. At 50-month follow-up, there was significant improvement in pain, range of motion, and outcome, with 89% able to return to their previous sport and 100% satisfied.

[24] Martinez AA, Calvo A, Domingo J, Cuenca J, Herrera A: Arthroscopic treatment for malunions of the proximal humeral greater tuberosity. *Int Orthop* 2010;34(8):1207-1211.

Eight patients underwent arthroscopic rotator cuff detachment, tuberoplasty, rotator cuff repair, and acromioplasty. All patients had improved pain, and seven returned to their previous occupations without restrictions.

[25] Gill TJ, Waters P: Valgus osteotomy of the humeral neck: A technique for the treatment of humerus varus. *J Shoulder Elbow Surg* 1997;6(3):306-310.

[26] Porcellini G, Campi F, Paladini P: Articular impingement in malunited fracture of the humeral head. *Arthroscopy* 2002;18(8):E39.

[27] Solonen KA, Vastamäki M: Osteotomy of the neck of the humerus for traumatic varus deformity. *Acta Orthop Scand* 1985;56(1):79-80.

[28] Neer CS II: Displaced proximal humeral fractures: I. Classification and evaluation. *J Bone Joint Surg Am* 1970;52(6):1077-1089.

[29] Park TS, Choi IY, Kim YH, Park MR, Shon JH, Kim SI: A new suggestion for the treatment of minimally displaced fractures of the greater tuberosity of the proximal humerus. *Bull Hosp Jt Dis* 1997;56(3): 171-176.

[30] Kim KC, Rhee KJ, Shin HD: Arthroscopic treatment of symptomatic malunion of the greater tuberosity of the humerus using the suture-bridge technique. *Orthopedics* 2010;33(4):242-245.

An arthroscopic technique for rotator cuff takedown, tuberoplasty, and double-row suture-bridge repair of symptomatic greater tuberosity malunion was described.

[31] Paavolainen P, Björkenheim JM, Slätis P, Paukku P: Operative treatment of severe proximal humeral fractures. *Acta Orthop Scand* 1983;54(3):374-379.

[32] Court-Brown CM, McQueen MM: Nonunions of the proximal humerus: Their prevalence and functional outcome. *J Trauma* 2008;64(6):1517-1521.

A prospective study of 1,027 consecutive proximal humeral fractures found a 1.1% nonunion rate. Risk factors included metaphyseal comminution and 33% to 100% surgical neck translation.

[33] Galatz LM, Iannotti JP: Management of surgical neck nonunions. *Orthop Clin North Am* 2000;31(1):51-61.

[34] Healy WL, Jupiter JB, Kristiansen TK, White RR: Nonunion of the proximal humerus: A review of 25 cases. *J Orthop Trauma* 1990;4(4):424-431.

[35] Lin JS, Klepps S, Miller S, Cleeman E, Flatow EL: Effectiveness of replacement arthroplasty with calcar grafting and avoidance of greater tuberosity osteotomy for the treatment of humeral surgical neck nonunions. *J Shoulder Elbow Surg* 2006;15(1):12-18.

[36] Ring D, McKee MD, Perey BH, Jupiter JB: The use of a blade plate and autogenous cancellous bone graft in the treatment of ununited fractures of the proximal humerus. *J Shoulder Elbow Surg* 2001;10(6):501-507.

[37] Badman BL, Mighell M, Kalandiak SP, Prasarn M: Proximal humeral nonunions treated with fixed-angle locked plating and an intramedullary strut allograft. *J Orthop Trauma* 2009;23(3):173-179.

Eighteen patients with a surgical neck proximal humeral nonunion were treated using internal fixation with a locked plate augmented with an intramedullary cortical allograft. At an average 26.5-month follow- up, 94% of the nonunions had healed.

［38］Goldstein C, Sprague S, Petrisor BA: Electrical stimulation for fracture healing: Current evidence. *J Orthop Trauma* 2010;24(suppl 1):S62-S65.

［39］Watanabe Y, Matsushita T, Bhandari M, Zdero R, Schemitsch EH: Ultrasound for fracture healing: Current evidence. *J Orthop Trauma* 2010;24(suppl 1):S56-S61.

［40］Zelle BA, Gollwitzer H, Zlowodzki M, Bühren V: Extracorporeal shock wave therapy: Current evidence. *J Orthop Trauma* 2010;24(suppl 1):S66-S70.

［41］Friedlaender GE, Perry CR, Cole JD, et al: Osteogenic protein-1 (bone morphogenetic protein-7) in the treatment of tibial nonunions. *J Bone Joint Surg Am* 2001;83(suppl 1 pt 2):S151-S158.

［42］Govender S, Csimma C, Genant HK, et al; BMP-2 Evaluation in Surgery for Tibial Trauma (BESTT) Study Group: Recombinant human bone morphogenetic protein-2 for treatment of open tibial fractures: A prospective, controlled, randomized study of four hundred and fifty patients. *J Bone Joint Surg Am* 2002;84-A(12):2123-2134.

［43］Izquierdo R, Voloshin I, Edwards S, et al; American Academy of Orthopedic Surgeons: Treatment of gleno- humeral osteoarthritis. *J Am Acad Orthop Surg* 2010;18(6):375-382.

The AAOS guidelines on the treatment of glenohumeral osteoarthritis were reviewed.

［44］Denard PJ, Wirth MA, Orfaly RM: Management of glenohumeral arthritis in the young adult. *J Bone Joint Surg Am* 2011;93(9):885-892.

Current management strategies for young, active patients with glenohumeral osteoarthritis include nonsurgical treatment, arthroscopic débridement, and arthroplasty.

［45］Silverstein E, Leger R, Shea KP: The use of intra-articular hylan G-F 20 in the treatment of symptomatic osteoarthritis of the shoulder: A preliminary study. *Am J Sports Med* 2007;35(6):979-985.

Thirty patients with glenohumeral osteoarthritis were treated with three weekly intra-articular hylan injections. At 6-month follow-up, there was significant improvement in UCLA and visual analog pain scores as well as sleeping ability.

［46］Blaine T, Moskowitz R, Udell J, et al: Treatment of persistent shoulder pain with sodium hyaluronate: A randomized, controlled trial. A multicenter study. *J Bone Joint Surg Am* 2008;90(5):970-979.

In a prospective randomized study, 456 patients with persistent shoulder pain of different etiologies were treated using sodium hyaluronate or saline. At 26- week follow-up, pain relief was significantly greater in the patients with glenohumeral osteoarthritis than in other patients.

［47］Weinstein DM, Bucchieri JS, Pollock RG, Flatow EL, Bigliani LU: Arthroscopic debridement of the shoulder for osteoarthritis. *Arthroscopy* 2000;16(5):471-476.

［48］Cameron BD, Galatz LM, Ramsey ML, Williams GR, Iannotti JP: Non-prosthetic management of grade IV osteochondral lesions of the glenohumeral joint. *J Shoulder Elbow Surg* 2002;11(1):25-32.

［49］Richards DP, Burkhart SS: Arthroscopic debridement and capsular release for glenohumeral osteoarthritis. *Arthroscopy* 2007;23(9):1019-1022.

After arthroscopic débridement and capsular release in eight patients, motion significantly improved in forward elevation (21°), external rotation (17°), and internal rotation (31°).

［50］Guyette TM, Bae H, Warren RF, Craig E, Wickiewicz TL: Results of arthroscopic subacromial decompression in patients with subacromial impingement and glenohumeral degenerative joint disease. *J Shoulder Elbow Surg* 2002;11(4):299-304.

［51］Kerr BJ, McCarty EC: Outcome of arthroscopic débridement is worse for patients with glenohumeral arthritis of both sides of the joint. *Clin Orthop Relat Res* 2008;466(3):634-638.

In 19 patients retrospectively reviewed at an average 20 months after arthroscopic débridement for glenohumeral osteoarthritis, the grade of the lesion was found not to influence outcome scores. Patients with unipolar lesions did better than those with bipolar lesions.

［52］Van Thiel GS, Sheehan S, Frank RM, et al: Retrospective analysis of arthroscopic management of glenohumeral degenerative disease. *Arthroscopy* 2010; 26(11):1451-1455.

In 81 patients retrospectively evaluated after arthroscopic débridement for glenohumeral osteoarthritis, the procedure was found to allow patients with residual joint space and no large osteophytes to avoid arthroplasty. The risks for failure included bipolar grade IV disease and a joint space of less than 2 mm.

[53] de Beer JF, Bhatia DN, van Rooyen KS, Du Toit DF: Arthroscopic debridement and biological resurfacing of the glenoid in glenohumeral arthritis. *Knee Surg Sports Traumatol Arthrosc* 2010;18(12):1767-1773.

Thirty-two patients underwent arthroscopic débridement and glenoid resurfacing with an acellular human dermal scaffold. At a minimum 2-year follow-up, the procedure was successful in 72% of patients. Five patients underwent conversion to arthroplasty.

[54] Savoie FH III, Brislin KJ, Argo D: Arthroscopic glenoid resurfacing as a surgical treatment for glenohumeral arthritis in the young patient: Midterm results. *Arthroscopy* 2009;25(8):864-871.

Twenty patients underwent arthroscopic glenoid resurfacing with a biologic patch for glenohumeral arthritis. At a minimum 3-year follow-up, 75% of patients were satisfied, with the other patients proceeding to shoulder replacement. Level of evidence: IV.

[55] Faraj D, Kooistra BW, Vd Stappen WA, Werre AJ: Results of 131 consecutive operated patients with a displaced proximal humerus fracture: An analysis with more than two years follow-up. *Eur J Orthop Surg Traumatol* 2011;21(1):7-12.

Ninety-two patients were treated with open reduction and internal fixation of a proximal humeral fracture with a locking proximal humeral plate or a PHILOS plate. At a median of 2.4 years after surgery, 39.1% of patients had a complication including loss of reduction or screw cutout (6.5%), impingement (11.9%), plate breakage (6.5%), and frozen shoulder (3.3%). Reoperations were required in 29% of patients due to a complication.

[56] Koval KJ, Gallagher MA, Marsicano JG, Cuomo F, McShinawy A, Zuckerman JD: Functional outcome after minimally displaced fractures of the proximal part of the humerus. *J Bone Joint Surg Am* 1997;79(2):203-207.

[57] Duralde XA, Leddy LR: The results of ORIF of displaced unstable proximal humeral fractures using a locking plate. *J Shoulder Elbow Surg* 2010;19(4):480-488.

Twenty-two patients underwent open reduction and internal fixation with a locking proximal humeral plate. At a minimum 2-year follow-up, all fractures had healed. Anatomic alignment was maintained in 72%, and osteonecrosis had developed in 9%. Level of evidence: IV.

[58] Hodgson SA, Mawson SJ, Saxton JM, Stanley D: Rehabilitation of two-part fractures of the neck of the humerus (two-year follow-up). *J Shoulder Elbow Surg* 2007;16(2):143-145.

In a prospective randomized study, patients treated with immediate therapy after a two-part humeral neck fracture had better function at 1-year follow-up than those treated with 3 weeks of immobilization, but there was no difference at 2-year follow-up.

[59] Lefevre-Colau MM, Babinet A, Fayad F, et al: Immediate mobilization compared with conventional immobilization for the impacted nonoperatively treated proximal humeral fracture: A randomized controlled trial. *J Bone Joint Surg Am* 2007;89(12):2582-2590.

Seventy-four patients with an impacted proximal humeral fracture were randomly assigned to early passive motion or 3 weeks of immobilization. Early mobilization led to better Constant scores, better active mobility, and less pain at 3-month follow-up, with no displacement or nonunion.

[60] Holloway GB, Schenk T, Williams GR, Ramsey ML, Iannotti JP: Arthroscopic capsular release for the treatment of refractory postoperative or postfracture shoulder stiffness. *J Bone Joint Surg Am* 2001;83-A(11):1682-1687.

[61] Levy O, Webb M, Even T, Venkateswaran B, Funk L, Copeland SA: Arthroscopic capsular release for posttraumatic shoulder stiffness. *J Shoulder Elbow Surg* 2008;17(3):410-414.

Twenty-one patients underwent arthroscopic capsular release for a posttraumatic stiff shoulder. At 33-month follow-up, the patients achieved a final mean net gain of 110% of motion compared with immediate postsurgical motion, and 95% were satisfied.

[62] Nicholson GP: Arthroscopic capsular release for stiff shoulders: Effect of etiology on outcomes. *Arthroscopy* 2003;19(1):40-49.

[63] Davis JJ, Swenson JD, Greis PE, Burks RT, Tashjian RZ: Interscalene block for postoperative analgesia using only ultrasound guidance: The outcome in 200 patients. *J Clin Anesth* 2009;21(4):272-277.

Two hundred patients undergoing shoulder or elbow surgery had ultrasonographically guided interscalene blocks. The success rate was 99%; 6% had needle paresthesia, and 1% had a transient neurologic deficit. There were no permanent deficits.

第三十六章 锁骨骨折

James M. Dunwoody, MD, FRCSC; Michael D. McKee, MD, FRCSC

流行病学

据报道，锁骨骨折每年的发病率为 29.14/10 万人。[1]男性更为常见。在锁骨骨折中，锁骨中 1/3 骨折占 80%，并通常伴有移位，锁骨远端骨折占 15%，内侧 1/3 骨折仅占 5%。

解剖学

锁骨紧靠胸膜顶部、臂丛神经、锁骨下动静脉的近端。这些结构可能会因骨折块或螺钉的放置而受损，在放置内固定物的过程中，锁骨下静脉的损伤风险最高。[2-3]在锁骨内 1/3 处，锁骨下静脉可与锁骨后方骨面紧密接触，这使得从前向后放置螺钉变得很危险。[2]在中 1/3，血管位于锁骨的后下方。在内固定过程中，将手臂外展 90° 可增加内固定放置的安全范围。[3]而在锁骨外 1/3 放置内固定是最安全的。

内侧、中间及外侧锁骨上神经的皮支呈扇形覆盖整个锁骨的皮下面，这些神经在采取横行切口及术中牵引的过程中有损伤的风险。切口下方的胸壁麻木在手术后很常见。[4-5]

分型

锁骨骨折最常用的分型是 Edinburgh 分型。该分型依据骨折的部位、移位、粉碎程度及关节内的受累情况对骨折进行分类，具有可靠性及可重复性。[1]应用相对较少的 AO 分型依据骨折的部位和特定的骨折模式细分为不同的组和亚组（图 36-1）。[6]

临床检查

开放性骨折和真正的皮肤顶起很少见，但可能发生在 65 岁以上或高能量创伤后的患者中（图 36-2）。[7]可以通过测量胸骨上切迹到肩锁关节的距离并将测量值与对侧的测量值进行比较，来评估锁骨短缩程度。锁骨骨折伴有短缩的畸形愈合可能导致肩胛骨的翼状凸起和运动障碍。[8]

必须进行仔细的神经血管检查，因为患者可能伴有锁骨下血管损伤和臂丛神经损伤，同时应该检查是否合并相关的肩带、胸壁和上肢损伤。[5]

影像学

需要常规拍摄前后位及头倾 20° 的 X 线片，CT 可能在内侧骨折中有助于诊断，但在其他部位骨折中并不常用。[9]如果怀疑有血管损伤，可进

Dr. Dunwoody or an immediate family member has stock or stock options held in Pfizer and Procter & Gamble. Dr. McKee or an immediate family member serves as a board member, owner, officer, or committee member of the American Shoulder and Elbow Surgeons, the Orthopaedic Trauma Society, and the Canadian Orthopedic Association; has received royalties from Stryker; is a member of a speakers' bureau or has made paid presentations on behalf of Synthes and Zimmer; serves as a paid consultant to or is an employee of Synthes and Zimmer; and has received research or institutional support from Wright Medical Technology and Zimmer.

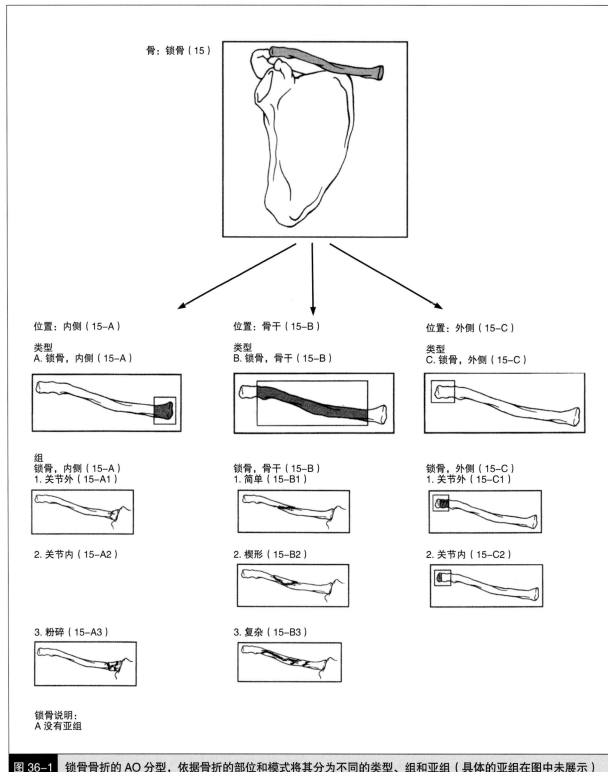

骨：锁骨（15）

位置：内侧（15-A）

类型
A. 锁骨，内侧（15-A）

组
锁骨，内侧（15-A）
1. 关节外（15-A1）

2. 关节内（15-A2）

3. 粉碎（15-A3）

锁骨说明：
A 没有亚组

位置：骨干（15-B）

类型
B. 锁骨，骨干（15-B）

锁骨，骨干（15-B）
1. 简单（15-B1）

2. 楔形（15-B2）

3. 复杂（15-B3）

位置：外侧（15-C）

类型
C. 锁骨，外侧（15-C）

锁骨，外侧（15-C）
1. 关节外（15-C1）

2. 关节内（15-C2）

图 36-1 锁骨骨折的 AO 分型，依据骨折的部位和模式将其分为不同的类型、组和亚组（具体的亚组在图中未展示）

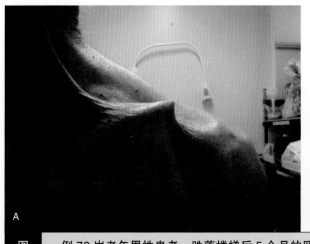
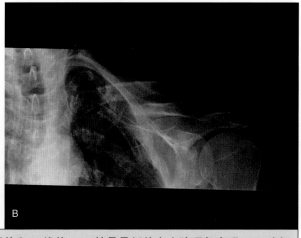

图 36-2　一例 79 岁老年男性患者，跌落楼梯后 5 个月的照片和 X 线片。A. 锁骨骨折伴有皮肤顶起表现。B. 头倾 20° 的前后位 X 线片显示伴有移位的锁骨中段骨折。该患者还合并有同侧第 2~10 肋骨骨折及血胸，因而需要胸腔置管引流。真正的皮肤顶起是很少见的，内侧骨折块尖端仅有最表层的皮肤覆盖，并有刺破皮肤的风险

行血管造影。

非手术治疗

在无移位的锁骨骨折中，大多数患者可以通过非手术治疗得到顺利的愈合。[10] 过去曾使用过 8 字绷带，但其与单纯使用吊带缓解疼痛相比没有任何优势。[11] 大多数患者可在 2~3 周后去除吊带，开始活动锻炼。

并非所有移位的骨折都需要手术干预。儿童具有比成年人更强的愈合潜能，而年龄超过 65 岁的患者在发生骨不连的情况下仍可获得令人满意的功能改善。据报道，对于移位的锁骨中段骨折，非手术治疗带来的功能障碍和发生并发症的风险较手术治疗更高。[10,13-14]

手术治疗

多项研究展示了切开复位内固定可给移位的锁骨中段骨折带来益处。对于 16~60 岁的患者，与非手术治疗相比，切开复位内固定可以带来更好的结果、更低的不愈合或畸形愈合的发生率。手术治疗患者的并发症发生率为 37%，非手术治疗患者为 63%。[13]

如果选择钢板内固定，则钢板可放置在上方或前下方（图 36-3）。前下位放置钢板的优点包括能够使用更长的螺钉、螺钉轨迹可能更安全、内固定物突出的发生率更低以及可能具有生物力学优势。[15-17] 应避免使用 3.5 mm 的重建钢板，尤其是在体型相对健壮且经常进行活动的患者中，因为与预塑形钢板或加压钢板相比，其抗弯曲和抗扭曲的能力较差。[8]

锁定钢板的使用目前已较普遍，但是其在锁骨骨折中的应用仍有争议。[17,19-20] 当施加轴向载荷时，锁定钢板的浅螺纹设计可能更容易失效。[19] 尚无前瞻性随机临床研究将锁定钢板与常规钢板进行比较，两者的临床效果尚不明确。

与切开复位钢板技术相比，髓内装置（图 36-4）具有理论上的优势，如软组织损伤更小、瘢痕较小及胸壁麻木的发生率更低。目前，正在使用的髓内植入物有 3 类。钛质弹性髓内钉通常会顺行插入。直的、较大直径的固定针采用逆行植入技术。尽管尚缺乏临床数据，但逆行弹性髓内钉已被引入使用。在生物力学上，非锁定的髓内装置劣于钢板，尤其是在抗旋转性能上。在大多数临床研究中，相较于钢板固定，使

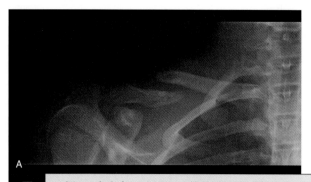
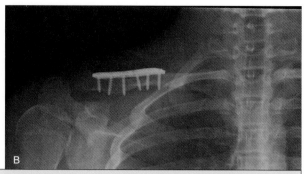

图 36-3　一例 16 岁患者，头倾 20° 的前后位 X 线片显示移位的锁骨中段骨折伴有明显的短缩。A. 术前 X 线片。B. 切开复位内固定，锁骨上方放置预塑形钢板的术后 X 线片

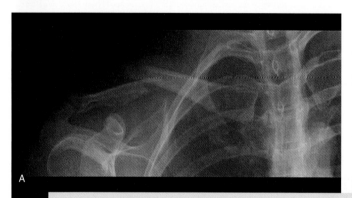
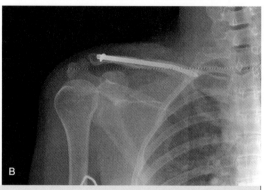

图 36-4　一例 28 岁女性患者，头倾 20° 的前后位 X 线片显示伴有移位的简单锁骨中段骨折。A. 术前 X 线片。B. 采用弹性、锁定髓内钉治疗的术后 X 线片。该技术较切开复位钢板内固定的优势包括切口小以及胸壁麻木和内固定物突出的发生率更低

用直的、大直径的固定针会带来更高的并发症发生率（5%~40%）。[18,21-22] 少数研究比较了钢板与髓内钉固定，结果表明髓内钉固定可能最适合简单骨折、粉碎性骨折较轻的患者。[23-25]

解剖板具有形态上的优势因而更常用。应尽可能保留锁骨上神经的分支，并尝试先用拉力螺钉固定，然后进行骨折的稳定固定，每个骨折块上最少固定 6 层皮质。伤口需进行仔细的两层缝合，术后手臂保持在吊带中以保持舒适，术后 3 个月内避免接触性运动。[9] 少数患者需要摘除钢板，但至少要推迟 1~2 年，以免发生再次骨折。[5]

畸形愈合

移位的锁骨中段骨折后畸形愈合的患者出现明显症状的情况并不常见。[8,26] 典型的畸形包括短缩、远端骨折块的下移和旋前。短缩具有最重要的临床意义，与肩部肌腱关系的改变和肋骨锁骨间隙的缩小有关。患者通常会感到疼痛、肩部肌肉容易疲劳和神经功能障碍。不能接受的外观改变可能是由锁骨的下垂和陷入导致的。

在手术计划中，将锁骨短缩的临床测量值与影像学重叠程度进行比较。如果临床短缩大于影像学重叠，则可能需要进行髂骨骨移植以恢复足够的长度。[8] 在大多数患者中，手术可成功恢复功能并缓解疼痛。锁骨在愈合的骨折平面内截骨、重建并矫正畸形。几乎所有的患者都可以使用局部骨移植，并不需要髂骨骨移植，除非临床短缩超过了影像学所见（例如，截骨和重建锁骨至其受伤前的位置后在截骨部位留下了明显的骨缺损）。优选的截骨稳定固定物为预塑形的锁骨钢板，放置在锁骨上方，如果可能的话每个骨折块至少固定 6 层皮质。尽可能通过钢板进行压缩。

在 6~8 周时允许加强和抵抗活动。在一项研究中，术前的平均短缩长度为 2.9 cm，术后为 0.4 cm。[8] 15 例患者中有 14 例在截骨处愈合，1 例患者有骨不连。均未进行髂骨骨移植。所有截骨愈合的患者对其手术和功能结局满意。

骨不连

骨不连被定义为在无手术干预的情况下的骨折不愈合。目前，对于进行手术干预矫正不愈合的确切时间尚存争议，有的老师定为 24 周也有的定为 1 年。[13,27] 据报道，在移位的锁骨中段骨折的非手术治疗中，骨不连的发生率约为 15%，相比之下，钢板固定的不愈合率为 1%~2%。[10,13] 与锁骨中段骨折骨不连发生相关的因素包括女性、高龄、骨折块移位和粉碎。[27] 尽管吸烟被认为是骨折后骨不连的危险因素，但关于吸烟对锁骨骨折影响的具体信息很少。

对于伴有疼痛症状的不愈合患者，手术有望获得很高的成功率。少数患者需要进行骨移植。[28-29] 仔细比较临床评估的短缩与影像学的重叠程度可能有助于预测患者是否需要在骨折块之间植入节段性的髂骨自体骨。骨折端的准备包括重新打通髓腔和羽化骨折断端。保存局部骨质并填充植入骨折不愈合部位。推荐使用上方固定的解剖板在每个骨折块上固定至少 6 层皮质。如果可以，使用拉力螺钉进行骨折块间的加压。

对于罕见的内固定失败的患者，必须考虑感染的可能性。可能需要进行分期手术：先根除感染，再进行确切的重建。这些具有挑战性的手术几乎总是需要自体骨移植，偶尔需要具有骨诱导性的生物学材料（骨形态发生蛋白）的增强。

锁骨远端骨折

锁骨远端骨折较中段骨折相对少见，并且往往发生在 65 岁以上的人群中。锁骨远端骨折不愈合的发生率为 28%~44%，其症状性不愈合的数量较中段骨折少。[1,12,30] 65 岁以上且功能需求低的患者在接受非手术治疗后可获得令人满意的功能改善。

锁骨远端骨折最常用的分型是改良的 Neer 分型。对于 Neer ⅡA 型、ⅡB 型及 Ⅴ 型的治疗是最具争议的。其他常见的分型为 AO 分型及 Edinburgh 分型。[1,6]

非移位性锁骨远端骨折可采取非手术治疗，而且可取得良好的效果。对于移位的骨折可采取手术治疗。尽管一些研究者更喜欢对所有骨折早期采用非手术治疗，但有证据表明，延迟固定将导致更多的并发症。[30] 已报道的固定方式非常多，最流行和研究最广泛的技术为在锁骨上方放置预塑形的锁定钢板和钩钢板的技术。[30-34]

自 1980 年代以来，钩钢板一直被用于远端骨折块较小、无法获得足够的螺钉把持的锁骨远端骨折。必须注意根据锁骨的形态调整钩的尺寸。在某些情况下，将钩向下弯曲几度可能更适配。将钩放置在肩峰下方、肩锁关节的后方。随着钢板复位至锁骨干，骨折也会被复位。该钢板需要在 6 个月内拆除。肩部疼痛、肩峰骨溶解以及钢板内侧锁骨干的骨折可能与钩钢板的使用有关。通常可通过去除钢板来缓解症状，并且可期望的骨折愈合率较高。[31,33-35] 尽管钩钢板可用于治疗极远端的骨折，但其并发症发生率很高，通常必须将钩钢板取出才能恢复肩部的全范围运动。

锁骨远端解剖锁定钢板技术也是一种常见的固定方法。远端骨折块较小或骨质较差时，将其固定在喙突上可能是有益的，尽管这种方式并不常见。该固定可以通过经钢板螺钉或围绕喙突的缝合实现。[32,34] 在骨量不佳的情况下，可以使用钩钢板进行固定（图 36-5）。在活跃、无其他疾病的人群中，绝大多数移位的锁骨远端骨折使用该内固定治疗是可行的。这种方法的愈合率超过 90%，而且可能获得满意的功能结果。需要告知患者不要期望在骨折愈合后至取出钢板之前可以进行正常的肩部运动。

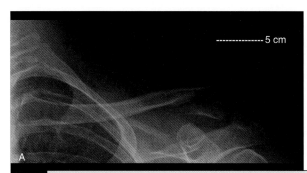
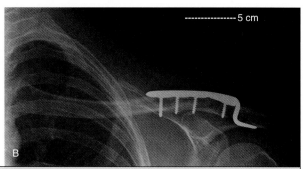

图 36-5 一例 26 岁男性患者，头倾 20° 的前后位 X 线片显示对有移位的锁骨远端 Ⅱ 型骨折采用切开复位，3.5 mm LCP 锁骨钩钢板（Synthes）内固定治疗。选用钩钢板是因为锁骨远端骨折块较小，无法获得足够的螺钉把持

喙突下固定是锁骨远端骨折中远端骨折块骨量不足或骨量不佳时的另一种选择。在该技术中，用粗线或肌腱（首选腘绳肌腱）将锁骨骨折块悬吊在喙突周围，并将锁骨干骨折块固定于喙突上以将其间接复位于远端骨折块上。或者，可将缝合锚钉埋入喙突中，并使其缝线绕锁骨边缘穿过固定。该技术可单独使用或与其他标准方法结合使用，均可实现较高的愈合率，并具有出色的肩部功能恢复效果和较低的内固定相关并发症的发生率。[36]

锁骨内侧骨折

内侧骨折是最不常见的锁骨骨折类型。这类骨折在锁骨骨折中的比例不到 5%，可能与高能量创伤有关。[1,37] 文献报道很少，主要为小型回顾性研究。内侧骨折通常伴有胸锁关节脱位。X 线片通常不能明确诊断，CT 有助于确定锁骨内侧骨折。对于移位的骨折可以考虑手术，特别是当邻近的重要结构受压时。从前向后放置螺钉可能导致锁骨下静脉受损。这些损伤必须根据患者的具体情况进行针对性的处理。

总结

大多数锁骨骨折可以采用非手术治疗。然而，有随机临床研究发现，在 60 岁以下无其他疾病的、活跃的个体中，完全移位的锁骨中段骨折初次手术治疗在功能结局和骨不连发生率这两方面均优于非手术治疗。至于其他骨折，要获得治疗的成功，必须谨慎筛选患者并注意手术技术。尽管髓内固定具有理论上的优势并且在某些研究中取得了良好的结果，但切开复位解剖钢板固定仍是目前最受欢迎的治疗方法。移位的锁骨外侧骨折的骨不连发生率很高，但 65 岁以上的患者通常很少出现症状。在对相对年轻的活跃患者的研究中，各种手术方式（包括预塑形的锁骨远端钢板固定、钩钢板固定以及经喙突下或经喙突修复）均已获得很高的成功率。

参考文献

[1] Robinson CM: Fractures of the clavicle in the adult: Epidemiology and classification. *J Bone Joint Surg Br* 1998;80(3):476-484.

[2] Sinha A, Edwin J, Sreeharsha B, Bhalaik V, Brownson P: A radiological study to define safe zones for drilling during plating of clavicle fractures. *J Bone Joint Surg Br* 2011;93(9):1247-1252.
Three-dimensional CT angiography was used to determine the relationship of vascular structures to the clavicle. The subclavian vein was most at risk, particularly with anterior-to-posterior screw placement in the medial third. Anteroinferior plating was considered safer than superior plating in the middle and lateral thirds.

[3] Werner SD, Reed J, Hanson T, Jaeblon T: Anatomic relationships after instrumentation of the midshaft clavicle with 3.5-mm reconstruction plating: An anatomic study. *J Orthop Trauma* 2011;25(11):657-660.
A cadaver study found increased distance of the sub-

clavian vein, the subclavian artery, and the brachial plexus from the clavicle when the arm was abducted to 90°.

[4] Wang K, Dowrick A, Choi J, Rahim R, Edwards E: Post-operative numbness and patient satisfaction following plate fixation of clavicular fractures. *Injury* 2010;41(10):1002-1005.

In a retrospective review of patients treated with plate fixation of a clavicle fracture using a horizontal or a vertical incision, less chest wall numbness occurred in those with a vertical incision. Level of evidence: IV.

[5] Hsu SH, Ahmad CS, Henry PD, McKee MD, Levine WN: How to minimize complications in acromioclavicular joint and clavicle surgery. *Instr Course Lect* 2012;61:169-183.

Complications related to clavicle fracture treatment and their avoidance are summarized.

[6] Marsh JL, Slongo TF, Agel J, et al: Fracture and dislocation classification compendium—2007: Orthopaedic Trauma Association classification, database and outcomes committee. *J Orthop Trauma* 2007;21(10, suppl):S1-S133.

The Orthopaedic Trauma Association classification of clavicle fractures is provided.

[7] Gottschalk HP, Dumont G, Khanani S, Browne RH, Starr AJ: Open clavicle fractures: Patterns of trauma and associated injuries. *J Orthop Trauma* 2012;26(2):107-109.

The largest study of open clavicle fractures found that these rare injuries may be associated with severe head injury and great vessel trauma. Level of evidence: IV.

[8] McKee MD, Wild LM, Schemitsch EH: Midshaft malunions of the clavicle. *J Bone Joint Surg Am* 2003;85-A(5):790-797.

[9] McKee MD, Hall JA: Open reduction and internal fixation of displaced clavicle fractures, in Schemitsch EH, McKee MD, eds: *Operative Techniques: Orthopaedic Trauma Surgery*. Philadelphia, PA, WB Saunders, 2010, pp 3-10.

The technical details of open reduction and internal fixation of midshaft clavicle fractures with a superior plate are described.

[10] McKee RC, Whelan DB, Schemitsch EH, McKee MD: Operative versus nonoperative care of displaced midshaft clavicular fractures: A meta-analysis of randomized clinical trials. *J Bone Joint Surg Am* 2012;94(8):675-684.

A meta-analysis of six randomized clinical studies

found a higher rate of symptomatic malunion and nonunion in nonsurgically treated patients. Functional outcomes at 1 year were only marginally better after surgery. Displaced midshaft clavicle fractures will heal with few consequences in approximately 75% of patients. Level of evidence: I.

[11] Andersen K, Jensen PO, Lauritzen J: Treatment of clavicular fractures: Figure-of-eight bandage versus a simple sling. *Acta Orthop Scand* 1987;58(1):71-74.

[12] Robinson CM, Cairns DA: Primary nonoperative treatment of displaced lateral fractures of the clavicle. *J Bone Joint Surg Am* 2004;86-A(4):778-782.

[13] Canadian Orthopaedic Trauma Society: Nonoperative treatment compared with plate fixation of displaced midshaft clavicular fractures: A multicenter, randomized clinical trial. *J Bone Joint Surg Am* 2007;89(1): 1-10.

A prospective, randomized clinical study compared plate fixation with nonsurgical treatment of displaced midshaft clavicle fractures. Open reduction and internal fixation led to better outcomes and a lower rate of complications at 1-year follow-up. Level of evidence: I.

[14] McKee MD, Pedersen EM, Jones C, et al: Deficits following nonoperative treatment of displaced midshaft clavicular fractures. *J Bone Joint Surg Am* 2006;88(1):35-40.

[15] Collinge C, Devinney S, Herscovici D, DiPasquale T, Sanders R: Anterior-inferior plate fixation of middle-third fractures and nonunions of the clavicle. *J Orthop Trauma* 2006;20(10):680-686.

[16] Favre P, Kloen P, Helfet DL, Werner CM: Superior versus anteroinferior plating of the clavicle: A finite element study. *J Orthop Trauma* 2011;25(11):661-665.

A finite element study found that anteroinferior plating had better resistance to cantilever bending than superior plating.

[17] Celestre P, Roberston C, Mahar A, Oka R, Meunier M, Schwartz A: Biomechanical evaluation of clavicle fracture plating techniques: Does a locking plate provide improved stability? *J Orthop Trauma* 2008;22(4):241-247.

A biomechanical comparison of plate position and locking used synthetic clavicle bones. Superior locking plates were found to have better properties than conventional or anteroinferiorly placed plates.

[18] Drosdowech DS, Manwell SE, Ferreira LM, Goel

DP, Faber KJ, Johnson JA: Biomechanical analysis of fixation of middle third fractures of the clavicle. *J Orthop Trauma* 2011;25(1):39-43.

A cadaver study compared the resistance to bending and torque of a clavicular pin and three superior plates. The 3.5-mm locking plate and dynamic compression plate were superior to the pin and 3.5-mm reconstruction plate, especially with simulated comminution.

[19] Brouwer KM, Wright TC, Ring DC: Failure of superior locking clavicle plate by axial pull-out of the lateral screws: A report of four cases. *J Shoulder Elbow Surg* 2009;18(1):e22-e25.

In a case study of four unsuccessful procedures using superiorly placed locking plates, failure was attributed to axial loading of screws and a shallow thread profile. The recommendations included using an anteroinferior plate position or conventional plating. Level of evidence: IV.

[20] Pai HT, Lee YS, Cheng CY: Surgical treatment of mid- clavicular fractures in the elderly: A comparison of locking and nonlocking plates. *Orthopedics* 2009;32(4).

In a prospective study, patients older than 60 years with a midshaft clavicle fracture were treated with locked or conventional plating. Patients in the locked plating group had a lower complication rate. Level of evidence: II.

[21] Millett PJ, Hurst JM, Horan MP, Hawkins RJ: Complications of clavicle fractures treated with intramedullary fixation. *J Shoulder Elbow Surg* 2011;20(1):86-91.

In a retrospective review of diaphyseal clavicle fractures treated with the Rockwood clavicle pin, all pins were removed at an average of 67 days. The rate of nonunion was 8.6%. Level of evidence: IV.

[22] Mudd CD, Quigley KJ, Gross LB: Excessive complications of open intramedullary nailing of midshaft clavicle fractures with the Rockwood Clavicle Pin. *Clin Orthop Relat Res* 2011;469(12):3364-3370.

In a retrospective review of clavicle fractures treated with the Rockwood clavicle pin, high rates of nonunion, repeat surgery, and soft-tissue complications were observed. Level of evidence: IV.

[23] Ferran NA, Hodgson P, Vannet N, Williams R, Evans RO: Locked intramedullary fixation vs plating for displaced and shortened mid-shaft clavicle fractures: A randomized clinical trial. *J Shoulder Elbow Surg* 2010;19(6):783-789.

A small, single-center, randomized controlled study compared intramedullary fixation with a Rockwood pin to open reduction and internal fixation with plates. The results were equivalent. All pins required removal, and 53% of the plates were removed. Level of evidence: I.

[24] Kleweno CP, Jawa A, Wells JH, et al: Midshaft clavicular fractures: Comparison of intramedullary pin and plate fixation. *J Shoulder Elbow Surg* 2011;20(7):1114-1117.

In a retrospective review of patients with an uncomminuted fracture who were treated with plating or intramedullary fixation using a Rockwood pin, comparable rates of complications were found. Level of evidence: III.

[25] Smekal V, Irenberger A, Attal RE, Oberladstaetter J, Krappinger D, Kralinger F: Elastic stable intramedullary nailing is best for mid-shaft clavicular fractures without comminution: Results in 60 patients. *Injury* 2011;42(4):324-329.

A prospective, randomized, single-center study recommended elastic stable intramedullary nailing over nonsurgical treatment of simple displaced midshaft clavicle fractures. Level of evidence: I.

[26] Hill JM, McGuire MH, Crosby LA: Closed treatment of displaced middle-third fractures of the clavicle gives poor results. *J Bone Joint Surg Br* 1997;79(4):537-539.

[27] Robinson CM, Court-Brown CM, McQueen MM, Wakefield AE: Estimating the risk of nonunion following nonoperative treatment of a clavicular fracture. *J Bone Joint Surg Am* 2004;86-A(7):1359-1365.

[28] Endrizzi DP, White RR, Babikian GM, Old AB: Nonunion of the clavicle treated with plate fixation: A review of forty-seven consecutive cases. *J Shoulder Elbow Surg* 2008;17(6):951-953.

In a large study of surgically treated clavicular nonunions, all patients were treated with a superiorly placed plate. Iliac crest autograft was rarely required. Level of evidence: IV.

[29] Rosenberg N, Neumann L, Wallace AW: Functional outcome of surgical treatment of symptomatic nonunion and malunion of midshaft clavicle fractures. *J Shoulder Elbow Surg* 2007;16(5):510-513.

A retrospective review of 11 patients with surgically treated symptomatic nonunion of midshaft clavicle fracture found that residual symptoms were common.

Bone graft was used in all patients. Level of evidence: IV.

[30] Banerjee R, Waterman B, Padalecki J, Robertson W: Management of distal clavicle fractures. *J Am Acad Orthop Surg* 2011;19(7):392-401.

Distal clavicle fractures were comprehensively reviewed.

[31] Tiren D, van Bemmel AJ, Swank DJ, van der Linden FM: Hook plate fixation of acute displaced lateral clavicle fractures: Mid-term results and a brief literature overview. *J Orthop Surg Res* 2012;7(1):2.

Complications of osteolysis around the tip of the hook and subacromial impingement were common but resolved with removal of the implant, typically at 6 months. A high rate of union was observed. Level of evidence: IV.

[32] Andersen JR, Willis MP, Nelson R, Mighell MA: Precontoured superior locked plating of distal clavicle fractures: A new strategy. *Clin Orthop Relat Res* 2011;469(12):3344-3350.

In a retrospective review of 20 patients treated with precontoured locked plating for distal clavicle fractures, approximately half of the patients required additional fixation to the coracoid. A high rate of union was observed. Level of evidence: IV.

[33] Good DW, Lui DF, Leonard M, Morris S, McElwain JP: Clavicle hook plate fixation for displaced lateralthird clavicle fractures (Neer type II): A functional outcome study. *J Shoulder Elbow Surg* 2012;21(8):1045-1048.

A review of hook plate fixation for displaced lateral clavicle fractures found predictable union and good functional outcomes. Plate removal before 6 months was recommended. Level of evidence: IV.

[34] Klein SM, Badman BL, Keating CJ, Devinney DS, Frankle MA, Mighell MA: Results of surgical treatment for unstable distal clavicular fractures. *J Shoulder Elbow Surg* 2010;19(7):1049-1055.

There was a higher complication rate after delayed treatment than after early treatment of distal clavicle fractures using a hook plate or a superior locking plate with suture augmentation. Level of evidence: IV.

[35] ElMaraghy AW, Devereaux MW, Ravichandiran K, Agur AM: Subacromial morphometric assessment of the clavicle hook plate. *Injury* 2010;41(6):613-619.

A cadaver study found that tip contact with the undersurface of the acromion, base-of-hook contact with the supraspinatus muscle, and penetration of the subacromial bursa were common after hook plate insertion.

[36] Shin SJ, Roh KJ, Kim JO, Sohn HS: Treatment of unstable distal clavicle fractures using two suture anchors and suture tension bands. *Injury* 2009;40(12):1308-1312.

A retrospective review of 19 patients treated with suture anchor fixation into the coracoid found that 18 had union, with a mean Constant Shoulder Score of 94. Level of evidence: IV.

[37] Throckmorton T, Kuhn JE: Fractures of the medial end of the clavicle. *J Shoulder Elbow Surg* 2007;16(1):49-54.

A retrospective review of medial clavicle fractures found that treatment usually was nonsurgical, and most patients had multisystem trauma. Level of evidence: IV.

第三十七章　肱骨干骨折

Robert M. Beer, MD; Robert V. O'Toole, MD

引言

最早的肱骨骨折治疗记录可追溯到公元前1600年，当时对3例患者用亚麻绷带复位和固定。[1]大多数肱骨干骨折仍需使用功能性支架进行非手术治疗，结果显示骨折愈合率较高，并发症较少。然而，手术治疗有许多相对适应证。手术治疗的支持者认为非手术治疗会导致更糟糕的功能结果和更高的不愈合率，尤其是对于某些特殊骨折类型。[2-8]到目前为止，还没有已发表的随机对照研究指出肱骨干骨折的手术或非手术治疗何者更优。理想的治疗方法仍然存在争议。[9]

流行病学

肱骨干骨折相对少见，据报道仅占所有骨折的1%~3%，具体取决于被研究人群的情况。[10]与许多骨折的典型情况一样，人群分布呈双峰形态，在30岁出现一个峰值，多为受到高能量创伤的男性，在80岁出现另一个峰值，为低能量损伤（摔倒）所致。肱骨近端骨折和中段骨干骨折的占比均在40%以上，而远端骨折占16%。[10]

Neither Dr. Beer nor any immediate family member has received anything of value from or owns stock in a commercial company or institution related directly or indirectly to the subject of this chapter. Dr. O'Toole or an immediate family member serves as a paid consultant to Synthes; has received research or institutional support from Synthes and Stryker; and serves as a board member, owner, officer, or committee member of the Orthopaedic Trauma Association.

分型

肱骨干骨折的分型可能具有一定的临床意义。某些类型的骨折经非手术治疗具有较高的骨折不愈合发生率，并且更有可能导致桡神经损伤。[4,11]AO-骨科创伤协会（AO-OTA）分类系统定义了3种骨折类型：A型骨折是简单的螺旋形、斜形或横断骨折；B型骨折骨折端有楔形碎片；C型骨折骨折端粉碎，近端和远端骨折之间分离移位。骨折常以位置（如近端、中段和远端）来描述。Holstein-Lewis骨折是肱骨远端1/3处的骨干骨折，其远端节段外侧移位，因为它被认为与桡神经麻痹有关，因此经常被讨论。[12]

非手术治疗

多项研究表明，使用支具对肱骨干骨折进行非手术治疗的骨折愈合率较高[2-3,5,7]（图37-1）。最近，一项对所有用英文发表的研究的系统综述发现，骨折后平均11周，使用功能性支具的不愈合率为5.5%（1438例骨折中存在79例）。[2]因为97%的患者为回顾性研究病例，所以需要谨慎对待这篇综述的结论。此外，该综述中最大的一项研究是对620例患者的单一回顾性病例研究，该研究报告的不愈合率非常低（2.6%），但随访率仅为67%。[2,13]排除该研究后，骨折不愈合率提高至10.7%，结果仍可接受。

一些研究者认为，非手术治疗某些类型的骨

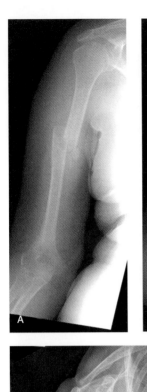
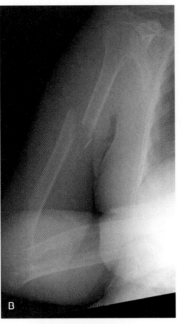
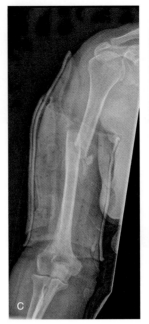
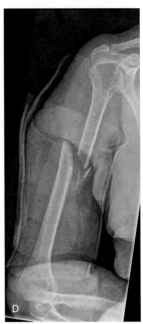

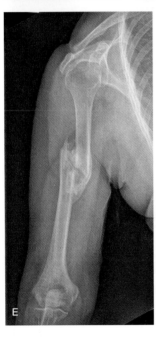
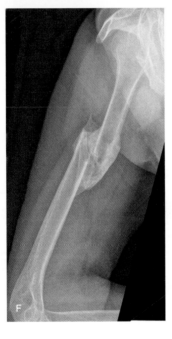

图
37-1

1 例患有多种内科疾病的老年女性患者的
X 线片。正位（A）和侧位（B）X 线片
显示右肱骨干闭合骨折。正位（C）和侧
位（D）X 线片显示了应用功能性支具固
定后的肱骨干骨折。正位（E）和侧位（F）
X 线片显示了应用功能性支具治疗后的骨
折情况。尽管畸形愈合，但功能恢复良好

折有较高的骨折不愈合的风险。有些研究认为，简单的螺旋形、斜形和横断骨折（AO-OTA 型 A 型）具有比粉碎性骨折（AO-OTA B 型和 C 型）更高的骨不连发生率，但并非所有研究都发现差异具有统计学意义。[2,5-7]尽管一些研究还发现近端 1/3 骨折发生骨不连的风险相对较高，发生率接近 32%，但尚无统一结果。[2-3,5,7]一项罕见的前瞻性研究发现，在 110 例骨折中，预测非手术治疗骨折不愈合的重要独立因素是近端骨干骨折

及在 8 周和 12 周时较低的 Neer 评分。[4]

最近，一项回顾性病例对照研究对肱骨远端 1/3 骨折的非手术治疗和手术治疗效果进行了比较，发现使用功能性支具治疗的效果良好，尽管之前有研究者认为这些骨折的非手术治疗更容易出现畸形愈合或肘关节功能差。这些数据表明，手术治疗肱骨远端 1/3 骨折的并发症发生率较高，包括感染和桡神经麻痹，而最终其肩关节或肘关节功能活动结果与非手术治疗相同。[14]

虽然使用功能性支具是目前最常见的肱骨干骨折的治疗方法，但需要注意的是，这种治疗方法需要患者有高度的依从性和参与性。痴呆患者或其他无法合作的患者的治疗可能比较困难。因为除了洗澡时，患者被要求一直悬吊制动，且要经常调整，最初往往要以直立的姿势睡觉，在许多治疗方案中，要避免主动的肩关节外展和前屈上举。通常情况下，夹板固定 1~2 周，然后应用一个功能性支具（包括一个预制的可调塑料套筒）或一个定制的热塑性支具。当肿胀消退时，收紧绑带。立即开始肘、腕和手指的活动练习，并制订一个渐进的肩关节主动活动锻炼计划。

功能性支具的并发症发生率很低。无法遵循支具说明的患者，尤其是痴呆患者，可能特别容易发生皮肤损伤，必须对其密切关注。最常见的皮肤并发症是轻微的皮肤刺激，发生率为 1%~5%。[2,13,15]

肱骨干骨折后最常发生内翻和后伸畸形。非手术治疗导致约 85% 的患者出现内翻或小于 10° 的矢状面畸形。[2] 通常认为骨干畸形的可接受极限是内翻或外翻 30°、前屈或后伸 20° 及短缩 2~3 cm。[16] 但这些观点仅基于较早的研究数据，并且很少有关于畸形与功能障碍的数据。肩关节的活动范围大，能够补偿肱骨干畸形而没有明显的功能限制。

据报道，80% 的患者可以恢复肩部活动范围。[2] 即使有一些肩部运动障碍，但一般屈伸和外旋或内旋活动范围减少在 10° 之内。这点仍然存在争论。一项前瞻性的非随机研究发现，肩关节功能不受畸形愈合程度的影响，但另一项研究发现，在使用功能性支具治疗肱骨干骨折后，受伤肩部的功能评分明显低于未受伤的肩部。[4,8]

需要进一步的研究来确定某些类型的骨折是否比其他类型的骨折更容易发生不愈合或延迟愈合，以及早期手术能否使这些骨折患者更早地恢复全部功能或得到更好的功能结果。大多数已

发表的非手术治疗结果评估集中在愈合、畸形以及肩关节和肘关节运动功能的丧失。不太常用标准化评分来评估肩关节功能。最近的一项 Cochrane 综述发现没有相关随机研究发表，只有一项前瞻性非随机研究比较了手术和非手术治疗。[9] 临床医师主要支持大多数肱骨干骨折接受非手术治疗，而手术治疗方面的证据并不充分。

手术治疗

肱骨干骨折的手术治疗适应证包括非手术治疗无效、开放性骨折、血管损伤、病理性骨折、严重的软组织损伤、同侧前臂或手部骨折、需要用拐杖承重的下肢骨折以及多发性创伤（例如，脑部或肺部受伤，非手术治疗困难）。闭合骨折手法复位导致的桡神经麻痹以前被认为是一种手术适应证，但现在不被认同。除了必要的手术修复血管外，上述所有手术适应证都是相对的。[3] 即使是开放性骨折，在适当的手术处理伤口后，也可以使用功能性支具成功地进行治疗，尽管这种治疗方法除了用于民用弹道损伤外很少被使用。在任何情况下都必须考虑患者的整体护理和功能，特别是非手术治疗对患者的影响。

目前尚无Ⅰ级研究结果用于决定手术治疗还是非手术治疗。[9] 肱骨干的手术固定方法包括外固定、髓内钉固定和钢板内固定。目前，对于钢板内固定和髓内钉固定是否能提供更好的结果尚有争议。

外固定

外固定很少用于肱骨干骨折治疗，通常用于伴有严重软组织损伤或缺损、需要修复血管损伤和在最终固定前需要暂时稳定骨折的患者（图 37-2）。[17] 在最近的一项对 84 例患者的研究中，外固定架被明确用于可能在其他医疗机构接受非手术治疗的患者，不愈合率为 0，肩肘关节功能恢复良好，该研究的结论是表面外固定可

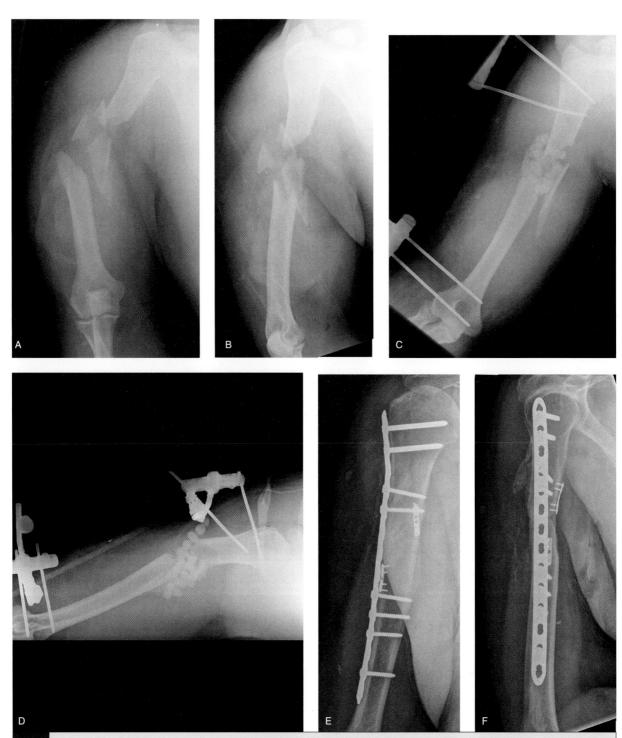

图 37-2

正位（A）和侧位（B）X线片显示，一例46岁男性患者右侧肱骨干开放性骨折。最初使用外固定架，后来更换为钢板内固定。正位（C）和侧位（D）X线片显示，应用外固定架和行骨折清创术后放置抗生素链珠。正位（E）和侧位（F）X线片显示，更换为钢板内固定治疗广泛应用。[18]

髓内钉

髓内钉常用于手术治疗肱骨干骨折，报告的愈合率高于90%。[19-20]该技术需要经皮切口和稳定的机械臂。一般来说，在病理性骨折中，髓内钉有利于稳定大部分骨。如果是软组织条件差而不适合钢板固定的手术入路，或者因软组织剥离多而手术并发症风险高，则首选髓内钉固定（图37-3）。

顺打固定技术比倒打固定技术更常被使用，因为与倒打的弹性髓内钉相比，顺打技术更容易操作，通过远近锁钉固定能提供更好的机械稳定性。顺打髓内钉可引起肩关节疼痛，倒打髓内钉可导致肘关节疼痛。[19]最近的一项前瞻性随机对照研究对92例患者进行了顺打髓内钉和倒打髓内钉的比较，发现在愈合时间和围手术期并发症方面没有差异。[19]顺打组的手术时间大约减少13分钟，但临床意义有限。顺打组患者的术后肩关节症状较多，尤其是年龄大于75岁的患者。该研究的作者认为这两种技术的临床结果大致相似。

肩关节疼痛是顺打髓内钉最常见的并发症，与切开复位和钢板内固定的结果相比较，肩关节疼痛是主要并发症。[21]最近的一项回顾性研究对33例肱骨干骨折患者在术后11天内进行了双侧MRI检查。[22]21例（64%）骨折侧出现异常，对侧无异常。尽管该研究的作者认为肱骨干骨折后肩痛的原因可能与髓内钉的放置无关，但一般认为顺打髓内钉比切开复位钢板内固定更容易引起肩关节疼痛。[23]

钢板固定

肱骨干骨折钢板内固定的愈合率一般高于90%。[20-21,24]切开复位和内固定的最重要风险是感染、医源性神经损伤和内固定失效。报道的并发症发生率是感染2%~4%，桡神经损伤2%~5%。[21]

选择前外侧入路还是后入路取决于骨折的位置、软组织的情况以及外科医师是否对桡神经进行探查。前外侧入路是胸大肌三角肌入路的延伸，提供进入肱骨近1/3的入路。因此，前外侧入路对肱骨近端骨折是有利的。患者取仰卧姿势，可在另一侧肢体上同时进行其他手术。缺点包括前方切口大和不美观、无法向后探及桡神经。后入路采用保留肱三头肌或分离肱三头肌的技术，当

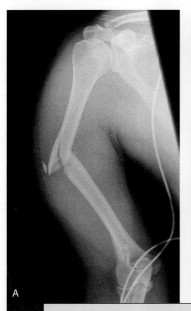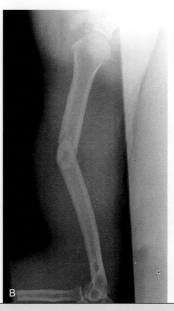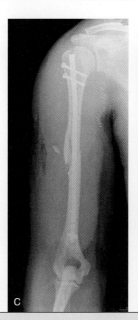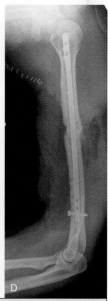

图 37-3　正位（A）和侧位（B）X线片显示，一例27岁男性患者肱骨干开放性骨折，腋动脉损伤需要血管修补。最初使用外固定架，后更换为髓内钉固定。正位（C）和侧位（D）X线片显示顺打髓内钉治疗后。（版权所有：Andrew Egleseder, MD, Baltimore, MD.）

游离出桡神经后，将肱三头肌自后外侧掀起到内侧，几乎可以到达整个肱骨干。[25] 如果骨折位于远端，则首选后入路，优点是有利于直视下显露桡神经，可隐藏切口瘢痕于手臂后方。后入路的主要缺点是需要解剖桡神经，且如果多发伤患者处于侧卧位，则难以对多处损伤同时进行手术。

为了尽量减少手术相关并发症的发生率，研究者们发展了固定肱骨的微创经皮钢板接骨（MIPPO）技术，主要操作是经肱骨干前方用近端和远端小切口插入钢板。解剖学研究发现，完全仰卧位时，桡神经距离放置在通常较宽的肱骨前表面的钢板至少 2.5 cm，并受到肱骨外侧半部分的保护。[26] 3 项回顾性研究报道了使用 MIPPO 的结果，发现总体上结果令人满意。[26-28] 但是，该技术在北美尚未普及。

钢板固定的生物力学

最有效的钢板 – 螺钉结构是最近许多生物力学研究的课题。加压钢板在治疗肱骨干骨折方面表现良好。尽管 3.5 mm 钢板也经常用于大型创伤中心，并取得了明显的成功，但是如果肱骨形态能够容纳一个较大的钢板，还是尽量使用宽的和窄的 4.5 mm 钢板（图 37-4）。对于同时伴有下肢骨折的患者，采用钢板固定肱骨干骨折的原则是，需要在早期活动时用带钢板的上臂使用拐杖负重行走（图 37-5）。最近的研究验证了这种做法的机械基础。对比 4.5 mm 和 3.5 mm 钢板后发现，在体重超过 50 kg 的患者中，两种非锁定结构在患者使用拐杖行走的过程中都发生了变形。[29] 在使用拐杖行走的负荷下，体重小于 90 kg 的患者应用较大钢板内固定没有发生灾难性的失效，体重小于 70 kg 的患者应用较小钢板没有失效。第二项研究使用合成骨和尸体骨模型来比较锁定和非锁定螺钉对 3.5 mm 钢板结构生物力学特性的影响。[30] 锁定螺钉在两种模型中都没有生物力学上的优势。两种钢板结构在承受远高于拐杖重量的预期生理负荷时都失效了。这项研究与早期的研究结果相矛盾，可能是因为失效的设置不同。两种研究模型都假设了最坏情况，即骨折节段之间没有皮质接触。在一个典型的应用中，钢板可能承受较小的极限载荷（图 37-6）。这一事实可以解释为什么使用 4.5 mm 甚至 3.5 mm 钢板的失效率很低。[31]

在骨质疏松骨中确定最佳的钢板 – 螺钉构型

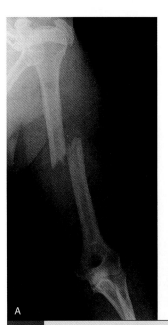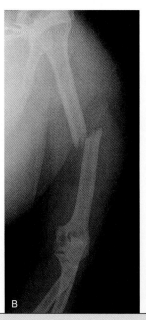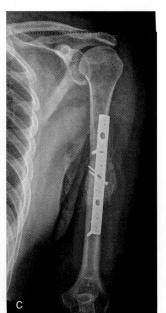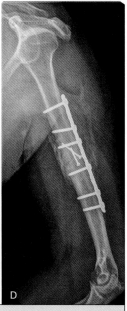

图 37-4　一例 62 岁男性患者正位（A）和侧位（B）X 线片显示左肱骨干闭合性骨折。正位（C）和侧位（D）X 线片显示，使用 4.5 mm 钢板固定

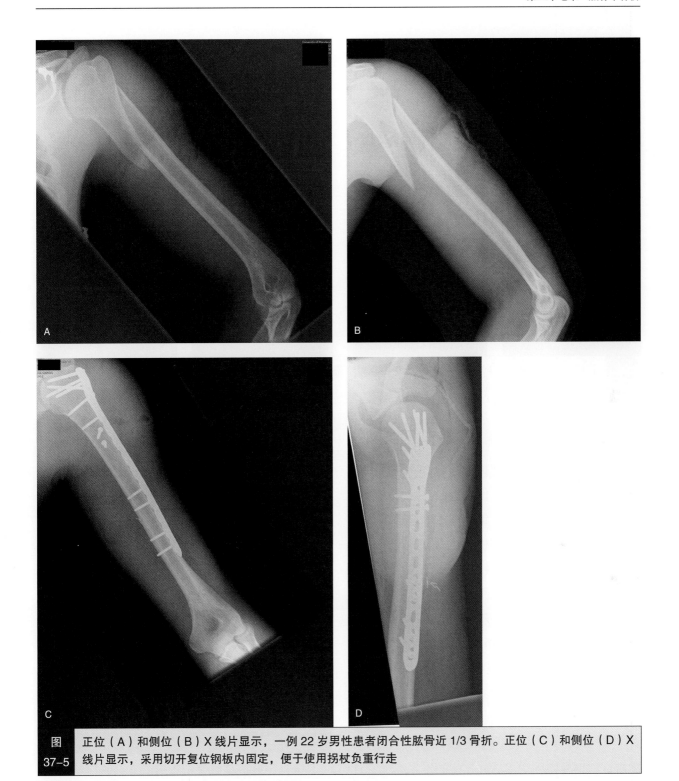

图
37-5

正位（A）和侧位（B）X线片显示，一例 22 岁男性患者闭合性肱骨近 1/3 骨折。正位（C）和侧位（D）X线片显示，采用切开复位钢板内固定，便于使用拐杖负重行走

变得越来越重要。最近的两项生物力学研究发现，在骨质疏松的尸体骨和合成骨模型中，锁定钢板具有生物力学上的优势。[32-33] 一项生物力学研究发现，在骨质疏松的尸体标本中，骨折部位两侧的第三枚锁定螺钉并没有增加轴向稳定性或弯曲载荷。[34] 基于生物力学的研究，一般的建议是，钢板应该尽可能长，以增加肱骨工作长度，每个骨折节段应至少有 3 枚双皮质螺钉，骨质疏松骨可能受益于锁定螺钉固定。

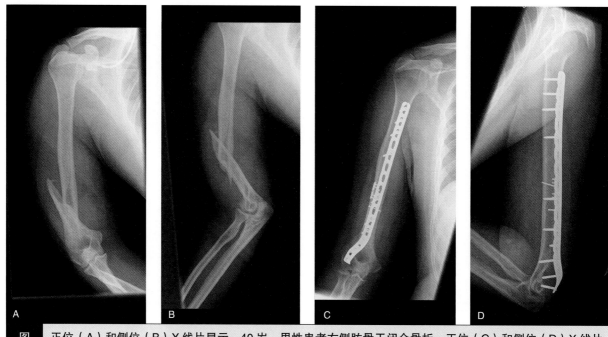

图 37-6　正位（A）和侧位（B）X线片显示，40岁，男性患者右侧肱骨干闭合骨折。正位（C）和侧位（D）X线片显示切开复位钢板内固定后

髓内钉与钢板

对于大多数肱骨干骨折，髓内钉固定和钢板内固定都是合理的选择，但理想的治疗方法仍存在争议。与髓内钉相比，钢板固定的优势是可对骨折解剖复位、直接显露桡神经以及对肩关节或肘关节的损伤更小。髓内钉的优点是生物力学稳定性好，对血供及软组织损伤小。

在最近的十几年，关于钢板与髓内钉治疗肱骨干骨折疗效的荟萃分析结论发生了变化。早期随机对照研究的数据表明钢板固定具有优势。2006年的一项荟萃分析发现，使用髓内钉时再手术、桡神经损伤、医源性骨折和肩痛的发生率更高。[35]2010年，一项更新的荟萃分析得出结论，髓内钉和钢板内固定术后并发症的发生率无统计学差异。这项分析增加了最新数据，扩大到4项研究和203名患者。[36-37]2010年的荟萃分析包括一项对33例患者的随机对照研究，发现髓内钉的并发症发生率更高。[20,37]目前相关文献的局限性在于，一项对34例患者的单一研究可能会使并发症发生率的平衡从"无差异"变为有利于钢板固定的0.52的风险比。最近的一项Cochrane综述对5项纳入了260例患者的随机对照研究进行了评估，结果发现两种固定方式的不愈合或手术并发症的发生率在统计学上无显著差异，但是该综述未纳入最新研究。[23]

2010年的荟萃分析指出，个别研究不完善，且研究人群的异质性很高。[37]该荟萃分析的作者计算出随机对照研究需要每组470例患者。文献支持以下结论：两种方法均有较高的骨折愈合率和较低的并发症发生率。但钢板和髓内钉治疗仍存在争论。

桡神经麻痹

桡神经麻痹是肱骨干骨折最常见的神经损伤。原发性桡神经麻痹约占所有肱骨干骨折的12%（在21项研究中，4517例骨折中有532例发生桡神经麻痹）。中远1/3骨折以及横断和螺旋形骨折与桡神经麻痹的相关性明显较高。Holstein-Lewis损伤模式（肱骨远端1/3的螺旋形骨折）也与桡神经麻痹有较大关系。医师对这些神经麻痹的治疗

正在形成共识。[11,12]

一项系统性回顾研究发现，采用早期观察的桡神经麻痹的自发恢复率为70.7%。对不能自行恢复的桡神经麻痹的晚期探查的恢复率达到69.2%。早期观察和晚期探查的总体恢复率为89%，与早期探查神经的84.7%的恢复率无显著差异。[11,38]

当结合决策模型对系统性回顾的数据进行分析时，早期观察被认为是闭合性骨折伴麻痹的最佳治疗方案。[39]在这个模型中，除非自然恢复率下降到40%（远低于目前71%的水平），否则早期探查将不会受到青睐。该研究的作者强调，如果神经恢复的可能性较低（如具有较高神经撕裂风险的开放性骨折），一些患者可能受益于早期手术。[39]

神经恢复所需的时间可能不同，临床症状可能持续6个月。肌电图和神经传导速度检查可能在临床症状好转前1个月就可见神经恢复的证据。肱桡肌和桡侧腕长伸肌是神经支配恢复最早的肌肉。功能完全恢复可能需要长达1年的时间。在没有临床康复迹象的情况下，一般建议在4~6个月后对神经进行探查。[40-41]

总结

大多数肱骨干骨折可以使用功能性支具进行非手术治疗。尽管最近的研究未能重现早期研究的高骨折愈合率，但这种方法确实会获得较高的骨折愈合率、较低的并发症发生率以及良好的功能恢复。肱骨近1/3骨折和简单的肱骨干骨折非手术治疗更容易导致不愈合，对于这些类型的骨折使用支具治疗的效果比手术治疗差。肱骨干骨折手术治疗的相对适应证多，绝对适应证少。文献支持使用髓内钉或钢板固定，效果良好。一些数据显示髓内钉固定后肩部症状的发生率更高。为了更充分地比较这两种固定方式，需要进行较大的随机对照研究。除神经断裂风险特别高的患者外，大多数肱骨干骨折后神经麻痹患者可以通过早期观察的非手术治疗恢复，这一点也得到了大量文献的支持。不过，仍然需要进一步研究以确定某些患者是否将从手术治疗中受益，以及哪种手术方法最有效。

参考文献

［1］ Brorson S: Management of fractures of the humerus in Ancient Egypt, Greece, and Rome: An historical review. *Clin Orthop Relat Res* 2009;467(7):1907-1914.
Early writings on the treatment of humeral shaft fractures are described.

［2］ Papasoulis E, Drosos GI, Ververidis AN, Verettas DA: Functional bracing of humeral shaft fractures: A review of clinical studies. *Injury* 2010;41(7):e21-e27.
A review of all published clinical studies of nonsurgical treatment of humeral shaft fractures found that the aggregate union rate is 94.5%. The nonunion rate rises to 10.7% if the largest study is excluded. Level of evidence: III.

［3］ Toivanen JA, Nieminen J, Laine HJ, Honkonen SE, Järvinen MJ: Functional treatment of closed humeral shaft fractures. *Int Orthop* 2005;29(1):10-13.

［4］ Broadbent MR, Will E, McQueen MM: Prediction of outcome after humeral diaphyseal fracture. *Injury* 2010;41(6):572-577.
In a prospective study of 110 patients with a fracture of the humeral shaft, a proximal third fracture and a poor Neer score at 8 and 12 weeks were significant predictors of nonunion. Level of evidence: II.

［5］ Rutgers M, Ring D: Treatment of diaphyseal fractures of the humerus using a functional brace. *J Orthop Trauma* 2006;20(9):597-601.

［6］ Ring D, Chin K, Taghinia AH, Jupiter JB: Nonunion after functional brace treatment of diaphyseal humerus fractures. *J Trauma* 2007;62(5):1157-1158.
A retrospective study found that short oblique fractures may have a higher rate of nonunion. A historical control group was used. Level of evidence: III.

［7］ Ekholm R, Tidermark J, Törnkvist H, Adami J, Ponzer S: Outcome after closed functional treatment of humeral shaft fractures. *J Orthop Trauma* 2006;20(9):591-596.

［8］ Rosenberg N, Soudry M: Shoulder impairment following treatment of diaphysial fractures of humerus by functional brace. *Arch Orthop Trauma Surg* 2006;126(7):437-440.

[9] Gosler MW, Testroote M, Moorenhof JW, Janzing HM: Surgical versus non-surgical interventions for treating humeral shaft fractures in adults. *Cochrane Database Syst Rev* 2012;1:D008832.

This review found insufficient evidence from randomized controlled studies to make recommendations regarding surgical or nonsurgical treatment of humeral shaft fractures. Level of evidence: III.

[10] Ekholm R, Adami J, Tidermark J, Hansson K, Törnkvist H, Ponzer S: Fractures of the shaft of the humerus: An epidemiological study of 401 fractures. *J Bone Joint Surg Br* 2006;88(11):1469-1473.

[11] Shao YC, Harwood P, Grotz MR, Limb D, Giannoudis PV: Radial nerve palsy associated with fractures of the shaft of the humerus: A systematic review. *J Bone Joint Surg Br* 2005;87(12):1647-1652.

[12] Ekholm R, Ponzer S, Törnkvist H, Adami J, Tidermark J: The Holstein-Lewis humeral shaft fracture: Aspects of radial nerve injury, primary treatment, and outcome. *J Orthop Trauma* 2008;22(10):693-697.

A retrospective analysis of 27 patients with the Holstein-Lewis fracture pattern found a higher rate of acute radial nerve palsy with these distal third humeral shaft fractures (22% versus 8%). Level of evidence: III.

[13] Sarmiento A, Zagorski JB, Zych GA, Latta LL, Capps CA: Functional bracing for the treatment of fractures of the humeral diaphysis. *J Bone Joint Surg Am* 2000;82(4):478-486.

[14] Jawa A, McCarty P, Doornberg J, Harris M, Ring D: Extra-articular distal-third diaphyseal fractures of the humerus: A comparison of functional bracing and plate fixation. *J Bone Joint Surg Am* 2006;88(11):2343-2347.

[15] Woon CY: Cutaneous complications of functional bracing of the humerus: A case report and literature review. *J Bone Joint Surg Am* 2010;92(8):1786-1789.

This is a case report of skin ulceration with bone protrusion during functional brace treatment of a closed humeral shaft fracture. A review of complications of functional bracing found low complication rates in earlier studies. Level of evidence: IV.

[16] Klenerman L: Fractures of the shaft of the humerus. *J Bone Joint Surg Br* 1966;48(1):105-111.

[17] Suzuki T, Hak DJ, Stahel PF, Morgan SJ, Smith WR: Safety and efficacy of conversion from external fixation to plate fixation in humeral shaft fractures. *J Orthop Trauma* 2010;24(7):414-419.

Conversion of external fixation to plate fixation in 17 patients led to few complications. Level of evidence: IV.

[18] Catagni MA, Lovisetti L, Guerreschi F, et al: The external fixation in the treatment of humeral diaphyseal fractures: Outcomes of 84 cases. *Injury* 2010;41(11):1107-1111.

Definitive external fixation led to few complications and no nonunions in humeral shaft fractures. Level of evidence: IV.

[19] Cheng H-R, Lin J: Prospective randomized comparative study of antegrade and retrograde locked nailing for middle humeral shaft fracture. *J Trauma* 2008;65(1):94-102.

Antegrade and retrograde nailing had similar outcomes, with antegrade nailing requiring an average 13 minutes less time to perform. Level of evidence: II.

[20] Putti AB, Uppin RB, Putti BB: Locked intramedullary nailing versus dynamic compression plating for humeral shaft fractures. *J Orthop Surg (Hong Kong)* 2009;17(2):139-141.

A randomized controlled study with 34 patients found a similar union rate but a higher complication rate in patients who received nailing compared with those who received plating. Level of evidence: II.

[21] McCormack RG, Brien D, Buckley RE, McKee MD, Powell J, Schemitsch EH: Fixation of fractures of the shaft of the humerus by dynamic compression plate or intramedullary nail: A prospective, randomised trial. *J Bone Joint Surg Br* 2000;82(3):336-339.

[22] O'Donnell TM, McKenna JV, Kenny P, Keogh P, O'Flanagan SJ: Concomitant injuries to the ipsilateral shoulder in patients with a fracture of the diaphysis of the humerus. *J Bone Joint Surg Br* 2008;90(1):61-65.

An MRI study found that the rate of ipsilateral shoulder injury is higher than previously known. This finding may explain some of the shoulder pain ascribed to nail insertion. Level of evidence: IV.

[23] Kurup H, Hossain M, Andrew JG: Dynamic compression plating versus locked intramedullary nailing for humeral shaft fractures in adults. [Review]. *Cochrane Database Syst Rev* 2011;6(6):CD005959.

This meta-analysis found no difference in outcomes after plating or nailing of humeral shaft fractures. Level of evidence: II.

[24] Denard A Jr, Richards JE, Obremskey WT, Tucker MC, Floyd M, Herzog GA: Outcome of nonoperative vs operative treatment of humeral shaft fractures: A retrospective study of 213 patients. *Orthopedics*

2010;33(8).

A nonrandomized study of surgical and nonsurgical treatment found no between-group difference in time to union or final range of motion. Nonsurgical treatment had a significantly higher rate of nonunion and malunion (20.6% versus 8.7% and 12.7% versus 1.3%, respectively). Level of evidence: III.

[25] Gerwin M, Hotchkiss RN, Weiland AJ: Alternative operative exposures of the posterior aspect of the humeral diaphysis with reference to the radial nerve. *J Bone Joint Surg Am* 1996;78(11):1690-1695.

[26] López-Arévalo R, de Llano-Temboury AQ, Serrano-Montilla J, de Llano-Giménez EQ, Fernández-Medina JM: Treatment of diaphyseal humeral fractures with the minimally invasive percutaneous plate (MIPPO) technique: A cadaveric study and clinical results. *J Orthop Trauma* 2011;25(5):294-299.

The results of the MIPPO technique were retrospectively reviewed in 86 patients, and the position of the radial nerve was examined in 10 arms in five cadavers. Three nonunions and three transitory radial nerve palsies were reported. The cadaver study found that with the extended arm in full supination, the radial nerve is located 2.5 cm from the center of the humerus on average. Level of evidence: IV.

[27] Zhiquan A, Bingfang Z, Yeming W, Chi Z, Peiyan H: Minimally invasive plating osteosynthesis (MIPO) of middle and distal third humeral shaft fractures. *J Orthop Trauma* 2007;21(9):628-633.

In a prospective study of 13 patients treated with minimally invasive plating osteosynthesis using a 4.5-mm plate, the time to union averaged 16 weeks, and no nonunions, radial palsies, or implant failures occurred. Level of evidence: IV.

[28] Kobayashi M, Watanabe Y, Matsushita T: Early full range of shoulder and elbow motion is possible after minimally invasive plate osteosynthesis for humeral shaft fractures. *J Orthop Trauma* 2010;24(4):212-216.

A study of minimally invasive plating osteosynthesis in 14 patients found that elbow motion took longer to return than shoulder motion. Level of evidence: IV.

[29] Patel R, Neu CP, Curtiss S, Fyhrie DP, Yoo B: Crutch weightbearing on comminuted humeral shaft fractures: A biomechanical comparison of large versus small fragment fixation for humeral shaft fractures. *J Orthop Trauma* 2011;25(5):300-305.

A synthetic bone model study found that the performance of 4.5-mm plates was superior to that of 3.5-mm

plates but questioned whether either is mechanically able to withstand crutch weight bearing after a comminuted fracture.

[30] O'Toole RV, Andersen RC, Vesnovsky O, et al: Are locking screws advantageous with plate fixation of humeral shaft fractures? A biomechanical analysis of synthetic and cadaveric bone. *J Orthop Trauma* 2008;22(10):709-715.

Locking screws offered no mechanical advantage over nonlocking screws in the plating of humeral shaft fractures in synthetic and cadaver fracture models.

[31] Sheerin DV, Sciadini MF, Halpern JL, Nascone JN, Eglseder WA: The use of locking small-fragment plates for treatment of humeral shaft fractures. *Final Program: 2004 Annual Meeting.* Rosemont, IL, Orthopaedic Trauma Association, 2004, poster 36. http://www.ota.org/education/archives.html. Accessed October 22, 2012.

[32] Davis C, Stall A, Knutsen E, et al: Locking plates in osteoporosis: A biomechanical cadaveric study of diaphyseal humerus fractures. *J Orthop Trauma* 2012;26(4):216-221.

A study of osteoporotic cadaver bone found that locking plates confer a mechanical advantage over nonlocking plates.

[33] Gardner MJ, Griffith MH, Demetrakopoulos D, et al: Hybrid locked plating of osteoporotic fractures of the humerus. *J Bone Joint Surg Am* 2006;88(9):1962-1967.

[34] Hak DJ, Althausen P, Hazelwood SJ: Locked plate fixation of osteoporotic humeral shaft fractures: Are two locking screws per segment enough? *J Orthop Trauma* 2010;24(4):207-211.

A biomechanical study found that the addition of a third locking screw on each side of a humeral shaft fracture may offer no mechanical advantage.

[35] Bhandari M, Devereaux PJ, McKee MD, Schemitsch EH: Compression plating versus intramedullary nailing of humeral shaft fractures: A meta-analysis. *Acta Orthop* 2006;77(2):279-284.

[36] Changulani M, Jain UK, Keswani T: Comparison of the use of the humerus intramedullary nail and dynamic compression plate for the management of diaphyseal fractures of the humerus: A randomised controlled study. *Int Orthop* 2007;31(3):391-395.

No difference was found in scores on the American Shoulder and Elbow Surgeons Shoulder Index after nail or plate fixation, but the average time to union was significantly lower after nailing. The infection rate was higher after plating. Shortening and shoulder pain were more likely after nailing.Level of evidence: II.

[37] Heineman DJ, Poolman RW, Nork SE, Ponsen K-J, Bhandari M: Plate fixation or intramedullary fixation of humeral shaft fractures. *Acta Orthop* 2010;81(2):216-223.

An addition of one study to a 2006 meta-analysis changed the conclusion so that similar outcomes were found after plate or nail fixation of humeral shaft fractures. Level of evidence: II.

[38] Ring D, Chin K, Jupiter JB: Radial nerve palsy associated with high-energy humeral shaft fractures. *J Hand Surg Am* 2004;29(1):144-147.

[39] Bishop J, Ring D: Management of radial nerve palsy associated with humeral shaft fracture: A decision analysis model. *J Hand Surg Am* 2009;34(6):991-996, e1.

Expected-value decision analysis was used to examine strategies for managing humeral shaft fractures. Initial observation was found to be the preferred option for radial nerve palsy with a closed humeral shaft fracture.

Early surgical exploration may be appropriate in some situations, such as an open fracture with a high risk of laceration.

[40] Shah A, Jebson PJ: Current treatment of radial nerve palsy following fracture of the humeral shaft. *J Hand Surg Am* 2008;33(8):1433-1434.

A literature review recommends initial nonsurgical management after closed primary or secondary radial nerve palsies. Initial exploration is recommended only for an open humerus fracture. Exploration at 6 months is recommended if clinical signs of function do not return.

[41] Venouziou AI, Dailiana ZH, Varitimidis SE, Hantes ME, Gougoulias NE, Malizos KN: Radial nerve palsy associated with humeral shaft fracture: Is the energy of trauma a prognostic factor? *Injury* 2011;42(11):1289-1293.

Eighteen patients with a humeral shaft fracture and associated radial nerve palsy underwent open reduction and internal fixation. Retrospective review found that a high-energy fracture mechanism is most likely to lead to laceration.

第三十八章　肩锁关节分离的分型与治疗

Steven Klepps, MD

损伤与分型的机制

　　肩锁关节损伤常发生于运动量大的人群，包括参加接触性运动的运动员。最常见的损伤机制是肩膀上方受到直接撞击。Rockwood 分型基于损伤所累及的解剖结构，是最常用的分型。Rockwood Ⅰ 型和 Ⅱ 型损伤累及肩锁关节囊；Ⅲ 型、Ⅳ 型和 Ⅴ 型损伤累及喙锁韧带和关节囊。Ⅲ 型损伤向上移位，Ⅳ 型损伤向后移位。而 Ⅴ 型损伤除了喙锁韧带和关节囊损伤外，还包括三角肌附丽点撕脱，导致分离增加，常造成锁骨嵌顿在三角肌筋膜中。导致锁骨向上移位的 Ⅲ 型和 Ⅴ 型损伤被认为是由上肢下坠引起的，而不是由锁骨上翘引起的。因此，使用吊带承担部分上肢重量通常可减少分离。Ⅵ 型损伤很少见，表现为锁骨移位至喙突下方。[1-2]

临床评估

病史和体格检查

　　患者通常主诉肩膀的上方受到直接创伤，如患者与地面强力撞击或从高处坠落。肩膀上方疼痛和肿胀。疼痛通常使患者无法抬起手臂或继续参与运动，也可能伴有颈部疼痛或麻木刺痛。

　　体格检查的发现取决于分离程度。Ⅰ 型或 Ⅱ

Neither Dr. Klepps nor any immediate family member has received anything of value from or has stock or stock options held in a commercial company or institution related directly or indirectly to the subject of this chapter.

型损伤的患者，触诊肩锁关节疼痛，交叉内收试验阳性，轻微肿胀是唯一的畸形。Ⅲ 型或 Ⅴ 型损伤，手臂下垂的力量导致患者出现锁骨远端高于肩峰的畸形并伴疼痛。当按压固定锁骨时直接将手臂向上推，或者当患者做耸肩动作时，Ⅲ 型损伤通常可以减轻。Ⅴ 型损伤的疼痛通常不能用这种手法减轻，因为锁骨通常嵌插于斜方肌内。[1-2] 这种区别有助于制订手术方案：Ⅴ 型损伤最好进行手术治疗，Ⅲ 型损伤则可进行非手术治疗。[3-4] 然而，Ⅲ 型损伤的首选治疗方法仍存在争议。Ⅳ 型损伤最显著的表现为锁骨后突出。通常，锁骨后突出较为轻微，可通过影像学检查发现，但在某些患者中，可以通过体格检查时仔细评估患者的锁骨水平不稳定性来发现。

影像学

　　肩锁关节损伤通常可以通过 X 线片确诊。肩锁关节位（也称为 Zanca 位）通常能很好地显示分离（图 38-1A）。此影像是在降低辐射量的条件下拍摄的，X 线向头侧倾斜 15° 以避免肩胛骨嵴和肩锁关节的影像重叠。腋位对于检测 Ⅳ 型损伤的向后移位至关重要（图 38-1B）。X 线片在排除主要的鉴别诊断时也很重要，如锁骨远端骨折与肩锁关节分离表现相似。在青少年患者中，只要在移位的锁骨远端附近的骨膜上观察到一条细的钙化线，就可以确定骨膜袖状骨折。应对整个锁骨和肩胛骨进行 X 线检查，以确保患者没有相关的胸锁关节损伤（双极锁骨脱位）、锁骨损伤或肩

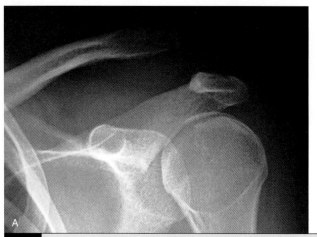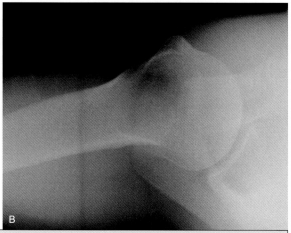

图 38-1　A. 肩锁关节位（Zanca 位）片显示Ⅲ型分离，锁骨相对肩峰向上方移位超过 100%。B. 肩胛骨腋位片显示锁骨相对肩峰前缘向后方移位

肿骨骨折（漂浮肩），尤其是在这些部位发现压痛或肿胀时。

在Ⅰ型损伤中，X 线片上没有分离的迹象。在Ⅱ型损伤中，常有轻微的增宽或上移，只能通过对患侧和对侧肩锁关节同时进行 X 线检查比较来评估。对于一个瘦弱的患者，一张 X 线片通常足以获得两个关节的图像。对于体型较健壮的患者，如果怀疑有Ⅱ型分离，通常需要通过双侧 X 线检查来评估。尽管通过双侧 X 线检查发现的Ⅱ型分离并不会明确影响治疗方案，但对确诊是有帮助的。持重 X 线检查因为通常没有帮助，已经很少采用。喙锁间隙的增加（最好与对侧位片对比）在Ⅲ型损伤中为 25%~100%，在Ⅴ型损伤中为 100%~300%。[1]Ⅳ型损伤最适合在腋位上评估，锁骨位于肩峰前缘的后方。

手术治疗与非手术治疗

Ⅰ型和Ⅱ型分离进行非手术治疗，可以缓解症状和逐渐恢复活动。一般来说，这些损伤在短时间的康复过程中可良好愈合。然而，Ⅱ型分离可能出现持续性疼痛，据报道，肩锁关节退行性改变可在受伤 5~10 年后逐渐发展，并表现出来。[5]患者应了解这些可能的预后，但通常这并不影响初始治疗。对于持续存在症状的Ⅱ型分离患者，可考

虑通过锁骨远端切除术来治疗。如果在手术时发现不稳定，肩锁关节重建也可能是必要的；单纯锁骨远端切除术与持续疼痛有关，也许是由潜在的不稳定引起的。[5]在Ⅱ型分离进行锁骨远端切除时，应考虑行切开式切除，因为这样可以在术中手法评估细微的不稳定。

虽然对Ⅲ型分离的治疗是有争议的，但在美国，除少数病例外，通常采用非手术治疗。[4]例如，对于过顶运动运动员和从事繁重体力劳动的患者，会考虑进行早期修复，但研究表明，即使是在这些患者中，非手术治疗也取得了良好的效果。[6-8]在包括德国和西班牙在内的一些国家，Ⅲ型分离通常进行手术治疗。[6-7]但目前仍没有明确的研究显示手术和非手术治疗哪一种的结果更好。最近的一项荟萃分析发现，手术治疗后的外观更美观，但在恢复投掷、缓解疼痛和改善功能方面并没有更好的结果。[9]另一项荟萃分析因没有找到足够的随机对照研究无法形成基于结果的结论。[10]在该荟萃分析所纳入的 6 项研究中，有一项研究发现，非手术治疗可以使患者更早地恢复运动或工作，降低并发症（如感染或假体失效）的发生率，但是手术治疗可获得更高的 Constant 肩关节评分。遗憾的是，这项荟萃分析的研究涉及使用克氏针（5 项研究）和钩钢板（1

项研究）治疗，这两种方法目前都不被认为是最佳的重建选择。现在的问题仍然为：对于Ⅲ型损伤，更为前沿的重建方法是否优于非手术治疗。

与Ⅰ型或Ⅱ型损伤患者相比，非手术治疗的Ⅲ型损伤患者通常需要更长的时间才能完全康复（恢复正常功能和恢复运动或工作），可能需要长达3个月的时间。因此，对于是否可对在赛季末受伤的运动员进行急性修复存在一些争论，因为患者需要在下个赛季开始前完成医师指导下的完整非手术治疗过程，这可能无法保证其有足够的时间来恢复。关节镜手术和不同修复方式的选择正在被采用，例如，使用环扎线或钩钢板比传统的重建创伤小，并可获得更早期的修复。

这些方法已经取代了用克氏针或Bosworth螺钉固定，尽管它们的工作原理相同。一般来说，无其他疾病的Ⅳ型和Ⅴ型分离患者在初始应进行手术治疗，因为非手术治疗往往会有症状残留。

手术治疗

曾有数百种手术技术被描述介绍，但很难确定哪种手术方法是最好的。外科医师应了解各种技术，以便更全面地为每个患者做出最佳选择。不管何种手术技术，外科医师都必须决定是否需要将锁骨远端切除作为重建的一部分。一般来说，锁骨远端在急性修复过程中应予以保留，因为它并没有出现明显的增生或不规则。一些研究者介绍应移除关节内软骨盘，特别是当它已经撕裂损伤时。[11]如果锁骨远端没有被切除，肩锁关节可能存在长期疼痛或骨关节炎的风险，但是在短期内，在重建时无论锁骨远端切除与否，患者似乎都恢复良好。锁骨远端切除被认为会增加修复后的水平不稳定性。[6,11]对于慢性分离，常常选择切除锁骨远端，特别是存在明显不规则或增生性改变时。

一些重要的技术要点适用于所有的肩锁关节重建技术；这些技术多是从最近的生物力学和临床研究中发展而来的。为了避免滑脱，应将环绕喙突的缝线或移植物放在喙突的底部而不是顶端。将缝合锚拧入喙突内或穿过喙突的骨道是一种避免滑脱的方法，但这种方法会因为缝合锚的使用而出现费用增加，并有导致喙突骨折的风险，因为骨道会降低喙突的强度。[12-13]在喙突周围置入缝线或移植物时，为了减少神经损伤的风险，从内侧到外侧穿出非常重要。[14]用suture tape（而不是缝线固定）增强已经变得很常见，但由于suture tape的强度比缝线的强度高，可能会切割骨质，导致喙突或锁骨骨折。可以使用多条缝线来降低缝合失败的风险；有研究报道对于急性损伤仅使用缝合方式修复的成功率达91%，其中缝线以环扎的方式放置在喙突下方，在锁骨远端则置于其上方或穿过锁骨远端。[11]

应用缝合加强方法时，所钻取的锁骨骨道不应太偏于锁骨远端，因为这样会将锁骨拉向内侧，从而导致肩锁关节间隙增宽。事实上，锁骨钻孔的位置应该与Weaver-Dunn和解剖重建的位置相同。锁骨过度复位有助于代偿重建过程中的牵拉。[2]广泛剥离锁骨骨膜和清除锁骨下瘢痕组织对于恢复修复前的活动和解剖复位至关重要。[2]在手术结束时牢固重叠缝合三角肌斜方肌筋膜对稳定性非常重要，因此，在显露过程中就应游离出大而厚的组织筋膜瓣。

改良的Weaver–Dunn重建

多年来，已有许多不同的肩锁关节重建技术被介绍，其中，改良Weaver-Dunn重建已经成为一种标准的手术方式。该方法包括将喙肩（CA）韧带从肩峰转移到锁骨远端，并辅助使用坚固的缝线或suture tape将喙锁韧带和锁骨连接在一起（图38-2）。改良的Weaver-Dunn重建效果良好，但因其易出现术后松动，故又发展了多种改良的技术，如Chuinard重建（肩峰骨块联合喙肩韧带移位）、联合腱移位和解剖重建（游离移植物移位）。[15]

利用周围组织进行重建有许多优点。例如，

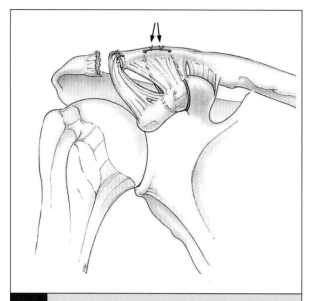

图 38-2　Weaver-Dunn 重建示意图，显示喙肩韧带转移固定至锁骨远端，缝线自喙突下方通过，再穿过锁骨骨道缝合加强（箭头）

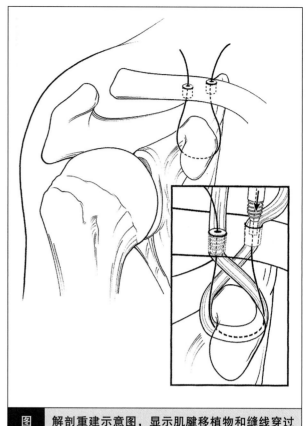

图 38-3　解剖重建示意图，显示肌腱移植物和缝线穿过喙突下方并通过锁骨远端骨道。固定是使用界面螺钉（嵌入）完成的

使用周围带血供的移植物重建，可以最大限度地发挥愈合潜力，创伤代价小。喙肩韧带经常被取下来治疗撞击，而不产生明显影响。Latarjet 肩关节稳定手术中应用联合腱移位，也没有明显影响。使用周围组织也避免了排异反应风险和使用异体材料的费用。

解剖重建

解剖重建在过去的 5~10 年中变得流行起来，主要是因为医师对 Weaver-Dunn 重建后松动风险的担忧。解剖重建多应用肌性移植物，如半腱肌或股薄肌，围绕喙突或穿过喙突并穿过锁骨的骨道（图 38-3）。放置在喙突下的移植物的主要优点是能提供比喙肩韧带移位更坚固的结构，并且在技术上比 Weaver-Dunn 重建更容易操作，因为游离喙肩韧带时，常无法保留足够的组织用于重建。可采用自体或异体移植物。移植物在锁骨内可以用缝线或界面螺钉固定。通常，将移植物与自身组织编织缝合从而避免置入螺钉。螺钉虽已被证明可提供更坚固的生物力学强度，但使用可吸收螺钉会导致骨道反应（骨溶解）从而引起骨折。一些医师考虑到这一因素所以只用缝线固定。[12,16]

通常，将肌腱延展到肩锁关节上方并附着于肩峰上以进一步增加强度，特别是在前后平面上。喙锁韧带重建可提供良好的上下稳定性，但仍残留前后不稳定性，这也是标准重建技术的缺点。一种新的技术应用髓内移植物将肩峰和锁骨固定，并与解剖重建相结合；该技术已被证明能够提供比解剖重建和 Weaver-Dunn 重建更好的前后稳定性。[16] 肩锁关节囊提供了大部分的前后稳定性，应用肩锁关节上方或髓内放置的移植物的目的是弥补这种关节囊损伤后的不稳定。

在 Weaver-Dunn 重建时，应避免锁骨螺钉孔位置过偏，以防引起肩锁关节间隙增宽。基于解剖学研究，将整个锁骨长度转化为直线来确定钻孔位置。这些钻孔位置与锁骨远端的距离为锁骨长度的 20% 和 30%。[17] 使骨道之间至少相距 15 mm 也有助于降低骨折风险。[12] 有些研究者提倡单隧道或无隧道重建，以进一步降低骨折风险。但是，这种技术可能导致肌腱松动或摆动切割。[2,18]也有研究者推荐仅使用缝合固定，从而减小锁骨骨道的直径。[12]虽然一些生物力学的尸体研究比较了解剖重建与Weaver-Dunn重建[1-2,16,19]但这些都是使用各种技术的时点研究，关于解剖重建是否比Weaver-Dunn重建更好这一问题，并没有得出明确结论。

一项纳入了24例患者的前瞻性临床研究直接比较了解剖重建和Weaver-Dunn重建。[20]其中12例经解剖重建治疗的患者获得了更高的ASES肩关节疼痛和功能障碍评分及Constant肩关节评分，以及更小的喙锁间隙。两个治疗组的患者都有很好的临床结果。尽管取得了不错的临床效果，但问题仍然存在：解剖重建所带来的临床效益与移植物和螺钉增加的费用、供区并发症以及可能的排斥反应相比是否值当。对比经典的Weaver-Dunn重建，在推荐解剖重建之前还需要进一步的研究。

关节镜重建

关节镜技术逐渐被应用于肩锁关节的修复和重建。急性修复固定使用牢固缝合和锁定金属夹，如Tightrope装置（Arthrex，Naples，FL），放置在锁骨和喙突之间。不同于刚性的螺钉固定，这种固定装置允许通过装置微动，而且不需要取出内固定物。操作的原理是将锁骨原位固定，使喙锁韧带能自行重建。这一概念类似Bosworth螺钉或克氏针固定，优点是不需要第二次手术。Bosworth螺钉和克氏针固定也存在螺钉失效、迁移、感染和拔出的风险。遗憾的是，类似Tightrope装置的装置断裂也时有发生。[14]因此，这些固定装置通过改变Button的形状（如狗骨形状）、大小或增加固定量（如双隧道技术）进行了改进。[21]一些厂家在flip-button装置上附着肌腱，依旧可以在关节镜下操作。[22]

关节镜下慢性分离的重建方法也已经被应用，包括GraftRope系统和肌腱或喙肩韧带移位（伴或不伴肩峰骨块）。[22-23]对10例使用关节镜下Weaver-Dunn手术治疗慢性不稳定的患者的研究显示成功率达90%。但并没有研究显示哪一种关节镜技术相对于其他技术存在显著优势。关节镜手术在移动锁骨远端或缝合固定三角肌斜方肌筋膜的能力方面不如开放手术，而这些恰是此类手术的关键内容，尤其在治疗慢性不稳定肩关节方面。关节镜技术的这些不足可能限制它们被更广泛地使用。

关节镜技术的一个优点是，在肩锁关节修复和重建时，可以评估肩关节内病变。一项研究发现15%的关节内病变，如肩袖和盂唇撕裂，可以在肩锁关节手术时进行修复。[24]

钩钢板

钩钢板已广泛用于治疗肩锁关节分离，虽然总体上它们更常被用于锁骨远端骨折。钩钢板与Bosworth螺钉固定相结合并短期留置可以使喙锁韧带和其他结构稳定愈合。[25]然而，与加强缝合修复相比，钩钢板没有明显改善结果，而且还需要二次手术取出。一项纳入了313例患者的研究所报道的钩钢板相关并发症，使其在治疗初次肩锁关节分离中的作用受到质疑。这些并发症包括钩钢板侵蚀肩峰（伴或不伴肩峰骨折，1例）、钩钢板骨折（4例）、感染（6例）和钩钢板取出后再脱位（7例）。[25-26]钩钢板与软组织移植物联合使用时表现更好。但这种方法似乎违背了微创钢板置入的目的。比较研究发现，Weaver-Dunn重建后的效果优于钩钢板治疗，前者休息时疼痛较轻且Constant肩关节评分更高。[27]

尽管钩钢板在急性单发的肩锁关节损伤中似乎没有重要的作用，但它们用于特定患者有一定的意义。例如，对于合并喙突或肩胛骨骨折的肩锁关节分离，若喙突和锁骨之间无法进行固定，可使用钩钢板进行固定（图38-4）。钩钢板沿着锁骨远端和肩峰嵴下方放置，此时稳定的基础是肩峰而不是喙突。钩钢板也被用于肩锁关节翻修重

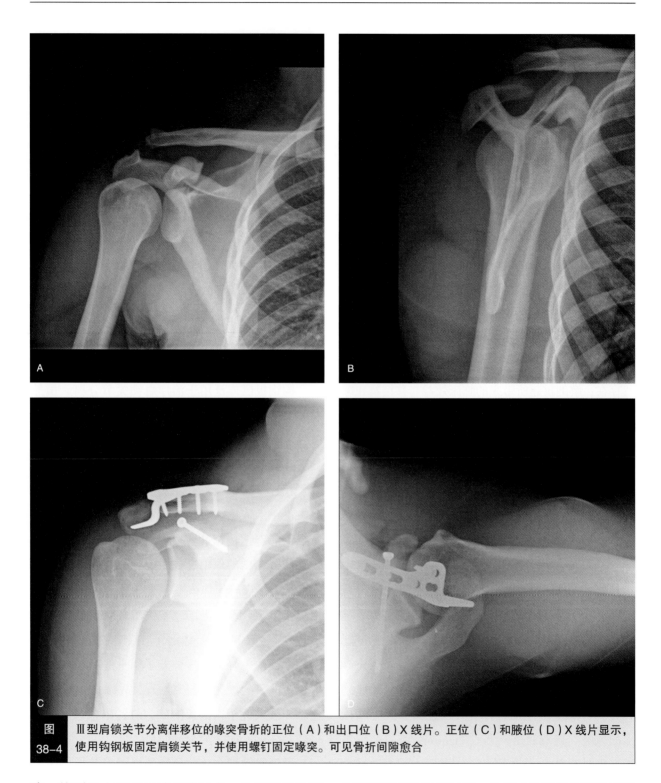

图 38-4　Ⅲ型肩锁关节分离伴移位的喙突骨折的正位（A）和出口位（B）X线片。正位（C）和腋位（D）X线片显示，使用钩钢板固定肩锁关节，并使用螺钉固定喙突。可见骨折间隙愈合

建，特别是在锁骨远端切除过多、软组织质量不佳时。

康复

在非手术治疗的患者中，级别较高的Ⅲ型、Ⅳ型和Ⅴ型损伤通常比级别较低的Ⅰ型和Ⅱ型损伤需要更多的恢复时间。Ⅰ型或Ⅱ型损伤通常需要 2~3 周的非手术治疗，然后逐渐恢复运动，Ⅲ型损伤通常需要 4~6 周。恢复运动需要全方位的运动和完全的力量恢复，以无及无疼痛的肩锁关节。如果患者在 3 个月后无法恢复运动或工作，则认为非手术治疗不成功；那么应该考虑手术。[28]

最近推广的渐进式康复计划分为四个阶段[29,30]。第一阶段，通过冰敷、非甾体抗炎药和最小限度的固定来减轻疼痛和肿胀。先进行肩胛骨稳定治疗和下肢力量训练。使用吊带仅为了舒适，Ⅲ型损伤患者通常需要比较低级别损伤患者更长时间的吊带使用。当患者恢复正常活动范围的 75% 时，进入第二阶段。第二阶段的治疗包括恢复全部活动范围，并允许进行早期力量训练。当力量恢复至 75% 时，进入第三阶段。第三阶段的目标是恢复全部力量，强调力量和耐力。当患侧手臂的力量与对侧手臂的力量相等时，进入第四阶段。第四阶段涉及运动专项训练。非手术治疗 6 周后未完全康复的患者比康复的患者更有可能需要手术。

目前已经有许多不同的术后康复方案。通常，肩部在最初的 6 周内需制动。在接下来的 6 周内，将进行全范围的主动和被动活动，避免持重。在 3 个月时开始力量训练，适度持重。从第 4 个月开始全范围活动和投掷，6 个月时恢复接触运动。

总结

肩锁关节损伤在运动量大的患者中很常见。大多数患者通过非手术治疗恢复良好，可恢复正常功能。逐步康复的方法往往能最有效地帮助患者恢复功能。然而，对于某些损伤类型，如Ⅳ型、Ⅴ型和Ⅵ型，最好选择手术治疗。此外，非手术治疗 3 个月后仍未恢复的患者也最好接受手术治疗。目前，对于最佳的手术方式仍存在争议，但只要按照相应的原则，包括充分活动、适当的骨道位置结合缝合或韧带加强固定以及适当的康复治疗，就可以获得良好的结果。解剖重建可提供更强的生物力学重建。一些外科医师报道了微创技术的应用，随着更好的固定物的应用和中期结果的报道，微创技术可能变得更加普遍。钩钢板作为一种逐渐被接受的固定装置，其在肩锁关节损伤治疗中的作用仍需要进一步探究。

参考文献

[1] Johansen JA, Grutter PW, McFarland EG, Petersen SA: Acromioclavicular joint injuries: Indications for treatment and treatment options. *J Shoulder Elbow Surg* 2011;20(2, suppl):S70-S82.
The management of AC joint injuries is summarized, with a focus on diagnosis and treatment. The role of surgical management is discussed, with indications for surgery based on current literature.

[2] Hsu SH, Ahmad CS, Henry PD, McKee MD, Levine WN: How to minimize complications in acromioclavicular joint and clavicle surgery. *Instr Course Lect* 2012;61:169-183.
The treatment of AC joint injuries is summarized, with a focus on avoiding complications of surgical treatment. Methods for managing and evaluating patients postoperatively are discussed in terms of complications and patient outcome.

[3] Nissen CW, Chatterjee A: Type III acromioclavicular separation: Results of a recent survey on its management. *Am J Orthop (Belle Mead NJ)* 2007;36(2):89-93.
Members of the American Orthopaedic Society for Sports Medicine and orthopedic residency directors were surveyed concerning treatment of type III AC joint separations. More than 80% of the respondents recommended nonsurgical treatment.

[4] Schlegel TF, Burks RT, Marcus RL, Dunn HK: A prospective evaluation of untreated acute grade IIIacromioclavicular separations. *Am J Sports Med* 2001;29(6):699-703.

[5] Mouhsine E, Garofalo R, Crevoisier X, Farron A: Grade I and II acromioclavicular dislocations: Results of conservative treatment. *J Shoulder Elbow Surg* 2003;12(6):599-602.

[6] Lizaur A, Sanz-Reig J, Gonzalez-Parreño S: Long-term results of the surgical treatment of type III acromioclavicular dislocations: An update of a previous report. *J Bone Joint Surg Br* 2011;93(8):1088-1092.
At an average 24-year follow-up of 38 patients treated with Kirschner wire fixation for acute AC joint separation, 35 patients were satisfied. Two patients had redisplacement, and 1 had osteoarthritis of the AC joint.

[7] Bäthis H, Tingart M, Bouillon B, Tiling T: The status of therapy of acromioclavicular joint injury: Results of a survey of trauma surgery clinics in Germany. *Unfallchirurg* 2001;104(10):955-960.

[8] Bannister GC, Wallace WA, Stableforth PG, Hutson

MA: The management of acute acromioclavicular dislocation: A randomised prospective controlled trial. *J Bone Joint Surg Br* 1989;71(5):848-850.

[9] Smith TO, Chester R, Pearse EO, Hing CB: Operative versus non-operative management following Rockwood grade III acromioclavicular separation: A meta-analysis of the current evidence base. *J Orthop Traumatol* 2011;12(1):19-27.

A meta-analysis of six studies attempted to determine whether surgical or nonsurgical treatment of type III AC separation was preferable. Only one study found better results with surgery. The older Kirschner wire technique was used in five studies. Surgical treatment had a better cosmetic result, but nonsurgical treatment was associated with less time to recovery. No difference was found related to strength, pain, or throwing.

[10] Ceccarelli E, Bondì R, Alviti F, Garofalo R, Miulli F, Padua R: Treatment of acute grade III acromioclavicular dislocation: A lack of evidence. *J Orthop Traumatol* 2008;9(2):105-108.

A literature review of the outcomes of surgical and nonsurgical treatment found only five randomized controlled studies. Patients had a similar result regardless of whether they were treated with or without surgery, but those treated surgically had a higher complication rate. Therefore, nonsurgical treatment was found to be valid for these patients.

[11] Lädermann A, Grosclaude M, Lübbeke A, et al: Acromioclavicular and coracoclavicular cECRLage reconstruction for acute acromioclavicular joint dislocations. *J Shoulder Elbow Surg* 2011;20(3):401-408.

An excellent result was reported for 34 of 37 patients who underwent AC and CC suture fixation using nonabsorbable sutures for acute AC separation, with no soft-tissue transfer. Isokinetic study found normal function. There was no need for hardware removal.

[12] Turman KA, Miller CD, Miller MD: Clavicular fractures following coracoclavicular ligament reconstruction with tendon graft: A report of three cases. *J Bone Joint Surg Am* 2010;92(6):1526-1532.

Three patients had clavicle fracture after CC ligament reconstruction with tendon graft. This complication may be avoidable with preoperative counseling to avoid postoperative overactivity, the use of small- diameter tunnels, maintenance of an adequate bone bridge, and avoidance of posterior cortical breach.

[13] Gerhardt DC, VanDerWerf JD, Rylander LS, McCarty EC: Postoperative coracoid fracture after transcoracoid acromioclavicular joint reconstruction. *J Shoulder Elbow Surg* 2011;20(5):e6-e10.

The risk of coracoid fracture after AC joint reconstruction using transcoracoid fixation should be considered in choosing the best reconstructive method.

[14] Motta P, Maderni A, Bruno L, Mariotti U: Suture rupture in acromioclavicular joint dislocations treated with flip buttons. *Arthroscopy* 2011;27(2):294-298.

Four of 20 patients undergoing acute AC joint repair using flip buttons had postoperative suture rupture. All patients had hyperlaxity. Horizontal instability of repair may lead to shearing of the suture and subsequent failure of repair.

[15] Jiang C, Wang M, Rong G: Proximally based conjoined tendon transfer for coracoclavicular reconstruction in the treatment of acromioclavicular dislocation: Surgical technique. *J Bone Joint Surg Am* 2008; 90(suppl 2, pt 2):299-308.

The lateral half of the conjoined tendon was used, rather than the CA ligament, for AC joint reconstruction in 38 patients. The results were good or excellent in 89% of the patients. The main advantage is adequate soft tissue, with no sacrifice of the CA arch or the need for soft-tissue transfer.

[16] Gonzalez-Lomas G, Javidan P, Lin T, Adamson GJ, Limpisvasti O, Lee TQ: Intramedullary acromioclavicular ligament reconstruction strengthens isolated coracoclavicular ligament reconstruction in acromioclavicular dislocations. *Am J Sports Med* 2010;38(10):2113-2122.

A cadaver study compared CC anatomic reconstruction alone and with intramedullary graft placement in the AC joint. The intramedullary graft improved horizontal stability.

[17] Rios CG, Mazzocca AD: Acromioclavicular joint problems in athletes and new methods of management. *Clin Sports Med* 2008;27(4):763-788.

The relevant anatomy, classification, evaluation, and treatment of AC joint pathology is systematically reviewed.

[18] Grutter PW, Petersen SA: Anatomical acromioclavicular ligament reconstruction: A biomechanical comparison of reconstructive techniques of the acromioclavicular joint. *Am J Sports Med* 2005;33(11):1723-1728.

[19] Thomas K, Litsky A, Jones G, Bishop JY: Biomechanical comparison of coracoclavicular reconstructive techniques. *Am J Sports Med* 2011;39(4):804-810.

A cadaver study compared Weaver-Dunn, nonanatomic allograft, anatomic allograft, anatomic suture, and GraftRope reconstructions. In comparison with native control shoulders, the anatomic allograft had the highest load to failure, which was significantly higher than those of the other subgroups. The nonanatomic allograft technique did not bring the tendon through the clavicle and did not weave the tendon on itself. No significant difference was found among other subgroups.

[20] Tauber M, Gordon K, Koller H, Fox M, Resch H: Semitendinosus tendon graft versus a modified Weaver-Dunn procedure for acromioclavicular joint reconstruction in chronic cases: A prospective comparative study. *Am J Sports Med* 2009;37(1):181-190.

A retrospective study of 24 patients compared the Weaver-Dunn and anatomic reconstructions. The 12 patients who received the anatomic reconstruction had superior clinical and radiographic outcomes.

[21] Scheibel M, Dröschel S, Gerhardt C, Kraus N: Arthroscopically assisted stabilization of acute high-grade acromioclavicular joint separations. *Am J Sports Med* 2011;39(7):1507-1516.

Arthroscopically assisted stabilization of acute AC separation using a double TightRope technique had excellent clinical results in 28 patients, despite greater CC distance compared with the contralateral side. Patients' fairly high rate of horizontal instability did not appear to affect the clinical results.

[22] DeBerardino TM, Pensak MJ, Ferreira J, Mazzocca AD: Arthroscopic stabilization of acromioclavicular joint dislocation using the AC graftrope system. *J Shoulder Elbow Surg* 2010;19(2, suppl):47-52.

Early results are reported for the AC flip button device with incorporated allograft as used for arthroscopic repair of acute AC joint separations. No complications were reported, and patients had an early return to function.

[23] Boileau P, Old J, Gastaud O, Brassart N, Roussanne Y: All-arthroscopic Weaver-Dunn-Chuinard procedure with double-button fixation for chronic acromioclavicular joint dislocation. *Arthroscopy* 2010;26(2):149-160.

Ten patients with chronic AC joint instability underwent arthroscopic CA ligament transfer along with a fleck of acromion. All patients were satisfied, and 9 re-turned to sport. One patient had a superficial infection. The bone fragment healed in 8 patients. Level of evidence: IV.

[24] Pauly S, Gerhardt C, Haas NP, Scheibel M: Prevalence of concomitant intraarticular lesions in patients treated operatively for high-grade acromioclavicular joint separations. *Knee Surg Sports Traumatol Arthrosc* 2009;17(5):513-517.

Forty patients underwent diagnostic arthroscopy during surgery for high-grade AC separation. Six patients (15%) were found to have pathology, including 2 with subscapularis tears, 3 with superior labrum anterior and posterior tears, and 1 with a combined supraspinatus-subscapularis tendon tear.

[25] Kienast B, Thietje R, Queitsch C, Gille J, Schulz AP, Meiners J: Mid-term results after operative treatment of Rockwood grade III-V acromioclavicular joint dislocations with an AC-hook-plate. *Eur J Med Res* 2011;16(2):52-56.

Midterm results were reported for an AC hook plate used to treat of 313 acute AC joint separations. The results were excellent in 89%, with an average Constant score of 92.4. The complication rate was 10.6%, with six infections, one acromial fracture, and seven redislocations.

[26] Chiang CL, Yang SW, Tsai MY, Kuen-Huang Chen C: Acromion osteolysis and fracture after hook plate fixation for acromioclavicular joint dislocation: A case report. *J Shoulder Elbow Surg* 2010;19(4):e13-e15.

Acromial osteolysis followed by fracture developed after hook plate placement for AC separation. The patient did not have the plate removed 4 months after surgery, as recommended, and the complication developed at 8 months. Early plate removal is recommended.

[27] Boström Windhamre HA, von Heideken JP, Une-Larsson VE, Ekelund AL: Surgical treatment of chronic acromioclavicular dislocations: A comparative study of Weaver-Dunn augmented with PDS-braid or hook plate. *J Shoulder Elbow Surg* 2010;19(7):1040-1048.

A retrospective study compared Weaver-Dunn reconstructions with polydioxanone braid or a hook plate for augmentation. The clinical results were similar, but the necessity of an additional surgical procedure for hook plate removal led to a recommendation for suture augmentation.

[28] Trainer G, Arciero RA, Mazzocca AD: Practical management of grade III acromioclavicular separations. *Clin J Sport Med* 2008;18(2):162-166.

A protocol is presented for the initial treatment of grade III AC joint separations depending on the timing of injury (in-season or off-season) and the response to initial nonsurgical treatment. Surgery was recommended after 3 months of unsuccessful nonsurgical treatment.

[29] Cote MP, Wojcik KE, Gomlinski G, Mazzocca AD: Rehabilitation of acromioclavicular joint separations: Operative and nonoperative considerations. *Clin Sports Med* 2010;29(2):213-228, vii.

The anatomy and biomechanics of the AC joint are considered in determining a rehabilitation protocol for patients treated nonsurgically or surgically.

[30] Lervick GN, Klepps SK: Shoulder dislocations, clavicle fractures, and acromioclavicular separations. *Orthopaedic Knowledge Online Journal*. March 1, 2011. http://orthoportal.aaos.org/oko/article.aspx?article=OKO_SHO042#abstract. Accessed September 6,2012.

A practical method is provided for enabling athletes to return to play after AC joint and clavicle injuries based on rehabilitation protocols and biomechanical studies.

第七部分

肘关节创伤、骨折与重建

栏目编委：
Mark S. Cohen, MD

第三十九章　肌腱损伤和肘关节疾病：肱二头肌损伤、肱三头肌损伤、外上髁及内上髁炎

Brandon Cincere, MD; Robert P. Nirschl, MD, MS

引言

　　肘部肌腱损伤通常可按病因分为：单次严重创伤（急性损伤、慢性合并急性损伤），作用于因过度使用而易受损伤的组织上；多次重复过度使用（慢性损伤）。从急性损伤到慢性损伤的许多病理状况，都可能发生在肘部周围。韧带功能障碍、神经功能障碍和骨软骨损伤都可能与该疾病有关。肘部肌腱过度使用损伤不是一种孤立的损伤，应该对从颈部和胸椎到肩和手的整个肢体进行评估。

肱二头肌损伤

评估

　　肱二头肌远端在桡骨结节上有两个止点。短头止点在结节的远端，使肱二头肌成为强有力的肘屈肌。长头止点更偏近端和尺骨，远离前臂的旋转轴。这种附着通过增加杠杆作用加强了旋后力量。肱二头肌腱呈带状螺旋，在左臂为顺时针方向，在右臂为逆时针方向。[1]

　　大多数肱二头肌远端损伤发生于肘关节处于中度屈曲位时，是由突然受到的偏心伸肘暴力所

致，常为桡骨结节的急性撕脱骨折。症状可能包括撕裂感和剧烈的疼痛。

　　大多数此类损伤发生在40~60岁男性的优势侧上肢。吸烟群体的撕裂风险是正常群体的7.5倍。[2] 肘窝区的疼痛和瘀斑是常见的体征，压痛以及旋后和屈肘力弱也可能发生。触诊肌腱处空虚、O'Driscoll-hook试验阳性或挤压试验阳性提示存在损伤，如肌腱部分撕裂、肱二头肌腱膜完全撕裂（纤维撕裂伤）及肱二头肌腱鞘炎。[3,4] O'Driscoll-hook试验有100%的敏感性和特异性。[3] 完全性撕裂如果发生在4周内，则诊断为急性撕裂；如果发生在更早期，则诊断为慢性撕裂。此类损伤的影像学检查通常显示不合并骨损伤，但偶尔可发现桡骨结节不规则增大或撕脱。[5] 无撕裂的肱二头肌腱腱鞘炎可单独发生，或与肘部滑囊炎或部分撕裂合并发生。部分撕裂不太常见，可发生在肌腱内或肌腱附丽点（图39-1）。前臂旋转时肌腱附丽点的弹响可能是由肌腱与结节之间的黏液囊炎症引起的。MRI有助于确认完整性和实质内部的变化，但这些变化并不总是明显的。[5] MRI在俯卧、屈肘、外展、旋后（FABS）位显示肱二头肌从粗隆到肌皮交界处的全长[6]（图39-2）。也可以考虑应用诊断性超声检查。

治疗

　　大多数急性完全肱二头肌远端断裂可通过止点重建治疗。各种手术技术的治疗效果明显优于非手术治疗。[5] 慢性撕裂的治疗具有挑战性，关

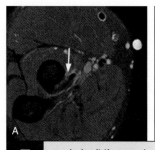
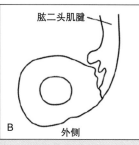

图
39-1
T2 加权成像 MRI（A）和线条图（B）显示肱二头肌远端肌腱桡侧附着处的部分厚度撕裂（箭头）。经允许引自 Sutton KM, Dodds SD, Ahmad CS, Sethi PM: Surgical treatment of distal biceps rupture. *J Am Acad Orthop Surg* 2010; 18(3): 139-148.

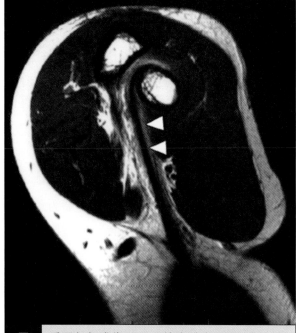

图
39-2
质子加权成像 MRI。检查时为 FABS 位，显示右肱二头肌远端部分撕裂（箭头，可见线性异常信号）。从 FABS 位可以看到整个肌腱。经允许引自 Giuffrè BM, Moss MJ: Optimal positioning for MRI of the distal biceps brachii tendon: Flexed abducted supinated view. *AJR Am J Roentgenol* 2004;182 (4): 944-946.

键是肱二头肌腱膜是撕裂的还是完整的。完整的肌腱膜可以防止向近端的挛缩。随着时间的推移，肱肌的挛缩和瘢痕可能限制手术恢复其足够长度的能力，难以获得满意的一期修复。半腱肌移植重建已被用于治疗长度不足的慢性损伤。[7] 在慢

性损伤中，桡骨粗隆的修复和重建结果并不确定，并且存在更高的神经血管损伤风险。在这种情况下，将软组织附着于肱肌的折中方法也可以考虑。

部分撕裂可能与肌腱炎和滑囊炎有关。MRI 上发现桡骨粗隆附着点部分撕裂，有助于进行诊断。[5] 关节镜检查已被用于评估修复部分撕裂的可能性。[8] 非手术治疗失败后的，可考虑对损伤进行手术治疗。多数部分撕裂可以通过肌腱的松解、清创及止点重建来成功治疗，特别是当撕裂超过 50% 时。单独清创一般不会有很好的结果。完全撕裂如果在伤后 2 周内进行修复，则恢复旋后和屈肘力量的可能性很高。[5]

经手术治疗的患者较非手术治疗患者的功能和客观结果更好。[2] 在接受修复的患者中，旋后力量而非屈肘力量会得到显著改善。[2] 非手术治疗患者活动时疼痛的发生率更高，并且旋后的力量和耐力较屈肘下降得更严重。一般来说，对于有慢性复杂撕裂、有其他严重合并症且久坐的患者，应考虑非手术治疗。[2] 单切口技术和双切口技术均有报道。

Boyd-Anderson 双切口技术可以避免单切口技术所引起的神经并发症。然而，这项技术的使用也导致了各种并发症，包括尺桡骨融合和异位骨化。将 Boyd-Anderson 双切口技术改良为不涉及尺骨骨膜的肌肉劈开入路，可降低并发症的发生率。[5] 用这种技术，屈肘和旋后力量基本恢复受伤前状态，且不伴有活动受限或再撕裂。[9] 其他几项研究均报告了这项技术取得良好的结果。[10-12] 一项系统综述表明，采用双切口技术的总并发症发生率为 16%，采用单切口技术的总并发症发生率为 18%。双切口手术患者相对于单切口手术患者，更容易出现较差的结果（分别为 31% 和 6%）[13]（表 39-1）。

随着技术、设备和修复方法的改进，单切口技术也在不断发展。与单切口技术相关的并发症包括骨间后神经和前臂外侧皮神经损伤。[2] 探查皮神经、保持前臂旋后和使用微创切口可降低

表 39-1

双切口及单切口肘关节修复术后并发症

	技术		
术后并发症	双切口（N=142）	单切口（N=165）	P
异位骨化（导致运动受限）	8 (6%)	5 (3%)	0.45
神经麻痹（暂时的或永久的）	10 (7%)	20 (12%)	0.12
前臂旋转受限	13 (9%)	3 (2%)	0.01
感染	0	3 (2%)	0.25
屈肘挛缩	2 (1%)	1 (1%)	0.61
出现并发症的肘关节	23 (16%)	29 (18%)	0.88

注：经允许引自 Chavan PR, Duquin TR, Bisson LJ: Repair of the ruptured distal biceps tendon: A systematic review. *Am J Sports Med* 2008;36:1618–1624.

神经损伤的风险。多项研究发现，采用单切口技术进行骨皮质襻固定的并发症风险最小，且效果良好。[14-16]荟萃分析发现，采用双切口技术的满意率为 69%，采用单切口技术的满意率为 94%。[13]双切口技术的满意率较低主要是由于前臂旋转活动范围小或旋转力量减弱。技术的选择应取决于外科医师的技术水平和经验。

诊断和治疗延误可能使解剖修复变得复杂。肱二头肌腱膜完整时可能掩盖急性撕裂，但也可以限制近端的挛缩，并可能完成直接修复。在慢性损伤中，应该预想到长度无法充分恢复，所以应准备好用于重建的移植物。半腱肌在解剖形态上与肱二头肌远端肌腱相似。[7]需要更充分地显露半腱肌，并游离和保护邻近半腱肌的神经血管结构。附着至肱肌的肌腱固定也应被视为一种治疗慢性损伤和活动性疼痛的合理备选方案，但应预期旋后力量将无法得到改善。[5]这种技术通常可以加速康复。在修复或重建时，应测试伸肘时的肌腱张力，以评估修复的安全性及与术后康复计划进展相关的任何可能的限制。

多项研究评价了桡骨结节的固定方法。其中一项研究比较了经骨隧道和缝合锚在循环载荷作用下的固定强度，在 50 N、3600 个循环中均没有样本失效；经骨隧道的平均失效载荷更高。[17]类似结果在第二项研究中也得到了证实。[18]比较使用界面螺钉修复完整肌腱和损伤肌腱的效果，没有发现显著差异，同时与骨道相比，界面螺钉的平均失效强度和刚度明显更高。[19]对几种固定技术的比较评估发现，使用骨皮质襻可获得最高的载荷、刚度和循环失效载荷，可能允许更早的和更积极的康复。[20-21]生物力学研究的系统综述发现，EndoButton（Smith 和 Nephew）是性能最好的固定装置[13]（表 39-2）。如果使用骨皮质襻和界面螺钉进行双重固定，采用更积极的康复方案，大多数患者可在手术后 4 周内恢复正常的日常活动。[22]

术后肘关节在屈曲 90° 和旋后位固定 7~10 天。根据术中确定的修复后张力，可以使用铰链式肘关节支具 6~8 周来保护修复部位和限制完全伸肘。此时，随着力量训练的开始，可以逐渐增加无活动限制的运动锻炼。患者通常能够在术后 5~6 个月恢复无限制的活动，这取决于患者的症状、力量和耐力。慢性损伤的患者在修复或重建后遵循类似的过程。接受过肱肌软组织肌腱固定的患者通常在术后 3~4 个月时能够恢复无限制的活动。

肱三头肌损伤

评估

大约 0.8% 的肌腱断裂涉及肱三头肌远端。[23]大多数肱三头肌远端断裂发生在男性，并与使用类

表 39-2

肱二头肌远端固定的生物力学研究

固定方法	单次失效载荷		循环载荷	
	极限抗拉载荷（N）	刚度（N/mm）	极限抗拉载荷（N）	位移（mm）
经骨隧道	125~210	15.9	195~310	3.55
界面螺钉	131~192	30.4	232	2.15
EndoButton	159	–	249~440	2.58~3.42
缝合锚	105~263	–	209~381	2.06~2.38

注：经允许引自 Chavan PR, Duquin TR, Bisson LJ: Repair of the ruptured distal biceps tendon: A systematic review. *Am J Sports Med* 2008;36:1618–1624.

固醇激素或举重运动等有关。这种情况还与代谢性骨疾病、肾性骨营养不良、鹰嘴滑囊炎、马方综合征、成骨不全、类风湿关节炎和糖尿病有关。肱三头肌的三个头会聚在尺骨鹰嘴的一个宽泛的止点（平均 466 mm²），大多数损伤发生在这个止点。[23]最常见的损伤机制是收缩的肱三头肌突然受到偏心载荷。患者有疼痛、肿胀、瘀斑以及明显的触诊缺损。并非所有的完全撕裂都会存在主动伸肘受限，也不是所有的主动伸肘都意味着完全撕裂。完整的外侧扩张部或腱膜可以代偿性主动伸肘。如果患者处于俯卧位，手臂悬在检查床边缘，则改良的汤普森挤压试验可能是阳性的。正位和侧位 X 线片可显示撕脱骨块。MRI 有助于判断完全撕裂和部分撕裂。[23]在 10 例患者中有 8 例受累的是内侧止点。[24]在连续的 801 个肘关节 MRI 检查中，28 例患者有肱三头肌撕裂，其中包括 5 例女性患者和 23 例男性患者。部分撕裂比完全撕裂更常见。[25]最常见的症状是疼痛，通常在运动损伤后。

治疗

肱三头肌撕裂的处理取决于患者的个体因素，以及撕裂的位置、完整性和患者的功能性伸肘力量。身体虚弱、运动需求低的部分撕裂患者可以选择非手术治疗。一般来说，小于 50% 的撕裂的非手术治疗结果令人满意。[24,26]一个非手术治疗的双侧部分撕裂的举重运动员在第 41 周时恢复正常功能，第 55 周时举重伴疲劳感。[27]运动需求高的

完全撕裂或超过 50% 的撕裂的患者最好进行手术治疗。而慢性撕裂（持续时间超过 6 周）的治疗更具挑战性，多种修复和重建技术都曾被应用。[23]

完全撕裂并严重失去力量的患者建议进行早期一期修复（在受伤后 2 周内）。最常见的方法是在钻取骨道后，将肱三头肌远端锁边缝合至骨桥上。作为替代方案，也可以考虑使用骨锚技术，也有文献提出使用类似肩袖缝合桥技术的解剖止点重建技术（图 39-3）。[28]与交叉缝合和缝合锚修复相比，当柱状缝合拉紧时，这种修复结构在

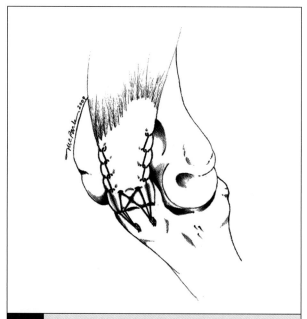

图 39-3 使用解剖技术修复肱三头肌的示意图。经允许引自 Yeh PC, Stephens KT, Solovyova O, et al: The distal triceps tendon footprint and a biomechanical analysis of 3 repair techniques. *Am J Sports Med* 2010; 38(5):1025–1033.

修复处的微动更少，从而使患者得以更早康复。

术后 2 周，肘关节固定于屈曲 30°~45°。在术后第 3 周时开始被动伸肘和主动指导下屈肘，在第 4 周时达到全范围的活动。术后 4~6 个月内应避免主动持重。并发症如滑囊炎、屈曲挛缩、再断裂等，均可能发生。

肘后（肱三头肌）肌腱炎

肱三头肌肌腱炎又称肘后网球肘或拳击肘。这种相对不常见的过度使用情况涉及肱三头肌肘后止点与鹰嘴窝滑膜炎。肘关节的重复性快速伸展，如投掷、拳击、拦截（橄榄球边锋）、网球发球和举重都与之有关。拳击和过顶运动中存在的迅速和激烈的伸肘撞击，使骨刺和游离体的形成常与鹰嘴窝滑膜炎并存。应注意鉴别诊断滑囊炎、后内侧撞击、尺骨鹰嘴应力性骨折和尺骨鹰嘴骨骺炎（青少年）。肱三头肌肌腱炎的组织病理学与肘关节内侧和外侧肌腱炎相同，可能伴有鹰嘴窝滑膜炎和游离体。患者可能出现伸直阻挡和屈曲挛缩。非手术治疗方法与肘关节外侧肌腱炎相似，但在伸直阻挡的情况下，治疗方案应包括尺骨在肱骨上向后侧、内侧和外侧滑动。[29-31]

肱三头肌肌腱炎的推荐手术入路是以触诊敏感区为中心的后方纵向小切口。对有血管成纤维细胞性肌腱炎改变的组织进行椭圆形切除。此外，也应该去掉在鹰嘴尖端的骨刺。在投掷运动员中，肱三头肌腱鞘炎最常合并鹰嘴窝滑膜炎、软骨病、骨刺和（或）游离体，应进行手术治疗。[32]术后处理类似肘关节外侧和内侧肌腱炎。

肘关节外侧肌腱炎

肘关节外侧肌腱炎又称网球肘，最常见的病因是肌腱过度使用和肌腱愈合失败。这种情况通常发生在 40~50 岁，影响优势侧肢体，男性和女性同样常见。病理解剖是一种非炎性、退行性血管成纤维细胞增生，可能是由微损伤后引起的愈

合不充分所致。肉眼下观察组织通常色泽灰暗，水肿易碎（图 39-4，39-5）。肘外侧的特定区域包括桡侧腕短伸肌（ECRB）和指总伸肌（EDC）复合体。ECRB 在该疾病中 100% 受累，EDC 的前缘有 35% 的可能性受累。非手术治疗的主要目的是使产生疼痛的不健康组织恢复健康从而不再产生疼痛。肌腱过度使用的患者的危险因素包括年龄大于 35 岁、活动水平高、运动要求高和锻炼水平不足等。表 39-3 列出了可能导致肘关节外侧肌腱炎的运动。相关疾病包括内上髁炎、肘管综合征、腕管综合征和肩袖肌腱炎。这些疾病共同被称为间充质综合征。在约 5% 的患者中，肘

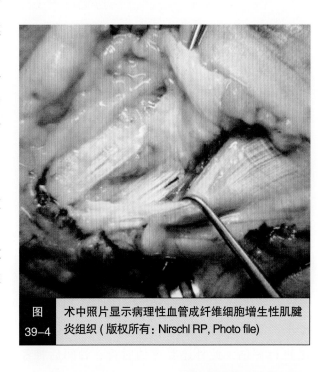

图 39-4　术中照片显示病理性血管成纤维细胞增生性肌腱炎组织（版权所有：Nirschl RP, Photo file）

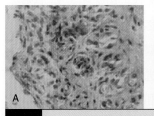
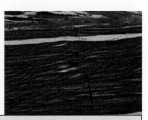

图 39-5　血管成纤维细胞增生性肌腱炎（A）和正常肌腱（B）的组织学表现。经允许引自 Nirschl RP, Ashman ES: Tennis elbow tendinosis (epicondylitis). *Clin Sports Med* 2003;22(4):813-836.

关节外侧肌腱炎会合并前外侧关节软骨软化和滑膜炎。[30,33-35]

表 39-3
导致内外上髁炎的常见因素

因素	外上髁炎	内上髁炎
体育运动	网球（落地球）	高尔夫球
	美式壁球	划艇
	壁球	棒球（投球）
	击剑	标枪投掷
		网球（发球）
职业或其他活动	切肉	瓦工
	水管工	锤击
	绘画	打字
	纺织	纺织品生产
	耙地	

注：经允许引自 Jobe FW, Ciccotti MG: Lateral and medial epicondylitis of the elbow. *J Am Acad Orthop Surg* 1994; 2(1): 1-8.

评估

随着病理性改变的加重，隐匿的活动性疼痛会逐渐发展至静息性疼痛及功能障碍。触诊时最明显的压痛点位于外上髁稍远处（5 mm）偏前方。肘部处于伸直和屈曲位置时，以及手腕和手指进行抗阻伸直时，患者会因应力试验而激发疼痛。肘部屈曲疼痛多表明存在严重的肌腱损伤。功能性力量损失可以使用测功仪进行测量。肘关节活动范围通常在正常范围内。也应对内侧和后侧肌腱进行评估，此外还要评估肘管、骨间后神经（远端 3~4 cm）、颈椎和腕管（10% 相关），这些部位都可能出现相关的并发症。[30]此外，还应该评估肩袖的强度，因为同侧肩袖力量减弱也较为常见，应在康复期间同时进行治疗。另外，也应对肘关节稳定性进行评估和治疗。应评估颈椎、胸椎、上肢和运动动力学。由于 20% 的患者存在肌腱钙化或外上髁反应性外生骨赘，建议进行影像学评估。[30]诊断时，很少需要 MRI 检查，但在 90% 有症状的患者中，MRI 可显示伸肌起点处水肿和增厚。而超声具有中等的敏感性和不确定的特异性，这主要取决于检查者。[34]

骨间后神经

一项 1972 年的研究描述了通过在 Froshe 弓处手术减压骨间后神经来治疗疑似肘关节外侧肌腱炎的病例，肘关节外侧肌腱炎可能与骨间后神经受压有关。[36]尽管如此，并没有确凿的证据表明骨间后神经受压是导致肘关节外侧肌腱炎的原因。尽管在解剖学上，骨间后神经与肘外侧肌腱的位置相邻，但更应考虑单发的骨间后神经损伤的可能性。骨间后神经压迫不易诊断；症状包括伸肌群隐约的疼痛感和抗阻旋后疼痛。肌电图和利多卡因阻滞可能有助于诊断。对神经进行手术减压常无效，部分原因可能是误诊。

非手术治疗

肘关节外侧肌腱炎的治疗应为自然生理愈合反应的辅助，遵循其本身的反应过程，增强血管新生和胶原有序形成。治疗应该从控制炎症渗出和出血开始，以减轻疼痛。然后，促进特定组织的愈合，适当锻炼并控制力量负荷和暴力。有些患者可能需要手术切除病变组织，但初始治疗应该包括保护、休息、冰敷、压迫、抬高、药物治疗（特别是非甾体抗炎药）和活动调整。肘关节外侧肌腱炎在组织学上不是一种炎症性疾病，但抗炎药物可以控制化学介质引起的疼痛，减轻周围脂肪和结缔组织的滑膜炎或炎症。[30,32]当将双氯芬酸组与安慰剂组做对比时，接受双氯芬酸治疗的患者疼痛程度较低。[37]萘普生组与安慰剂组相比并无显著差异。[38]非手术治疗包括同心性和偏心性康复运动、高压经皮神经电刺激、有氧和常规锻炼运动、不滥用药物，还可辅以超声波治疗。全身调理可以保持或改善身体健康，刺激受伤组织的愈合。力量负荷控制可以减少潜在的可能造成损伤的运动，包括使用支具保护、改进运动技术、控制活动强度和持续时间，以及应用设备评估等。[30]

类固醇注射多被用于缓解疼痛，但并不具有促进组织愈合的能力。尽管类固醇注射可获得良好的早期疗效，但在 1 年的随访中，结果并不比使用非甾体抗炎药或物理治疗的结果好，效果甚至更差。[39] 过量使用类固醇注射（超过 3 次局灶注射）可对其下方的组织造成损害，导致进一步的力弱和肌腱断裂。此外，注射技术也很重要，针头应该置于 ECRB 下方，而不是在外上髁处。A 型肉毒毒素在用于镇痛治疗时的 3 个月的效果存在争议，患者握力也没有显著改善。[40] 因为使用 A 型肉毒毒素可能出现肌肉萎缩，导致失用和症状恶化。最近，一项 I 级研究发现，与注射类固醇相比，使用富血小板血浆（PRP）后，DASH评分和视觉模拟评分法评分均有显著改善。[41] 类固醇注射治疗患者的早期疗效得到改善，但无法持续；PRP 治疗患者的效果则为进行性改善，1 年随访时结果持续改善，且无并发症。另一项类似的I 级研究在 2 年的随访中也报告了类似的结果。[42] 也有研究指出 PRP 比自体全血的治疗结果有更明确的改善。[43] 长期的生物治疗方法还有待研究。

体外冲击波技术已被应用于治疗各种肌腱病，但纳入 9 项安慰剂对照研究的荟萃分析发现，与安慰剂相比，效果仍存在争议，并没有显著的益处。[44] 超声引导下经皮射频消融可减少 78% 的患者的症状。[45] 在一项 5 年的前瞻性研究中，硝酸甘油贴剂提供的一氧化氮与安慰剂相比没有任何益处。[46] 非手术治疗的整体研究报道，83% 的患者在 1 年的随访中有改善，但 40% 的患者在 5 年的随访中仍然有轻微的不适。[47-48] 不良预后指标包括体力劳动受限和较严重的初始疼痛。

手术治疗及其适应证

存在疼痛的肘关节外侧肌腱炎是手术的主要适应证。但还需考虑以下 3 个问题，疼痛强度是否显著限制功能；疼痛是否影响患者的日常活动或工作；疼痛和压痛是否位于靠近外上髁的 ECRB 起点处。通常经过持续约 6 个月的高质量

非手术治疗后，才应考虑手术治疗。如果非手术治疗并不充分，则患者不符合要求，若患者有工伤索赔需求，并有二次收益成分，则需要仔细重新评估。该情况可能是手术禁忌证。[35]

Nirschl Miniopen 技术自 1979 年被首次提出以来，已不断得到改进[35,49]（图 39-6）。在外上髁的前方做一个 2.5 cm 长的直切口。应注意避免比较常见的太偏远和太偏内侧的切口。在切开滑囊和脂肪组织后找到桡侧腕长伸肌（ECRL）与 EDC 腱膜之间的间隔；ECRL 通常没有伸肌腱膜牢固，且 ECRL 肌纤维的倾斜角度更大。沿 ECRL-EDC 间隔垂直切开 1~2 mm 的深度，切开的间隙恰位于外上髁前内侧，并与 EDC 肌纤维走行一致。然后，沿着更为水平的方向进行锐性分离，以便找到病变组织。该操作的一个常见错误是分离 ECRL-EDC 间隔的垂直深度超过 1~2 mm，这样会阻碍对 ECRB 的清晰显露和识别。将 ECRL 向前内侧牵拉，可以看到 ECRB 的斜向纤维与 EDC 结合处和外上髁的前内侧缘。ECRB 中的病变组织呈暗灰色，易碎，常伴有水肿。将病变组织呈椭圆形切开，保留 ECRB 起点的远端附着处。ECRB 保留着起点远端与关节囊、环状韧带、伸肌腱膜前远端和 ECRL 下方的附着，收缩不超过 1~2 mm。因此，基本上 ECRB 的正常生物力学工作长度被保留。任何有疑虑的组织都可以用 Nirschl 划痕法进行评估，正常组织看起来有光泽且坚固，并且呈黄白色，35% 的患者 EDC 前内下侧边缘有病变，大概占 EDC 总体积的 15%。在任何情况下，都不应从外上髁上完全游离 EDC 的起点。大概 20% 的患者存在外上髁骨刺，且几乎都在前内侧；因此，不需要切除大部分外上髁。当所有的病变组织都被切除后，可以在已显露的外上髁远端皮质骨上钻一个小孔，但不能在外上髁本身钻一个小孔，这样有利于增强血供。如怀疑关节内病变，切口可向远端延伸 0.5 cm，在桡侧副韧带前方关节囊处做一个小的纵向切口。

大约有 5% 肘关节外侧肌腱炎合并关节内病

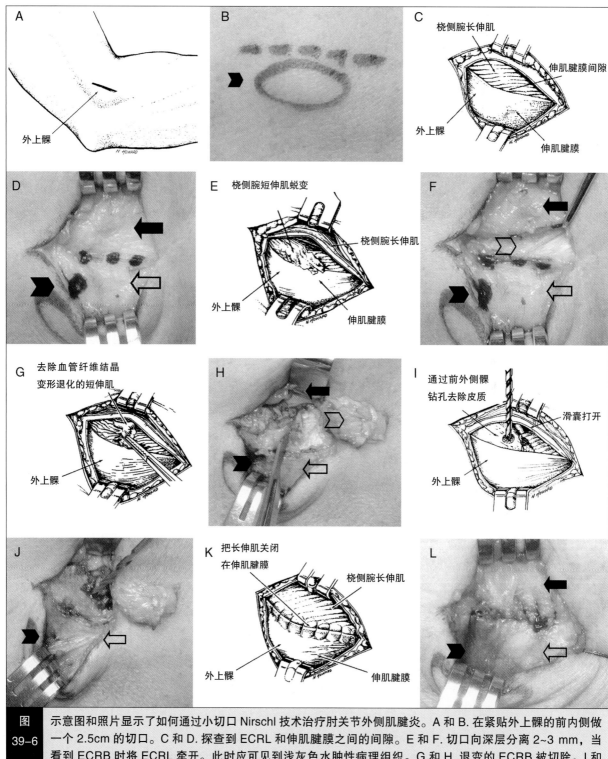

图
39-6
示意图和照片显示了如何通过小切口 Nirschl 技术治疗肘关节外侧肌腱炎。A 和 B. 在紧贴外上髁的前内侧做一个 2.5cm 的切口。C 和 D. 探查到 ECRL 和伸肌腱膜之间的间隙。E 和 F. 切口向深层分离 2~3 mm，当看到 ECRB 时将 ECRL 牵开。此时应可见到浅灰色水肿性病理组织。G 和 H. 退变的 ECRB 被切除。I 和 J. 通过前外上髁皮质骨向松质骨水平钻孔，以增强血运。K 和 L. ECRL 被牢固地修复至 EDC 的前缘。因为 ECRB 仍然附着在邻近组织上，所以不必缝合短肌远端。黑色箭 = 外上髁；黑色箭头 =ECRL；透明箭 = 腱肌组织；透明箭头 = 伸肌腱膜。经允许引自 Nirschl RP, Ashman ES: Tennis elbow tendinosis (epicondylitis). *Clin Sports Med* 2003:22（4）:813–836.

变（最常见的是滑膜炎或皱襞）。偶尔，ECRB 的全层撕裂会延伸到关节内。如果出现这种情况，可以在直视下评估关节内的病变。注意缝合修复关节囊以防止术后关节液外渗。ECRB 远端仍与骨骼有牢固的连接附着，因此无须修复。对 ECRL 和 EDC 进行侧对侧缝合修复，将线结埋入或使用 Quill 无线结缝合装置（Angiotech）。在少见的肘关节囊撕裂的情况下，用可吸收缝线修复关节囊。然后，进行皮下闭合，并使用无菌敷料覆盖。[35] 术后处理与肘关节外侧、内侧或后侧肌腱炎类似。

关节镜的作用

与切开或小切口手术相比，关节镜下清创和松解需要的术后物理治疗更少，可以使患者更早地恢复工作，并具有治疗相关关节内病变的优势。[50-54] Baker 等对外侧关节囊的关节镜下外观进行了分类。[55] 利用刨刀将退变的关节囊和 ECRB 从外上髁上游离。关节镜技术的主要缺点在于医源性软骨损伤、神经血管损伤和无法彻底清除病变组织。关节镜清理术后的切开探查显示，18 例患者中有 10 例在研究的第 1 年时仍残留肉眼可见的病变组织，而另外有 4 例残留有显微镜下观察到的病变组织。[56] 因此，该技术转变为使用弯曲的射频探头代替刨刀。[57] 与切开式或小切口切开式技术相比，关节镜技术的其他缺点包括器械成本较高，以及设置时长、手术时间和学习曲线较长。与微创技术相比，关节镜技术在疗效和康复时间方面没有明显的优势。

手术结果

在 ECRB 切开式病灶清除术后，85% 的患者疼痛可以完全缓解，并恢复前臂的全部肌力，另外有 12% 的患者也有明显的疼痛缓解。[49] 其余 3% 的患者疼痛没有缓解或力量无改善，包括那些有工伤赔偿要求的患者。并发症的发生率为 1%。ECRB 清理术后随访 10~14 年，成功率为 97%。[58] 一项纳入 19 例行切开式 EDC 松解、清理和止点重建患者的研究发现，18 例患者的疗效有所改善。但是，60% 的

高需求运动员和 15% 的高需求工作者在术后改变了他们的运动或工作。[59] 一项关于外侧 EDC 松解的长期前瞻性研究发现，40% 的患者术后 6 周有持续性疼痛，24% 的患者术后 1 年有持续性疼痛，9% 的患者在术后 5 年时有持续性疼痛。[60] 比较切开式 Nirschl 手术与经皮 EDC 松解术后发现，经皮松解术后 DASH 评分的改善更为明显，患者能更快地重返工作岗位。[61] 3 项对关节镜手术的研究发现，93%~100% 的患者在第 2 年随访时有改善，但只有 62%~80% 的患者疼痛完全缓解。[51-52,54] 一项研究将患者分为关节镜手术组（44 例）、切开手术组（41 例）、经皮松解术组（24 例），在至少 2 年的随访中，结果比较无统计学意义；5.8% 的复发患者包括经皮松解术组 3 例，关节镜手术组 1 例，切开手术组 2 例。[62] 比较切开手术与关节镜手术后发现，术后 6 个月随访无统计学差异；70% 的患者术后效果好或良好。[53] 关节镜手术患者术后恢复快，术后物理治疗少。

手术失败和持续疼痛的最常见原因是术者未能充分切除病变的肌腱组织。这种情况在伸肌腱松解术中很常见，其作用更像是减弱了伸肘启动力，而不是切除病变组织。在 35 例切除残余 ECRB 肌腱病变组织的翻修手术中，其成功率为 83%。[63] 其他因手术技术不完善而导致的并发症包括过度清创损伤侧副韧带（影响稳定性）、桡侧皮支神经瘤（其恰好走行于外上髁前 1.5 cm 处）、反应性骨形成及与外上髁切除相关的外上髁疼痛。[33]

肘关节内侧肌腱炎

肘关节内侧肌腱炎（高尔夫球肘）是由过度使用导致的腕屈肌 - 旋前肌群损伤。疼痛和压痛集中在屈肌总腱的内上髁起点处，腕屈肌 - 旋前肌群和尺侧副韧带的附着点。病理学上主要累及的肌腱是桡侧腕屈肌腱、旋前圆肌腱和尺侧腕屈肌腱（5% 的患者）。[33,35] 这 3 个肌腱有共同汇合的起点。组织学改变与肘关节外侧肌腱炎相同。肘关节内侧肌

腱炎的发生率约为外侧肌腱炎的 1/5。青壮年运动员易受到影响，这种情况通常在 40~50 岁时出现高峰。

评估

当肘关节伸直且腕关节处于伸直旋后位时，可通过腕关节抗阻屈曲旋前来诱发肘关节内侧肌腱炎的疼痛。在内上髁处及稍远区会有明显的触痛。通常活动范围是不受限的，但可能会出现轻微的伸肘受限。与肘外侧肌腱炎一样，肘内侧损伤也是由肌腱不能适应过度的活动所致。合并的损伤可能包括尺侧副韧带损伤伴外翻不稳，这多发生于过顶投掷运动员和肘管综合征患者。尺神经受累大多数发生于内上髁沟的第 3 区，多达 40% 的患者会出现症状，应该予以仔细评估。[33,35] 过度使用的机制包括反复的手腕屈曲和前臂旋前，这在球拍类运动和投掷运动及高尔夫球运动中常见，患者挥击侧手臂受到影响。旋前综合征和骨间前神经压迫综合征相对少见，但鉴别诊断时也应考虑。青少年运动员肘内侧疼痛应评估为小球队员肘（内侧骨骺炎和外侧桡骨头压迫）。X 线片通常是正常的，但也可能发现关节内病变，如在一个高需求运动员的检查中发现骨刺等。MRI 检查通常是不必要的，但如果怀疑有尺侧副韧带异常则可能有帮助。[30,33,35]

非手术治疗

肘关节内侧肌腱炎的初始非手术治疗与外侧肌腱炎相似，其成功率为 88%~96%。[64] 在一项 I 级对比研究中，与接受生理盐水治疗的患者相比接受类固醇注射的患者在 6 周的随访中疼痛明显缓解，但在 3 个月或 1 年时二者没有差异。[65] 超声引导自体血液注射结果显示 4 周和 10 个月随访时的 VAS 评分和改良 Nirschl 评分有改善。[66]

手术治疗

如果 6 个月的高质量非手术治疗对患者没有效果，可以考虑手术治疗。手术治疗通过小切口手术来切除退变组织并将健康组织重新缝合（图 39-7）。

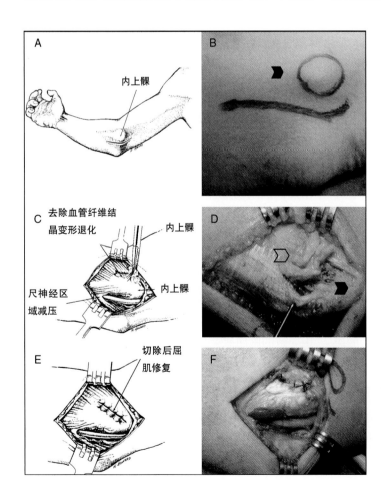

图 39-7 示意图和照片显示了小切口 Nirschl 技术治疗内侧肌腱炎。A 和 B. 从内上髁尖向远端切开 3~4 cm，小心操作以避免损伤内上髁正前方的皮神经感觉支（前臂内侧皮神经）。C 和 D. 血管成纤维细胞性肌腱切除术。血管成纤维细胞的改变通常位于旋前圆肌和桡侧腕屈肌的起点。将病理组织纵向、椭圆形切除，使正常组织附着完整。60% 的患者临床上存在尺神经功能障碍，需接受 3 区的尺神经减压。E 和 F. 修复屈肌总腱的起点。正常内上髁附着组织不受干扰。黑色箭头 = 内上髁；透明箭头 = 腱组织。经允许引自 Nirschl RP, Ashman ES: Tennis elbow tendinosis (epicondylitis). *Clin Sports Med* 2003;22（4）:813-836.

图内标注：
内上髁
去除血管纤维结晶变形退化
内上髁
尺神经区域减压
内上髁
切除后屈肌修复

皮肤切口长约 4 cm，平行于内上髁后的内上髁沟，从近端 1 cm 处延伸至远端 3 cm 处。这个切口避开了前臂内侧皮神经的分支。通过分离皮下组织到达覆盖尺侧腕屈肌尺侧头的深筋膜，然后转向前外侧剥离，使用拉钩牵拉皮肤和皮下组织，显露屈肌总腱的起点。此时大多数情况下都无法观察到肌腱病变，因为其通常位于肌腱内部。然而，有一些肌腱炎和软化病灶可以在表层被探及。最常见的病变区域多位于旋前圆肌和桡侧腕屈肌的交界处，从内上髁尖向远端延伸 2~3 cm 处。在麻醉前确认患者的主要触痛点非常重要，因为这有助于确定可能的肌腱病变部位。从肌腱的起点处将肌腱纵向劈开，并沿纤维走行向远端延伸 2~3 cm。肌腱分离后可观察到隐匿的病变组织。椭圆形切除病变组织，并使用划痕试验评估周围的组织。屈肌总腱的起点是维持肘关节内侧稳定性的关键结构，所以应避免对正常屈肌总腱的剥离。为了促进新生血管的发生潜力，使用 2.0 mm 或更小的钻头，在内上髁远端的皮质骨钻孔。因在内上髁上钻孔可能导致术后疼痛加剧，所以应避免。

40% 的患者因伴有肘管综合征，进行了内上髁尺神经沟第 3 区的减压。第 3 区位于内上髁远端，压迫性神经功能障碍最常见于该区域（图 39-8）。神经压迫很少发生在第 1 区（内上髁近端）或第 2 区（内上髁处）。肘管支持带和尺侧腕屈肌腱弓的松解对第 3 区的充分减压至关重要。减压后，应对肘关节进行屈伸检查，以确保尺神经不会滑脱出尺神经沟且张力正常。如果出现不常见的肘关节不稳定或继发于高张力的神经功能障碍，可以考虑尺神经完全前置。[33] 使用边对边缝合来修补病变肌腱切除后的椭圆形缺损，并将线结留在缝合的组织中。这种闭合方式有助于加强第 3 区尺神经的减压。最后进行皮下缝合，并使用无菌敷料覆盖。

内上髁切除术和完全的屈肌总腱起点松解术是备选方案之一，但对于大多数患者都不推荐这

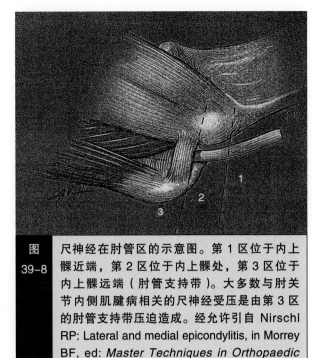

图 39-8　尺神经在肘管区的示意图。第 1 区位于内上髁近端，第 2 区位于内上髁处，第 3 区位于内上髁远端（肘管支持带）。大多数与肘关节内侧肌腱病相关的尺神经受压是由第 3 区的肘管支持带压迫造成。经允许引自 Nirschl RP: Lateral and medial epicondylitis, in Morrey BF, ed: *Master Techniques in Orthopaedic Surgery*: The Elbow.New York, NY, Raven, 1994, pp 129–148.

种方法。

关于肘关节内侧肌腱炎手术结果的报道相对较少，一项研究发现 23% 的患者有尺神经受累，20% 的患者伴有外上髁炎。术后客观功能评分由 38% 提高到 98%。在 86% 的患者中，肘关节进行日常活动或体育活动不受限制。[67] 也有 90% 的患者得到改善。[33] 在 7 年的随访中，87% 的患者在屈肌总腱清创和尺神经减压术后（53% 受累）有好或良好的效果；在手术前，这些患者中的 62% 有过度使用综合征的倾向，如伴发肌肉肌腱功能障碍或有此类功能障碍的病史。[64] 这些研究发现强调了评估和治疗患者整体，特别是整个上肢的重要性。

术后处理

肘关节内侧和外侧肌腱炎与肘后肌腱炎的术后处理类似。上肢在肘关节 90° 屈曲和旋转中立位固定 48 小时，此后开始主动运动练习。在接下来的 3~5 天内，根据需要使用肘关节支具，第 3~4 天开始日常活动。无阻力的主动活动锻炼在

第 3~4 天内开始，颈部和肩部的运动也是如此。3 周后，从 0.45 kg 的力量开始抗阻运动锻炼。在接下来的 2 个月内使用支具保护，随后由患者自行决定是否继续使用。术后 6~8 周逐渐恢复高需求活动。通常在 4~6 个月内可以完全恢复不受限制的活动。表 39-4 显示了肘关节肌腱炎手术后康复的三个阶段。

合并性肘关节内侧和外侧肌腱炎

肘关节肌腱炎的症状和体征也可能同时包括内侧和外侧肌腱炎，这种情况最常见于业余高尔夫球运动员和网球运动员，也被称为乡村俱乐部肘。在非手术治疗失败后，53 例患者的肘关节接受手术治疗，平均随访 11.7 年（最少 5 年）。[68] Nirschl 网球肘量表、数值疼痛强度量表及 ASES 肩关节疼痛和功能障碍评分的平均分均有显著提高，96% 的患者已恢复运动，没有患者需要行翻修手术，1 例术后感染在治疗后 1 个月痊愈。

总结

随着对急性和慢性肘部肌腱损伤的认识越来越全面，治疗方法也在不断发展，最终可取得令人满意的结果，且并发症发生率低。微创小切口手术技术的发展就是这一进展的实例。成功的腱鞘炎非手术治疗始于正确的诊断、对损伤的理解以及适当的康复恢复组织的活力。手术成功的关键在于确定病变组织并进行适当的切除。对 PRP 和聚多卡醇硬化作用的基础科学研究和深入探索，可将治疗提升到细胞水平上，并为肌腱炎患者带来更好的结果。

参考文献

[1] Kulshreshtha R, Singh R, Sinha J, Hall S: Anatomy of

表 39-4

肘关节内侧和外侧肌腱炎的物理治疗方案

第一阶段

肘关节位置：患者屈肘至 90° 并以下肢为支撑

频率：每天 1 次

练习：等张腕部屈曲，伸展和旋前 – 旋后

进阶：在可耐受的情况下逐渐增加重复次数和阻抗，若有症状出现则停止，直到可以连续两天进行 1.36 kg 抗阻重复 30 次的锻炼，且未出现新的症状

第二阶段

肘关节位置：增大伸肘角度，减少下肢支撑

频率：每天 1 次

练习：等张腕部屈曲，伸展和旋前 – 旋后。根据患者的承受能力，阻力可从 1.36 kg 降低到 0.91 kg 或 0.45 kg

进阶：在可耐受的情况下逐渐增加次数和阻抗，若有症状出现则停止，直到可以连续两天进行 1.36 kg 抗阻重复 30 次的锻炼，且未出现新的症状

第三阶段

肘关节位置：完全伸肘且不需支撑

频率：每天 1 次

练习：腕部屈伸、伸直和旋前。根据患者的承受能力，阻力可从 1.36 kg 降低到 0.91 kg 或 0.45 kg

进阶：在可耐受的情况下逐渐增加重复次数和阻抗，若有症状出现则停止，直到可以连续两天进行 1.36 kg 抗阻重复 30 次的锻炼，且未出现新的症状。此时，频率可以减少到每周 3~4 次

补充运动

手指外展（张开）以抵抗橡皮筋的阻力，在可耐受的情况下全天频繁挤压鸡蛋、绷带或压力球。建议从中等挤压力开始，并随着患者承受能力的提高逐渐加强挤压力

调整

如果患者在运动期间或运动后出现疼痛并持续 24 小时以上，则应减少重复次数，或减小阻力或活动范围

注：经允许引自 Johnson B, Nirschl RP: Overuse injuries of the elbow. *Orthop Phys Ther Clin N Am* 2001;10[4]:617–634.

the distal biceps brachii tendon and its clinical relevance. *Clin Orthop Relat Res* 2007;456:117-120.

An anatomic cadaver study analyzed the complex fiber arrangement of the distal biceps.

[2] Miyamoto RG, Elser F, Millett PJ: Distal biceps tendon injuries. *J Bone Joint Surg Am* 2010;92(11):2128-2138.

This is a current concepts review of distal biceps tendon injuries.

[3] O'Driscoll SW, Goncalves LB, Dietz P: The hook test for distal biceps tendon avulsion. *Am J Sports Med* 2007;35(11):1865-1869.

A cohort study evaluated the hook test for complete distal biceps injuries, finding that it is more sensitive and specific than MRI. Level of evidence: II.

[4] Ruland RT, Dunbar RP, Bowen JD: The biceps squeeze test for diagnosis of distal biceps tendon ruptures. *Clin Orthop Relat Res* 2005;437:128-131.

[5] Ramsey ML: Distal biceps tendon injuries: Diagnosis and management. *J Am Acad Orthop Surg* 1999;7(3):199-207.

[6] Giuffrè BM, Moss MJ: Optimal positioning for MRI of the distal biceps brachii tendon: Flexed abducted supinated view. *AJR Am J Roentgenol* 2004;182(4):944-946.

[7] Hang DW, Bach BR Jr, Bojchuk J: Repair of chronic distal biceps brachii tendon rupture using free autogenous semitendinosus tendon. *Clin Orthop Relat Res* 1996;323:188-191.

[8] Bain GI, Johnson LJ, Turner PC: Treatment of partial distal biceps tendon tears. *Sports Med Arthrosc* 2008;16(3):154-161.

Partial tears of the biceps were described and defined, with treatment options.

[9] Morrey BF, ed: *Master Techniques in Orthopaedic Surgery: The Elbow*. New York, NY, Raven, 1994, pp 115-128.

[10] D'Alessandro DF, Shields CL Jr, Tibone JE, Chandler RW: Repair of distal biceps tendon ruptures in athletes. *Am J Sports Med* 1993;21(1):114-119.

[11] Baker BE, Bierwagen D: Rupture of the distal tendon of the biceps brachii: Operative versus non-operative treatment. *J Bone Joint Surg Am* 1985;67(3):414-417.

[12] Davison BL, Engber WD, Tigert LJ: Long term evaluation of repaired distal biceps brachii tendon ruptures. *Clin Orthop Relat Res* 1996;333:186-191.

[13] Chavan PR, Duquin TR, Bisson LJ: Repair of the rup-tured distal biceps tendon: A systematic review. *Am J Sports Med* 2008;36(8):1618-1624.

A systematic review evaluated the outcomes of single- and two-incision distal biceps injury treatment. EndoButton fixation performed best in biomechanical studies. The eight studies reported comparable complication rates. Each technique had specific complications. Level of evidence: IV.

[14] Bain GI, Prem H, Heptinstall RJ, Verhellen R, Paix D: Repair of distal biceps tendon rupture: A new technique using the Endobutton. *J Shoulder Elbow Surg* 2000;9(2):120-126.

[15] Greenberg JA, Fernandez JJ, Wang T, Turner C: EndoButton-assisted repair of distal biceps tendon ruptures. *J Shoulder Elbow Surg* 2003;12(5):484-490.

[16] Peeters T, Ching-Soon NG, Jansen N, Sneyers C, Declercq G, Verstreken F: Functional outcome after repair of distal biceps tendon ruptures using the endobutton technique. *J Shoulder Elbow Surg* 2009;18(2):283-287.

A retrospective clinical study found that EndoButton fixation of distal biceps repairs is safe and efficacious, with 80% flexion and 91% supination strength regained. Level of evidence: IV.

[17] Berlet GC, Johnson JA, Milne AD, Patterson SD, King GJ: Distal biceps brachii tendon repair: An in vitro biomechanical study of tendon reattachment. *Am J Sports Med* 1998;26(3):428-432.

[18] Pereira DS, Kvitne RS, Liang M, Giacobetti FB, Ebramzadeh E: Surgical repair of distal biceps tendon ruptures: A biomechanical comparison of two techniques. *Am J Sports Med* 2002;30(3):432-436.

[19] Idler CS, Montgomery WH III, Lindsey DP, Badua PA, Wynne GF, Yerby SA: Distal biceps tendon repair: A biomechanical comparison of intact tendon and 2 repair techniques. *Am J Sports Med* 2006;34(6):968-974.

[20] Kettler M, Lunger J, Kuhn V, Mutschler W, Tingart MJ: Failure strengths in distal biceps tendon repair. *Am J Sports Med* 2007;35(9):1544-1548.

A controlled laboratory study compared 13 fixation options for the distal biceps and found that the EndoButton had a substantially higher load to failure.

[21] Mazzocca AD, Burton KJ, Romeo AA, Santangelo S, Adams DA, Arciero RA: Biomechanical evaluation of 4 techniques of distal biceps brachii tendon repair. *Am J Sports Med* 2007;35(2):252-258.

A controlled cadaver laboratory study compared the dualincision bone tunnel, suture anchor repair, interference screw, and EndoButton techniques for distal biceps repair. The load to failure was substantially greater with the EndoButton technique than with the other options.

[22] Heinzelmann AD, Savoie FH Ⅲ, Ramsey JR, Field LD, Mazzocca AD: A combined technique for distal biceps repair using a soft tissue button and biotenodesis interference screw. *Am J Sports Med* 2009;37(5):989-994.

A clinical study found that dual fixation of the distal biceps tendon with a soft-tissue button and biotenodesis screw may allow earlier return to function, with minimal complications. Level of evidence: Ⅳ.

[23] Yeh PC, Dodds SD, Smart LR, Mazzocca AD, Sethi PM: Distal triceps rupture. *J Am Acad Orthop Surg* 2010;18(1):31-40.

Distal triceps injuries were reviewed.

[24] Mair SD, Isbell WM, Gill TJ, Schlegel TF, Hawkins RJ: Triceps tendon ruptures in professional football players. *Am J Sports Med* 2004;32(2):431-434.

[25] Koplas MC, Schneider E, Sundaram M: Prevalence of triceps tendon tears on MRI of the elbow and clinical correlation. *Skeletal Radiol* 2011;40(5):587-594.

An MRI-based retrospective study found a 3.8% prevalence of triceps tendon tearing. The most common was a partial tear from an athletic injury. Pain was the initial symptom.

[26] Vidal AF, Drakos MC, Allen AA: Biceps tendon and triceps tendon injuries. *Clin Sports Med* 2004;23(4):707-722, xi.

[27] Harris PC, Atkinson D, Moorehead JD: Bilateral partial rupture of triceps tendon: Case report and quanti-tative assessment of recovery. *Am J Sports Med* 2004;32(3):787-792.

[28] Yeh PC, Stephens KT, Solovyova O, et al: The distal triceps tendon footprint and a biomechanical analysis of 3 repair techniques. *Am J Sports Med* 2010;38(5):1025-1033.

A controlled cadaver laboratory study described the 466-mm^2 footprint anatomy of the triceps insertion on the olecranon. An anatomic footprint repair using the suture bridge technique, similar to the rotator cuff repair technique, was compared with two other techniques and found to better restore anatomy and allow less repair site motion when cyclically loaded.

[29] Johnson B, Nirschl RP: Overuse injuries of the elbow. *Orthop Phys Ther Clin N Am* 2001;10(4):617-634.

[30] Nirschl RP, Ashman ES: Tennis elbow tendinosis (epicondylitis). *Instr Course Lect* 2004;53:587-598.

[31] Ellenbecker TS, Mattalino AJ: *The Elbow in Sport: Injury Treatment and Rehabilitation.* Champaign, IL, Human Kinetics, 1997.

[32] Nirschl RP: Elbow tendinosis/tennis elbow. *Clin Sports Med* 1992;11(4):851-870.

[33] Nirschl RP, Davis L: *Wrist and Elbow Reconstruction and Arthroscopy.* Rosemont, IL, American Society for Surgery of the Hand, 2006, pp 513-521.

[34] Calfee RP, Patel A, DaSilva MF, Akelman E: Management of lateral epicondylitis: Current concepts. *J Am Acad Orthop Surg* 2008;16(1):19-29.

This is a current concepts review of the management of lateral epicondylitis.

[35] Nirschl RP: *Master Techniques in Orthopaedic Surgery: The Elbow.* New York, NY, Raven, 1994, pp 129-148.

[36] Roles NC, Maudsley RH: Radial tunnel syndrome: Resistant tennis elbow as a nerve entrapment. *J Bone Joint Surg Br* 1972;54(3):499-508.

[37] Labelle H, Guibert R: The University of Montreal Orthopaedic Research Group: Efficacy of diclofenac in lateral epicondylitis of the elbow also treated with immobilization. *Arch Fam Med* 1997;6(3):257-262.

[38] Hay EM, Paterson SM, Lewis M, Hosie G, Croft P: Pragmatic randomised controlled trial of local corticosteroid injection and naproxen for treatment of lateral epicondylitis of elbow in primary care. *BMJ* 1999;319(7215):964-968.

[39] Smidt N, van der Windt DA, Assendelft WJ, Devillé WL, Korthalsde Bos IB, Bouter LM: Corticosteroid injections, physiotherapy, or a wait-and-see policy for lateral epicondylitis: A randomised controlled trial. *Lancet* 2002;359(9307):657-662.

[40] Wong SM, Hui AC, Tong PY, Poon DW, Yu E, Wong LK: Treatment of lateral epicondylitis with botulinum toxin: A randomized, double-blind, placebo-controlled trial. *Ann Intern Med* 2005;143(11):793-797.

[41] Peerbooms JC, Sluimer J, Bruijn DJ, Gosens T: Positive effect of an autologous platelet concentrate in lateral epicondylitis in a double-blind randomized controlled trial: Platelet-rich plasma versus corticosteroid injection with a 1-year follow-up. *Am J Sports Med* 2010;38(2):255-262.

Both corticosteroid injection and PRP use led to lateral epicondylitis improvement. Improvement was progressive in patients treated with PRP but declined over time in those treated with corticosteroid. Level of evidence: I.

[42] Gosens T, Peerbooms JC, van Laar W, den Oudsten BL: Ongoing positive effect of platelet-rich plasma versus corticosteroid injection in lateral epicondylitis: A double-blind randomized controlled trial with 2-year follow-up. *Am J Sports Med* 2011;39(6):1200-1208.
At 2-year follow-up, patients treated with PRP had greater improvement than those treated with corticosteroid. Level of evidence: I.

[43] Thanasas C, Papadimitriou G, Charalambidis C, Paraskevopoulos I, Papanikolaou A: Platelet-rich plasma versus autologous whole blood for the treatment of chronic lateral elbow epicondylitis: A randomized controlled clinical trial. *Am J Sports Med* 2011;39(10):2130-2134.
A comparison of PRP and autologous whole blood treatments of chronic lateral epicondylitis found PRP to be effective and superior to whole blood at 6-week follow-up. Level of evidence: I.

[44] Buchbinder R, Green SE, Youd JM, Assendelft WJ, Barnsley L, Smidt N: Shock wave therapy for lateral elbow pain. *Cochrane Database Syst Rev* 2005;4(4): CD003524.

[45] Lin CL, Lee JS, Su WR, Kuo LC, Tai TW, Jou IM: Clinical and ultrasonographic results of ultrasonographically guided percutaneous radiofrequency lesioning in the treatment of recalcitrant lateral epicondylitis. *Am J Sports Med* 2011;39(11):2429-2435.
An evaluation of a new, minimally invasive procedure for recalcitrant lateral epicondylitis found improvement of 78% at an average 14.3-month follow-up, with no major complications. Level of evidence: IV.

[46] Bokhari AR, Murrell GA: The role of nitric oxide in tendon healing. *J Shoulder Elbow Surg* 2012;21(2):238-244.
The basic science of nitric oxide use is reviewed for various tendinopathies.

[47] Haahr JP, Andersen JH: Prognostic factors in lateral epicondylitis: A randomized trial with one-year follow-up in 266 new cases treated with minimal occupational intervention or the usual approach in general practice. *Rheumatology (Oxford)* 2003;42(10):1216-1225.

[48] Binder AI, Hazleman BL: Lateral humeral epicondylitis—a study of natural history and the effect of conservative therapy. *Br J Rheumatol* 1983;22(2):73-76.

[49] Nirschl RP, Pettrone FA: Tennis elbow: The surgical treatment of lateral epicondylitis. *J Bone Joint Surg Am* 1979;61(6):832-839.

[50] Kuklo TR, Taylor KF, Murphy KP, Islinger RB, Heekin RD, Baker CL Jr: Arthroscopic release for lateral epicondylitis: A cadaveric model. *Arthroscopy* 1999;15(3):259-264.

[51] Owens BD, Murphy KP, Kuklo TR: Arthroscopic release for lateral epicondylitis. *Arthroscopy* 2001;17(6):582-587.

[52] Mullett H, Sprague M, Brown G, Hausman M: Arthroscopic treatment of lateral epicondylitis: Clinical and cadaveric studies. *Clin Orthop Relat Res* 2005;439:123-128.

[53] Peart RE, Strickler SS, Schweitzer KM Jr: Lateral epicondylitis: A comparative study of open and arthroscopic lateral release. *Am J Orthop (Belle Mead NJ)* 2004;33(11):565-567.

[54] Baker CL Jr, Baker CL III: Long-term follow-up of arthroscopic treatment of lateral epicondylitis. *Am J Sports Med* 2008;36(2):254-260.
After 42 elbow arthroscopies for lateral epicondylitis, 77% of patients had improvement, and the satisfaction rating was 87%. Level of evidence: IV.

[55] Baker CL Jr, Murphy KP, Gottlob CA, Curd DT: Arthroscopic classification and treatment of lateral epicondylitis: Two-year clinical results. *J Shoulder Elbow Surg* 2000;9(6):475-482.

[56] Cummins CA: Lateral epicondylitis: In vivo assessment of arthroscopic debridement and correlation with patient outcomes. *Am J Sports Med* 2006;34(9):1486-1491.

[57] Baker CL Jr, Baker CL III: Arthroscopy remains a viable, reliable method for treating lateral epicondylitis. *OrthopedicsToday* February 2012. http://www.helio.com/orthopedics/arthroscopy/news/print/orthopedics-today. Accessed October 1, 2012.
Enhancements to the arthroscopic technique for lateral epicondylitis were described.

[58] Dunn JH, Kim JJ, Davis L, Nirschl RP: Ten-to 14-year follow-up of the Nirschl surgical technique for lateral epicondylitis. *Am J Sports Med* 2008;36(2):261-266.
A clinical study with long-term follow-up found an

overall improvement rate of 97% and patient satisfaction of 8.9 out of 10 when the Nirschl technique for lateral epicondylitis was used; 93% of the patients returned to their sport. Level of evidence: Ⅳ.

[59] Rosenberg N, Henderson I: Surgical treatment of resistant lateral epicondylitis: Follow-up study of 19 patients after excision, release and repair of proximal common extensor tendon origin. *Arch Orthop Trauma Surg* 2002;122(9-10):514-517.

[60] Verhaar J, Walenkamp G, Kester A, van Mameren H, van der Linden T: Lateral extensor release for tennis elbow: A prospective long-term follow-up study. *J Bone Joint Surg Am* 1993;75(7):1034-1043.

[61] Dunkow PD, Jatti M, Muddu BN: A comparison of open and percutaneous techniques in the surgical treatment of tennis elbow. *J Bone Joint Surg Br* 2004;86(5):701-704.

[62] Szabo SJ, Savoie FH Ⅲ, Field LD, Ramsey JR, Hosemann CD: Tendinosis of the extensor carpi radialis brevis: An evaluation of three methods of operative treatment. *J Shoulder Elbow Surg* 2006;15(6):721-727.

[63] Organ SW, Nirschl RP, Kraushaar BS, Guidi EJ: Salvage surgery for lateral tennis elbow. *Am J Sports Med* 1997;25(6):746-750.

[64] Gabel GT, Morrey BF: Operative treatment of medical epicondylitis: Influence of concomitant ulnar neuropathy at the elbow. *J Bone Joint Surg Am* 1995;77(7): 1065-1069.

[65] Stahl S, Kaufman T: The efficacy of an injection of steroids for medial epicondylitis: A prospective study of sixty elbows. *J Bone Joint Surg Am* 1997;79(11):1648-1652.

[66] Suresh SP, Ali KE, Jones H, Connell DA: Medial epicondylitis: Is ultrasound guided autologous blood injection an effective treatment? *Br J Sports Med* 2006;40(11):935-939, discussion 939.

[67] Vangsness CT Jr, Jobe FW: Surgical treatment of medial epicondylitis: Results in 35 elbows. *J Bone Joint Surg Br* 1991;73(3):409-411.

[68] Schipper ON, Dunn JH, Ochiai DH, Donovan JS, Nirschl RP: Nirschl surgical technique for concomitant lateral and medial elbow tendinosis: A retrospective review of 53 elbows with a mean follow-up of 11.7 years. *Am J Sports Med* 2011;39(5):972-976.

At long-term follow-up, a combined surgical procedure for concurrent lateral and medial epicondylitis was found to improve surgical outcome scores, with 85% good to excellent results and 96% of the patients returning to their sport. Level of evidence: Ⅳ.

第四十章　肘关节损伤和投掷

James Hammond, DO, ATC; Brian J. Cole, MD, MBA

引言

过顶投掷运动会给肘关节带来巨大的压力，并可能造成特殊的损伤。生物力学和临床研究已经阐明了这些损伤的原因，并指导了预防和治疗策略的演变。特殊的检查手法有助于肘关节疾病的诊断，X 线检查有助于明确诊断。为了降低年轻运动员受伤的风险，医师们已经制订了预防策略，如监测投球次数。外科手术策略的持续发展也促使治疗投掷运动员某些疾病的技术发生了变化。

投掷相关的肘关节解剖和生物力学

内侧副韧带或尺侧副韧带（UCL）是对治疗投掷运动员而言最具临床意义的肘关节解剖结构。UCL 是由前斜韧带、后斜韧带和横韧带组成的复合体。前斜韧带是复合体中最强壮的韧带，也是投掷运动员抵抗肘关节外翻应力最重要的稳定结构。前斜韧带起源于内上髁。最近一项针对前斜韧带尺骨止点的研究发现，它沿着一个之前并未命名的

Dr. Cole or an immediate family member has received royalties from Arthrex and DJ Orthopaedics; is a member of a speakers' bureau or has made paid presentations on behalf of Genzyme; serves as a paid consultant to or is an employee of Zimmer, Arthrex, Carticept, Biomimmetic, Allosource, and DePuy; and has received research or institutional support from Regentis, Arthrex, Smith & Nephew, and DJ Orthopaedics. Neither Dr. Hammond nor any immediate family member has received anything of value from or has stock or stock options held in a commercial company or institution related directly or indirectly to the subject of this chapter.

嵴延伸到结节的远端，并存在于所有尸体骨骼标本上。[1] 构成前斜韧带的前束和后束在肘关节屈伸过程中交替地成为外翻应力的主要稳定结构：前束在伸肘时是紧张的，后束在屈肘时是紧张的。

UCL 接受来自周围肌肉组织的动态支持。尺侧腕屈肌是肘部外翻稳定性的主要动力稳定结构，指浅屈肌是第二动力稳定结构。[2] 这两块肌肉有助于在投掷运动中分散肘关节的大量应力，从而起到保护 UCL 的作用。他们之间的关系对预防和治疗 UCL 损伤具有重要意义。

投掷运动会产生巨大的能量和随之而来的应力，都由肘关节周围的结构所传递。在投掷运动的加速阶段，肘关节运动的角速度高达 3000° /s，这个速度转化为外翻力矩则高达 64 N/m。由于 UCL 的抗扭强度仅为 34 N/m，所以肘关节的其他稳定结构对于避免或尽量减少损伤也至关重要。[3] 外翻负荷会在肘关节的其他方面产生应力：肘关节内侧出现张力，当肘关节伸直时，鹰嘴窝会产生剪切力和压力；外侧则产生压力，主要在肱桡关节。最近的一项尸体研究发现，切断 UCL 后，外侧接触压力增加了 67%。[4] 了解这些应力有助于理解肘关节周围损伤之间的关系。

临床评估

病史

要了解投掷运动员的肘关节病变，具体的、详细的病史是至关重要的。应注意优势侧手臂和症状的持续时间、强度和位置，以及引起症状的活动类

型（例如，疼痛是在休息时、日常生活活动中出现，还是只在投掷运动时出现）。还应注意相关的其他关节，尤其是肩部合并的运动症状、感觉异常或疼痛的信息。重要的是要确定投掷动作中出现症状的时间（准备期、挥臂早期、挥臂晚期、加速期、减速期和跟随期），此外还应确定投球类型、每次出局的投球次数和投球时间。曲线球在肘部产生的外翻应力最大，快球和滑球产生的力量最大，而变速球在肘部产生的应力较小，被认为是对各年龄段运动员都相对安全的投球方式。然而，与其他投掷运动员相比，技术熟练的投掷运动员更有可能投出快球或曲线球，参加更多的比赛，投球频率也更高。[5]

体格检查

在评估肘部时，一般检查很容易被省略，但它们可以为深入检查肘部应力提供线索。例如，通过观察患者的双侧肘关节评估双侧提携角差异。一般检查还可以确定疼痛的确切位置和内侧、外侧或后方疼痛特征。此外，还应评估肘关节活动范围，投掷运动员普遍存在肘关节伸直受限。

一般来说，投掷运动员的体格检查重点是肘关节内侧。UCL 急性撕脱伤通常在内上髁近端发生，应确定该位置或沿前斜韧带全长有无压痛。对屈曲 – 旋前肌群进行抗阻应力试验。并在屈曲 0° 和 30° 时评估外翻应力情况，但在投掷运动员中，不稳定往往更隐匿。这项体格检查在识别慢性损伤方面缺乏可靠的敏感性。挤奶试验和活动外翻应力试验也被用来评估外翻不稳定性和 UCL 损伤。挤奶试验是在前臂旋后、肘部屈曲超过 90° 的情况下拉动患者拇指。活动外翻应力试验是从同一体位开始，牵拉患者拇指使肩关节也达到外旋极限。通过恒定的力量拉动拇指，在一定的活动范围内检查肘关节。在肘部处于外翻 70° ~120° 时，疼痛通常最剧烈（图 40-1）。据报道，活动外翻应力试验的敏感性为 100%，特异性为 75%。[6]

应对怀疑存在 UCL 损伤的患者进行尺神经病变评估。当存在尺神经半脱位、Tinel 征阳性，或

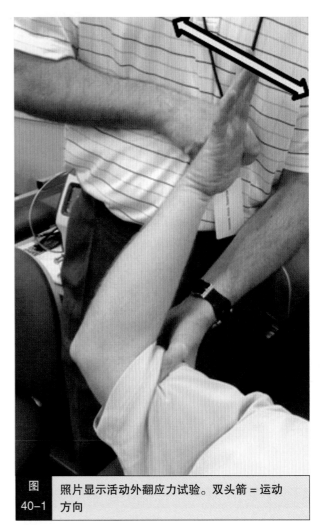

图 40-1　照片显示活动外翻应力试验。双头箭 = 运动方向

在肘关节过度屈曲时存在症状，应特别注意。与屈曲 – 旋前肌群损伤相关的疼痛，表现为抗阻试验疼痛，应将其与内上髁炎相关的疼痛区分，其表现为正常活动外翻应力试验时仅在内上髁上有压痛。

影像学检查

最初始的影像学检查包括正位、侧位、桡骨头位和腋位 X 线检查。外翻应力 X 线片可用于识别内侧关节间隙增宽，大于 3 mm 的增宽具有诊断意义。[7] X 线片可评估是否存在骨刺、关节间隙变窄、游离体和骨软骨缺损。MRI 可用于确诊多种肘关节的损伤，包括剥脱性骨软骨炎、UCL 损伤、屈曲 – 旋前肌群撕脱伤和 UCL 慢性增厚等。最近的一项研究发现，MRI 上的信号强度可以用来预测康复结果；完全或高度的 UCL 撕裂患者可能更需要手术治疗[8]（图 40-2）。

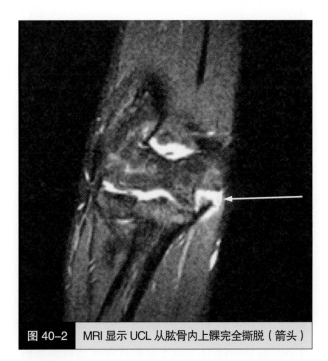

图 40-2　MRI 显示 UCL 从肱骨内上髁完全撕脱（箭头）

已有介绍使用超声和动态超声检查来评估 UCL 损伤，但大多数有价值的研究都是小样本病例研究或个案报道。有些研究发现，投掷运动员 UCL 松弛度存在差异，投掷侧和非投掷侧的 UCL 松弛度也有所不同。[9~10]

关节镜也可作为一种诊断工具，主要用于直接评估应力下的内侧关节间隙增宽，1~2 mm 的增宽提示韧带部分撕裂，4~10 mm 的增宽提示全层撕裂。关节镜于肘关节屈曲 65°~70° 时应力下，从前外侧入路观察肱尺关节。[11]

引起肘关节内侧疼痛的疾病

内上髁炎

内上髁炎并不像外上髁炎那么常见，通常由反复的前臂强力旋前和腕关节屈曲运动如高尔夫球、球拍类运动或过顶运动导致。疼痛通常位于肘关节内侧，并在前臂抗阻屈伸和旋前时加剧。诊断以临床为主，但有研究表明超声和 MRI 也有一定作用。[12] 标准的非手术治疗方案包括使用非甾体抗炎药、柔韧性练习、冰敷以及物理治疗。[13] 有时也可使用激素注射。一项对比研究发现，使用离子电渗法可以使疼痛缓解。[14] 超声引导自体血液注射可以改善 VAS 评分和改良的 Nirschl 疼痛分级评分。[15] 手术干预通常包括通过切开、小切口和关节镜技术切除病变部分的肌腱。如果手术达到目标，疼痛可以预期得到缓解，但仍可能存在肌力损失。

UCL 损伤

非手术治疗应是过顶投掷运动员 UCL 损伤的初步处理方案。该方案包括一个 6 周的休息期，期间避免进行投掷运动以及屈曲 – 旋前肌群发力。[2] 运动员只有在症状消失且体格检查正常后，才能恢复投掷活动。此时，运动员应优化改良投掷动作以抵消肘关节内侧的应力。躯干旋转延迟、肩关节外旋减少及肘关节屈曲增加，都会增加肘部外翻应力。[16] 在平均 24.5 周的随访中，42% 的投掷运动员正重返运动。[17]

在最早的 Jobe 重建 UCL 技术中，8 字形肌腱移植物穿过骨道并与自身相缝合。这项技术需要松解屈曲 – 旋前肌群，显露肱骨后方皮质以钻取其中一个骨道。通常需要进行尺神经前置。显露手术区所导致的大量并发症促使此项技术不断改进及发展新技术。改良 Jobe 技术包含肌肉劈开入路（以减少屈曲 – 旋前肌群损伤的并发症）、改变肱骨骨道方向以及仅在患者有术前症状时才对尺神经进行前置。将肱骨骨道置于稍偏前处，以避免移植物通过时损伤尺神经，并减少剥离暴露。改良 Jobe 技术的结果和生物力学强度已成为评价其他技术的标准。研究显示过顶投掷运动员的运动恢复率为93%。[7] 另一项研究显示，在使用改良的 Jobe 技术后至少 2 年的随访中，投掷运动的恢复率为 83%。[18]

通常所描述的对接技术也使用肌肉劈开入路和尺骨上两个汇聚通道。在肱骨上只钻一个主要的骨道，另外在肱骨上钻两个较小的骨道以便缝合。肌腱移植物的一支穿入肱骨骨道。在评估肌腱移植物另一支的长度和张力后，将其修剪至适当的长度，并固定至肱骨窝中。最终将肌腱移植物两端的缝线在骨桥上拉紧打结。使用对接技术治疗的 21 名运动员中，19 名（90%）取得了良好或优秀的结果。[19]优秀结果被定义为至少 1 年内恢复到以前的水平，良好结果被定义为至少 1 年内投掷运动恢复到较低水平或恢复进行日常击球练习的能力。在使用对折两次后的移植物进行对接技术移植后的 11.5 个月的随访中，92% 的患者投掷运动恢复到损伤前水平。[20]

还有几种方法可以归类为混合技术。其中一种相对较新的技术为在高耸结节钻一个孔，在内上髁钻一个孔，在高耸结节处使用界面螺钉，在肱骨骨道处使用对接技术。术后 3 年随访，22 例患者中有 19 例（86%）取得良好疗效。[21]另一种术式为在高耸结节和内上髁上钻取相同的单钻孔，在移植物两端都使用界面螺钉。在一项生物力学研究中，这项技术的稳定性与完整的 UCL 标本相似。[3]

尺神经炎

约 40% 的 UCL 损伤患者有尺神经炎。巨大的外翻应力会对神经产生牵拉、摩擦和压迫，并诱发神经炎。此外，粘连和（或）骨刺、神经半脱位、肱三头肌内侧增厚和 UCL 损伤也会增加神经的应力，可能导致尺神经分布区的夜间痛和感觉异常。尺神经症状可能由投掷动作引起。在体格检查中，可以发现肘管 Tinel 征阳性、肘关节过屈试验阳性和（或）存在尺神经半脱位。非手术治疗方式包括使用夜间支具、冰敷、使用非甾体抗炎药和活动矫正，都可以取得好的治疗效果。手术治疗通常包括将尺神经进行皮下前置。手术治疗结合适当的康复治疗和逐步恢复投掷运动可取得很好的效果。单独的尺神经前置术后恢复运动的时间约为 12 周。[22]如果患者存在尺神经症状且合并需要重建的 UCL 损伤，则应在重建时进行尺神经前置。

引起肘关节后方疼痛的疾病

后内侧撞击或外翻伸直过载

外翻伸直过载在过顶投掷运动员中是一种比较常见的损伤，通常为后方和内侧骨赘在肘关节伸直时撞击鹰嘴窝所致。一项纳入 72 例接受过肘部手术的职业棒球运动员的回顾研究发现，65% 的运动员存在鹰嘴后方骨赘。[23]运动员通常主诉在投球过程中肘关节伸直时后方疼痛，这就是鹰嘴骨赘在鹰嘴窝内的撞击点。患者在检查时通常会有一些终点时的伸直受限。当肘关节在外翻应力下由屈曲 20°~30° 位快速伸直时，肘关节后内侧疼痛诱发试验通常为阳性。必须注意确定是否合并 UCL 损伤，因为这些疾病之间有密切的联系。X 线片则可显示后方骨赘。

非手术治疗首先为休息及 10~14 天内避免投掷，然后进行间歇投掷训练，以逐步恢复投掷运动。在间歇投掷训练中，应改良投掷动作以尽量减小肘关节的应力。如果症状持续或患者无法恢复到伤前水平，建议休息更长的时间。关节内注射对后内侧撞击的患者没有特别的帮助，不建议重复进行。

应慎重考虑手术治疗。在投掷运动员中，肘关节内侧承受着巨大的外翻应力，鹰嘴与鹰嘴窝的对合为肘关节提供了次级稳定结构，特别是在伸直时。UCL 任何细微的松弛都可能将应力转移到尺骨鹰嘴后内侧，并导致其在肘关节伸直时撞击鹰嘴窝。这种应力会引起骨赘形成，然后又会因为剪切效应增加撞击。后内侧鹰嘴的过度切除可能使 UCL 损伤的症状显现或加重。25% 的职业棒球运动员在接受骨赘切除术后会出现外翻不稳，需要进行 UCL 重建。[23]研究显示，在 UCL 出现可见的应变增加之前，可被去除的鹰嘴骨量的结果并不一致，是否应该去除部分正常的鹰嘴也存在争议。切除可以在关节镜下或切开手术下进行。在切开手术中，用骨刀去除一部分尺骨鹰嘴尖端、并切除内侧部分尺骨鹰嘴。关节镜手术可以使用后外侧入路进行探查，从后正中入路进行操作。必须注意只去除骨赘，尽量避免切除正常的鹰嘴。此外，切除内侧骨赘时，在尺神经进入肘管的部位必须注意避免尺神经损伤。最近的一项研究显示，在 9 例关节镜下治疗外翻伸直过载的患者中，有 7 例患者疗效良好。[24]

鹰嘴应力性骨折

标枪运动员和其他投掷运动员的尺骨鹰嘴应力性骨折已有报道。[25-26] 这些骨折最早被描述为横向或斜向骨折，其损伤机制类似外翻伸直过载。当肘关节承受外翻负荷并接近伸直时，鹰嘴会承受更大的应力。肱三头肌伸展时的巨大力量也与此有关。

在体格检查中，运动员的鹰板（如果是张开的）及鹰嘴后方或后内侧可能有压痛，可能是由用力伸肘或肱三头肌抗阻试验引起的。通常情况下，患者的患侧伸肘范围会比对侧小。如果是慢性损伤，X 线片可能显示出骨折重塑的硬化线。如果鹰板是张开的，那么可以通过对比双侧肘关节 X 线片检测是否存在鹰板增宽。骨扫描会显示该区域的吸收增加。MRI 将显示骨髓内水肿，并显示骨折线的特征。如果怀疑合并 UCL 损伤，MRI 也有助于评估。

鹰嘴应力性骨折的治疗有些争议。非手术治疗包括避免投掷运动和必要时的临时支具保护。间歇投掷训练应在症状消失后开始，并且需要有骨折愈合的影像学证据。因此，避免进行投掷运动的时间可能需要长达 6 个月。应力性骨折可能对骨刺激因子有反应，但这种治疗方法尚未明确。

一些专家建议早期手术治疗，以减短恢复投掷的时间。[27] 如果非手术治疗不成功，也建议手术治疗，包括使用张力带、张力带联合加压螺钉以及仅使用加压螺钉。通常使用 6.5 mm 或 7.3 mm 空心加压螺钉。最近的一个病例研究报道了一个大学投手内固定术后仍存在持续性骨折，最终需要进行植骨以帮助愈合。[28]

持续性尺骨鹰嘴骺线

持续性尺骨鹰嘴骺线类似于尺骨鹰嘴应力性骨折，可能是运动员肘后疼痛的原因。尺骨鹰嘴有两个骨化中心：后方骨化中心垂直于尺骨纵轴并纵向生长；第二中心在尺骨鹰嘴尖端前方，向关节面生长而不是纵向生长。这两个中心融合成为一个单一的骨骺，一直持续到大约女性 14 岁时和男性 16 岁时。形成的骺线在闭合过程中会硬化，宽度可达 5 mm。

肘后方疼痛通常发生在青春期。疼痛发生在投掷动作的后期跟随阶段肘关节伸直时，休息可以减轻疼痛。体格检查可能是正常的：运动正常、肘关节稳定、触诊无压痛。X 线片显示尺骨鹰嘴有一个连续的骺线，患侧可能比对侧宽。X 线片可能发现与患者年龄不相符的骺线硬化。T2 加权成像 MRI 可显示骺线水肿，但该发现并不具有诊断价值。

治疗由非手术方案开始，包括一段时间的相对休息和停止投掷运动。必要时可使用非甾体抗炎药和冰敷。非手术治疗在大多数患者中可以取得好的治疗效果，但可能需要长达 4 个月的时间。手术治疗的选择包括切开复位内固定、植骨、切开复位内固定联合植骨。固定技术包括张力带线缆、加压螺钉及螺钉联合张力带线缆。现有的研究大多局限于病例报道和小样本的病例研究。[29-30] 植骨联合（或不联合）内固定的患者，愈合成功率是最高的。单独进行固定的患者约有 66% 的失败率。最近的一项研究发现，那些有连续性鹰嘴骺线和硬化征象的患者，非手术治疗的失败率为 100%。[31]

引起肘关节外侧疼痛的疾病

肱骨小头剥脱性骨软骨炎

剥脱性骨软骨炎（OCD）是软骨下骨的一种局灶疾病，导致关节软骨及软骨下骨的分离和碎裂。应注意将此病与 Panner 病相鉴别，Panner 病多发生于年轻患者，是特发性的，通常具有自限性，在没有手术干预的情况下会改善。OCD 通常发生在需进行高强度重复过顶投掷动作的年轻运动员的肘关节。其发病机制尚未完全清楚。遗传因素、血供、重复性创伤和脆弱的骨骺都与此有关。软骨下骨的退化会削弱上覆软骨的稳定性。多种因素都可能参与到病变的形成过程。

一般来说，运动员在运动中会有肘部疼痛。疼痛在开始时是轻微的，可以通过休息缓解，如果休息后继续活动，疼痛也会持续。疼痛很难定位，经常伴有运动障碍。偶尔会出现机械性症状，如肘关节卡住或交锁。检查中最常见的体征是肱桡关节处压痛。旋前和旋后可诱发关节外侧弹响，并有 15°~30° 的活动范围丧失。在主动肱桡关节压迫试验中，肘部完全伸直，而患者主动内旋和外旋前臂，并收缩肘部周围的肌肉。阳性结果为患者的症状重现。

X 线检查是初始的影像学检查。在肘关节伸直的标准正位及屈曲 90° 的侧位 X 线片中，可以看到典型的肱骨小头透亮和关节表面扁平（图 40-3）。病损通常发生在肱骨小头的前外侧面。在 Minami 分型中，1 级病变是肱骨小头中央的透光囊性阴影，2 级病变为病变与其软骨下骨之间有分裂线或透亮带，3 级病变为存在游离体。[32]

MRI 为评价这些病变的首选方法。在 MRI 上可以发现 X 线片上无法发现的早期改变，并且可以评估病变的大小、位置和稳定性。制订治疗策略的关键就是确定关节面是否完整，以及根据 MRI 判断病变是否稳定。关节面周围环状液体或关节面下方液体提示病变不稳定，这些表现与身体其他部位的 OCD 相似。关节造影或静脉注射钆有时有助于诊断。

如果 OCD 病灶愈合倾向大，则可以选择非手术治疗。初始治疗为肘关节避免投掷运动休息 6 个月。使用消炎药物，并实施物理治疗，以改善运动和力量。每 6 周进行一次 X 线检查，以评估病灶的愈合情况。必要时在大约 3 个月时复查 MRI，并与最初的影像相对比。如果患者活动范围良好、无症状且有愈合迹象，则在 6 个月时开始间歇投掷训练。[33] 肱骨小头透亮或扁平的 33

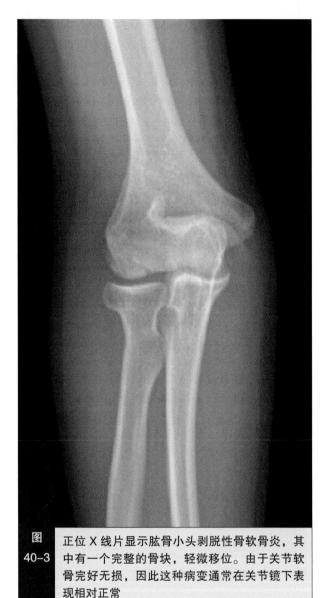

图 40-3　正位 X 线片显示肱骨小头剥脱性骨软骨炎，其中有一个完整的骨块，轻微移位。由于关节软骨完好无损，因此这种病变通常在关节镜下表现相对正常

例患者的治愈率为 88%~91%。[34-35] 肱骨小头骨骺未闭合患者的治愈率较高。严重病变的非手术治疗愈合能力较低。稳定病变的特征是肱骨小头生长板未闭合，软骨下骨局限性扁平或透光，肘关节活动良好。在不稳定的病变中，骺线是闭合的，影像学上可见游离体及超过 20° 的肘关节活动范围丧失。[36]

如果患者有不稳定的病变或游离体，或非手术治疗失败，则应进行手术治疗。目前有几种外科手术方式。对于肱骨小头关节面受累不及 50% 的局限性病变，单纯的清理是有效的。在骨块切除及骨床清理准备好后，可在软骨下骨基底处使用克氏针制造微骨折或进行环形钻孔（图40-4）。可以通过不同的方法固定相对较大的、未游离的病灶。外拉线、植骨和Herbert螺钉都已被成功应用。软骨替代有几种选择，类似膝关节和其他关节的方案。镶嵌成形术、异体骨软骨移植和自体移植均被用于治疗相对较大的OCD病损或无连接的病变（如失去外侧柱支撑）。

肱桡关节皱襞

肱桡关节皱襞，最早被视为导致肘关节弹响的原因，本质上是肥大增生的滑膜皱襞，当肘关节从屈曲到伸直时，与桡骨头的边缘撞击弹响。鉴别诊断包括关节内游离、不稳定、外上髁炎和内上髁上方的肱三头肌内侧半脱位。可以根据病变区域排除某些疾病。肘关节检查通常是正常的，稳定性存在、全范围活动及力量正常。患者的压痛可能以肘关节为中心出现在外上髁后方。X线片通常不能提供有效的信息，MRI也常会遗漏皱襞。

应考虑非手术治疗，包括相对的休息、使用非甾体抗炎药和柔和运动。关节内激素注射用于减轻炎症和疼痛。关节镜手术的治疗效果良好。通常情况下，在关节镜检查时可以重现皱襞的弹

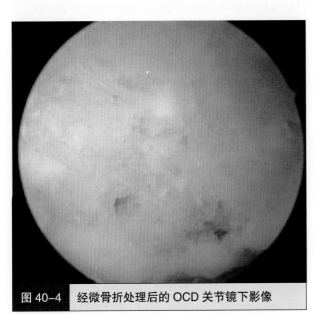

图40-4 经微骨折处理后的OCD关节镜下影像

响，术者可以一次定位需要松解的位置。其目的为充分松解滑膜皱襞，使其不再卡到桡骨头上。注意重复检查以确保松解完成。术后康复允许早期关节活动和力量锻炼。间歇投掷训练通常在术后第8周时，患者没有症状后开始进行。

总结

投掷运动员的肘关节在投掷运动的各个阶段都承受着巨大的应力。肘关节损伤的正确诊断的关键是按肘关节部位分析病情，获得详细的病史，应用特定的检查手法，以及进行合适的影像学检查。在疾病发展的特定阶段，非手术治疗可以取得好的治疗效果，手术技术的进步也改善了患者的预后。关节镜技术对许多疾病的治疗作用越来越大，其疗效和恢复率都令人满意。术后康复是逐步且个性化的，以恢复受累肌肉群的最佳机制、柔韧性和力量。

参考文献

[1] Farrow LD, Mahoney AJ, Stefancin JJ, Taljanovic MS, Sheppard JE, Schickendantz MS: Quantitative analysis of the medial ulnar collateral ligament ulnar footprint and its relationship to the ulnar sublime tubECRLe. *Am J Sports Med* 2011;39(9):1936-1941.

The anterior band of the UCL was evaluated in 10 fresh-frozen cadaver specimens. The mean length was 53.0 mm, and the mean length of the footprint on the ulna was 29.2 mm. The ridge was present in all specimens and had a mean measurement of 24.5 mm.

[2] Park MC, Ahmad CS: Dynamic contributions of the flexor-pronator mass to elbow valgus stability. *J Bone Joint Surg Am* 2004;86-A(10):2268-2274.

[3] Ahmad CS, Lee TQ, ElAttrache NS: Biomechanical evaluation of a new ulnar collateral ligament reconstruction technique with interference screw fixation. *Am J Sports Med* 2003;31(3):332-337.

[4] Duggan JP Jr, Osadebe UC, Alexander JW, Noble PC, Lintner DM: The impact of ulnar collateral ligament tear and reconstruction on contact pressures in the lateral compartment of the elbow. *J Shoulder Elbow*

Surg 2011;20(2):226-233.

Six cadaver specimens were tested under a valgus load of 1.75 N/m and 5.25 N/m torque to simulate late cocking and the release phase. The average valgus laxity was doubled after UCL transection and restored after reconstruction.

[5] Fleisig GS, Kingsley DS, Loftice JW, et al: Kinetic comparison among the fastball, curveball, change-up, and slider in collegiate baseball pitchers. *Am J Sports Med* 2006;34(3):423-430.

[6] O'Driscoll SW, Lawton RL, Smith AM: The "moving valgus stress test" for medial collateral ligament tears of the elbow. *Am J Sports Med* 2005;33(2):231-239.

[7] Thompson WH, Jobe FW, Yocum LA, Pink MM: Ulnar collateral ligament reconstruction in athletes: Muscle-splitting approach without transposition of the ulnar nerve. *J Shoulder Elbow Surg* 2001;10(2):152-157.

[8] Kim NR, Moon SG, Ko SM, Moon WJ, Choi JW, Park JY: MR imaging of ulnar collateral ligament injury in baseball players: Value for predicting rehabilitation outcome. *Eur J Radiol* 2011;80(3):e422-e426.

Thirty-nine baseball players with clinical evidence of UCL injury were evaluated with MRI. After nonsurgical treatment, 27 required surgery. The patients who responded to nonsurgical treatment had a less severe injury on MRI, and those with a higher-grade injury required surgery.

[9] Nazarian LN, McShane JM, Ciccotti MG, O'Kane PL, Harwood MI: Dynamic US of the anterior band of the ulnar collateral ligament of the elbow in asymptomatic major league baseball pitchers. *Radiology* 2003;227(1):149-154.

[10] Sasaki J, Takahara M, Ogino T, Kashiwa H, Ishigaki D, Kanauchi Y: Ultrasonographic assessment of the ulnar collateral ligament and medial elbow laxity in college baseball players. *J Bone Joint Surg Am* 2002;84-A(4):525-531.

[11] Field LD, Altchek DW: Evaluation of the arthroscopic valgus instability test of the elbow. *Am J Sports Med* 1996;24(2):177-181.

[12] Park GY, Lee SM, Lee MY: Diagnostic value of ultrasonography for clinical medial epicondylitis. *Arch Phys Med Rehabil* 2008;89(4):738-742.

An ultrasonographic assessment of 21 elbows with a clinical diagnosis of medial epicondylitis had sensitivity, specificity, accuracy, positive predictive value, and negative predictive value > 90%. This study reinforced the value of the physical examination and moved toward validating ultrasonography for diagnosing medial epicondylitis.

[13] Kijowski R, De Smet AA: Magnetic resonance imaging findings in patients with medial epicondylitis. *Skeletal Radiol* 2005;34(4):196-202.

[14] Nirschl RP, Rodin DM, Ochiai DH, Maartmann- Moe C; DEX-AHE-01-99 Study Group: Iontophoretic administration of dexamethasone sodium phosphate for acute epicondylitis: A randomized, double-blinded, placebo-controlled study. *Am J Sports Med* 2003;31(2):189-195.

[15] Suresh SP, Ali KE, Jones H, Connell DA: Medial epicondylitis: Is ultrasound guided autologous blood injection an effective treatment? *Br J Sports Med* 2006;40(11):935-939, discussion 939.

[16] Aguinaldo AL, Chambers H: Correlation of throwing mechanics with elbow valgus load in adult baseball pitchers. *Am J Sports Med* 2009;37(10):2043-2048.

Three-dimensional motion analysis was used to evaluate 69 adult baseball pitchers at an indoor mound. The variables most associated with elbow valgus included late trunk rotation, reduced shoulder external rotation, and increased elbow flexion. Sidearm pitchers were less susceptible to elbow valgus than those with a higher arm slot.

[17] Rettig AC, Sherrill C, Snead DS, Mendler JC, Mieling P: Nonoperative treatment of ulnar collateral ligament injuries in throwing athletes. *Am J Sports Med* 2001;29(1):15-17.

[18] Cain EL Jr, Andrews JR, Dugas JR, et al: Outcome of ulnar collateral ligament reconstruction of the elbow in 1281 athletes: Results in 743 athletes with minimum 2-year follow-up. *Am J Sports Med* 2010;38(12):2426-2434.

Prospective data were collected for a 2-year minimum on 942 patients, most of whom underwent UCL reconstruction with a palmaris longus or gracilis graft using the modified Jobe technique. All patients underwent subcutaneous nerve transposition. The rate of re- turn to previous level of function was 83%. The average time to return to throwing was 4.4 months, and the average return to competition was 11.6 months.

[19] Bowers AL, Dines JS, Dines DM, Altchek DW: Elbow medial ulnar collateral ligament reconstruction: Clinical relevance and the docking technique. *J Shoulder El- bow Surg* 2010;19(2, suppl):110-117.

Of 21 overhead athletes who underwent UCL reconstruction with a modified docking technique using a three-strand graft, 90% had a good or excellent result. This technique is acceptable for UCL reconstruction.

[20] Paletta GA Jr, Wright RW: The modified docking procedure for elbow ulnar collateral ligament reconstruction: 2-year follow-up in elite throwers. *Am J Sports Med* 2006;34(10):1594-1598.

[21] Dines JS, ElAttrache NS, Conway JE, Smith W, Ahmad CS: Clinical outcomes of the DANE TJ technique to treat ulnar collateral ligament insufficiency of the elbow. *Am J Sports Med* 2007;35(12):2039-2044.

Twenty-two athletes underwent UCL reconstruction with a hybrid variation of the docking technique in which an interference screw is used in a single tunnel on the ulna to avoid the fracture risk of the two-tunnel technique. Nineteen patients had an excellent result, as did patients requiring revision for sublime tubECRLe avulsions.

[22] Rettig AC, Ebben JR: Anterior subcutaneous transfer of the ulnar nerve in the athlete. *Am J Sports Med* 1993;21(6):836-839, discussion 839-840.

[23] Andrews JR, Timmerman LA: Outcome of elbow surgery in professional baseball players. *Am J Sports Med* 1995;23(4):407-413.

[24] Cohen SB, Valko C, Zoga A, Dodson CC, Ciccotti MG: Posteromedial elbow impingement: Magnetic resonance imaging findings in overhead throwing athletes and results of arthroscopic treatment. *Arthroscopy* 2011;27(10):1364-1370.

After unsuccessful nonsurgical treatment, nine patients with posteromedial impingement underwent arthroscopy followed by rehabilitation and an interval throwing program. The results were excellent at a mean 68-month follow-up.

[25] Hulkko A, Orava S, Nikula P: Stress fractures of the olecranon in javelin throwers. *Int J Sports Med* 1986;7(4):210-213.

[26] Nuber GW, Diment MT: Olecranon stress fractures in throwers: A report of two cases and a review of the lit- erature. *Clin Orthop Relat Res* 1992;278:58-61.

[27] Suzuki K, Minami A, Suenaga N, Kondoh M: Oblique stress fracture of the olecranon in baseball pitchers. *J Shoulder Elbow Surg* 1997;6(5):491-494.

[28] Stephenson DR, Love S, Garcia GG, Mair SD: Recurrence of an olecranon stress fracture in an elite pitcher after percutaneous internal fixation: A case report. *Am J Sports Med* 2012;40(1):218-221.

A collegiate pitcher with an olecranon stress fracture was successfully treated nonsurgically but had a recurrence on return to full activity. Seven months after surgical treatment with a single cannulated screw, he had posterior elbow pain with bullpen throwing. Revision fixation was with repeat screw fixation and a second smaller screw. After an interval throwing program, the patient returned to pitching without symptoms at 17-month follow-up.

[29] Charlton WP, Chandler RW: Persistence of the olecranon physis in baseball players: Results following operative management. *J Shoulder Elbow Surg* 2003;12(1):59-62.

[30] Skak SV: Fracture of the olecranon through a persistent physis in an adult: A case report. *J Bone Joint Surg Am* 1993;75(2):272-275.

[31] Matsuura T, Kashiwaguchi S, Iwase T, Enishi T, Yasui N: The value of using radiographic criteria for the treatment of persistent symptomatic olecranon physis in adolescent throwing athletes. *Am J Sports Med* 2010;38(1):141-145.

In a retrospective analysis of persistent olecranon physis in 16 male baseball players, the lesions were classified as stage I (a widened physis compared with the contralateral elbow) or stage II (radiographic lesion). Nonsurgical treatment was successful in 92% of those with a stage I lesion but none with a stage II lesion.

[32] Minami M, Nakashita K, Ishii S, et al: Twenty-five cases of osteochondritis dissecans of the elbow. *Rinsho Seikei Geka* 1979;14(8):805-810.

[33] Baker CL III, Romeo AA, Baker CL Jr: Osteochondritis dissecans of the capitellum. *Am J Sports Med* 2010;38(9):1917-1928.

OCD of the capitellum was reviewed, including pathoanatomy, clinical presentation, diagnostic studies, nonsurgical and surgical treatments, and a rehabilitation program.

[34] Mihara K, Tsutsui H, Nishinaka N, Yamaguchi K: Nonoperative treatment for osteochondritis dissecans of the capitellum. *Am J Sports Med* 2009;37(2):298-304.

Retrospective review of 39 patients with OCD of the capitellum who were treated nonsurgically led to the recommendation that patients with an advanced lesion undergo surgical intervention because of poor healing rates and evidence of progression with nonsurgical management.

[35] Matsuura T, Kashiwaguchi S, Iwase T, Takeda Y, Yasui N: Conservative treatment for osteochondrosis of the humeral capitellum. *Am J Sports Med* 2008;36(5):868-872.

Retrospective review of 176 patients with OCD of the humeral capitellum found that 90.5% of stage I and 53% of stage II lesions healed with nonsurgical measures. Mean time to healing was 14.9 months and 12.3 months for stage I and II lesions, respectively, and return-to-throwing rates were 78.6% and 52.9%, respectively.

[36] Takahara M, Mura N, Sasaki J, Harada M, Ogino T: Classification, treatment, and outcome of osteochondritis dissecans of the humeral capitellum. *J Bone Joint Surg Am* 2007;89(6):1205-1214.

In a retrospective review of 106 patients with OCD of the humeral capitellum, treatment was nonsurgical or surgical fragment removal, fragment fixation with bone grafting, or mosaicplasty with plugs from the lateral femoral condyle. Lesions were classified as stable or unstable at 7.2-year follow-up. Stable lesions responded well to nonsurgical measures, and unstable lesions responded to surgical intervention.

第四十一章 复发性肘关节内侧和外侧不稳定

April D. Armstrong, BSc(PT), MSc, MD, FRCSC

引言

复发性肘关节内侧和外侧不稳定并不常见。患者的主诉常为肘部疼痛，而并非不稳定，这给诊断造成了困难。与静态的影像学检查相比，患者的病史、体格检查结果和高度怀疑指数对准确诊断更为重要，因为静态影像学检查的结果通常是正常的。外侧副韧带功能不全的耐受性较差，因为大多数日常生活活动需要肘内翻负荷。相比之下，大多数患者可耐受内侧副韧带（MCL）功能不全，因为外翻负荷在日常生活中并不常见。过顶投掷运动员，特别是棒球投手，往往无法承受 MCL 功能不全，需要进行重建手术。

肘外翻不稳定

在最近的 5~10 年间，骨科医师对肘关节内侧不稳定的认识有了很大的提高。MCL 损伤最常见的原因是过顶投掷运动时的重复性过高负荷，而此类损伤大多发生在棒球运动员身上。在投球的挥臂晚期（即肩关节外旋到最大程度时）和加速期，肘关节外翻负荷超过了 MCL 前束的拉伸强度。[1-2] 投球速度高的职业运动员发生 MCL 损伤

的风险相对较高。[3] 一名身材高大的高中棒球运动员可能由于具有更强的肘关节外翻力量，导致更容易出现 MCL 损伤。[4] 与棒球投手相比，标枪投手的投掷动作明显不同，术后康复需求也会不同。[5] 因为标枪比棒球重，所以 10 名标枪投手在接受 MCL 重建手术后需要比棒球投手更长的康复时间才能开始间歇投掷训练，恢复期为 15 个月（传统上棒球投手的恢复期为 1 年）。标枪运动员应该被提前告知会经历一个漫长的恢复期。[5] 也有报道称橄榄球四分卫易出现 MCL 损伤，但最近一项对美国国家橄榄球联盟损伤监测系统的研究显示，1994—2008 年，仅报告了 10 个 MCL 损伤运动员接受了成功的非手术治疗。[6] 相比之下，棒球运动员经常需要行重建手术。MCL 损伤也可能在创伤后发生，如肘关节脱位。这种损伤通常可以进行非手术治疗，因为在大多数患者的日常生活活动中，肘部外翻负荷很小。

生物力学研究已经证实，MCL 前束是肘关节外翻的主要稳定结构。[7-9] 最近的一项生物力学尸体研究测试了在模拟投球运动的两个关键阶段中肱桡关节的接触压力。[10] MCL 重建使肱桡关节的平均关节压力恢复至全部肘关节值的 20% 以内。这项研究支持了 MCL 前束和 MCL 重建在维持外翻稳定性方面的主要作用。

存在肘关节外翻不稳定的过顶投掷运动员，常主诉投掷时肘关节内侧疼痛。他们可能描述投掷过程中有明显的弹响，或者在投掷过程中出现

Dr. Armstrong or an immediate family member has received nonincome support (such as equipment or services), commercially derived honoraria, or other non–research-related funding (such as paid travel) from Zimmer and serves as a board member, owner, officer, or committee member of the American Shoulder and Elbow Surgeons.

隐匿性的疼痛加剧和力度及准确性的降低。偶尔，患者也会出现短暂的尺神经症状。一些运动员描述的肘关节后方疼痛与后内侧骨刺或外翻伸展应力过高有关（图 41-1）。运动员可能主诉在减速期和球脱手时疼痛加剧。一些外科医师认为，后内侧撞击发生在肘关节小角度屈曲的情况下，外翻不稳定导致了肘关节后内侧间室接触应力增加。[11-12] 最近的生物力学研究提出，这种撞击发生在整个肘关节活动范围中，不仅在小角度屈曲时，而且与肱尺关节软骨损伤并发。[13]

肘关节外翻不稳定的诊断具有挑战性，体格检查的结果也可能是隐匿性的。患者常有内上髁和屈曲-旋前肌群的点状压痛。如果患者有外翻伸直过载且伴后方骨赘，则触诊鹰嘴后内侧可能引起疼痛。患者也可能主诉肘关节用力伸展时疼痛。有时投掷运动员有轻微的屈曲挛缩，因此尽管存在后方骨赘也可能无疼痛症状。应记录体格

检查结果和尺神经症状，特别是神经半脱位。激发性试验应包括外翻应力试验、挤奶试验和活动性外翻应力试验。[14] 外翻应力试验在肘关节屈曲 30° 的情况下进行，从而将鹰嘴从鹰嘴窝中解锁。应控制肩部旋转，与对侧肢体比较关节间隙大小。在外翻应力试验中触诊关节内侧可以引起疼痛，并且可以更好地评估关节间隙。挤奶试验使 MCL 受到静态负荷。在控制肩部旋转的同时，患者的肘部屈曲至 90°，前臂完全旋后。然后，牵拉动患者的拇指并施加外翻压力。MCL 处疼痛为阳性结果。活动性外翻应力试验是一项动态试验，在肘关节活动过程中施加恒定的外翻负荷。[14] MCL 损伤的患者通常主诉屈曲 70°~120° 时肘关节内侧疼痛（图 41-2）。

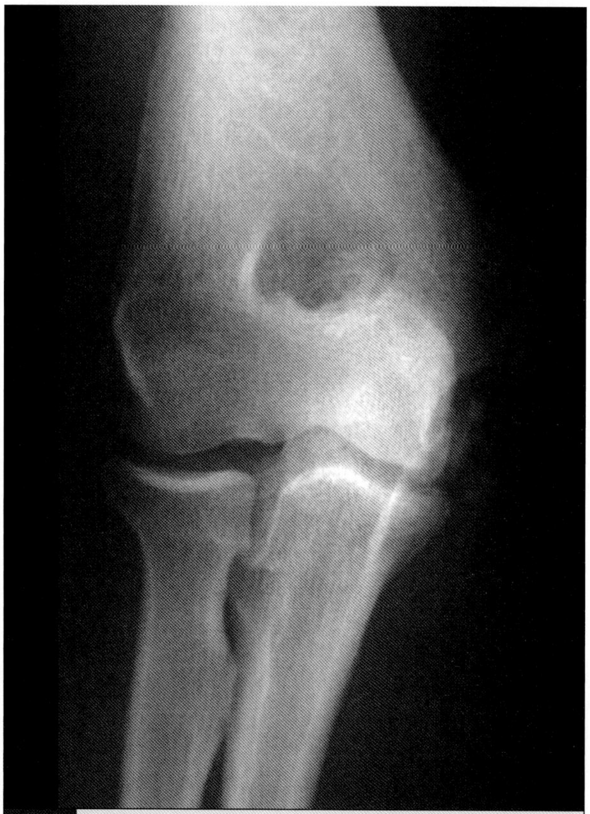

肘关节外翻不稳定的体格检查不应只局限于肘关节。应检查同侧肩关节是否有相关的肩袖疾病或由后方关节囊紧张引起的盂肱关节内旋不足。MCL 损伤后功能不全的投掷运动员比未受伤的运动员更容易出现肩关节旋转受限。[15] 评估运动员的核心肌肉力量也很重要。投掷时的力学机制包括力量从腿到躯干及上肢的转移，而核心力量较

图41-1 退役棒球投手肘关节的正位 X 线片显示后内侧骨赘，这与慢性外翻伸直过载有关

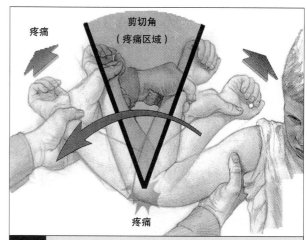

图41-2 活动外翻应力试验的示意图，在该试验中，在肘关节整个运动弧中施加外翻负荷。MCL 损伤的患者会在运动弧中段时主诉疼痛，通常是在屈肘 70°~120° 时（剪切角）。经允许引自 The Mayo Foundation for Medical Education and Research, Rochester, MN.

低可能增加上肢的负荷。单腿站立可以快速方便地测试核心力量水平。当患者单腿站立并进行深蹲屈膝时，核心无力的患者会失去平衡，或者必须向支撑腿侧倾斜以保持平衡。[16]对运动员投球力学的规范评估也可以提供信息。尤其是年轻的投手在投球时往往过早地打开躯干，将肘关节留在身体后方。这种"肘关节掉落"会增加肘关节的外翻负荷。

肘关节外翻不稳定的诊断主要依赖于患者的病史和体格检查结果，但影像学检查也对诊断有所帮助。肘关节静态 X 线片常显示正常，但应力 X 线片可显示肱尺关节间隙不对称增宽 2~3 mm。常规或联合关节造影的 MRI 检查以及关节造影 CT 检查有助于鉴别骨软骨损伤等合并病变。一项研究发现，即使在无症状的高中投手中，MCL 增厚和滑车后内侧软骨下骨硬化也很常见，这些情况可能是投掷造成的正常适应性变化。[17]较高的肘关节内收力矩峰值与 MRI 上 MCL 增厚有关。[18] MCL 动态超声评估正变得越来越普遍。[19]

运动员 MCL 功能障碍的初始治疗包括针对性的 3~6 个月的休息和康复期。非手术治疗 MCL 损伤后，42% 的患者恢复运动。[20]康复应重点关注提高屈曲–旋前肌群的力量和耐力，减少肩关节后方关节囊的紧张，增加核心力量和稳定性。

韧带重建是投掷运动员 MCL 功能障碍的经典手术治疗方法。对相对年轻的运动员来说，MCL 修复可能是一种合理的选择，因为他们具有更好的韧带组织质量和较低的韧带慢性病变的可能性。[21]对于局限于近端或远端的损伤，有研究报道，修复后有 91% 的运动恢复率；97% 的患者在 6 个月内可完全恢复运动，而重建手术后则需要 1 年。治疗年轻运动员时，MCL 手术是一项可考虑的重要技术。

在非手术治疗失败后，韧带重建仍然是投掷运动员的首选治疗方法。MCL 重建的重点是 MCL 前束的重建。研究表明，MCL 前束为几乎等长的

纤维，起点位于肱骨侧的旋转解剖轴。[22]最近的一项研究表明，MCL 前束包含 4 个单独的等长韧带，起点在冠状面上广泛分布于旋转解剖轴。[23]等长纤维在冠状面上比以前认为的更靠近内侧，且更具主导作用，几乎占 MCL 前束纤维的一半。与过去的研究一样，MCL 前束的等长性更容易在肱骨侧被观察到，而不是在尺骨侧。[22]

许多 MCL 韧带重建技术被介绍，大多都基于双束或单束结构。[24-34]两种方式均被报道有良好的临床效果。平均的运动恢复率为 83%（68%~95%），[35]单束重建可能更适用于 MCL 重建失败后的翻修手术。[36-37]在患者数最多的 MCL 重建研究中，使用改良的 Jobe（8 字形）技术，显露时将屈曲–旋前肌群牵开而不游离，并进行尺神经皮下前置。[38]743 例患者随访 2 年后，运动恢复率为 83%，平均完全恢复的时间为 11.6 个月，20% 出现并发症（16% 轻微，4% 严重）。尺神经症状是最常见的轻微并发症，主要是短暂性神经麻痹。将尺神经皮下前置术从双悬吊改为单悬吊，以及使用肌间隔而不是屈肌筋膜制作软组织床可以改善手术效果。尺神经移位的绝对指征尚不明确。此外，还有 5 例治疗肱骨内上髁骨折的报道，对肱骨骨道的位置进行了改良，使其在内上髁上的位置更深（更外侧）。34% 的患者需要行开放手术切除后内侧鹰嘴骨赘。

MCL 重建的最新进展包括尺神经不前置的屈曲–旋前肌群劈开技术，据报道该技术可降低尺神经病变的发生率。[39] MCL 重建的对接技术具有相对较高的运动恢复率[28-30,34]（图 41-3、41-4）。30 岁以上的患者发生 MCL 损伤和屈曲–旋前肌群联合损伤的风险较高，从而导致较低的运动恢复率（12.5%）。[40]

MCL 损伤发生率的增长引起了更多的关注，尤其是在大学生运动员和高中运动员中。预防是关键，特别是对于年轻运动员。适当的康复是必要的，同样，限制投手的投球次数和制订

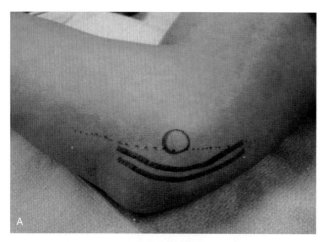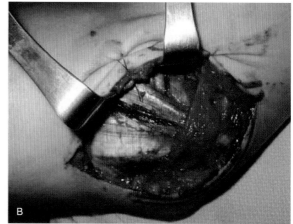
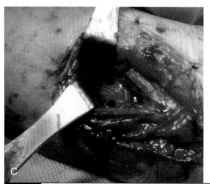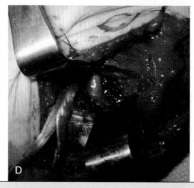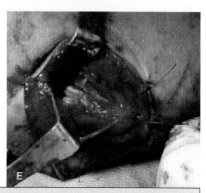

图 41-3 MCL 重建的对接技术。A. 分别标记内侧切口（虚线）、内上髁（圆圈）和尺神经走行（实线）。B. 肌肉劈开入路需要注意保护前臂内侧皮神经。C. 在尺骨上钻了两个孔来桥接高耸结节。D. 显露内上髁并在等长点钻孔，肌腱移植物通过尺骨骨道。E. 在完全重建中，移植物两个肌腱端都被插入到肱骨中，肌腱端的缝线通过等长点孔以近的钻取的两个较小骨道穿出

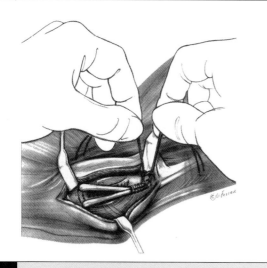

图 41-4 MCL 重建的对接技术最早被提出时的示意图。肌腱移植物通过尺骨的两个钻孔和肱骨等长点的一个对接钻孔。而缝线则通过更偏近端的两个较小的孔引出 (© Hospital for Special Surgery, New York, NY.)

投手的绝对休息期也是有必要的。美国棒球医疗与安全咨询委员会发布的《限制投球次数和累积投球次数指南》强调，这些因素与受伤风险呈线性关系。[41] 研究表明，投球次数是比投球种类更显著的受伤风险因素。[42] 该指南还提供棒球赛季结束后的建议，包括改善的投球技术和至少3 个月的不投掷休息期。疲劳是与手臂损伤最密切相关的因素。[41]

后外侧旋转不稳定

与肘关节外翻不稳定不同，后外侧旋转不稳定（PLRI）并非仅发生在运动员身上。PLRI 会使外侧副韧带复合体（LCLC）处于持续的应激状态，即使是只需要常规日常生活活动的患者，也可能出现不适。通常，发生在肘关节脱位或

摔倒时上肢外展撑地后的 LCLC 愈合不充分是导致 PLRI 的原因。有多种机制描述，其中，肘关节脱位的经典机制是肘关节的轴向压迫、外旋和外翻负荷。[43-44]一项关于单纯肘关节脱位的 MRI 研究表明，后外侧脱位更容易发生 LCLC 的愈合，因为外侧的损伤往往是脱套损伤。肘关节复位后，损伤的 LCLC 会回复至原位，靠近骨骼的位置，此处的愈合率更高，因此，PLRI 的发生率较低。肩关节后内侧脱位导致牵拉伤伴内侧骨挫伤，从而造成更严重的外侧软组织损伤。一项 2012 年的研究显示，肩关节后内侧脱位可能与 PLRI 和复发性不稳定的风险更高有关，这是由于外侧损伤本身的牵张作用。[45]PLRI 也可能由医源性因素导致，例如，广泛的外上髁松解或多次激素注射治疗顽固性外上髁炎。[46]其他报道的原因有慢性肘内翻畸形，如儿童髁上骨折后畸形愈合以及桡骨头切除，因为桡骨头 LCLC 上的张力会减弱。[47-49]

LCLC 由尺侧副韧带（LUCL）、桡侧副韧带（RCL）、环状韧带和副韧带组成。通常，LUCL 被认为是限制 PLRI 的主要结构，但生物力学研究表明 RCL 也对 PLRI 的稳定性有显著作用。[43,50-51]有研究指出，RCL 是等长束，而 LUCL 不是。[52]另一项研究发现，LCLC 并没有真正的等距点，在 LCLC 重建中等长度移植物的最佳植入点位置在肘关节中存在显著的个体差异。[53]对抗 PLRI 的力最有可能由 LUCL 和 RCL 联合提供。最近有报道称，为处理 PLRI，应进行 LUCL 和 RCL 的双重重建。[54]

PLRI 的诊断较为困难。患者通常只主诉肘部疼痛或"不对劲"的非特异性感觉。一些患者会描述有疼痛、交锁或弹响出现，并在肘关节伸直或通过手臂持重时发生肘关节半脱位。PLRI 的经典检查方法是外侧轴移试验。该试验通常在麻醉下进行，因为患者无法耐受检查手法[55]（图 41-5）。在患者仰卧、手臂过顶弯曲、前臂最大旋后的状态下，于肘关节伸直过程中施加轴向和外翻负荷，此时出现肘关节半脱位。透视分析显示桡骨

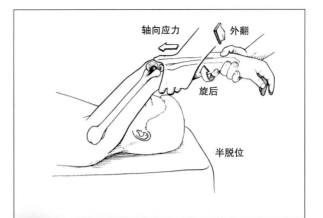

图 41-5 外侧轴移试验示意图，是检查 PLRI 的经典不稳定试验。在对肘关节施加轴向负荷的同时，施以旋后和外翻力量。肘关节在伸直时是半脱位的，肘关节在屈曲过程中复位，此过程经常可以通过视觉和听觉感受到。经允许引自 O'Driscoll SW, Bell DF, Morrey BF: Posterolateral rotatory instability of the elbow. *J Bone Joint Surg Am* 1991;73(3):440–446.

头位于肱骨小头后，肱尺关节间隙变宽。将肘关节屈曲，则会诱使肘关节出现明确的落槽和复位感。外侧轴移试验具有很高的可重复性，不依赖于检查者的技术水平或经验。[56]

后外侧抽屉试验、撑椅俯卧撑试验、地板俯卧撑试验和撑桌复位试验更容易被患者接受。[57-58]这些试验都模拟了外侧轴移试验，通过产生伸直、旋后、轴向和外翻的肘关节载荷，从而引起半脱位。如果结果呈阳性，患者就会感知到体征再现或对此产生恐惧。

PLRI 是一个临床诊断。静态影像学图像通常是正常的，但更进一步的影像学检查可能会有所帮助，特别是医源性 PLRI。如果 LCLC 功能受损的原始病因不是不稳定，那么按照典型的不稳定去检查可能比较困难。MRI（加或不加关节造影）和超声都有应用。[59-60]肱骨小头后方压缩骨折可能与肘关节脱位并发，类似肩关节的 Hill-Sachs 损伤。[61]MRI 可能显示肱骨小头假性缺损，这可能预示着存在 PLRI，不应与肱骨小头后方压缩骨折相混淆，也不应误诊为 Osborne-

Cotterill 损伤（一种类似肩关节盂 Bankart 损伤的肱骨小头后外侧软骨骨折）。[62-64]

症状性 PLRI 最常应用的治疗方法是肌腱移植重建 LCLC。然而，手术修复的效果通常较差，可能是因为韧带强度经常减弱。[65-66] 经典的 LCLC 重建包括采用 8 字形结构连接肱骨到尺骨，在尺骨旋后嵴上钻 2 个孔，在肱骨上钻 3 个孔，并在 LCLC 的起点等距点处钻 1 个皮质孔。[55] 肌腱移植物以 8 字形通过皮质孔并缝合到自身。在一项研究中，12 例患者直接修复，33 例采用 8 字形重建术，平均随访 6 年，86% 的患者对手术结果主观满意，7 例患者仍存在不稳定。[66] 重建效果优于韧带修复。创伤导致的和有主观不稳定症状的患者也有较好的疗效。小规模的研究报道了其他重建方案，如使用肱三头肌腱、关节镜技术和界面固定单束结构等。[67-71]

类似 MCL 重建技术中的对接技术，在 LCLC 重建中的应用也在增加（图 41-6）。通过 Kocher

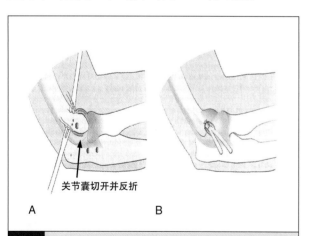

关节囊切开并反折

A　　　　　　　　B

图 41-6　对接技术进行外侧副韧带复合体重建的示意图。A. 在尺骨上钻取 2 个孔，在肱骨等距点上钻取 1 个孔，在该孔向肱骨近端钻取 2 个较小的孔用于缝线穿出。B. 在完整的重建中，修复附着的关节囊肌腱复合体，肌腱移植物穿过 2 个尺骨钻孔后对接固定于肱骨等距点钻孔内。经允许引自 Jones KJ, Dodson CC, Osbahr DC, et al: The docking technique for lateral ulnar collateral ligament reconstruction: Surgical technique and clinical outcomes. *J Shoulder Elbow Surg* 2012;21(3):389–395.

入路显露肘关节。在尺骨上钻两个骨道，用约 2 cm 的骨桥桥接旋后肌嵴，一个骨道位于旋后嵴上，另一个骨道更偏向近端，靠近环状韧带的基底处。肌腱移植物穿过骨道，移植物的两端都与肱骨等长点处骨道对接。由肱骨等长点向近端钻取两个较小的骨道出口，使缝线从等距点骨道分别穿出，并在大于 1 cm 的骨桥上拉紧打结。将薄弱的关节囊韧带复合体与肌腱移植物缝线缝合在一起，以加强修复。肱骨等长骨道的定位是韧带重建手术的关键环节之一。后侧的骨道应放置在肱骨小头的中心，即肘关节的旋转轴中心处。由于肘关节在旋后位和伸直位会变得不稳定，所以重建的韧带在该位置时为最大张力置管。为此，需要对肱骨等长点处进行偏心钻孔。生物力学研究发现，在 LCLC 重建中，无法确定真正的等长骨道位置，并且尸体标本之间存在显著差异。[53] 3 点到 4 点 30 分之间的位置被认为是肱骨骨道定位的理想位置。肱骨侧的骨道钻取应比等距点稍偏前和近端，使肱骨后侧的骨道可以保持等距，特别是在肘关节伸直时。在一个纳入 8 例患者的平均 7 年的随访研究中，75%（6 例）的患者无复发性不稳定，25%（2 例）在日常生活活动中偶尔出现不稳定。[72] 所有患者均对治疗结果满意。

总结

肘关节内侧或外侧复发性不稳定虽不常见，但可能致残。非手术治疗通常是无效的。诊断依赖于高度怀疑的临床表现和针对性的临床体格检查。韧带重建是首选治疗方法且成功率高。

参考文献

[1] Fleisig GS, Andrews JR, Dillman CJ, Escamilla RF: Kinetics of baseball pitching with implications about injury mechanisms. *Am J Sports Med* 1995;23(2):233-239.

[2] Dillman CJ, Fleisig GS, Andrews JR: Biomechanics of pitching with emphasis upon shoulder kinematics. *J Orthop Sports Phys Ther* 1993;18(2):402-408.

［3］ Bushnell BD, Anz AW, Noonan TJ, Torry MR, Hawkins RJ: Association of maximum pitch velocity and elbow injury in professional baseball pitchers. *Am J Sports Med* 2010;38(4):728-732.

A significant association was found between maximum pitch velocity and elbow injury in 23 professional baseball pitchers. Level of evidence: III.

［4］ Han KJ, Kim YK, Lim SK, Park JY, Oh KS: The effect of physical characteristics and field position on the shoulder and elbow injuries of 490 baseball players: Confirmation of diagnosis by magnetic resonance imaging. *Clin J Sport Med* 2009;19(4):271-276.

An analysis of baseball-related injuries in 490 baseball players referred to a shoulder and elbow institute for rehabilitation revealed that high school and collegiate players were more likely to have an MCL injury or superior labrum anterior to posterior injury than junior high school players. Pitchers and outfielders were more likely to have MCL injury than infielders. Players who were relatively tall and heavy had a higher incidence of MCL injury.

［5］ Dines JS, Jones KJ, Kahlenberg C, Rosenbaum A, Osbahr DC, Altchek DW: Elbow ulnar collateral ligament reconstruction in javelin throwers at a minimum 2-year follow-up. *Am J Sports Med* 2012;40(1):148-151.

MCL reconstruction in 10 javelin throwers highlighted that the rehabilitation needs of javelin throwers are different from those of baseball players. Level of evidence: IV.

［6］ Dodson CC, Slenker N, Cohen SB, Ciccotti MG, DeLuca P: Ulnar collateral ligament injuries of the elbow in professional football quarterbacks. *J Shoulder Elbow Surg* 2010;19(8):1276-1280.

A review of the National Football League Injury Surveillance System found that MCL injuries are uncommon in quarterbacks, and most are treated nonsurgically. Level of evidence: IV.

［7］ Hotchkiss RN, Weiland AJ: Valgus stability of the elbow. *J Orthop Res* 1987;5(3):372-377.

［8］ Søjbjerg JO, Ovesen J, Nielsen S: Experimental elbow instability after transection of the medial collateral ligament. *Clin Orthop Relat Res* 1987;218:186-190.

［9］ Morrey BF, An KN: Articular and ligamentous contributions to the stability of the elbow joint. *Am J Sports Med* 1983;11(5):315-319.

［10］ Duggan JP Jr, Osadebe UC, Alexander JW, Noble PC, Lintner DM: The impact of ulnar collateral ligament tear and reconstruction on contact pressures in the lateral compartment of the elbow. *J Shoulder Elbow Surg* 2011;20(2):226-233.

A biomechanical cadaver study found that MCL reconstruction restored valgus stability and decreased radiocapitellar contact pressures almost to normal levels.

［11］ Ahmad CS, Park MC, ElAttrache NS: Elbow medial ulnar collateral ligament insufficiency alters postero- medial olecranon contact. *Am J Sports Med* 2004;32(7):1607-1612.

［12］ Kamineni S, ElAttrache NS, O'Driscoll SW, et al: Medial collateral ligament strain with partial posteromedial olecranon resection: A biomechanical study. *J Bone Joint Surg Am* 2004;86-A(11):2424-2430.

［13］ Osbahr DC, Dines JS, Breazeale NM, Deng XH, Altchek DW: Ulnohumeral chondral and ligamentous overload: Biomechanical correlation for posteromedial chondromalacia of the elbow in throwing athletes. *Am J Sports Med* 2010;38(12):2535-2541.

The authors examine, using a biomechanical model, the contact area and pressure across the posteromedial elbow before and after sectioning the anterior bundle of the medial collateral ligament. They reported that valgus laxity increased contact pressures, with the elbow held at 90 degrees, across the posteromedial elbow. They suggested that posteromedial impingement and the potential for chondral damage is possible throughout the entire arc of flexion and not just in extension.

［14］ O'Driscoll SW, Lawton RL, Smith AM: The "moving valgus stress test" for medial collateral ligament tears of the elbow. *Am J Sports Med* 2005;33(2):231-239.

［15］ Dines JS, Frank JB, Akerman M, Yocum LA: Glenohumeral internal rotation deficits in baseball players with ulnar collateral ligament insufficiency. *Am J Sports Med* 2009;37(3):566-570.

In a comparison of 29 baseball players with MCL insufficiency with a matched control group of 29 baseball players with no insufficiency, the injured players were found to have significantly less glenohumeral internal rotation motion. Level of evidence: III.

［16］ Ben Kibler W, Sciascia A: Kinetic chain contributions to elbow function and dysfunction in sports. *Clin Sports Med* 2004;23(4):545-552, viii.

［17］ Hurd WJ, Kaufman KR, Murthy NS: Relationship between the medial elbow adduction moment during pitching and ulnar collateral ligament appearance during magnetic resonance imaging evaluation. *Am J Sports Med* 2011;39(6):1233-1237.

A comparison of elbow MRI with three-dimensional

motion analysis testing in 20 uninjured, asymptomatic high school baseball pitchers found that MCL thickening was associated with higher peak internal elbow adduction moments. Level of evidence: II.

[18] Hurd WJ, Eby S, Kaufman KR, Murthy NS: Magnetic resonance imaging of the throwing elbow in the uninjured, high school-aged baseball pitcher. *Am J Sports Med* 2011;39(4):722-728.

Thickening of the anterior band of the MCL and posteromedial subchondral sclerosis was found in 23 uninjured, asymptomatic high school baseball pitchers. These findings may be considered normal or warn of risk for injury. Level of evidence: III.

[19] Smith W, Hackel JG, Goitz HT, Bouffard JA, Nelson AM: Utilization of sonography and a stress device in the assessment of partial tears of the ulnar collateral ligament in throwers. *Int J Sports Phys Ther* 2011;6(1):45-50.

An ultrasonographic technique for assessing valgus elbow instability is described.

[20] Rettig AC, Sherrill C, Snead DS, Mendler JC, Mieling P: Nonoperative treatment of ulnar collateral ligament injuries in throwing athletes. *Am J Sports Med* 2001;29(1):15-17.

[21] Savoie FH III, Trenhaile SW, Roberts J, Field LD, Ramsey JR: Primary repair of ulnar collateral ligament injuries of the elbow in young athletes: A case series of injuries to the proximal and distal ends of the ligament. *Am J Sports Med* 2008;36(6):1066-1072.

Acute repair of the MCL is proposed as a viable alternative to reconstruction in young nonprofessional athletes. Level of evidence: IV.

[22] Armstrong AD, Ferreira LM, Dunning CE, Johnson JA, King GJ: The medial collateral ligament of the elbow is not isometric: An in vitro biomechanical study. *Am J Sports Med* 2004;32(1):85-90.

[23] Miyake J, Moritomo H, Masatomi T, et al: In vivo and 3-dimensional functional anatomy of the anterior bundle of the medial collateral ligament of the elbow. *J Shoulder Elbow Surg* 2012;21(8):1006-1012.

Four unique isometric bands of the anterior bundle of the MCL were found to broadly align along the axis of rotation in the coronal plane.

[24] Jobe FW, Stark H, Lombardo SJ: Reconstruction of the ulnar collateral ligament in athletes. *J Bone Joint Surg Am* 1986;68(8):1158-1163.

[25] Conway JE, Jobe FW, Glousman RE, Pink M: Medial instability of the elbow in throwing athletes: Treatment by repair or reconstruction of the ulnar collateral ligament. *J Bone Joint Surg Am* 1992;74(1):67-83.

[26] Azar FM, Andrews JR, Wilk KE, Groh D: Operative treatment of ulnar collateral ligament injuries of the elbow in athletes. *Am J Sports Med* 2000;28(1):16-23.

[27] Thompson WH, Jobe FW, Yocum LA, Pink MM: Ulnar collateral ligament reconstruction in athletes: Muscle-splitting approach without transposition of the ulnar nerve. *J Shoulder Elbow Surg* 2001;10(2):152-157.

[28] Rohrbough JT, Altchek DW, Hyman J, Williams RJ III, Botts JD: Medial collateral ligament reconstruction of the elbow using the docking technique. *Am J Sports Med* 2002;30(4):541-548.

[29] Paletta GA Jr, Wright RW: The modified docking procedure for elbow ulnar collateral ligament reconstruction: 2-year follow-up in elite throwers. *Am J Sports Med* 2006;34(10):1594-1598.

[30] Koh JL, Schafer MF, Keuter G, Hsu JE: Ulnar collateral ligament reconstruction in elite throwing athletes. *Arthroscopy* 2006;22(11):1187-1191.

[31] Dines JS, ElAttrache NS, Conway JE, Smith W, Ahmad CS: Clinical outcomes of the DANE TJ technique to treat ulnar collateral ligament insufficiency of the elbow. *Am J Sports Med* 2007;35(12):2039-2044.

Patients who underwent a single-strand MCL ligament reconstruction technique had an 86% rate of return to sport. Level of evidence: IV.

[32] Bowers AL, Dines JS, Dines DM, Altchek DW: Elbow medial ulnar collateral ligament reconstruction: Clinical relevance and the docking technique. *J Shoulder Elbow Surg* 2010;19(suppl 2):110-117.

A modified docking technique for MCL reconstruction had an excellent result in 90% of patients. Level of evidence: IV.

[33] Hechtman KS, Zvijac JE, Wells ME, Botto-van Bemden A: Long-term results of ulnar collateral ligament reconstruction in throwing athletes based on a hybrid technique. *Am J Sports Med* 2011;39(2):342-347.

At an average follow-up of 6.9 years, patients treated with a hybrid technique for MCL reconstruction had an 85% recovery to preinjury level of performance. Level of evidence: IV.

[34] Dodson CC, Thomas A, Dines JS, Nho SJ, Williams RJ III, Altchek DW: Medial ulnar collateral ligament reconstruction of the elbow in throwing athletes. *Am J Sports Med* 2006;34(12):1926-1932.

[35] Vitale MA, Ahmad CS: The outcome of elbow ulnar collateral ligament reconstruction in overhead athletes:

A systematic review. *Am J Sports Med* 2008;36(6):1193-1205.

Articles published from 1950 to 2007 on ulnar collateral ligament reconstruction were systematically reviewed.

[36] Dines JS, Yocum LA, Frank JB, ElAttrache NS, Gambardella RA, Jobe FW: Revision surgery for failed elbow medial collateral ligament reconstruction. *Am J Sports Med* 2008;36(6):1061-1065.

A retrospective review of 15 patients who required a revision MCL reconstruction procedure found that the rate of return to sport was lower and the complication rate was higher than after the initial procedure. Level of evidence:IV.

[37] Lee GH, Limpisvasti O, Park MC, McGarry MH, Yocum LA, Lee TQ: Revision ulnar collateral ligament reconstruction using a suspension button fixation technique. *Am J Sports Med* 2010;38(3):575-580.

A cadaver biomechanical study found successful restoration of elbow kinematics using a suspension button fixation technique.

[38] Cain EL Jr, Andrews JR, Dugas JR, et al: Outcome of ulnar collateral ligament reconstruction of the elbow in 1281 athletes: Results in 743 athletes with minimum 2-year follow-up. *Am J Sports Med* 2010;38(12):2426-2434.

At a minimum follow-up of 2 years of 743 patients who underwent MCL reconstruction using a modified Jobe technique with subcutaneous ulnar nerve transposition, the rate of return to sport was 83%, the average time to competition was 11.6 months, and the rates of complications were 16% minor (mostly related to ulnar neuropathy) and 4% major. Level of evidence: IV.

[39] Smith GR, Altchek DW, Pagnani MJ, Keeley JR: A muscle-splitting approach to the ulnar collateral ligament of the elbow: Neuroanatomy and operative technique. *Am J Sports Med* 1996;24(5):575-580.

[40] Osbahr DC, Swaminathan SS, Allen AA, Dines JS, Coleman SH, Altchek DW: Combined flexor-pronator mass and ulnar collateral ligament injuries in the elbows of older baseball players. *Am J Sports Med* 2010;38(4):733-739.

A study of 187 baseball players age 14 to 42 years who had undergone MCL reconstruction found that 4% were treated for a combined flexor-pronator and MCL injury. These patients were older and had a poorer prognosis than other patients; their rate of return to sport was only 12.5%. Level of evidence: IV.

[41] Kerut EK, Kerut DG, Fleisig GS, Andrews JR: Prevention of arm injury in youth baseball pitchers. *J La State Med Soc* 2008;160(2):95-98.

Concern exists about the increasing number of injuries in youth baseball pitchers. The injury prevention recommendations of the USA Baseball Medical and Safety Advisory Committee are described.

[42] Dun S, Loftice J, Fleisig GS, Kingsley D, Andrews JR: A biomechanical comparison of youth baseball pitches: Is the curveball potentially harmful? *Am J Sports Med* 2008;36(4):686-692.

A three-dimensional motion analysis system was used during different types of pitches thrown by 29 youth baseball pitchers. The shoulder and elbow loads were greatest during the fastball pitch and least during the change-up. The type of pitch was found to affect the risk of injury less than the number of pitches.

[43] O'Driscoll SW, Morrey BF, Korinek S, An KN: Elbow subluxation and dislocation: A spectrum of instability. *Clin Orthop Relat Res* 1992;(280):186-197.

[44] Deutch SR, Jensen SL, Olsen BS, Sneppen O: Elbow joint stability in relation to forced external rotation: An experimental study of the osseous constraint. *J Shoulder Elbow Surg* 2003;12(3):287-292.

[45] Rhyou IH, Kim YS: New mechanism of the posterior elbow dislocation. *Knee Surg Sports Traumatol Arthrosc* 2012;20(12):2535-2541.

Soft-tissue injury after simple elbow dislocation is described, with the mechanisms of injury. Level of evidence: IV.

[46] Kalainov DM, Cohen MS: Posterolateral rotatory instability of the elbow in association with lateral epicondylitis: A report of three cases. *J Bone Joint Surg Am* 2005;87(5):1120-1125.

[47] O'Driscoll SW, Spinner RJ, McKee MD, et al: Tardy posterolateral rotatory instability of the elbow due to cubitus varus. *J Bone Joint Surg Am* 2001;83-A(9):1358-1369.

[48] Beuerlein MJ, Reid JT, Schemitsch EH, McKee MD: Effect of distal humeral varus deformity on strain in the lateral ulnar collateral ligament and ulnohumeral joint stability. *J Bone Joint Surg Am* 2004;86-A(10):2235-2242.

[49] Hall JA, McKee MD: Posterolateral rotatory instability of the elbow following radial head resection. *J Bone Joint Surg Am* 2005;87(7):1571-1579.

[50] Dunning CE, Zarzour ZD, Patterson SD, Johnson JA, King GJ: Ligamentous stabilizers against posterolateral

rotatory instability of the elbow. *J Bone Joint Surg Am* 2001;83-A(12):1823-1828.

［51］McAdams TR, Masters GW, Srivastava S: The effect of arthroscopic sectioning of the lateral ligament complex of the elbow on posterolateral rotatory stability. *J Shoulder Elbow Surg* 2005;14(3):298-301.

［52］Moritomo H, Murase T, Arimitsu S, Oka K, Yoshikawa H, Sugamoto K: The in vivo isometric point of the lateral ligament of the elbow. *J Bone Joint Surg Am* 2007;89(9):2011-2017.

　　The three-dimensional kinematics of the normal elbow were studied. The radial collateral ligament was found to be isometric, and the lateral collateral ligament was not. The isometric point for a graft origin was 2 mm proximal to the center of the capitellum.

［53］Goren D, Budoff JE, Hipp JA: Isometric placement of lateral ulnar collateral ligament reconstructions: A biomechanical study. *Am J Sports Med* 2010;38(1):153-159.

　　A cadaver study found that the isometric position for LUCL reconstruction on the humerus is between the 3-o'clock and 4:30 positions on the lateral epicondyle for the posterior distal wall of the tunnel.

［54］Rhyou IH, Park MJ: Dual reconstruction of the radial collateral ligament and lateral ulnar collateral ligament in posterolateral rotator instability of the elbow. *Knee Surg Sports Traumatol Arthrosc* 2011;19(6):1009-1012.

　　A dual reconstruction technique is described for LCLC reconstruction. Level of evidence: IV.

［55］O'Driscoll SW, Bell DF, Morrey BF: Posterolateral rotatory instability of the elbow. *J Bone Joint Surg Am* 1991;73(3):440-446.

［56］Lattanza LL, Chu T, Ty JM, et al: IntECRLinician and intraclinician variability in the mechanics of the pivot shift test for posterolateral rotatory instability (PLRI) of the elbow. *J Shoulder Elbow Surg* 2010;19(8):1150-1156.

　　Pivot-shift testing performed by three clinicians on five cadaver elbows was consistent and reproducible.

［57］Regan W, Lapner PC: Prospective evaluation of two diagnostic apprehension signs for posterolateral instability of the elbow. *J Shoulder Elbow Surg* 2006;15(3):344-346.

［58］Arvind CH, Hargreaves DG: Tabletop relocation test: A new clinical test for posterolateral rotatory instability of the elbow. *J Shoulder Elbow Surg* 2006;15(6):707-708.

［59］Teixeira AA, Buffani A, Tavares A, et al: Effects of fluvastatin on insulin resistance and cardiac morphology in hypertensive patients. *J Hum Hypertens* 2011;25(8):492-499.

　　The authors reported their technique and findings when imaging the LCLC in 10 cadaver elbows.

［60］Stewart B, Harish S, Oomen G, Wainman B, Popowich T, Moro JK: Sonography of the lateral ulnar collateral ligament of the elbow: Study of cadavers and healthy volunteers. *AJR Am J Roentgenol* 2009;193(6):1615-1619.

　　This effectiveness of ultrasonography was investigated for detecting LCLC in four cadaver elbows and subsequently in 35 healthy individuals. Level of evidence: IV.

［61］Faber KJ, King GJ: Posterior capitellum impression fracture: A case report associated with posterolateral rotatory instability of the elbow. *J Shoulder Elbow Surg* 1998;7(2):157-159.

［62］Rosenberg ZS, Blutreich SI, Schweitzer ME, Zember JS, Fillmore K: MRI features of a posterior capitellar impaction injuries. *AJR Am J Roentgenol* 2008;190(2):435-441.

　　The distinguishing features of posterior capitellar impression fracture and a pseudodefect of the capitellum are described. Level of evidence: IV.

［63］Jeon IH, Micic ID, Yamamoto N, Morrey BF: Osborne-Cotterill lesion: An osseous defect of the capitellum associated with instability of the elbow. *AJR Am J Roentgenol* 2008;191(3):727-729.

　　An association was proposed between the Osborne-Cotterill lesion and PLRI. Level of evidence: IV.

［64］Jeon IH, Min WK, Micic ID, Cho HS, Kim PT: Surgical treatment and clinical implication for posterolateral rotatory instability of the elbow: Osborne- Cotterill lesion of the elbow. *J Trauma* 2011;71(3): E45-E49.

　　A study of five patients with an Osborne-Cotterill lesion found that LCLC reconstruction may not be successful for such patients. Level of evidence: IV.

［65］Lee BP, Teo LH: Surgical reconstruction for posterolateral rotatory instability of the elbow. *J Shoulder Elbow Surg* 2003;12(5):476-479.

［66］Sanchez-Sotelo J, Morrey BF, O'Driscoll SW: Ligamentous repair and reconstruction for posterolateral rotatory instability of the elbow. *J Bone Joint Surg Br* 2005;87(1):54-61.

［67］Savoie FH III, O'Brien MJ, Field LD, Gurley DJ: Arthroscopic and open radial ulnohumeral ligament reconstruction for posterolateral rotatory instability of the elbow. *Clin Sports Med* 2010;29(4):611-618.

　　The authors' experience with open and arthroscopic

LCLC reconstruction was described. Level of evidence:Ⅴ.

［68］ Gong HS, Kim JK, Oh JH, Lee YH, Chung MS, Baek GH: A new technique for lateral ulnar collateral ligament reconstruction using the triceps tendon. *Tech Hand Up Extrem Surg* 2009;13(1):34-36.
A technique for LCLC reconstruction uses a portion of the triceps tendon. Level of evidence: Ⅴ.

［69］ Eygendaal D: Ligamentous reconstruction around the elbow using triceps tendon. *Acta Orthop Scand* 2004;75(5):516-523.

［70］ Lehman RC: Lateral elbow reconstruction using a new fixation technique. *Arthroscopy* 2005;21(4):503-505.

［71］ King GJ, Dunning CE, Zarzour ZD, Patterson SD, Johnson JA: Single-strand reconstruction of the lateral ulnar collateral ligament restores varus and posterolateral rotatory stability of the elbow. *J Shoulder Elbow Surg* 2002;11(1):60-64.

［72］ Jones KJ, Dodson CC, Osbahr DC, et al: The docking technique for lateral ulnar collateral ligament reconstruction: Surgical technique and clinical outcomes. *J Shoulder Elbow Surg* 2012;21(3):389-395.
The docking technique for LCLC reconstruction led to complete resolution in 75% of patients; 25% had occasional instability. Level of evidence: Ⅳ.

第四十二章　肘关节僵硬：发病机制、评估和开放治疗

Rudy Kovachevich, MD; Hill Hastings Ⅱ, MD

引言

上肢的功能很大程度上取决于肘关节对手部的定位能力。因此，肘关节活动障碍会严重影响日常生活。外伤、异位骨化、烧伤、神经麻痹、制动时间过长或术后瘢痕均可导致肘关节挛缩和僵硬。导致肘关节僵硬的原因有很多，这和肘关节的结构有关，关节腔内包含 3 个关节，且关节面、关节囊、囊内韧带和囊外肌肉之间的间距很小。[1]肘关节僵硬的病因可分为关节外、关节内及混合型病因[2]（表 42-1）。

病因学

肘关节僵硬的治疗效果和预后由其解剖结构和病理生理机制决定。肘关节周围的软组织结构，尤其是关节囊和侧副韧带在关节纤维化发展过程中发挥了重要作用。这种纤维化主要是结构和生化成分改变导致的软组织增厚、活动范围减小和组织容受性减低。[3]动物实验发现，兔僵硬的肘关节囊中转化生长因子－β（TGF-β）表达增加。[4]TGF-β 可能通过提高肌原纤维细胞水平、增加细胞外基质、提高胶原交联水平等使肘关节周围组织形成纤维瘢痕。[5-7]

Dr. Hastings or an immediate family member has received royalties from Biomet and serves as a paid consultant to or is an employee of Biomet. Neither Dr. Kovachevich nor any immediate family member has received anything of value from or has stock or stock options held in a commercial company or institution related directly or indirectly to the subject of this chapter.

表 42-1

肘关节僵硬的病因

类别	种类
外源性（关节外）	皮肤挛缩
	皮下组织挛缩
	关节囊挛缩
	内/外侧副韧带挛缩
	肌肉挛缩
	关节外骨折畸形愈合
	异位骨化
内源性（关节内）	关节对合不齐
	骨关节不匹配
	关节炎
	关节内粘连
	肢体松弛
	骨赘撞击
	鹰嘴、鹰嘴窝、冠突及冠突窝纤维化
混合性	同时存在内源性和外源性病因

异位骨化是指成熟的骨组织在非骨性部位的异常形成，可在遭受创伤等情况下导致肘关节僵硬。异位骨化必须和关节周围钙化相区分，关节周围钙化是未定型的钙沉积于软组织，通常发生在损伤后，但不一定影响关节活动。[8-9]异位骨化的原因尚不完全清楚，但它涉及多能间充质干细胞的成骨分化，因为它通常在外伤、手术或其他炎症状态之后出现。异位骨化骨在组织学上和天然骨大致相同，但它的代谢更活跃，且没有真正的骨膜层。

评估

肘关节僵硬的治疗极具挑战性，因此预防很重要。对于僵硬患者，应先进行非手术治疗，必要时可进行手术治疗。若要了解肘关节活动范围丢失的原因，需要完整病史、体格检查及影像学资料。应关注肘关节活动终末位置的抵抗，如果突然出现强有力的终末位置抵抗，表明存在骨性阻挡，若终末位置抵抗较弱，表明存在软组织挛缩。

在标准正侧位 X 线片中能够很好地查看冠突和肱桡关节的情况。观察屈曲状态的肘关节需要把正位片分成两部分，一部分垂直于肱骨，另一部分垂直于尺骨和桡骨。完全屈曲状态的侧位片对判断是否存在骨性阻挡很重要。透视检查可作为一种辅助手段来区分运动的骨性阻挡和单纯的软组织挛缩。医师可以通过先进的影像学检查，如二维或三维重建 CT，辨别关节内阻挡对活动范围的影响，进而制订相应的手术计划。通常不必应用 MRI。

治疗方法

肘关节僵硬的治疗目的是缓解疼痛、提高功能，以及维持关节稳定。僵硬发生后 3~6 个月可以进行非手术治疗，包括物理治疗、静态可调夹板、动态夹板、连续性适模固定和麻醉后关节被动活动。

如果患者非手术治疗失败，或体格检查、影像学检查证明存在典型的骨性阻挡，应该考虑进行手术治疗。手术适应证包括肘关节屈曲挛缩超过 30°或者不能屈曲到 130°。患者如果有较高的运动需求，希望获得更大的活动范围，可扩大适应证范围。

肘关节松解的先决条件包括充足的关节腔容量、手术部位足够的软组织覆盖、创伤后软组织炎症消退、异位骨化成熟以及患者术后有较好的康复锻炼依从性。关节对合不好、关节腔容量不足是松解手术的禁忌证，因为松解可能使疼痛加重，且对活动范围改善不明显。严重的创伤性关节炎可以行肘关节置换术，如半肘关节置换术和全肘关节置换术。

开放治疗

肘关节松解术已被证明是提高活动范围的有效措施，可通过切开手术或关节镜手术完成。关节镜下松解将在本书第四十六章和四十七章中讨论。切开松解手术通常采用超声引导下区域麻醉阻滞（留或不留置导管），或使用可提供术后镇痛和肌肉松弛的长效药物。

切开松解手术应该根据每个患者的具体情况进行，例如，患者存在屈曲受限、伸直受限，还是两者皆有。如果想要提高屈曲角度，则应该松解后侧挛缩的软组织（包括后方关节囊和肱三头肌伸肌）。应该切除前方限制屈曲的骨性结构，包括松质体、异位骨化和过度生长的冠突及填在冠突窝和桡骨头窝的瘢痕或骨块（图 42-1）。后内侧关节囊（尺侧副韧带后束）可能增厚或挛缩，松解后可以改善屈肘。提高肘关节伸直角度与之类似。在前方（例如，前外侧关节囊和肱二头肌附着点处）进行松解，后方的鹰嘴和鹰嘴窝间的软组织可通过鹰嘴部分切除和（或）鹰嘴窝清理术进行改善。

松解时需要特别注意尺神经。对于僵硬的肘关节，应重视屈曲时尺神经受到的拉力和压力。如果患者术前就有尺神经症状，如 Tinel 征、肘屈曲试验阳性或尺神经压迫试验阳性，则应通过前置或非前置尺神经的方法进行尺神经减压。

松解有多种手术方式。可选择限制性内外侧联合切口或单纯的后正中切口（能提供肘双侧的入路）。选择什么方法主要取决于术者习惯、以前切口的位置、神经减压需要及异位骨化的位置和量。如果最终需要置换肘关节，可能要做一个后侧切口。游离皮瓣所获得的内侧或外侧更深的暴露通常比内外侧联合切口更容易引起皮下血肿。无论什么方法，一定要在松解术中保护并避免损伤前臂内侧皮神经、正中神经以及尺侧、中间、桡侧、后部骨间神经。

深外侧入路，也被称为外侧副韧带保护入路或外侧柱入路，主要构建方法是在标准 Kocher 入路的近端做一个 6 cm 左右的切口[10-12]（图 42-2）。经外侧入路逐层切开，随后剥离肱三头肌和肘肌近端以显

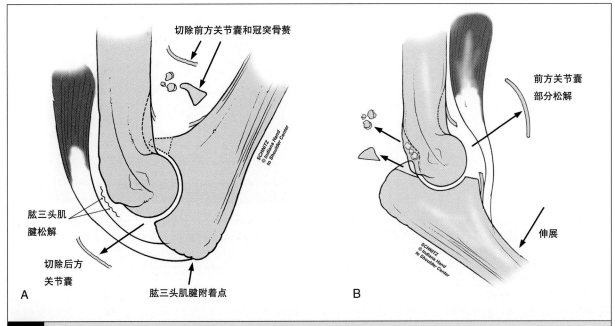

图
42-1 原理图展示了前方（A）和后方（B）关节囊切除术和异位骨化清除术 (© G. Schnitz, Indiana Hand to Shoulder Center, Indianapolis, IN.)

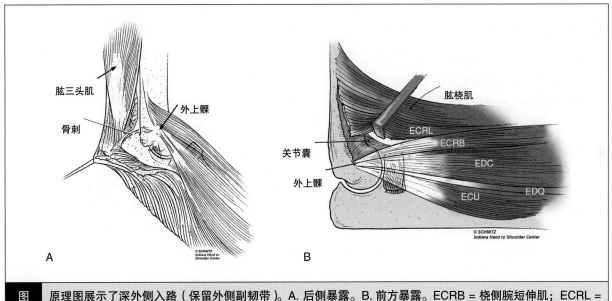

图
42-2 原理图展示了深外侧入路（保留外侧副韧带）。A. 后侧暴露。B. 前方暴露。ECRB = 桡侧腕短伸肌；ECRL = 桡侧腕长伸肌；ECU = 尺侧腕伸肌；EDC = 指总伸肌；EDQ = 小指固有伸肌（© G. Schnitz, Indiana Hand to Shoulder Center, Indianapolis, IN.）

露鹰嘴、鹰嘴窝及外侧肱尺关节。切除后侧关节囊及瘢痕，清除鹰嘴窝中的游离体、骨、瘢痕和肱骨、鹰嘴上可能存在的骨过度增长区域。可以切除从软组织近端外侧到肱桡关节的关节囊，以探查桡骨头和切除增生的滑囊。肱骨小头和外侧鹰嘴的任何可能影响肘关节伸直的骨化都应被去除（图42-3）。

前外侧入路，从肱骨髁上嵴向远端沿桡侧腕长伸肌和肱桡肌起点切开，远端在桡侧腕长伸肌和桡侧腕短伸肌之间分离 2~3 cm 至外上髁。这种远端延伸位有利于暴露及在必要时松解近端旋后肌，为骨间后神经减压。在这种情况下，冠突、鹰嘴和桡骨窝的异位骨化以及松质体均被切除。

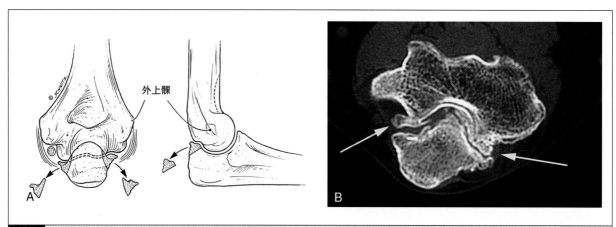

图 42-3　关节间隙异位骨化清除术。A. 原理图展示了鹰嘴内、外、后侧典型骨化形成。B.CT 展示了较大的鹰嘴内、外侧异位骨化（箭头）。(© G. Schnitz, Indiana Hand to Shoulder Center, Indianapolis, IN.)

恢复冠状窝和桡骨窝的容积，尤其是恢复其深度和宽度非常重要。向前臂近端施加压力，在直视下伸肘和屈肘。在长期的僵硬中，肱肌和肱三头肌通常发生了肌挛缩，可能限制肘部的终末位置的屈伸，在手术松解时可以对其进行拉伸。

外侧入路的优点包括操作相对简单，操作平面避开了浅表感觉神经，可以进入 3 个关节。但是，外侧入路也有其局限性，例如，无法处理后内侧关节囊和尺神经。对某些患者来说，要完全松解或单纯尺神经减压，可能需要再使用一个限制性内侧入路。这种方法通常需要做一个 3~5 cm 的后内侧切口，用于肘管原位松解。如果尺神经未移位，则通过尺神经后 1.5 cm 的内侧肱三头肌上的纵向切口暴露并清除后内侧鹰嘴残余骨化。

如果存在严重的病变需要尺神经向前移位，则选择概念上相似的内侧入路（Hotchkiss）。做一内侧或后侧切口以暴露屈肌 – 旋前肌起点（图42-4）。保护前臂内侧皮神经，松解并前移尺神经。将肱三头肌从肌间隔和肱骨向后游离，显露后内侧关节。松解后方关节囊及内侧副韧带后束，以保留并保护内侧副韧带较重要的前束。然后，可以进一步清理关节后部和鹰嘴窝。将屈肌起点纵向切开，前 2/3 从内髁分离。使肱肌和前屈肌群的前部从肱骨内侧分开从而露出前方关节囊。

切开关节囊，清理冠突和桡骨窝，切除冠突过度生长的部分。此时，可以进行被动屈肘和伸肘。

内侧入路的优点包括术后瘢痕不明显、尺神经更易暴露和减压以及可直接松解尺侧副韧带后束。但内侧入路不便于暴露常见的外侧骨化。因为内侧入路和外侧入路均存在局限性，所以对于异位骨化严重的患者，常需使用内外侧联合入路。如果患者存在机械性运动障碍（骨性阻挡），而非单纯的软组织挛缩，则肘关节松解的效果会更好。[13-14]

异位骨化

肘部异位骨化最常见于肘关节外伤、手术、烧伤和头部创伤后。它的发生与损伤的严重程度及损伤至手术之间的时间有部分相关性。有研究表明，3% 的简单肘关节脱位患者和 20% 的肘关节周围骨折脱位患者会产生异位骨化。[15] 而肘关节创伤合并颅脑损伤时，75%~89% 的患者发生异位骨化。[11]尽管肘关节的异位骨化始于创伤刺激，但在 2~12 周后才会出现相关症状和体征。最初的表现包括局部红肿热痛，随后肘关节活动范围逐步减小。初期异位骨化可能被误认为是围手术期感染，但其局部病变或扩散形式可能不遵循解剖组织平面。异位骨化患者屈肘终末或伸肘时疼痛较明显，这表明关节运动不协调。Hastings 和 Graham 的分级系统对制订

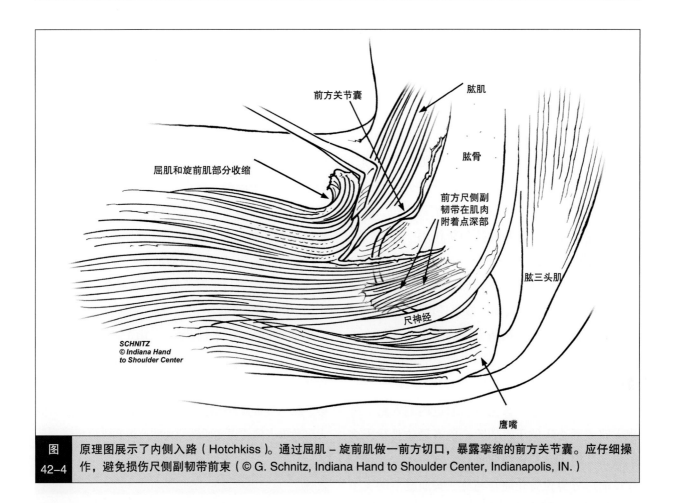

前方关节囊

肱肌

屈肌和旋前肌部分收缩

肱骨

前方尺侧副韧带在肌肉附着点深部

肱三头肌

尺神经

SCHNITZ
© Indiana Hand
to Shoulder Center

鹰嘴

图 42-4	原理图展示了内侧入路（Hotchkiss）。通过屈肌 - 旋前肌做一前方切口，暴露挛缩的前方关节囊。应仔细操作，避免损伤尺侧副韧带前束（© G. Schnitz, Indiana Hand to Shoulder Center, Indianapolis, IN.）

手术计划和治疗计划很有帮助[16]（表 42-2）。

表 42-2　异位骨化的分级

分级	特点
I	临床症状不明显，无肘关节活动范围减小
II	肘关节活动障碍
IIA	肘关节活动范围小于 100°，屈伸范围为 30°~130°
IIB	前臂旋转范围小于 100°
IIC	屈伸、旋转均受限
III	肘关节僵硬
IIIA	屈伸活动范围丧失
IIIB	旋转活动范围丧失
IIIC	屈伸和旋转活动范围均丧失

　　骨化成熟度和开始产生骨质的时间是评估异位骨化和考虑手术干预的重要因素。过去常采用实验室检查（血清钙、无机磷酸和碱性磷酸酶）和锝骨扫描追踪异位骨化的进展。这些检查的预后价值尚未得到证实，因此现在不再用于评估。[17-18]

X 线片是评估异位骨化及其进展的最有效手段。对于广泛异位骨化患者，CT 对于观察异位骨化的形状、评估肱尺关节的对合程度以及规划手术入路非常重要。在异位骨化发生的 4~6 周内，可以通过影像学检查发现不清晰的关节周围松质骨，随后其边缘愈发清晰，并出现骨小梁。异位骨化成熟的影像学定义是骨质边缘平滑、界限清楚，其通常在异位骨化出现 3~6 个月后才会出现。[8]大多数患者只要可以通过影像学明确异位骨化范围，就可以安全地进行手术切除，没有必要等到其完全成熟。早期手术治疗能够改善关节囊、韧带挛缩、肌肉萎缩和软骨变性，并且手术难度比后期干预更低。

　　因为没有有效的治疗用药，所以异位骨化的预防非常重要。以前常使用双膦酸盐进行预防，但后来有研究发现其只能延迟异位骨化的矿化。[11]现在常用的预防措施主要是 NSAIDs（如吲哚美辛、布洛芬、萘普生和阿司匹林）以及低剂量放疗。创伤发生后的 3~5 天内使用 NSAIDs 已被证明能够很好地发挥预防作用。其治疗持续时间目前还没有定论，从 5 天至 6 周不等。[19]这些药物通过抑制前列腺素的形成发挥预防作用，而且实验室研究发现，它们可以抑制干细胞的分化和迁移。低剂量放疗是通过有限场技术在手术或创伤后 72 小时内以 600~700 cGy 的单剂量给药。放疗通过抑制干细胞的分化发挥预防作用。[16]放疗、NSAIDs 或两者结合预防异位骨化已被证明是安全有效的，可在松解术后预防异位骨化。[16]但是，对于急性肘部创伤，其预防效果还没有得到证实。多项研究证实了这些预防方法的安全性，但由于骨折和鹰嘴截骨部位的骨不连概率的增高，[20-21]最近的一项相关前瞻性随机研究被中止。[22]

位于前方的异位骨化可以通过内侧入路、外侧入路或联合入路手术切除。前方异位骨化大多形成于肱肌下，似乎与前关节面被一个透光区隔开；而后方异位骨化通常与肱三头肌腱下的关节面连续形成。切除时必须注意识别和保护附近的桡神经、骨间后神经和正中神经。通常使用毛刺、刮匙、截骨刀和咬骨钳来切除骨头。由于后方骨与关节面的连续性，需要部分或完全剥离肱三头肌。尺神经可密切累及，必须注意和保护。由异位骨化导致的广泛活动受限不一定是一个负面的预后因素。最近的一项研究发现，完全强直性肘关节和部分活动受限肘关节的术后活动相当。[23]

治疗措施

如果患者的肘关节僵硬与关节不协调或关节炎有关，则不应进行肘关节松解术。对于这些患者，通常需要修复或更换受损的关节面，可以采用肘关节置换术，以恢复肘关节活动范围并减轻疼痛。肘关节置换术的目的是通过在肘关节骨折断端间放置表面重铺材料以改善和保持功能稳定性并防止再僵硬。已有多种材料被用于重塑肱尺关节，包

括自体或同种异体筋膜、跟腱、再生组织基质、牛胶原蛋白、可吸收明胶泡沫和硅树脂。肘关节不稳定的患者即使采用侧副韧带重建，松解术预后仍然较差。[24-25]对于这类患者，可以在术后使用铰链式外固定架，其可在保证功能锻炼的同时，为软组织愈合提供足够的稳定性。[26]外固定架在 69%~92% 的松解患者中取得了满意的效果。[24-25,27]但其可能有较严重的并发症，包括骨吸收、神经功能障碍、异位骨化、肱三头肌断裂、肘关节不稳定和感染。

对于年龄超过 60 岁且对活动范围要求较低的患者，可以考虑进行半肘关节置换术或全肘关节置换术。由于此类患者的骨储备、畸形和囊膜韧带不稳定，因此建议使用半限制性假体。[28]由于患者通常具有关节畸形，因此这类手术的难度较大，并且可能发生多种并发症，包括假体损坏、松动、伤口愈合不良、感染、肱三头肌破裂和骨折。[26]尽管存在上述问题，但大多数患者能获得实质性的功能改善和疼痛缓解。[27]

术后护理

对于接受肘关节松解的患者，已知多种有效的术后康复方案。其总体目标是保持功能性的活动范围，增强肘关节周围肌肉，使患肢重新融入日常功能活动。[1]术后早期就应开始进行活动范围锻炼，可以配合使用局部麻醉阻滞、进行持续被动运动以及使用静态运动夹板。局部麻醉阻滞对术后疼痛控制非常有用，并且可以促使患者早期开始进行活动范围锻炼。持续被动运动仍存在争议，尽管支持这种治疗方法的科学证据等级很低，但许多研究者还是推荐了这种治疗方法。最近的一项研究统计了 32 例肘关节切开松解患者进行持续被动运动的情况。[29]持续被动运动在 6 个月或最后的随访中对松解的术后效果没有明显的益处。与未进行此类功能锻炼的患者相比，两组肘关节屈伸活动范围在统计学上无明显差异（分别为 96° 和 101°）。

术后康复方案应持续进行 3~6 个月，直到运动达到平稳。如果患者仍然活动受限，则应在麻

醉下行屈伸活动范围及关节稳定性评估。最近的一项研究在松解术后平均 40 天，对 51 例患者进行了麻醉下肘关节屈伸活动范围检查，以评估是否出现骨性阻挡、关节不匹配等问题。[30]患者的活动范围平均改善了 36°，且无永久性并发症。麻醉下肘关节屈伸检查的目的是克服粘连和挛缩，从而改善去除外固定架的患者和松解术后最初几周活动范围提高有限的患者的肘部运动。

总结

肘关节对于整个上肢功能至关重要，其解剖结构和功能特点决定了其创伤后容易僵硬和挛缩。尽管仍有许多问题未能解决，但最近很多实验室研究和临床研究阐明了肘关节僵硬的病因和治疗选择。肘关节僵硬的预防至关重要。在考虑进行手术干预时，患者的主观需求至关重要，因为手术结果部分取决于患者的意愿及其进行术后康复的依从性。对于合适的患者，肘关节松解术可以显著提高其肘关节活动范围。

参考文献

[1] Modabber MR, Jupiter JB: Reconstruction for post-traumatic conditions of the elbow joint. *J Bone Joint Surg Am* 1995;77(9):1431-1446.

[2] Morrey BF: Post-traumatic contracture of the elbow: Operative treatment, including distraction arthroplasty. *J Bone Joint Surg Am* 1990;72(4):601-618.

[3] Cohen MS, Schimmel DR, Masuda K, Hastings H II, Muehleman C: Structural and biochemical evaluation of the elbow capsule after trauma. *J Shoulder Elbow Surg* 2007;16(4):484-490.

Contractures around the elbow, particularly capsular and ligamentous, play a critical role in the develop- ment of arthrofibrosis secondary to structural and bio- chemical alterations. Traumatic injury was found to lead to capsular thickening, collagen fiber disorganization, and increased cytokine levels.

[4] Hildebrand KA, Zhang M, Hart DA: Myofibroblast upregulators are elevated in joint capsules in posttrau-matic contractures. *Clin Orthop Relat Res* 2007;456:85-91.

Growth factor mRNA levels in joint capsules of pa-tients with posttraumatic elbow contracture were com-pared with those of organ donor control tissues. In-creased myofibroblast upregulator levels (transforming growth factor–β1, connective tissue growth factor, and α-smooth muscle actin) were found.

[5] Hildebrand KA, Zhang M, van Snellenberg W, King GJ, Hart DA: Myofibroblast numbers are elevated in human elbow capsules after trauma. *Clin Orthop Relat Res* 2004;419:189-197.

[6] Unterhauser FN, Bosch U, Zeichen J, Weiler A: Alpha-smooth muscle actin containing contractile fibroblastic cells in human knee arthrofibrosis tissue: Winner of the AGA-DonJoy Award 2003. *Arch Orthop Trauma Surg* 2004;124(9):585-591.

[7] Hildebrand KA, Zhang M, Hart DA: High rate of joint capsule matrix turnover in chronic human elbow contractures. *Clin Orthop Relat Res* 2005;439:228-234.

[8] Viola RW, Hastings H II: Treatment of ectopic ossification about the elbow. *Clin Orthop Relat Res* 2000;370:65-86.

[9] Summerfield SL, DiGiovanni C, Weiss AP: Heterotopic ossification of the elbow. *J Shoulder Elbow Surg* 1997;6(3):321-332.

[10] Cohen MS, Hastings H II: Post-traumatic contracture of the elbow: Operative release using a lateral collat-eral ligament sparing approach. *J Bone Joint Surg Br* 1998;80(5):805-812.

[11] Cohen MS, Hastings H II: Operative release for elbow contracture: The lateral collateral ligament sparing technique. *Orthop Clin North Am* 1999;30(1):133-139.

[12] Mansat P, Morrey BF: The column procedure: A lim-ited lateral approach for extrinsic contracture of the el-bow. *J Bone Joint Surg Am* 1998;80(11):1603-1615.

[13] Jupiter JB, O'Driscoll SW, Cohen MS: The assessment and management of the stiff elbow. *Instr Course Lect* 2003;52:93-111.

[14] Kasparyan NG, Hotchkiss RN: Dynamic skeletal fixation in the upper extremity. *Hand Clin* 1997;13(4):643-663.

[15] Thompson HC III, Garcia A: Myositis ossificans: Aftermath of elbow injuries. *Clin Orthop Relat Res* 1967;50:129-134.

[16] Hastings H II, Graham TJ: The classification and treatment of heterotopic ossification about the elbow and forearm. *Hand Clin* 1994;10(3):417-437.

[17] Lindenhovius AL, Linzel DS, Doornberg JN, Ring DC, Jupiter JB: Comparison of elbow contracture release in elbows with and without heterotopic ossification restricting motion. *J Shoulder Elbow Surg* 2007;16(5):621-625.

Sixteen patients with elbow contracture and posttraumatic heterotopic ossification were compared with 21 patients with capsular contracture alone. The average flexion-extension arc for contractures with associated heterotopic bone was 116° compared with 98° for capsular contracture alone. Level of evidence: III.

[18] Park MJ, Kim HG, Lee JY: Surgical treatment of posttraumatic stiffness of the elbow. *J Bone Joint Surg Br* 2004;86(8):1158-1162.

[19] McAuliffe JA, Wolfson AH: Early excision of heterotopic ossification about the elbow followed by radiation therapy. *J Bone Joint Surg Am* 1997;79(5):749-755.

[20] Ellerin BE, Helfet D, Parikh S, et al: Current therapy in the management of heterotopic ossification of the elbow: A review with case studies. *Am J Phys Med Rehabil* 1999;78(3):259-271.

[21] Strauss JB, Wysocki RW, Shah A, et al: Radiation therapy for heterotopic ossification prophylaxis afer high- risk elbow surgery. *Am J Orthop (Belle Mead NJ)*2011;40(8):400-405.

A retrospective study analyzed the outcomes of prophylactic single-fraction radiotherapy and NSAID use for preventing heterotopic ossification in high-risk elbow surgery. At a mean 136-day follow-up, radiographic heterotopic ossification that was small and not functionally significant had developed in 48% of the patients. No complications were noted. Level of evidence: IV.

[22] Hamid N, Ashraf N, Bosse MJ, et al: Radiation ther- apy for heterotopic ossification prophylaxis acutely af- ter elbow trauma: A prospective randomized study. *J Bone Joint Surg Am* 2010;92(11):2032-2038.

A multicenter prospective randomized study compared prophylactic radiotherapy with no treatment after intraarticular distal humerus or elbow fracture- dislocation. The study was terminated early because of the high nonunion rate in the treated patients (38%) versus the control group patients (4%).

[23] Brouwer KM, Lindenhovius AL, de Witte PB, Jupiter JB, Ring D: Resection of heterotopic ossification of the elbow: A comparison of ankylosis and partial restriction. *J Hand Surg Am* 2010;35(7):1115-1119.

Eighteen patients with surgical release of complete elbow ankylosis were compared with 27 matched patients with partial restriction of motion by heterotopic bone. At an average 22-month follow-up, range of motion and outcomes scores were similar. Level of evidence: III.

[24] Larson AN, Morrey BF: Interposition arthroplasty with an Achilles tendon allograft as a salvage procedure for the elbow. *J Bone Joint Surg Am* 2008;90(12):2714-2723.

Thirty-four elbows were evaluated at a mean 6-year follow-up after interposition arthroplasty for treatment of inflammatory or posttraumatic elbow arthritis. Patients with preoperative instability had a poor result. Thirteen patients had a good or excellent result, 14 had a fair result, and 11 had a poor result. Seven underwent revision. Level of evidence: IV.

[25] Cheng SL, Morrey BF: Treatment of the mobile, painful arthritic elbow by distraction interposition arthroplasty. *J Bone Joint Surg Br* 2000;82(2):233-238.

[26] Ring D, Jupiter JB: Operative release of complete ankylosis of the elbow due to heterotopic bone in patients without severe injury of the central nervous system. *J Bone Joint Surg Am* 2003;85(5):849-857.

[27] Nolla J, Ring D, Lozano-Calderon S, Jupiter JB: Interposition arthroplasty of the elbow with hinged external fixation for post-traumatic arthritis. *J Shoulder Elbow Surg* 2008;17(3):459-464.

In a review of 13 patients with posttraumatic elbow arthritis treated with interposition arthroplasty and hinged external fixation, 2 patients had early instability. The remaining 11 were followed for a mean of 4 years. Mean range of motion improved 48° to 110°, with five good or excellent, four fair, and four poor results. The poor results were secondary to severe postoperative instability. Level of evidence: IV.

[28] Mansat P, Morrey BF: Semiconstrained total elbow arthroplasty for ankylosed and stiff elbows. *J Bone Joint Surg Am* 2000;82(9):1260-1268.

[29] Lindenhovius AL, van de Luijtgaarden K, Ring D, Jupiter J: Open elbow contracture release: Postoperative management with and without continuous passive motion. *J Hand Surg Am* 2009;34(5):858-865.

A retrospective study compared 16 patients who received continuous passive motion after open elbow contracture release with 16 patients who did not use continuous passive motion. At an average 6-month follow-up, there was no difference in range of motion or other benefits. Level of evidence: III.

[30] Araghi A, Celli A, Adams RA, Morrey BF: The outcome of examination (manipulation) under anesthesia on the stiff elbow after surgical contracture release. *J Shoulder Elbow Surg* 2010;19(2):202-208.

In 51 patients who underwent elbow examination under anesthesia a mean 40 days after open elbow contracture release, the range-of-motion arc improved an average of 38°, with 44 patients showing improvement, 3 with no change, and 1 with loss of motion. Level of evidence: IV.

第四十三章　肘关节炎

Julie Adams, MD; Scott P. Steinmann, MD

引言

　　肘关节炎的治疗仍然极具挑战性。类风湿关节炎和其他炎症性关节炎是最常见的需经手术治疗的关节炎。由于控制这类疾病的抗风湿药物的出现和广泛应用，多数患者的关节损坏已明显减轻，所以针对这类疾病的手术治疗越来越少。但是，骨关节炎和创伤后关节炎在治疗上仍然存在一些问题。血友病患者也会继发肘关节炎。虽然血液成分置换疗法明显提高了血友病患者的寿命，但是肘部持续的亚临床或临床出血可能引起关节病变。

　　肘关节炎流行病学的改变引发了一个难题。之前，多数需手术治疗的伴肘关节病变的类风湿关节炎患者的年龄较大，对术后肘关节运动功能的恢复要求较低。如今，很多肘关节炎患者相对

Dr. Adams or an immediate family member has received royalties from DePuy; serves as a paid consultant to or is an employee of Arthrex, DePuy, and Articulinx; serves as an unpaid consultant to Synthes; and serves as a board member, owner, officer, or committee member of the American Association for Hand Surgery, the Minnesota Orthopaedic Society, the American Shoulder and Elbow Surgeons, the American Society for Surgery of the Hand, and the Arthroscopy Association of North America. Dr. Steinmann or an immediate family member has received royalties from DePuy; serves as a paid consultant to or is an employee of Arthrex, DePuy, and Articulinx; serves as an unpaid consultant to Synthes; and serves as a board member, owner, officer, or committee member of the American Association for Hand Surgery, the Minnesota Orthopaedic Society, the American Shoulder and Elbow Surgeons, the American Society for Surgery of the Hand, and the Arthroscopy Association of North America.

年轻，对术后肘关节运动功能要求更高。这些患者不能接受全肘关节置换（TEA）带来的局限性。既往治疗类风湿关节炎的肘关节假体的活动范围较小，对要求较高的患者可能不是最佳选择。最近，已有研究者开始研究适用于这类患者的替代手术方案或替代假体。

非手术治疗

　　肘关节炎的非手术治疗包括休息、支持疗法、使用非甾体抗炎药或口服镇痛药以及注射皮质类固醇或透明质酸。其中，向肘关节注射透明质酸6个月之后患者未见明显获益。[1]与其他关节内注射一样，注射透明质酸获得的短期疗效可能仅因为其抗炎作用。

　　在过去的几十年中，疾病干预措施改变着类风湿关节炎的治疗状况。以前联合应用非甾体抗炎药和镇痛药以减轻症状。如今，干预疾病进程的抗风湿药物使疾病治疗有所改变。这些药物能有效减轻滑膜炎和全身炎症，改变关节损害的进程。通常，在确诊关节炎后应尽快单独或联合应用甲氨蝶呤、磺胺嘧啶和来氟米特。糖皮质激素能在短期内改善关节炎症，或作为长期辅助用药。最近，生物制剂的引入改变了类风湿关节炎的炎症级联，其通过靶向细胞因子加强疾病治疗，彻底改变了这种疾病的治疗状况。生物制剂包括肿瘤坏死因子抑制剂（如阿达木单抗、伊那西普、英夫利昔单抗、赛妥珠单抗、戈利木单抗）、白介

素 –6 抑制剂（如托珠单抗）、B 细胞抑制剂（如利妥昔单抗）以及 T 细胞协同刺激抑制剂（如阿巴西普）。这些药物可以改变患者对感染产生免疫反应的能力。但是，需要关注免疫原性的长远影响、潜在病毒感染以及恶性肿瘤发生的风险。为了促进手术愈合，大多数专家建议在原计划手术前几个半衰期时间停用这些生物制剂。[2]

血友病性关节炎患者可通过按需预防性补充血液因子的方法来降低肘关节内出血的频率和严重程度。这种治疗可能长期控制滑膜炎和关节损害的进程，并使症状短期缓解。[3]

肘关节退行性骨关节炎主要发生于有体力劳动史的男性。使用拐杖行走或使用轮椅也增加了原发性退行性肘关节炎的风险。大多数患者的发病年龄在 40 岁以上，并具有机械症状，包括关节交锁、有症状的游离体及运动受限，特别是在伸肘终末时。患者通常在运动弧的终末出现疼痛，疾病晚期疼痛则会遍布运动弧，这表明发生了严重的关节病变，这种情况无法通过简单的关节内清除术进行治疗。

评估

肘关节炎患者通常会伴有肘管综合征。对于这种患者，仔细询问症状、对患者进行详细的体格检查非常重要。患者的症状有时与神经相关，而没有明显的影像学证据。肘关节三位（正位、侧位、斜位）平片有助于诊断。骨性解剖和软骨下囊肿可在 CT 图像中显示。CT 三维重建有助于理解三维解剖结构，制订手术计划，选择治疗区域。

手术选择

对于非手术治疗失败后功能受限的患者，可以考虑手术干预。决定是否手术治疗的因素包括患者的活动水平、年龄和期望值，外科医师的经验和习惯，以及病理变化的程度。

开放手术、关节镜清除术和滑膜切除术是类

风湿关节炎、骨关节炎、创伤后关节炎和血友病性关节炎的有效治疗方法。这些手术在疾病早期阶段最有效，即在关节间隙和软骨完全消失之前。滑膜切除术可以延缓疾病的进展，并减少炎症性关节炎或血友病症状性出血发作中疼痛性滑膜炎的发生。关节镜下清除术因为微创、恢复期短、痛苦少，所以被认为是理想的治疗手段。然而，肘关节镜手术的预后与开放手术的预后相比无明显优势，并且关节镜手术的风险可能大于传统的开放手术。如果外科医师缺乏关节镜经验，患者运动受限严重或需要进行开放手术（尽管有证据表明某些患者可以通过关节镜对尺神经减压），则应首选开放手术。[4-5]

开放松解术的入路包括内侧切口、外侧切口和联合切口，具体取决于病变情况和外科医师的习惯。可以使用单个后侧切口，在内侧和外侧留存全层皮瓣。该方法所需要的切口较大，可能导致血肿或伤口并发症。

TEA 是改善肘关节炎疼痛和功能的重要手段。但是，TEA 后手臂只能进行轻度活动，这对年轻或活动需求较高的患者来说很不适合。因此，TEA 不能应用于这类患者。

目前研究者正在探索其他减轻疼痛、保持手臂功能的治疗手段，有研究者建议采用内固定关节置换术。多种材料已被用于这种手术，包括同种异体移植物以及自体真皮、跟腱和筋膜。一项对肘关节成形术平均 6 年的随访研究报道，45 例患者中有 32 例后续需要翻修手术或预后很差。[6]术前稳定性与预后相关。这项研究论述了几种关节置换术的成功因素，包括保留肘关节稳定性、保持相对良好的骨解剖结构、术中关节充分松解、牢固的关节面重建以及细致的伤口缝合和处理。[7]患者应了解这类手术的目标是改善运动和减轻疼痛，但不能有太高的期望值。

半肘关节置换术和全肘关节置换术

某些患者可考虑行半肘关节置换术（图 43–1）。

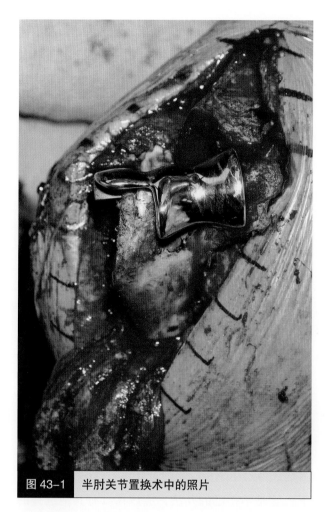

图 43-1 半肘关节置换术中的照片

大多数已发表的文献都是针对单例患者或小型研究的。但是，随着这项技术热度的升高，最近有许多新的研究结果即将产生。半肘关节置换术的适应证包括希望保持关节活动范围并保留肱骨、尺骨的类风湿关节炎患者，肱骨远端骨折无法重建且保留了尺骨关节的患者，以及肱骨远端骨折骨不连或内固定失败的患者。一项使用 Kudo 肱骨假体（Biomet）治疗 4 例无法重建的肱骨远端骨折患者（平均年龄为 80 岁）的研究显示，这种半肘关节置换术的早期结果很好。[8] 在一项对半肘关节置换患者评价随访 4 年的研究中，8 例女性患者（平均年龄为 79 岁）的 Mayo 肘关节功能评分为优秀或良好，一例患者在术后 3 年出现了假体周围骨折，另一例患者肘关节活动范围较小。[9] X 线片显示这些患者尺骨关节发生了炎症性改变，但这与关节功能并不相关。一项对 10 例

肱骨远端粉碎性骨折行半肘关节置换的女性患者（平均年龄为 75 岁）的研究显示，在 1 年的随访中，有 9 例患者的 Mayo 肘关节功能评分由良转为优，这些患者一共出现了 5 种并发症，其中大多数程度较轻，包括短暂的尺神经刺激、异位骨化和尺骨关节炎。[10] 此外，在半肘关节置换术中，没有尺骨组件的肱骨假体尚未获得 FDA 的批准。

部分肘关节炎患者采用了外侧的半肘关节置换术（图 43-2）。这种手术可用于 Essex-Lopresti 损伤、桡骨头骨折伴关节嵌插以及肱骨小头剪切损伤的患者。[11] 发生 Essex-Lopresti 损伤后，肱骨小头软骨可能无法承受桡骨颈手术带来的影响，因此可换用人工关节。但关于应用此类手术的报道很少。[11-12]

可转换假体最近成功问世。这种假体可以把肱骨远端半肘关节置换术转换为非铰链型或铰链型 TEA，而无须去除肱骨组件。对这种方法的研究较少，但已有针对非铰链型 TEA 翻修的研究发表。[12] 该研究显示，将半肘关节置换假体翻修为铰链型假体的效果优于翻修为非铰链型假体，且初次手术使用铰链型假体时，翻修成功率更高。但是，该研究所用假体并非当前使用的最新型的假体。[12-13]

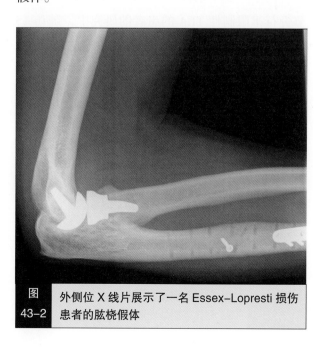

图 43-2 外侧位 X 线片展示了一名 Essex-Lopresti 损伤患者的肱桡假体

对于能够严格限制手臂活动的患者，铰链型TEA是可接受的选择（图43-3）。对于年轻的患者，必须预见到假体需要翻修的可能，并且所有患者都必须认识到手术相关并发症的发生率较高。[14-15]

对TEA并发症的研究主要基于美国加利福尼亚州出院数据库中的患者。[16]已有研究报道，在TEA术后，10%的患者因短期并发症需要住院治疗，8%的患者植入假体后的90天内需要再次手术。在一项平均4年的随访中，170例患者中有120例接受了翻修、截肢或肘关节融合术。这些患者中有48例在12个月内行翻修术。这些研究结果表明，行全肘关节置换术应谨慎。尽管如此，最近美国纽约州的一项研究报道TEA的使用在逐步增长。[17]1997—2006年，TEA在创伤患者中的应用有所增加，而在炎症性关节炎患者中的使用则大大减少。在术后的90天内，有5.6%的患者因假体并发症而需要再次入院。其中骨关节炎患者的翻修率（14.7%）高于创伤患者（4.8%）和炎症性关节炎患者（8.3%）。患者多是因为发生感染、套管失效、骨折或无菌松动等情况进行翻修。铰链型（半限制）假体失效可能与假体的固定要求高有关，其中，创伤后关节炎或骨关节炎患者的手术要求最高。[18]在一项对因创伤后关节炎行半限制性TEA的患者的研究中，随访15年后发现成功率为70%；在失败的TEA病例中，

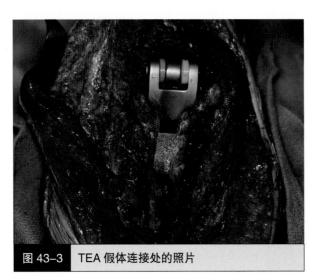

图43-3　TEA假体连接处的照片

65%为60岁以下的患者。使用无铰链型假体有可能提高肘关节置换假体的耐久性，但仍需进一步研究证明。[13,19]

肘关节融合术

如果骨关节炎患者不适宜行关节置换术，或者肘关节置换术失败后需行补救治疗，则可以选择肘关节融合术。现有研究病例数均较少。肘关节融合术会造成很大的功能局限性，一些研究者认为肘关节融合不存在合适的固定位置。预先制订计划、铸型模拟可能的融合位置、帮助患者选择能够发挥最佳功能的固定位置，这样进行的选择性肘关节融合术通常是可行的。患者必须在手臂的功能定位方面做出选择，是要保有进行手臂一般活动的功能还是要能够将手放在嘴上的能力。一位经验丰富的外科医师在对急性创伤或创伤后关节炎患者进行肘关节融合的研究时发现，在12例患者中，有10例需要进行额外手术，其中42%的患者肘关节不愈合或延迟愈合，并且33%的患者肘关节发生感染。该研究指出："在大多数情况下，这是不得已的办法，应该在没有其他选择的情况下执行。"[20]

总结

肘关节炎的治疗具有挑战性。尽管治疗技术飞速发展，但是许多手术仍是以牺牲关节的稳定性或功能为代价来减轻疼痛的。仔细考虑每例患者的特异性和疾病的特异性因素对成功治疗肘关节炎至关重要。

参考文献

[1] van Brakel RW, Eygendaal D: Intra-articular injection of hyaluronic acid is not effective for the treatment of post-traumatic osteoarthritis of the elbow. *Arthroscopy* 2006;22(11):1199-1203.

[2] Scott DL: Biologics-based therapy for the treatment of rheumatoid arthritis. *Clin Pharmacol Ther* 2012;91(1):30-43.

The medical treatment options for rheumatoid arthritis were reviewed, including an overview of current therapies and recent advances in treatment.

[3] Adams JE, Reding MT: Hemophilic arthropathy of the elbow. *Hand Clin* 2011;27(2):151-163, v.
Nonsurgical and surgical experience at a large center was described for treatment of the elbow in patients with hemophilia.

[4] Kovachevich R, Steinmann SP: Arthroscopic ulnar nerve decompression in the setting of elbow osteoarthritis. *J Hand Surg Am* 2012;37(4):663-668.
Outcomes were described for arthroscopic ulnar nerve decompression in patients with elbow arthritis. This technique, although technically challenging, was effective for treating symptomatic ulnar neuritis.

[5] Adams JE, Wolff LH III, Merten SM, Steinmann SP: Osteoarthritis of the elbow: Results of arthroscopic osteophyte resection and capsulectomy. *J Shoulder Elbow Surg* 2008;17(1):126-131.
Outcomes were described for elbow arthroscopy in patients with primary osteoarthritis of the elbow. Improvement in range of motion and pain was noted, with a low complication rate.

[6] Larson AN, Morrey BF: Interposition arthroplasty with an Achilles tendon allograft as a salvage procedure for the elbow. *J Bone Joint Surg Am* 2008;90(12):2714-2723.
At a mean 6-year follow-up of interposition arthroplasty with Achilles tendon allograft in 45 elbows with posttraumatic or inflammatory arthritis, the average arc of motion had increased from 51° to 97° in surviving implants. Seven patients (15.5%) required revision surgery; 11 of the remaining patients (29%) had a poor result, and 14 (37%) had a fair result. Preoperative instability should be an exclusion criterion.

[7] Chen DD, Forsh DA, Hausman MR: Elbow interposition arthroplasty. *Hand Clin* 2011;27(2):187-197, vi.
Interposition arthroplasty of the elbow with a biologic material was described, with tips and techniques for the procedure as well as a discussion of patient selection factors.

[8] Adolfsson L, Hammer R: Elbow hemiarthroplasty for acute reconstruction of intra-articular distal humerus fractures: A preliminary report involving 4 patients. *Acta Orthop* 2006;77(5):785-787.

[9] Adolfsson L, Nestorson J: The Kudo humeral component as primary hemiarthroplasty in distal humeral fractures. *J Shoulder Elbow Surg* 2012;21(4):451-455.
Eight women were treated with elbow hemiarthroplasty for distal humerus fracture. At a mean 4-year follow-up, all patients had a good or excellent outcome with an average range of motion of 31° to 126°. Radiographic changes occurred in the ulna but were not correlated with symptoms.

[10] Burkhart KJ, Nijs S, Mattyasovszky SG, et al: Distal humerus hemiarthroplasty of the elbow for comminuted distal humeral fractures in the elderly patient. *J Trauma* 2011;71(3):635-642.
Satisfactory short-term outcomes were described for hemiarthroplasty in 10 elderly women to treat osteoporotic or unreconstructable distal humerus fracture or failed fixation. Complications frequently occurred.

[11] Heijink A, Morrey BF, Cooney WP III: Radiocapitellar hemiarthroplasty for radiocapitellar arthritis: A report of three cases. *J Shoulder Elbow Surg* 2008;17(2):e12-e15.
Radiocapitellar replacement arthroplasty was performed in three patients, with an acceptable complication rate.

[12] Steinmann SP: Hemiarthroplasty of the ulnohumeral and radiocapitellar joints. *Hand Clin* 2011;27(2):229-232, vi.
The author's experience with hemiarthroplasty of the distal humerus and the radiocapitellar joint was described, with a literature review and discussion of the available evidence.

[13] Levy JC, Loeb M, Chuinard C, Adams RA, Morrey BF: Effectiveness of revision following linked versus unlinked total elbow arthroplasty. *J Shoulder Elbow Surg* 2009;18(3):457-462.
The outcomes of unlinked and linked arthroplasty were compared. Primary linked arthroplasty implants had longer survival than unlinked implants, but the unlinked implants were mostly of older designs.

[14] Celli A, Morrey BF: Total elbow arthroplasty in patients forty years of age or less. *J Bone Joint Surg Am* 2009;91(6):1414-1418.
At 7-year follow-up, a 22% revision rate was found in young patients undergoing TEA for posttraumatic or inflammatory arthritis. Those with posttraumatic arthritis had a poorer result than those with inflammatory arthritis.

[15] Leclerc A, King GJ: Unlinked and convertible total elbow arthroplasty. *Hand Clin* 2011;27(2):215-227, vi.

The indications and techniques for linked and un- linked arthroplasty were described.

[16] Krenek L, Farng E, Zingmond D, SooHoo NF: Complication and revision rates following total elbow arthroplasty. *J Hand Surg Am* 2011;36(1):68-73.

A comprehensive look at complication and revision rates after TEA was provided in this study of a statewide database.

[17] Gay DM, Lyman S, Do H, Hotchkiss RN, Marx RG, Daluiski A: Indications and reoperation rates for total elbow arthroplasty: An analysis of trends in New York State. *J Bone Joint Surg Am* 2012;94(2):110-117.

An analysis of TEA performed in New York state suggested increasing use for patients with trauma or osteoarthritis and decreasing use for those with inflammatory arthritis. Complication and revision rates were high.

[18] Throckmorton T, Zarkadas P, Sanchez-Sotelo J, Morrey B: Failure patterns after linked semiconstrained total elbow arthroplasty for posttraumatic arthritis. *J Bone Joint Surg Am* 2010;92(6):1432-1441.

TEA with a semiconstrained device was studied in patients with posttraumatic arthritis. The revision rate was high, and revisions were more common in patients younger than 60 years, probably because they placed relatively high demands on the arm. The 15-year survival rate was 70%.

[19] Ring D, Kocher M, Koris M, Thornhill TS: Revision of unstable capitellocondylar (unlinked) total elbow replacement. *J Bone Joint Surg Am* 2005;87(5):1075-1079.

[20] Reichel LM, Wiater BP, Friedrich J, Hanel DP: Arthrodesis of the elbow. *Hand Clin* 2011;27(2):179-186, vi.

The results and complications of elbow arthrodesis were discussed.

第四十四章 桡骨头骨折、桡骨颈骨折

Albert Yoon, MBChB; Graham J.W. King, MD, MSc, FRCSC

引言

桡骨头骨折和桡骨颈骨折是肘部骨折最常见的类型，每年发病率为 55.4/10 万。桡骨头骨折比桡骨颈骨折更为常见。尽管较早的研究发现桡骨骨折在男性中更为常见，但最新的流行病学研究发现，桡骨骨折的发病率基本无性别差异（男女比例为 3：2）。[1-2] 以往的研究称桡骨头骨折患者的平均年龄为 30~40 岁，但最近的研究认为平均年龄为 43~48 岁。[1-2]

无移位的桡骨头骨折和桡骨颈骨折可以进行非手术治疗，但桡骨头及桡骨颈的移位和粉碎性骨折的治疗尚存争议。目前已有大量关于不同治疗方案的长期预后的研究正在运行，将来的随机对照研究可能进一步指导患者治疗。

解剖和生物机制

桡骨头近端凹陷的关节面为椭圆形，在此处

与凸起的肱骨形成肱桡关节，在桡骨头的边缘处，稍扁平的部分与较小的乙状凹接合而形成近端的桡尺关节。桡骨头的非圆形解剖结构以及桡骨头相对于桡骨颈的可变偏移意味着在旋转过程中两个关节都会发生少量平移。[3-5] 在桡骨头骨折修复或置换术中需要考虑这些解剖特征。金属内固定物应放置在桡骨头较圆的非关节边缘上，即安全区，其大致为在前臂旋转中立位的以桡骨头前外侧 10° 为中心的 110° 圆弧。[6]

桡骨头有助于维持肘关节的内外翻和后外侧旋转稳定性，在存在相关肘部损伤的情况下，其作用更明显。此外，桡骨头还是前臂的轴向稳定器。切除桡骨头骨折碎片会降低桡骨头维持稳定的能力，而全部切除会将正常的肱桡关节负荷转移到剩余的肱尺关节。[7-8]

桡骨头的主要骨外供血是由桡侧返动脉（供应掌侧、外侧和背侧）及尺动脉分支在桡骨颈周围形成的颈周动脉环提供的。顺行血管塑形技术表明，使用钢板内固定比单独使用螺钉更容易损坏这种血供。[9]

与其他骨骼一样，桡骨头的微结构也会经历与年龄和性别相关的变化。[10] 骨质疏松症可能是造成女性和 50 岁以上患者的比例较高，以及由性别导致的损伤机制和严重程度差异的原因。桡骨头骨折的女性患者的平均年龄为 52 岁，其中 73% 由单纯跌倒导致。[1-2] 这些人群因素意味着桡骨头骨折符合脆性骨折的标准，因此对骨质疏松症的调查和管理也很重要。而桡骨头损伤的男性患者中有 60% 具有高能量损伤机制，并且该损伤发生在较年轻的年龄（平均 40 岁）。[1-2]

评估

患者病史应包括损伤机制、涉及的能量水平及并发损伤的可能性。应询问患者肩部或腕部是否疼痛，以及受伤时肘关节脱位或半脱位的感觉。应通过病史和体格检查来评估神经血管损伤的可能性。由于疼痛，在早期很难进行肘部的稳定性测试。肘部骨突出和侧副韧带标志的触诊可提供与相关损伤有关的线索。对前臂运动范围的评估很重要，可指导移位或无移位的桡骨头骨折的治疗。如果肘部不能进行完全旋转运动，那么应确定这是由关节内血肿导致的还是由机械性阻滞导致的。可以在 1 周内重新评估或在注射局部麻醉药的情况下吸出关节内血肿，可以检查是否有弹响、骨擦音和骨性阻挡。

普通 X 线片可用于评估桡骨头或桡骨颈骨折。如有前方或后方脂肪垫征应高度怀疑未移位的骨折。根据患者的病史和体格检查的结果，可能需要进行肩部、前臂和腕部 X 线检查。与普通的 X 线检查相比，CT 可以更准确地发现骨折特征和并发的骨损伤，而 MRI 可用于检查相关的韧带损伤。[11-12] 尚未证明 MRI 对治疗其他方面有帮助，所以常规不需要进行 MRI 检查。[13]

分型

尽管引入了 CT 和三维重建技术，但对于桡骨头骨折的分类，研究者依然不能达成共识。Mason 在 1954 年描述了 3 种类型的桡骨头骨折。[14] I 型骨折是无移位的边缘骨折，II 型骨折是有移位的边缘骨折，III 型骨折是包括整个桡骨头的粉碎性骨折。Johnston 在 1962 年将桡骨头骨折合并肘关节脱位定义为 IV 型骨折。[15] 但 IV 型骨折并不是对桡骨头本身所造成的损伤进行的分类。Broberg 和

Morrey 修改了原始的 Mason 分型，定义 II 型骨折移位超过 2 mm 并累及关节表面 30%，以此来阐明 I 型和 II 型之间的区别。[16] 桡骨颈骨折的分型也包含在这种修改中。在进一步的修改中（Mayo-Mason 分类），这种分型用于表示相关的骨、韧带或脱位损伤。[17]

相关损伤

相关损伤可能与患者年龄、受伤机制和骨折复杂性有关。[1] 最近的一项研究发现，在 46 例桡骨头骨折患者中，有 35 例（76%）MRI 提示存在相关损伤。[12] 全部 6 例 Mason III 型桡骨头骨折 [6 例外侧副韧带（LCL）损伤，1 例内侧副韧带（MCL）损伤和 2 例肱骨小头损伤]、23 例 Mason II 型骨折中的 17 例和 17 例 Mason I 型骨折中的 12 例存在相关损伤，其中以 LCL 损伤和肱骨小头损伤最常见。尽管这些相关损伤很重要，但并不会改变治疗策略，需要手术干预的情况通常可以在术中发现。[13] 尽管肱骨小头软骨损伤的概率随着桡骨头骨折的移位程度的增高而增高，但其通常不如移位较少的骨折的软骨损伤严重。[18] 在 Mason I 型和 II 型骨折的桡骨头碎片间发现的肱骨小头软骨碎片，可能限制前臂旋转。[18-19] 在 Mason II 型骨折中，骨折碎片的皮质接触完全丧失预示了可能存在相关的肘部骨折或韧带损伤。[20] 有研究表明，在 12.4% 的桡骨头骨折患者中发现了相关的骨损伤，多达 10% 的患者发生了肘关节脱位，如果其伴有冠突骨折，则称为恐怖三联征。[2] 这种损伤预后通常较差。[21]

治疗

非手术治疗

不移位或移位较小的桡骨头和桡骨颈骨折可以采用非手术治疗，对大多数患者而言，长期预后较好。[22] Mason II 型桡骨头骨折适度移位（2~5 mm）且无旋转障碍的患者，非手术治疗

的长期预后也较好，其中 12% 的患者早期预后较差，随后行桡骨头切除术。[23]受伤后 1 周内肘部制动可显著减轻疼痛，改善肘关节活动范围及关节功能，尚未发现与之相关的明显副作用。[24]有研究报道，对 Mason Ⅰ 型桡骨头骨折患者行血肿抽吸，可将视觉模拟评分法评分从平均 5.5 降低至平均 2.5。[25]一项随机临床研究比较了无移位桡骨头骨折患者接受单独血肿抽吸与血肿抽吸联合丁哌卡因注射治疗的临床疗效。从术后第 1 天至术后 1 年，使用局部麻醉药的患者未见明显功能获益。[26]

切开复位内固定

目前还没有研究比较切开复位内固定（ORIF）和非手术治疗对没有骨性阻挡的涉及关节面的有移位的桡骨头骨折的疗效。如果因为存在骨性阻挡或相关的肘部损伤而选择手术干预，则只要固定稳定，其预后通常较好。[27-28]简单的部分关节骨折的预后要优于完全关节骨折或具有 3 个以上移位碎片的骨折，因此粉碎性桡骨头骨折建议行桡骨头置换术。[29-30]在一项非随机对照研究中，桡骨头切除患者的预后比 ORIF 患者的预后差，而且前者的骨关节炎发生率更高。[28,31]

如果条件允许，桡骨头骨折可以使用埋头螺钉进行固定，效果优于钢板螺钉固定，因为后者更容易发生肘关节僵硬，且行内固定取出术的患者更多。[32-33]所有桡骨头手术均可以使用后侧皮肤切口，同时行外侧全厚度皮瓣游离或直接做一外侧皮肤切口。如果在压力检查或软组织损伤检查中怀疑存在 LCL 损伤，则可在手术完成时使用 Kocher 法对 LCL 进行修复。在 LCL 完整的情况下，首选普通的伸肌起点 – 分离方法，因为它可以进入桡骨头骨折常见的前外侧节段。在深入过程中使前臂保持在旋前状态，并避免在桡骨颈前方使用牵开器，以降低骨间后神经麻痹的可能。在保留周围软组织以保持血供的同时，应尽可能减少骨折碎片，并用克氏针或复位钳临时固定骨折块。随后可以使用埋头螺钉来固定部分骨折

（图 44-1）。在非粉碎性的完全关节骨折或桡骨颈骨折中，埋头空心螺钉可以从桡骨头到桡骨颈倾斜地穿过多个平面，达到稳定固定的效果（图 44-2）。空心螺钉的导丝有助于防止螺钉在倾斜放置时从桡骨颈的皮质骨穿过。如果桡骨颈严重粉碎并且需要放置钢板来维持稳定，则应在桡骨头的非关节部分放置一块短小的钢板并尽量减少软组织剥离。桡骨头和桡骨颈的解剖结构复杂且易变，任何解剖学上预先成型的钢板都无法实现完美贴合。但术者可以在手术期间通过调整钢板形状实现较好的贴合。[34]

桡骨头置换

如果粉碎性桡骨头骨折不能进行稳定的内固定，则桡骨头置换术比 ORIF 更为可取。随着多种人工桡骨头的问世，桡骨头置换取得了较好的早、中期预后。[35-39]生物力学测试表明，单极桡骨头置换可稳定肱桡关节，而双极假体容易导致半脱位。[40]非骨水泥假体光滑的柄部会形成 X 线透亮带，这与患者的症状无关[41]（图 44-3）。非光滑设计的假体柄部出现 X 线透亮带常与疼痛有关，是再次手术的常见原因。[42]当使用完全喷砂处理的非骨水泥假体时，可观察到桡骨近端由于应力屏蔽而发生明显的骨溶解。[43]一项术后 8 年的随访研究报道，骨水泥双极桡骨头置换术后发生的进行性骨溶解很可能是聚乙烯磨损造成的。在 24~48 个月的随访中，非骨水泥双极桡骨头置换的治疗效果良好，没有聚乙烯磨损的证据，也没有桡骨头颈分离的报道。[44]金属桡骨头置换失败的其他原因包括肘关节僵硬、肘关节不稳定、假体过长和感染。

碳纤维具有与骨相似的弹性模量，是金属桡骨头假体的新替代品。尽管早期这种假体的头颈交界处发生过几次严重事故，但一项 21 个月的随访研究显示其预后良好。[45]需要进一步长期随访以确定碳纤维假体的理论优势是否可带来更好的临床疗效。

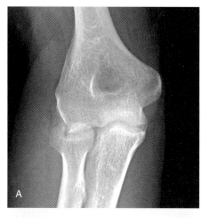
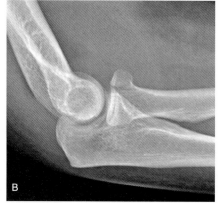
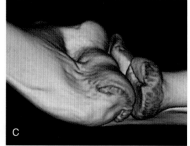
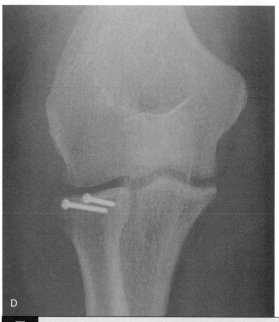
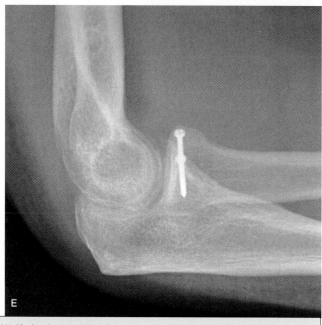

图 44-1　一例 31 岁男性患者桡骨头骨折的正位片（A）、侧位片（B）及三维重建 CT（C）。患者行切开复位内固定。术中观察到其肱骨小头有明显的慢性损伤，伴有外侧副韧带撕裂，均在术中予以修复。术后 3 个月拍摄 X 线平片（D）和侧位片（E）。患者肘关节偶有不适，但已顺利重返工作，肘部屈伸角度为 0°~135°，旋前旋后均为 70°

最近的研究提高了对桡骨头置换术中假体尺寸的理解。假体的直径和厚度应基于天然桡骨头的大小。为了避免外侧滑车磨损，假体的直径应与天然桡骨头的较小直径相似，假体直径通常比桡骨头的最大直径小 2 mm。假体应与关节相对合，其近端应与尺骨近端距冠突尖端约 2 mm 处齐平[46]（图 44-4）。如果 LCL 因原始骨折或手术损伤，则不应使用肱骨与桡骨头假体之间的间隙来判断桡骨头假体的最佳厚度。术中透视和术后 X 线片可用于判断桡骨长度。在健康的肘关节中，影像学上肱尺关节外侧间隙通常比内侧间隙更宽，并且可能不平行（横向变得更宽）。因此，肱尺关节外侧间隙不是衡量桡骨头置换术后桡骨长度的可靠指标。[47] 肱尺关节内侧间隙通常在未受伤的肘部平行，但在肘关节正位片上，除非桡骨增长至少 6 mm，否则关节间隙可能不明显。在手术过程中可以使用牙镜来评估肱尺关节外侧间隙的不对称性增宽，而桡骨头的增长仅为 2 mm。[48] 侧位片可用于量化桡骨头置换术后桡骨增长，因为测量值前后左右一致。最近的研究报道影像学测量桡骨头假体的误差在 1 mm 以内，灵敏性为 98%。[49]

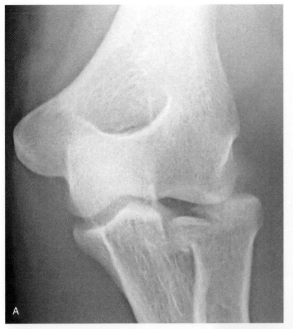
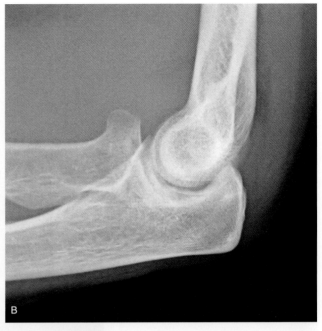
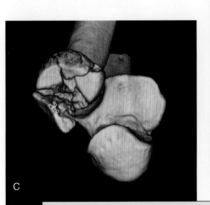
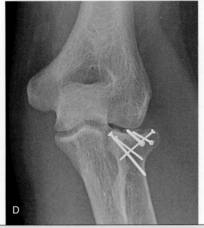
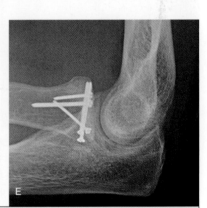

图 44-2　一例 31 岁重体力劳动者的桡骨头骨折的正位片（A）、侧位片（B）及三维重建 CT（C）。患者行切开复位内固定，术后 5 个月拍摄正位片（D）及侧位片（E）。患者肘关节屈伸角度为 17°~144°，旋前 70°，旋后 85°

桡骨头切除术

一期切除不可修复的桡骨头骨折较少见，因为伴有韧带损伤的复杂桡骨头骨折较常见，这促使医师对桡骨头功能的认识较透彻：可维持韧带缺损的肘关节稳定，传递肘关节负荷。在理论上，切除桡骨头可能出现一些并发症，但最近的一些长期临床研究发现，对桡骨头骨折患者行桡骨头切除术的功能预后良好，大多数患者的肘关节在 X 线片上呈现退行性改变，提携角增加 7°~11°。[50-52] 桡骨头切除后桡骨向近端移位较常

见，可能导致腕部发生尺骨撞击综合征。[53] 由于延迟桡骨头切除术可以取得良好预后，因此在初始治疗失败后可以将桡骨头切除术视为晚期治疗选择。[54]

康复

非手术治疗的患者应在受伤后 1 周内开始主动的屈伸、旋转锻炼。[24] 手术后也应尽早进行主动训练，以减少僵硬的发生。关节活动范围可能受到相关的骨骼或韧带肘关节损伤的限制。如果肘关节存在伸直时半脱位的情况，则应在安全范

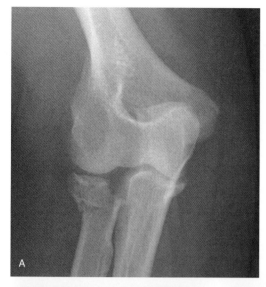
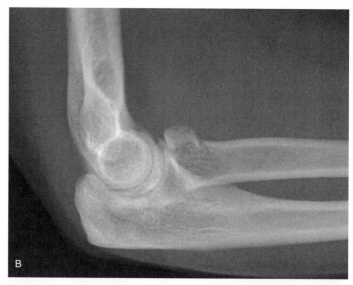
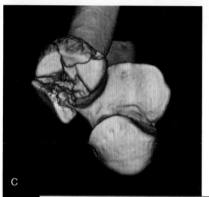
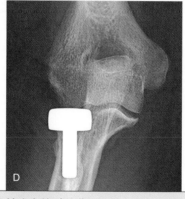
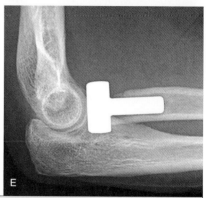

图 44-3　一例粉碎性桡骨头骨折的 60 岁女性患者的肘关节正位片（A）、侧位片（B）及三维重建 CT（C）。其行桡骨头置换术后 3 个月随访拍摄肘关节正位片（D）及侧位片（E）。根据假体关节面对合情况，肱尺关节内侧间隙平行且肱尺关节外侧间隙未见增宽，可知假体的植入深度和尺寸均较为合适。假体柄周围可见透亮带。患者现在可进行正常日常活动，肘关节活动范围正常，未诉疼痛

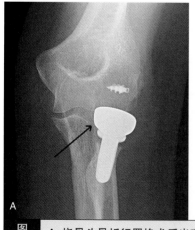
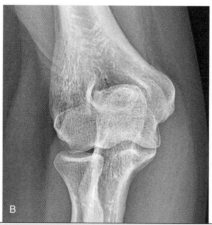
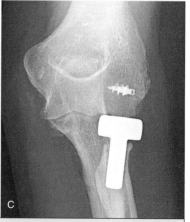

图 44-4　A. 桡骨头骨折行置换术后出现明显疼痛和肘关节僵硬的患者的正位片，可见假体明显过长，假体近端接近桡窝近端和冠突。肱尺关节外侧间隙可见增宽，内侧间隙未见明显增宽。B. 对侧肘关节正位片显示了患者正常的桡骨头。C. 患者二次手术后 3 个月的肘关节正位片，假体位置良好，肱尺关节序列以及假体和桡切迹、冠突的关系均得到修复

围内进行康复，并且随着肌肉张力的改善和韧带的愈合，每周可将伸直范围增加 10°~15°。[55] 鼓励进行肌肉等长收缩训练。如果 LCL 有缺损，则应避免旋后位，肘关节可旋前和 90° 屈曲，只能在旋前位伸直。应避免因重力在肘关节屈曲内旋时产生肘内翻应力。[56] 如果 MCL 缺损，则应避免旋前位，肘关节可旋后和 90° 屈曲，只能在旋后位伸直。[57] 应避免肘外翻应力。如果肘关节内外侧均存在缺损，则可在中立位屈曲 90°，只能在旋转中立位伸直。对于任何韧带缺损的患者，首先应在屈肘的情况下进行可接受的旋转活动。

X 线检查可用于观察运动过程中碎片的位移，并确定何时骨愈合足以承受被动拉伸，这通常需要 6 周左右。[58] 遗留肘关节不稳定或关节活动范围小的患者应接受正规的物理治疗和夹板治疗，以降低半脱位和僵硬的风险。

并发症

肘关节僵硬是桡骨头骨折后最常见的手术并发症，可能与 ORIF 的内固定植入、桡骨头假体的尺寸不当、术者技术水平较低以及患者术后康复治疗不规范有关。即使骨折得到了适当处理，进行了规范的康复治疗，但由于关节囊挛缩、异位骨化形成，部分患者仍会发生肘关节僵硬。软组织僵硬通常可以使用物理疗法及静态或动态夹板治疗，但是如果活动中发生明显骨性阻挡则可能需要手术治疗。[58]

骨折畸形愈合和骨不连在非手术治疗后很常见，在 ORIF 术后较少见，通常无症状，仅在影像学上可观察到。对于有明显的疼痛或机械症状的患者，桡骨头切除术和桡骨头置换术是公认的治疗选择，其预期结果较好[53,59]。据报道，在没有明显退行性改变的情况下，关节内截骨术可安全有效地治疗部分桡骨头骨折的症状性畸形愈合。[60]

一些长期临床研究发现，影像学骨关节炎性改变在桡骨头骨折后很常见，但与功能不良不相关。[23] 如果肱尺关节未受累，可以通过桡骨头

切除术治疗临床症状明显的骨关节炎。如果正确处理了相关的肘关节损伤且未切除桡骨头，则肘关节不稳定的情况很少见。桡骨头切除后桡骨向近端移位会引起腕肘关节症状。这种并发症很复杂，且没有简单可靠的治疗方法。

总结

桡骨头和桡骨颈骨折很常见，通常与其他肘关节损伤相关，部分需要进行治疗。非移位性骨折可以使用非手术治疗，效果极佳。没有明显粉碎性的移位骨折可以选择非手术治疗或 ORIF，具有良好的预后，但是最佳治疗方法仍然未知。粉碎性骨折可通过桡骨头置换术治疗，中期效果良好，但还需要长期随访研究。桡骨头切除术似乎是一种较好的挽救方法，但应让患者充分了解切除桡骨头后可能出现提携角增大以及影像学上的退行性改变等风险。

最近的长期随访研究增进了医师对某些治疗方案的了解。需要进行随机对照临床研究以指导对桡骨头和桡骨颈移位的粉碎性骨折的治疗方案。

参考文献

[1] Duckworth AD, Clement ND, Jenkins PJ, Aitken SA, Court-Brown CM, McQueen MM: The epidemiology of radial head and neck fractures. *J Hand Surg Am* 2012;37(1):112-119.

A prospective trauma database containing 199 radial head fractures and 86 radial neck fractures revealed that male patients were younger on average than female patients, women commonly sustained their fracture from a low-energy fall, and 99% of radial neck fractures were nondisplaced or noncomminuted. Level of evidence: IV.

[2] Kaas L, van Riet RP, Vroemen JP, Eygendaal D: The epidemiology of radial head fractures. *J Shoulder Elbow Surg* 2010;19(4):520-523.

A retrospective database contained 328 radial head fractures. The incidence was calculated at 2.8 per 10,000 population per year. In patients older than 50 years, the number of women was significantly higher than the number of men. Level of evidence: IV.

［3］ King GJ, Zarzour ZD, Patterson SD, Johnson JA: An anthropometric study of the radial head: Implications in the design of a prosthesis. *J Arthroplasty* 2001;16(1):112-116.

［4］ van Riet RP, Van Glabbeek F, Neale PG, Bortier H, An KN, O'Driscoll SW: The noncircular shape of the radial head. *J Hand Surg Am* 2003;28(6):972-978.

［5］ Galik K, Baratz ME, Butler AL, Dougherty J, Cohen MS, Miller MC: The effect of the annular ligament on kinematics of the radial head. *J Hand Surg Am* 2007;32(8):1218-1224.

In a cadaver study, the radial head was found to translate an average 2.1 mm in the anteroposterior plane and 1.6 mm in the mediolateral plane. Resection of the annular ligament increased the translation in both planes but did not change the location of the pronation-supination axis.

［6］ Smith GR, Hotchkiss RN: Radial head and neck fractures: Anatomic guidelines for proper placement of in- ternal fixation. *J Shoulder Elbow Surg* 1996;5(2, pt 1):113-117.

［7］ Beingessner DM, Dunning CE, Gordon KD, Johnson JA, King GJ: The effect of radial head fracture size on elbow kinematics and stability. *J Orthop Res* 2005;23(1):210-217.

［8］ Beingessner DM, Dunning CE, Gordon KD, Johnson JA, King GJ: The effect of radial head excision and arthroplasty on elbow kinematics and stability. *J Bone Joint Surg Am* 2004;86(8):1730-1739.

［9］ Koslowsky TC, Schliwa S, Koebke J: Presentation of the microscopic vascular architecture of the radial head using a sequential plastination technique. *Clin Anat* 2011;24(6):721-732.

Seventeen fresh human cadaver elbows were sequentially plastinated. The blood supply to the radial head was found to come from branches of the radial recurrent artery and a branch of the ulnar artery (ramus periostalis ulnaris), both of which form a pericervical arterial ring. A branch of the interosseus artery supports the neck, and the nutrient artery provides intraosseous blood supply.

［10］ Gebauer M, Barvencik F, Mumme M, et al: Microarchitecture of the radial head and its changes in aging. *Calcif Tissue Int* 2010;86(1):14-22.

An equal number of left-side and right-side radial head cadaver specimens were examined from an equal number of males and females in three age categories. Age-

and sex-related changes in bone structure were observed, with significantly worse trabecular parameters in older women compared with men.

［11］ Guitton TG, Ring D: Science of Variation Group: Interobserver reliability of radial head fracture classification: Two-dimensional compared with three- dimensional CT. *J Bone Joint Surg Am* 2011;93(21):2015-2021.

Eighty-five orthopaedic surgeons evaluated and classified 12 radial head fractures with radiographs and two-dimensional or three-dimensional CT scans. Although three-dimensional CT led to a slightly more accurate classification, there is still considerable disagreement regarding classification of radial head fractures.

［12］ Kaas L, Turkenburg JL, van Riet RP, Vroemen JP, Eygendaal D: Magnetic resonance imaging findings in 46 elbows with a radial head fracture. *Acta Orthop* 2010;81(3):373-376.

An associated elbow injury was found in 35 of 46 patients with a radial head fracture who underwent MRI within 16 days of injury, including 28 LCL and 1 MCL injuries, 18 capitellar injuries, and 1 coronoid fracture.

［13］ Kaas L, van Riet RP, Turkenburg JL, Vroemen JP, van Dijk CN, Eygendaal D: Magnetic resonance imaging in radial head fractures: Most associated injuries are not clinically relevant. *J Shoulder Elbow Surg* 2011;20(8):1282-1288.

Retrospective review of 40 patients (42 radial head fractures) at a mean 13 months after injury found clinical MCL or LCL laxity in three elbows, which was not detected on initial MRI in two of the elbows. One patient had infrequent elbow locking.

［14］ Mason ML: Some observations on fractures of the head of the radius with a review of one hundred cases. *Br J Surg* 1954;42(172):123-132.

［15］ Johnston GW: A follow-up of one hundred cases of fracture of the head of the radius with a review of the literature. *Ulster Med J* 1962;31:51-56.

［16］ Broberg MA, Morrey BF: Results of treatment of fracture-dislocations of the elbow. *Clin Orthop Relat Res* 1987;216:109-119.

［17］ van Riet RP, Morrey BF: Documentation of associated injuries occurring with radial head fracture. *Clin Orthop Relat Res* 2008;466(1):130-134.

Associated injury was seen in 88 of 333 radial head fractures at one institution. A expansion of the Mason classification was devised in which associated injuries were designated by a suffix (c for coronoid fracture, *o* for olecranon fracture, *m* for MCL injury, *l* for LCL injury, *d* for distal radioulnar disruption).

[18] Nalbantoglu U, Gereli A, Kocaoglu B, Aktas S, Turkmen M: Capitellar cartilage injuries concomitant with radial head fractures. *J Hand Surg Am* 2008;33(9):1602-1607.

Of 51 consecutive patients with Mason type II or type III fracture who were surgically treated, 10 had a capitellar cartilage injury. Although this injury was more common with higher grade radial head fracture, injury severity was worse in lower grade fractures because the more intact radial head was able to cause more damage to the capitellum. Level of evidence: IV.

[19] Caputo AE, Burton KJ, Cohen MS, King GJ: Articular cartilage injuries of the capitellum interposed in radial head fractures: A report of ten cases. *J Shoulder Elbow Surg* 2006;15(6):716-720.

[20] Rineer CA, Guitton TG, Ring D: Radial head fractures: Loss of cortical contact is associated with concomitant fracture or dislocation. *J Shoulder Elbow Surg* 2010;19(1):21-25.

A retrospective review of 121 consecutive radial head fractures with displacement of more than 2 mm found that in 91 (75%), there was complete cortical loss of contact of a fracture fragment with the rest of the proximal radius. Only 6% of the fractures were isolated. In the fractures classified as having cortical contact, 88% had no other injuries or dislocation.

[21] Regan W, Morrey B: Fractures of the coronoid process of the ulna. *J Bone Joint Surg Am* 1989;71(9):1348-1354.

[22] Herbertsson P, Josefsson PO, Hasserius R, Karlsson C, Besjakov J, Karlsson MK: Displaced Mason type I fractures of the radial head and neck in adults: A fifteen-to thirty-three-year follow-up study. *J Shoulder Elbow Surg* 2005;14(1):73-77.

[23] Akesson T, Herbertsson P, Josefsson PO, Hasserius R, Besjakov J, Karlsson MK: Primary nonoperative treatment of moderately displaced two-part fractures of the radial head. *J Bone Joint Surg Am* 2006;88(9):1909-1914.

[24] Liow RY, Cregan A, Nanda R, Montgomery RJ: Early mobilisation for minimally displaced radial head fractures is desirable: A prospective randomised study of two protocols. *Injury* 2002;33(9):801-806.

[25] Ditsios KT, Stavridis SI, Christodoulou AG: The effect of haematoma aspiration on intra-articular pressure and pain relief following Mason I radial head fractures. *Injury* 2011;42(4):362-365.

Intra-articular pressure monitoring was done before and after aspiration in 16 patients with a Mason type I radial head fracture. A mean 2.75 mL was aspirated, and intra-articular pressure was found to drop from between 49 and 120 mm Hg to between 9 and 25 mm Hg. Reported pain decreased from a mean 5.5 to 2.5 on the visual analog scale.

[26] Chalidis BE, Papadopoulos PP, Sachinis NC, Dimitriou CG: Aspiration alone versus aspiration and bupivacaine injection in the treatment of undisplaced radial head fractures: A prospective randomized study. *J Shoulder Elbow Surg* 2009;18(5):676-679.

A prospective randomized controlled study of 40 patients with Mason type I radial head fracture found no difference in range of motion, pain, and elbow function based on treatment with aspiration of hematoma alone or with aspiration and intra-articular local anesthetic injection. Level of evidence: I.

[27] Lindenhovius AL, Felsch Q, Ring D, Kloen P: The long-term outcome of open reduction and internal fixation of stable displaced isolated partial articular fractures of the radial head. *J Trauma* 2009;67(1):143-146.

Sixteen patients with a stable Mason type II radial head fracture received ORIF with screws (11 patients) or plate and screws (5 patients). At an average 22-year follow-up, 14 patients were found to have undergone routine removal of hardware an average 14 months after surgery. The average Disabilities of the Arm, Shoulder, and Hand (DASH) score was 12. Level of evidence: IV.

[28] Lindenhovius AL, Felsch Q, Doornberg JN, Ring D, Kloen P: Open reduction and internal fixation compared with excision for unstable displaced fractures of the radial head. *J Hand Surg Am* 2007;32(5):630-636.

Fifteen patients with an unstable displaced radial head fracture treated with excision were compared with 13 patients with a similar fracture treated with ORIF. There was no difference in range of motion at 1 year or 17 years after injury. At long-term follow, up the average DASH score was 5 in patients treated with ORIF and 15 in those treated with excision. Level of evidence: III.

[29] Ring D, Quintero J, Jupiter JB: Open reduction and internal fixation of fractures of the radial head. *J Bone Joint Surg Am* 2002;84(10):1811-1815.

At 2-year follow-up of 56 patients treated with ORIF for a radial head fracture, patients with a comminuted fracture with more than three fragments had a relatively poor result. Level of evidence: III.

[30] Chen X, Wang SC, Cao LH, Yang GQ, Li M, Su JC: Comparison between radial head replacement and open reduction and internal fixation in clinical treatment of unstable, multi-fragmented radial head fractures. *Int Orthop* 2011;35(7):1071-1076.

A randomized controlled study of 45 patients with a Mason type III fracture compared ORIF and radial head replacement. Severely comminuted fractures were excluded. At 2-year follow-up, 91% of patients with arthroplasty had a good or excellent result, compared with 65% of those with ORIF. Level of evidence: II.

[31] Ikeda M, Sugiyama K, Kang C, Takagaki T, Oka Y: Comminuted fractures of the radial head: Comparison of resection and internal fixation. *J Bone Joint Surg Am* 2005;87(1):76-84.

[32] Smith AM, Morrey BF, Steinmann SP: Low profile fixation of radial head and neck fractures: Surgical technique and clinical experience. *J Orthop Trauma* 2007;21(10):718-724.

A retrospective review of 19 patients who underwent ORIF using a technique for low-profile fixation of radial head fracture found a trend toward reduced forearm rotation. Heterotopic ossification occurred in five patients who received ORIF with plate fixation and one with low-profile fixation. Level of evidence: III.

[33] Neumann M, Nyffeler R, Beck M: Comminuted fractures of the radial head and neck: Is fixation to the shaft necessary? *J Bone Joint Surg Br* 2011;93(2):223-228.

A retrospective review of 25 patients with Mason type III radial head fracture identified two groups at a mean 4-year follow-up, based on whether the radial head rotated as one with the neck and shaft after the head fracture was fixed with ORIF or required a plate to fix the head to the neck. Hardware was removed in 7 of 13 patients requiring plate fixation and 1 of 12 patients without plate fixation. Level of evidence: III.

[34] Burkhart KJ, Nowak TE, Kim YJ, Rommens PM, Müller LP: Anatomic fit of six different radial head plates: Comparison of precontoured low-profile radial head plates. *J Hand Surg Am* 2011;36(4):617-624.

Twenty-two human cadaver proximal radius specimens were used in assessing the fit and profile of six precontoured radial head plates. Although two plates appeared to have a better fit and lower profile than the others, none of the plates had a reproducibly perfect fit because of the complexity and variability of the proximal radius. The surgeon's ability to modify a plate may be important in achieving optimal fit.

[35] Popovic N, Lemaire R, Georis P, Gillet P: Midterm re- sults with a bipolar radial head prosthesis: Radiographic evidence of loosening at the bone-cement interface. *J Bone Joint Surg Am* 2007;89(11):2469-2476.

At a mean 8.4-year follow-up of 51 patients with a cemented bipolar radial head replacement, the outcome on the Mayo Elbow Performance Index (MEPI) was excellent in 14, good in 25, fair in 9, and poor in 3. Osteolysis was seen on radiographs in 37 patients, and there were 10 complications. Level of evidence: IV.

[36] Grewal R, MacDermid JC, Faber KJ, Drosdowech DS, King GJ: Comminuted radial head fractures treated with a modular metallic radial head arthroplasty: Study of outcomes. *J Bone Joint Surg Am* 2006;88(10):2192-2200.

[37] Dotzis A, Cochu G, Mabit C, Charissoux JL, Arnaud JP: Comminuted fractures of the radial head treated by the Judet floating radial head prosthesis. *J Bone Joint Surg Br* 2006;88(6):760-764.

[38] Doornberg JN, Parisien R, van Duijn PJ, Ring D: Radial head arthroplasty with a modular metal spacer to treat acute traumatic elbow instability. *J Bone Joint Surg Am* 2007;89(5):1075-1080.

At a mean 40-month follow-up of 27 patients with an uncemented smooth-stem modular radial head replacement, the average range of motion was from 20° of flexion to 131° of flexion, 73° of pronation, and 57° of supination. Seventeen patients had lucency around the neck of the prosthesis not associated with pain. Nine patients had radiographic changes around the capitellum. Level of evidence: IV.

[39] Chapman CB, Su BW, Sinicropi SM, Bruno R, Strauch RJ, Rosenwasser MP: Vitallium radial head prosthesis for acute and chronic elbow fractures and fracture-dislocations involving the radial head. *J Shoulder Elbow Surg* 2006;15(4):463-473.

[40] Moon JG, Berglund LJ, Zachary D, An KN, O'Driscoll SW: Radiocapitellar joint stability with bipolar versus monopolar radial head prostheses. *J Shoulder Elbow Surg* 2009;18(5):779-784.

Bipolar and monopolar radial head prosthesis designs were tested using 12 human cadaver elbow specimens. The monopolar radial head replacement and the native radial head both resisted radiocapitellar subluxation. The bipolar radial head replacement facilitated subluxation.

[41] Fehringer EV, Burns EM, Knierim A, Sun J, Apker KA, Berg RE: Radiolucencies surrounding a smooth-

stemmed radial head component may not correlate with forearm pain or poor elbow function. *J Shoulder Elbow Surg* 2009;18(2):275-278.

Radiolucency around the stem was detected in 16 of 17 patients assessed clinically and radiographically at a minimum 2 years after surgery. All elbows were stable, and radiolucency was not correlated with proximal forearm pain. Level of evidence:IV.

[42] van Riet RP, Sanchez-Sotelo J, Morrey BF: Failure of metal radial head replacement. *J Bone Joint Surg Br* 2010;92(5):661-667.

In 44 patients (47 elbows) who had removal of a metal radial head replacement, the most common indication for removal was painful loosening (31 elbows). The implant was revised for stiffness in 18 elbows and instability in 9 elbows. Overlengthening was seen before removal in 11 elbows. Degenerative changes were found in all but one elbow. Level of evidence: IV.

[43] Chanlalit C, Fitzsimmons JS, Moon JG, Berglund LJ, An KN, O'Driscoll SW: Radial head prosthesis micromotion characteristics: Partial versus fully grit-blasted stems. *J Shoulder Elbow Surg* 2011;20(1):27-32.

In a human cadaver biomechanical study, micromotion was comparable in partially and fully grit-blasted radial head replacement stems. Less stress shielding with a partially grit-blasted uncemented stem was believed to be advantageous.

[44] Zunkiewicz MR, Clemente JS, Miller MC, Baratz ME, Wysocki RW, Cohen MS: Radial head replacement with a bipolar system: A minimum 2-year follow-up. *J Shoulder Elbow Surg* 2012;21(1):98-104.

The results of using 30 smooth stem and telescoping radial neck bipolar radial head replacements were assessed a mean 34 months after surgery. The mean MEPI score was 92.1, and the DASH score was 13.8. Level of evidence: IV.

[45] Sarris IK, Kyrkos MJ, Galanis NN, Papavasiliou KA, Sayegh FE, Kapetanos GA: Radial head replacement with the MoPyC pyrocarbon prosthesis. *J Shoulder Elbow Surg* 2012;21(9):1222-1228.

At a mean 27-month follow-up of 32 patients with a pyrocarbon uncemented radial head replacement, the mean arc of flexion-extension was 130°, mean pronation was 74°, and mean supination was 72°. Broberg and Morrey scores were excellent in 33% of patients, good in 44%, and fair in 23%. Six patients had osteolysis, and 2 had early catastrophic failure at the stemneck junction. Level of evidence: IV.

[46] Doornberg JN, Linzel DS, Zurakowski D, Ring D: Reference points for radial head prosthesis size. *J Hand Surg Am* 2006;31(1):53-57.

[47] Rowland AS, Athwal GS, MacDermid JC, King GJ: Lateral ulnohumeral joint space widening is not diagnostic of radial head arthroplasty overstuffing. *J Hand Surg Am* 2007;32(5):637-641.

Evaluation of 50 AP radiographs of the elbow revealed that the lateral ulnohumeral joint space often is wider than the medial ulnohumeral joint space in a normal elbow. The medial joint space usually is parallel, but the lateral joint space can be nonparallel and wider laterally.

[48] Frank SG, Grewal R, Johnson J, Faber KJ, King GJ, Athwal GS: Determination of correct implant size in radial head arthroplasty to avoid overlengthening. *J Bone Joint Surg Am* 2009;91(7):1738-1746.

After implantation of a radial head replacement of a varying thickness in seven human cadaver specimens, a significant incongruity of the medial ulnohumeral joint appeared radiographically only after overlengthening of the radius by more than 6 mm. Overlengthening of 2 mm or more could be detected by intraoperative assessment of a lateral ulnohumeral joint space gap.

[49] Athwal GS, Rouleau DM, MacDermid JC, King GJ: Contralateral elbow radiographs can reliably diagnose radial head implant overlengthening. *J Bone Joint Surg Am* 2011;93(14):1339-1346.

Examination of 100 radiographs of 50 elbow pairs revealed no difference in same-patient radiographic measurements. A measurement technique tested on a cadaver model was found to reliably predict overlengthening of as little as 1 mm (sensitivity, 98%).

[50] Iftimie PP, Calmet Garcia J, de Loyola Garcia Forcada I, Gonzalez Pedrouzo JE, Giné Gomà J: Resection arthroplasty for radial head fractures: Long-term follow-up. *J Shoulder Elbow Surg* 2011;20(1):45-50.

Radial head excision was reviewed in 27 patients at an average 17-year follow-up. On the MEPI, the outcome was excellent in 81%, good in 15%, and fair in 4%. The mean DASH score was 4.9. Eighty-five percent of patients reported no pain. Their mean range of motion was 5° to 135°, mean pronation was 83°, and mean supination was 79°. Almost all patients had radiographic degenerative changes. Level of evidence: IV.

[51] Antuña SA, Sánchez-Márquez JM, Barco R: Long-term results of radial head resection following isolated radial head fractures in patients younger than forty years old. *J Bone Joint Surg Am* 2010;92(3):558-566.

At a mean 25-year follow-up, radial head excision was retrospectively reviewed in 26 patients younger than 40 years at surgery. Eighty-one percent of patients reported no pain. Their mean arc of flexion was 9° to 139°. Mean pronation was 84°, and mean supination was 85°. The mean MEPI was 92, and 92% were classified as good or excellent. The mean DASH score was. The mean carrying angle of the elbow had increased by 11°. Level of evidence: IV.

[52] 52. Karlsson MK, Herbertsson P, Nordqvist A, Hasserius R, Besjakov J, Josefsson PO: Long-term outcome of displaced radial neck fractures in adulthood: 16-21 year follow-up of 5 patients treated with radial head excision. *Acta Orthop* 2009;80(3):368-370.

At a mean 18-year follow-up, retrospective review of three women and two men treated with radial head excision for a comminuted radial neck fracture found occasional weakness in two patients, a mean loss of 10° of terminal extension, and a mean loss of less than 5° of flexion, pronation, and supination. The mean difference in carrying angle was 2° between the injured and uninjured sides. Level of evidence: IV.

[53] Schiffern A, Bettwieser SP, Porucznik CA, Crim JR, Tashjian RZ: Proximal radial drift following radial head resection. *J Shoulder Elbow Surg* 2011;20(3):426-433.

At a mean 72-month follow-up, 13 patients treated with radial head excision were retrospectively reviewed. The proximal radial stump had migrated medially and posteriorly, and resection of more than 2 cm resulted in increased posterior drift. Level of evidence: IV.

[54] Broberg MA, Morrey BF: Results of delayed excision of the radial head after fracture. *J Bone Joint Surg Am* 1986;68(5):669-674.

[55] Coonrad RW, Roush TF, Major NM, Basamania CJ: The drop sign, a radiographic warning sign of elbow instability. *J Shoulder Elbow Surg* 2005;14(3):312-317.

[56] Dunning CE, Zarzour ZD, Patterson SD, Johnson JA, King GJ: Muscle forces and pronation stabilize the lateral ligament deficient elbow. *Clin Orthop Relat Res* 2001;388:118-124.

[57] Armstrong AD, Dunning CE, Faber KJ, Duck TR, Johnson JA, King GJ: Rehabilitation of the medial collateral ligament-deficient elbow: An in vitro biomechanical study. *J Hand Surg Am* 2000;25(6):1051-1057.

[58] Szekeres M, Chinchalkar SJ, King GJ: Optimizing elbow rehabilitation after instability. *Hand Clin* 2008;24(1):27-38.

[59] Shore BJ, Mozzon JB, MacDermid JC, Faber KJ, King GJ: Chronic posttraumatic elbow disorders treated with metallic radial head arthroplasty. *J Bone Joint Surg Am* 2008;90(2):271-280.

At a mean 8-year follow-up, 32 patients treated with a metallic radial head arthroplasty on a delayed basis for a variety of indications had an average MEPI score of 83, with 53% of patients rated as excellent, 13% as good, 22% as fair, and 13% as poor. Posttraumatic arthritis was found in 74% on radiographs. None of the implants required revision. Level of evidence: IV.

[60] Rosenblatt Y, Young C, MacDermid JC, King GJ: Osteotomy of the head of the radius for partial articular malunion. *J Bone Joint Surg Br* 2009;91(10):1341-1346.

Five patients were treated with intra-articular osteotomy for a malunited partial articular radial head fracture a mean 8 months after injury. At a mean 5.5-year follow-up, MEPI scores had improved from 74 to 88, and four patients had a good or excellent outcome. All osteotomies healed, and there were no complications. Level of evidence: IV.

第四十五章　肱骨远端骨折

David Ring, MD, PhD

引言

肱骨远端骨折是一种复杂的损伤，治疗难度大且容易发生并发症。对双柱骨折和肱骨小头－滑车骨折患者进行的长期评估表明，手术治疗的结果较好，并且症状和功能障碍与关节炎无关。

在 2007—2011 年，已发表的研究证实了许多肱骨小头－滑车骨折的复杂性长期以来未得到充分认识，讨论了肱骨远端半肘关节置换的使用，并对 65 岁以上的全肘关节置换与双柱骨折的钢板内固定的患者进行了比较。一些固定技术或手术的案例研究发现，尺神经损伤的发病率比以前认为的要高。3 项已发表的研究专门报道了尺神经病变：1 项赞成尺神经前移，1 项不赞成，1 项没有发现差异。目前，这些问题仍然具有争议。

柱状骨折

肱骨远端的单柱骨折很少见。在一些较大的内固定临床研究中，几乎没有报道过 AO B 型骨折，在过去的 5 年中，只有一项研究评估了单柱骨折。[1]一项临床研究回顾了近年来内侧柱骨折的相关病例，发现 14 例患者中有 10 例（71%）

发生了复杂的关节破坏（图 45-1）。平均屈伸活动角度为 92°，10 例患者的 Broberg-Morrey 功能评定指数良好或优异。[1]

大多数涉及肱骨远端柱（冠状鹰嘴窝两侧的骨，在鹰嘴窝底部与肱骨干之间）的骨折为双柱骨折或髁上骨折。与肱骨远端双柱骨折相关的研究热点包括采用平行板与垂直板固定的选择，角度稳定固定的作用（用螺钉锁定板）、获得最佳的暴露同时减少相关风险的方法以及最佳的尺神经处理方式。

钢板螺钉固定的生物力学机制

在两个正交平面垂直双钢板内固定是一个基本的工程概念，长期以来一直应用于肱骨远端骨折的固定。但是，将钢板彼此平行放置在肱骨远端的内侧和外侧表面上，可以使用更多的螺钉和更长的螺钉来接合远端骨折块。这些螺钉中的每一个都可以穿过一块板并有助于稳定整个柱及固定骨折块。随着配备较小的远端螺钉的接骨板的出现，一些外科医师认为平行双钢板为固定骨折块提供了更多选择。直到 2007 年，生物力学测试依然没有阐明垂直和平行双钢板哪种方法具有更明显的优势。在过去的几年中，一些生物力学研究比较了垂直板和平行板，均认为平行板的优势更明显，[2-6]平行双钢板可以使用更长的螺钉和更多的金属材料，从而使固定更牢固。

一项使用了 14 具尸体构建 AO C 2.3 型骨折模型的研究，该研究中的模型模拟了完整肘关节

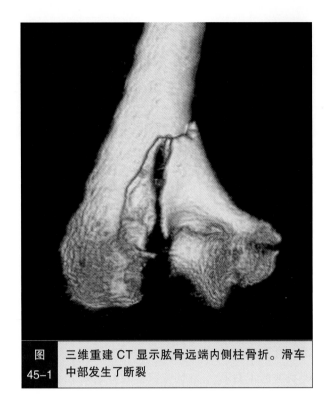

图 45-1　三维重建 CT 显示肱骨远端内侧柱骨折。滑车中部发生了断裂

好接触，则切除部分外侧滑车影响不大。肘关节正常运动需要完整的内侧肱尺关节或完整的外侧滑车和肱桡关节，两者不一定必须同时存在。

一项对 14 具尸体肱骨远端的定量 CT 研究发现，外侧髁后部的骨量和皮质厚度最低。[10]这一发现与以下事实相对应：在外侧后柱远端从前向后的定向螺钉必须短且穿透单皮层。与之相符，根据临床观察，外侧髁是用后外侧接骨板固定肱骨远端的潜在弱固定点，在骨质疏松症患者尤为明显。如果准备使用后外侧钢板，应考虑到在日常活动中肘关节处于内翻状态（如倒牛奶）时，肘关节会受到较大的内翻应力。

一项对 141 名肱骨远端骨折患者术后随访 6 个月的临床研究发现，以肱骨干直径的百分比表示，肘关节屈曲角度与滑车前移之间存在有限但显著的相关性[11]（图 45-2）。这项研究发现，滑车正常前移的丧失可阻碍肘关节屈曲，这种阻碍无法通过功能锻炼或关节囊松解来缓解。这种前移丧失导致冠

所承受的应力。[2]一项研究使用了 AO C 2.3 型骨折的人工骨模型来研究屈伸单平行钢板和垂直双钢板的屈伸应力。[3]一项研究使用了 AO C 2.3 型骨折的尸体，比较了平行双钢板与垂直锁定钢板。[4]一项研究使用了环氧树脂肱骨，并测试了矢状面剪切力的破坏作用[5]。还有一项研究使用了 AO C 2.3 型骨折的尸体，对垂直和平行锁定钢板的生物力学进行了比较。[6]

此外，一项生物力学研究使用具有垂直钢板的髁上截骨尸体骨模型，发现将内侧六孔锁定板向远端移动能获得更大的刚度，虽然这样多个远端螺钉会更短，但远端骨折块中的螺钉也更多了（由 1 个变为 3 个）。[7]一项研究在 AO C 2.3 型尸体模型中比较了常规和锁定接骨板及肱骨远端特异性锁定板，结果唯一区别是，在骨质疏松的骨中，非锁定板容易发生螺钉松动。[8]

其他相关研究

在一项对 8 具尸体的连续切除肱骨小头和滑车的研究中，直到滑车的一部分被切除后肘关节运动才受到显著影响。[9]如果维持肱桡关节的良

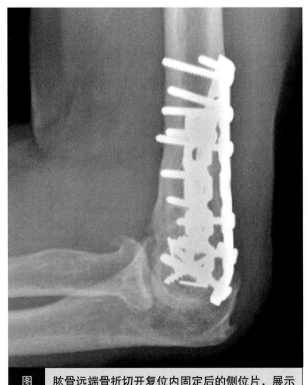

图 45-2　肱骨远端骨折切开复位内固定后的侧位片，展示了肱骨远端正常的前移消失，患者只能屈曲 90°

突在屈曲时更早地与肱骨干接触，并且前臂肌肉组织的空间减少。一项针对 9 个新鲜冷冻尸体的灌注研究发现，肱骨远端由单支营养动脉供应，而肱骨远端的外侧柱主要由后段血管供应。[12] 这一发现部分解释了最近观察到的后柱粉碎性骨折和肱骨 – 滑车骨折不愈合的关系。[13]

双柱骨折：案例研究

在过去的 5 年中，已经发表了许多回顾性病例研究，这些病例通过手术治疗了肱骨远端的柱状骨折。从长远来看，已愈合的骨折最终会发展为骨关节炎，但可以保持良好的功能，不需要二次手术。一项研究对 30 例肱骨远端 AO C 型骨折行切开复位内固定的患者进行了平均 19 年的随访，平均屈伸活动范围为 106°，其中 26 例取得了良好或优异的结果，预后与是否发生关节炎无关。[14]

患者的年龄和骨质疏松不是切开复位内固定的禁忌证。根据现有观点，在考虑治疗方案时，患者的健康和功能需求比年龄更重要。在一项对 14 例年龄大于 65 岁的肱骨远端骨折行切开复位内固定的患者的随访研究中，所有（14 例）骨折均愈合，Mayo 肘关节功能评分的平均值为 83；DASH 评分平均得分为 34.7；肘关节平均屈伸活动范围为 20° ~120°。[15] 在一项研究中，65 岁以上行 ORIF 的 32 例患者骨折愈合后均功能良好，平均运动范围为 22° ~125°。[16]

根据已发表的研究，Y 形钢板固定的长期预后较好。但这种方法具有一些风险，例如，许多髁上部位发生了骨不连。一项研究随访了 34 例肱骨远端骨折的患者，其中 13 例采用 Y 形钢板，21 例采用双钢板固定，71% 的患者预后较好，但 65 岁以上患者的并发症更多，功能更差。[17] 另一项研究显示，所有（17 例）AO C 型骨折患者接受 Y 形钢板治疗后均愈合；平均屈伸活动范围为 13° ~112°，有 14 例患者的结果良好或优秀。[18]

有许多临床试验研究了传统的双柱钢板固定的功能预后。在一项研究中，60 例相对年轻的肱骨远端骨折患者（平均年龄为 30 岁）均在双钢板固定后加用第三块管状钢板和 3.5 mm 重建钢板或动力加压钢板；术后 1 年随访时的平均屈伸活动范围为 20° ~110°。[19] 一项针对 184 例患者的研究发现所有患者骨折均愈合，平均屈曲活动范围为 20° ~110°，并且 72% 的患者功能良好或优秀。[20] 在垂直钢板内固定治疗的 22 例肱骨远端骨折中，有 86.4% 的结果为优秀或良好，Quick-DASH 评分平均得分为 36.1，平均屈伸活动范围为 11° ~128°。[21] 一项研究对 56 例骨折患者使用双钢板固定，有 16% 存在并发症。[22] 在年龄超过 60 岁（平均 77.6 岁）接受手术治疗的 AO C 型骨折的 34 例患者（24 例使用了钢板，10 例使用了钢针、螺钉、或外固定）中，Mayo 肘关节功能评分平均得分为 73.3。21 例患者的结果优秀或良好，平均屈伸活动范围为 80°。[23]

目前许多研究着眼于在肱三头肌的一侧操作而不剥离肱三头肌或不进行鹰嘴截骨。一项回顾性临床研究回顾了 34 例使用肱三头肌保留方法治疗的患者和 33 例使用鹰嘴截骨术治疗的患者，发现运动功能无明显差异。然而，据报道，在未进行鹰嘴截骨的 60 岁以上患者中，较差结果的百分比更高。[24] 一项研究随访了 22 例采用了肱三头肌旁入路进行钢板固定的 AO C 型骨折患者，86% 的患者结果良好或优秀，平均屈伸活动范围为 120°，其中一例发生深部感染，没有骨不连发生。[25] 一项研究采用肱三头肌旁入路治疗了 7 例 AO C 型骨折，所有骨折均已治愈，肘关节活动范围的中值为 90°，所有患者的 Mayo 肘关节功能评分均优秀或良好，DASH 评分平均为 17.9。[26] 当使用肱三头肌旁入路时，如果发现未预见的粉碎性骨折或由患者的肱骨尺寸及骨骺丢失导致可视化或复位困难，应采用辅助鹰嘴截骨入路。肱骨远端骨折很复杂，二次手术去除鹰嘴截骨术内固定可能是最佳骨折修复和避免并发症的方法。

最新的关于平行钢板固定的临床数据并不差

于垂直钢板固定。在 16 例接受等高平行钢板固定的骨折患者中，骨折 100% 愈合，平均屈伸活动范围为 29°~132°，Mayo 肘关节功能评分平均得分为 72.3，平均 DASH 评分为 46.1。[27]在一项对 37 例经平行钢板治疗的 AO C 型肱骨远端骨折的研究中，所有骨折愈合，肘关节平均屈伸活动范围为 97°，Mayo 肘关节功能评分平均为 82，DASH 评分平均为 24，5 例（16%）患者伴有神经功能障碍，总共 17 例患者发生了 24 例（53%）并发症。[28]在 32 例经平行钢板修复的 AO C 型骨折患者中，有 1 例不愈合，有 5 例因肘关节僵硬而接受了二次手术，其中 1 例为深层感染，平均屈伸活动范围为 99°，平均 Mayo 肘关节功能评分为 85，有 27 例患者功能结果良好或优秀。[29]一项来自中国的临床研究比较了 17 例垂直钢板治疗的患者和 18 例平行钢板治疗的患者，发现功能预后无明显差异，但有 2 例接受垂直钢板治疗的患者发生了骨不连。[30]

也有一些研究讨论了肱骨远端锁定钢板或角度稳定钢板固定的结果。一项研究回顾了 40 例接受肱骨远端特异性锁定钢板治疗的患者，有 29 例（72.5%）的预后良好或优秀。Mayo 肘关节功能评分的中位数为 84，平均屈伸活动范围为 100°。[31]在另一项对锁定钢板的临床研究中，1 例患者发生内固定失效，相对年轻和受伤但关节面未粉碎的患者的功能结果更好，5 例（12.5%）患者出现尺神经症状，所有患者（14 例，其中 12 例为 AO 型 C 骨折，2 例为远端肱骨 B 型骨折）均在 ORIF 后愈合。平均屈伸活动范围为 121°，所有患者的 Mayo 肘关节功能评分良好或优秀（平均 91 分），DASH 评分平均为 18.5。[32]

开放双柱骨折

一项对肱骨远端开放性骨折的研究比较了 8 例一期行外固定治疗、二期行钢板螺钉固定的患者与 6 例一期进行钢板螺钉固定的患者。[33]前者的肘关节平均屈伸活动范围（74°）小于后者的（94°），Mayo 肘关节功能评分也较低（分别为 56

和 84），功能障碍也更明显（平均肌肉骨骼功能评分为 33 和 12）。在这项小型回顾性研究中，接受外固定治疗的患者很可能初始受伤更严重。

肱骨小头–滑车骨折

肱骨小头骨折通常累及一部分外侧滑车、前滑车、外侧柱的后部，甚至是滑车的后部和内侧，以上骨折称为典型的肱骨小头骨折或肱骨小头–滑车骨折。这种骨折在 X 线上看起来相对较轻，但其具有潜在复杂性（图 45-3）。最近的研究证实了这些损伤的复杂性，并证明了如果同时存在肱骨小头–滑车骨折和侧柱后侧骨折及滑车后部骨折，发生骨不连或骨坏死的可能性将大大提高。

研究者在苏格兰爱丁堡皇家医院的骨折数据库中对肱骨小头–滑车骨折进行了回顾研究，确定了 79 例患者，估计每年的发病率为 1.5/10 万。[34]24% 的患者伴有桡骨头骨折，59% 的患者骨折不单单局限于肱骨小头。

一项纳入了 27 例肱骨小头–滑车骨折切开复位内固定患者的 1 年随访和 14 例患者的长期随

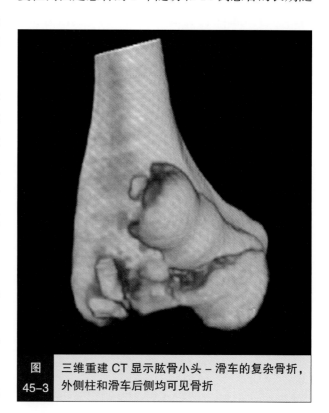

图 45-3　三维重建 CT 显示肱骨小头–滑车的复杂骨折，外侧柱和滑车后侧均可见骨折

访（中位随访时间为 17 年）的研究发现，有 4 例患者伴肘关节脱位，3 例患者伴尺骨近端骨折，2 例患者伴桡骨头骨折，8 例患者需要进行二次手术。[35] 在 14 例长期随访的患者中，屈伸活动范围中位值从骨折后 1 年的 106° 提高到 119°，Broberg-Morrey 评分中值分别为 93 和 95。末次随访 DASH 平均分数为 8。9 例患者出现了关节炎影像学表现。如果患者为后部骨折（Dubberley 3 型骨折）或肱骨小头 – 滑车粉碎性骨折，则预后相对较差。[36]

在一项对 30 例肱骨小头 – 滑车骨折患者行切开复位内固定后平均随访 34 个月的研究中，18 例 Dubberley 3B 型骨折（肱骨小头 – 滑车粉碎性和后部骨折）中有 8 例发生骨不连[13]（图 45-4）。其他简单骨折患者未出现骨不连。26 例患者中有 8 例（31%）肱骨小头 – 滑车骨折伴后部粉碎，这些患者在切开复位内固定后取得了满意的结果。[37] 手术治疗 11 例 Dubberley 1A 型骨折和 7 例 2A 型骨折（肱骨小头 – 滑车骨折）后，取得了较好的

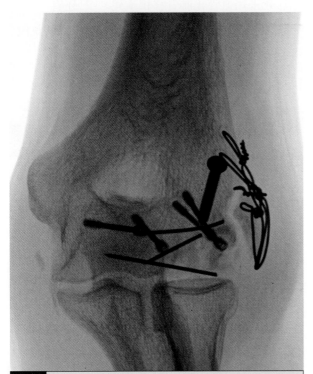

图 45-4 肘关节正位片显示了复杂的 Dubberley 3B 型肱骨小头 – 滑车骨折切开复位内固定后肱骨小头处的骨不连

效果，1 例结果不理想，3 例发生骨坏死。[38]

关节置换术

半肘关节置换术

对于活动量较小的老年患者的复杂性肱骨小头 – 滑车骨折，半肘关节置换术是一种治疗选择。在这类骨折中，肱骨双柱、内侧副韧带、内侧髁上都是完整的，外侧髁上骨折可以得到修复，从而恢复外侧副韧带复合体的功能。一些医师还考虑对可修复的柱状骨折行半肘关节置换术，以恢复侧副韧带功能。在一项对 8 例平均年龄为 79 岁的肱骨远端骨折的女性患者行 Kudo 半肘关节置换术的临床研究中，平均随访 4 年，平均屈曲活动范围为 31°~126°，根据 Mayo 肘关节功能评分，所有患者获得了良好或优秀的结果。[39] 在一项对 10 例平均年龄为 75 岁的接受肱骨远端肱骨置换术治疗的骨折患者的临床研究中，有 9 例 Mayo 肘关节功能评分良好或优秀，平均屈曲活动范围为 18°~125°，平均 DASH 评分为 11。[40]

全肘关节置换术

肱骨远端骨折行全肘关节置换术通常需要去除整个肱骨远端，包括肱骨髁和侧副韧带起点。在过去的 5 年，多项临床试验（包括 1 项随机对照临床研究）研究了使用铰链式全肘关节置换术治疗肱骨远端骨折的效果。

加拿大骨伤学会完成了一项前瞻性随机研究，比较了 42 例 65 岁及以上的 AO C 型骨折患者切开复位内固定与一期半限制性全肘关节置换的预后。有 2 例患者在进行充分评估之前死亡，有 5 例本计划行切开复位内固定的患者最后进行了全肘关节置换。一项对 25 例全肘关节置换患者与 15 例开放复位内固定患者进行的分析发现，全肘关节置换患者的手术时间更短，Mayo 肘关节功能评分更高，但二者关节活动范围及 DASH 评分无显著差异，组间再手术率相似。[41]

在一项回顾性研究中，所有患者均为肱骨远

端的 AO B 型或 AO C 型骨折，年龄均超过 60 岁，平均随访 15 个月，将 9 例全肘关节置换术后的结果与 11 例钢板螺钉固定后的结果进行比较。平均屈伸活动范围分别为 92° 和 98°，Mayo 评分分别为 79 和 85，DASH 评分分别为 30 和 32，每组中有 2 例患者死亡，1 例患者骨折未愈合，4 例患者关节假体松动。[42]

在一项对 26 例行肘关节置换术的肱骨远端骨折患者（手术时平均年龄为 72 岁）的随访研究中，平均随访时间为 63 个月，其中 3 例死亡，1 例严重痴呆，2 例无法联系，其余 4 例男性患者和 16 例女性患者在手术时的平均年龄为 72 岁，Mayo 肘关节功能评分平均得分为 92，平均屈伸活动范围为 27°~125°，2 例患者发生异位骨化，1 例患者影像学上观察到假体松动。[43] 在另一项平均随访 2.8 年的对全肘关节置换治疗肱骨远端骨折的研究中，年龄在 75 岁或 75 岁以上的 11 例患者平均屈伸活动范围为 107°，Mayo 肘关节功能评分平均得分为 90，8 例患者影像学上观察到假体松动。[44] 在一项对 32 例行全肘关节置换术的肱骨远端骨折患者（早期治疗 15 例，延迟治疗 17 例）的随访研究中，平均随访 56 个月，两组间 Mayo 肘关节功能评分、满意度和假体成功率无显著差异。延迟治疗的 17 例患者中有 2 例感染较重。[45]

一项独特的研究报道了在北美洲以外地区普遍采用的无铰链全肘关节置换术治疗肱骨远端骨折的预后。该研究中的骨折类型主要是肱骨小头 – 滑车骨折，可以选择半肘关节置换术。平均随访 3.5 年，研究中的 9 例患者（平均年龄 73 岁）的 Mayo 肘关节功能评分平均得分为 95（65~100）。[46]

并发症

在过去的 5 年中，已经有研究报道了一些与平行钢板有关的罕见并发症。一项研究报道了 4 例肱骨远端骨折患者在行平行钢板内固定后发生骨坏死[47]（图 45–5）。另一项研究报道了肱骨远

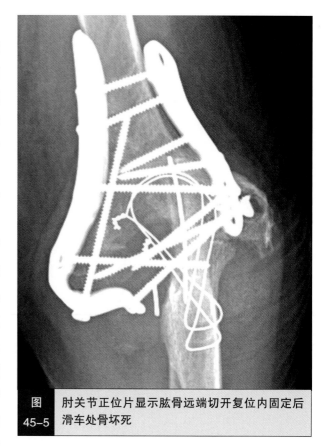

图 45–5 肘关节正位片显示肱骨远端切开复位内固定后滑车处骨坏死

端坏死采用血管化腓骨移植重建。[48] 还有一项研究报道了 3 例双柱骨折钢板固定后肘关节脱位，可能与侧副韧带起点损伤有关。[49]

一项对肘关节损伤的长期随访研究发现，肱骨远端双柱骨折和肱骨小头 – 滑车骨折比其他肘关节损伤更容易发生创伤性关节炎。[50] 这种关节炎无症状，也不会引起功能障碍，通常不需要额外手术治疗。一项通过放疗预防异位骨化的随机对照临床试验因为肱骨远端骨折患者放疗后骨不连率过高而被终止。[51]

三项针对尺神经病变的研究相对复杂。尺神经病变的定义、诊断及其在手术期间所需要的处理存在差异，在回顾性研究中差异更大。第一项研究随访了 69 例 ORIF 治疗肱骨远端双柱骨折的患者，尺神经功能障碍的发生率为 16%，但没有人口学统计表明损伤或治疗因素与术后尺神经功能障碍的风险相关[52]。第二项研究随访了 48 例肱骨远端骨折 ORIF 时进行尺神经旷置的患者，有

16 例（33%）发生尺神经病变，而未经旷置治疗的 89 例患者中有 8 例（9%）发生尺神经病变。[53] 在这项回顾性研究中，有可能实行尺神经旷置治疗的患者在内侧进行了更复杂的手术操作，对神经的处理更多，假体需要进入肘管，因此才进行了旷置。第三项研究报道了术前尺神经功能异常的发生率很高，但其不常被诊断。117 例肱骨远端 AO C 型骨折中有 29 例术前出现尺神经症状，117 例患者被随机分组并分别进行筋膜下尺神经移位或尺神经原位减压。88 例无术前症状的患者未报告新的尺神经病变，尺神经移位患者比尺神经原位减压患者尺神经恢复得更好。[54]

　　一项纳入 59 例患者的随访研究发现，不稳定的肘关节损伤（如远端移位的骨折）合并肱骨和桡骨远端骨折（9 例）的风险比单纯桡骨远端骨折发生前臂骨筋膜室综合征的风险高 50 倍。[55]

总结

　　肱骨远端骨折的大多数数据来自小型回顾性案例研究。这些研究得出了许多有意义的结果。例如，肱骨小头-滑车骨折比看起来复杂得多。将来的研究领域应包括平行和垂直钢板固定的预后比较、锁定螺钉的作用、尺神经损伤的危险因素以及处理尺神经的最佳方法。肱骨远端骨折很少见，因此多中心参与注册和随机临床研究（与加拿大骨伤学会的研究一样）对于改善治疗很重要。

参考文献

[1] Brouwer KM, Guitton TG, Doornberg JN, Kloen P, Jupiter JB, Ring D: Fractures of the medial column of the distal humerus in adults. *J Hand Surg Am* 2009;34(3):439-445.
　　Medial column fractures are uncommon in adults and often feature complex articular comminution.

[2] Zalavras CG, Vercillo MT, Jun BJ, Otarodifard K, Itamura JM, Lee TQ: Biomechanical evaluation of parallel versus orthogonal plate fixation of intra-articular distal humerus fractures. *J Shoulder Elbow Surg* 2011;20(1):12-20.
　　Parallel plates were found to be stronger than perpendicular plates in a bicolumnar metaphyseal defect model.

[3] Penzkofer R, Hungerer S, Wipf F, von Oldenburg G, Augat P: Anatomical plate configuration affects mechanical performance in distal humerus fractures. *Clin Biomech (Bristol, Avon)* 2010;25(10):972-978.
　　Three different plate configurations offered adequate stability for active motion after open reduction and internal fixation of bicolumnar fractures.

[4] Windolf M, Maza ER, Gueorguiev B, Braunstein V, Schwieger K: Treatment of distal humeral fractures using conventional implants: Biomechanical evaluation of a new implant configuration. *BMC Musculoskelet Disord* 2010;11:172.
　　A cadaver study found that a new method of interlocking parallel plates was slightly stronger than conventional methods.

[5] Arnander MW, Reeves A, MacLeod IA, Pinto TM, Khaleel A: A biomechanical comparison of plate configuration in distal humerus fractures. *J Orthop Trauma* 2008;22(5):332-336.
　　Parallel plates were found to be stronger than perpendicular plates in certain bending modes.

[6] Stoffel K, Cunneen S, Morgan R, Nicholls R, Stachowiak G: Comparative stability of perpendicular versus parallel double-locking plating systems in osteoporotic comminuted distal humerus fractures. *J Orthop Res* 2008;26(6):778-784.
　　A biomechanical study found greater stability with parallel plating than with perpendicular plating.

[7] Mehling I, Schmidt-Horlohé K, Müller LP, Sternstein W, Korner J, Rommens PM: Locking reconstruction double plating of distal humeral fractures: How many screws in the distal ulnar column segment in A3 fracture provide superior stability? A comparative biomechanical in vitro study. *J Orthop Trauma* 2009;23(8):581-587.
　　Based on biomechanical analysis, the use of more than one locked screw was recommended in the distal humerus was recommended by the authors.

[8] Schuster I, Korner J, Arzdorf M, Schwieger K, Diederichs G, Linke B: Mechanical comparison in cadaver specimens of three different 90-degree double-plate osteosyntheses for simulated C2-type distal humerus fractures with varying bone densities. *J Orthop Trauma* 2008;22(2):113-120.

Locking screws were found to make a difference only in distal humerus fractures in cadavers with poor quality bone.

[9] Sabo MT, Fay K, McDonald CP, Ferreira LM, Johnson JA, King GJ: Effect of coronal shear fractures of the distal humerus on elbow kinematics and stability. *J Shoulder Elbow Surg* 2010;19(5):670-680.

Excision of the capitellum did not destabilize the elbow if the ligaments were intact, but any loss of the trochlea destabilized the elbow.

[10] Park SH, Kim SJ, Park BC, et al: Three-dimensional osseous micro-architecture of the distal humerus: Implications for internal fixation of osteoporotic fracture. *J Shoulder Elbow Surg* 2010;19(2):244-250.

The lowest quality bone was found in the posterolateral distal humerus.

[11] Brouwer KM, Lindenhovius AL, Ring D: Loss of anterior translation of the distal humeral articular surface is associated with decreased elbow flexion. *J Hand Surg Am* 2009;34(7):1256-1260.

Relative straightening of the distal humerus in the sagittal plane hindered flexion after distal humeral fracture.

[12] Kimball JP, Glowczewskie F, Wright TW: Intraosseous blood supply to the distal humerus. *J Hand Surg Am* 2007;32(5):642-646.

The blood supply to the distal humerus was found to be limited.

[13] Brouwer KM, Jupiter JB, Ring D: Nonunion of operatively treated capitellum and trochlear fractures. *J Hand Surg Am* 2011;36(5):804-807.

Thirty patients underwent open reduction and internal fixation of a capitellum-trochlea fracture. At an average follow-up of 34 months, 8 of the 18 patients with a Dubberley type 3B fracture had nonunion. No patient with a simpler fracture had nonunion.

[14] Doornberg JN, van Duijn PJ, Linzel D, et al: Surgical treatment of intra-articular fractures of the distal part of the humerus: Functional outcome after twelve to thirty years. *J Bone Joint Surg Am* 2007;89(7):1524-1532.

At an average follow-up of 19 years after plate-and-screw fixation of an AO type C fracture of the distal humerus in 30 patients, the average arc of flexion was 106°, the average DASH score was 7, and the average Mayo score was 91, with 26 good or excellent results. The results were not correlated with arthrosis.

[15] Huang JI, Paczas M, Hoyen HA, Vallier HA: Functional outcome after open reduction internal fixation of intra-articular fractures of the distal humerus in the elderly. *J Orthop Trauma* 2011;25(5):259-265.

Distal humeral fracture was found to be an elbow-changing injury that causes pain and disability in the elderly.

[16] Liu JJ, Ruan HJ, Wang JG, Fan CY, Zeng BF: Double-column fixation for type C fractures of the distal humerus in the elderly. *J Shoulder Elbow Surg* 2009;18(4):646-651.

A retrospective study found acceptable results after open reduction and internal fixation of double-column fractures.

[17] Frattini M, Soncini G, Corradi M, Panno B, Tocco S, Pogliacomi F: Mid-term results of complex distal humeral fractures. *Musculoskelet Surg* 2011;95(3):205-213.

Another retrospective study found acceptable results after open reduction and internal fixation of double-column fractures.

[18] Luegmair M, Timofiev E, Chirpaz-Cerbat JM: Surgical treatment of AO type C distal humeral fractures: Internal fixation with a Y-shaped reconstruction (Lambda) plate. *J Shoulder Elbow Surg* 2008;17(1):113-120.

The functional outcome of fixation of distal humeral fractures with a Y-shaped plate was analyzed.

[19] Bhattacharyya A, Jha AK, Chatterjee D, Ghosh B, Roy SK, Banerjee D: Operative management of closed intra-articular fractures of distal end of humerus in adults. *J Indian Med Assoc* 2011;109(6):418-423, 423.

The fixation of type C distal humeral fractures using older methods had acceptable outcomes in India.

[20] Babhulkar S, Babhulkar S: Controversies in the management of intra-articular fractures of distal humerus in adults. *Indian J Orthop* 2011;45(3):216-225.

The use of three different dual-plate configurations for distal humeral fractures had comparably good results.

[21] Puchwein P, Wildburger R, Archan S, Guschl M, Tanzer K, Gumpert R: Outcome of type C (AO) distal humeral fractures: Follow-up of 22 patients with bicolumnar plating osteosynthesis. *J Shoulder Elbow Surg* 2011;20(4):631-636.

A retrospective study found acceptable outcomes after open reduction and internal fixation of bicolumnar fractures using dual plates.

[22] Li SH, Li ZH, Cai ZD, et al: Bilateral plate fixation for type C distal humerus fractures: Experience at a single institution. *Int Orthop* 2011;35(3):433-438.

A retrospective study found acceptable outcomes after

open reduction and internal fixation of bicolumnar fractures using a transolecranon approach.

[23] Proust J, Oksman A, Charissoux JL, Mabit C, Arnaud JP: [Intra-articular fracture of the distal humerus: Outcome after osteosynthesis in patients over 60]. *Rev Chir Orthop Reparatrice Appar Mot* 2007;93(8):798-806.

Open reduction and internal fixation of bicolumnar fractures had a good or very good outcome in 59% of patients older than 60 years.

[24] Chen G, Liao Q, Luo W, Li K, Zhao Y, Zhong D: Triceps-sparing versus olecranon osteotomy for ORIF: Analysis of 67 cases of intercondylar fractures of the distal humerus. *Injury* 2011;42(4):366-370.

Olecranon osteotomy was found to lead to better results than a triceps-sparing approach in patients older than 60 years.

[25] Ali AM, Hassanin EY, El-Ganainy AE, Abd-Elmola T: Management of intercondylar fractures of the humerus using the extensor mechanism-sparing paratricipital posterior approach. *Acta Orthop Belg* 2008;74(6):747-752.

The use of the paratricipital approach in patients with an interarticular fracture of the distal humerus led to satisfactory results.

[26] Ek ET, Goldwasser M, Bonomo AL: Functional outcome of complex intercondylar fractures of the distal humerus treated through a triceps-sparing approach. *J Shoulder Elbow Surg* 2008;17(3):441-446.

The use of the paratricipital approach in patients with an interarticular fracture of the distal humerus led to satisfactory results.

[27] Theivendran K, Duggan PJ, Deshmukh SC: Surgical treatment of complex distal humeral fractures: Functional outcome after internal fixation using precontoured anatomic plates. *J Shoulder Elbow Surg* 2010;19(4):524-532.

The use of anatomic precontoured plates led to acceptable functional outcomes with complex distal humeral fractures.

[28] Athwal GS, Hoxie SC, Rispoli DM, Steinmann SP: Precontoured parallel plate fixation of AO/OTA type C distal humerus fractures. *J Orthop Trauma* 2009;23(8):575-580.

The use of anatomic precontoured plates was effective, but more than one half of the patients experienced a complication.

[29] Sanchez-Sotelo J, Torchia ME, O'Driscoll SW: Complex distal humeral fractures: Internal fixation with a principle-based parallel-plate technique. *J Bone Joint Surg Am* 2007;89(5):961-969.

After 32 AO type C fractures were repaired with parallel plates, 1 patient had nonunion, 5 underwent subsequent surgery for elbow stiffness, and 1 had a deep infection. The mean arc of flexion was 99°, and the mean Mayo score was 85, with 27 patients with good or excellent results.

[30] Shin SJ, Sohn HS, Do NH: A clinical comparison of two different double plating methods for intraarticular distal humerus fractures. *J Shoulder Elbow Surg* 2010;19(1):2-9.

Perpendicular plating was less successful than parallel plating in achieving bony union for supracondylar fractures of the distal humerus.

[31] Reising K, Hauschild O, Strohm PC, Suedkamp NP: Stabilisation of articular fractures of the distal humerus: Early experience with a novel perpendicular plate system. *Injury* 2009;40(6):611-617.

The use of locking precontoured plates led to stable fixation for articular fractures of the distal humerus.

[32] Greiner S, Haas NP, Bail HJ: Outcome after open reduction and angular stable internal fixation for supra-intercondylar fractures of the distal humerus: Preliminary results with the LCP distal humerus system. *Arch Orthop Trauma Surg* 2008;128(7):723-729.

The use of locking precontoured plates led to stable fixation for supracondylar fractures of the distal humerus.

[33] Min W, Ding BC, Tejwani NC: Staged versus acute definitive management of open distal humerus fractures. *J Trauma* 2011;71(4):944-947.

Patients with open distal humeral fractures who were treated with temporary external fixation and staged open reduction and internal fixation had worse results than those who underwent early definitive fixation, probably because these patients had more severe fractures.

[34] Watts AC, Morris A, Robinson CM: Fractures of the distal humeral articular surface. *J Bone Joint Surg Br* 2007;89(4):510-515.

This recent case study reported that fractures of the capitellum and the trochlea are more common than previously recognized.

[35] Guitton TG, Doornberg JN, Raaymakers EL, Ring D, Kloen P: Fractures of the capitellum and trochlea. *J Bone Joint Surg Am* 2009;91(2):390-397.

This case study provides data on long-term outcomes of fractures of the capitellum and the trochlea.

[36] Dubberley JH, Faber KJ, Macdermid JC, Patterson SD,

King GJ: Outcome after open reduction and internal fixation of capitellar and trochlear fractures. *J Bone Joint Surg Am* 2006;88(1):46-54.

［37］ Ashwood N, Verma M, Hamlet M, Garlapati A, Fogg Q: Transarticular shear fractures of the distal humerus. *J Shoulder Elbow Surg* 2010;19(1):46-52.

The treatment of patients with a capitellum-trochlea fracture is described.

［38］ Mighell M, Virani NA, Shannon R, Echols EL Jr, Badman BL, Keating CJ: Large coronal shear fractures of the capitellum and trochlea treated with headless compression screws. *J Shoulder Elbow Surg* 2010;19(1):38-45.

The treatment of patients with a capitellum-trochlea fracture is described.

［39］ Adolfsson L, Nestorson J: The Kudo humeral component as primary hemiarthroplasty in distal humeral fractures. *J Shoulder Elbow Surg* 2012;21(4):451-455.

Eight women (average age, 79 years) who were evaluated at a mean 4-year follow-up after Kudo hemiarthroplasty for fracture of the distal humerus had an average flexion from 31° to 126°. All patients had good or excellent Mayo scores.

［40］ Burkhart KJ, Nijs S, Mattyasovszky SG, et al: Distal humerus hemiarthroplasty of the elbow for comminuted distal humeral fractures in the elderly patient. *J Trauma* 2011;71(3):635-642.

Hemiarthroplasty for distal humeral fracture had good results in 10 patients (mean age, 75.2 years).

［41］ McKee MD, Veillette CJ, Hall JA, et al: A multicenter, prospective, randomized, controlled trial of open reduction—internal fixation versus total elbow arthroplasty for displaced intra-articular distal humeral fractures in elderly patients. *J Shoulder Elbow Surg* 2009;18(1):3-12.

A Canadian Orthopaedic Trauma Society prospective randomized study compared open reduction and internal fixation with primary semiconstrained total elbow arthroplasty in 42 patients (minimum age, 65 years) with AO type C fracture. Total elbow arthroplasty was associated with shorter surgical times and better Mayo scores but not better motion or DASH scores.

［42］ Egol KA, Tsai P, Vazques O, Tejwani NC: Comparison of functional outcomes of total elbow arthroplasty vs plate fixation for distal humerus fractures in osteoporotic elbows. *Am J Orthop (Belle Mead NJ)* 2011;40(2):67-71.

A retrospective study found that both open reduction and internal fixation and total elbow arthroplasty had good results in patients with an osteoporotic elbow.

［43］ Ali A, Shahane S, Stanley D: Total elbow arthroplasty for distal humeral fractures: Indications, surgical approach, technical tips, and outcome. *J Shoulder Elbow Surg* 2010;19(Suppl 2):53-58.

Total elbow arthroplasty was described for patients with a bicolumnar fracture.

［44］ Chalidis B, Dimitriou C, Papadopoulos P, Petsatodis G, Giannoudis PV: Total elbow arthroplasty for the treatment of insufficient distal humeral fractures: A retrospective clinical study and review of the literature. *Injury* 2009;40(6):582-590.

The treatment and outcomes of total elbow arthroscopy for distal humeral fracture were described.

［45］ Prasad N, Dent C: Outcome of total elbow replacement for distal humeral fractures in the elderly: A comparison of primary surgery and surgery after failed internal fixation or conservative treatment. *J Bone Joint Surg Br* 2008;90(3):343-348.

A small comparative study found that delayed total elbow arthroscopy had less satisfactory outcomes than early arthroplasty, but the difference was not significant.

［46］ Kalogrianitis S, Sinopidis C, El Meligy M, Rawal A, Frostick SP: Unlinked elbow arthroplasty as primary treatment for fractures of the distal humerus. *J Shoulder Elbow Surg* 2008;17(2):287-292.

The use of an unlinked total elbow prosthesis is described.

［47］ Wiggers JK, Ring D: Osteonecrosis after open reduction and internal fixation of a bicolumnar fracture of the distal humerus: A report of four cases. *J Hand Surg Am* 2011;36(1):89-93.

Some patients experienced a complication related to osteonecrosis in the articular surface after open reduction and internal fixation.

［48］ Vigler M, Gargano F, Hausman MR: Trochlear reconstruction using vascularized lateral clavicle bone graft for posttraumatic osteonecrosis of the distal humerus. *J Shoulder Elbow Surg* 2008;17(5):e4-e8.

The treatment of osteonecrosis of the distal humerus was reported.

［49］ Lu HT, Guitton TG, Capo JT, Ring D: Elbow instability associated with bicolumnar fracture of the distal humerus: Report of three cases. *J Hand Surg Am* 2010;35(7):1126-1129.

Instability, presumably related to lateral collateral ligament injury during fixation, was found to be a complication of open reduction and internal fixation.

［50］Guitton TG, Zurakowski D, van Dijk NC, Ring D: Incidence and risk factors for the development of radiographic arthrosis after traumatic elbow injuries. *J Hand Surg Am* 2010;35(12):1976-1980.

Distal humeral fractures were found to be more likely to lead to arthritis than other elbow trauma.

［51］Hamid N, Ashraf N, Bosse MJ, et al: Radiation therapy for heterotopic ossification prophylaxis acutely after elbow trauma: A prospective randomized study. *J Bone Joint Surg Am* 2010;92(11):2032-2038.

A randomized study was abandoned because preventive radiation for heterotopic ossification was causing nonunion of osteotomies and fractures.

［52］Vazquez O, Rutgers M, Ring DC, Walsh M, Egol KA: Fate of the ulnar nerve after operative fixation of distal humerus fractures. *J Orthop Trauma* 2010;24(7):395-399.

After 69 bicolumnar distal humeral fractures were treated with plate and screw fixation, ulnar nerve dysfunction occurred in 16%, but no demographic, injury, or treatment factors were associated with a risk of postoperative ulnar nerve dysfunction.

［53］Chen RC, Harris DJ, Leduc S, Borrelli JJ Jr, Tornetta P III, Ricci WM: Is ulnar nerve transposition beneficial during open reduction internal fixation of distal humerus fractures? *J Orthop Trauma* 2010;24(7):391-394.

A study of plate fixation of the distal humerus documented ulnar neuropathy in 33% (16 of 48) treated with transposition of the ulnar nerve and 9% (8 of 89) treated without.

［54］Ruan HJ, Liu JJ, Fan CY, Jiang J, Zeng BF: Incidence, management, and prognosis of early ulnar nerve dysfunction in type C fractures of distal humerus. *J Trauma* 2009;67(6):1397-1401.

This randomized study found a high rate of preoperative ulnar nerve symptoms (25%) in patients with a distal humeral fracture. Transposition wa considered preferable to in situ release.

［55］Hwang RW, de Witte PB, Ring D: Compartment syndrome associated with distal radial fracture and ipsilateral elbow injury. *J Bone Joint Surg Am* 2009;91(3):642-645.

Ipsilateral unstable wrist and elbow injuries were found to have an increased risk for acute forearm compartment syndrome.

第四十六章　肘关节镜：适应证和手术考量

Aaron Chamberlain, MD; Ken Yamaguchi, MD

引言

1931 年，Burman 根据尸体研究，认为肘关节不适合进行关节镜操作。[1] 1985 年，Andrews 和 Carson 描述了 12 例成功进行肘关节镜手术的案例，并得出结论：如果外科医师密切注意手术细节及安全性，则肘关节镜手术是可行的。虽然手术技术和设备的进步显著提高了肘关节镜的实用性，但是对手术适应证的严格把握，以及术者的关节镜操作经验，对于安全、有效地进行肘关节镜手术至关重要。

适应证

肘关节镜手术的适应证范围随着手术技术和设备的进步已大大拓宽。1985 年，作为一种诊断和治疗工具，肘关节镜被用于去除游离体及进行桡骨头和肱骨小头软骨成形术。[2] 时至今日，肘关节镜的适应证已包括类风湿关节炎、肘关节炎、肘关节僵硬、剥脱性骨软骨炎、肱骨外上髁炎、部分骨折及有临床症状的关节挛缩。目前已有较高质量的证据证实肘关节镜可用于治疗类风湿关节炎及肱骨外上髁炎。

Dr. Yamaguchi or an immediate family member has received royalties from Tornier. Neither Dr. Chamberlain nor any immediate family member has received anything of value from or has stock or stock options held in a commercial company or institution related directly or indirectly to the subject of this chapter.

只有少部分低质量的证据支持使用肘关节镜进行挛缩关节囊和环状韧带的切除，以及治疗肘关节炎、剥脱性骨软骨炎、后外侧旋转不稳定、游离体、创伤后关节纤维化及骨折。[3] 总体来说，肘关节镜仍是一种相对较新的技术，需要更多高质量的研究来确定其有效性。

游离体切除

游离体切除是肘关节镜检查的最常见适应证。[4] Andrews 和 Carson 发现，与软骨成形术等操作相比，松质体切除术是肘关节镜最成功的临床应用。在一项对 33 例肘关节镜切除游离体的研究中，有 85% 的患者的疼痛得到缓解，92% 的患者的交锁症状得到缓解，71% 的患者的肿胀得到改善。[5] 大量病例研究报告了肘关节镜下切除游离体的临床结果。近期 12 项关于关节镜下游离体清除的病例研究发现，在 109 例患者中，有98 例（90%）预后优异或良好的，或获得了症状的显著改善。[3] 在对 9 项通过肘关节镜行软骨成形术或骨赘清创术的临床研究中，150 例患者中有 110 例（73%）预后良好或优异。但是，目前尚无关于比较关节镜和开放式手术的游离体切除效果的研究发表。

滑膜切除术

多项研究证明使用肘关节镜行滑膜切除术治疗类风湿关节炎可获得良好的预后。[6-8] 与开放式滑膜切除术相比，关节镜滑膜切除术的侵入性较小，有助于早期恢复活动，并且具有较低的术后僵硬风险。但是，由于该手术的局限性和技术挑战，有两篇文献强调了滑膜切除不完全的风险。[6,9]与开放式滑膜切除术相比，行不完全的关节镜下滑膜切除术后，患者恶化得更快。14例因类风湿关节炎或幼年特发性关节炎而接受关节镜滑膜切除术的患者在术后早期随访时疼痛程度较轻，但只有8例（57%）在最终随访时（平均42个月）获得了较好的功能恢复。[6]

技术的进步使医师在关节镜下能够更完整地切除滑膜。接受关节镜滑膜切除术的26例类风湿关节炎病例使用了软点入路和外侧入路来进入肱桡关节后侧和近端桡尺关节。此外，标准的前正中入路和前外侧入路被用来进入前方关节间隙，后外侧入路和后正中入路被用来进入后方关节间隙。[10]在一项使用肘关节镜切除滑膜的平均34个月的随访研究中，患者视觉模拟评分法的平均得分从6.5改善到3.1，平均屈伸活动范围从98°增加到113°。19例（73%）患者的功能结果良好或优异，4例患者滑膜炎复发，其中2例需要再次行滑膜切除术，1例需行全肘关节置换术，1例拒绝进一步手术。

相比较而言，肘关节镜滑膜切除术的总体效果不如其他关节镜滑膜切除术。目前仅有有限的病例研究提供了一些薄弱的证据支持行关节镜滑膜切除术，医师在操作过程中一定要将滑膜彻底切除。

肘关节僵硬

肘关节僵硬相对比较常见，且治疗手段有限。导致肘关节僵硬的原因很多，可分为内在因素和外在因素。内在因素包括关节炎、骨折等引起关节不匹配的情况，外在因素包括关节囊紧张或挛缩、异位骨化及皮肤或肌肉挛缩。关节镜可用于治疗关节囊挛缩及伴有骨化形成的关节炎等。

目前，肘关节镜治疗肘关节僵硬仍具有一定挑战性。一项关于肘关节镜学习曲线的研究发现，外科医师完成15次肘关节镜手术后，手术时间没有明显减少。[11]尽管如此，关节镜下处理肘关节

僵硬的应用仍越来越广泛。[11-20]一项回顾性研究随访了14例创伤后肘关节僵硬行关节镜下松解的患者，发现在至少1年的随访中，有6例主诉疼痛，视觉模拟评分法平均得分为4.6。[12]肘关节平均伸直角度术前为35.4°，术后提高到9.3°，屈曲角度从117.5°提高到133°。总活动范围从82°提高到123.6°（平均改善41.6°）。最近的一项研究报道了27例创伤后肘关节僵硬行肘关节镜下松解的结果[13]。术前伸直角度和屈曲角度分别为24°和123°，术后伸直角度提高到7°，屈曲角度提高到133°，总活动范围从99°提高到125°，没有发现神经损伤等并发症。

只有一项已发表的研究直接比较了关节镜和开放式肘关节松解术。对Outerbridge-Kashiwagi手术（开放松解和鹰嘴窝开窗术）和关节镜下肘关节松解的非随机对照研究发现，这两种方法均有效且无严重并发症。[21]关节镜松解术对疼痛的减轻更明显（$P<0.10$），而开放式Outerbridge-Kashiwagi手术患者的屈曲活动范围更大（$P<0.05$）。一项对20例肘关节僵硬患者行关节镜下松解术的平均2年的回顾性临床研究发现，这些患者的肘关节活动范围从94°提高至123°，视觉模拟评分法评分从5.8提高至1.8，总体结果令人满意，其中有16例预后评级为优秀，2例一般，2例较差。[14]

大多数关于关节镜下肘关节僵硬松解的研究包括了具有内在因素和外在因素的患者，排除了关节不匹配和明显异位骨化的患者。还没有关于此类手术的一级研究。尽管证据存在局限性，但现有已发表的案例研究表明，对有经验的外科医师来说，关节镜下松解是一种安全、有效的方法，可处理非手术治疗难以改善的肘关节僵硬。

剥脱性骨软骨炎

肘部的OCD病变通常是局部病变，影响肱骨头的关节面。这种损伤在年轻运动员中并不罕见。手术治疗需考虑的主要因素包括关节面的完整性、病变的稳定性以及骨骺是否闭合。如果患者的病灶

不稳定，有游离体和（或）非手术治疗不成功，则可能需要手术干预。[22] 完整的关节镜手术步骤主要包括经关节钻孔、松质体摘除、钻孔、微骨折和镶嵌成形术。[23] 目前有许多关于关节镜下 OCD 治疗的案例研究。[22, 24-32] 最近一项纳入 9 项研究的系统综述，评估了运动员肘关节 OCD 关节镜手术的治疗效果。[33] 手术干预措施包括松解术、骨折块固定、微骨折和骨软骨自体移植。手术干预后，81%~100% 的患者重返赛场，89%~100% 的患者未诉疼痛。但是，评估肘关节 OCD 关节镜手术的治疗效果时使用了多种临床结果指标，因此难以进行直接的研究比较。目前还没有比较非手术治疗预后和关节镜治疗预后的研究。

肱骨外上髁炎

两项回顾性队列研究比较了开放式和关节镜下松解桡侧腕短伸肌（ECRB）对顽固性肱骨外上髁炎的治疗效果。[34-35] 两项研究均未发现开放式和关节镜手术治疗效果存在显著差异。预后良好或优异的患者占患者总数的 60%~75%。一项研究发现，与开放式手术相比，经关节镜治疗的患者较早恢复工作（分别为 1.7 周或 2.5 周）[34]。在最近一项对 36 例因持续性外上髁炎症状接受关节镜下 ECRB 松解治疗的患者的研究中，有 31% 的患者在平均 3.5 年的随访中报告了剧烈运动时的轻度疼痛。[36] 有 2 例（6%）患者没有从该手术中获益。

总体而言，现有研究表明关节镜 ECRB 松解与开放式手术的结果无明显差异。虽然，在多数研究中关节镜下 ECRB 松解的治疗效果很好，但尚无高质量的临床研究，也没有比较关节镜治疗预后和非手术治疗预后的研究。尽管如此，现有研究仍为关节镜治疗肱骨外上髁炎提供了有力支持。[34-37]

骨折

关节镜治疗肘关节骨折是肘关节镜手术的一个相对较新的发展方向。大多数已有的关于关节镜治疗骨折的研究为小型的病例研究和病例报告，

已经描述了肱骨小头（切除和固定）、冠突（切除和固定）和桡骨头骨折的关节镜下治疗。[38-43] 但是，尚未有比较这些骨折的开放式手术治疗效果和关节镜手术治疗效果的研究发表。目前，尚无证据表明关节镜手术的治疗效果是否优于开放手术。

尺神经

对于肘部屈曲角度限制在 90°~100° 的患者，必须进行预防性尺神经处理，以防止松解和改善屈曲后神经受压。[15] 尺神经位于肘管内，其底部为尺侧副韧带后束，随着肘部屈曲超过 90°，肘管的空间减小，这增加了对尺神经的压力。[44] 如果不治疗后束挛缩，则屈曲活动范围大幅减小（保持屈曲角度小于 90°）的肘关节无法恢复屈曲。此外，随着后束拉紧，将肘关节放置到更屈曲的位置时，可能发生尺神经损伤。

之前的尺神经移位，尤其是肌肉下移位，被认为是肘关节镜检查的相对禁忌证。[45-46] 值得关注的是，在尺神经移位后，尺神经相对于其正常的解剖位置在肘关节前部，并且紧邻通常用于关节镜治疗的前内侧入口。然而，凭借经验和标准化的方法，近端正中入口可以安全地用于尺神经已移位的肘关节镜手术。一项纳入 59 例肘关节半脱位或尺神经前移病例的研究发现，使用标准的前内侧入口进行关节镜检查，如果移位的神经的位置是明确的，则从神经对应的皮肤切开一个 1 cm 的切口；如果神经的位置是模棱两可的，则在距神经较明显的位置约 1 cm 处做切口，钝性分离至关节囊，并穿透关节囊；如果无法定位神经，则切开 2~4 cm 的切口，确定神经位置并建立入口。目前还没有与使用前内侧入口相关的手术性尺神经损伤报道。[47]

禁忌证

关节镜治疗的相对禁忌证包括肘关节对合严重不良、解剖结构变形、异位骨化和肌肉挛缩。在这些情况下最好采用开放式手术进行治疗。[15]

由于邻近周围神经，如果预计手术难度较大，则手术经验不足可能是最重要的手术禁忌证。严重的肘关节挛缩常与大量的软组织粘连和关节外软组织挛缩有关，这在关节镜下难以处理。肘关节严重挛缩时，可能难以进行关节腔充气，这大大增加了关节镜检查的难度和危险性。之前提到的尺神经移位，尤其是肌肉下移位是相对禁忌证，需要对手术方法进行修正以避免神经损伤。

手术考量

术前准备和定位

肘关节镜检查有可能对周围神经血管结构和关节软骨造成严重伤害。在术前准备和定位时必须特别注意细节，以最大限度地降低此类并发症的发生。

一些外科医师在局部麻醉下进行肘关节镜检查。但是，没有特殊情况还是应首选全身麻醉，因为医师可以即刻和反复进行术后神经系统评估。另外，局部麻醉不能使患者完全放松，进而不容易让患者处于侧卧位或俯卧位，而且局部麻醉可能无法预防手术过程中止血带引起的疼痛。

预防性应用抗生素是肘关节镜的关键考虑因素。据报道，肘关节镜检查后严重的深部关节感染发生率为0.8%，长期引流和浅表感染的发生率为7%。[48] 在止血带充气之前可使用第一代头孢

菌素。如果头孢过敏，可以用克林霉素或万古霉素代替。手术结束时，用水平褥式缝合封闭进镜部位，以防止术后入口渗出和（或）瘘管形成。术后，患者预防性应用口服抗生素2周，直到伤口完全闭合且渗出的风险很小。

肘关节镜检查可在侧卧位、俯卧位或仰卧位进行。[2,49-50] 侧卧位的优点是在手术过程中易于进行气道管理，术中肘关节活动范围更大，以及肘关节镜可以更好地进入关节腔后部。当进行关节松解时，肘关节镜易于接近关节腔后部，便于从鹰嘴尖端切除骨化组织。

将患者置于侧卧位后，应放置腋窝卷或凝胶垫。在近端绑扎非无菌带状止血带。患肢置于带衬垫的固定式手臂支架中，肘关节固定在约90°的屈曲位。为确保肘关节和胸部之间有足够的空间容纳器械，手臂应与身体至少保持90°的外展角度，肘关节的位置应略高于肩关节。此外，应确保患者的前胸壁在床的边缘。这种定位方法可以方便术者在手术过程中完全屈曲和伸展患者的肘关节[51]（图46-1）。

液体管理

正确的液体管理对于肘关节镜手术的成功和安全至关重要。液体扩张对于增加关节腔的操作空间非常重要。在进镜之前，通过由外侧髁、桡骨头和鹰嘴形成的三角形中心的入口，注射

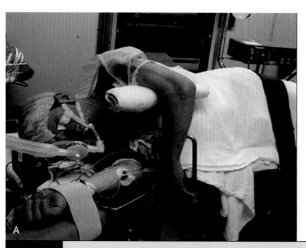
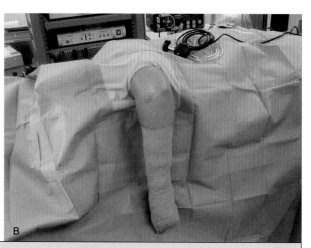

图46-1　术中照片展示了肘关节镜手术铺巾前（A）和铺巾后（B）的患者体位

20~30 ml 的生理盐水使关节扩张（图 46-2）。扩张关节囊时可通过增加肱骨与关节囊及附近神经血管结构之间的距离来提高安全性。非常僵硬的肘关节的关节囊顺应性可低至正常肘关节的 15%。这意味着关节间隙的容积大大减小，受伤的风险增加。[52] 关节囊扩张不足（无法注射超过 10 ml 生理盐水）表明该手术危险性很高，只能由经验丰富的外科医师进行。该手术可以使用泵控制系统或重力流体系统。

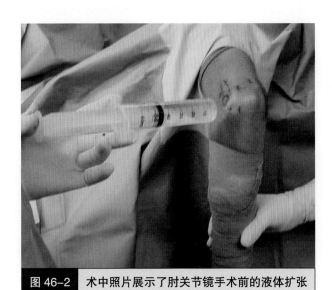

图 46-2 术中照片展示了肘关节镜手术前的液体扩张

建议使用泵控制系统，将流体泵压力设置为 35 mmHg。应注意，实际泵压在不同制造商的产品之间会有所不同。通常，肘关节镜手术的泵压设定为比肩关节镜手术的泵压低约 30% 的水平。应使用低泵压最大限度地减少软组织肿胀，肘关节软组织肿胀可迅速发生，并严重阻碍肘关节镜手术进行。手术时间在肘关节镜手术中很重要，因为关节囊组织会迅速变得肿胀并影响关节内的观察和工作空间。因此，在肘关节镜手术中，手术效率比在其他主要关节的关节镜手术中更为重要。

手术工具发展

使用现代仪器有助于安全、有效地进行肘关节镜操作。尽管可以考虑使用较小的 2.7 mm 关节镜，但常用的肘关节镜还是标准的 4.5 mm 关节镜。标准的 30° 镜头适用于大多数手术。但是，使用 70° 镜头可以更完整地显示冠突窝深度以及一些隐蔽的游离体和软骨损伤。[53] 尽管不一定必须使用引流管，但引流管可用于操作时引流，这有助于减少周围软组织充气和水肿。如果使用引流管，则应使用无侧窗的低流量引流管，以最大程度地减少软组织充气。有多种型号的引流管可供选择，通常直径应小于 5.5 mm。

与其他主要关节的关节镜手术相比，肘关节镜对进镜口位置偏差的敏感性要高得多，而且不精确的进镜口选择将阻碍术者的有效地操作。导丝和空心扩张器用于准确、安全地创建进镜口。使用这些器械避免了引流管和手术器械反复通过周围的软组织，从而减少了神经血管损伤的机会。将关节镜放置在近端前内侧入路观察肱桡关节时，将导丝在直视下放置在关节中。用手术刀切开导丝周围的皮肤，然后用空心扩张器形成精确的进镜口。导丝和扩张器的放置必须精确，因为桡神经平均距离近端前入路 5~10 mm。建立了近端前内侧和前外侧入路后，可以使用钝的套管针松解关节内粘连并从肱骨前方抬起前方关节囊，从而增加操作空间。

4.0 规格的刨削器可用于去除滑膜和粘连组织。应注意不要将刨削器直接对准关节囊。应小心抽吸，防止关节囊组织被吸入，进而损坏邻近的神经血管结构。前关节腔很少使用抽吸操作。

小口径刨削器可用于切除较大的骨化或进行骨囊置换术。经过特殊设计的截骨器可用于在肘关节后部及鹰嘴尖端进行骨化切除。

可以使用 15° 篮剪在肱肌和前方关节囊之间剪切一个平面，随后使用篮剪从外向内分隔前方关节囊。如有必要，可以将关节镜切换到近端前外侧入路，并且可以从近端前内侧入路完成关节囊切开术，直至暴露肱骨深表面。关节囊切开术应在完成前方关节囊所有操作后进行，因为切开后，会迅速发生软组织肿胀，从而减少关节内的操作空间。

特殊设计的肘关节镜牵开器可用于安全牵开软组织（如前方关节囊）和保护神经血管结构（如尺神经）。

总结

肘关节镜曾经被认为不可能被成功应用，但其目前已经发展成为一种治疗各种肘关节病变的有价值的技术。虽然技术上的进步和改进已使肘关节镜技术具有了很高的安全性和可靠性，但仍需要较高水平的操作技术。为了肘关节镜向安全、有效的方向持续发展，未来应专注于外科医师的教育和技术进步。

参考文献

[1] Burman MS: Arthroscopy or the direct visualization of joints: An experimental cadaver study. *J Bone Joint Surg* 1931;13:669-695.

[2] Andrews JR, Carson WG: Arthroscopy of the elbow. *Arthroscopy* 1985;1(2):97-107.

[3] Yeoh KM, King GJ, Faber KJ, Glazebrook MA, Athwal GS: Evidence-based indications for elbow arthroscopy. *Arthroscopy* 2012;28(2):272-282.

A recent review of the outcomes of elbow arthroscopy makes evidence-based recommendations for or against elbow arthroscopy for the treatment of various conditions. Level of evidence: IV.

[4] Baker CL, Brooks AA: Arthroscopy of the elbow. *Clin Sports Med* 1996;15(2):261-281.

[5] Ogilvie-Harris DJ, Schemitsch E: Arthroscopy of the elbow for removal of loose bodies. *Arthroscopy* 1993;9(1):5-8.

[6] Lee BP, Morrey BF: Arthroscopic synovectomy of the elbow for rheumatoid arthritis: A prospective study. *J Bone Joint Surg Br* 1997;79(5):770-772.

[7] Nemoto K, Arino H, Yoshihara Y, Fujikawa K: Arthroscopic synovectomy for the rheumatoid elbow: A short-term outcome. *J Shoulder Elbow Surg* 2004;13(6):652-655.

[8] Tanaka N, Sakahashi H, Hirose K, Ishima T, Ishii S: Arthroscopic and open synovectomy of the elbow in rheumatoid arthritis. *J Bone Joint Surg Am* 2006;88(3):521-525.

[9] Horiuchi K, Momohara S, Tomatsu T, Inoue K, Toyama Y: Arthroscopic synovectomy of the elbow in rheumatoid arthritis. *J Bone Joint Surg Am* 2002;84-A(3):342-347.

[10] Kang HJ, Park MJ, Ahn JH, Lee SH: Arthroscopic synovectomy for the rheumatoid elbow. *Arthroscopy* 2010;26(9):1195-1202.

Management of the rheumatoid elbow with an arthroscopic total synovectomy is described, with multiple portals and division of the elbow into the anterior, posterior, and radiocapitellar compartments. Level of evidence: IV.

[11] Kim S-J, Moon H-K, Chun Y-M, Chang J-H: Arthroscopic treatment for limitation of motion of the elbow: The learning curve. *Knee Surg Sports Traumatol Arthrosc* 2011;19(6):1013-1018.

A learning curve for elbow arthroscopy was assigned in the setting of the stiff elbow by comparing mean surgical times, mean improvement in motion, and clinical scores. Level of evidence: IV.

[12] Ball CM, Meunier M, Galatz LM, Calfee R, Yamaguchi K: Arthroscopic treatment of post-traumatic elbow contracture. *J Shoulder Elbow Surg* 2002;11(6):624-629.

[13] Cefo I, Eygendaal D: Arthroscopic arthrolysis for post-traumatic elbow stiffness. *J Shoulder Elbow Surg* 2011;20(3):434-439.

The outcomes of 27 patients with posttraumatic elbow stiffness treated with arthroscopic capsular release were assessed. Level of evidence: IV.

[14] DeGreef I, Samorjai N, De Smet L: The Outerbridge-Kashiwaghi procedure in elbow arthroscopy. *Acta Orthop Belg* 2010;76(4):468-471.

The results of the arthroscopic Outerbridge-Kashiwaghi procedure were evaluated at a mean 2-year follow-up in a retrospective review of 20 elbows in 19 patients. Level of evidence: IV.

[15] Keener JD, Galatz LM: Arthroscopic management of the stiff elbow. *J Am Acad Orthop Surg* 2011;19(5):265-274.

This review article discusses intrinsic and extrinsic causes of elbow stiffness as well as the arthroscopic management of these causes of elbow stiffness.

[16] Singh H, Nam KY, Moon YL: Arthroscopic management of stiff elbow. *Orthopedics* 2011;34(6):167.

Functional results after arthroscopic management of the stiff elbow were evaluated in a case study. Level of evidence: IV.

[17] Van Zeeland NL, Yamaguchi K: Arthroscopic capsular release of the elbow. *J Shoulder Elbow Surg* 2010;19(2, suppl):13-19.

The reviewed technical advances and modifications have allowed arthroscopic capsular release of the elbow to emerge as a safe and reliable although technically demanding method to restore elbow motion.

[18] Lapner PC, Leith JM, Regan WD: Arthroscopic debridement of the elbow for arthrofibrosis resulting from nondisplaced fracture of the radial head. *Arthroscopy* 2005;21(12):1492.

[19] Nguyen D, Proper SI, MacDermid JC, King GJ, Faber KJ: Functional outcomes of arthroscopic capsular release of the elbow. *Arthroscopy* 2006;22(8):842-849.

[20] Savoie FH III, Nunley PD, Field LD: Arthroscopic management of the arthritic elbow: Indications, technique, and results. *J Shoulder Elbow Surg* 1999;8(3):214-219.

[21] Cohen AP, Redden JF, Stanley D: Treatment of osteoarthritis of the elbow: A comparison of open and arthroscopic debridement. *Arthroscopy* 2000;16(7):701-706.

[22] Yadao MA, Field LD, Savoie FH III: Osteochondritis dissecans of the elbow. *Instr Course Lect* 2004;53:599-606.

[23] Ahmad CS, Vitale MA, ElAttrache NS: Elbow arthroscopy: Capitellar osteochondritis dissecans and radiocapitellar plica. *Instr Course Lect* 2011;60:181-190.

Available arthroscopic treatment options are described for capitellar OCD and radiocapitellar plica, including mosaicplasty and transarticular drilling or removal of detached fragments or loose bodies, followed by drilling.

[24] Brownlow HC, O'Connor-Read LM, Perko M: Arthroscopic treatment of osteochondritis dissecans of the capitellum. *Knee Surg Sports Traumatol Arthrosc* 2006;14(2):198-202.

[25] Jones KJ, Wiesel BB, Sankar WN, Ganley TJ: Arthroscopic management of osteochondritis dissecans of the capitellum: Mid-term results in adolescent athletes. *J Pediatr Orthop* 2010;30(1):8-13.

The mid-term results of 25 consecutive patients who underwent arthroscopic treatment of OCD of the capitellum are described. Level of evidence: IV.

[26] Micheli LJ, Luke AC, Mintzer CM, Waters PM: Elbow arthroscopy in the pediatric and adolescent population. *Arthroscopy* 2001;17(7):694-699.

[27] Mihara K, Suzuki K, Makiuchi D, Nishinaka N, Yamaguchi K, Tsutsui H: Surgical treatment for osteo-

chondritis dissecans of the humeral capitellum. *J Shoulder Elbow Surg* 2010;19(1):31-37.

Arthroscopic management of OCD of the capitellum was described in 27 male baseball players. Management consisted of drilling, fragment fixation, fragment excision, and reconstruction with osteochondral autograft. Level of evidence: IV.

[28] Miyake J, Masatomi T: Arthroscopic debridement of the humeral capitellum for osteochondritis dissecans: Radiographic and clinical outcomes. *J Hand Surg Am* 2011;36(8):1333-1338.

A retrospective review evaluated the radiographic and clinical outcomes of arthroscopic débridement of the humeral capitellum for OCD in 106 patients. Level of evidence: IV.

[29] Nobuta S, Ogawa K, Sato K, Nakagawa T, Hatori M, Itoi E: Clinical outcome of fragment fixation for osteochondritis dissecans of the elbow. *Ups J Med Sci* 2008; 113(2):201-208.

A case study assessed the efficacy of fragment fixation for OCD of the humeral capitellum. Level of evidence: IV.

[30] Rahusen FT, Brinkman J-M, Eygendaal D: Results of arthroscopic debridement for osteochondritis dissecans of the elbow. *Br J Sports Med* 2006;40(12):966-969.

[31] Takeda H, Watarai K, Matsushita T, Saito T, Tera- shima Y: A surgical treatment for unstable osteochon- dritis dissecans lesions of the humeral capitellum in adolescent baseball players. *Am J Sports Med* 2002;30(5):713-717.

[32] Tis JE, Edmonds EW, Bastrom T, Chambers HG: Short-term results of arthroscopic treatment of osteochondritis dissecans in skeletally immature patients. *J Pediatr Orthop* 2012;32(3):226-231.

A retrospective review evaluated a treatment regimen using arthroscopic-assisted treatments for pediatric capitellar OCD, including the removal of loose bodies, antegrade or retrograde drilling, and chondroplasty. Level of evidence: IV.

[33] de Graaff F, Krijnen MR, Poolman RW, Willems WJ: Arthroscopic surgery in athletes with osteochondritis dissecans of the elbow. *Arthroscopy* 2011;27(7):986-993.

A systematic review evaluated studies on the results of arthroscopic surgery, including débridement, fragment fixation, microfracture, and osteochondral autografting, in athletes with OCD of the elbow. Level of evidence: III.

[34] Peart RE, Strickler SS, Schweitzer KM Jr: Lateral epicondylitis: A comparative study of open and arthro-

scopic lateral release. *Am J Orthop (Belle Mead NJ)* 2004;33(11):565-567.

[35] Rubenthaler F, Wiese M, Senge A, Keller L, Wittenberg RH: Long-term follow-up of open and endoscopic Hohmann procedures for lateral epicondylitis. *Arthroscopy* 2005;21(6):684-690.

[36] Lattermann C, Romeo AA, Anbari A, et al: Arthroscopic debridement of the extensor carpi radialis brevis for recalcitrant lateral epicondylitis. *J Shoulder Elbow Surg* 2010;19(5):651-656.

The outcome of arthroscopic release of the ECRB tendon was assessed in a consecutive series of patients. Level of evidence: IV.

[37] Savoie FH III, VanSice W, O'Brien MJ: Arthroscopic tennis elbow release. *J Shoulder Elbow Surg* 2010;19(2, suppl):31-36.

The management of lateral epicondylitis with arthroscopic tennis elbow release was reviewed.

[38] Feldman MD: Arthroscopic excision of type II capitellar fractures. *Arthroscopy* 1997;13(6):743-748.

[39] Hardy P, Menguy F, Guillot S: Arthroscopic treatment of capitellum fracture of the humerus. *Arthroscopy* 2002;18(4):422-426.

[40] Adams JE, Merten SM, Steinmann SP: Arthroscopic-assisted treatment of coronoid fractures. *Arthroscopy* 2007;23(10):1060-1065.

Coronoid fractures were arthroscopically treated with screw fixation, threaded Steinmann pin fixation, and fracture débridement. Level of evidence: IV.

[41] Hausman MR, Klug RA, Qureshi S, Goldstein R, Parsons BO: Arthroscopically assisted coronoid fracture fixation: A preliminary report. *Clin Orthop Relat Res* 2008;466(12):3147-3152.

A preliminary report investigated the feasibility of arthroscopically assisted reduction and fixation of small coronoid fractures and the anterior capsule for treatment of patients with Regan-Morrey type or O'Driscoll type I or II coronoid fracture with instability of the ulnohumeral joint. Level of evidence: IV.

[42] Michels F, Pouliart N, Handelberg F: Arthroscopic management of Mason type 2 radial head fractures. *Knee Surg Sports Traumatol Arthrosc* 2007;15(10):1244-1250.

Mid-to-long-term results were presented for an arthroscopic technique for reduction and percutaneous fixation of Mason type II radial head fractures. Level of evidence: IV.

[43] Rolla PR, Surace MF, Bini A, Pilato G: Arthroscopic treatment of fractures of the radial head. *Arthroscopy* 2006;22(2):e1-e6.

[44] Gelberman RH, Yamaguchi K, Hollstien SB, et al: Changes in interstitial pressure and cross-sectional area of the cubital tunnel and of the ulnar nerve with flexion of the elbow: An experimental study in human cadavera. *J Bone Joint Surg Am* 1998;80(4):492-501.

[45] Dodson CC, Nho SJ, Williams RJ III, Altchek DW: Elbow arthroscopy. *J Am Acad Orthop Surg* 2008;16(10):574-585.

The indications for elbow arthroscopy were reviewed, with the technical advances that have expanded its indications.

[46] Gramstad GD, Galatz LM: Management of elbow osteoarthritis. *J Bone Joint Surg Am* 2006;88(2):421-430.

[47] Sahajpal DT, Blonna D, O'Driscoll SW: Anteromedial elbow arthroscopy portals in patients with prior ulnar nerve transposition or subluxation. *Arthroscopy* 2010;26(8):1045-1052.

Management strategies and complications related to the use of anteromedial portals for elbow arthroscopy were documented in a case study of patients with subluxating or previously transposed ulnar nerves. Level of evidence: IV.

[48] Kelly EW, Morrey BF, O'Driscoll SW: Complications of elbow arthroscopy. *J Bone Joint Surg Am* 2001;83-A(1):25-34.

[49] O'Driscoll SW, Morrey BF: Arthroscopy of the elbow: Diagnostic and therapeutic benefits and hazards. *J Bone Joint Surg Am* 1992;74(1):84-94.

[50] Poehling GG, Whipple TL, Sisco L, Goldman B: Elbow arthroscopy: A new technique. *Arthroscopy* 1989;5(3):222-224.

[51] Yamaguchi K, Tashjian RZ: *Advanced Reconstruction: Elbow*. Rosemont, IL, American Academy of Orthopaedic Surgeons, 2007, pp 3-11.

The setup and portals used to perform elbow arthroscopy were described.

[52] Gallay SH, Richards RR, O'Driscoll SW: Intraarticular capacity and compliance of stiff and normal elbows. *Arthroscopy* 1993;9(1):9-13.

[53] Bedi A, Dines J, Dines DM, et al: Use of the 70° arthroscope for improved visualization with common arthroscopic procedures. *Arthroscopy* 2010;26(12):1684-1696.

A technique is described for using the 70° arthroscope, with the circumstances in which it offers visualization superior to that of a 30° arthroscope.

第四十七章　高级肘关节镜

James A. Hurt Ⅲ , MD; Felix H. Savoie Ⅲ , MD

引言

最初，肘关节镜只是被用于在切开手术之前对肘关节内部的解剖和病理结构进行可视化检查，以及辅助取出关节内游离体。近些年，肘关节镜治疗的适应证范围大大增加，已经被广为接受的包括关节炎、肘关节僵硬、关节纤维化、肱骨外上髁炎、后外侧旋转不稳定（PLRI）、后内侧旋转不稳定、剥脱性骨软骨炎（OCD）、肘关节后方撞击、关节内骨折、肱三头肌修复及化脓性关节炎。尽管肘关节镜在上述情况中的应用都有文献支持，但其证据质量级别普遍较低。[1]肘关节镜在操作技术上的要求很高，需要操作者熟知关节周围的解剖及神经血管结构。

Dr. Savoie or an immediate family member serves as a board member, owner, officer, or committee member of the Arthroscopy Association of North America, the American Shoulder and Elbow Surgeons, the American Academy of Orthopaedic Surgeons, the American Orthopaedic Society for Sports Medicine, and the International Society of Arthroscopy, Knee Surgery, and Orthopaedic Sports Medicine; serves as a paid consultant to or is an employee of Mitek, Smith & Nephew, and Exactech; serves as an unpaid consultant to Cayenne Medical; and has received research or institutional support from Mitek, Smith & Nephew, and Amp Orthopedics, Inc. Neither Dr. Hurt nor any immediate family member has received anything of value from or has stock or stock options held in a commercial company or institution related directly or indirectly to the subject of this chapter.

病史及检查

对于每个有肘关节疼痛或功能障碍的患者都应该询问完整的病史并进行体格检查。要确定患者的年龄、优势手、职业、参与体育运动的情况、活动水平及外伤史。应询问发病时间、症状何时最严重及症状的具体性质（疼痛、不稳定、僵硬及机械性症状）。疼痛部位（前方、后方、内侧或外侧）及病史甚至可以使检查者在进行体格检查或影像学检查之前就能明确诊断。

详尽的体格检查应包括对颈部、同侧肩关节、患侧肘关节及对侧肘关节的检查。肢体的血管神经检查应包括脉搏、神经反射及感觉和运动功能的测试。需要测量并记录活动范围（屈曲、伸直、旋前和旋后）。对肘关节稳定性的测试应该以在其屈伸活动弧中施加内翻或外翻应力为前提下进行。其他诱发试验则可根据患者所述病史以及体格检查结果酌情进行。

X线检查包括拍摄正侧位片及斜位片，这对于判断肘关节的整体力线以及发现骨折、OCD损伤和退行性关节病都有帮助。CT能够帮助明确骨折类型并发现游离体的存在。MRI对于软组织（软骨及韧带等结构）的评估则要远优于CT。

肘关节镜的操作需要医师掌握技巧、经验并对肘关节及其解剖深入透彻地了解。周围神经损伤是最常见、最令人担忧的肘关节并发症。因此，术者必须熟悉肘关节解剖，并且确信找到正确的入路通道。对大多数肘关节镜手术而言，建议将患者置于俯卧位。尽管侧卧位也同样合适，但需要配备一个稳定上臂的特殊装置。

可使用关节镜治疗的疾病

肱骨外上髁炎

对肱骨外上髁炎的描述最早见于 1873 年。该疾病因与草地网球运动相关而通常被称为网球肘。[2]在 140 多年后的今天，对于这种疾病的最佳手术治疗方法与非手术治疗方法依然缺乏共识。多数肱骨外上髁炎患者对各种非手术治疗方法反应良好，但有 4%~11% 的患者因为症状持续而需要手术干预[3]（图 47-1）。

关于肱骨外上髁炎，最为广泛接受的理论是肘关节的反复使用造成了桡侧腕短伸肌（ECRB）肌腱的细微撕裂。由于这种疾病缺少炎症的组织学改变，因此描述时常常使用血管成纤维细胞性增生或血管成纤维细胞性肌腱变性这类术语。[4-5]另一种理论则认为疼痛是由滑膜皱襞与肱桡关节发生撞击所致。在一项尸体研究中发现，滑膜皱襞是独立于环状韧带存在的，但是与伸肌总腱起点有着极为密切的关系。[6]也有观点认为肱骨外上髁炎是由关节内病变和关节外病变共同导致的。

近期的一项尸体研究表明，ECRB 肌腱的确切起点恰好位于肱骨外侧髁上嵴最远端的前方。[6-7]研究发现肌腱起点呈钻石形，平均长度为 13 mm（±2 mm），平均宽度在近端为 3 mm（±1 mm），在中部为 7 mm（±2 mm），在远端为 4 mm（±1 mm）。[6-7]

手术治疗肱骨外上髁炎的方法有很多，包括经皮手术、关节镜手术及切开手术。非手术治疗无效即为手术治疗适应证，常用的非手术治疗方法包括调整运动方式、物理治疗、使用非甾体抗炎药物、注射皮质类固醇及富血小板血浆以及使用反作用力支具制动。

采用关节镜手术治疗肱骨外上髁炎时，于外上髁尖端前方 2 mm 处另外建立一个入路很有帮助。这条通道横贯 Nirschl 病变，允许自上而下而非自中向上切除病变，这样可使切除范围限于病变组织，还可减小损伤桡神经的风险。当各入路均已建立后，可用刨削器先切除一部分外侧关节囊以显露其下方的伸肌总腱起点。用刨削器或电刀彻底松解 ECRB 起点。外侧的韧带结构位于桡骨头等分线的后方，松解操作不要越过这条线。用一个 70° 的关节镜就可以很清楚地在肱骨小头拐角处看到 ECRB 附着点及外侧韧带

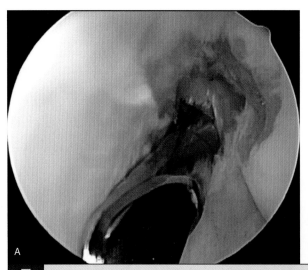
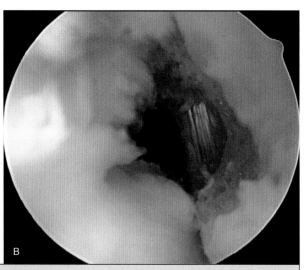

图 47-1　近端前内侧入路的关节镜图像，显示肱骨外上髁炎的治疗。A. 可见灰色不规则的 ECRB 肌腱血管纤维化结构不良。B. 结构不良的病变已被切除，保留正常的肌腱组织

结构。[8]经由中部前外侧入路可以进行外侧的关节外松解，此操作仅需在关节囊上开一个小口即可完成。将关节镜退到关节外便可以直视病变组织，还可以看到经近端前外侧入路进入的刨削器对病变组织进行清理的过程。[9]

在整个病变被切除之后，被破坏的肌腱便可以直接在骨或肌间隔上进行修复了。这一步骤可以通过经标准前外侧入路在前方外上髁上打入一枚小的缝合锚钉，并将锚线穿过 ECRB 带出完成。此外，ECRB 也可以采用针带线技术折叠缝合在其上方的桡侧腕长伸肌上。[10]历来的观点认为将下方骨质做去皮质化处理能够增加愈合潜力。然而，近期的一项研究发现，与仅接受 ECRB 松解的患者相比，同时接受松解和去皮质化处理的患者的术后疼痛更明显，恢复工作所需的时间也更长。[3]

一项病例研究显示，36 例接受关节镜治疗的难治性肱骨外上髁炎患者的疼痛均有所缓解，表明该治疗方法安全并且有效。[3]另一项长期随访研究结果显示，30 例接受关节镜治疗的肱骨外上髁炎患者中无一人需要进一步行手术治疗，其中 87% 的患者对治疗结果表示满意。[11]

尽管多数研究得到了不错的结果，但也不是所有患者都对治疗效果感到满意。ECRB 病变组织清理的效果有时不可预测，有些患者仍存在包括疼痛在内的肘关节外侧症状。[7]研究发现，有工伤赔偿要求的患者以及从事高要求、需承受重复性应力工作的患者的治疗结果都比较差。

关节纤维化

肘关节极容易发生僵硬，尤其是在创伤之后，而活动范围丢失也是肘关节受伤后最常见的并发症。包含 3 个关节的肘关节是一个非常匹配、协调的整体。哪怕一点微小的改变都常常被放大成导致关节僵硬的原因。一点轻微损伤就可能使肘关节囊增厚并丧失顺应性。鹰嘴窝或冠突窝如果被游离体或瘢痕组织充填，则伸肘或屈肘的终末期将分别受限。肌肉挛缩也有可能限制肘关节周围的活动。疼痛常会加剧创伤后肘关节僵硬，因为疼痛所引起的自主性和非自主性肌抵抗会加重关节囊及肌肉的挛缩。[12]伸肘终末期丧失远比屈肘终末期丧失多见。正常的肘关节活动范围为屈曲 0°~145°，旋前和旋后各 90°。功能活动范围为屈曲 30°~130°，旋前和旋后各 50°。[13]适合手术治疗的患者应该是伸肘终末期丧失达到 25°~30° 和（或）屈肘小于 110°~115° 的人群。在手术松解之前，患者应该接受为期数月的术前物理治疗，并明确记录关节活动范围所能增加到的稳定水平。记录术前关节的顺应性非常重要，因为术后治疗时顺应性对于保持术中所增加的活动范围十分关键。过于激进的物理治疗和手法操作可能加重患者的症状，甚至会加重组织的挛缩。[12]

创伤后肘关节僵硬的关节镜下松解十分复杂，在保护好血管神经组织的同时改善活动范围需要高超的关节镜操作技巧。异位骨化是关节镜下松解的相对禁忌证。与切开手术治疗相比，关节镜治疗的优点包括更好地显现关节内结构、对周围组织的创伤更小以及术后有可能更早地活动和接受康复治疗。进行肘关节镜操作必须了解尺神经所在位置。如果肘关节屈曲明显丧失，或者对尺神经的位置有任何疑问，都应单独切口探查，明确尺神经的位置并对其予以保护。[14]

创伤后肘关节僵硬关节镜下松解的核心原则如表 47-1 所示。手术操作从前方还是后方间室开始取决于术者的习惯。多数术者习惯从前方间室开始，随着肿胀程度的增高，前方间室的显现和与血管神经结构的极度贴近都可能限制术者的操作。在前方间室中，可进行滑膜清理和切除，并取出所有游离体。关节囊要从肱骨前方剥离。应去除冠突、冠突窝及桡骨头上的骨赘。在不抽吸的情况下用咬钳和（或）刨削器彻底清除前方关节囊。必须小心避免于肱肌外侧缘处损伤骨间后神经。[15]于后方间室中可行滑膜切除并取出所有游离体。在近端，可用拉钩将关节囊剥离，肱三头肌和肱骨之间的所有粘连均可得以松解。根据需要去除鹰嘴尖及鹰嘴窝内的骨赘。对于内外侧沟处的关节囊应予以小心松解。内侧沟和内侧尺骨副韧带后束的松解对改善屈肘非常重要。

表 47-1
创伤后肘关节僵硬关节镜下松解的核心原则
采用标准且可重复的技术
进行预防性尺神经减压
控制液体流入量以避免关节过度肿胀
去除骨质以重建相互匹配的关节面
进行关节囊切除
常规使用拉钩
实践水平要低于理论水平

高度挛缩是关节镜下松解的相对禁忌证，因为可供器械使用的操作空间非常小，关节囊的顺应性也比较差。对于超过 50° 的挛缩病例，有文献报道了囊外的关节囊切除方法，该方法是将骨膜剥离器自近端内侧入路插入，在肱骨前方皮质与前方的肱肌之间建立一个操作空间。[12] 随后，可在直视下进行前方关节囊的切除。

近期，一些证据水平为 IV 级的采用关节镜治疗肘关节纤维化的病例研究报道了良好的功能结果。[14-16] 其中能够恢复体育运动或工作，并且能够在 24 个月的时间内维持手术成果的患者占比很高。术前症状持续时间较短的创伤患者的治疗结果优于其他患者。

肘关节切开手术和关节镜手术的并发症发生率大致相当。与切开手术相比，关节镜手术造成永久性损伤的风险更高。一些关节镜手术中发生血管神经损伤的情况也有所报道。[17] 为应对这种风险，需要在所有肘关节镜手术中，尤其是操作空间有所改变或者减小时，采取常规步骤，按部就班地谨慎操作。[17]

退行性关节病

肘关节骨性关节炎并不常见，通常表现为活动至极限位置时的疼痛、无力及活动范围丧失。

肘关节炎与其他关节的关节炎类似，通常都会伴有骨赘和游离体形成，使关节活动范围减小，同时可合并（或不合并）如关节交锁之类的机械性症状。与其他关节的关节炎不同的是，肘关节炎一般不会出现关节间隙变窄和关节软骨丢失。[18]

肘关节的退行性关节病通常是由类风湿关节炎和创伤导致的。肘关节原发性骨关节炎几乎仅见于男性运动员和男性重体力劳动者。患有类风湿关节炎的患者常在活动全程伴有疼痛，而不仅限于活动的终末期。X 线检查对确诊肘关节炎很有帮助，通常可以发现关节间隙变窄、骨刺形成及关节内游离体。当考虑进行手术治疗的时候，CT 对于制订关节清理、游离体取出及肱尺关节置换术或骨关节囊成形术的手术计划有所帮助。

在手术治疗之前，一般应该先尝试非手术治疗。应用 NSAIDs 药物或病症缓解性抗风湿药物（针对患有类风湿关节炎的患者）、皮质类固醇注射、支具制动、物理治疗以及调整活动方式都是手术治疗的替代方案。如果非手术治疗不能缓解疼痛或确保肘关节的功能性活动范围，使患者的工作能力或日常活动能力受到限制，则应该考虑手术治疗。在关节镜下清理骨赘，取出游离体，同时进行选择性的关节囊松解可以获得较好的短期和中期效果。[12]

在建立入路之前，应该先找到尺神经的走行路径。通常在前方间室内有一些游离体，如果较小可立即取出。假如游离体较大，则可以晚些取出以保持关节的膨大状态。可以从内侧入路进行滑膜切除，而经此入路使用刨削器切除冠突骨赘则最为简便。如果患者存在肱桡关节症状，则由术者决定是否行桡骨头切除。然后，便可以钻孔开窗将冠突窝和鹰嘴窝打通。[19]

在后方间室内，需要切除鹰嘴及鹰嘴窝里的骨赘，清理内外侧沟，取出游离体。随后扩大开窗孔洞至 1~2 cm，广泛切除鹰嘴尖以获得充足的伸肘活动范围，从而完成 Outerbridge-Kashiwagi

手术的所有步骤。[19]术前即有显著活动范围丧失的患者应行尺神经减压或移位。术后即刻开始进行肘关节活动。在术后48小时内还可以让患者接受700 cGY的放疗以预防异位骨化的形成。

Outerbridge-Kashiwagi手术最初是切开进行的，不过在关节镜下操作用于治疗肘关节炎时也可以得到很好的效果。[20-21]在一项回顾性研究中，19名轻中度肘关节炎患者接受了关节镜下的Outerbridge-Kashiwagi手术。术后平均2年的随访显示，患者在活动范围和疼痛评分上均有改善。一项回顾性病例研究发现，41例接受关节镜下骨赘切除和关节囊切除的患者经过平均176.3周的随访，疼痛均有所减轻，而关节活动范围均有所增加。[22]另一项研究表明，经过平均47个月的随访，13例肘关节炎合并尺神经压迫的患者，在接受关节镜下尺神经松解、骨赘切除及关节囊切除后，有12例获得了优良的结果。[23]

剥脱性骨软骨炎

尚未发育完全的肘关节外侧间室的反复损伤在参与棒球和体操运动的儿童中很常见，而OCD则常见于参与过顶运动的青少年（年龄为11~15岁）。疾病的进程很可能受多方面因素影响。该疾病是由反复的微创伤和血管的易感性共同导致的，但是确切的病因尚不明确。肱骨小头的血供来自两支带有极少量侧支循环的终末动脉，而在反复承受微创伤的肘关节中，这种结构很有可能处于一种缺血的状态。患者经常感到肘关节外侧隐隐作痛，并且有些僵硬。15°~20°的屈曲挛缩并不少见。OCD病变和内侧尺骨副韧带（MUCL）撕裂都可由外翻负荷过大导致。应该检查MUCL的完整性。肘关节的影像学检查应该包括完全伸肘和屈肘45°时的正位片、斜位片和标准侧位片。如果X线检查怀疑存在OCD病变，则应行MRI检查以进一步明确病变的特点。

OCD病变的治疗取决于其大小和位置，以及其上所覆盖的软骨的稳定性。例如，累及肱骨小头外侧面（非约束性或肩部病变）需行更广泛的手术，并且与仅累及肱骨小头中部的病变相比预后较差。I期OCD病变是稳定的，骨软骨病灶完整且无移位。I期病变通常在3~6个月后愈合，可以采取非手术治疗。投掷及其他可能给患肢造成压力的活动都应该中止。每2~3个月进行一次MRI检查有助于监测愈合的进程。II期病变不稳定，存在软骨骨折但尚有连接。II期病变应该采取手术治疗，决定手术治疗方式的是病变的大小。相对小的病变可以进行清理，可立即缓解疼痛，且效果很好。

对于II期病变或更大病变的治疗究竟是采取清理、修复还是自体骨软骨移植尚存争议。肱骨小头上病变的位置可影响治疗结果，累及外侧柱的病变预后较差。骨块可使用无头钉固定，关于可吸收针的应用也有报道。[24]III期病变是不稳定且完全移位的，必须采取手术治疗。和II期病变类似，钻孔清理、微骨折和自体骨软骨移植都是可选择的方案。[25]微骨折适用于非手术治疗无效的较小的I期病变和不累及外侧柱的II期病变。较大的病变、累及外侧柱超过6~7 mm的病变和由桡骨头撞击导致的病变，都应该采用自体骨软骨移植的方法治疗。OCD病变的手术治疗后的近期效果通常不错，但II期和III期病变的手术治疗远期效果就不如人意。[26]

为了全面彻底地清理、钻孔或放置骨软骨栓，入口的角度极其重要。使用直接外侧双入路不会破坏外侧韧带复合体，并且在器械的辅助下能够对肱骨小头的78%进行操作。[27]远端尺侧入路也能很好地显示肱骨小头，在关节镜下进行钻孔、磨削和清理都很简单。[28]有一种对OCD病变进行钻孔的新方法是使用1.8 mm克氏针自远端3 cm处钻入桡骨头。通过旋前、旋后、屈肘和伸肘，可以在不做很大的关节切开的前提下对病变实施钻孔操作。[29]一般情况下，经近端后外侧入路以70°插入关节镜可以最清楚地看到病变，而中间和远端薄弱部位的入路则用于放置器械。

一篇证据等级为Ⅲ级的文献综述认为，非手术治疗未获成功是手术适应证，不过这些发表了的研究所用的方法都不太经得起推敲。[25]病灶清理、固定、微骨折及自体移植的近期效果尚能令人满意，但远期效果不明确。尽管缺乏证据，但从长期来看，自体移植的效果似乎比其他手术治疗方法的效果更好。

一项回顾性研究的结果表明，在106例在肱骨小头骨骺闭合以后接受关节镜下OCD病变清理的患者中，病变较大且桡骨骨骺未闭合者的X线片和临床结果均较差。[25,27-30]其他患者的短期结果则非常好。在另一项回顾性研究中，13例患者在OCD病变清理后随访至少1年的结果显示，主观症状均有所缓解，肘关节功能也得到改善，尽管很多患者都表示已经终止了从前的体育活动。[30]在一项研究中，有25例连续病例对OCD病变采用了关节镜下清理和钻孔治疗；其中12例为了植骨还做了很小的关节切开。[26]这些患者术后肘关节屈曲和伸直角度的增加（分别为10°和17°）都具有统计学意义，随访到的21例患者中有18例已经恢复了受伤前的运动水平。

肱三头肌损伤

肱三头肌的功能是伸直肘关节。肱三头肌腱止于尺骨近端鹰嘴的近侧和后方。很多老年人仍然保持活跃状态，这使肱三头肌腱止点损伤的发生率有所增加，但这种损伤还是更常见于需要举起重物的人群。患者经常在做推的动作时感到肱三头肌腱止点处一阵突然的疼痛，例如，从坐位站起时用手臂支撑身体或者进行卧推运动。肌腱部分撕裂时疼痛的发作往往更为隐匿，当从完全屈肘位开始伸直时疼痛变得更加明显。

体格检查常可于肱三头肌腱止点处发现肿胀和瘀斑。肌腱完全撕裂时伸肘活动彻底丧失，部分撕裂时伸肘活动力量减弱。行肱三头肌应力试验时能够发现，当患者试图从完全屈肘位做伸肘动作时，在伤处可以引出疼痛。如果非手术治疗无效则可行手术治疗。

与切开肱三头肌腱修复术相比，关节镜下固定是一种损伤更小的治疗方法。将患者置于俯卧位或侧卧位，进行诊断性关节镜操作。如果是为了修复，可先建立后侧正中入路（图47-2），该入路常穿过肱三头肌腱撕裂处。再建立一个后外侧入路，当关节镜移到这个入路时可以看到肱三头肌腱的撕裂。清理其在鹰嘴上的止点，将双缝线的缝合锚拧入鹰嘴尖端，以两个褥式缝合来修复撕裂的近端。于鹰嘴更远端的地方拧入第二个缝合锚，这些缝线也都要穿过肌腱缝合，从而完成修复。

进行任何肘关节镜手术时，在建立通道之前，都应该先明确尺神经的体表投影（图47-3）。鹰嘴的骨质有可能极其坚硬，因此在置入缝合锚的时候必须小心勿使缝合锚折断。如果肿胀过于严重，关节镜下修复无法完成，应该改为切开手术进行修复。术后，肘关节应该保持在完全伸肘位。应限制肘关节活动，屈肘角度可以在术后6~8周内缓慢增加。[31]

骨折

肘关节镜的新兴用途之一就是用于骨折的复位和固定。很多治疗骨折的新技术得到了发展，这些技术采用微创方法，保护了软组织，减少了剥离。关节镜辅助骨折固定已经被用于桡骨头骨折、冠突骨折、儿童肱骨外髁骨折、肱骨小头骨折以及髁上和髁间骨折。患者的疼痛常常使X线检查和体格检查受到限制。抽吸关节内的积血并在关节腔内注射麻醉药物，既能够让医师在患者感觉更舒适的情况下进行准确的体格检查，也便于在X线检查时摆放肢体的位置。由术者决定是否行CT和MRI检查以明确骨折的类型及合并的软组织损伤，以便确定术前计划。

未能发现的软骨损伤及其他关节内异常情况可以在关节镜下得以发现。关节镜下可以直观评

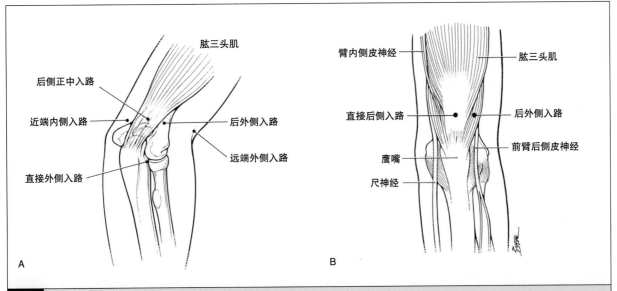

图 47-2 肱三头肌修复时肘关节镜通道定位示意图（后前位）。A. 后侧正中入路可能穿过肱三头肌腱撕裂处。B. 当关节镜移至后外侧入路后，便可以看到肱三头肌腱的撕裂

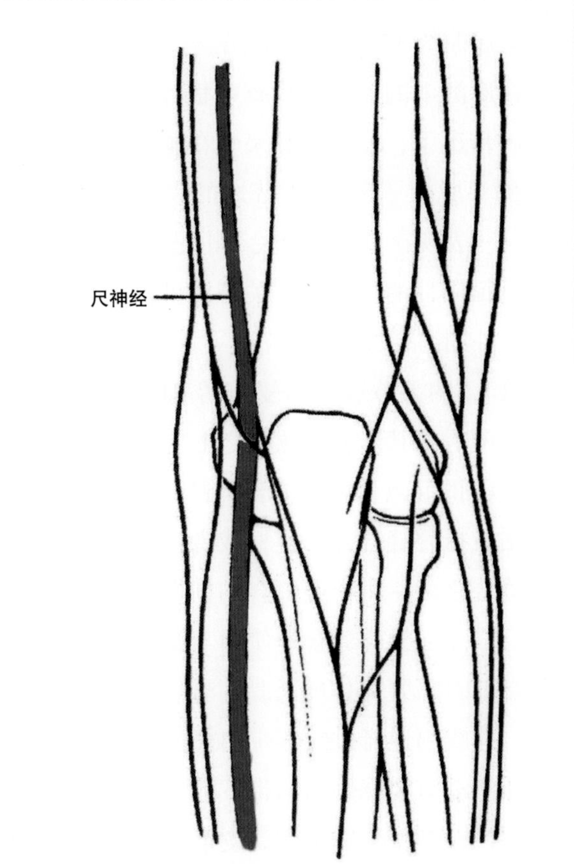

图 47-3 肘关节示意图显示入路建立之前尺神经的体表投影

估骨折的复位情况，这增加了复位的准确性，并且能够减少对术中透视的需求。

存在严重感染或污染、神经血管损伤或严重骨质疏松的患者应行切开手术治疗。桡骨头骨折穿破前方关节囊和肱肌的患者应该切开探查骨间后神经。[32]

桡骨头骨折

桡骨头骨折是肘关节周围最常见的骨折。无移位或移位很小的 Mason Ⅰ型骨折常常可以采取非手术治疗，并且可以早期进行关节活动练习。Mason Ⅱ型和Ⅲ型骨折通常移位明显并且在关节活动时有阻挡，最好行手术治疗。在关节镜下，移位的两部分骨折通过近端前内侧入路或后外侧入路能够显示得最清楚。骨折块复位之后，可以通过前外侧入路或薄弱部位入路置入克氏针临时固定，然后使用经皮置入无头螺钉或可吸收针的技术对骨折进行最终固定。在一项病例研究中，对 14 例 Mason Ⅱ型桡骨头骨折采取关节镜下复位、经皮穿针并打入 1~2 枚无头螺钉固定的方法进行治疗，全部患者在 5.5 年的随访中取得了优良的结果。[33]

冠突骨折

冠突在维持肘关节的骨性稳定性中扮演了很重要的角色。冠突骨折常与肘关节的轴向负荷及后脱位有关。对于 Regan-Morrey Ⅲ 型骨折和任何影响关节活动及稳定性的骨折类型，通常都建议手术治疗。小骨块或无法使用螺钉固定的粉碎骨块可以清除或在骨折部位使用缝合锚固定。较大的冠突骨块通常可以借助前交叉韧带经骨导向器进行复位。骨块可以经此导向器钻入导针临时固定，接着用小空心钉进行最终固定。一项回顾性研究的结果显示，全部（7 例）这类用关节镜辅助冠突骨折复位的患者，骨折得到愈合，肘关节具有功能性活动范围并且没有疼痛。[34] 在一项病例研究中，4 例患者采用了关节镜辅助下的螺钉固定或缝合治疗，结果表明，全部患者骨折愈合且关节稳定，肘关节都到了可以进行功能性活动的范围。[35]

外髁骨折

外髁骨折常见于儿童患者，通常采取长臂石膏固定（无移位骨折）、闭合复位穿针固定或经 Kocher 入路切开复位经皮穿针固定。这类骨折通常可采用关节镜评估及辅助复位，随后再行经皮穿针和长臂石膏固定。与切开手术相比，关节镜下操作避免了大范围的软组织剥离，减少了骨块血供破坏的风险。两项小的病例研究结果显示，应用这种技术可以得到非常好的近期结果。[36-37]

后外侧旋转不稳定

对后外侧旋转不稳定（PLRI）的描述最早见于 1991 年，主要包含了外侧韧带结构的功能障碍，尤其是桡侧肱尺韧带（RUHL）。[38] RUHL 是前臂旋后和伸肘过程中重要的轴关节稳定结构。它的损伤会使很简单的日常生活动作变得困难重重。RUHL 包括 3 个部分：桡侧副韧带、外侧尺骨副韧带及环状韧带。PLRI 和明确的肘关节脱位之间似乎仅有一步之遥。[39] 通常疼痛伴肘关节外侧不稳定的表现很像肱骨外上髁炎，

PLRI 可能增加伸肌上的张力，引起肱骨外上髁炎的症状。[40] ECRB 止点与 RUHL 紧邻的特点可能在切开行 ECRB 清理的时候导致医源性 PLRI。

最初使用关节镜治疗 PLRI 的报道见于 2001 年，近年来又可见到一些相关报道。[39,41-42] 治疗方法的选择取决于患者究竟是急性脱位、复发性脱位还是 PLRI。在单纯脱位中，RUHL 复合体通常会从肱骨上的附着点撕脱，通过非手术治疗也可以愈合。在建立肘关节前内侧通道后可行诊断性关节镜检查。应清除血肿，缝合撕裂的环状韧带。建立后侧正中入路可以清除后方的血肿。应确认肱骨外髁上的撕脱部位并进行清理，然后，于肱骨上打入 1 枚缝合锚钉，使之位于肱桡关节中线上，再于更近端的 RUHL 起点撕脱位置上打入第二枚缝合锚钉。缝线均穿过韧带复合体进行缝合。为防止缝合过紧，水平褥式缝合线应该在肘关节屈曲约 45°~60° 时打结。

在麻醉下的关节镜检查中很容易发现 PLRI，在这种情况下，桡骨头和尺骨在轴移试验中会向后外侧半脱位。PLRI 很普遍的表现之一是穿越征，这一表现在稳定的肘关节中是不可能见到的。在穿越征阳性的情况下，关节镜可以经后正中入路从后外侧沟穿过肱尺关节。

PLRI 的关节镜下修复包括 RUHL 的折叠缝合以及随后将其修复在肱骨之上。肱骨端于 RCL 和 RUHL 的起点处打入缝合锚钉，韧带端则使用这些锚线折叠缝合并修复，或者将韧带另以缝线折叠缝合之后，将折叠缝合的韧带复合体与肱骨端进行修复。折叠缝合是使用 4~7 根可吸收缝线自远端 RUHL 复合体的尺骨附着点开始向近端进行的。缝线用逆行过线器带出。过线器位于外上髁后外侧沟，在桡侧副韧带下方。通过已存在的皮肤切口，缝线分别被带到皮下并依次打结。在调整好张力之后，穿越征即应彻底消失。[42] 关节镜下治疗 PLRI 的结果可以等同于切开手术修复。[41]

后内侧撞击

从事过顶运动的运动员在投掷过程中其肘关节会承受很大的外翻应力和伸肘应力。限制肘部外翻应力的最主要结构是 MUCL 前束。MUCL 失去功能会导致肘关节外翻不稳定。长此以往，肘关节外翻不稳定的患者就会出现后内侧撞击（又称为投掷肘）、尺神经症状、尺骨应力骨折、OCD 病变，甚至关节囊挛缩。这些症状组成了外翻伸展超负荷。在投掷动作不同阶段所出现的疼痛可以提醒医师注意可能对应的病理过程。如果症状发展到使患者功能丧失（运动员无法继续从事体育运动）且非手术治疗无效，应该考虑手术干预。做术前计划时需要进行 X 线检查及 MRI 检查。在一项包含 9 例后内侧撞击患者的病例研究中，当把术前 MRI 结果和术中关节镜所见相比较时，可以发现相应的病理改变。[43]

在关节镜下，应该检查前方间室中的骨刺、软骨损伤及肱骨小头的 OCD 病变。患者如果存在伸肘终末期丧失，还应该检查前方关节囊。伴有伸肘终末期丧失的运动员在接受关节镜下挛缩松解之后能够恢复到伤前运动水平。[44]应在关节镜下进行外翻应力试验以检查内侧副韧带。在后方间室中，可以看到鹰嘴及鹰嘴窝，并可对骨赘进行清理。经常可以在鹰嘴的后内侧面发现骨刺。在一项研究中，16 例存在后方撞击的运动员接受了关节镜下鹰嘴窝的清理，伸肘受限从 8° 减小至 2°。[45]如果 MUCL 已经撕裂，则应在关节镜操作之后行切开手术重建。

总结及未来方向展望

肘关节镜操作需要具备高超的技巧和对肘关节周围解剖的深入理解。肘关节镜的适应证范围似乎也正不断地扩展着。其他已经可以应用肘关节镜处理的情况还包括肘关节的软骨瘤病、类风湿关节炎、骨样骨瘤、感染性关节炎及肱骨内上髁炎。[46-47]

参考文献

[1] Yeoh KM, King GJ, Faber KJ, Glazebrook MA, Athwal GS: Evidence-based indications for elbow arthroscopy. *Arthroscopy* 2012; 28(2): 272-282.

A systematic review of therapeutic studies that investigated the indications and outcomes of elbow arthroscopy found that the evidence supports elbow arthroscopy but that the quality of the evidence is poor. Level of evidence: IV.

[2] Morris HP: Lawn-tennis elbow. *BMJ* 1883; 2: 557.

[3] Kim JW, Chun CH, Shim DM, et al: Arthroscopic treatment of lateral epicondylitis: Comparison of the outcome of ECRB release with and without decortication. *Knee Surg Sports Traumatol Arthrosc* 2011; 19(7): 1178-1183.

A nonrandomized clinical study compared arthroscopic ECRB release with and without decortication. Pain and return-to-work time were greater in patients undergoing decortication, without improvement in clinical results. Level of evidence: IV.

[4] Nirschl RP, Pettrone FA: Tennis elbow: The surgical treatment of lateral epicondylitis. *J Bone Joint Surg Am* 1979; 61(6A): 832-839.

[5] Nirschl RP: Elbow tendinosis/tennis elbow. *Clin Sports Med* 1992; 11(4): 851-870.

[6] Ando R, Arai T, Beppu M, Hirata K, Takagi M: Anatomical study of arthroscopic surgery for lateral epicondylitis. *Hand Surg* 2008; 13(2): 85-91.

The anatomic and histologic relationships among the ECRB, articular capsule, and lateral collateral ligament complex, along with the number and location of synovial fringes, was studied in 100 elbows in 50 cadavers. Both extra- and intra-articular lesions were found to have a role in lateral epicondylitis.

[7] Cohen MS, Romeo AA: Open and arthroscopic management of lateral epicondylitis in the athlete. *Hand Clin* 2009; 25(3): 331-338.

The authors compared open and arthroscopic treatment of lateral epicondylitis and described surgical techniques. The results of surgical intervention for lateral epicondylitis can be less predictable than those of other procedures about the elbow.

[8] Arrigoni P, Zottarelli L, Spennacchio P, Denti M, Cabitza P, Randelli P: Advantages of 70° arthroscope in management of ECRB tendinopathy. *Musculoskelet Surg* 2011; 95(Suppl 1): S7-S11.

A technique for arthroscopic ECRB release was described, including the use of a 70° arthroscope to visualize the tendon insertion and lateral collateral ligament during the procedure.

[9] Brooks-Hill AL, Regan WD: Extra-articular arthroscopic lateral elbow release. *Arthroscopy* 2008; 24(4): 483-485.

The arthroscopic treatment of lateral epicondylitis is described, with the use of an extra-articular technique with a smaller capsulectomy.

[10] Savoie FH III, VanSice W, O'Brien MJ: Arthroscopic tennis elbow release. *J Shoulder Elbow Surg* 2010; 19(2, Suppl): 31-36.

A review article outlined the history of tennis elbow and an arthroscopic release procedure that uses a modified lateral portal (the tennis elbow portal). Two additional arthroscopic repair techniques were described: plication of the ECRB to the extensor carpi radialis longus and suture anchor repair of the ECRB.

[11] Baker CL Jr, Baker CL III: Long-term follow-up of arthroscopic treatment of lateral epicondylitis. *Am J Sports Med* 2008; 36(2): 254-260.

A case study outlined the long-term results of 30 patients who underwent arthroscopic treatment of lateral epicondylitis. No patient required further surgery, and 87% were satisfied with their outcome. Level of evidence: IV.

[12] Tucker SA, Savoie FH III, O'Brien MJ: Arthroscopic management of the post-traumatic stiff elbow. *J Shoulder Elbow Surg* 2011; 20(2, suppl): S83-S89.

A review outlined a technique for arthroscopic management of the posttraumatic stiff elbow. The authors cautioned against overly aggressive therapy and manipulation, which can worsen the symptoms and subsequently worsen the contracture.

[13] Morrey BF, Askew LJ, Chao EY: A biomechanical study of normal functional elbow motion. *J Bone Joint Surg Am* 1981; 63(6): 872-877.

[14] Van Zeeland NL, Yamaguchi K: Arthroscopic capsular release of the elbow. *J Shoulder Elbow Surg* 2010; 19(2, suppl): 13-19.

A review provided an overview of arthroscopic capsular release of the stiff elbow as well as the history of the stiff elbow, physical examination and workup, surgical technique, and preferred postoperative protocols.

[15] Sahajpal D, Choi T, Wright TW: Arthroscopic release of the stiff elbow. *J Hand Surg Am* 2009; 34(3): 540-544.

A technique for arthroscopic release of the stiff elbow is described. The anatomy of the surgical portals and the release in a stepwise fashion are included. The focus is on safe surgical technique to avoid nerve injury.

[16] Degreef I, De Smet L: Elbow arthrolysis for traumatic arthrofibrosis: A shift towards minimally invasive surgery. *Acta Orthop Belg* 2011; 77(6): 758-764.

The results of 12 patients who underwent arthroscopic elbow arthrolysis were reported. On average, the patients gained 38° in range of motion. A literature review found that open and arthroscopic arthrolysis yielded gains of 44° and 31.25°, respectively. Level of evidence: IV.

[17] Park JY, Cho CH, Choi JH, Lee ST, Kang CH: Radial nerve palsy after arthroscopic anterior capsular release for degenerative elbow contracture. *Arthroscopy* 2007; 23(12): 1360, e1-e3.

A case report documented radial nerve palsy after an arthroscopic anterior capsular release. A 3-mm ball-tipped cautery was used instead of a 0.5-mm sharp-tipped cautery. The nerve fully recovered by one year.

[18] Cheung EV, Adams R, Morrey BF: Primary osteoarthritis of the elbow: Current treatment options. *J Am Acad Orthop Surg* 2008; 16(2): 77-87.

The treatment options for primary osteoarthritis of the elbow were outlined.

[19] Savoie FH III, O'Brien MJ, Field LD: Arthroscopy for arthritis of the elbow. *Hand Clin* 2011; 27(2): 171-178, v-vi.

The use of arthroscopy for arthritis of the elbow were outlined, including the preoperative workup and spur excision and ulnohumeral arthroplasty for elbow arthritis after unsuccessful nonsurgical treatment.

[20] Kashiwagi D: Intra-articular changes and the special operative procedure, Outerbridge-Kashiwagi method, in Kashiwagi D, ed: *Elbow Joint*. Amsterdam, The Netherlands, Elsevier Science, 1985, pp 177-178.

[21] Degreef I, De Smet L: The arthroscopic ulnohumeral arthroplasty: From mini-open to arthroscopic surgery. *Minim Invasive Surg* 2011; 2011: 798084.

A literature review described the transition of the ulnohumeral Outerbridge-Kashiwagi procedure from open to arthroscopic, with good results.

[22] Adams JE, Wolff LH III, Merten SM, Steinmann SP: Osteoarthritis of the elbow: Results of arthroscopic osteophyte resection and capsulectomy. *J Shoulder Elbow Surg* 2008; 17(1): 126-131.

A retrospective chart review of 42 elbows in 41 patients at an average 176.3-week follow-up after arthroscopic osteophyte resection and capsulectomy found decreased pain and increased range of motion.

[23] Kovachevich R, Steinmann SP: Arthroscopic ulnar nerve decompression in the setting of elbow osteoarthritis. *J Hand Surg Am* 2012; 37(4): 663-668.

A retrospective chart review of 15 elbows in 13 patients with concurrent symptoms of arthritis and ulnar nerve compression at an average 47-month follow-up after arthroscopic ulnar nerve decompression, osteophyte resection, and capsulectomy found a good to excellent result in 12 elbows. Level of evidence: IV.

[24] Takeba J, Takahashi T, Hino K, Watanabe S, Imai H, Yamamoto H: Arthroscopic technique for fragment fixation using absorbable pins for osteochondritis dissecans of the humeral capitellum: A report of 4 cases. *Knee Surg Sports Traumatol Arthrosc* 2010; 18(6): 831-835.

A case study described four patients with an OCD lesion of the humeral capitellum who were treated using absorbable pins for fragment fixation. Posterolateral portals were used, and the elbow was held maximally flexed during the procedure.

[25] Gonzalez-Lomas G, Ahmad C, Wanich T, ElAttrache N: Osteochondritis dissecans of the elbow, in Ryu RKN, ed: *AANA Advanced Arthroscopy: The Elbow and Wrist.* Philadelphia, PA, Saunders Elsevier, 2010, pp 40-54.

Current treatment options for OCD lesions and Panner's disease were presented, with anatomy, patient history, and physical examination as well as treatment algorithms.

[26] Jones KJ, Wiesel BB, Sankar WN, Ganley TJ: Arthroscopic management of osteochondritis dissecans of the capitellum: Mid-term results in adolescent athletes. *J Pediatr Orthop* 2010; 30(1): 8-13.

A retrospective study of 25 consecutive patients treated with arthroscopic débridement and drilling for capitellar OCD lesions found a statistically significant increase in both flexion and extension. Eighteen of the 21 patients available for follow-up returned to their sport at the preinjury level.

[27] Davis JT, Idjadi JA, Siskosky MJ, ElAttrache NS: Dual direct lateral portals for treatment of osteochondritis dissecans of the capitellum: An anatomic study. *Arthroscopy* 2007; 23(7): 723-728.

An anatomic cadaver study examined the relationship and distance of dual direct lateral portals to the lateral ligamentous complex and determined on dissection that the ligamentous complex was not damaged by dual lateral portals. Seventy-eight percent of the capi- tellum

was accessible for instrumentation with these portals.

[28] van den Ende KI, McIntosh AL, Adams JE, Steinmann SP: Osteochondritis dissecans of the capitellum: A review of the literature and a distal ulnar portal. *Arthroscopy* 2011; 27(1): 122-128.

The diagnosis and current treatment options for OCD of the capitellum were discussed. A new distal ulnar portal allows good in-line visualization of the OCD lesion.

[29] Arai Y, Hara K, Fujiwara H, Minami G, Nakagawa S, Kubo T: A new arthroscopic-assisted drilling method through the radius in a distal-to-proximal direction for osteochondritis dissecans of the elbow. *Arthroscopy* 2008; 24(2): 237, e1-e4.

A novel treatment of OCD lesions is described, in which a 1.8-mm Kirschner wire is drilled from 3 cm distal to the humeroradial joint through the radial head and into the lesion. By pronating-supinating and flexing-extending, multiple holes can be drilled into the lesion without creating an arthrotomy.

[30] Schoch B, Wolf BR: Osteochondritis dissecans of the capitellum: Minimum 1-year follow-up after arthroscopic débridement. *Arthroscopy* 2010; 26(11): 1469-1473.

A retrospective study examined the results of 13 patients who underwent arthroscopic débridement of an OCD lesion. Débridement led to a functional elbow with subjective symptom relief, but many patients ceased some sports activity. Level of evidence: IV.

[31] Savoie F III, Field L, O'Brien M: *AANA Advanced Arthroscopy: The Elbow and Wrist.* Philadelphia, PA, Saunders Elsevier, 2010, pp 132-135.

An arthroscopic method of repairing partial and full-thickness triceps tendon tears using suture anchors was described.

[32] Peden JP, Savoie F III, Field L: Arthroscopic treatment of elbow fractures, in Ryu RKN, ed: *AANA Advanced Arthroscopy: The Elbow and Wrist.* Philadelphia, PA, Saunders Elsevier, 2010, pp 136-143.

An arthroscopic method of assisted fracture fixation was described for a variety of intra-articular fractures about the elbow.

[33] Michels F, Pouliart N, Handelberg F: Arthroscopic management of Mason type 2 radial head fractures. *Knee Surg Sports Traumatol Arthrosc* 2007; 15(10): 1244-1250.

A treatment technique for Mason type II radial head fractures was described, involving arthroscopic reduction and percutaneous pinning to stabilize the fracture, followed by placement of one or two headless screws. All 14 patients had a good to excellent result at an average 5.5-year follow-up. Level of evidence: IV.

[34] Adams JE, Merten SM, Steinmann SP: Arthroscopic-assisted treatment of coronoid fractures. *Arthroscopy* 2007; 23(10): 1060-1065.

A case study examined seven coronoid fractures reduced with arthroscopic assistance and fixed using an anterior cruciate ligament guide for directional guidance and screw fixation. All patients healed with a functional range of motion and were pain free. Level of evidence: IV.

[35] Hausman MR, Klug RA, Qureshi S, Goldstein R, Parsons BO: Arthroscopically assisted coronoid fracture fixation: A preliminary report. *Clin Orthop Relat Res* 2008; 466(12): 3147-3152.

A case study of arthroscopically assisted coronoid fracture fixation found all four consecutive patients had a stable elbow with a functional range of motion.

[36] Hausman MR, Qureshi S, Goldstein R, et al: Arthroscopically-assisted treatment of pediatric lateral humeral condyle fractures. *J Pediatr Orthop* 2007; 27(7): 739-742.

Six skeletally immature patients with a lateral condyle fracture were treated with arthroscopic reduction and percutaneous pinning. All patients healed within 4 weeks with full range of motion. There were no malunions or nonunions. Level of evidence:IV.

[37] Perez Carro L, Golano P, Vega J: Arthroscopic-assisted reduction and percutaneous external fixation of lateral condyle fractures of the humerus. *Arthroscopy* 2007; 23(10): 1131, e1-e4.

Arthroscopic lateral condyle fracture reduction followed by percutaneous Kirschner wire fixation was described in an 11-year-old girl.

[38] O'Driscoll SW, Bell DF, Morrey BF: Posterolateral rotatory instability of the elbow. *J Bone Joint Surg Am* 1991; 73(3): 440-446.

[39] Smith JP III, Savoie FH III, Field LD: Posterolateral rotatory instability of the elbow. *Clin Sports Med* 2001; 20(1): 47-58.

[40] Kalainov DM, Coehn MS: Posterolateral rotatory instability of the elbow in association with lateral epicondylitis: A report of three cases. *J Bone Joint Surg Am* 2005; 87(5): 1120-1125.

[41] Savoie FH III, Field LD, Gurley DJ: Arthroscopic and open radial ulnohumeral ligament reconstruction for posterolateral rotatory instability of the elbow. *Hand Clin* 2009; 25(3): 323-329.

A retrospective chart review of 61 patients treated surgically for posterolateral rotatory instability found improvement of both subjective and objective symptoms after open or arthroscopic treatment.

[42] Savoie F III, Field L, Gurley DJ: Arthroscopic and open radial ulnohumeral ligament reconstruction for posterolateral rotatory instability of the elbow, in Ryu RKN, ed: *AANA Advanced Arthroscopy: The Elbow and Wrist*. Philadelphia, PA, Saunders Elsevier, 2010, pp 94-100.

Open and arthroscopic techniques for PLRI are presented, with satisfactory results.

[43] Cohen SB, Valko C, Zoga A, Dodson CC, Ciccotti MG: Posteromedial elbow impingement: Magnetic resonance imaging findings in overhead throwing athletes and results of arthroscopic treatment. *Arthroscopy* 2011; 27(10): 1364-1370.

A case study correlated MRI findings in overhead throwing athletes with posteromedial impingement findings during arthroscopy. Reproducible pathology was seen in all nine patients, including articular surface changes at the posterior trochlea and anterior medial olecranon on MRI and posteromedial synovitis and olecranon spurring during arthroscopy. Level of evidence: IV.

[44] Blonna D, Lee GC, O'Driscoll SW: Arthroscopic restoration of terminal elbow extension in high-level athletes. *Am J Sports Med* 2010; 38(12): 2509-2515.

In 26 elbows in 24 athletes, loss of terminal elbow extension adversely affected performance. All patients underwent arthroscopic contracture release, and 22 patients returned to the preinjury sport at the same level of intensity and performance. Level of evidence: IV.

[45] Rahusen FT, Brinkman JM, Eygendaal D: Arthroscopic treatment of posterior impingement of the elbow in athletes: A medium-term follow-up in sixteen cases. *J Shoulder Elbow Surg* 2009; 18(2): 279-282.

A retrospective case study evaluated the results of 16 elbows in athletes who underwent arthroscopic débridement of the posterior fossa for posterior impingement. The average extension deficit decreased from 8° preoperatively to 2° postoperatively. Level of evidence: IV.

[46] Flury MP, Goldhahn J, Drerup S, Simmen BR: Arthroscopic and open options for surgical treatment of chondromatosis of the elbow. *Arthroscopy* 2008; 24(5): 520-525, e1.

A retrospective study compared arthroscopic and open surgical treatment options for chondromatosis of the elbow. Both approaches led to satisfactory results, but the arthroscopically treated patients tended to have a shorter rehabilitation time and higher satisfaction. Level of evidence: III.

[47] Kang HJ, Park MJ, Ahn JH, Lee SH: Arthroscopic synovectomy for the rheumatoid elbow. *Arthroscopy* 2010; 26(9): 1195-1202.

Twenty-six rheumatoid elbows in 25 patients were treated with arthroscopic synovectomy using multiple portals. Overall, patients had decreased pain and increased range of motion, and 19 had a good to excellent result. Four patients had a recurrence of synovitis. Level of evidence: IV.

第八部分

其他肩肘相关问题

栏目编委：
Edward G. McFarland, MD

第四十八章　肩胛上神经疾病

Umasuthan Srikumaran, MD; Nicholas Jarmon, MD

引言

　　肩胛上神经疾病是由肩胛上神经受到牵拉、卡压或压迫所导致的。肩胛上神经疾病最常被认为是肩胛上神经冈下支的异常，但冈下支和冈上支可能单独或同时受累。患者通常表现为肩后方疼痛，伴（或不伴）肩关节前屈或外旋无力。肩胛上神经疾病在英文文献中的报道最早见于 1959 年，其真实的发病率及流行程度均不明确。[1]近年的一篇荟萃分析显示，1959—2001 年仅有 88 例被文献报道。[2]到 2011 年为止，最大的一宗病例报道包含 53 例患者。[3]

解剖

　　肩胛上神经接受来自 C5 和 C6 神经根的神经纤维，偶尔也有来自 C4 的神经纤维加入。肩胛上神经自臂丛神经上干发出，经过锁骨后方，越过肩胛骨上缘并向肩胛上切迹走行（图 48-1）。

　　肩胛上神经走行于肩胛横韧带下方，肩胛横韧带通常构成肩胛上切迹的封顶，该切迹是位于喙突基底部内侧的骨性凹陷结构，肩胛上动脉则

Dr. Srikumaran or an immediate family member is a member of a speakers' bureau or has made paid presentations on behalf of Norvartis and serves as a paid consultant to or is an employee of Abbott. Neither Dr. Jarmon nor any immediate family member has received anything of value from or has stock or stock options held in a commercial company or institution related directly or indirectly to the subject of this chapter.

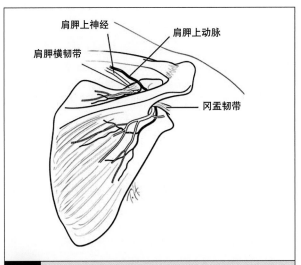

图 48-1　肩胛上神经的解剖。经允许引自 Safran MR: Nerve injury about the shoulder in athletes: Part 1. Suprascapular nerve and axillary nerve. *Am J Sports Med* 2004;32:803–819.

通常走行于韧带的上方。对此切迹形态的描述多种多样，从细微的骨性凹陷到伴有骨化的肩胛横韧带的骨性隧道都可见到。[4]在穿出这个隧道之后，神经向后外侧走行，跨过冈上窝的底部并在这里发出支配冈上肌的运动支和支配肩锁关节及盂肱关节的感觉支。研究发现，支配冈上肌的运动支自距盂上结节平均 3 cm 处发出，而支配冈下肌的运动支则是自距肩胛盂后缘平均 2 cm 处发出。[5]神经在冈上窝后外侧角处进入冈盂切迹，自冈盂韧带（肩胛下横韧带）下方通过。解剖学分析已经表明，此韧带存在与否有着很大的变异，[6]但近期的一项研究显示，在 58 例连续的尸体标本中均有此韧带存在（图 48-2）。[7]此

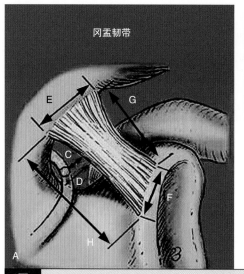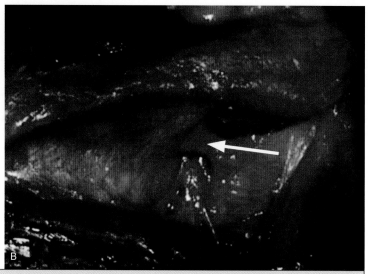

图 48-2 冈盂韧带解剖的后面观。A. 手绘简图。图中所示标线分别表示：C，韧带到神经的最短距离；D，韧带到骨的最长距离；E，肩胛冈附着点；F，肩胛盂附着点；G，上缘；H，下缘。B. 尸体标本，箭头所示为自肩胛冈至后关节囊的冈盂韧带（可以看到肩胛上神经走行于韧带下方）。经允许引自 Plancher KD, Peterson RK, Johnston JC, Luke TA: The spinoglenoid ligament: Anatomy, morphology, and histological findings. *J Bone Joint Surg Am* 2005;87（2）:361–365.

韧带的一部分止于后方关节囊，在肩关节内收及内旋时绷紧。[8]这种姿势被认为与投掷运动的后续顺势动作一致。[8]在从冈盂切迹出来之后，神经绕过肩胛冈基部向内侧走行，同时发出支配冈下肌的运动支。

损伤机制

有很多种机制被认为可以导致肩胛上神经疾病，包括反复的牵拉和微小创伤、压迫性疾病、局部解剖变异、盂肱关节脱位、肩胛骨骨折及手术创伤。[9]

多项研究提示，在从事过顶运动的运动员中，肩胛上神经疾病是反复的牵拉和微小创伤的结果，[10-11]这可能与投掷运动的后续顺势动作中冈盂韧带绷紧导致神经上的压力增加有关。[8]对神经的压迫可发生在其走行过程中的任何部位。在肩胛上切迹和锁骨远端骨折后可以发现肩胛上神经受压。[12-13]肩胛上神经在冈盂切迹处被盂唇旁囊肿卡压也很常见。[14]尽管被认为相对少见，但盂唇旁囊肿可以向内侧延伸得更远，

越过冈盂切迹，在肩胛上切迹处对神经造成压迫。[15]某些解剖学变异，如狭窄的肩胛上或冈盂切迹、[16]前方的喙肩韧带、[17]骨化的肩胛横韧带、[16]以及肌纤维向上方走行的肩胛下肌，[18]都有可能使患者易于患肩胛上神经疾病。软组织肿瘤及骨肿瘤也与肩胛上神经疾病有关。[19-20]行肌电图（EMG）检查发现在肱骨近端骨折或盂肱关节脱位的患者，肩胛上神经损伤的发生率达到 29%。[21]

肩胛上神经还可在肩胛上切迹或肩胛冈基部被回缩的撕裂肩袖卡压。[22]由于神经的运动支在肌肉中比较固定，因此回缩的撕裂肩袖在神经穿过肩胛上切迹和绕过冈盂切迹的部位时可能增加神经内侧的张力。[22]尸体研究同样表明，肌腱的过度移动（>3 cm）会使运动支产生张力。[5]

除直接损伤外，肩胛上神经疾病还被描述成一种手术并发症。近期一项研究的作者报道了 1 例使用 2 枚缝合锚进行 II 型 SLAP 损伤修复的患者。[23]在手术之后，患者出现持续性疼痛。再次行 MRI 检查显示后方的缝合锚穿透了

骨皮质，紧邻着肩胛上神经，而 EMG 检查则证实肩胛上神经的部分失神经支配。在第二次手术中，可以看到缝合锚直接压迫着神经，将其取出后患者的症状得以缓解。[23]在 2007 年的一篇个案报道中，描述了一例 Latarjet 手术中由于螺钉穿入冈盂切迹导致的肩胛上神经疾病。[24] CT 可以证实螺钉的穿出，EMG 则证实了神经疾病的存在。螺钉后来被取出，在最近的一次随访中，患者的症状已经彻底缓解，EMG 检查结果也已恢复正常。在需要使用肩胛骨后方入路的手术中，肩胛上神经也同样存在受损的风险。[25]

病史和体格检查

肩胛上神经损伤的患者可能自诉有创伤史或疼痛和（或）过顶运动无力。疼痛通常并不局限，患者经常描述为肩关节后外侧、上方或前方的钝痛或烧灼样痛。由于这种疼痛常为非局限的弥漫性疼痛，所以考虑这些患者是否存在其他导致疼痛的潜在疾病或合并疾病十分重要。颈部的 C5 或 C6 神经根受累也可能在此区域产生类似的疼痛，并且可能与更多的肩胛上神经或其分支外周压迫或牵拉损伤同时存在。肩胛上神经没有负责皮肤感觉的感觉支，所以肩部或上肢的任何皮肤感觉异常都不应归因于肩胛上神经损伤，而应该寻找其他可能导致感觉异常的原因。

在检查肩关节疼痛患者，尤其是肩胛上神经或肩袖损伤患者时，让患者双肩完全暴露以便从前后方分别对比检视，这一操作十分重要且有益处。对比双侧，尤其是从后方，可以让检查者看出冈上肌或冈下肌的萎缩。单纯地从肩后方检视有时可以在某种程度上提醒检查者肩胛上神经受累的可能。由于肩胛上神经疾病的疼痛变化多端，有可能沿着上臂向远端放射或向颈部放射，因此也有可能出现颈部疼痛，应该检查颈椎的活动范围以评估是否存在颈椎受累。同样，如果存在任何神经损伤的迹象，就需要对整个上肢进行包括感觉、运动及反射在内的神经检查。进行上肢神经系统检查的时候与对侧对比会有帮助，因为很多情况都可能与肩胛上神经疾病相混淆。

肩胛上神经疾病的最佳检查是受累肌肉对抗徒手应力试验。对神经在肩胛上切迹水平受累的最佳检查是肩关节抗阻力外展试验。有研究表明，如果冈上肌和冈下肌受累，肩关节外展和外旋的力量将降低 75%。[26]有些患者可能出现外旋滞后征阳性，不过尽管这一检查对于冈上肌和冈下肌无力非常敏感，但对检查神经损伤并无特异性，其他可以导致肌肉严重无力的原因也需要考虑。上肢置于体侧的抗阻力外旋是检查冈下肌力量的最佳试验。[27]

肩关节的其他诱发试验也可以为确定疼痛的来源提供一些线索，不过其中大多数试验对肩胛上神经单独受累的情况既无特异性也不够敏感。肩胛上神经冈下支单独受累的患者可能表现出合并 SLAP 损伤的体征，不过目前对于 SLAP 损伤的检查仍然不够准确且存在争议。一项尸体研究结果提示症状可能在做交臂内收和内旋动作时加剧，但这种说法尚未得到临床证实。[8]

详尽的体格检查有助于分辨出病变的位置。单纯的冈下肌萎缩与冈盂切迹处的损伤有关。体格检查中，冈盂切迹部位的肩胛上神经疾病会导致单独的体侧外旋力弱。这种力弱可能与其他体格检查（甚至影像学检查）结果不相称；也就是说，并不存在腱鞘囊肿或肩袖撕裂的证据。冈上肌与冈下肌萎缩的患者有可能存在肩胛上切迹部位的损伤（图 48-3）。肩关节周围肌肉的整体萎缩则提示患者的症状是由其他异常所引起的。在巨大肩袖撕裂的病例中，仅凭体格检查发现的肌肉无力并不能确定神经是否受到了牵拉张力。对于这种病例，EMG 和神经传导速度检查能够对诊断有所帮助。

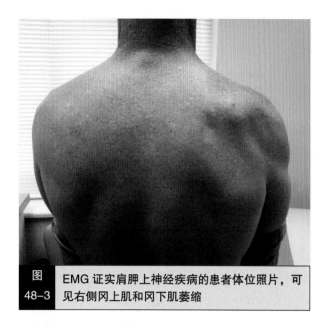

图
48-3 EMG 证实肩胛上神经疾病的患者体位照片，可见右侧冈上肌和冈下肌萎缩

诊断性检查

任何肩关节痛的患者最初评估时都建议行常规 X 线检查。常规 X 线检查可以帮助评价疼痛的肩关节是否存在骨折、既往手术导致的骨性改变、肿瘤、发育异常和其他骨性异常，这些异常都可导致神经受到压迫。CT 则能比 X 线片更精确地显示可能导致神经卡压的骨性异常（如韧带骨化和骨痂形成）。

考虑肩关节痛与肩胛上神经疾病有关时，MRI 被认为是下一步最佳的检查方法。MRI 检查能够最精确地评估肩袖肌腱撕裂的情况，同时也能为肌肉萎缩的存在及其分布状况提供重要信息。此外，它还有可能提供关于腱鞘囊肿和其他可能压迫神经的占位病变的相关信息。不过，MRI 并不能分辨出肩胛上切迹，除非有对获得该部位影像的特殊要求。[28]

很多研究采用超声检查来判别肩胛上神经的异常。[29-30]这种方法具有以下几个优点：①可以将诊断与治疗性注射相结合；②可以看到块状的病变，包括腱鞘囊肿、肿瘤及骨性异常；③对于较瘦的患者，可以沿其走行看到神经本身，而对于较胖的患者，则可以看到与神经相邻的血管结构。这种方法的缺点则在于其高度依赖检查者的经验，而且

对于体重较重的患者的可靠性欠佳。

确诊任何水平的肩胛上神经疾病最重要的标准方法是上肢 EMG/ 神经传导速度检查。EMG/ 神经传导速度检查应包括整个上肢，以便排除可能导致患者症状的其他潜在原因，如颈神经根病、臂丛神经病变、肌肉病和其他周围神经疾病。当要求进行此项检查以评估肩胛下神经时，检查肩胛骨周围肌肉，尤其是冈下肌、冈上肌及三角肌通常有所帮助。[31] EMG 能够协助定位压迫发生的部位。除 EMG 波幅降低之外，潜伏期延长和出现纤颤电位也同样提示神经受压和失神经支配。评价感觉传导速度并不可靠，因为感觉神经的支配很不分明。肩胛上神经运动文传导速度检查的正常值已经明确，目前仍未明确的是这项检查对发现肩胛上神经疾病的敏感性和特异性。[32]

治疗方案

肩胛上神经疾病的治疗取决于其症状的严重程度以及医师对于患者症状是否由该病因所致的判断。很多患者同时存在其他疾病，如有症状的肩锁关节炎或颈椎病，都可能有相似症状。治疗方法还取决于患者的疼痛及不能进行日常活动或参加体育运动的程度。

在不存在占位性病变的前提下，非手术治疗方法（包括改变活动方式、应用 NSAID 及物理治疗）作为肩胛上神经疾病的标准初始治疗已经被广为接受。有研究对 15 例经临床和电诊断方法确诊的肩胛上神经疾病患者采取非手术治疗的结果进行了评估。[33]其中 5 例结果优秀，7 例良好，仅有 3 例因症状持续存在而需行手术治疗。[33]

然而，对于已经证实存在神经压迫及占位性病变或囊肿的患者，随着时间的推移，非手术治疗（尽管通常还是建议作为最初的治疗方法）的效果可能没有那么令人满意。在 19 例已知存在冈盂切迹囊肿并采取非手术治疗的肩胛上神经疾病患者中，只有 10 例对结果满意，而在另外 27 例

具有同样病因而行囊肿切除手术的患者中，对结果表示满意的患者达到了 26 例。[34]

在不存在占位性病变的前提下，如果非手术治疗失败则可考虑手术治疗。理想情况下，为优化治疗结果，应该对存在压迫或异常的区域进行定位。关于判定没有占位性病变的患者在非手术治疗失败后接受手术治疗的转归的相关数据十分有限。在前文提及的那项研究中，3 例非手术治疗无效的患者接受了减压手术治疗，最终结果为 1 例优秀，1 例良好，1 例较差。[33]在有巨大肩袖撕裂的情况下，修补撕裂肌腱后的 EMG/ 神经传导速度检查显示肩胛上神经疾病会出现转归。[22]目前尚不明确在肩袖修补的同时于肩胛上切迹行神经减压是否会有额外的益处。

肩胛上神经减压可以采取关节镜下或切开手术进行，取决于压迫的部位及原因，也取决于术者的经验。

进行肩胛上切迹切开减压时，可以采用沿肩胛冈的军刀状切口或横行切口（图 48-4）。[35]然后，将斜方肌沿其肌纤维方向分开，将冈上肌拉向后方。随后，可确认横韧带的位置并进行松解（图 48-5），应注意保护在韧带上方走行的血管结构及在韧带下方走行的神经。除了松解韧带之

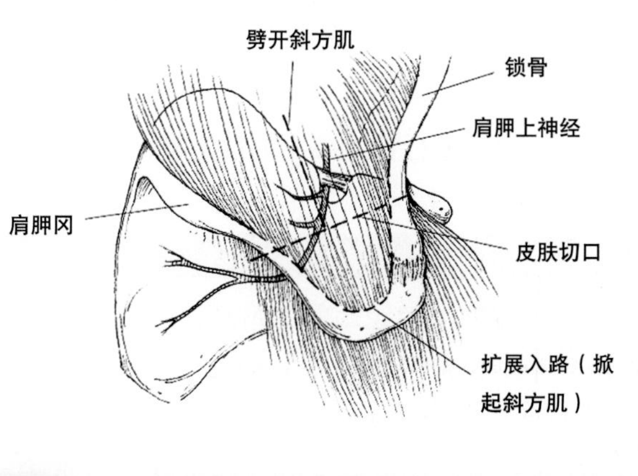

图 48-4 肩胛上切迹切开手术入路。经允许引自 Romeo AA, Rotenberg DD, Bach BR Jr: Suprascapular neuropathy. *J Am Acad Orthop Surg* 1999;7(6):358–367.

外，如果有指征，也可以使用磨钻扩大切迹。

采用关节镜在肩胛上切迹处松解肩胛上神经的方法也已见诸报道。[36-38]该手术从建立常规诊断性关节镜的标准入路开始。当从外侧入路或前外侧入路进入检视时，在切除肩峰下滑囊之后，需要辨认冈上肌的前缘并向内侧追踪。随后，可辨认出喙锁韧带，在沿着喙锁韧带向内侧和下方进一步剥离时，喙锁韧带可作为前方的标志。用脊椎穿刺针于肩锁关节内侧 1~2 cm 处的皮肤上定位一个上方通道。脊椎穿刺针应直接朝向喙突基底，紧邻肩胛上横韧带。接着，将钝性套管针自此通道置入，以将组织沿横韧带方向向内侧拉开，从而显露肩胛上神经及血管（图 48-6）。还可以在第一个通道的外侧再建立第二个通道，以便使用一些附加器械松解横韧带。钝性套管针可以放置在韧带下方，用于在松解韧带的时候保护神经。如果肩胛上横韧带部分或完全骨化，可以使用小骨凿进行神经松解。Kerrison 咬骨钳也可以用来去除神经上方的骨质。这种方法对不熟悉这种技术或周围解剖的外科医师来说可能比较费时费力。

在行冈盂切迹切开减压时可采用后方切口，例如，在肩峰后外侧角以内 3 cm 处做一纵形切口或垂直于皮纹做一切口。沿肌纤维方向劈开三角肌，注意劈开的范围不要过于靠近远端，以免损伤腋神经。随后，辨认冈下肌筋膜并切开，可以将冈下肌拉向下方。然后，继续向深部切开至肩胛冈的外侧面，找到冈盂韧带并松解。[39]切开减压也可以与关节镜检查同时进行，关节镜可用来明确是否存在需要处理的关节内异常，例如，SLAP 损伤和肩袖问题。

采用关节镜技术在冈盂切迹处行肩胛上神经松解最早见于 2007 年的一项研究。[40]操作步骤从建立常规诊断性关节镜的标准入路开始。在切除肩峰下滑囊后即可从肩峰下间隙看到冈盂切迹。再从后方建立第二个入路，用小 Langenbeck 拉钩将冈下肌肌腹轻轻地拉向下方，这样可以更清楚地看到肩胛上神经和盂唇旁囊肿。然后，将囊肿

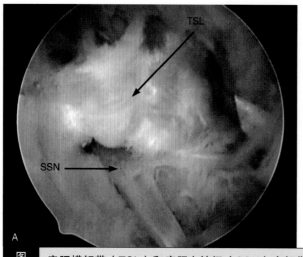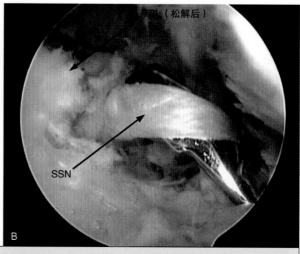

图
48-5 肩胛横韧带（TSL）和肩胛上神经（SSN）在韧带松解之前（A）和之后（B）的关节镜术中图像。经允许引自 Boykin RE, Friedman DJ, Higgins LD, Warner JJ: Suprascapular neuropathy. *J Bone Joint Surg Am* 2010;92(13):2348–2364.

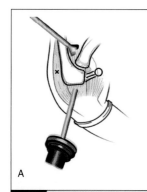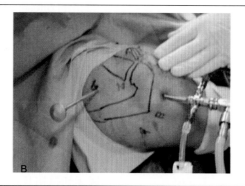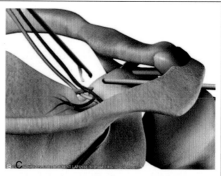

图
48-6 右侧肩胛上神经关节镜下松解入路的建立。A. 手绘简图，上面观。B. 临床照片，上面观。C. 电脑生成图像，后面观。经允许引自 Boykin RE, Friedman DJ, Higgins LD, Warner JJ: Suprascapular neuropathy. *J Bone Joint Surg Am* 2010;92(13):2348–2364.

切开，其内容物可使用刨削器吸除。这一技术的潜在优点是可以评估关节内的异常，而这些异常通常与局部的囊肿相关。有观点认为在某些情况下，当发现冈盂囊肿与 SLAP 损伤或后方盂唇撕裂有关时，可以单独采取盂唇修复的方法进行治疗。[41] 在 10 例冈盂切迹囊肿伴上方盂唇撕裂接受盂唇修复但未行囊肿减压的患者中，4 例术前EMG 检查确认存在肩胛上神经疾病，这 4 例患者术后 EMG 检查结果均显示功能恢复正常。8 例患者术后进行了 MRI 检查，结果全部显示囊肿问题得以解决。[41]

当 MRI 上无法明确辨认单一的压迫部位时，一些研究者推荐对两个切迹一起进行经验性减压。[42-43] 使用关节镜[43] 和切开手术[5] 在两个部位同时进行神经减压的技术都已见诸报道。

临床结果

对于肩胛上神经疾病的最佳治疗方法，想要给出一个结论性的建议十分困难，因为这类疾病并不常见，诊断的标准各异，诊断又常常缺少EMG/ 神经传导速度检查结果的确认，也没有前瞻性随机研究分析各种不同治疗方法的结果优劣。2002 年的一项荟萃分析确认了 1959—2001 年的88 例肩胛上神经卡压病例。[2] 遗憾的是，报道了临床治疗结果的研究不足 50%。尽管这篇荟萃分析指出，早期手术干预可能有助于限制可见的肌肉萎缩程度，但由于缺乏治疗结果的报道，无法得出更多的结论。

有报道称，在 31 例于肩胛上切迹处切开减压的患者中，有 28 例疼痛得到了缓解，肌肉力量也得以改善。[44] 2011 年，有研究者[45]报道了对 27 例患者行关节镜下肩胛上和（或）冈盂切迹减压治疗的结果：在随访到的 24 例患者中，71% 的患者自诉疼痛缓解，75% 的患者 ASES 肩关节疼痛和功能障碍评分显著提高并有统计学意义，71% 的患者肩关节主观评分显著提高并有统计学意义，71% 的患者愿意再次接受这种手术（表 48-1）。[3,33,38,44-47]

表 48-1

临床结果

研究发表（年份）	病例数	平均年龄（岁）	平均随访（范围）	治疗
Martin 等[33]（1997）	15	35	47 个月（15~54 个月）	物理治疗：关节活动范围改善以及肩胛骨周围力量强化
Antoniou 等[3]（2001）	53	38	28 个月（12~91 个月）	手术，36 例；非手术，17 例
Kim 等[44]（2005）	42	41	18 个月（12~48 个月）	切开减压
Mallon 等[46]（2006）	8	68	24 个月（16~36 个月）	非手术治疗，4 例；用边缘重叠法部分修复巨大肩袖撕裂，4 例
Westerheide 等[47]（2006）	14	41	51 个月（24~73 个月）	关节镜下减压
Lafosse 等[38]（2007）	10	50	15 个月（6~27 个月）	关节镜下减压
Shah 等[45]（2011）	27	49.3	22.5 个月（3~44 个月）	关节镜下减压

表 48-1

临床结果（续）

术前 EMG	术后 EMG	结果衡量标准	临床结果
非手术治疗组 10 例中有 4 例有异常发现	治疗后恢复正常	活动范围、疼痛、力量	5 例优，7 例良，3 例因持续疼痛需要手术（1 例良，1 例优，1 例差）
有	无	改良 ASES	压迫性病变手术治疗有效；过度使用性损伤对手术及非手术治疗的反应同等良好
有	无	疼痛及力量分级	8 例持续性疼痛患者中有 7 例疼痛缓解。术前所有病例冈上肌肌力均为 0~2 级；术后 90% 的患者冈上肌肌力为 4 级以上，10% 的患者冈上肌肌力为 2~3 级
所有病例 SS±IS 均失神经支配	手术组中 2 例随访时 EMG 显示神经部分恢复	临床检查	非手术治疗组，无变化；手术治疗组，全部 4 例患者肩上举改善，临床上冈上肌、冈下肌萎缩依然存在
11 例显示 IS 失神经支配	无	SST、Constant 肩关节评分、力量	SST 改善（从 4.3 到 11.5），术后 Constant 肩关节评分为 94；所有病例均力量增强
10 例发现慢性压迫	8 例中有 7 例恢复至完全正常，1 例部分恢复	Constant 肩关节评分、力量、VAS、患者满意度	Constant 肩关节评分和外旋外展肌力提高，10 例中 9 例为优秀，疼痛彻底缓解，1 例满意，疼痛中度缓解
27 例中有 24 例有阳性发现	无	VAS、肩关节主观评分、ASES	24 例有阳性发现的病例中 17 例疼痛缓解，17 例主观评分改善，18 例 ASES 改善

注：EMG = 肌电图；ASES = ASES 肩关节疼痛和功能障碍评分；VAS = 视觉模拟评分法；SS = 冈上肌；IS = 冈下肌；SST = 肩关节简明测试。

总结

尽管尚不清楚真实的发病率，但肩胛上神经疾病依然是一种不常见的诊断。为了能够准确识别这种异常，同时排除其他可能情况，需要进行细致的临床评估。在确认疾病过程并排除占位性病变之后，非手术治疗依然是首选的治疗方法。如果非手术治疗失败，采取切开手术或关节镜技术进行减压的方法也有报道。能用以指导治疗的随机对照研究仍很缺乏，尚需要进一步的研究以建立理想的治疗流程。

参考文献

［1］ Kopell HP, Thompson WA: Pain and the frozen shoulder. *Surg Gynecol Obstet* 1959;109(1):92-96.

［2］ Zehetgruber H, Noske H, Lang T, Wurnig C: Suprascapular nerve entrapment: A meta-analysis. *Int Orthop* 2002;26(6):339-343.

［3］ Antoniou J, Tae SK, Williams GR, Bird S, Ramsey ML, Iannotti JP: Suprascapular neuropathy: Variability in the diagnosis, treatment, and outcome. *Clin Orthop Relat Res* 2001;386:131-138.

［4］ Edelson JG: Bony bridges and other variations of the suprascapular notch. *J Bone Joint Surg Br* 1995;77(3):505-506.

［5］ Warner JP, Krushell RJ, Masquelet A, Gerber C: Anatomy and relationships of the suprascapular nerve: Anatomical constraints to mobilization of the supraspinatus and infraspinatus muscles in the management of massive rotator-cuff tears. *J Bone Joint Surg Am* 1992; 74(1):36-45.

［6］ Rengachary SS, Burr D, Lucas S, Brackett CE: Suprascapular entrapment neuropathy: A clinical, anatomical, and comparative study. Part 3: Comparative study. *Neurosurgery* 1979;5(4):452-455.

［7］ Plancher KD, Peterson RK, Johnston JC, Luke TA: The spinoglenoid ligament: Anatomy, morphology, and histological findings. *J Bone Joint Surg Am* 2005;87(2):361-365.

［8］ Plancher KD, Luke TA, Peterson RK, Yacoubian SV: Posterior shoulder pain: A dynamic study of the spinoglenoid ligament and treatment with arthroscopic release of the scapular tunnel. *Arthroscopy* 2007; 23(9):991-998.
This cadaver study sought to determine the pressure exerted on the suprascapular nerve by compression of the spinoglenoid ligament during glenohumeral range of motion. The most pressure was noted with the arm in full adduction and internal rotation.

［9］ Boykin RE, Friedman DJ, Higgins LD, Warner JJ: Suprascapular neuropathy. *J Bone Joint Surg Am* 2010; 92(13):2348-2364.
This review article details the anatomy, the pathophysiology, the diagnosis, and the treatment of suprascapular neuropathy. More research is needed to determine proper etiology and treatment.

［10］ Ferretti A, Cerullo G, Russo G: Suprascapular neuropathy in volleyball players. *J Bone Joint Surg Am* 1987; 69(2):260-263.

［11］ Lajtai G, Pfirrmann CW, Aitzetmüller G, Pirkl C, Gerber C, Jost B: The shoulders of professional beach volleyball players: High prevalence of infraspinatus muscle atrophy. *Am J Sports Med* 2009;37(7):1375-1383.
This cross-sectional study of 84 professional volleyball players found a 30% prevalence of infraspinatus muscle atrophy. Fully competitive players typically had subjectively unrecognized weakness in external rotation and frequent unspecific shoulder pain. Level of evidence: III.

［12］ Huang KC, Tu YK, Huang TJ, Hsu RW: Suprascapular neuropathy complicating a Neer type I distal clavicular fracture: A case report. *J Orthop Trauma* 2005; 19(5):343-345.

［13］ Solheim LF, Roaas A: Compression of the suprascapular nerve after fracture of the scapular notch. *Acta Orthop Scand* 1978;49(4):338-340.

［14］ Tirman PF, Feller JF, Janzen DL, Peterfy CG, Bergman AG: Association of glenoid labral cysts with labral tears and glenohumeral instability: Radiologic findings and clinical significance. *Radiology* 1994;190(3): 653-658.

［15］ Moore TP, Fritts HM, Quick DC, Buss DD: Suprascapular nerve entrapment caused by supraglenoid cyst compression. *J Shoulder Elbow Surg* 1997;6(5): 455-462.

［16］ Ticker JB, Djurasovic M, Strauch RJ, et al: The incidence of ganglion cysts and other variations in anatomy along the course of the suprascapular nerve. *J Shoulder Elbow Surg* 1998;7(5):472-478.

［17］ Avery BW, Pilon FM, Barclay JK: Anterior coracoscapular ligament and suprascapular nerve entrapment. *Clin Anat* 2002;15(6):383-386.

［18］ Bayramoglu A, Demiryürek D, Tüccar E, et al:

Variations in anatomy at the suprascapular notch possibly causing suprascapular nerve entrapment: An anatomical study. *Knee Surg Sports Traumatol Arthrosc* 2003; 11(6):393-398.

[19] Hazrati Y, Miller S, Moore S, Hausman M, Flatow E: Suprascapular nerve entrapment secondary to a lipoma. *Clin Orthop Relat Res* 2003;411:124-128.

[20] Yi JW, Cho NS, Rhee YG: Intraosseous ganglion of the glenoid causing suprascapular nerve entrapment syndrome: A case report. *J Shoulder Elbow Surg* 2009; 18(3):e25-e27.

A case report of an intraosseous ganglion causing a suprascapular neuropathy treated with diagnostic arthroscopy and needle aspiration of the cyst is discussed. The patient presented with pain, weakness, and tenderness to palpation at the infraspinatus fossa, all symptoms resolved at early follow-up.

[21] de Laat EA, Visser CP, Coene LN, Pahlplatz PV, Tavy DL: Nerve lesions in primary shoulder dislocations and humeral neck fractures: A prospective clinical and EMG study. *J Bone Joint Surg Br* 1994;76(3):381-383.

[22] Costouros JG, Porramatikul M, Lie DT, Warner JJ: Reversal of suprascapular neuropathy following arthroscopic repair of massive supraspinatus and infraspinatus rotator cuff tears. *Arthroscopy* 2007; 23(11):1152-1161.

A case series of seven patients with massive rotator cuff tears and isolated suprascapular neuropathy who underwent arthroscopic rotator cuff tear repair is discussed. EMG/nerve conduction velocity studies 6 months postoperatively demonstrated partial or full recovery of suprascapular nerve palsy that correlated with pain relief and functional improvement. Level of evidence: IV.

[23] Kim SH, Koh YG, Sung CH, Moon HK, Park YS: Iatrogenic suprascapular nerve injury after repair of type II SLAP lesion. *Arthroscopy* 2010;26(7):1005-1008.

A case report of suprascapular nerve injury at the spinoglenoid notch after repair of a type II SLAP lesion caused by improperly inserted suture anchor is discussed.

[24] Maquieira GJ, Gerber C, Schneeberger AG: Suprascapular nerve palsy after the Latarjet procedure. *J Shoulder Elbow Surg* 2007;16(2):e13-e15.

A case report of suprascapular neuropathy after a Latarjet procedure is discussed. The diagnosis was confirmed by abnormal EMG and CT scan showing screw penetration into the spinoglenoid notch. After screw removal, the clinical and EMG findings returned to normal.

[25] Wijdicks CA, Armitage BM, Anavian J, Schroder LK, Cole PA: Vulnerable neurovasculature with a posterior approach to the scapula. *Clin Orthop Relat Res* 2009; 467(8):2011-2017.

A cadaver study of 24 specimens that defines the location of the suprascapular nerve and the circumflex scapular artery with respect to various osseous landmarks in the posterior shoulder is discussed.

[26] Gerber C, Blumenthal S, Curt A, Werner CM: Effect of selective experimental suprascapular nerve block on abduction and external rotation strength of the shoulder. *J Shoulder Elbow Surg* 2007;16(6):815-820.

The authors performed nerve blocks of the suprascapular nerve in healthy volunteers. Infraspinatus paralysis caused a loss of 70% external rotation and 45% abduction strength. Infraspinatus-supraspinatus paralysis caused a loss of 80% external rotator and 75% abduction strength.

[27] Kelly BT, Kadrmas WR, Speer KP: The manual muscle examination for rotator cuff strength: An electromyographic investigation. *Am J Sports Med* 1996;24(5): 581-588.

[28] Inokuchi W, Ogawa K, Horiuchi Y: Magnetic resonance imaging of suprascapular nerve palsy. *J Shoulder Elbow Surg* 1998;7(3):223-227.

[29] Martinoli C, Bianchi S, Pugliese F, et al: Sonography of entrapment neuropathies in the upper limb (wrist excluded). *J Clin Ultrasound* 2004;32(9):438-450.

[30] Yücesoy C, Akkaya T, Ozel O, et al: Ultrasonographic evaluation and morphometric measurements of the suprascapular notch. *Surg Radiol Anat* 2009;31(6):409-414.

Both shoulders of each of 50 volunteers were evaluated by ultrasound to measure the width and the depth of the suprascapular notch. The skin-notch base interval and the neighboring vasculature were also imaged. Variations between the sexes are discussed.

[31] Bredella MA, Tirman PF, Fritz RC, Wischer TK, Stork A, Genant HK: Denervation syndromes of the shoulder girdle: MR imaging with electrophysiologic correlation. *Skeletal Radiol* 1999;28(10):567-572.

[32] Buschbacher RM, Weir SK, Bentley JG, Cottrell E: Normal motor nerve conduction studies using surface electrode recording from the supraspinatus, infraspinatus, deltoid, and biceps. *PM R* 2009;1(2):101-106.

One hundred volunteers were recruited and completed bilateral testing using simple surface electrodes. Normal values for distal latency, amplitude, duration, and area were developed for proximal nerve conductions to the axillary, musculocutaneous, and suprascapular nerves.

[33] Martin SD, Warren RF, Martin TL, Kennedy K, O'Brien SJ, Wickiewicz TL: Suprascapular neuropathy: Results of non-operative treatment. *J Bone Joint Surg Am* 1997;79(8):1159-1165.

[34] Piatt BE, Hawkins RJ, Fritz RC, Ho CP, Wolf E, Schickendantz M: Clinical evaluation and treatment of spinoglenoid notch ganglion cysts. *J Shoulder Elbow Surg* 2002;11(6):600-604.

[35] Post M: Diagnosis and treatment of suprascapular nerve entrapment. *Clin Orthop Relat Res* 1999;368: 92-100.

[36] Bhatia DN, de Beer JF, van Rooyen KS, du Toit DF: Arthroscopic suprascapular nerve decompression at the suprascapular notch. *Arthroscopy* 2006;22(9): 1009-1013.

[37] Lafosse L, Tomasi A: Technique for endoscopic release of suprascapular nerve entrapment at the suprascapular notch. *Tech Shoulder Elbow Surg* 2006;7:1-6.

[38] Lafosse L, Tomasi A, Corbett S, Baier G, Willems K, Gobezie R: Arthroscopic release of suprascapular nerve entrapment at the suprascapular notch: Technique and preliminary results. *Arthroscopy* 2007; 23(1):34-42.
A prospective series (Level IV) of 10 patients with EMG findings consistent with chronic suprascapular notch compression, posterior shoulder pain, and subjective weakness were treated with a novel arthroscopic suprascapular notch decompression. All patients had improved pain, function, and EMG findings. Level of evidence: IV.

[39] Piasecki DP, Romeo AA, Bach BR Jr, Nicholson GP: Suprascapular neuropathy. *J Am Acad Orthop Surg* 2009;17(11):665-676.
This review article details the anatomy, the pathophysiology, the diagnosis, and the treatment of suprascapular neuropathy.

[40] Werner CM, Nagy L, Gerber C: Combined intra- and extra-articular arthroscopic treatment of entrapment neuropathy of the infraspinatus branches of the suprascapular nerve caused by a periglenoidal ganglion cyst. *Arthroscopy* 2007;23(3):e1-e3.
A case report of an arthroscopic technique for exposure of the spinoglenoid notch with débridement of paralabral cysts causing suprascapular neuropathy is discussed.

[41] Youm T, Matthews PV, El Attrache NS: Treatment of patients with spinoglenoid cysts associated with superior labral tears without cyst aspiration, debridement, or excision. *Arthroscopy* 2006;22(5):548-552.

[42] Sandow MJ, Ilic J: Suprascapular nerve rotator cuff compression syndrome in volleyball players. *J Shoulder Elbow Surg* 1998;7(5):516-521.

[43] Soubeyrand M, Bauer T, Billot N, Lortat-Jacob A, Gicquelet R, Hardy P: Original portals for arthroscopic decompression of the suprascapular nerve: An anatomic study. *J Shoulder Elbow Surg* 2008;17(4): 616-623.
A cadaver study of 30 specimens is discussed. Suprascapular nerve decompressions were performed using various portals to determine the efficacy and the safety of each portal.

[44] Kim DH, Murovic JA, Tiel RL, Kline DG: Management and outcomes of 42 surgical suprascapular nerve injuries and entrapments. *Neurosurgery* 2005;57(1): 120-127, discussion 120-127.

[45] Shah AA, Butler RB, Sung SY, Wells JH, Higgins LD, Warner JJ: Clinical outcomes of suprascapular nerve decompression. *J Shoulder Elbow Surg* 2011;20(6): 975-982.
A case series of 27 patients without rotator cuff pathology who underwent suprascapular nerve decompression is presented. At final follow-up, 71% had pain relief, 75% had an improved American Shoulder and Elbow Surgeons score, and 71% had an improved subjective shoulder value score. Level of evidence: IV.

[46] Mallon WJ, Wilson RJ, Basamania CJ: The association of suprascapular neuropathy with massive rotator cuff tears: A preliminary report. *J Shoulder Elbow Surg* 2006;15(4):395-398.

[47] Westerheide KJ, Dopirak RM, Karzel RP, Snyder SJ: Suprascapular nerve palsy secondary to spinoglenoid cysts: Results of arthroscopic treatment. *Arthroscopy* 2006;22(7):721-727.

第四十九章　肩胛骨的运动学、动力障碍及损伤

W. Ben Kibler, MD

肩胛骨的运动学

作为肩胛盂和肩峰解剖结构不可分割的部分，肩胛骨在肩关节与上肢发挥正常功能的过程中扮演着举足轻重的角色。肩胛骨能影响盂肱关节和肩锁关节的活动，并且通过肩肱节律与上肢的活动结合在一起，从而产生高效的运动。传统上，肩胛骨的运动被描述成一种二维单平面模式的活动，运动时肩胛骨向上旋转，以肩峰抬高为终点。[1-2]上部斜方肌收缩拉动肩峰上抬，同时前锯肌收缩使肩胛骨下缘向外侧运动，这一对肌肉的力偶被认为至关重要。[1]在不同的研究中，肩胛骨上旋的幅度各异，不过平均值为60°，这也为整体肩肱节律确立了1∶2的肩胛骨–肱骨运动比。

研究发现，肩胛骨的运动实际上是三维多平面的。[3]使用运动跟踪系统和骨内留置针的研究结果表明，肩胛骨的全部运动是一种由旋转（围绕不同轴线的旋转运动）和平移（沿着一个表面的滑行运动）复合而成的运动（图49–1）。3种能观察到的旋转运动分别是围绕沿着肩胛冈的水平轴线的前后倾运动、围绕沿着肩胛骨内侧缘垂向轴线的内外旋运动以及围绕垂直于肩胛骨体部轴

Dr. Kibler or an immediate family member serves as an unpaid consultant to Alignmed; has stock or stock options held in Alignmed; and serves as a board member, owner, officer, or committee member of the International Society of Arthroscopy, Knee Surgery, and Orthopaedic Sports Medicine and the American Orthopaedic Society for Sports Medicine.

线的上下旋运动。[3]在锁骨支柱和肩锁关节完整的情况下，可以发生两种平移运动：在胸壁上的向上–向下滑动（由锁骨在胸锁关节处发生的上下运动所引起）；绕着胸壁侧方弧度的前后滑动（由锁骨在胸锁关节处发生的前后运动所引起）。

与肩胛骨相邻的骨性结构和肌肉结构决定了肩胛骨的运动。锁骨、胸锁关节和肩锁关节对肩胛骨位置、旋转运动和平移运动的形成十分重要。[4]若想有正常的肩胛骨运动，锁骨、胸锁关节和肩锁关节的解剖必须几乎完全正常。锁骨是肩胛骨与中轴骨之间唯一的骨联结。为使肩胛骨和肩肱关节的运动在上肢完全上举过程中最大化，锁骨需要回收16°，上抬6°，并沿其长轴向后旋转31°。[4]上述所有运动都以胸锁关节为基础进行。肩锁关节的运动是由肩峰在锁骨上的运动形成的，包括8°的内旋、11°的上旋及19°的后倾。[4]这些受限的运动通过肩锁关节在锁骨和肩胛骨之间创造出一个可复制的螺旋运动轴，从而使肩胛骨可以产生三维运动。[5]

参与肩胛骨运动的主要肌肉包括上部斜方肌、下部斜方肌、前锯肌和菱形肌。伴随着上肢上举的肩胛骨上抬是通过上部斜方肌、下部斜方肌、前锯肌及菱形肌的激活与力偶来完成的。[6]在这一活动中，下部斜方肌通过其附着于内侧肩胛冈上来帮助维持肩胛骨的瞬时旋转中心。[2]当上肢上举和肩胛骨上旋时，下部斜方肌在肩胛冈上的附着能产生一个直线拉力，从而形成维持这种位置

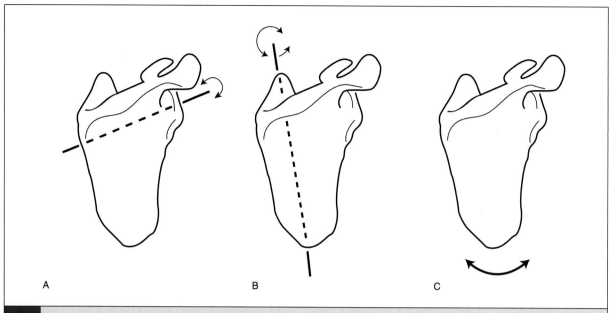

图 49-1　肩胛骨三维运动示意图。A. 围绕水平轴线（虚线所示）的前后倾运动（双头箭头所示）。B. 围绕垂直轴线（虚线所示）的内外旋运动（双头箭头所示）。C. 围绕矢状面轴线的上下旋运动（双头箭头所示）。经允许引自自 McClure PW, Bialker J, Neff N, Williams G, Karduna A: Shoulder function and 3-dimensional kinematics in people with shoulder impingement syndrome before and after a 6-week exercise program. *Phys Ther* 2004;84(9):832-848.

的力学优势。当上肢从上举位置放下时，下部斜方肌同时也发挥着稳定肩胛骨的作用。前锯肌由多部分多层面肌束组成，肩胛骨三维运动中的所有部分都有其参与，它能在稳定肩胛骨内侧缘和下角的同时帮助肩胛骨上旋、后倾及外旋。[6]

因为这些负责稳定性和运动的肌肉全部都附着于中轴骨，所以控制身体核心的姿势和稳定性对于最大限度地激活这些肌肉非常重要，就像控制肩胛骨对于最大限度地激活肩袖非常重要一样。肌肉及其力偶的最大限度激活只能通过自核心开始到肢体末端的激活方式来进行。这些方式将肌肉的协同收缩、力偶及协同激活整合在一起，使得所产生的肌肉力量最大化。当肌肉的募集处于对角线方向，例如，从对侧髋关节经腰背筋膜至下部斜方肌时，下部斜方肌和前锯肌能够获得最大化的激活。[7] 肩胛骨发挥其功能最稳定且高效的位置是回收的位置。[8-10] 在此位置上，肩峰下间隙是最宽的，肩袖的激活是最大的，内部撞击是最小的，发生损伤的概率则是最低的。[8-13]

多数与肩胛骨相关的功能障碍追溯其原因都能够发现肩胛骨正常休息位置与动态运动的失控，这会造成其位置和活动的改变，从而导致肩胛骨在静息与运动时都过度前伸。[14] 这种前伸的位置会导致与加重功能障碍的症状（图 49-2）。

改变后的肩胛骨休息位置被描述为 SICK 肩胛骨，意为肩胛骨位置不正 - 内下缘突出 - 喙突痛 - 肩胛骨动力障碍合并存在。[15] SICK 肩胛骨的特征是明显的下垂，这实际上代表着肩胛骨的前倾。这种改变后的位置提示了胸小肌的柔韧性及前锯肌和下部斜方肌肌力的改变，应该引起检查者对可能存在的与肩胛骨相关的病情的警惕。

肩胛骨动力障碍

改变后的动态运动被称为肩胛骨动力障碍（scapular dyskinesis），这个词结合了 dys（改变）和 kinesis（运动）二者的含义。肩胛骨动力障碍的特征是肩胛骨内侧缘或内下缘凸起，当上肢上举时肩胛骨早期上抬或耸肩，当上肢放下时

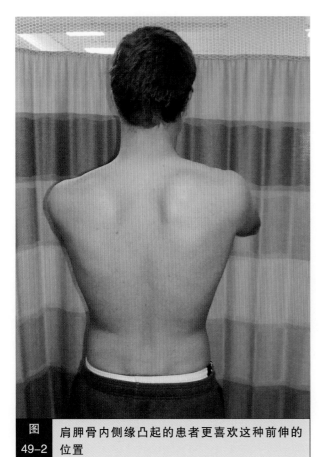

图
49-2 | 肩胛骨内侧缘凸起的患者更喜欢这种前伸的位置

肩胛骨快速下旋。[14-16]存在动力障碍的肩胛骨最突出的临床特征是前伸,具体表现为肩胛骨内侧缘的不对称性突起。已经确认了3种单平面类型:内下角突起(I型)、内侧缘整体突起(II型)及内上缘突起(III型)。[17]具体是哪种类型往往会在上肢活动时显现出来。每种类型确切的病理生理及其与特定的肩关节异常有何关系仍待阐明。普遍认为各型动力障碍产生的运动方式改变了肩胛骨在高效的肩肱节律中扮演的角色及结果。

肩胛骨动力障碍可见于67%~100%的肩部损伤患者,其病因有很多。[12-13]在大多数情况下,肩胛骨动力障碍是由力偶肌激活的改变所导致的。神经源性病因则包括胸长神经和副神经的损伤,这种情况相对少见。肌肉激活的改变更为常见的原因包括盂肱关节损伤引起的疼痛所导致的神经激活受到抑制、肩胛骨稳定肌群力量的失衡、肌肉激活的疲劳以及激活方式的变化。在几乎所有患

者中都能发现前锯肌与下部斜方肌无力,激活强度低于正常或激活时间延迟,而上部斜方肌的激活增强,激活时间呈现异常。[18]这种模式导致了肩胛骨的后倾、外旋和上旋运动少于正常,而上抬和平移运动则多于正常。这些结果在存在撞击、不稳定及盂唇撕裂的患者中都能见到。[19-21]

肩胛骨动力障碍还可能由肌肉或盂肱关节的僵硬引起。在几乎所有肩关节严重退行性关节炎或粘连性关节囊炎的患者中都可以发现肩胛骨动力障碍。在部分患者中,胸小肌过紧而缺乏柔韧性被认为是造成肩胛骨后倾、上旋及外旋运动减少的原因。在投掷过程中,当上肢进入顺势动作阶段时,与后方肌肉僵硬和关节囊过紧相关的盂肱关节内旋不足会使肩胛骨随同肱骨头的内旋而产生前伸,进而造成动力障碍。[20]

锁骨骨折后如果其解剖结构没能恢复到几乎完全正常也可能导致动力障碍。伴有短缩的畸形愈合或不愈合会使锁骨支柱的长度变短,尤其是在短缩超过2 cm时,会改变肩胛骨的位置,使肩胛骨更为内旋和前倾。[22]与之类似,显著成角的锁骨骨折也会导致功能性的短缩及旋转活动的丢失。锁骨中段骨折时远端常处于外旋位,这会使在上肢上举过程中必然发生的锁骨后旋和肩胛骨后倾变小,从而影响正常的动力学。

III型、IV型和V型肩锁关节损伤常会导致动力障碍。这些较严重的肩锁关节分离会破坏锁骨的支柱功能,使第三种平移运动得以发生,即肩胛骨向锁骨的下方和胸壁的内侧平移。[23]由锁骨远端切除过多和肩锁韧带剥离导致的医源性肩锁关节损伤会使骨性支柱变短,由于肩锁关节处的前后方向活动过度,肩胛骨也可能过度内旋。

几乎所有这些致病因素导致的最终结果就是肩胛骨在休息时处于前伸位或在上肢运动时过度前伸。通常,这种由于肩胛骨内旋和前倾增大而形成的位置几乎不利于肩关节的所有功能,只有在举重运动中的附加位置除外。肩胛骨的位置不

良造成了肩峰下间隙的减小，因此可能增加撞击症状的发生。[11] 此外，位置不良会使肩袖的力量降低，盂肱前韧带的张力、肩胛骨稳定肌群的张力及内部撞击的风险则均会增加。[24] 多数针对肩胛骨动力障碍治疗的主要目标都与恢复其功能性回收能力相关。

动力障碍与肩关节症状之间的关系并不总是非常清楚。对于神经损伤、骨折、肩锁关节分离和肌肉剥离的患者，损伤会造成动力障碍，从而影响肩关节功能。在部分存在肩袖疾病、盂唇损伤或肩关节多向不稳定的患者中，动力障碍可能是致病原因，它产生的病理力学会使上肢更容易受到损伤。而在另一些患者中，动力障碍则可能是对损伤的一种反应，导致会加剧功能障碍的病理力学所产生。无论哪种情况，动力障碍都是存在的，必须与患者的其他病理状态一起得到治疗。

这些发病机制往往不是孤立出现的，在同一个患者身上可能同时存在几种病因。对于肩关节损伤的患者，仔细检查是否存在肩胛骨动力障碍以及每种致病机制都应该作为综合评价的一部分。肩胛骨的临床评估应该包括所有可能导致动力障碍的局部与远隔因素，评估还应该包含动态检查，因为肩胛骨的运动是动力障碍的关键组成部分。

临床上，一项有用且可靠的检查能够分辨出动力障碍，并且可以作为治疗的基础。[14,16,25] 对肩胛骨进行体格检查的目的在于确定是否存在SICK肩胛骨，是否存在动力障碍，评估关节、肌肉及骨性致病因素，并且用动态的纠正手法来评价纠正动力障碍后对患者的症状能起到何种效果。[16] 体格检查的结果有助于确定功能障碍各个方面的完整诊断，并可指导治疗和康复。

大多数肩胛骨的检查都应该从后面进行，并且暴露肩胛骨使其能被完全看到。应检查患者的休息姿势，观察是否存在两侧不对称，尤其注意有无SICK体位、有无内下角或内侧缘突起。如果在判断内下角或内上角的骨性标志时有困难，在上缘和内下缘做出标记可能有所帮助。

应该检查胸锁关节和肩锁关节是否不稳定，对于锁骨则应评价其成角、短缩或旋转异常的情况。肩锁关节前后方向松弛性的检查可以通过用一只手稳定锁骨，另一只手抓住并在前后方向上活动肩峰来进行（图49-3）。

临床上对肩胛骨的动态检查比较可靠的方法是从患者后方观察，观察其上肢上举和落下时肩胛骨的运动。这种运动需要激活能够保持肩肱节律闭链机制的肌肉。不能保持这种节律就会导致肩胛骨的内旋增加，从而造成肩胛骨内侧缘突出。临床上检查有症状的患者时，观察其肩胛骨内侧缘突出情况，这与从生物力学角度上明确的动力

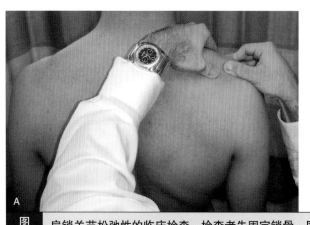
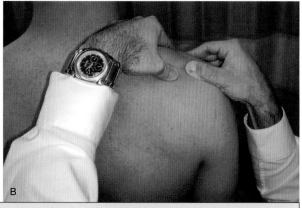

图 49-3 肩锁关节松弛性的临床检查。检查者先固定锁骨，同时抓住肩峰（A），然后尝试向前和向后平移肩峰来判断是否存在关节松弛及松弛的程度（B）

障碍相关，应用这种方法判断是否存在肩胛骨动力障碍具有足够的可靠性。[25]检查时嘱患者双手各持 1.4~2.3 kg 的物品，双上肢前屈上举至最大程度后再放下，如此重复 3~5 次。[26-27]有症状侧的肩胛骨内侧缘任何地方突出都应被记录下来。

肩胛骨协助试验（SAT）、肩胛骨回收试验（SRT）及肩胛骨复位试验是能够改变损伤症状、提供关于肩胛骨动力障碍在伴随肩关节损伤产生的功能障碍中所扮演角色的信息的纠正性手法。[28]SAT 能够用来评估肩胛骨在撞击症状和肩袖力量中所起的作用，而 SRT 则可以用来评估其在肩袖力量和盂唇症状中所起的作用。在 SAT 中，检查者在患者一侧上肢上举时柔缓施压以辅助肩胛骨上旋和后倾（图 49-4）。SAT 最重要的生物力学作用是在整个上肢上举运动弧中增加了 7°~10° 的肩胛骨后倾。这个试验的检查者间可信度是令人满意的。[29]撞击症状的疼痛弧得以缓解、活动范围增大为阳性结果。在 SRT 中，

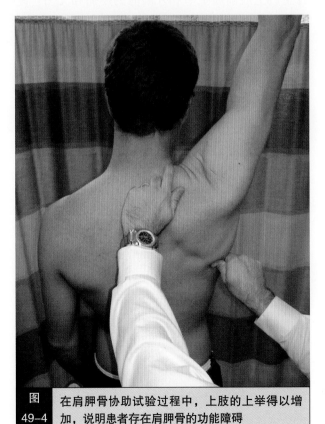

图 49-4　在肩胛骨协助试验过程中，上肢的上举得以增加，说明患者存在肩胛骨的功能障碍

检查者用标准的徒手肌力测试方法来评估冈上肌肌力，以及与动态盂唇剪切试验相关的盂唇损伤（图 49-5）。[9]随后检查者将患者肩胛骨置于回收位并用手固定住。其生物力学作用是使肩胛骨的外旋和后倾一起增加。肩胛骨在回收位置上表现出冈上肌肌力增加，或与盂唇损伤相关的内部撞击症状减轻为阳性结果。尽管 SAT 或 SRT 阳性并不具有对某种特定肩关节疾病的诊断意义，但还是能证明肩胛骨动力障碍与症状的产生直接相关，并且意味着需要早期进行肩胛骨康复锻炼以改善对肩胛骨的控制。

肩部损伤中涉及肩胛骨的情况

翼状肩

翼状肩通常是形容肩胛骨内侧缘在休息或上肢活动时存在不对称突起情况。由于肩胛骨不稳定，患者一般都有肩关节功能的欠缺。以往，多数病例被认为是由支配肩胛骨稳定肌群的神经受到损伤，或某种潜在的神经肌肉疾病（如肌营养不良）所造成的。[30-32]近来的研究结果显示，与这种生物力学位置或运动相关的最常见因素包括支撑骨结构的改变，胸肩肱复合体相互之间连接的改变和（或）稳定肌群的肌力、柔韧性、激活次序及其附着的改变。[23]因此，对翼状肩患者的评估必须充分全面，以便发现导致其位置及运动发生改变的因素。

基于神经源性因素导致的翼状肩胛，其确切发生率尚不明确。损伤有可能是创伤性、医源性或特发性的，若想解释清楚需要对患者进行仔细的病史询问和体格检查。胸长神经和副神经最常牵涉其中。胸长神经损伤和前锯肌功能丧失会导致肩胛骨向上方和内侧移位，正常的肩肱关节运动受到阻碍。临床上，这种旋转造成肩胛骨下角在静态及动态检查中都显著突出。肌电图检查可以在大约 6 周时确诊。最初的治疗措施包括支持治疗并观察、康复治疗以及每 3 个月随访复查一

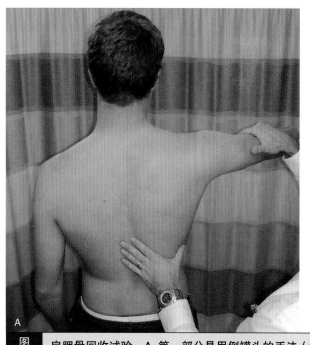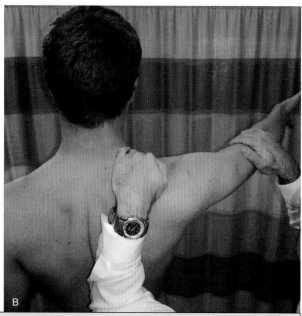

图 49-5　肩胛骨回收试验。A. 第一部分是用倒罐头的手法（译者注：即 Jobe 试验）进行徒手肌力测试。B. 第二部分是用手稳定住肩胛骨后进行的上肢肌力测试

次肌电图。康复治疗重点集中在通过激活菱形肌和下部斜方肌来维护盂肱关节的活动及肩胛骨的稳定。如果没有明显的神经恢复，则肩关节很难获得最大的功能，因为没有其他肌肉能够代替前锯肌的功能。

胸长神经麻痹的患者如果症状及功能缺陷持续达 1 年且没有恢复的迹象，则为手术治疗适应证。胸大肌的胸骨肋骨头转位是最成功的术式，一般来说效果很好。[31] 将所选择的部分肌腱自其在肱骨上的附着点切断并向后折转，通过隧道抵达肩胛骨，之后采取任意一种固定技术将其固定在肩胛骨下角上。肌腱的长度一般需要使用阔筋膜或其他移植物进行延长。

翼状肩也可由副神经损伤所导致，副神经很容易因钝性外力、牵拉或穿透伤而受到创伤。医源性损伤有可能在颈淋巴结活检或根治性颈淋巴结清扫过程中发生。缺少了斜方肌的作用，肩胛骨会呈现一种更为靠下和靠外（下垂）的姿态。翼状突起常常不像前锯肌麻痹导致的那样明显，不过上部斜方肌的萎缩、肌张力的丧失及无法耸

肩可以很容易地被识别出来。下部斜方肌无法使肩胛骨达到并维持回收的功能位，这样会造成患者主诉上肢前屈上举和外展时的疼痛和无力。菱形肌和肩胛提肌的代偿性肌痉挛很常见。肌电图检查可以用来确认诊断，不过检查结果必须仔细解读。有时候，当记录电极没有插在浅层菲薄萎缩的斜方肌内，而是插入了深层正常的菱形肌时，也可能导致出现假阴性的结果。治疗必须针对具体病因，对于神经炎或医源性原因，建议采取支持治疗并观察 1 年。

当非手术治疗不成功时，可以考虑手术治疗副神经麻痹。Eden-Lange 转位术是为了提供肩胛骨内侧与上方动力性限制而设计的术式，术中将肩胛提肌和菱形肌外移大约 5 cm 后通过钻孔固定来提高其力学效益，并以此作为斜方肌功能的替代。据报道，术后患者的平均 ASES 肩关节疼痛和功能障碍评分及 Constant 肩关节评分都有切实的改善。[33]

弹响肩胛

弹响肩胛是形容在上肢活动过程中肩胛骨内侧缘出现痛性捻发音的情况。传统上，这类症状

被认为由骨软骨瘤或其他骨性病变，或肩胛胸壁间隙中增厚的滑囊炎组织所导致，但近来的研究发现，正常肩肱节律的改变是大多数弹响肩胛发病的基础。[32]这些改变造成了沿着肩胛骨内侧缘的压力增高，从而导致症状的发生。为了辨别致病原因，必须仔细评估检查周围所有肌肉组织的柔韧性和肌力。

弹响肩胛的诊断和治疗在临床上具有挑战性。弹响肩胛通常提示肩胛骨在胸廓及其周围肌肉上的平滑滑动受到破坏。上肢上举时肩胛骨正常的后倾 - 外旋耦合运动会减少。因此，肩胛骨瞬时旋转中心自内上缘至肩锁关节的正常移动也被破坏，造成肩胛骨发生围绕内侧缘的旋转，形成了过高的压力，从而导致了症状的产生。[23]

患者通常会主诉在过顶运动过程中肩胛骨周围疼痛。在投掷动作中肩胛骨的行程比较长，因此该动作尤其受影响。患者在进行主动的肩关节活动或仅仅做出耸肩动作时，常会突然注意到一种可以听到的研磨或弹响声，该声响还可能被胸腔放大。多数情况下，疼痛被定位于肩胛骨的内上缘。因为这种异常的力学表现，很多人认为捻发音产生的原因在于慢性滑囊炎症。在少数患者中，解剖上的异常（如骨软骨瘤或畸形愈合的肋骨骨折）有可能破坏肩胛胸壁联合，使患者容易出现弹响肩胛。

弹响肩胛的治疗应该从针对患者个体病因的综合性非手术治疗开始。其中最重要的部分通常是旨在恢复正常姿势和肩胛骨周围生物力学的物理治疗方法。可以通过等长收缩与动态耐力训练来强化下部斜方肌和前锯肌。前方紧缩的肌肉应该通过按摩和拉伸使其活跃调动起来。此外，还包括活动方式的调整和各种物理治疗方法。对有些患者而言，肩胛骨支具可能有效。滑囊炎症可以采取精准的注射进行治疗，但一定要谨慎并使用正确的技术。

经历过全面彻底但不成功的非手术治疗计划、功能障碍非常严重并且愿意遵从术后护理的患者，可以考虑行手术治疗。见诸报道的手术治疗方法千差万别，但无论采用哪种方法，治疗的成功率都能令人满意。[31-32]目前，切开手术和关节镜手术都已获得了成功，但是有些学者会担心切开手术的并发症发生率和美观问题。关节镜手术恢复起来更为迅速，但是对技术的要求较高，并且会带来更高的血管神经损伤风险。无论采用哪种技术，术者都可以选择进行一个简单的滑囊切除或肩胛骨部分切除。

撞击和肩袖疾病

很多研究针对肩袖无力、肩袖肌腱病、肩袖撞击和肩袖撕裂患者的肩胛骨运动学进行了评估。大多数研究都发现了肩胛骨运动学的改变。[34]目前还不清楚观察到的肩胛骨动力障碍究竟是原因还是结果，亦或是对病理状态的一种代偿。如果是原因，则肩胛骨的上旋和后倾减少可能改变肩峰下空间的大小以及喙肩弓下的肩袖间隙，从而造成机械性的磨损。其他情况则包括肩胛骨前倾和内旋的增加可能造成在上肢活动过程中肩胛盂的前倾，使肩袖肌腱易于发生内部撞击；或者肌肉激活的减少造成肩袖肌腱内部的张力增加，使肌腱细胞内部能观察到的凋亡性改变也相应增加。如果动力障碍是结果，则个别肌肉的激活可能因疼痛而受到抑制，正常的激活模式被破坏，并且运动方式也会因避痛而发生改变。[34]一种结果是，肩袖撕裂患者肩胛骨的上旋会增大，这可能代表着患者在面对肩袖激活无力甚至缺失时，试图使上肢上举幅度增大或最大化所做的代偿。无论二者关系如何，肩胛骨动力障碍经常在肩袖疾病患者中出现，并且与功能障碍有关。

SAT 检查阳性能够表明患者肩胛骨的过度前倾是产生外部撞击症状的部分病理生理学因素。治疗不仅要强化前锯肌作为肩胛骨外旋肌和下部斜方肌作为肩胛骨回收肌的力量，还应该包括增加胸小肌和肱二头肌短头腱的柔韧性。加强肩胛骨稳定性的系列练习对达到这一目标切实有效（图49-6）。SRT检查阳性表明患者肌肉无力的症状有一部分是由肩胛骨造成的，就像康复训练的第一步一样，治疗方法直接针对的是肩胛骨回收时的稳定性而不是肩袖本身。

盂唇损伤

在一种病理性级联模型中，肩胛骨动力障碍被发现与盂唇损伤有关。[20]肩胛骨的位置和运动变成内旋和前倾可能改变盂肱关节的对线，增大前方韧带所承受的张力，从而使肩胛盂上肱二头肌腱 – 盂唇复合体对肩胛盂的回削作用增强，造成病理性的内部撞击，也减小了肩袖协同收缩的力量。如果存在盂肱关节内旋不足的情况，上述效应还会被进一步放大，因为在投掷运动的后续顺势动作阶段，紧张的后方结构被绷得更紧，导致了肩胛骨的前伸增加。对怀疑盂唇损伤的患者来说，评估是否存在肩胛骨动力障碍是康复的关键。若在动态盂唇剪切试验中引出的疼痛常能被SRT手法所消除或缓解，则说明动力障碍是盂唇损伤病理生理学机制的一部分。为了改善肩胛骨的回收需要进行肩胛骨康复训练，包括对前方紧张僵硬肌肉的动员及强化肩胛骨稳定性的系列练习。另外，判断是否存在肩胛骨动力障碍也是预防盂唇损伤的重要部分。

肩锁关节疾病

肩关节要想达到最理想的功能状态，其骨性组成部分必须完整。伴不稳定或高等级肩锁关节分离的肩锁关节疾病会改变锁骨对于肩胛骨的支柱功能，同时改变肩肱节律的生物力学螺旋运动轴线，使得肩胛骨过度前伸，上肢上举时的肩峰上抬减少。[5,23]这个所谓的肩胛骨第三种平移运动使肩胛骨相对于锁骨向内下方移动，最常见于高等级的肩锁关节分离（Ⅲ型、Ⅳ型或Ⅴ型）。肩胛骨的前伸位置会产生很多与慢性肩锁关节分离相关的功能障碍，包括撞击症状及能够表现出来的肩袖力量减弱。Ⅲ型损伤患者临床检查时如果发现存在肩胛骨动力障碍，表现为上肢上举或前屈时出现第三种平移运动，可以帮助医师做出手术治疗的决定。

锁骨骨折

锁骨骨折不愈合或短缩旋转畸形愈合会改变锁骨的支柱功能，导致较差的功能结果。肌肉无力和活动范围丧失是与锁骨骨折畸形愈合或不愈合相关的最为常见的功能障碍。[22]锁骨支柱功能被改变会使肩胛骨过度前伸，这一位置会限制肩袖发挥功能并使肱骨完全上举的能力受限。对于新鲜或陈旧性锁骨骨折的患者，评估其肩胛骨的位置有助于决定是否需要手术治疗以恢复锁骨体的对位对线及锁骨作为支柱的功能。

多向不稳定

肩关节多向不稳定最显著的特征之一是症状和不稳定发生在盂肱关节活动的中段（在这一阶段，凹面 – 压缩机制、骨骼对线及肌肉的激活最为重要），而非关节活动的终末段（在这一阶段，关节囊韧带的限制作用最为重要）。很多存在多向不稳定的患者同时也存在肩胛骨前伸的增大及上肢运动时肱骨头从关节中心的迁移。[19-35]当患者上举上肢时，肩胛骨的运动背离了正常的模式，从上旋、后倾及轻度内旋变成了上旋、前倾及过度内旋。这种状态使肱骨头能够向下平移出肩胛盂窝，从而形成不稳定。肩胛下肌、下部斜方肌和前锯肌的抑制以及胸小肌和背阔肌激活的增强，共同使肩胛骨处于这种前伸的位置之上。

仔细观察肩胛骨的静息位置及在上肢活动时的肩胛骨的运动，可以发现很多肩关节多向不稳定的患者的肩胛骨前伸，尤其是在与不稳定症状相关的位置上。通过把肩胛骨稳定在回收的位置上，SRT检查能够改变肩胛盂的位置，减少背阔肌的激活，并由此减少或消除伴随着上肢运动出现的不稳定症状。SRT检查阳性能够使治疗方案指向强化前锯肌和下部斜方肌，同时增加胸小肌和背阔肌的柔韧性。肩关节多向不稳定的患者如

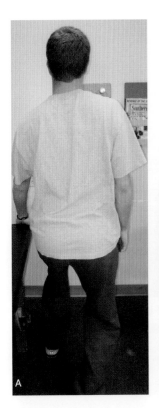
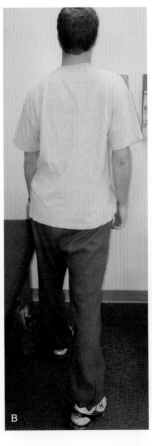
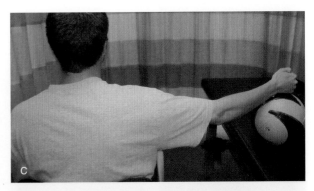
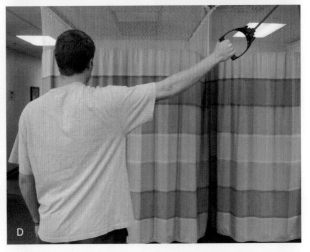
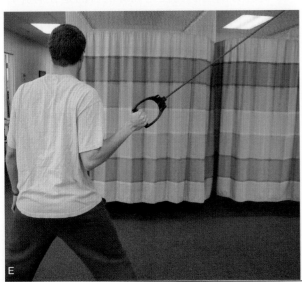
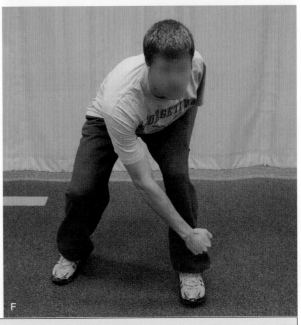

图
49-6

肩胛骨稳定性系列练习。低位划船练习的起始姿势（A）以及伸直髋关节和躯干以利于肩胛骨回收（B）。在主动下滑练习中，肩关节和肩胛骨的肌肉协同收缩能够帮助压低肱骨和肩胛骨（C）。击剑式练习的起始动作，上肢在冠状面上外展上举超过 90°（D），之后在侧跨步的同时回收肩胛骨并内收上肢（E）。割草机式练习（为了兼顾下肢、躯干和上肢的运动而设计的动作）的起始位置（F）

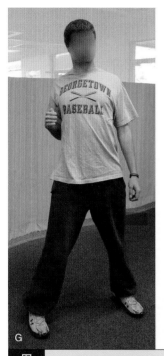
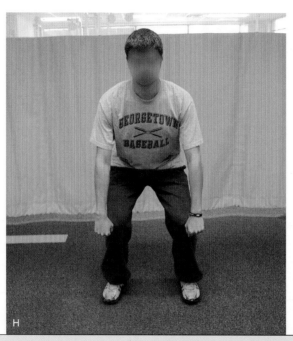
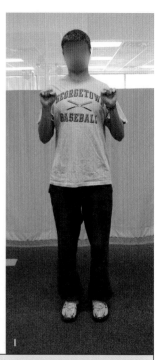

图 49-6 肩胛骨稳定性系列练习（续）。割草机式练习，伸直髋关节和躯干，随后旋转躯干以便回收肩胛骨（G）。抢劫手法式练习的起始位置，膝关节屈曲且躯干前屈，双上肢离开身体（H）。伸直髋关节和躯干，同时要求患者尝试做"将双肘放入后兜"的动作（I）

果有恢复正常肌肉激活模式的能力，就说明与创伤后肩关节不稳定的患者相比，前者能够成功康复的可能性更大。

肩胛骨动力障碍的康复

针对肩胛骨控制的康复训练有 3 种，分别为能够增强肩胛部肌肉力量的近端运动链训练、使影响肩胛骨姿态的牵拉力最小化的柔韧性训练以及专门针对肩胛骨周围肌肉激活的训练。躯干和髋关节运动链训练最理想的开始位置和结束位置是伸髋和躯干伸直，包括躯干及髋的屈伸、旋转和对角线运动。训练的过程应包括上下台阶及逐渐增加负重。这些训练在手术之前发现功能缺陷的时候即应开始，在肩关节受到保护的情况下也可以进行。

柔韧性训练的目标应该集中在前方的喙突周围肌肉（胸小肌和肱二头肌短头）及肩关节的旋转。这些部位过于紧张会增加肩胛骨的前伸。训练包括针对喙突肌肉的开书样拉伸和拐角拉伸，以及针对肩关节旋转的睡眠者拉伸和横向交叉拉伸（图 49-7）。

肩胛骨周围肌肉强化训练的目的是让肩胛骨能够回到回收的位置上，因为这是能使肩胛骨发挥最大功能的最有效位置。肩胛骨回收练习可以在站立位进行，以刺激正常的肌肉激活顺序并让运动链能够按序运转。肩胛骨挤压和躯干伸展－回收训练在康复早期肩关节还处于保护之下时即可开始，因为这种训练作用于盂肱关节上的拉伸负荷与剪切负荷非常小。

有些特定的训练方法对激活稳定肩胛骨的关键肌肉（下部斜方肌和前锯肌）并使上部斜方肌的激活最小化非常有效。[36] 低位划船练习、主动下滑练习、击剑式练习、割草机式练习及抢劫手法式练习，这些统称为肩胛骨稳定性系列练习，能够激活目标肌肉，使其达到最大激活程度的 18%~30%[36]（图 49-6）。上肢外展角度限制在 90° 之内的这种激活，表明肩胛骨稳定性练习在创伤或术后康复的早期阶段尤其有效。

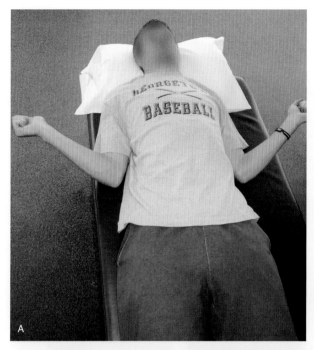
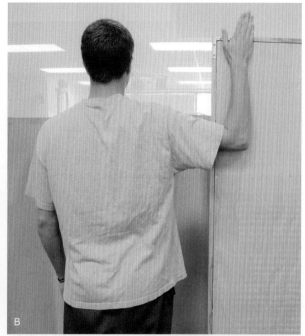
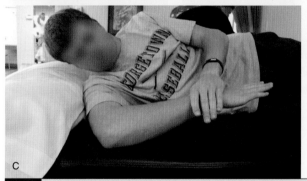
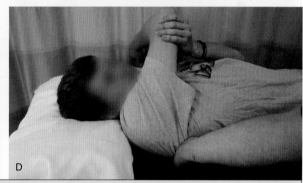

图
49-7
柔韧性训练。开书样拉伸（A）及拐角拉伸（B）针对紧张的前方软组织结构。睡眠者拉伸（C）和横向交叉拉伸（D）针对紧张的后方肩袖肌肉。当肩胛骨固定时，横向交叉拉伸最为有效

随着愈合过程的进展及肩关节负重能力的提高，也应该开始强调闭链训练以恢复用来稳定肩关节的闭链机制的正常激活。[37]在这些训练中，手撑在一个稳定或能活动的平面上，上肢和肩胛骨自远端向近端施加负荷。节奏性稳定训练和摸墙训练即为闭链训练的两个实例（图49-8）。

当肩胛骨的控制能力已经能够达到时，可以增加肩胛骨－肩袖结合训练内容，如出拳和甩肩练习，在稳定的肩胛骨基础上刺激肩袖的激活。这些训练可以在内收和屈曲的不同平面上进行，配合不同大小和不同类型的阻力，也可以改进为针对某种体育项目的训练。

运动链的最大化整合——肩胛骨－肩关节协作发生在强调对角线形式的激活和负荷时。可以采用四点式训练、站立位对角线式训练及旋转式训练。

总结

肩胛骨在肩关节和上肢功能的各个方面都处于十分关键的位置，扮演着十分重要的角色。正常的肩胛骨运动学能够使盂肱关节处于最为稳定的骨性架构之上，使能量和力自核心传导到手部，最大限度地激活肌肉以使上肢移动，并稳定关节。

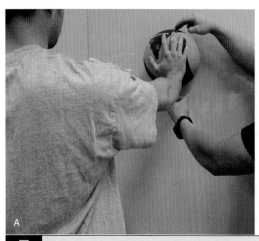
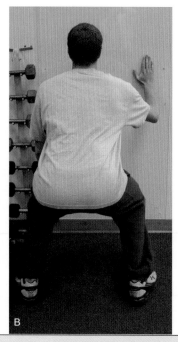
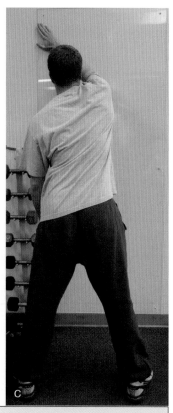

图 49-8 闭链训练，可以用来辅助肌肉再教育，也可用于上肢功能性姿势的训练。在节奏性稳定训练中，患者要尝试稳定住图中所示的球，同时医师从不同方向对球施加外力（A）。在摸墙训练中，患者初始时取半蹲或全蹲姿势，患肢手部置于墙上（B），随后用腿部和躯干发力站起，带动上肢在不同范围和不同平面内运动（C）

肩胛骨动力障碍（肩关节正常活动的改变）被发现与几乎所有肩关节异常状态都有关。目前还不清楚动力障碍究竟是肩关节异常的原因还是结果。动力障碍往往是导致临床功能障碍的原因之一，但是，对它的评估和治疗应该作为对肩关节异常状态综合评估与治疗的一部分。动力障碍可以通过临床上有效且可靠的检查方法发现，而致病因素也可以查明。随后针对这一功能缺陷就可以制订相应的治疗和康复计划了。

参考文献

[1] Bagg SD, Forrest WJ: Electromyographic study of the scapular rotators during arm abduction in the scapular plane. *Am J Phys Med* 1986;65(3):111-124.

[2] Bagg SD, Forrest WJ: A biomechanical analysis of scapular rotation during arm abduction in the scapular plane. *Am J Phys Med Rehabil* 1988;67(6):238-245.

[3] McClure PW, Michener LA, Sennett BJ, Karduna AR: Direct 3-dimensional measurement of scapular kinematics during dynamic movements in vivo. *J Shoulder Elbow Surg* 2001;10(3):269-277.

[4] Ludewig PM, Phadke V, Braman JP, Hassett DR, Cieminski CJ, LaPrade RF: Motion of the shoulder complex during multiplanar humeral elevation. *J Bone Joint Surg Am* 2009;91(2):378-389.

Bone pin placement was used to accurately categorize the exact three-dimensional motions of the clavicle, the SC and AC joints, the scapula, and the humerus. The important roles of clavicle movement and SC and AC joint motion in scapular motion were documented.

Disruptions anywhere along the clavicle have deleterious effects on scapular motion and arm function.

[5] Sahara W, Sugamoto K, Murai M, Yoshikawa H: Three-dimensional clavicular and acromioclavicular rotations during arm abduction using vertically open MRI. *J Orthop Res* 2007;25(9):1243-1249.

The screw axis is the three-dimensional guide motion

that defines AC motions and thereby controls coupled scapuloclaviculohumeral movement.

［6］Speer KP, Garrett WE: Muscular control of motion and stability about the pectoral girdle, in Matsen FA III, Fu F, Hawkins RJ (eds): *The Shoulder: A Balance of Mobility and Stability*. Rosemont, IL, American Academy of Orthopaedic Surgeons, 1994, pp 159-173.

［7］Cools AM, Dewitte V, Lanszweert F, et al: Rehabilitation of scapular muscle balance: Which exercises to prescribe? *Am J Sports Med* 2007;35(10):1744-1751.
Some of the rehabilitation parameters that guide the restoration of muscular balance for scapular control are defined.

［8］Smith J, Kotajarvi BR, Padgett DJ, Eischen JJ: Effect of scapular protraction and retraction on isometric shoulder elevation strength. *Arch Phys Med Rehabil* 2002;83(3):367-370.

［9］Kibler WB, Sciascia AD, Dome DC: Evaluation of apparent and absolute supraspinatus strength in patients with shoulder injury using the scapular retraction test. *Am J Sports Med* 2006;34(10):1643-1647.

［10］Tate AR, McClure PW, Kareha S, Irwin D: Effect of the scapula reposition test on shoulder impingement symptoms and elevation strength in overhead athletes. *J Orthop Sports Phys Ther* 2008;38(1):4-11.
The use of a position of scapular retraction during clinical manual muscle testing improved rotator cuff strength. This finding confirmed earlier work by other researchers.

［11］Solem-Bertoft E, Thuomas KA, Westerberg CE: The influence of scapular retraction and protraction on the width of the subacromial space: An MRI study. *Clin Orthop Relat Res* 1993;296:99-103.

［12］Warner JJ, Micheli LJ, Arslanian LE, Kennedy J, Kennedy R: Patterns of flexibility, laxity, and strength in normal shoulders and shoulders with instability and impingement. *Am J Sports Med* 1990;18(4):366-375.

［13］Warner JJ, Micheli LJ, Arslanian LE, Kennedy J, Kennedy R: Scapulothoracic motion in normal shoulders and shoulders with glenohumeral instability and impingement syndrome: A study using Moiré topographic analysis. *Clin Orthop Relat Res* 1992;285:191-199.

［14］Kibler WB, Sciascia AD: Current concepts: Scapular dyskinesis. *Br J Sports Med* 2010;44(5):300-305.
This is a concise review of scapular dyskinesis, including its definition, effects on shoulder function and dysfunction, relationship to all types of shoulder injuries, clinical evaluation, and treatment guidelines.

［15］Burkhart SS, Morgan CD, Kibler WB: The disabled throwing shoulder: Spectrum of pathology part III. The SICK scapula, scapular dyskinesis, the kinetic chain, and rehabilitation. *Arthroscopy* 2003;19(6):641-661.

［16］Kibler WB, Ludewig PM, McClure P, Uhl TL, Sciascia A: Scapular summit 2009: Introduction. July 16, 2009, Lexington, Kentucky. *J Orthop Sports Phys Ther* 2009;39(11):A1-A13.
The results of a consensus meeting on the basic science and the clinical application of research on the scapula were presented, including current knowledge of scapular motion and dyskinesis, rehabilitation, and an evidence-based recommendation for clinical evaluation of the scapula in patients with shoulder injury.

［17］Kibler WB, Uhl TL, Maddux JW, Brooks PV, Zeller B, McMullen J: Qualitative clinical evaluation of scapular dysfunction: A reliability study. *J Shoulder Elbow Surg* 2002;11(6):550-556.

［18］Cools AM, Witvrouw EE, Declercq GA, Danneels LA, Cambier DC: Scapular muscle recruitment patterns: Trapezius muscle latency with and without impingement symptoms. *Am J Sports Med* 2003;31(4):542-549.

［19］Ogston JB, Ludewig PM: Differences in 3-dimensional shoulder kinematics between persons with multidirectional instability and asymptomatic controls. *Am J Sports Med* 2007;35(8):1361-1370.
Altered scapular position was found to exacerbate the symptoms typically associated with multidirectional instability. Rehabilitation for patients with this condition should focus on scapular strengthening.

［20］Burkhart SS, Morgan CD, Kibler WB: The disabled throwing shoulder: Spectrum of pathology part I. Pathoanatomy and biomechanics. *Arthroscopy* 2003;19(4):404-420.

［21］Michener LA, McClure PW, Karduna AR: Anatomical and biomechanical mechanisms of subacromial impingement syndrome. *Clin Biomech (Bristol, Avon)* 2003;18(5):369-379.

［22］McKee MD, Pedersen EM, Jones C, et al: Deficits following nonoperative treatment of displaced midshaft clavicular fractures. *J Bone Joint Surg Am* 2006;88(1):35-40.

［23］Gumina S, Carbone S, Postacchini F: Scapular dyskinesis and SICK scapula syndrome in patients with chronic type III acromioclavicular dislocation. *Arthroscopy* 2009;25(1):40-45.
A high percentage of patients with a type III AC separation were found to have clinical evidence of scapular

dyskinesis, indicating the third translation of the scapula in conjunction with AC separation.

[24] Smith J, Dietrich CT, Kotajarvi BR, Kaufman KR: The effect of scapular protraction on isometric shoulder rotation strength in normal subjects. *J Shoulder Elbow Surg* 2006;15(3):339-343.

[25] Uhl TL, Kibler WB, Gecewich B, Tripp BL: Evaluation of clinical assessment methods for scapular dyskinesis. *Arthroscopy* 2009;25(11):1240-1248.

A yes-no assessment system for clinical observation of scapular dyskinesis was correlated with biomechanical evaluation of scapular motion and found to have clinically relevant utility, with sensitivities, specificities, and positive predictive values between 0.64 and 0.84.

[26] McClure PW, Tate AR, Kareha S, Irwin D, Zlupko E: A clinical method for identifying scapular dyskinesis, part 1: Reliability. *J Athl Train* 2009;44(2):160-164.

This is the first part of a two-part article on a method of visual observation found to help clinicians distinguish between the presence and the absence of scapular dyskinesis in a general population.

[27] Tate AR, McClure P, Kareha S, Irwin D, Barbe MF: A clinical method for identifying scapular dyskinesis, part 2: Validity. *J Athl Train* 2009;44(2):165-173.

This is the second part of a two-part article on a method of visual observation found to help clinicians distinguish between the presence and the absence of scapular dyskinesis in a general population.

[28] Kibler WB: The role of the scapula in athletic shoulder function. *Am J Sports Med* 1998;26(2):325-337.

[29] Rabin A, Irrgang JJ, Fitzgerald GK, Eubanks A: The intertester reliability of the scapular assistance test. *J Orthop Sports Phys Ther* 2006;36(9):653-660.

[30] Kuhn JE, Plancher KD, Hawkins RJ: Scapular winging. *J Am Acad Orthop Surg* 1995;3(6):319-325.

[31] Steinmann SP, Wood MB: Pectoralis major transfer for serratus anterior paralysis. *J Shoulder Elbow Surg* 2003;12(6):555-560.

[32] Kuhne M, Boniquit N, Ghodadra N, Romeo AA, Provencher MT: The snapping scapula: Diagnosis and treatment. *Arthroscopy* 2009;25(11):1298-1311.

This review (and a subsequent letter to the editor) discussed pathophysiology, clinical presentation, and treatment guidelines related to snapping scapula.

[33] Romero J, Gerber C: Levator scapulae and rhomboid transfer for paralysis of trapezius: The Eden-Lange procedure. *J Bone Joint Surg Br* 2003;85(8):1141-1145.

[34] Ludewig PM, Reynolds JF: The association of scapular kinematics and glenohumeral joint pathologies. *J Orthop Sports Phys Ther* 2009;39(2):90-104.

The literature on scapular motion and position in relation to pathologic conditions in the shoulder shows how scapular dysfunction can influence the clinical presentation of the shoulder pathology.

[35] Morris AD, Kemp GJ, Frostick SP: Shoulder electromyography in multidirectional instability. *J Shoulder Elbow Surg* 2004;13(1):24-29.

[36] Kibler WB, Sciascia AD, Uhl TL, Tambay N, Cunningham T: Electromyographic analysis of specific exercises for scapular control in early phases of shoulder rehabilitation. *Am J Sports Med* 2008;36(9):1789-1798.

A series of rehabilitation exercises was described as capable of activating scapular muscles in the early stages of rehabilitation with minimal stress on injured tissues.

[37] Kibler WB, Livingston B: Closed-chain rehabilitation for upper and lower extremities. *J Am Acad Orthop Surg* 2001;9(6):412-421.

第五十章　肩肘关节的复杂区域疼痛综合征

Paul J. Christo, MD, MBA; Brian G. Wilhelmi, MD, JD

引言

复杂区域疼痛综合征（CRPS）是一种罕见的、使人衰弱的神经病学疾病，症状为过度疼痛，伴随感觉、自主神经、运动和营养方面的功能障碍。[1]CRPS 一般表现为局限于患肢的慢性疼痛，诱因可能是轻伤、创伤及手术，发病后临床表现不断进展。CRPS 可能发生于术后，并使患肢术后剧烈疼痛。CRPS 不仅降低生活质量，还给个人和社会带来了巨大的医疗卫生费用负担。[2]对骨科医师来说，认识并分诊 CRPS 患者是必要的能力。早期治疗会带来最大的收益，包括药物治疗、物理治疗、职业疗法及介入性疼痛治疗。

定义和流行病学

CRPS 过去被称为肩手综合征、反射性交感神经性营养不良、灼痛（causalgia）、骨痛退化症（allodystrophy）。国际疼痛研究学会（International Society for the Study of Pain）为 CRPS 制定了诊断标准，该标准整合了一组互不相干、各具特性的症状。[1]CRPS 的诊断标准包

含了与诱发事件不相符的剧烈疼痛，伴随感觉、血管舒缩、泌汗、运动、营养方面的改变（表 50-1，50-2）。[3-4]根据是否有明确的神经损伤，CRPS 分为两型（1 型、2 型）。

在已有的流行病学研究中，CRPS 定义不统一。在明确的诊断标准建立后，未来对 CRPS 的流行病学一定会有更深的理解。CRPS 是一种罕见病，年发病率估计为 5.46~26.2/100 000。一项包含 596 例患者的前瞻性研究使用修订版布达佩斯临床诊断标准，结果显示骨折后 CRPS 发病率高达 7%。[6]女性的发病率更高，是男性的 2.3~5 倍。[5]对于哪个年龄段最易受 CRPS 影响，几乎没有一致的研究结果。[6]起病年龄越大，临床症状越轻。[7]虽然单中心或多中心的流行病学数据较难获得，但是像电子网络调查或宣传组网址这样的新工具可能会促进未来的研究。[7]

Dr. Christo or an immediate family member serves as a paid consultant to or is an employee of Ameritox, Actavis, Quadrant Healthcom, Perrigo, and Cattem and has received research or institutional support from Medtronic. Neither Dr. Wilhelmi nor any immediate family member has received anything of value from or has stock or stock options held in a commercial company or institution related directly or indirectly to the subject of this chapter.

表 50-1

国际疼痛研究学会复杂区域疼痛综合征奥兰多标准

1. 存在有害的诱发事件或导致制动的原因
2. 持续疼痛、痛觉超敏或痛觉过敏，疼痛严重程度与诱发事件不相符
3. 出现疼痛区域水肿、皮肤血运改变或泌汗异常的证据（症状或体征）
4. 排除其他可解释疼痛或功能障碍程度的状况

注：经允许引自 Merskey H, Bogduk N: *Classification of Chronic Pain: Descriptions of Chronic Pain Syndrome and Definitions of Pain Terms*, ed 2. Seattle, WA, IASP Press, 1994.

表 50-2

CRPS^a 布达佩斯临床诊断标准

1. 持续疼痛，严重程度与诱发事件不相符
2. 必须有下列 4 类症状中的至少 3 类（每类至少 1 个表现）
   感觉：痛觉过敏、痛觉超敏
   血管舒缩：皮温不对称、皮肤颜色改变、皮肤颜色不对称
   泌汗 / 水肿：水肿、泌汗改变、泌汗不对称
   运动 / 营养：活动范围减小、运动障碍（力弱、震颤、肌张力障碍）、营养状况改变（毛发、指甲、皮肤）
3. 检查时，必须有下列 4 类体征中的至少 2 类（每类至少 1 个表现）
   感觉：痛觉过敏（针刺）、痛觉超敏（轻触、温度感觉、躯体深压、关节运动）
   血管舒缩：皮温不对称（> 1℃）、皮肤颜色改变、皮肤颜色不对称
   泌汗 / 水肿：水肿、泌汗改变、泌汗不对称
   运动 / 营养：活动范围减小、运动障碍（力弱、震颤、肌张力障碍）、营养状况改变（毛发、指甲、皮肤）
4. 没有其他可以更好地解释症状、体征的诊断。

　　注：^a 描述一系列疼痛表现，特点是持续（自发或诱发）的区域疼痛，疼痛时间或程度与任何已知的创伤或其他损伤的疾病过程不符。疼痛是区域性的（不符合特定神经支配或皮节分布），主要表现为肢体远端的感觉、运动、泌汗、血管舒缩及营养状况改变。CRPS 表现随时间而变化。经允许引自 Harden RN, Bruehl S, Perez RS, et al: Validation of proposed diagnostic criteria (the "Budapest Criteria") for complex regional pain syndrome. *Pain* 2010;150(2):268-274.

病理生理学

　　虽然 CRPS 发生的确切机制还没研究清楚，但过去十几年中，研究者们对 CRPS 的病理生理学基础的理解已有很大进步。[8]研究认为，可能有多种病理机制参与 CRPS 的发生和发展，这些机制在不同患者身上的不同表现造成 CRPS 的不同临床表现。[1]

　　即使是微不足道的神经损伤都可能诱发 CRPS 的发展（包括 1 型）。因此，神经损伤是修订版诊断标准的一部分。[8]考虑到 CRPS 患者受累区域与未受累区域相比几乎没有 C 型和 A δ 型皮肤传入神经纤维，这种作为诱因的神经损伤有可能改变外周神经系统。肢体的创伤也可以导致外周神经释放更多神经肽（如 P 物质、缓激肽、谷氨酸），激活局部外周痛觉神经元和次级中枢痛觉神经元，并增加疼痛。

　　外周神经系统痛觉感受器（nociceptor）的重复刺激和敏化导致中枢神经系统的痛觉加工过程改变。CRPS 患者表现为数量动态变化的中枢神经元关闭（wind-up）或兴奋性增强。中枢神经元关闭使患者因非伤害性刺激产生疼痛（痛觉超敏）以及因伤害性刺激产生过度疼痛（痛觉过敏）。几种脑皮质活动显像技术已经证明了 CRPS 患者脑皮质存在改组，这些技术包括功能磁共振成像（fMRI）。[9]研究显示，负责拇指和小指触觉的脑皮质区域间距离减小，并且针刺痛觉过敏和机械痛觉超敏后出现脑皮质广泛激活。通过随访脑皮质改变的患者，研究人员发现，治疗后疼痛减轻的患者的脑皮质改变是可逆的。

　　根据 CRPS 急性期的临床表现，研究者们提出了一些关于炎症通路在 CRPS 发展中的作用的假说。[10]起初，肢体的红、肿、热可能由血管扩张、血浆和蛋白外渗造成。这一组织过程可能由促炎细胞因子（白介素 -1 β、白介素 -2、白介素 -6 和 TNF-α）和神经多肽［降钙素基因相关肽（CGRP）、缓激肽、P 物质］诱导。研究已经证明，CRPS 患者的水泡液、血浆和脑脊液中促炎细胞因子的含量增加。促炎神经多肽可能在炎性疼痛中有特定作用，不仅直接增加痛觉发动（nociceptive firing），也刺激血管扩张、蛋白外渗和其他促炎细胞因子的进一步释放。

　　交感神经系统（SNS）功能障碍很久以来一直被认为是 CRPS 病理生理学的核心部分。[8]在临床表现的急性期或温暖期（warm phase），患肢血管扩张，受到低温刺激亦无法收缩，并且泌汗量下降。同时，去甲肾上腺素的血浆浓度下降。当临床表现转变为慢性期或冰凉期（cold phase）时，即使血浆去甲肾上腺素水平下降，患肢依然出现血管收缩且泌汗量增加。这样的表现说明，在病程从急性期转变为慢性期的过程中，肾上腺素能受体表达上调，慢性期患肢对肾上腺素能刺激过度反应。CRPS 的疼痛可以在寒冷或极端情绪的刺

激下加重，也可以通过交感神经阻滞来缓解，因而看起来像是 SNS 介导的。动物实验证明，痛觉神经纤维在神经创伤后表达肾上腺素能受体，这表明这种受体表达可能也是人类 SNS 介导性疼痛的发生机制。

关于 CRPS 发病因素的研究仍在继续，研究者们希望用这些因素找出易患 CRPS 的人群。[8]最近，关于 CRPS 家族病例的遗传学研究聚焦于 HLA（主要组织相容性复合体）分子，关于 HLA 基因和 TNF-α 炎症细胞因子的启动子区域。其他研究已经聚焦于血管紧张素转化酶成功转录的基因抑制（血管紧张素转化酶帮助降解缓激肽）。目前，还没有任何遗传因素被证实与 CRPS 有确定的联系。

研究发现，CRPS 患者血浆中存在直接与自主神经元表面抗原结合的自身抗体。[10]在一项小规模的预实验中，静脉免疫球蛋白与安慰剂相比使 CRPS 患者疼痛症状明显缓解。[11]这些发现和潜在的 HLA 易患基因型都支持了 CRPS 有自身免疫病理机制的假说。

焦虑和抑郁在 CRPS 患者中很普遍，这表明 CRPS 的产生和发展也有心理病理学因素。[8]目前还没发现明确的病因。

临床特点

CRPS 是临床诊断，过去研究者们已对其病程进行了分期。[12]然而，最近有一项研究表明不同患者的初始临床表现和后续临床过程均不同。[7]即使如此，经典的分期也可以根据表现型将患者进行分类，并对患者当前的病理和症状进行针对性治疗。[7]

神经损伤后，CRPS 最初为急性期或温暖期，患肢表现为过度疼痛（痛觉超敏和痛觉过敏）、热、红、泌汗较少和关节外水肿。[12]接下来是营养不良期，患肢表现为疼痛增加、感觉功能障碍、持续的血管舒缩功能障碍、明显的运动和营养状况改变（皮肤闪亮或增厚、指甲增厚或出现条纹、毛发生长加快或减慢）。[12]最后是慢性期、冰凉

期或萎缩期，患肢的典型表现为血流减少、皮肤变薄、肌肉萎缩、关节活动范围减小并挛缩、骨质脱钙（图 50-1）。[12]

神经损伤后 CRPS 症状出现，神经损伤可能为机械性、温度性、化学性、缺血性。[13]外科医师很难预料哪些情况会导致上肢更易发生 CRPS，应该考虑到任何手术或损伤都可能诱发 CRPS。起始症状表现为温度改变、水肿、皮肤颜色质地改变、泌汗量改变、毛发或指甲质地改变及力弱。几乎所有 CRPS 患者都经历过持续性疼痛，疼痛性质可表现为灼烧痛、撕裂痛、针刺痛、酸痛及跳痛。[7]生理和情绪的压力、寒冷的天气、活动患肢和工作都会使持续性疼痛加重。这种疼痛与定义这种疾病的症状、体征相关，即诱发痛（包括痛觉超敏和痛觉过敏）、温度改变和水肿。患者的临床症状常常是进展性的。疼痛的位置和范围趋于扩大。临床症状也进展为诱发痛、温度改变及颜色变化。在患肢活动减弱和不能活动的同时，水肿可能减轻。有报道称，一部分患者症状缓解，但这些患者大多会复发。

约 1/3 的患者有 SNS 介导性疼痛，这种疼痛随 SNS 儿茶酚胺释放的增加而加重。[14]可能的机制是躯体传入神经系统与 SNS 发生病理性偶联，如前文所讨论。这些患者在冰冷、轻微机械刺激、激动情绪的诱发下出现疼痛。因为药物或交感神经溶解术可以缓解 SNS 介导性疼痛，所以 SNS 介导性疼痛已是一个单独的研究领域。

CRPS 给患者个体带来了严重的心理、社会、经济负担。[7]疼痛对睡眠、活动、自理和日常生活均造成不良影响。CRPS 的诊断和治疗花费不菲，平均每例患者确诊前要就诊至少 4 名医师，还可能需要使用费用昂贵的检查来辅助诊断和治疗。患者常出现工作业绩下滑和接连被解雇，因而收入大减，这使治疗的花费更难以承受。包括焦虑、抑郁在内的精神科疾病比较常见。据报道，多达一半的患者在病程中曾有过自杀的想法。

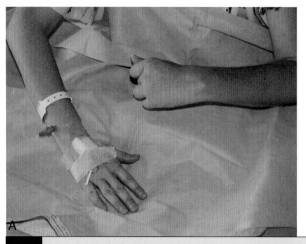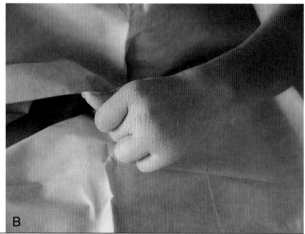

图 50-1 照片显示左手处于 CRPS 冰凉期。可以看到关节挛缩、皮肤颜色改变、肌肉萎缩和皮肤及指甲的营养状态改变

疑似上肢 CRPS 患者的评估

骨科医师要评估各种病因的上肢疼痛，识别 CRPS 并且开始基础治疗很重要。CRPS 是罕见病，初始症状可能很细微。如果在有害事件（如创伤、手术）或外周神经损伤后出现过度疼痛，就要高度怀疑 CRPS。CRPS 是一个临床诊断，完整的病史和体格检查是诊断 CRPS 的基础。诊断试验为 CRPS 的后遗症提供额外证据，也可以用于排除其他病理情况。

上肢 CRPS 体格检查的目的是将 CRPS 与损伤、手术造成的炎症、神经及骨科改变相鉴别。在检查上肢损伤、术后过度疼痛和疼痛没有按预期缓解的患者时，临床医师应高度怀疑 CRPS。骨科医师应进行完整的患肢体格检查，记录感觉障碍、运动减弱、水肿、自发疼痛或痛觉超敏的情况。骨科医师应记录患处远、近端关节的活动范围和关节畸形。应双侧对比检查皮肤颜色及质地、毛发及指甲的表现，应询问泌汗改变。

CRPS 最简单的诊断试验是冰块试验。发生 CRPS 的肢体常对冰冷敏感，患肢受凉会使灼痛加重。[1]冰块试验是简单、快捷、有效的诊断试验，应该在首次评估时进行。

肌电图（EMG）和神经传导速度（NCS）检查可量化神经信号的振幅和传输速度。EMG/NCS 可以将 CRPS 与糖尿病外周神经病、尺神经卡压、重症肌无力、Lambert-Eaton 综合征相鉴别。肩肘手术后神经损伤（即使是神经麻痹）可能诱发 CRPS，神经损伤的患者应被视为高危人群。

肢体疼痛患者一般都会行 X 线检查，慢性 CRPS 患者可表现为骨量减少。颈椎 CT 或 MRI 可能发现其他原因造成的上肢神经性疼痛，如椎管狭窄和神经根型颈椎病。[7]痛肢 MRI 可能发现臂丛神经病、粘连性关节囊炎或其他损伤。患肢 MRI 可能发现急性 CRPS 造成的软组织或骨髓水肿以及慢性 CRPS 相关的萎缩。

有很多方法可以检查 CRPS 患者的自主神经和泌汗功能障碍。红外热成像使用红外线摄像机生成皮肤的温度分布图，以此对比患侧与健侧温度。[15]健侧和患侧温度差达 1℃ 就是有意义的。定量泌汗运动神经轴突反射试验（quantitative sudomotor axon reflex test）是评估泌汗的定量试验，该试验可测定局部使用泌汗诱导制剂（如乙酰胆碱）后的泌汗量。

SNS 介导性疼痛可能提示 CRPS，但并非绝对。α-肾上腺素受体阻滞剂静脉区域封闭或局部麻醉药封闭星状神经节、腰交感链、胸交感链后疼痛缓解，是 SNS 介导性疼痛的阳性试验结果。

三期骨扫描（TPBS）是注射放射性核素示踪

剂后的按时间顺序得到的一系列放射性图像，依次显示动脉血的放射性浓聚、局部淤滞血的放射性浓聚、骨摄取的放射性浓聚。[15]急性期 CRPS 表现为关节周围放射性浓聚增加。这是因为 CRPS 急性期的血流和骨转化增加。TPBS 可以支持 CRPS 的诊断，但不能用来确诊 CRPS。

尽管这些诊断试验的潜在获益很大，但它们应该作为确诊的补充手段。[15]最近，一项包含了 158 例桡骨骨折的前瞻性研究分析了伤后 16 周内的各种检查方法，发现热成像、X 线检查、MRI 和 TPBS 都缺乏足够的敏感性和特异性，无法提供恰当的阳性预测值和阴性预测值（表 50-3）。[15]

治疗

CRPS 是一种复杂的疾病，可能包含多种病理机制，因而需要使用物理治疗、药物治疗、心理治疗、外科治疗等多学科治疗手段（表 50-4）。[2-3, 13, 16-40]所有医师都应该努力尽早与患者建立密切的治疗关系，因为长期治疗需要以医患间的信任为基础。治疗的目标是重建肢体功能，关键是早治疗。应该鼓励没有直接被手术影响的关节进行早期全范围活动（ROM）（如肩部手术后鼓励肘、腕、指关节的早期 ROM）。延迟治疗超过 6 个月的患者长期预后更差，而且早

期的 CRPS 症状一般被认为是可逆的。[41]

物理治疗和职业治疗

为确保良好的功能结果，包括物理治疗和职业治疗在内的物理医学是康复的核心。活动患肢造成的疼痛会给 CRPS 患者造成心理上的恐惧，这种状况被称为运动恐惧症（kinesophobia）。物理治疗和职业治疗的目标是克服这种对疼痛的恐惧，并且使患肢回到最佳功能状态。为实现这一目标，物理治疗师发展了一套渐进的程序使患肢脱敏，并且增加 ROM、灵活性、姿势和肌肉力量。[3]常见形式包括对比浴（contrast baths）、冷热交替浸泡、等长肌肉收缩训练和应力载荷。[13]职业治疗师鼓励患者在日常活动中每天使用患肢。专门的衣服和绷带可能有助于减少患肢水肿和感觉超载。镜像疗法（mirror box therapy）在减少神经性疼痛上有发展前景。物理医学应该考虑到逐渐增加的压力，并根据需要中断治疗以阻止极度难忍的疼痛。

心理治疗

最好的治疗有时仍不能缓解慢性疼痛，这给 CRPS 患者带来很大的情绪负担，这种情况需要心理治疗。[28]至少，新诊断为 CRPS 的患者应该和心理健康工作者讨论，了解该病的病理生理学原理和病程，并理解主动自我管理和参与护理计划的必要性。心理治疗旨在重建功能失调的疼痛

表 50-3

桡骨远端骨折后诊断方法的敏感性、特异性、阳性预测值、阴性预测值

桡骨远端骨折后诊断方法	敏感性（%）	特异性（%）	阳性预测值（%）	阴性预测值（%）
创伤后 2 周				
热成像	45	50	17	79
创伤后 8 周				
热成像	50	67	26	85
双侧 X 线检查	36	94	58	86
MRI	43	78	31	85
三期骨扫描	19	96	58	86
创伤后 16 周				
热成像	29	89	38	84
MRI	13	98	60	83
TPBS	14	100	100	83

注：经允许引自 Schurmann M, Zaspel J, Löhr P, et al: Imaging in early posttraumatic complex regional pain syndrome: A comparison of diagnostic methods *Clin J Pain* 2007;23(5):449–457.

表 50-4

CRPS 的治疗策略和可获得的证据

治疗分类	方式	证据
药物（口服、经静脉和经皮给药）[16-27]	多种	见表 50-5
物理治疗和职业治疗[3, 13]	对比浴 应力载荷 等长肌肉收缩训练 冷热交替浸泡、弹力袜	物理治疗和职业治疗可改善生活质量和患肢功能
心理治疗[28]	放松 生物反馈	证据不足以推荐，但是专家鼓励以此治疗由非器质性病因引起的慢性疼痛
交感封闭和区域麻醉[29-33]	星状神经节阻滞 斜角肌间阻滞	小规模回顾性研究证实配合物理治疗使用有益处
静脉区域阻滞[34]	胍乙啶 利多卡因 可乐定 氟哌利多 利血平	与安慰剂相比无优势
神经调制[35-36]	脊髓刺激器 经皮电神经刺激疗法 （transcutaneous electrical nerve stimulation，TENS）	对于实验性刺激有效的难治性患者，可以减轻疼痛、改善生活质量 TENS 治疗 CRPS 的证据不足以推荐
蛛网膜下腔用药[37-39]	巴氯芬	有些证据表明，对治疗与 CRPS 相关的肌张力障碍有效，可以改善患肢功能
外科消融[26, 40]	交感神经手术切除 交感神经射频消融 交感神经化学消融	用于缓解 CRPS 疼痛的证据不足以推荐 有可能缓解疼痛，但是有文献称交感神经切除后可能出现新的神经性疼痛

认知模式和行为，使其成为促进康复的思维模式（认知 – 行为治疗）。下一步目标包括恢复放松和生物反馈的功能，这些可以在疼痛发作时使用。评价和治疗伴发的轴 I 障碍（axis I disorders）也很重要，如抑郁、广泛焦虑障碍及创伤后应激障碍，这类障碍阻碍功能恢复。

药物治疗

如果 CRPS 的疼痛严重到限制功能康复的程度，则应该使用药物治疗。药物制剂的使用还缺乏前瞻性随机对照试验（RCT）的支持。[16]临床医师最近以 CRPS 的临床试验数据和神经性疼痛的 RCT 数据为指导，进行了有序的药物试验。

目前，皮质类固醇和 NSAID 已经被用于治疗 CRPS 相关的炎症，而且有 RCT 证明口服皮质类固醇在损害发生后的急性期有积极的临床效果。[17]用皮质类固醇治疗 CRPS 的控制实验只有 1 项，该实验的药物剂量为每日口服 30 mg 泼尼松（10 mg，TID）12 周。[17]在开放实验中，临床医师起初使患者口服 40~60 mg 泼尼松，在 4 周内快速减量。[18]还没有研究证明 NSAID 能明显减轻神经性疼痛。[16]

炎症产生的氧自由基可能是 CRPS 发展的关键组分，抗氧化剂的使用就是基于这一观点。实验发现腕部骨折后使用维生素 C 可以减小骨折后 CRPS 发病率。[19]回顾性实验已经证明二甲基亚砜（DMSO）和 N– 乙酰半胱氨酸局部使用 17 周和 52 周可以明显缓解疼痛。[20]

有较高等级的证据显示，抗惊厥药物（如加巴喷丁、普瑞巴林）可有效治疗神经性疼痛疾病，这促进了此类药物在 CRPS 中的应用。一项前瞻性研究显示，加巴喷丁不能明显缓解 1 型 CRPS 患者的疼痛，但是可以改善感觉障碍。[21]另一项研究显示，加巴喷丁可以明显减轻 CRPS 患者的自发性和诱发性疼痛，平均病程 2.7 个月。[22]

炎症通路上调激活兴奋性痛觉通路，兴奋性痛觉通路以 N- 甲基 -D- 天冬氨酸（NMDA）为神经递质。[23]氯胺酮（NMDA 受体阻滞剂）因有可能逆转中枢敏化和改变神经元可塑性而引起关注。亚麻醉剂量氯胺酮静脉注射、氯胺酮诱导的昏迷、局部氯胺酮软膏已经被证明可以有效降低疼痛数值评分，但药效持续时间不确定。[23]局部和皮下使用氯胺酮最近已被证明至少有同样的效果，且入血量更少。[23]

肾上腺素能受体拮抗剂（如酚苄明和酚妥拉明）可以封闭 SNS 介导性疼痛，已经被用于治疗 CRPS。回顾性研究已经显示出口服肾上腺素能拮抗剂对缓解疼痛的作用，但尚缺乏前瞻性研究。[24]静脉区域性使用酚妥拉明可能用于诊断 SNS 介导性疼痛。局部使用可乐定（一种 α2 肾上腺素能激动剂）已被证明可以缓解 SNS 介导性疼痛患者的局部痛觉过敏。[25]

在 CRPS 进展过程中，通过 TPBS 可发现患肢局部骨质吸收。双膦酸盐和降钙素抑制破骨细胞介导的骨质吸收，临床有效。[26]在预实验中，双膦酸盐缓解主观疼痛的效果优于安慰剂。降钙素降低平均疼痛分数的实验数据不一致。[26]

治疗 CRPS 可能需要使用阿片类药物，这是内科医师争论的一个话题。虽然阿片类药物在组织损伤的急性期可能有用，但是长期使用阿片类药物治疗外周或中枢神经性疼痛的效果差，或者说所需剂量大。[27]大剂量使用阿片类药物时，诸如药物耐受、药物成瘾、免疫抑制或内分泌功能障碍等不良反应的发生率可能更高（表 50–5）。[17–21, 26–27, 37–39, 42–48]

交感神经阻滞和区域麻醉

上肢的初级交感神经节是星状神经节。SNS 介导性疼痛的提出使研究者们开始使用星状神经节阻滞来诊断和治疗 SNS 介导性疼痛。最近的前瞻性研究支持用局部麻醉药或肉毒毒素阻滞星状神经节来减轻疼痛和促进康复，尤其是发病早期（＜ 16 周）。星状神经节阻滞有几个问题待研究，包括：疼痛缓解持续时间，以及间断单剂量给药和持续性给药哪个更有效。[29]目前通过交感神经阻滞诊断 SNS 介导性疼痛已经导致大量假阳性和假阴性结果。[30]虽然没有预测交感神经阻滞成功的方法，但是痛觉超敏和感觉减退意味着交感神经阻滞失败。[31]

已经有研究证明，臂丛神经阻滞可以通过封闭躯体 Aδ 和 C 型传入神经纤维来减轻疼痛，使药物难治性 CRPS 患者得以进行肩部康复治疗。[32]持续注射大约 1 周有效。虽然存在臂丛神经阻滞用于交感神经阻滞失败的患者，但最近的预实验证明持续性星状神经节阻滞和持续性锁骨下臂丛神经阻滞均可明显减轻基础神经性疼痛和疼痛发作。[33]

用 Bier 麻醉技术实现区域交感神经阻滞已有研究。已经用过的药物包括胍乙啶、酮色林、溴苄铵、阿托品、氟哌利多和利血平，但是在荟萃分析后很长一段时间内，这些药物在减轻疼痛方面都没有显著的临床效果。[34]

外科治疗

通过在硬膜外植入脊髓刺激器进行神经调制可以有效缓解慢性 CRPS 相关的灼痛（成功率 70%），长期随访已证实其有效性。[35]永久性脊髓刺激器植入的非预期结果发生率高达 34%。[36]最常见的翻修原因是电极移位，其他并发症包括植入物失效和感染。[36]长期随访已经证实其镇痛效果在大约 5 年内逐渐减弱。[35]

椎管内药物已经被证明是一种针对中枢神经系统机制治疗 CRPS 疼痛的可靠方法。前瞻性实验已经证明，一种 γ- 氨基丁酸 -β 受体激动剂（巴氯芬）可

表 50-5

CRPS 的药物治疗

药物	作用机制	剂量	疗效证据
抗炎药			
皮质类固醇[17-18]	减少炎症细胞因子转录	泼尼松 10 mg PO TID；甲泼尼龙 32 mg PO QID 14 天，后接 14 天减量	CRPS 分级改善 6 个月随访时 CRPS 分级改善
帕瑞昔布[43]	抑制环氧酶 2，减少前列腺素形成	5 mg IV 联合 1 mg/kg 体重利多卡因或 30 mg 可乐定 IV 区域阻滞，每周一次，使用 3 周	比对照组日常急救用药少且 VAS 评分低
自由基清除剂			
维生素 C[19]	清除自由基	每日 500 mg PO，使用 50 天	降低 CRPS 发病率
二甲基亚砜[20]	清除自由基	患处每日涂抹 5 次 50% 二甲基亚砜乳剂，使用 52 周	对急性期 CRPS 比 N- 乙酰半胱氨酸的效果好 比 N- 乙酰半胱氨酸总治疗费用低 改善 ROM 和血管舒缩不稳定
N- 乙酰半胱氨酸[20]	清除自由基	600 mg PO TID，使用 52 周	对慢性期 CRPS 比二甲基亚砜的效果好
镇痛药			
加巴喷丁[21]	封闭神经元钙离子通道	每日 600 mg PO，使用 2 天，再 600 mg BID，使用 2 天，然后 600 mg TID，使用 17 天	3 周后治疗组和安慰剂组的疼痛评分无差异，但是治疗组对整体感知到的疼痛改善效果更佳
阿片类[27,44]	激活阿片受体	吗啡缓释片每日 90 mg PO；每日大约 8.9 mg 左吗喃 PO	没有数据证明能显著缓解疼痛 大剂量可显著缓解神经性疼痛
氯胺酮[45-47]	NMDA 受体拮抗剂	10% 氯胺酮乳剂，经皮给药 静脉氯胺酮亚麻醉 30 mg/h，使用 4.2 天 静脉氯胺酮麻醉 7 mg/（kg·h）+ 咪达唑仑 IV 0.15-0.4 mg/（kg·h），使用 5 天	减轻机械性痛觉超敏和痛觉过敏 11 周随访时仍可显著缓解疼痛 治疗后 10 年 50% 的患者症状完全缓解
抗痉挛制剂			
巴氯芬[37-39]	抑制 GABA-β 受体	椎管内巴氯芬注射可高达 450 µg/d	改善肌张力障碍和缓解疼痛，提高生活质量
破骨细胞抑制剂			
双膦酸盐[26,48]	抑制破骨细胞 / 骨重塑	伊班膦酸盐每日 6 mg IV，使用 3 天 阿仑膦酸钠每日 40 mg PO，使用 8 周；每日 7.5 mg IV，使用 3 天 帕米膦酸二钠 60 mg IV，使用 1 次 氯膦酸二钠每日 300 mg IV，使用 10 天	改善平均和最差疼痛分级 改善自发疼痛、压力耐受和关节活动 第 2 周和第 4 周时，明显缓解自发疼痛、压痛、肿胀，改善受累肢体活动 改善疼痛评分、疾病严重程度评分和生理功能 40 天时，改善疼痛评分和提高临床整体评估
降钙素[26]	释放 β- 内啡肽 抑制破骨细胞 / 骨重塑	每日 200 IU 鼻内给药 100 IU 肌内注射 100 IU TID，使用 3 周 100 IU BID，使用 4 周 100 IU TID，使用 3 周	统计学上没有显著益处 显著改善疼痛评分和 ROM 显著改善疼痛和增加 ROM，水肿程度无改善 不能改善疼痛评分、僵硬、水肿和血管活动 1 周时，改善疼痛评分

注：IV（intravenous）：静脉注射。PO（by mouth）：口服。ROM：活动范围。BID（twice daily）：每日 2 次。TID（three times daily）：每日 3 次。QID（four times daily）：每日 4 次。

以改善肌张力障碍和缓解慢性 CRPS 相关性疼痛。[37-39]

外科交感神经切除使用化学消融、射频消融和开放手术切断交感神经干或破坏星状神经节，以此来缓解 SNS 介导性疼痛。这些技术是暂时性交感神经阻滞技术的扩展，可以延长疼痛缓解持续的时间。一项回顾性研究发现，射频消融破坏星状神经节后大约 1 年，40% 的患者疼痛缓解大于 50%。[40]尽管得到了不错的结果，但外科交感神经切除的长期效果仍有争议[26]。

预防

预防术后 / 创伤后 CRPS 的发生或复发是目前正在研究的领域。有研究者研究了腕部骨折后使用维生素 C 50 天的效果，发现维生素 C 可以明显降低 CRPS 的发病率（维生素 C 组 7%，对照组 22%）。[19]对过去发生过 CRPS 的肢体再手术可导致症状加重或复发。研究显示，围手术期使用降钙素、星状神经节阻滞、静脉阻滞和多模式联合麻醉初期都可以减少复发。[16]最近，专家建议推迟手术至 CRPS 体征尽可能轻微。[16]

总结

CRPS 是一种病理生理学机制复杂的疾病，可导致患者的痛苦不断增加。骨科医师应该在肩肘手术术前或术后尽早识别 CRPS，并给予正确的治疗。早诊断、早治疗、多学科团队合作治疗可以带来最好的长期结果。

参考文献

[1] Marinus J, Moseley GL, Birklein F, et al:Clinical features and pathophysiology of complex regional pain syndrome. *Lancet Neurol* 2011;10(7):637-648.
This review article summarizes the basic and clinical research into the epidemiology and pathophysiological mechanisms of CRPS. The authors emphasize multiple mechanisms to explain the complex clinical presentation of CRPS.

[2] Goebel A:Complex regional pain syndrome in adults. *Rheumatology (Oxford)* 2011;50(10):1739-1750.
This review article summarizes the epidemiology, pathophysiology, clinical presentation, and treatment of CRPS. It provides additional information on the economics of CRPS, initiatives for treatment, and opportunities for future research.

[3] Merskey H, Bogduk N:*Classification of Chronic Pain. Descriptions of Chronic Pain Syndromes and Definitions of Pain Terms*, ed 2. Seattle, WA, IASP Press, 1994.

[4] Harden RN, Bruehl S, Perez RS, et al:Validation of proposed diagnostic criteria (the "Budapest Criteria") for complex regional pain syndrome. *Pain* 2010;150(2):268-274.
This study applied the older Orlando criteria and the more recent Budapest criteria to a cohort of 113 CRPS and 47 non-CRPS neuropathic pain patients to compare specificity and sensitivity. The Orlando criteria had a sensitivity of 1.0 and a specificity of 0.41 while the Budapest criteria had a sensitivity of 0.99 and a specificity of 0.68.

[5] Sethna NF, Meier PM, Zurakowski D, Berde CB:Cutaneous sensory abnormalities in children and adolescents with complex regional pain syndromes. *Pain* 2007;131(1-2):153-161.
This study examined 42 patients with CRPS for standardized neurologic examination and quantitative sensory testing. Twenty-one patients exhibited allodynia in response to cold, and 26 patients exhibited allodynia in response to dynamic and static mechanical stimulation.

[6] Beerthuizen A, Stronks DL, Van't Spijker A, et al:Demographic and medical parameters in the development of complex regional pain syndrome type 1 (CRPS1):Prospective study on 596 patients with a fracture. *Pain* 2012;153(6):1187-1192.
This study reviewed 596 patients with a single fracture. There were 7% in whom CRPS was later diagnosed. An analysis of these patients demonstrated they more often had intra-articular fracture, fracture-dislocations, rheumatoid arthritis, or musculoskeletal comorbidities.

[7] Sharma A, Agarwal S, Broatch J, Raja SN:A web-based cross-sectional epidemiological survey of complex regional pain syndrome. *Reg Anesth Pain Med* 2009;34(2):110-115.
This study was a survey of 75 questions posted on the Reflex Sympathetic Dystrophy Syndrome Association of America website. There were 888 responses that were accepted for analysis of demographic and symptomatic

review.

［8］ Bruehl S:An update on the pathophysiology of complex regional pain syndrome. *Anesthesiology* 2010;113(3):713-725.

This review article summarizes the basic and clinical research into the epidemiology and pathophysiologic mechanisms of CRPS. The authors emphasize multiple mechanisms to explain the complex clinical presentation of CRPS.

［9］ Cappello ZJ, Kasdan ML, Louis DS:Meta-analysis of imaging techniques for the diagnosis of complex regional pain syndrome type I. *J Hand Surg Am* 2012; 37(2):288-296.

The results of MRI, plain films, and TPBS were examined by meta-analysis. TPBS was found to have greatest sensitivity and higher negative predictive value.

［10］ Kohr D, Tschernatsch M, Schmitz K, et al:Autoantibodies in complex regional pain syndrome bind to a differentiation-dependent neuronal surface autoantigen. *Pain* 2009;143(3):246-251.

Serum of the patients with CRPS and control patients were screened for the presence of autoantibodies. Thirteen of 30 patients with CRPS demonstrated specific surface binding to autonomic neurons.

［11］ Goebel A, Baranowski A, Maurer K, Ghiai A, Mc- Cabe C, Ambler G:Intravenous immunoglobulin treatment of the complex regional pain syndrome:A randomized trial. *Ann Intern Med* 2010;152(3):152-158.

A randomized, double-blind, placebo-controlled crossover trial of 12 patients is presented. The average pain intensity score was 1.55 units lower on the visual analog scale following intravenous immunoglobulin treatment.

［12］ Bonica JJ:*The Management of Pain, With Special Emphasis on the Use of Analgesic Block in Diagnosis, Prognosis and Therapy.* Philadelphia, PA, Lee and Feibeger;1953.

［13］ Patterson RW, Li Z, Smith BP, Smith TL, Koman LA:Complex regional pain syndrome of the upper extremity. *J Hand Surg Am* 2011;36(9):1553-1562.

This review article summarizes the epidemiology, pathophysiology, clinical presentation, and treatment of CRPS. It emphasizes the viewpoint of the hand surgeon in describing potential functional limitations to the hand and therapeutic surgical interventions.

［14］ Drummond PD:Sensory disturbances in complex regional pain syndrome:Clinical observations, autonomic interactions, and possible mechanisms. *Pain Med* 2010;11(8):1257-1266.

This review article describes the sensory disturbances found in CRPS and potential pathophysiologic mechanisms. A special focus of the article involves the clinical presentation of sensory disturbances.

［15］ Schürmann M, Zaspel J, Löhr P, et al:Imaging in early posttraumatic complex regional pain syndrome:A comparison of diagnostic methods. *Clin J Pain* 2007;23(5):449-457.

One hundred fifty-eight consecutive patients were followed for 16 weeks following trauma with bilateral thermography, plain films, MRI, and TPBS. All studies were demonstrated to have a low positive predictive value (17% to 60%) and moderate negative predictive value (79% to 86%).

［16］ Perez RS, Zollinger PE, Dijkstra PU, et al: CRPS I task force:Evidence based guidelines for complex regional pain syndrome type 1. *BMC Neurol* 2010;10:20.

This article presents a multidisciplinary task force's review of the literature to provide evidence-based recommendations for care. It classifies the evidence found in the literature according to objective standards.

［17］ Christensen K, Jensen EM, Noer I:The reflex dystrophy syndrome response to treatment with systemic corticosteroids. *Acta Chir Scand* 1982;148(8):653-655.

［18］ Kozin F, Ryan LM, Carerra GF, Soin JS, Wortmann RL:The reflex sympathetic dystrophy syndrome (RSDS):III. Scintigraphic studies, further evidence for the therapeutic efficacy of systemic corticosteroids, and proposed diagnostic criteria. *Am J Med* 1981;70(1):23-30.

［19］ Zollinger PE, Tuinebreijer WE, Kreis RW, Breederveld RS:Effect of vitamin C on frequency of reflex sympathetic dystrophy in wrist fractures:A randomised trial. *Lancet* 1999;354(9195):2025-2028.

［20］ Perez RS, Zuurmond WW, Bezemer PD, et al:The treatment of complex regional pain syndrome type I with free radical scavengers:A randomized controlled study. *Pain* 2003;102(3):297-307.

［21］ van de Vusse AC, Stompvan den Berg SG, Kessels AH, Weber WE:Randomised controlled trial of gabapentin in complex regional pain syndrome type 1 [IS-RCTN84121379]. *BMC Neurol* 2004;4:13-22.

［22］ Tan AK, Duman I, Tas̗kaynatan MA, Hazneci B, Kalyon TA:The effect of gabapentin in earlier stage of reflex sympathetic dystrophy. *Clin Rheumatol* 2007;26(4):561-565.

Twenty-two patients with CRPS were enrolled to take

an average of 1,145 mg of gabapentin daily. At 6 weeks, there was statistically significant improvement in spontaneous and provoked pain.

[23] Schwartzman RJ, Alexander GM, Grothusen JR:The use of ketamine in complex regional pain syndrome:Possible mechanisms. *Expert Rev Neurother* 2011;11(5):719-734. This review article describes the clinical experience using differing protocols of ketamine dosing for the treatment of chronic pain in CRPS. It provides possible explanations of the physiological mechanism of the relief provided by ketamine to patients with CRPS.

[24] Muizelaar JP, Kleyer M, Hertogs IA, DeLange DC:Complex regional pain syndrome (reflex sympathetic dystrophy and causalgia):Management with the cal- cium channel blocker nifedipine and/or the alpha- sympathetic blocker phenoxybenzamine in 59 patients. *Clin Neurol Neurosurg* 1997;99(1):26-30.

[25] Davis KD, Treede RD, Raja SN, Meyer RA, Campbell JN:Topical application of clonidine relieves hyperalgesia in patients with sympathetically maintained pain. *Pain* 1991;47(3):309-317.

[26] Sharma A, Williams K, Raja SN:Advances in treatment of complex regional pain syndrome:Recent insights on a perplexing disease. *Curr Opin Anaesthesiol* 2006;19(5):566-572.

[27] Rowbotham MC, Twilling L, Davies PS, Reisner L, Taylor K, Mohr D:Oral opioid therapy for chronic peripheral and central neuropathic pain. *N Engl J Med* 2003;348(13):1223-1232.

[28] Bruehl S, Chung OY:Psychological and behavioral aspects of complex regional pain syndrome management. *Clin J Pain* 2006;22(5):430-437.

[29] Yucel I, Demiraran Y, Ozturan K, Degirmenci E:Complex regional pain syndrome type I:Efficacy of stellate ganglion blockade. *J Orthop Traumatol* 2009;10(4):179-183.
The authors discuss a prospective study of 22 patients following administration of three stellate ganglion blocks separated by 1-week intervals. A significant decrease in VAS pain scores and increased range of motion were documented.

[30] Krumova EK, Gussone C, Regeniter S, Westermann A, Zenz M, Maier C:Are sympathetic blocks useful for diagnostic purposes? *Reg Anesth Pain Med* 2011;36(6):560-567.
The authors discuss a pilot study of 19 patients with chronic neuropathic pain where sympathetic block was used in diagnosis. Of the 12 with sufficient temperature change following sympathetic block, 3 were diagnosed with CRPS.

[31] van Eijs F, Geurts J, van Kleef M, et al:Predictors of pain relieving response to sympathetic blockade in complex regional pain syndrome type 1. *Anesthesiology* 2012;116(1):113-121.
The authors discuss a prospective study of 49 patients with CRPS for less than 1 year duration before stellate ganglion block. Allodynia and hypoesthesia were negative predictors for treatment success.

[32] Detaille V, Busnel F, Ravary H, Jacquot A, Katz D, Allano G:Use of continuous interscalene brachial plexus block and rehabilitation to treat complex regional pain syndrome of the shoulder. *Ann Phys Rehabil Med* 2010;53(6-7):406-416.
The authors present a prospective trial of a 1-week continuous interscalene brachial plexus on 59 patients with treatment-refractory CRPS type 1.

[33] Toshniwal G, Sunder R, Thomas R, Dureja GP:Management of complex regional pain syndrome type I in upper extremity-evaluation of continuous stellate ganglion block and continuous infraclavicular brachial plexus block:A pilot study. *Pain Med* 2012;13(1):96-106.
The authors present a randomized prospective trial of 1 week of either continuous stellate ganglion block or continuous infraclavicular block. At 4-week follow-up, both groups demonstrated improvement in edema and range of motion.

[34] Kingery WS:A critical review of controlled clinical trials for peripheral neuropathic pain and complex regional pain syndromes. *Pain* 1997;73(2):123-139.

[35] Kemler MA, de Vet HC, Barendse GA, van den Wildenberg FA, van Kleef M:Effect of spinal cord stimulation for chronic complex regional pain syndrome Type I:Five-year final follow-up of patients in a randomized controlled trial. *J Neurosurg* 2008;108(2):292-298.
A randomized controlled trial involving 36 patients with implanted spinal cord stimulators with 5-year follow-up is discussed. Despite diminishing efficacy at 5 years, 19 patients indicated a willingness to repeat treatment of the same result.

[36] Turner JA, Loeser JD, Deyo RA, Sanders SB:Spinal cord stimulation for patients with failed back surgery syndrome or complex regional pain syndrome:A systematic review of effectiveness and complications. *Pain* 2004;108(1-2):137-147.

[37] van Rijn MA, Munts AG, Marinus J, et al:Intrathecal baclofen for dystonia of complex regional pain syndrome. *Pain* 2009;143(1-2):41-47.

A single-blind, placebo-run-in, dose-escalation study enrolling 36 patients is presented. Intention-to-treat analysis revealed a substantial improvement in dystonia, pain, disability, and quality of life.

[38] van der Plas AA, van Rijn MA, Marinus J, Putter H, van Hilten JJ:Efficacy of intrathecal baclofen on different pain qualities in complex regional pain syndrome. *Anesth Analg* 2013;116(1):211-215.

A prospective study examining the effects of intrathecal baclofen infusion pumps in 6 women. Three of six women had complete resolution of hand dystonia, 4 women had reduced painful muscle spasms, and 2 had marked reduction in myoclonic jerks.

[39] van Hilten BJ, van de Beek WJ, Hoff JI, Voormolen JH, Delhaas EM:Intrathecal baclofen for the treatment of dystonia in patients with reflex sympathetic dystrophy. *N Engl J Med* 2000;343(9):625-630.

The authors present a prospective study of 42 patients with intrathecal baclofen pumps and one or more limbs affected by CRPS for 1 year. Of these patients, more than 60% had a reduction in pain score and global dystonia severity.

[40] Forouzanfar T, van Kleef M, Weber WE:Radiofrequency lesions of the stellate ganglion in chronic pain syndromes:Retrospective analysis of clinical efficacy in 86 patients. *Clin J Pain* 2000;16(2):164-168.

A retrospective review of 86 patients treated with radiofrequency ablation of the stellate ganglion is discussed. There were 40.7% of patients who experienced > 50% reduction of pain, 54.7% who noted no effect, and 4.7% who experienced worsening of pain.

[41] Varitimidis SE, Papatheodorou LK, Dailiana ZH, Poultsides L, Malizos KN:Complex regional pain syndrome type I as a consequence of trauma or surgery to upper extremity:Management with intravenous regional anaesthesia, using lidocaine and methylprednisolone. *J Hand Surg Eur Vol* 2011;36(9):771-777.

One hundred sixty-eight patients with CRPS-1 of the upper extremity were treated with intravenous lidocaine and methylprednisolone. The reported results were 88% of patients with minimal or no pain, and a complete absence of pain in 92% of patients at 5-year follow-up.

[42] Braus DF, Krauss JK, Strobel J:The shoulder-hand syndrome after stroke:A prospective clinical trial. *Ann Neurol* 1994;36(5):728-733.

[43] Frade LC, Lauretti GR, Lima IC, Pereira NL:The antinociceptive effect of local or systemic parecoxib combined with lidocaine/clonidine intravenous regional analgesia for complex regional pain syndrome type I in the arm. *Anesth Analg* 2005;101(3):807-811.

Thirty patients with CRPS were randomized into either intravenous regional analgesia with lidocaine/ clonidine or intravenous regional analgesia with oral parecoxib. Patients on intravenous regional analgesia/ parecoxib consumed less rescue medication.

[44] Harke H, Gretenkort P, Ladleif HU, Rahman S, Harke O:The response of neuropathic pain and pain in complex regional pain syndrome I to carbamazepine and sustained-release morphine in patients pretreated with spinal cord stimulation:A double-blinded randomized study. *Anesth Analg* 2001;92(2):488-495.

[45] Finch PM, Knudsen L, Drummond PD:Reduction of allodynia in patients with complex regional pain syndrome:A double-blind placebo-controlled trial of topical ketamine. *Pain* 2009;146(1-2):18-25.

Twenty patients received 10% topical ketamine on two occasions separated by 1 week. Ketamine was found to inhibit allodynia to light brushing and hyperalgesia punctate stimuli.

[46] Sigtermans M, Dahan A, Mooren R, et al:S(+)-ketamine effect on experimental pain and cardiac output:A population pharmacokinetic-pharmacodynamic modeling study in healthy volunteers. *Anesthesiology* 2009;111(4):892-903.

Sixty CRPS type 1 patients were administered subanesthetic ketamine for 4.2 days. Significant pain relief was demonstrated against placebo at up to 11 weeks follow-up.

[47] Kiefer RT, Rohr P, Ploppa A, et al:Efficacy of ketamine in anesthetic dosage for the treatment of refractory complex regional pain syndrome:An openlabel phase II study. *Pain Med* 2008;9(8):1173-1201.

A prospective study of 20 American Society of Anesthesiologists I-III patients using anesthetic dosage ketamine is presented. Significant pain relief was observed at 1, 3, and 6 months following treatment.

[48] Breuer B, Pappagallo M, Ongseng F, Chen CI, Goldfarb R:An open-label pilot trial of ibandronate for complex regional pain syndrome. *Clin J Pain* 2008;24(8):685-689.

An open-label three day trial of ibandronate is presented. A significant improvement in average and worst pain ratings was observed.

第五十一章 冻结肩

Douglas Scott, MD; Andrew Green, MD

引言

冻结肩一词常被医学专业人士和普通人用于描述肩部疼痛、僵硬的状况。肩关节周围炎一词在1872年首次出现，用来描述肩关节主被动活动受限。[1]Codman在1934年引入冻结肩一词，用来描述一系列症状，而不是一种特定疾病。[2]许多情况可以造成肩部疼痛和活动受限。粘连性关节囊炎，基于冻结肩的手术所见和尸检结果由Neviaser推广。[3]研究者们强调冻结肩各种病因间的差异。特发性粘连性关节囊炎被定义为肩关节主被动活动明显受限，而未发现肩关节本身有任何病变。[4]尽管这种状况很常见且相关研究很多，但全科医师甚至骨科医师常对其诊断和治疗毫无头绪，而且其病理生理学机制还未研究清楚。

Dr. Green or an immediate family member has received royalties from Tornier; is a member of a speakers' bureau or has made paid presentations on behalf of DJ Orthopaedics; serves as a paid consultant to or is an employee of Tornier; has stock or stock options held in IlluminOss Medical and Pfizer; has received research or institutional support from DJ Orthopaedics and Synthes; has received nonincome support (such as equipment or services), commercially derived honoraria, or other non–research-related funding (such as paid travel) from Arthrex and Smith & Nephew; and serves as a board member, owner, officer, or committee member of the American Academy of Orthopaedic Surgeons and the American Shoulder and Elbow Surgeons. Neither Dr. Scott nor any immediate family member has received anything of value from or has stock or stock options held in a commercial company or institution related directly or indirectly to the subject of this chapter.

按冻结肩治疗患者前，要考虑到各种可能引起肩关节疼痛和僵硬的原因。冻结肩主要采用非手术治疗，对于难治性病例，手术治疗可以改善结果。

流行病学

冻结肩的发病率很难评估，因为其缺乏严格的诊断标准，通常隐匿起病、易与其他肩关节疾病相混淆。大多数研究报道，冻结肩在人群中的发病率为2%~5%，这个数字可能有些夸大。[5]一项研究报道，女性患病率为10%~12%。[6]虽然同侧肩的复发罕见，但是冻结肩患者对侧发病率高达20%。大约60%~80%的患者是女性，大部分患者的年龄为40~60岁。[7]60%的冻结肩累及非主力侧，左肩受累约60%。

病因和病理生理学

许多肩部原发病最终引起疼痛和活动障碍。肩袖疾病、原发性盂肱关节炎、创伤后挛缩（软组织损伤或骨折后）、术后挛缩、炎性关节、全身疾病、神经系统疾病后遗症等均是肩关节僵硬的原因。相比之下，特发性粘连性关节囊炎没有重大创伤、手术或其他疾病的病史。诱发特发性粘连性关节囊炎的疾病很难被发现，因此其潜在病因未知。

分析关节镜下得到的组织，其含有成纤维细胞、增生的成纤维细胞和肌成纤维细胞。[8]有些研究者认为，该病在组织学上和掌腱膜挛缩（Dupuytren 病）相似，二者发生挛缩和纤维化的生化途径相同。肩关节囊中沉积致密的Ⅲ型胶原基质。在一项 2007 年的研究中，于病变组织中发现了慢性炎症细胞浸润和血管新生，慢性炎症细胞包括肥大细胞、T 细胞、B 细胞、巨噬细胞，血管新生通过 CD34 抗体染色发现。[8] 该研究还发现了 S100 蛋白染色阳性物质，与神经细胞一样。与其他研究相比，该研究几乎没有发现肌成纤维细胞群。

患者所处的临床分期可能影响冻结肩病理生理学研究的结果。因为这些研究所取得的病理组织一般源自早期非手术治疗无效的晚期患者，所以研究结果可能无法直接体现粘连性关节囊炎病理生理学过程的真实病因。有关特发性粘连性关节囊炎自然病程的基础科学研究结果总结如下：某个诱发事件或过程导致最初的进行期（freezing phase），这个时期表现为疼痛、炎症反应，随后逐渐进展为慢性的、挛缩性的冻结期（frozen phase）。

已经有研究者进行过冻结肩病理解剖的尸体研究。通过选择性折叠缝合关节囊可以模拟局部关节囊挛缩，最终表现为盂肱关节被动活动受限。[9] 该研究发现关闭肩袖间隙（包括喙肱韧带和盂肱上韧带）可以限制外旋，尤其当肩关节处于内收位时。该研究还发现紧缩关节囊的前下部（包括前下盂肱韧带复合体）可以限制上臂外展时的肩关节活动。这些发现与粘连性关节囊炎和肩关节挛缩患者的术中发现一致，并且为选择性手术松解特定解剖结构提供了依据。

通过对比女性同卵双生和异卵双生双胞胎中冻结肩的患病率，可以研究冻结肩的遗传性。[6] 同卵双生与异卵双生双胞胎相比，两人同患冻结肩的概率更大，这说明冻结肩的发生是有遗传因素的。

临床评估

冻结肩是基于病史和体格检查做出的临床诊断。典型情况是，患者经历过微不足道的创伤事件或根本回忆不起来任何相关事件。疼痛是最初的主诉，随后出现肩关节活动受限逐渐加重。夜间痛是常见的主诉。疼痛在休息或静止时缓解消失，在任何方向上肩关节活动达极限时出现。大多数患者最终表现为患肩主被动活动与对侧相比明显受限，尤其当肩关节处于外展 90° 时。经常出现外旋受限达到或超过 50%。体格检查发现肩关节活动达极限时有明确的终点（firm end point）并且出现疼痛。与此类似，关节囊挛缩导致肩关节平移活动整体受限。

完整的评估包括肩关节标准 X 线检查（正位、腋位、出口位），以排除肩关节疼痛和僵硬的其他原因，（如盂肱关节炎、肩锁关节炎和钙化性肌腱炎）。评估早期冻结肩一般不需要高级影像学检查。影像学文献中描述了 MRI 和增强 MRI 的典型表现。[10-11] 冻结肩患者表现为喙肱韧带增厚、腋隐窝中关节囊增厚和钆元素增强、关节腔总容积减小、肩袖间隙中出现喙突下脂肪填充。需要特殊说明的是，喙肱韧带增厚已经被证明和内外旋受限相关。[10] 应避免过度使用高级影像学检查，因为冻结肩通常可以通过病史、体格检查和 X 线检查明确诊断。非必要的高级影像学检查可能造成有害的临床结果。最近，有一项研究报道，冻结肩患者关节囊松解后的 MRI 检查结果有很高的肩袖撕裂假阳性率。[12]

近期的文献报道显示，冻结肩可出现喙突和肩锁关节疼痛。通过连续评估 830 名患者，研究者发现喙突压痛敏感性和特异性很高，研究者假设这种疼痛源自附近的喙肱韧带和肩袖间隙组织。[13] 一项 2011 年的研究提出假设：盂肱关节活动受限导致病理性的肩胛胸壁和肩锁关节代偿性活动，是导致肩锁关节疼痛的原因。[14] 当冻结肩治疗后且盂肱关节活动恢复后，大多数患者的肩锁关节疼痛会自行消失。

临床上，冻结肩的自然病程被分成 3 期（表 51-

1）。表现经常延迟、起病隐匿、病程和严重程度多变，这些因素使这个分期不太准确。虽然有时候很难确切指出患者病程进展到哪一期，但是这个分期仍是预期临床过程的重要指导。

表 51-1	
冻结肩的分期	
分期	特点
进行期	严重的急性疼痛和僵硬
冻结期	疼痛缓解但僵硬持续
解冻期	症状逐渐缓解消失

伴随疾病

为发现原发性冻结肩的伴随疾病，一定要全面地采集病史。在冻结肩的伴随疾病中，糖尿病是最值得注意的，也是研究最广泛的。许多不同的研究均已证明糖尿病患者冻结肩的发病率高达 10%~36%，并且糖尿病对冻结肩的自然病程和手术、非手术治疗结果均能产生深远影响。[15-16] 人们普遍相信糖尿病患者非手术治疗的失败风险更高，且手术或被动活动治疗后复发风险也更高，常迁延不愈。然而，一项 2012 年的研究称，麻醉下被动活动的疗效在糖尿病患者和非糖尿病患者中无显著性差异，事实上，糖尿病患者的复发率更高，更频繁地要求重复被动活动。[17]

虽然一项近期的研究阐述了糖尿病和冻结肩常同时发生，但研究者没能找到血糖控制和冻结肩实际患病率的直接相关性（用糖化血红蛋白 A1c 评估血糖的控制情况）。[18] 然而，1 型糖尿病冻结肩的患病率几乎是 2 型糖尿病患者的 2 倍，且糖尿病的患病时间与冻结肩的发展相关。

其他与冻结肩相关的内科疾病包括甲状腺疾病、卒中、外周神经病、臂丛损伤及心肺疾病。几乎 10% 的患者有甲状腺功能减退。[7] 另外，神经疾病和同侧上肢非肩部创伤的患者都可能发生冻结肩。肱骨近端骨折和相关腋神经或臂丛神经损伤患者有发生肩关节僵硬的倾向。

非手术治疗

非手术治疗是治疗冻结肩的主要方法，得到了许多研究的支持。包括随机对照实验在内的许多研究已经研究了各种冻结肩的非手术疗法——与安慰剂和其他治疗做对比。特发性粘连性关节囊炎是最常见的问题，大部分研究专注于其治疗。

皮质类固醇激素

很多研究支持用皮质类固醇激素（下文简称激素）治疗冻结肩。一项随机临床实验对比了关节内激素注射联合理疗与单独激素注射、盐水注射联合理疗、单独盐水注射，治疗 6 周后的随访时，用肩关节疼痛和残疾指数评分（Shoulder Pain and Disability Index scores）和活动范围作为评价指标，发现关节内激素注射联合理疗的疗效显著优于其他 3 种。[19] 3 个月后，激素组的肩关节疼痛和残疾指数评分更高。但是，12 个月后组间没有差异。最近的一项前瞻性研究对比了一组口服激素的患者和一组疗程为 3 次的透视引导下的关节内激素注射的患者。[20] 这两组患者都联合使用了物理治疗。在长达 1 年的随访中，关节内注射组的 Constant-Murley 评分始终优于另一组。8 周内，关节内注射组的活动范围优于另一组，8 周后结果各不相同。两组的疼痛和功能的视觉模拟量表评分无差异，关节内注射组的满意度评分更优。一项 2012 年的随机临床实验专门研究了 45 例预后不良的糖尿病患者对激素注射的反应。[21] 虽然治疗 4 周后注射组患者的疼痛改善，且治疗 12 周后注射组患者的功能改善，但是治疗 24 周后两组间无显著差异。

一项 2010 年的随机实验的系统综述对比了激素注射和物理治疗，结论是激素注射在短期内有中等疗效，其疗效随时间延长而不断减弱。[22] 另一项研究分析了多次激素注射的益处。[23] 在 4 个被认为高质量的研究中，有 3 项显示多次激素注射有利于减轻疼痛、改善功能和增加肩关节活动。但研究证明，超过 3 次的激素注射是无益的。

多个研究强调，临床实践中无法保障将激素精确地注射到盂肱关节内。一项研究的结果提示，在没有透视引导的情况下，从前入路注射到盂肱关节内的精度仅为 26%。[24]一项研究报道，盂肱关节内注射的精度分别为：前入路 65%、后入路 46%、上入路 46%。[25]一项研究对比了超声引导下盂肱关节和肩峰下激素注射的短期疗效，结果发现，虽然治疗 3 周后盂肱关节注射的疼痛缓解更明显，但是治疗 6 周后、12 周后两组无显著差异。[26]另外，盂肱关节和肩峰下激素注射的 Constant-Murley 评分和活动范围在任何时间点都没有显著差异。还有一项研究对比了激素注射治疗关节内病变（包括粘连性关节囊炎）的效果，发现短期疗效与注射位置无关（关节内对比关节外）。[27]该研究没有评估长期疗效。

有证据支持通过盂肱关节内激素注射短期内缓解症状。然而，如果疗效的确依赖于注射位置的精度，那么应该用影像辅助引导来确保注射位置正确。但是，激素注射没有表现出可以治疗特发性粘连性关节囊炎的效果，也没有表现出对该病的自然病程有长期的好处。

物理治疗

除了传统的物理治疗活动，冻结肩的仪器治疗（modalities）和其他治疗已经引起了越来越多研究者的兴趣。一篇 2011 年的文献总结了 2008 年的 Cochrane 综述和其他新的关于非手术和手术治疗的随机临床实验。[28]该文献的作者发现，在短期和长期随访中，中等质量的证据支持关节松动技术。此外，作者还发现，与安慰剂相比，激光疗法、电针针刺和干扰波针灸对缓解疼痛、改善功能和活动范围都有显著的短期积极影响。

一项 2009 年的研究探讨了动态夹板治疗粘连性关节囊炎的效果。[29]该项研究的规模相对较小，研究结果证明动态夹板的疗效与激素注射和标准理疗的疗效相当。但因相关数据过少而无法下结论。

以家中自行肩关节拉伸活动为主的理疗是冻结肩的常用疗法。一项前瞻性研究报道，钟摆式环转运动和被动肩关节拉伸活动（包括前举、外旋、水平内收和内旋）的长期随访满意率达 90%。糖尿病和男性是不良结果的相关因素。虽然还没有研究对比过拉伸活动和不特殊处理该病的结果有无差别，但是尝试活动对于冻结肩似乎仅有极小的风险和不利。

一项回顾性研究报道了 89 例患肩在医师监督下接受拉伸活动，其中 47 例患肩还需要接受激素注射。[30]23 例患者的 25 例患肩接受了麻醉下拉伸活动联合关节镜下关节囊松解。逐步逻辑回归分析显示，患者的发病年龄越轻、起始内旋受限越严重，越需要外科治疗。另外，这个研究结果提示，有糖尿病不意味着一定需要手术。

滑液补充

透明质酸（hyaluron）是关节内透明软骨和滑液的主要成分，FDA 已批准将其用于膝关节骨性关节炎。透明质酸治疗肩关节疾病的应用还不广泛。基础科学研究证明了通过补充滑液来治疗粘连性关节囊炎的可能性。有研究人员从特发性或继发性粘连性关节囊炎患者的盂肱关节囊提取成纤维细胞，再将透明质酸用于这些成纤维细胞，发现透明质酸对细胞增生和与粘连相关的前胶原及细胞因子的 mRNA 的表达有明显的抑制作用，这种抑制作用具有剂量依赖性。[31]

一项 2012 年的前瞻性随机临床实验评估了关节内透明质酸注射的疗效，研究包含 70 例粘连性关节囊炎患者。[32]3 个月后，实验组和对照组患者的疼痛、残疾、生活质量均得到明显改善，主被动活动范围呈线性改善。

一篇系统综述总结了关于透明质酸治疗冻结肩的 4 项 Ⅰ 级研究和 3 项 Ⅳ 级研究，发现在短期随访（平均 9 周）时，肩关节活动范围、Constant 肩关节评分明显改善、疼痛明显缓解。[33]该综述还报道，单独使用关节内透明质酸注射与关节内激素注射有相同的临床效果和活动范围改善。

关节扩张

关节腔扩张（arthrodilatation 或 arthrographic distention）的目标是通过向挛缩的肩关节内注入高渗液体以提高关节内压力、撑开关节囊。多项研究支持这种治疗。最近的 Cochrane 综述得出结论：有些不是很强的证据支持使用盐水和激素进行关节腔扩张，这样可以为粘连性关节囊炎提供短期的疼痛缓解、活动范围改善和功能改善。但是，这种方法是否优于其他方法还未可知。[34]

肩胛上神经阻滞

肩胛上神经除了支配冈上肌和冈下肌的运动，还支配盂肱关节囊的感觉。

最近的研究方向包括用肩胛上神经阻滞来缓解疼痛和提高对拉伸活动的耐受性。[35]近期有限的数据证明了这种方法缓解疼痛的短期效果，未来还需要进一步研究证明其缓解疼痛、治疗肩关节功能障碍的长期效果及患者的满意度。

手术治疗

麻醉下被动活动

非手术治疗可以成功治疗至少 95% 的特发性粘连性关节囊炎患者。大多数医师推荐非手术治疗至少 6 个月，若效果不佳再考虑手术治疗。许多研究阐述了麻醉下被动活动治疗非手术治疗无效的冻结肩。大多数文献报告被动活动的短期和中期效果。美国梅奥诊所的一项研究称，疼痛、活动范围和满意度的改善可以持续 15 年。[36]非手术治疗对糖尿病冻结肩患者的疗效不如非糖尿病冻结肩患者。一项回顾性病例对照研究对比了麻醉下被动活动对于糖尿病和非糖尿病冻结肩患者的疗效。[17]该项研究包含了原发性和继发性冻结肩患者，发现 50% 的糖尿病原发性冻结肩患者需要额外的被动活动，与此相比，只有 14% 的非糖尿病患者需要该治疗。虽然糖尿病组需要二次被动活动的比例很高，但是其中 85% 的患者对最终结果和活动范围满意，结局评分和非糖尿病组无统计学差异。

当非手术治疗失败后，病程进展到冻结期再开始麻醉下被动活动是很重要的。进行期被动活动会加重患者的症状。被动活动最近大多数在区域神经阻滞下进行，这样可以确保肌肉松弛并提供术后镇痛。被动活动时应该固定肩胛骨，以隔离盂肱关节，然后逐渐拉伸。小心预防医源性损伤，包括盂肱关节脱位、肩袖撕裂、骨折，尤其在治疗老年患者和骨质疏松患者时。按下列顺序进行被动活动是安全的，并且能够可靠地测量治疗前后的被动活动范围：牵拉和屈曲、内收、外旋、外展位外旋和内旋。治疗后继续努力拉伸非常重要。麻醉下被动活动后应进行 X 线检查排除骨性损伤。在一项前瞻性研究中，30 例原发性冻结肩患者在麻醉下被动活动后进行了关节镜检查。[37]所有患者均成功恢复肩关节被动活动范围。11 例患者关节囊上方撕裂，24 例患者关节囊前方撕裂至肩胛盂下，16 例患者关节囊后方撕裂。18 例患者未发现新发的关节损伤。医源性损伤包括 4 例上盂唇损伤、3 例肩胛下肌部分新鲜撕裂、4 例前盂唇撕脱（其中一例有小的骨软骨缺损）、2 例盂肱中韧带撕裂。该研究得出结论：麻醉下被动活动可以有效地恢复肩关节活动范围，但是有医源性损伤的风险，操作时要小心。

关节囊松解

关节镜下关节囊松解是一种比较成熟的治疗难治性冻结肩的方法，临床效果稳定。目前，这种方法逐渐取代了单纯被动活动，因为它可以提供直观的诊断、更精确的关节囊切开，并减小医源性损伤的风险。当关节挛缩时，关节镜下操作会很困难。因为关节囊增厚和挛缩，以及关节腔容积减小，进入盂肱关节变得更困难。减小的关节腔容积和滑膜炎使标准诊断性关节镜检查操作困难。在这个过程中，要先切开肩袖间隙的滑膜，以便看到肱二头肌腱、肩胛下肌腱和前方关节囊。

关节囊松解可以使用关节镜打孔器或烧灼装置。可以通过被动活动证明关节囊已完全松解，被动活动中可以触及残余的挛缩关节囊。一项 2012 年的研究描述了改良的关节囊松解常用技术，从肩峰下间隙开始松解而不是从盂肱关节[38]。关于是否应该常规松解后方关节囊和后下方肱骨韧带以达到 360° 松解，不同的文献持不同的观点。[39-40]

有了关节镜后，治疗特发性粘连性关节囊炎已不需要切开关节囊松解。然而，在一些外在因素（如肩关节不稳定修复后关节囊过紧、肱骨近端骨折）导致的继发性肩关节僵硬病例的治疗中，切开松解仍有一席之地。如果需要延长肩胛下肌腱以实现外旋，那么行切开手术还是有必要的。另外，关节镜下关节囊松解无法治疗广泛的三角肌下瘢痕形成。切开手术的缺点包括需要保护修复或延长后的肩胛下肌腱，这导致术后不能充分锻炼，从而影响活动范围。

有一项关于关节镜下关节囊松解的前瞻性研究，纳入了 73 例患者，术后随访 1 年。[41]平均 2.24 周后疼痛消失，平均 5.5 周后患肩活动范围限制不小于对侧的 10%，平均 8.9 周治疗完成。然而，37% 的患者术后接受了激素注射，11% 的患者最终症状复发，复发率与许多其他研究一致。关节镜下关节囊松解长期效果的回顾性研究显示，疼痛缓解、功能和活动范围明显改善。患侧活动范围与健侧相同。[42]

虽然肩关节僵硬和活动障碍是创伤性肩关节损伤和肩关节手术的常见后遗症，但是并不经常需要手术松解。有一项研究报道，345 例肩袖撕裂修复后的患者中有 3 例接受了关节镜下关节囊松解。[43]还有一项研究报道了 21 例创伤（其中 14 例为肱骨近端骨折）后冻结肩的患者接受了关节镜下关节囊和肩峰下松解。[44]肩关节活动和临床效果有明显改善。单纯软组织损伤而没有骨折的患者临床效果更好。一项 2010 年的研究探讨了关节镜下关节囊松解对不同病因引起的冻结肩的

疗效，发现其治疗特发性和创伤后僵硬的效果无差异。[5]与此不同的是，其治疗术后关节囊挛缩的效果明显比前两者差。

证据回顾

已经有很多分析粘连性关节囊炎治疗的系统综述和荟萃分析。在过去几年内，这类文献的数量超过了各种治疗方法的原始调查。这些综述将过去发表的研究以一种有序的方式呈现出来，评价这些研究的质量，并且总结了结果。

有一篇 2011 年的综述讨论了冻结肩的非手术治疗和手术治疗的有效性，这篇综述纳入了 5 篇 Cochrane 综述和 18 项随机对照实验。[28]注射激素、激光治疗、关节松动技术、关节腔扩张及肩胛上神经阻滞均可以改善冻结肩患者的短期疼痛、活动范围和总体疗效。物理治疗有长期效果。该综述的作者得出结论，缺乏高等级的文献和研究方法不一致这两个因素限制了对许多现有治疗方法的有效性的评估。

粘连性关节囊炎非手术治疗的证据表明，口服和注射激素对缓解疼痛和恢复功能有很好的短期效果，但是长期随访未发现任何效果。手术治疗的证据只有病例系列报道，这些证据表明手术治疗可以明显改善肩关节活动、缓解疼痛、改善功能，没有很大的并发症风险。

总结

特发性粘连性关节囊炎的特点是肩关节疼痛和盂肱关节活动受限。虽然研究者们已经知道了该病的自然史，但对其病因和病理生理学理解不足。大部分患者可以通过非手术治疗恢复，但该病通常病程迁延。各种非手术治疗的效果还不明确。难治性病例可以通过手术治疗（包括关节镜下关节囊松解）得到可靠的疗效。该病的自然史和相应的基础科学发现仍然存在争议，这使医师很难预测非手术治疗对哪些患者无效。研究者希望通过研究冻结肩的特点和后遗症来更好地理解

它的病因。

参考文献

[1] Duplay S:De la péri-arthrite scapula-humérale et des raideurs de l'épaule qui en sont al consequence. *Arch gen méd* 1872;20:513-542.

[2] Codman EA:*The Shoulder:Rupture of the Supraspinatus Tendon and Other Lesions in or About the Subacromial Bursa.* Boston, MA, Thomas Todd and Co, 1934, pp 216-224.

[3] Neviaser JS:Adhesive capsulitis of the shoulder:A study of pathological findings in periarthritis of the shoulder. *J Bone Joint Surg Am* 1945;27-A(2):211-222.

[4] Zuckerman JD, Cuomo F:Frozen shoulder, in Matsen FA III, Fu FH, Hawkins RJ, eds:*The Shoulder:A Balance of Mobility and Stability.* Rosemont, IL, American Academy of Orthopaedic Surgeons. 1993, pp 253-267.

[5] Elhassan B, Ozbaydar M, Massimini D, Higgins L, Warner JJ:Arthroscopic capsular release for refractory shoulder stiffness:A critical analysis of effectiveness in specific etiologies. *J Shoulder Elbow Surg* 2010;19(4):580-587.

This retrospective case series found that arthroscopic capsular release is an effective treatment of refractory shoulder stiffness and showed that patients with idiopathic and posttraumatic shoulder stiffness have better outcomes than patients with postsurgical stiffness. Level of evidence:IV.

[6] Hakim AJ, Cherkas LF, Spector TD, MacGregor AJ:Genetic associations between frozen shoulder and tennis elbow:A female twin study. *Rheumatology (Oxford)* 2003;42(6):739-742.

[7] Griggs SM, Ahn A, Green A:Idiopathic adhesive capsulitis:A prospective functional outcome study of nonoperative treatment. *J Bone Joint Surg Am* 2000;82-A(10):1398-1407.

[8] Hand GC, Athanasou NA, Matthews T, Carr AJ:The pathology of frozen shoulder. *J Bone Joint Surg Br* 2007;89(7):928-932.

Biopsies obtained from tissues of the rotator cuff interval during arthroscopic release were analyzed and found to include fibroblasts, proliferating fibroblasts, and chronic inflammatory cells, including mast cells, T cells, B cells, and macrophages. In addition, the authors found increased vascularity from angiogenesis and positive results from S100 staining consistent with the presence of nerve cells.

[9] Gerber C, Werner CM, Macy JC, Jacob HA, Nyffeler RW:Effect of selective capsulorrhaphy on the passive range of motion of the glenohumeral joint. *J Bone Joint Surg Am* 2003;85-A(1):48-55.

[10] Lee SY, Park J, Song SW:Correlation of MR arthrographic findings and range of shoulder motions in patients with frozen shoulder. *AJR Am J Roentgenol* 2012;198(1):173-179.

The thickness of the coracohumeral ligament and the capsule in axillary recess seen with MR arthrography were significantly greater in patients with frozen shoulder than patients in a control group. Additionally, coracohumeral ligament thickness correlated with clinical range-of-motion limitations. Level of evidence:IV.

[11] Song KD, Kwon JW, Yoon YC, Choi SH:Indirect MR arthrographic findings of adhesive capsulitis. *AJR Am J Roentgenol* 2011;197(6):W1105-9.

An abundance of enhancing tissue in the rotator cuff interval and thickening and enhancement of the axillary recess were found to be signs suggesting adhesive capsulitis on indirect magnetic resonance arthrography. Level of evidence:IV.

[12] Loeffler BJ, Brown SL, D'Alessandro DF, Fleischli JE, Connor PM:Incidence of false positive rotator cuff pathology in MRIs of patients with adhesive capsulitis. *Orthopedics* 2011;34(5):362.

MRI interpretation of the rotator cuff was compared with the rotator cuff status intraoperatively for patients who underwent capsular release for frozen shoulder. MRI interpretations predicted a 57.9% incidence of rotator cuff pathology compared with a true incidence of 13.2%. Level of evidence:IV.

[13] Carbone S, Gumina S, Vestri AR, Postacchini R:Coracoid pain test:A new clinical sign of shoulder adhesive capsulitis. *Int Orthop* 2010;34(3):385-388.

Patients with adhesive capsulitis were clinically evaluated to establish whether pain elicited by pressure on the coracoid may be considered a sign of this condition. With respect to patients in a control group, the sensitivity and the specificity were 0.99 and 0.98, respectively. Level of evidence:IV.

[14] Anakwenze OA, Hsu JE, Kim JS, Abboud JA:Acromioclavicular joint pain in patients with adhesive capsulitis:A prospective outcome study. *Orthopedics* 2011;34(9):e556-e560.

In adhesive capsulitis, there is not only compensatory

scapulothoracic motion but also acromioclavicular motion. The authors hypothesized this would result in transient symptoms at the acromioclavicular joint, which abated as the adhesive capsulitis resolved and glenohumeral motion improved. Level of evidence:III.

[15] Bridgman JF:Periarthritis of the shoulder and diabetes mellitus. *Ann Rheum Dis* 1972;31(1):69-71.

[16] Walker-Bone K, Palmer KT, Reading I, Coggon D, Cooper C:Prevalence and impact of musculoskeletal disorders of the upper limb in the general population. *Arthritis Rheum* 2004;51(4):642-651.

[17] Jenkins EF, Thomas WJ, Corcoran JP, et al:The outcome of manipulation under general anesthesia for the management of frozen shoulder in patients with diabetes mellitus. *J Shoulder Elbow Surg* 2012;21(11):1492-1498.

This retrospective case-control study showed improvement, including no difference between patients with and without diabetes treated with manipulation for frozen shoulder. However, a repeat procedure was required in 36% of the patients with diabetes compared with 15% of the control patients. Level of evidence:III.

[18] Yian EH, Contreras R, Sodl JF:Effects of glycemic control on prevalence of diabetic frozen shoulder. *J Bone Joint Surg Am* 2012;94(10):919-923.

This retrospective analysis with statistical review showed no association between the hemoglobin A1c level and the prevalence of frozen shoulder in the studied diabetic population. Level of evidence:II.

[19] Carette S, Moffet H, Tardif J, et al:Intraarticular corticosteroids, supervised physiotherapy, or a combination of the two in the treatment of adhesive capsulitis of the shoulder:A placebo-controlled trial. *Arthritis Rheum* 2003;48(3):829-838.

[20] Lorbach O, Anagnostakos K, Scherf C, Seil R, Kohn D, Pape D:Nonoperative management of adhesive capsulitis of the shoulder:Oral cortisone application versus intra-articular cortisone injections. *J Shoulder Elbow Surg* 2010;19(2):172-179.

Intra-articular injections of glucocorticoids showed superior results in shoulder outcome scores, range of motion, and patient satisfaction compared with a short course of oral corticosteroids for the treatment of adhesive capsulitis in this randomized controlled trial. Level of evidence:I.

[21] Roh YH, Yi SR, Noh JH, et al:Intra-articular corticosteroid injection in diabetic patients with adhesive capsulitis:A randomized controlled trial. *Knee Surg Sports Traumatol Arthrosc* 2012;20(10):1947-1952.

This randomized clinical trial concluded that a corticosteroid injection decreased pain and functional outcome scores in the early treatment of adhesive capsulitis in patients with diabetes compared with a control group of patients. Level of evidence:II.

[22] Blanchard V, Barr S, Cerisola FL:The effectiveness of corticosteroid injections compared with physiotherapeutic interventions for adhesive capsulitis:A systematic review. *Physiotherapy* 2010;96(2):95-107.

Six studies were included in this systematic review, which suggests that corticosteroid injections have greater effect compared with physical therapy interventions in short-term treatments of adhesive capsulitis. This finding decreased over time, however, with only a small effect in favor of injections at longer time points studied.

[23] Shah N, Lewis M:Shoulder adhesive capsulitis:Systematic review of randomised trials using multiple corticosteroid injections. *Br J Gen Pract* 2007;57(541):662-667.

This systematic review of randomized clinical trials concluded that multiple additional corticosteroid injections provided pain reduction, improved function, and increased range of shoulder motion in the treatment of adhesive capsulitis for up to 16 weeks after the initial injection. Level of evidence:I.

[24] Sethi PM, Kingston S, ElAttrache N:Accuracy of anterior intra-articular injection of the glenohumeral joint. *Arthroscopy* 2005;21(1):77-80.

[25] Tobola A, Cook C, Cassas KJ, et al :Accuracy of glenohumeral joint injections:Comparing approach and experience of provider. *J Shoulder Elbow Surg* 2011;20(7):1147-1154.

The accuracies of posterior, supraclavicular, and anterior approaches used for glenohumeral injections were compared in a case-controlled study. The anterior approach was the most accurate, but neither provider experience nor confidence was associated with success. Level of evidence:III.

[26] Oh JH, Oh CH, Choi JA, Kim SH, Kim JH, Yoon JP:Comparison of glenohumeral and subacromial steroid injection in primary frozen shoulder:A prospective, randomized short-term comparison study. *J Shoulder Elbow Surg* 2011;20(7):1034-1040.

This randomized controlled trial showed that although patients with frozen shoulder treated with intraarticular glenohumeral injection showed lower pain visual analog scale scores at 3 weeks, no difference was seen at 6 and 12 weeks between these patients and those being administered subacromial injections. Level of evidence:I.

[27] Hegedus EJ, Zavala J, Kissenberth M, et al:Positive outcomes with intra-articular glenohumeral injections are independent of accuracy. *J Shoulder Elbow Surg* 2010;19(6):795-801.

This prospective cohort demonstrated that despite documented inaccuracy of glenohumeral injections, short-term follow-up showed improvement in pain and Disabilities of the Arm, Shoulder and Hand scores in patients with various shoulder pathologies. Level of evidence:II.

[28] Favejee MM, Huisstede BM, Koes BW:Frozen shoulder:The effectiveness of conservative and surgical interventions—systematic review. *Br J Sports Med* 2011;45(1):49-56.

This review found strong evidence for the short-term effectiveness of steroid injections and laser therapy in frozen shoulder. Moderate evidence was found for steroid injections in midterm follow-up, mobilization techniques in the long term, and the effectiveness of arthrographic distension. Level of evidence:III.

[29] Gaspar PD, Willis FB:Adhesive capsulitis and dynamic splinting:A controlled, cohort study. *BMC Musculoskel Disord* 2009;10:111.

This controlled cohort study showed the efficacy of dynamic splinting as an effective home therapy adjunct to physical therapy. This additional end-range stretching combined with standardized physical therapy was considered to be responsible for the greatest change in external rotation. Level of evidence:II.

[30] Rill BK, Fleckenstein CM, Levy MS, Nagesh V, Hasan SS:Predictors of outcome after nonoperative and operative treatment of adhesive capsulitis. *Am J Sports Med* 2011;39(3):567-574.

This cohort study concurrently evaluated patients with adhesive capsulitis who were treated surgically and nonsurgically. The two cohorts showed similar improvement in final outcomes scores, illustrating that although most patients improved with nonsurgical treatment, refractory cases responded well to surgical intervention. Level of evidence:III.

[31] Nago M, Mitsui Y, Gotoh M, et al:Hyaluronan modulates cell proliferation and mRNA expression of adhesion-related procollagens and cytokines in glenohumeral synovial/capsular fibroblasts in adhesive cap-

sulitis. *J Orthop Res* 2010;28(6):726-731.

This in vitro study examined the effects of hyaluronan on glenohumeral synovial and capsular fibroblasts from patients with frozen shoulder. Hyaluronan modulated cell proliferation and the expression of adhesion-related procollagens and cytokines, suggesting it may prevent the progression of adhesion formation.

[32] Hsieh LF, Hsu WC, Lin YJ, Chang H-L, Chen C-C, Huang V:Addition of intra-articular hyaluronate injection to physical therapy program produces no extra benefits in patients with adhesive capsulitis of the shoulder:A randomized controlled trial. *Arch Phys Med Rehabil* 2012;93(6):957-964.

This randomized clinical trial found that hyaluronate injections did not significantly change active or passive range of motion, pain, disability, or quality of life outcomes for adhesive capsulitis patients treated with physical therapy. Level of evidence:I.

[33] Harris JD, Griesser MJ, Copelan A, Jones GL:Treatment of adhesive capsulitis with intra-articular hyaluronate:A systematic review. *Int J Shoulder Surg* 2011;5(2):31-37.

This systematic review concluded that short-term clinical outcomes for patients with adhesive capsulitis treated with hyaluronate injections are better than control groups but equivalent to intra-articular corticosteroid injection. Level of evidence:IV.

[34] Buchbinder R, Green S, Youd JM, Johnston RV, Cumpston M:Arthrographic distension for adhesive capsulitis (frozen shoulder). *Cochrane Database Syst Rev* 2008;1:CD007005.

[35] Dahan TH, Fortin L, Pelletier M, Petit M, Vadeboncoeur R, Suissa S:Double blind randomized clinical trial examining the efficacy of bupivacaine suprascapular nerve blocks in frozen shoulder. *J Rheumatol* 2000;27(6):1464-1469.

[36] Farrell CM, Sperling JW, Cofield RH:Manipulation for frozen shoulder:Long-term results. *J Shoulder Elbow Surg* 2005;14(5):480-484.

[37] Loew M, Heichel TO, Lehner B:Intraarticular lesions in primary frozen shoulder after manipulation under general anesthesia. *J Shoulder Elbow Surg* 2005;14(1):16-21.

[38] Lafosse L, Boyle S, Kordasiewicz B, Guttierez-Arramberi M, Fritsch B, Meller R:Arthroscopic arthrolysis for recalcitrant frozen shoulder:A lateral approach. *Arthroscopy* 2012;28(7):916-923.

The authors describe a technique for arthroscopic capsular release that begins in the subacromial space followed by intra-articular entry to perform a 360° capsular release. Level of evidence:IV.

[39] Chen J, Chen S, Li Y, Hua Y, Li H:Is the extended release of the inferior glenohumeral ligament necessary for frozen shoulder? *Arthroscopy* 2010;26(4):529-535.
This randomized controlled study compared arthroscopic capsular with and without posterior capsular release. The addition of posterior release did not improve patient function or range of motion at 6 months. However, extended release did improve range of motion more rapidly in the short term. Level of evidence:I.

[40] Jerosch J:360 degrees arthroscopic capsular release in patients with adhesive capsulitis of the glenohumeral joint—indication, surgical technique, results. *Knee Surg Sports Traumatol Arthrosc* 2001;9(3):178-186.

[41] Watson L, Dalziel R, Story I:Frozen shoulder:A 12-month clinical outcome trial. *J Shoulder Elbow Surg* 2000;9(1):16-22.

[42] Le Lievre HM, Murrell GA:Long-term outcomes after arthroscopic capsular release for idiopathic adhesive capsulitis. *J Bone Joint Surg Am* 2012;94(13):1208-1216.
Patients with idiopathic adhesive capsulitis treated with an arthroscopic capsular release had significant improvements in shoulder range of motion, pain frequency and severity, and function. These improvements were maintained and/or enhanced at 7-year follow-up. Level of evidence:IV.

[43] Namdari S, Green A:Range of motion limitation after rotator cuff repair. *J Shoulder Elbow Surg* 2010;19(2):290-296.
This case-control study followed patients after rotator cuff repair and found that preoperative limited range of motion, diabetes, and worker's compensation claims were all associated with postoperative loss of motion. Level of evidence:III.

[44] Levy O, Webb M, Even T, Venkateswaran B, Funk L, Copeland SA:Arthroscopic capsular release for posttraumatic shoulder stiffness. *J Shoulder Elbow Surg* 2008;17(3):410-414.
This study reports the results of arthroscopic capsular release in 21 patients who presented with posttraumatic stiff shoulders resistant to nonsurgical therapy. Improvements were observed in range of motion and patient satisfaction. Level of evidence:IV.

第五十二章　肩关节和肘关节手术的麻醉和镇痛

E. David Bravos, MD

引言

肩关节和肘关节手术围术期管理有几个挑战。鉴于患者年龄分布广泛、合并症多、可能合并神经系统疾病，因此术者和麻醉科医师共同制订手术计划是必要的。术后疼痛治疗是最重要的问题之一。除了使用传统的阿片类和非阿片类镇痛药物，臂丛神经的外周神经阻滞（PNB）也是术后镇痛非常有效的方法，因为大多数手术可以通过单一入路的臂丛神经阻滞覆盖。在过去几年内，随着超声引导技术的进步，PNB 的应用越来越多。作为一种镇痛方法，与单用静脉内阿片类药物相比，PNB 镇痛效果佳、减少了阿片类药物相关的不良反应、患者满意度更高。[1-2] 在某些肘关节手术中，PNB 可能被用作术中麻醉，但在肩关节手术中，PNB 通常被用作术后镇痛，常联合全身麻醉或深度镇静。预计术后会出现中、重度疼痛时，可以使用持续外周神经阻滞（CPNB）。最近，CPNB 也被用于门诊和住院患者的早期理疗辅助和冻结肩的被动活动。

术前管理的一般原则

鉴于肩肘手术患者可能涵盖各类人群，从年轻健壮的运动员，到有重大合并症的老年人，因此医师术前必须仔细评估。除了众所周知的 PNB 禁

忌证，某些合并症患者也不宜使用 PNB。因为臂丛神经阻滞可以引起膈神经麻痹，所以患有重大肺部疾病的患者可能不宜接受 PNB。研究显示，斜角肌间阻滞 100% 会引起膈神经阻滞，锁骨上阻滞 80% 会引起膈神经阻滞。[3-5] 这可能导致肺功能下降 27%（如用力肺活量和第一秒用力呼气量）。[6] 另外，对侧膈肌轻瘫（diaphragmatic paresis）的患者不能使用影响膈神经的臂丛神经阻滞。其他禁忌证还包括喉返神经麻痹，因为斜角肌间阻滞和锁骨上神经阻滞可能导致喉返神经麻痹。

已患有神经损伤的患者必须评估是否适合PNB。如果 PNB 过程中可能伤到了神经或者需要立刻或持续术后神经检查，麻醉医师必须和术者沟通。

术前还应考虑患者是否需要预防性使用镇痛药，可以使用塞来昔布、加巴喷丁和对乙酰氨基酚。

术中管理的一般原则

肩肘手术的术中麻醉可以采用全身麻醉、区域麻醉或两者联合。有几个因素决定患者术中是否可以单用区域麻醉或必须联合全身麻醉，后者需要气道管理、气管内插管、喉罩通气或深度镇静。麻醉医师必须理解上肢的解剖和神经支配，以及不同的臂丛神经阻滞方法的麻醉范围。

选择合适的 PNB 方法

主要的臂丛神经阻滞方法有 4 种，根据阻滞

的解剖位置而命名（图 52-1）。这 4 种方法阻滞臂丛神经的不同水平，因而有不同的上肢麻醉和镇痛分布范围。肩部和肱骨近端的手术最好用斜角肌间阻滞。斜角肌间阻滞可以阻滞 C3、C4 神经根。C3、C4 神经根虽然不参与臂丛神经的组成，但参与组成颈丛浅支。颈丛浅支包含锁骨上神经，锁骨上神经支配肩胛角的感觉。在 C6 水平阻滞时，需要提高局部麻醉药浓度以使其扩散。这样可以覆盖至肩角的切口。如果局部麻醉药体积足够，可以用单次锁骨上阻滞满足肩部手术要求；但是，如果需要 CPNB，那么最好不要选择锁骨上阻滞。因为 CPNB 通常需要术后小剂量使用局部麻醉药。锁骨下和腋窝阻滞不适合肩部和肱骨近端的手术。对于肱骨远端和肘部的手术，可选择锁骨下或锁骨上阻滞。而斜角肌间阻滞可能不

是最好的选择，因为斜角肌间阻滞会遗留 C8 和 T1 神经根，这使尺神经没有被阻滞。然而，低位斜角肌间阻滞配合足够容量的局部麻醉药可能覆盖到 C8、T1 水平。腋窝阻滞最好用于肘关节以下的手术。

其他局部麻醉技术

除了臂丛的 PNB，其他局部麻醉技术包括肩峰下（滑囊）或关节内局部麻醉药浸润，以及肩胛上神经阻滞联合或不联合腋神经阻滞。最近有一篇系统综述研究了不同局部麻醉技术的效果和减少阿片类药物使用的潜能。[7]

目前，肩峰下 / 关节内浸润的镇痛效果尚不明确。重要的是，对于持续注入局部麻醉药引起医源性软骨溶解的担忧已经导致这种方法被弃用。肩胛上神经阻滞与安慰剂相比可以提供显著的镇痛效

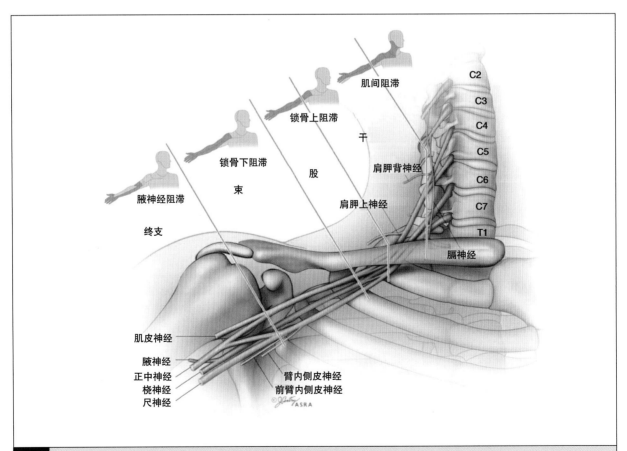

图 52-1 理想化的臂丛神经分布图。各种入路决定各种臂丛神经阻滞方法及其预期皮肤麻醉分布范围。经允许引自 Neal JM: Upper extremity regional anesthesia: Essentials of our understanding. *Reg Anesth Pain Med* 2009;34(2):134–170.

果。联合腋神经阻滞可能提高肩胛上神经阻滞的镇痛效果。虽然这种方法不及斜角肌间阻滞有效，但是可以用于患有重大肺部疾病的患者，对于这类患者，要优先考虑避免膈神经麻痹。肩部手术最有效的局部麻醉技术是基础小剂量持续注入的斜角肌间阻滞联合患者操控的即刻大剂量注入。

术中麻醉技术

在肩关节手术中，单纯臂丛神经阻滞可能不足以覆盖皮肤和骨结构，所以 PNB 常用于术后镇痛，且常联合全身麻醉或深度镇静。这通常取决于患者体位（沙滩椅位或侧卧位）和麻醉医师控制气道的能力。

在肘关节手术中，臂丛神经阻滞可以完全满足所有手术的要求，因而可单独用作麻醉，这同样取决于患者的体位。需要的话，这种方法可以

让患者保持清醒或轻度镇静。侧卧位或仰卧位的患者需要更完备的气道管理。

体位

肩部手术的典型体位是沙滩椅位或侧卧位。无论什么技术，小心地摆放体位和理解潜在并发症都是最重要的。沙滩椅位的优点包括：便于摆放、减小牵拉造成神经损伤的风险、便于转换为开放手术。[8]沙滩椅位是仰卧位的一种，床头根据需要抬高 20°~30° 到 80°。可以使用手术台，使髋关节屈曲 45°~60°、膝关节屈曲 30°。此外，也可以伸直膝关节，减少下肢静脉充血、增加回心血量。沙滩椅位的患者可能突然出现明显的低血压和心动过缓，有心血管衰竭（cardiovascular collapse）的报道。[9-10]这是由 Bezold–Jarisch 反射造成的（图 52-2），源于血液淤积在下肢静脉造成

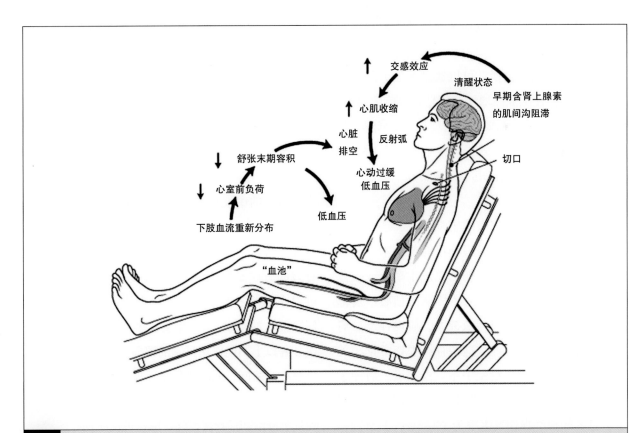

图 52-2 低血压 / 心动过缓的机制。接受斜角肌间臂丛神经阻滞联合深度镇静且处于沙滩椅位的患者，在麻醉中可能出现低血压和心动过缓。这种现象的假设机制是前负荷相对不足，这源于坐位（导致回心血量不足）和内源性、外源性肾上腺素导致的心室过度收缩。猛烈收缩的"空"心脏导致反射性心动过缓和低血压。经允许引自 Neal JM: Essentials of our understanding. *Reg Anesth Pain Med* 2009;34（2）:134-170.

静脉回流减少。心率和心脏收缩的代偿性增加导致心脏内受体激活，从而造成矛盾性地副交感神经兴奋性增加及交感神经兴奋性下降，最终导致心动过缓、血管舒张、血压下降和心血管衰竭。PNB 使用的局部麻醉药中包含的肾上腺素可能加剧这种情况。[11]治疗包括充足补液，如果患者出现反射性心动过速，则使用 β 受体阻滞剂，如果患者出现严重心动过缓，则使用阿托品或肾上腺素。[12]另外，使用沙滩椅位还应提防中枢神经系统终末器官缺血，包括脑缺血、眼肌麻痹和视野缺损。[13-14]其确切机制未知，有研究称这源于体位性低血压，术中小腿血压监测不能发现这种低血压。[15]因为头部和下肢的静水压差大，所以脑灌注压可能和术中监测的血压大相径庭。而关节镜手术中为了获得清晰的术野需要进一步降低血压，因此在关节镜手术中这种情况更严重。其他原因可能还包括被动活动头部导致颈部血管机械性梗阻。

侧卧位的优点包括：可以通过牵拉上肢获得更好的视野，使脑灌注增加、更易获得前后通道。侧卧位的缺点包括：需要气道管理和全身麻醉、有拉伤神经的风险、难以转为切开手术。[8]肘关节手术可以根据需要使用仰卧位、侧卧位、俯卧位。

神经系统并发症

神经损伤可以是细微的感觉异常，也可以是运动功能完全丧失。神经损伤可能与手术、患者本人和麻醉相关。神经损伤的总发生率低，一旦发生，会严重影响患者和手术团队的信心。肩部手术最常损伤的神经包括腋神经、肌皮神经、肩胛上神经和肩胛下神经。这些神经损伤常见于关节置换和关节前方不稳定手术。据报道，肩袖手术患者的神经损伤发生率为 1%~2%，前方不稳定手术患者的神经损伤发生率为 1%~8%，关节置换患者的神经损伤发生率为 1%~4%。[16-19]使用 PNB 后，神经系统并发症是来源于手术还是麻醉将难以判断。具体来说，斜角肌间阻滞通常在 C6 水平。

肩部手术最易损伤的神经源自 C5、C6 及 C7 神经根。PNB 造成神经损伤的发生率小于 3%。[20]因此，如果患者神经损伤风险高，那么术者和麻醉医师必须与其坦诚沟通。术前应该进行完善的神经系统检查。虽然可以术后使用单次神经阻滞或术前外周神经置管，但是如果有神经损伤的可能或需要术后监测神经，那么术后神经系统检查恢复正常前不能给药。

术后镇痛

镇痛不足不仅会造成不良的心理和生理影响，还会干扰早期理疗和康复，可能增加慢性术后疼痛的风险。[21-23]虽然阿片类药物有很多众所周知的不良反应，包括恶心、呕吐、瘙痒、淡漠、便秘和呼吸抑制，但是阿片类药物仍是围术期治疗疼痛的重要药物。除了这些众所周知的不良反应，术后有中重度疼痛的手术使用大剂量阿片类药物后，可以延长住院时间或增加门诊患者意外住院的概率。为了减少不良反应的发生，可以联合使用多种不同机制的镇痛药、使用预防性和多模式镇痛策略。

预防性和多模式镇痛

预防性镇痛指的是预防和减弱创伤及随后的炎症带来的中枢感受。[24]虽然研究者们最初认为伤害前给药比伤害后给药更有效，但临床实验并不都支持这一观点。[25-26]最近，研究者们认为最有效的方法是整个围术期使用多模式镇痛，这样可以在术前、术中、术后减少传入中枢的伤害性信息传入的触发。[27]相反，多模式镇痛使用 2 种或 2 种以上不同作用机制的镇痛药，这些药物的效果叠加或协同，同时降低了任何一种药物的不良反应。[28]更多研究者强调区域麻醉技术用阿片类或非阿片类麻醉药治疗爆发痛（breakthrough pain）。[29]

阿片类药物

阿片类药物是最常用的麻醉药之一，可以通过多途径给药（口服、静脉注射、肌内注射、皮下注射、肛门给药、黏膜给药和神经轴索给药）。阿片类药物没有镇痛天花板效应（ceiling effect），但是其镇痛效果被不良反应（恶心、呕吐、瘙痒、淡漠、便秘、呼吸抑制）所限制。肩肘手术术后患者一般通过静脉注射、口服或肌内注射给药。

肠外给药

与其他途径相比，静脉给药起效快，镇痛效果可靠，可以快速达到有效药物浓度。中重度疼痛患者可能需要静脉注射阿片类药物，最常用的给药途径是静脉内患者自控镇痛（IV PCA）。与护士给药相比，这种给药方式在缓解疼痛、改善患者满意度方面的效果可能更好。[30]

IV PCA 的程序需要的变量包括单次给药剂量（bolus）或需要量（demand dose）、锁定间隔（lockout interval）、基础输注量（background infusion）（表 52-1）。最理想的设置还不清楚，但是遵守几个基础原则可能增加镇痛效果并减小潜在的超量风险。理想的单次给药剂量或需要量取决于阿片类药物的效能，应该在几次患者控制给药后足够减轻疼痛。剂量太小会导致镇痛不足，剂量太大会导致包括呼吸抑制在内的不良反应增加。锁定间隔取决于阿片类药物的阵痛起效（analgesic onset）和峰值效应（peak effect），应该在患者前次给药起效后才能再次给药。锁定间隔太长会导致镇痛不足，太短会导致药效叠加。

持续或基础输注不推荐用于首次使用阿片类药物的患者（opiate-naïve patients）。过去认为，患者睡眠不能自行给药时，持续输注可以改善镇痛。然而，持续输注可能导致不良反应（如呼吸抑制）增加，且没有发现持续输注可以改善镇痛。[31-32]持续输注可能对阿片类药物耐药的患者有益处。

使用 IV PCA 时要知道的一个重要概念是，同一剂量不能用于所有患者。[33]疼痛的治疗是一个动态过程。[31-32]不同个体可能有不同的镇痛要求，同一个个体在围术期不同时间的镇痛要求可能改变，术后 24~48 小时尤其如此。需要经常评估患者的疼痛以调整镇痛方案。

表 52-1

阿片类药物的静脉内患者自控镇痛

药物	单次给药剂量	锁定间隔	基础输注量 a
吗啡	0.5~2.5 mg	5~10 min	1~10 mg/h
芬太尼	10~20 μg	5~10 min	20~100 μg/h
盐酸氢吗啡酮	0.1~0.2 mg	5~10 min	0.1~0.2 mg/h

注：a 持续输注不推荐用于首次使用阿片类药物的患者。

肠内给药

只要患者可以耐受口服给药，口服阿片类药物可以用来治疗中重度疼痛，但是口服给药不如静脉给药可靠和便于控制剂量。口服剂型包括速释剂型和控释剂型（表 52-2）。即刻释放剂型可以

表 52-2

口服阿片类药物

药物	单次剂量	间隔时间	评价
羟考酮（速释）	5~10 mg	4~6 h	24 小时内用药不超过 4 次，否则易出现药效叠加，阿片类药物不良反应风险增加
羟考酮（控释）	10~20 mg	12 h	可联合使用对乙酰氨基酚或阿司匹林
吗啡（控释）	15~30 mg	8~12 h	24 小时内用药不超过 4 次，否则易出现药效叠加，阿片类药物不良反应风险增加
氢可酮	5~10 mg	4~6 h	可联合使用对乙酰氨基酚
盐酸氢吗啡酮	2~4 mg	4~6 h	
可待因	30~60 mg	4 h	可联合使用对乙酰氨基酚或阿司匹林
曲马多	50~100 mg	6 h	

治疗中重度疼痛，但需要每 4~6 小时给药 1 次以维持血药浓度。不按时给药会导致不必要的疼痛。使用速释剂型时，有指南给出固定剂量。[34] 控释剂型可以使血药浓度更稳定、作用时间更长和波动更少。有研究者在使用控释剂型的同时使用速释剂型来缓解爆发痛。

曲马多

曲马多是一种人工合成的镇痛药，其结构与可待因和吗啡相关。曲马多直接作用于 μ 受体，并阻止去甲肾上腺素和 5- 羟色胺的摄取，参与疼痛的脊髓抑制。[35-36] 曲马多虽然不如吗啡有效，但其呼吸抑制、便秘、药物依赖等不良反应的发生率更低。[37-38] 与其他阿片类药物相比，曲马多在治疗中度术后疼痛方面效果不错。曲马多可用于多模式镇痛，也可用于不能耐受阿片类药物的患者。

非阿片类镇痛药

非阿片类镇痛药在治疗术后疼痛方面有重要地位，是多模式镇痛方案的一部分。恰当使用非阿片类镇痛药可以减少阿片类药物的用量，在减少阿片类药物不良反应的同时增强了镇痛效果（表 52-3）。

非甾体抗炎药

非甾体抗炎药（NSAIDs）有镇痛、抗炎、退热的效果，能有效治疗非手术原因造成的疼痛。随着酮咯酸和双氯芬酸这样的静脉 NSAIDs 制剂的

出现，NSAIDs 越来越多地应用于术后患者，研究显示其镇痛效果与阿片类药物相似。[39-40] 前列腺素是急性炎症和疼痛反应的化学介质，NSAIDs 的作用机制就是通过抑制环氧化酶（COX）来减少前列腺素分泌。NSAIDs 主要作用于外周神经系统，但是也作用于中枢的伤害性感受（nociception）。[41] COX-1 是结构性表达的，通过产生前列腺素 E_2 参与胃黏膜的保护，并通过血栓素（thromboxane）参与血小板的聚集。COX-2 是诱导性表达的，在炎症和发热时产生。非特异性 COX 抑制剂（如酮咯酸）抑制 COX-1 和 COX-2 同工酶，选择性 COX 抑制剂（塞来昔布）仅抑制 COX-2 同工酶。COX-2 对凝血系统的影响很小，围术期可以安全使用，很少需要担心出血。

虽然 NSAIDs 可以有效镇痛，但是不良反应限制了它的使用。围术期最令人担心的并发症是血小板功能障碍、肾功能不全及胃肠道出血。另外，也有研究者担心 NSAIDs 用于骨科手术会影响骨愈合，因为炎症反应和前列腺素参与骨愈合过程。[42] 不良反应是由于 COX 被抑制引起的。血栓素合成被抑制会导致血小板聚集受限，增加手术出血的风险。前列腺素合成被抑制会导致胃肠道黏膜保护丧失而出血，也会导致肾小动脉血管收缩从而引起肾功能障碍。所有 COX 抑制剂都会影响肾功能，但是选择性 COX-2 抑制剂可以减小血小板功能障碍和胃肠道出血的风险。NSAIDs

表 52-3

非阿片类镇痛药

镇痛药	单次剂量	间隔	24 小时最大剂量	评价
阿司匹林	325~1000 mg	4~6 h	4000 mg	
对乙酰氨基酚	500~100 mg	4~6 h	4000 mg	
布洛芬	200~800 mg	4~6 h	3200 mg	
萘普生	500 mg	12 h	1000 mg	
塞来昔布	200~400 mg	12 h	800 mg	
酮咯酸	15~30 mg	6 h	60~120 mg	如果患者体重 < 50 kg 或年龄 > 65 岁，则 15 mg；如果患者体重 > 50 kg 或年龄 < 65 岁，则 30 mg；疗程不应超过 5 天
加巴喷丁	300~1200 mg			理想的镇痛剂量未知
普瑞巴林	150~ 300 mg			理想的镇痛剂量未知

的使用应该根据患者自身情况和手术具体分析。

对乙酰氨基酚

对乙酰氨基酚是一种非阿片类镇痛药，通过抑制 COX，减少中枢前列腺素分泌。[43]在美国，对乙酰氨基酚过去只有口服和直肠给药两种剂型，最近刚出现静脉剂型。对乙酰氨基酚虽然抗炎效果差，但是镇痛和退热效果显著，且胃肠道、肾、血小板不良反应少。对乙酰氨基酚已经在很多类型的手术（如骨折手术）中做过研究。与安慰剂组相比，对乙酰氨基酚组的 24 小时吗啡总用量减少，疼痛评分和患者满意度得到改善。[44-45]另外，对乙酰氨基酚和 NSAIDs 联合使用的效果比单独使用对乙酰氨基酚或 NSAIDs 的效果好，[46]按计划定时给药的效果比按需给药的效果更好。[47]虽然对乙酰氨基酚有镇痛效果且减少了阿片类药物的用量，但是其减少阿片类药物不良反应的作用并未得到公认。[48-49]

加巴喷丁和普瑞巴林

加巴喷丁和普瑞巴林是 γ- 氨基丁酸类似物，作用于电压门控钙离子通道，真实镇痛效果未知。有多项研究显示，术前给 1 次加巴喷丁可以减少阿片类药物的用量，并且可以改善休息和运动时的疼痛评分。[50-53]另外，有一项研究显示加巴喷丁可以减少阿片类药物相关的不良反应（如呕吐），但其他研究没有得出这样的结果。与之类似，用普瑞巴林、安慰剂、400mg 布洛芬治疗拔牙引起的疼痛时，普瑞巴林组与另两组相比，疼痛缓解、疼痛强度差异和疼痛缓解强度差异显著降低。[54-55]

氯胺酮

氯胺酮是一种 N- 甲基 -D- 天冬氨酸受体拮抗剂，手术室中用作麻醉药。在发现 N- 甲基 -D- 天冬氨酸受体及其在中枢致敏和慢性术后疼痛中的作用后，研究者们重新开始了将氯胺酮用于术后镇痛的研究。[56]然而，因为麻醉中可能出现的致幻作用和心血管作用，氯胺酮的使用受到了限制。[57]全身麻醉下人工全膝关节置换的患者，术

中或术后 48 小时内用小剂量氯胺酮与用安慰剂相比，前者的休息和运动时的疼痛评分更低，且膝关节能屈曲到 90° 所用的时间更短。[58]

总结

肩肘手术的麻醉和镇痛有多种途径。麻醉医师和术者之间的持续沟通是提供良好术中、术后护理的基础。使用局部麻醉药（以 PNB 的形式）、非阿片类镇痛药的多模式镇痛方案效果理想，可以减小阿片类药物的用量。多模式镇痛使患者获得更佳的镇痛效果、更少的阿片类药物相关的不良反应及更好的最终满意度。这些优点可以帮助患者获得最好的功能结果和临床结果。

参考文献

［1］ Richman JM, Liu SS, Courpas G, et al:Does continuous peripheral nerve block provide superior pain control to opioids? A meta-analysis. *Anesth Analg* 2006;102(1):248-257.

［2］ Pogatzki-Zahn EM, Zahn PK:From preemptive to preventive analgesia. *Curr Opin Anaesthesiol* 2006;19(5):551-555.

［3］ Urmey WF, Talts KH, Sharrock NE:One hundred percent incidence of hemidiaphragmatic paresis associated with interscalene brachial plexus anesthesia as diagnosed by ultrasonography. *Anesth Analg* 1991;72(4):498-503.

［4］ Knoblanche GE:The incidence and aetiology of phrenic nerve blockade associated with supraclavicular brachial plexus block. *Anaesth Intensive Care* 1979;7(4):346-349.

［5］ Dhuner KG, Moberg E, Onne L:Paresis of the phrenic nerve during brachial plexus block analgesia and its importance. *Acta Chir Scand* 1955;109(1):53-57.

［6］ Urmey WF, McDonald M:Hemidiaphragmatic paresis during interscalene brachial plexus block:Effects on pulmonary function and chest wall mechanics. *Anesth Analg* 1992;74(3):352-357.

［7］ Fredrickson MJ, Krishnan S, Chen CY:Postoperative analgesia for shoulder surgery:A critical appraisal and review of current techniques. *Anaesthesia* 2010;65(6):608-624.
This review critically assesses the evidence relating

to the efficacy of different local anesthetic-based techniques for postoperative analgesia following shoulder surgery.

［8］Peruto CM, Ciccotti MG, Cohen SB:Shoulder arthroscopy positioning:Lateral decubitus versus beach chair. *Arthroscopy* 2009;25(8):891-896.

The authors review the advantages and the disadvantages of the lateral decubitus and beach chair positions, including setup, surgical visualization, access, and patient risk.

［9］Aviado DM, Guevara Aviado D:The Bezold-Jarisch reflex:A historical perspective of cardiopulmonary reflexes. *Ann N Y Acad Sci* 2001;940:48-58.

［10］Campagna JA, Carter C:Clinical relevance of the Bezold-Jarisch reflex. *Anesthesiology* 2003;98(5):1250-1260.

［11］D'Alessio JG, Weller RS, Rosenblum M:Activation of the Bezold-Jarisch reflex in the sitting position for shoulder arthroscopy using interscalene block. *Anesth Analg* 1995;80(6):1158-1162.

［12］Liguori GA, Kahn RL, Gordon J, Gordon MA, Urban MK:The use of metoprolol and glycopyrrolate to prevent hypotensive/bradycardic events during shoulder arthroscopy in the sitting position under interscalene block. *Anesth Analg* 1998;87(6):1320-1325.

［13］Bhatti MT, Enneking FK:Visual loss and ophthalmoplegia after shoulder surgery. *Anesth Analg* 2003;96(3):899-902.

［14］Pohl A, Cullen DJ:Cerebral ischemia during shoulder surgery in the upright position:A case series. *J Clin Anesth* 2005;17(6):463-469.

［15］Rains DD, Rooke GA, Wahl CJ:Pathomechanisms and complications related to patient positioning and anesthesia during shoulder arthroscopy. *Arthroscopy* 2011;27(4):532-541.

The authors comprehensively review case reports and studies looking at complications related to patient positioning (lateral decubitus versus beach chair) for shoulder surgery and the possible pathophysiologic mechanisms associated with them.

［16］Boardman ND III, Cofield RH:Neurologic complications of shoulder surgery. *Clin Orthop Relat Res* 1999; 368:44-53.

［17］Wirth MA, Rockwood CA Jr:Complications of shoulder arthroplasty. *Clin Orthop Relat Res* 1994;307:47-69.

［18］Wirth MA, Rockwood CA Jr:Complications of total

shoulder-replacement arthroplasty. *J Bone Joint Surg Am* 1996;78(4):603-616.

［19］Zanotti RM, Carpenter JE, Blasier RB, Greenfield ML, Adler RS, Bromberg MB:The low incidence of suprascapular nerve injury after primary repair of massive rotator cuff tears. *J Shoulder Elbow Surg* 1997;6(3):258-264.

［20］Brull R, McCartney CJ, Chan VW, El-Beheiry H:Neurological complications after regional anesthesia:Contemporary estimates of risk. *Anesth Analg* 2007;104(4):965-974.

The authors report an estimate for risk of neurologic complications associated with regional anesthetic techniques by retrospectively reviewing 32 studies over a 10-year period.

［21］Perkins FM, Kehlet H:Chronic pain as an outcome of surgery:A review of predictive factors. *Anesthesiology* 2000;93(4):1123-1133.

［22］Wu CL, Fleisher LA:Outcomes research in regional anesthesia and analgesia. *Anesth Analg* 2000;91(5):1232-1242.

［23］Wu CL, Rowlingson AJ, Partin AW, et al:Correlation of postoperative pain to quality of recovery in the immediate postoperative period. *Reg Anesth Pain Med* 2005;30(6):516-522.

［24］Kissin I:Preemptive analgesia. *Anesthesiology* 2000;93(4):1138-1143.

［25］Woolf CJ, Chong MS:Preemptive analgesia—treating postoperative pain by preventing the establishment of central sensitization. *Anesth Analg* 1993;77(2):362-379.

［26］Kissin I:Preemptive analgesia:Why its effect is not always obvious. *Anesthesiology* 1996;84(5):1015-1019.

［27］Pogatzki-Zahn EM, Zahn PK:From preemptive to preventive analgesia. *Curr Opin Anaesthesiol* 2006;19(5):551-555.

［28］Buvanendran A, Kroin JS:Multimodal analgesia for controlling acute postoperative pain. *Curr Opin Anaesthesiol* 2009;22(5):588-593.

The authors review and evaluate recent studies that explore new and improved methods of multimodal anesthesia for relieving moderate to severe postoperative pain.

［29］Elvir-Lazo OL, White PF:The role of multimodal analgesia in pain management after ambulatory surgery. *Curr Opin Anaesthesiol* 2010;23(6):697-703.

This review article discusses the role of multimodal analgesia in the ambulatory setting and, more specifically, the role and use of nonopioid analgesic agents.

[30] Rathmell JP, Wu CL, Sinatra RS, et al:Acute postsurgical pain management:A critical appraisal of current practice, December 2-4, 2005. *Reg Anesth Pain Med* 2006;31(4, suppl 1):1-42.

[31] Macintyre PE:Safety and efficacy of patient-controlled analgesia. *Br J Anaesth* 2001;87(1):36-46.

[32] Smythe MA, MB Zak, O'Donnell MP, Schad RF, Dmuchowski CF:Patient-controlled analgesia versus patient-controlled analgesia plus continuous infusion after hip replacement surgery. *Ann Pharmacother* 1996;30(3):224-227.

[33] Etches RC:Patient-controlled analgesia. *Surg Clin North Am* 1999;79(2):297-312.

[34] *Acute Pain Management:Operative or Medical Procedures and Trauma*. (Clinical Practice Guideline). Publication No. AHCPR 92-0032. Rockville, MD:Agency for Health Care Policy and Research, Public Health Service, U.S. Department of Health and Human Services, February 1992.

[35] Halfpenny DM, Callado LF, Hopwood SE, Bamigbade TA, Langford RM, Stamford JA:Effects of tramadol stereoisomers on norepinephrine efflux and uptake in the rat locus coeruleus measured by real time voltammetry. *Br J Anaesth* 1999;83(6):909-915.

[36] Bamigbade TA, Davidson C, Langford RM, Stamford JA:Actions of tramadol, its enantiomers and principal metabolite, O-desmethyltramadol, on serotonin (5- HT) efflux and uptake in the rat dorsal raphe nucleus. *Br J Anaesth* 1997;79(3):352-356.

[37] Scott LJ, Perry CM:Tramadol:A review of its use in perioperative pain. *Drugs* 2000;60(1):139-176.

[38] Edwards JE, McQuay HJ, Moore RA:Combination analgesic efficacy:Individual patient data metaanalysis of single-dose oral tramadol plus acetaminophen in acute postoperative pain. *J Pain Symptom Manage* 2002;23(2):121-130.

[39] Ding Y, White PF:Comparative effects of ketorolac, dezocine, and fentanyl as adjuvants during outpatient anesthesia. *Anesth Analg* 1992;75(4):566-571.

[40] McLoughlin C, McKinney MS, Fee JP, Boules Z:Diclofenac for day-care arthroscopy surgery:Comparison with a standard opioid therapy. *Br J Anaesth* 1990;65(5):620-623.

[41] Møiniche S, Kehlet H, Dahl JB:A qualitative and quantitative systematic review of preemptive analgesia for postoperative pain relief:The role of timing of analgesia. *Anesthesiology* 2002;96(3):725-741.

[42] Harder AT, An YH:The mechanisms of the inhibitory effects of nonsteroidal anti-inflammatory drugs on bone healing:A concise review. *J Clin Pharmacol* 2003;43(8):807-815.

[43] Duggan ST, Scott LJ:Intravenous paracetamol (acetaminophen). *Drugs* 2009;69(1):101-113.
This article discusses the analgesic efficacy of acetaminophen when given in single or multiple doses compared with that of placebo.

[44] Sinatra RS, Jahr JS, Reynolds LW, Viscusi ER, Groudine SB, Payen-Champenois C:Efficacy and safety of single and repeated administration of 1 gram intravenous acetaminophen injection (paracetamol) for pain management after major orthopedic surgery. *Anesthesiology* 2005;102(4):822-831.

[45] Sinatra RS, Jahr JS, Reynolds L, et al:Intravenous acetaminophen for pain after major orthopedic surgery:An expanded analysis. *Pain Pract* 2012;12(5):357-365.
This article reexamines the analgesic efficacy of intravenous acetaminophen since its approval by the FDA showing a statistically significant difference compared with that of placebo.

[46] Ong CK, Seymour RA, Lirk P, Merry AF:Combining paracetamol (acetaminophen) with nonsteroidal antiinflammatory drugs:A qualitative systematic review of analgesic efficacy for acute postoperative pain. *Anesth Analg* 2010;110(4):1170-1179.
This systematic review looks at the efficacy of combining paracetamol with NSAIDs and comparing the analgesic efficacy of the combination of each alone. The review suggests that a combination of paracetamol and an NSAID may offer superior analgesia compared with either drug alone.

[47] Sutters KA, Miaskowski C, Holdridge-Zeuner D, et al:A randomized clinical trial of the efficacy of scheduled dosing of acetaminophen and hydrocodone for the management of postoperative pain in children after tonsillectomy. *Clin J Pain* 2010;26(2):95-103.
This study shows the increased analgesic efficacy of around-the-clock dosing of acetaminophen compared with as-needed dosing in children after tonsillectomy.

［48］Remy C, Marret E, Bonnet F:Effects of acetaminophen on morphine side-effects and consumption after major surgery:Meta-analysis of randomized controlled trials. *Br J Anaesth* 2005;94(4):505-513.

［49］Maund E, McDaid C, Rice S, Wright K, Jenkins B, Woolacott N:Paracetamol and selective and non-selective non-steroidal anti-inflammatory drugs for the reduction in morphine-related side-effects after major surgery:A systematic review. *Br J Anaesth* 2011;106(3):292-297.

This systematic review shows that the addition of paracetamol or other NSAIDs decreases opioid consumption after major surgery. There was not a significant difference between the different classes of these analgesic adjuncts in doing so.

［50］Dirks J, Fredensborg BB, Christensen D, Fomsgaard JS, Flyger H, Dahl JB:A randomized study of the effects of single-dose gabapentin versus placebo on postoperative pain and morphine consumption after mastectomy. *Anesthesiology* 2002;97(3):560-564.

［51］Dierking G, Duedahl TH, Rasmussen ML, et al:Effects of gabapentin on postoperative morphine consumption and pain after abdominal hysterectomy:A randomized, double-blind trial. *Acta Anaesthesiol Scand* 2004;48(3):322-327.

［52］Rorarius MG, Mennander S, Suominen P, et al:Gabapentin for the prevention of postoperative pain after vaginal hysterectomy. *Pain* 2004;110(1-2):175-181.

［53］Dahl JB, Mathiesen O, Møiniche S:"Protective premedication":An option with gabapentin and related drugs? A review of gabapentin and pregabalin in in the treatment of postoperative pain. *Acta Anaesthesiol Scand* 2004;48(9):1130-1136.

［54］Hill CM, Balkenohl M, Thomas DW, Walker R, Mathé H, Murray G:Pregabalin in patients with postoperative dental pain. *Eur J Pain* 2001;5(2):119-124.

［55］Agarwal A, Gautam S, Gupta D, Agarwal S, Singh PK, Singh U:Evaluation of a single preoperative dose of pregabalin for attenuation of postoperative pain after laparoscopic cholecystectomy. *Br J Anaesth* 2008;101(5):700-704.

This study shows that a single preoperative dose of pregabalin decreases both static and dynamic pain as well as opioid consumption after laparascopic surgery.

［56］Schmid RL, Sandler AN, Katz J:Use and efficacy of low-dose ketamine in the management of acute postoperative pain:A review of current techniques and outcomes. *Pain* 1999;82(2):111-125.

［57］Subramaniam K, Subramaniam B, Steinbrook RA:Ketamine as adjuvant analgesic to opioids:A quantitative and qualitative systematic review. *Anesth Analg* 2004;99(2):482-495.

［58］Aveline C, Gautier JF, Vautier P, et al:Postoperative analgesia and early rehabilitation after total knee replacement:A comparison of continuous low-dose intravenous ketamine versus nefopam. *Eur J Pain* 2009;13(6):613-619.

This study shows that ketamine produces opioid sparing, decreases pain intensity, and improves mobilization after total knee replacement to a greater degree than that of nefopam.

第五十三章　肩关节和肘关节的高级影像学检查

John A. Carrino, MD, MPH; Rashmi S. Thakkar, MD

引言

肩关节和肘关节的各种异常情况都会造成疼痛或功能异常。因此，过去几年中，这些复杂关节成像的需求与日俱增。标准 X 线检查是所有影像学检查的基础。因为 X 线检查价格低廉，容易获得，还可以发现骨折、钙化性肌腱炎、中重度退变性疾病和某些肿瘤性疾病，所以 X 线检查是首选检查方式。然而，如果想得到更详细的诊断，尤其是关于软组织的，就需要进行高级的影像学检查。

本章节主要讨论肩关节和肘关节的高级影像学检查，包括 MRI、MRA，CT、计算机断层扫描关节造影（CTA，以及各种肩关节和肘关节疾病）。

MRI 和 MRA

在过去几年内，3.0 T 肌肉骨骼 MRI 已经从研究阶段进入了常规临床应用阶段。与低磁场 MRI

Dr. Carrino or an immediate family member serves as a paid consultant to or is an employee of Quality Medical Metrics, Medtronic, General Electric Healthcare, Vital Images, and Siemens Medical Systems; serves as an unpaid consultant to General Electronic Healthcare, Carestream Health, and Siemens Medical Systems; has stock or stock options held in Merge; and has received research or institutional support from Siemens Medical Systems, Carestream Health, and Toshiba Medical. Neither Dr. Thakkar nor any immediate family member has received anything of value from or has stock or stock options held in a commercial company or institution related directly or indirectly to the subject of this chapter.

相比，高磁场 MRI 最重要的优势是更高的信号噪声比（SNR），这使其在相同的扫描时间内可以得到空间分辨率更高的图像。[1] SNR 的增高使肌肉骨骼和神经结构的图像分辨率更高且扫描速度更快。最大的对比噪声比（CNRs）依赖于磁场强度。研究显示，与 1.5T MRI 的图像相比，3.0 TMRI 的图像的肌肉和骨、骨和软骨、软骨和液体间的 CNRs 更高。更高的图像质量的优势引起了人们对更高的诊断精度的期待。分辨率的提高有益于观察肘关节等小关节及肩肘关节的纤维软骨解剖和病理。

大多数医疗机构使用的肌肉骨 MRI 包括多平面的二维快速 / 涡轮自旋回波序列。这些序列具有良好的 SNR、高组织对比度和高平面内分辨率。然而，它们的切片相对较厚，切片之间的间隙较小，这可能因部分体积平均（partial volume averaging）而掩盖病变。而三维序列可以获得通过关节的连续的薄切片，这样就降低了部分体积平均。[2] 此外，三维序列也可以用来创建多平面重建图像。这样，仅进行一次检查就能从所有方向对关节进行评估。

肩关节

MRI 是许多疾病的首选影像学检查，主要原因是它可以自由选择成像平面，而且有极好的软组织对比分辨率。MRI 为许多病变提供了最详细的诊断，包括肩袖、关节囊盂唇结构、肌腱、肌肉的异常，隐匿性骨折，关节面异常，以及肩关节不稳定性疾病。MRI 可以帮助检查与肩部卡压相关的骨和软组织异常。MRI 可以发现冈上肌腱、肩峰下滑囊和肱二头肌腱的病变，以及肩峰、肩锁关节、喙肩韧带的形态异常。

在非增强 MRI 上，正常情况下肩袖、盂唇、关节囊和皮质骨在所有脉冲序列上均为黑色。由于这些结构在位置上相互毗邻，所以很难把它们区别开。关节积液或关节内钆造影剂有助于分离这些结构和改善组织对比度，勾勒出不同物质的结构，这些物质本质上有不同的信号特征。[3]

最近，有一项研究探讨了在相同患者群体中肩部 3.0 T 常规 MRI 与 MRA 诊断的敏感性。[4] 常规 MRI 与关节镜检查相比，敏感性和特异性分别为：前盂唇撕裂 83%，100%；后盂唇撕裂 84%，100%；SLAP 损伤 83%，99%；冈上肌腱撕裂 92%，100%；冈上肌腱关节面部分撕裂 68%，100%；冈上肌腱滑膜面部分撕裂 84%，100%。MRA 与关节镜检查相比，敏感性和特异性分别为：前盂唇撕裂 98%，100%；后盂唇撕裂 95%，100%；SLAP 损伤 98%，99%；冈上肌腱撕裂 100%，100%；冈上肌腱关节面部分撕裂 97%，100%；冈上肌腱滑膜面部分撕裂 84%，100%。3.0 T MRA 对下列疾病诊断的敏感性优于 3.0 T 常规 MRI（$P < 0.05$）：冈上肌腱关节面部分撕裂、前盂唇撕裂、SLAP 损伤。

在肩关节，二维快速自旋回波序列是非增强 MRI 的首选序列。然而，许多机构已经尝试过三维序列，如梯度回波稳态自由旋进（gradient echo steady-state free precession）。近年来，三维各向同性分辨率快速自旋回波序列已被用于肩关节的非增强 MRI，并减少了检查所需的时间。此外，三维 T1 加权各向同性分辨率序列已被用于 MRA，这使肩关节的检查快速而全面。

肩袖

肩袖成像通常选用轴位、矢状斜位和冠状斜位。矢状斜位和冠状斜位与冈上肌腱有关，而与解剖轴无关。常规肩关节 MRI 采用组合序列。一般来说，短回波时间序列（T1 和质子密度加权）描述解剖细节和帮助量化脂肪萎缩，而液敏序列（质子密度压脂、T2 压脂像）对水信号异常增加最敏感，大多数肌腱病变都有水信号异常增加。常规 MRI 可准确识别肩袖肌腱全层撕裂，具有较高的敏感性和特异性。信号强度从肌腱下表面到肌腱上表面均增加是全层肩袖肌腱撕裂的准确征象。肩袖撕裂相关的形态学改变包括肌腱回缩、肌肉萎缩和脂肪浸润，这些也是重要的预后因素（图 53-1）。这类信息有利于治疗决策的制订，例如，采用非手术治疗还是手术修复、决定手术修复的类型（开放或关节镜，肌腱重建或肌腱转位），也有利于对预后的判断。

如果对全层和部分撕裂的鉴别有疑问，那么建议进行 MRA 检查。[5] 异常信号强度沿肌腱下表面延伸的征象尤其重要。特定角度的图像可以帮助检测这些部分撕裂。首先，外展和外旋位可以将肌腱从肱骨头上提起，减小关节面纤维的压迫，这可以使肌腱关节面部分撕裂显示得更清晰，而且这种体位可以使前方稳定结构紧张。其次，

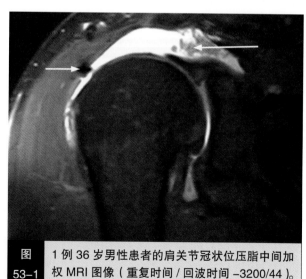

图 53-1　1 例 36 岁男性患者的肩关节冠状位压脂中间加权 MRI 图像（重复时间 / 回波时间 –3200/44）。该患者 1 年前接受过肩袖修复手术，受伤后再次出现疼痛。图像显示复发性冈上肌全层、全宽断裂，肌腱纤维回缩至盂肱关节（长箭头），存在疑似既往手术遗留下来的人工材料（短箭头）

肱骨外旋可以使冠状斜位与肌腱走行一致，这减小了与肌腱走行相关的部分体积平均。

一项 2009 年发表的荟萃分析对比了 MRI、MRA 和超声诊断肩袖撕裂的准确度。[6]65 篇文章满足纳入标准。在全层和部分肩袖撕裂的诊断中，MRA 比 MRI 和超声检查更敏感、更特异（$P < 0.05$）。在全层和部分肩袖撕裂的诊断中，MRI 和超声检查的敏感性和特异性无显著差异（$P > 0.05$）。总结所有肩袖撕裂的 MRA、MRI 和超声的受试者操作特征（ROC）曲线，发现 ROC 曲线下面积 MRA 最大（0.935）、超声其次（0.889）、MRI 最小（0.878）；然而，单独对比 MRI 和超声检查时，其 ROC 曲线无显著差异（$P > 0.05$）。

关节囊盂唇病变

进行直接 MRA 时，关节内注射稀释钆溶液可以扩张关节腔。直接 MRA 可以帮助描绘盂唇和关节囊结构，辅助诊断、制订治疗计划和随访（图 53-2）。

如果怀疑前盂唇撕裂、SLAP 损伤及部分冈上肌撕裂，那么给患者进行 3.0 T MRA 检查。MRA 可以帮助精确地识别和描述盂肱韧带、关节囊和盂唇的完整性，还有助于疾病分期。[7]MRA 发现盂唇撕脱、盂唇退变、盂唇下部和下盂肱韧带病变的敏感性和特异性都不错。

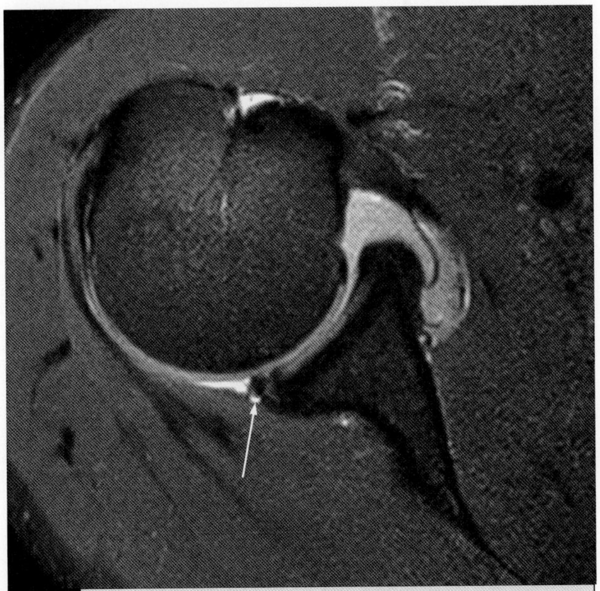

冠状斜位最适合显示上盂唇的 SLAP 损伤。盂唇和肩胛盂上部之间有液体或造影剂是诊断 SLAP 损伤的征象。支持真实 SLAP 损伤诊断的辅助征象包括异常信号强度向外扩展至盂唇实质、盂唇边缘不规则及信号扩展至肱二头肌腱近端。鉴别真实 SLAP 损伤与正常变异（如盂唇下孔）的方法：在正常变异中，盂唇下隐窝比 SLAP 损伤更靠内侧，位于肱二头肌腱和肩胛盂关节软骨之间。与此相反，SLAP 损伤常常延伸至肱二头肌腱后方，比盂唇下隐窝更靠外侧。SLAP 损伤在冠状斜位表现为向外突出的弧形高信号强度，在轴位上表现为前后延伸。

轴位最适合显示盂唇的前部和后部。盂唇撕裂的 MRI 表现包括盂唇内异常信号或盂唇和肩胛盂之间异常信号。前方关节囊的撕脱很难评估，因为正常关节囊沿前方肩胛盂附着的位置变异性极大。

肩关节的软骨

理想的软骨评估是有挑战性的，尤其是肩关节的软骨。改善二维序列的空间分辨率，通过扫描不同平面或改变上肢体位来更好地看清弧形肱骨头的不同区域，都有助于评估软骨。某些序列可以改善组织对比度，如中间加权质子密度序列，这是专为软骨成像设计的。

肘关节

拍摄肘关节 MRI 的患者可以取仰卧位双臂置于身体两侧，或者俯卧位双臂伸直举过头顶。俯卧位通常更好，因为肘关节靠近等中心点，信号均匀、压脂一致，但有时候患者难以耐受俯卧位。

肘关节 MRI 方案包括快速自旋回波 T1 加权或质子密度序列，使用快速自旋回波 T2 加权序列或短 T1 反向恢复序列的液敏序列。诊断肘关节外侧和内侧间室的病变需要轴位和冠状位图像，而诊断

图 53-2　1 例 40 岁肩部疼痛的男性患者的肩关节 MRI 图像。本例为直接 MRA 压脂轴位 T1 加权成像（重复时间／回波时间 –850/18），图像显示后方盂唇撕裂伴小的盂唇旁囊肿（箭头）

前方、后方间室的病变需要轴位和矢状位图像。[8]

肘关节三维序列既可以得到比二维序列更薄的切片，又可以从冠状位更好地看清侧副韧带。此外，三维序列也可以获得多平面重建图像，可以从任何方向评估侧副韧带。这对于评估外侧尺骨副韧带尤其重要，在向后斜 20° 的冠状位图像上可以看到外侧尺骨副韧带全长。最新发展的三维各向同性分辨率快速自旋回波序列不仅有最理想的组织对比度，还可以获得肘关节的连续薄层切片，这使得侧副韧带撕裂更容易被发现。这些序列的中间加权组织对比和多平面重建能力也有利于评估肘关节的肌腱、肌肉及骨性结构，尤其在联合压脂改善液体敏感的时候。

骨软骨损伤

肘关节的 Panner 病（骨软骨病）是一类疾病，MRI 可以很好地评估这类疾病。Panner 病病因不明，可能源于重复外翻应力导致的压缩和剪切力，这使投掷运动员（通常是青少年运动员）局部血管损伤。在 X 线片上，骨骺显示出斑驳和碎裂。在 MRI 上，Panner 病表现为 T1 加权序列上的斑片状高信号强度。游离体不是 Panner 病的突出特征。

肱骨小头剥脱性骨软骨炎一般发生于青少年运动员（12~16 岁），在棒球和体操运动员中更常见。他们受到慢性的外侧压缩力，局部反复发生微创伤，这导致病变累及软骨和软骨下骨。起初，X 线片表现正常，但 MRI 可以更早发现异常。关节内注入造影剂的 MRA 尤其适用于定位缺损和描述骨折块不稳定。下列征象表明骨折块不稳定：骨折块周围 T2 高信号强度、骨折块深部囊性变、骨折块内部 T2 高信号强度水肿。CT 上也可以发现骨性缺损（图 53-3）。

侧副韧带损伤的 MRI

尺侧副韧带在尺骨上的附着点撕脱是投掷运动员慢性肘关节内侧疼痛的原因之一，最好同时用 X 线检查和 MRI 进行评估。[9]MRI 显示韧带信号强度增加，如果韧带完全撕裂，则显示信号连

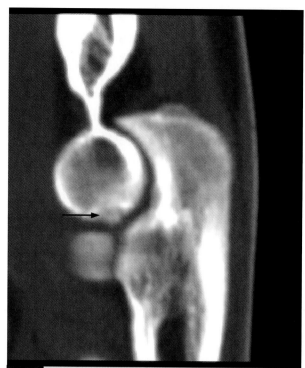

图 53-3　1 例肘关节疼痛的男性患者的肘关节矢状位 CT 图像显示肱骨小头的小块骨软骨缺损（箭头）

续性中断（图 53-4）。此外，MRI 也可以看到相关损伤，如外侧间室骨挫伤和（或）伸肌总腱损伤。慢性损伤时可以看到韧带增厚或变薄，可能伴随异常内在信号强度及钙化或骨化。MRA 在鉴别尺侧副韧带的部分或全部撕裂方面表现卓越。诊断尺侧副韧带部分撕裂的 MRA 征象是 "T" 字征，即造影剂、生理盐水或关节液沿着冠突内侧缘线性延伸，穿过撕裂的尺侧副韧带深层，但是被完整的关节囊限制。MRA 也可以帮助识别肘关节的软骨异常（图 53-5）。

桡侧副韧带复合体包括桡侧固有副韧带、环状韧带、外侧尺骨副韧带和侧副韧带。桡侧副韧带复合体损伤比尺侧副韧带损伤少。如果桡侧副韧带复合体扭伤或部分撕裂，MRI 显示高信号强度，表现为完整的韧带周围水肿和出血。韧带撕裂可能表现为韧带纤维不连续。

肌肉和肌腱损伤的 MRI

正常肌腱在所有脉冲序列上均表现为均匀的

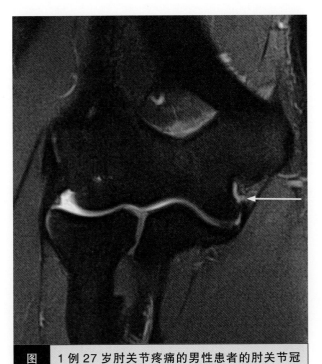

图 53-4　1 例 27 岁肘关节疼痛的男性患者的肘关节冠状位压脂质子密度 MRI（重复时间 / 回波时间 –2210/52）显示尺侧副韧带在肱骨附着点部分撕裂（箭头）

低信号强度。病变肌腱通常表现为增厚和 T1、T2 中等信号强度。急性创伤事件和慢性进展性肌腱病变均可造成肌腱部分或全部撕裂。部分撕裂表现为肌腱变细，周围 T2 高强度液体信号。完全撕裂表现为撕裂的肌腱被 T2 高强度液体信号分隔。

肱骨外上髁炎是一种过度使用综合征，受累肌腱发生病变。最初受累的肌腱是伸肌腱，桡侧腕短伸肌腱第一个受累。指总伸肌前缘在 50% 的情况下受累，受累概率仅次于它的包括桡侧腕长伸肌和尺侧腕伸肌。随着损伤程度增加，深层的侧副韧带也可能受累，尤其要注意外侧尺骨副韧带。

肘关节内侧最常见的疾病是肱骨内上髁炎（也被称为内侧网球肘、肱骨内上髁炎及投手肘）。受累肌腱起自旋前圆肌、桡侧腕屈肌和（或）掌长肌。尺侧腕屈肌和指浅屈肌可能出现继发性受累。

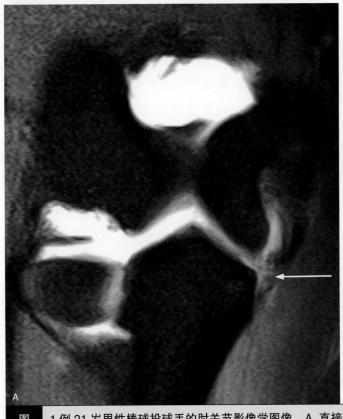
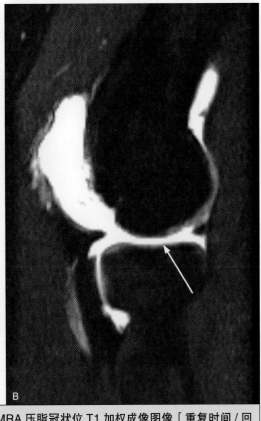

图 53-5　1 例 21 岁男性棒球投球手的肘关节影像学图像。A. 直接 MRA 压脂冠状位 T1 加权成像图像 [重复时间 / 回波时间（TR/TE）–800/21] 显示尺侧副韧带前束全层从尺骨附着处撕裂（箭头）。B. 压脂矢状位图像（TR/TE–1020/60）显示肱桡关节高度软骨缺损

随着损伤程度增加，深层的内侧副韧带前束也可能受累。

对于骨骼不成熟的运动员，如果出现肘关节内侧疼痛，MRI 是重要的检查方法。内上髁骺板的强度比内侧副韧带前束差，再加上肘关节外翻应力下屈肌总腱起点产生的张力，使骺板损伤，这就是小球员肘（little leaguer's elbow）。MRI 表现为骺板形态不规则，伴骺板增宽和周围骨水肿（图 53-6）。

在肘关节前方，肱二头肌腱远端断裂罕见，占肱二头肌腱损伤的 5% 以下。部分撕裂可以表现为肌腱异常增厚或变细，肌腱内部 T2 信号增加，伴随桡骨结节内骨水肿和肱桡滑囊内液体聚集。完全撕裂伴断端回缩表现为撕裂的肌腱松弛，断端被 T2 高信号液体分隔。如果评估肱二头肌腱在桡骨结节的止点比较困难，那么可以屈肘、外展肩关节、旋后前臂。这样，从肱骨延伸到前臂的矢状位图像可以显示包括止点在内的肱二头肌腱远端的纵向全长。单发肱肌撕裂极其罕见。肱

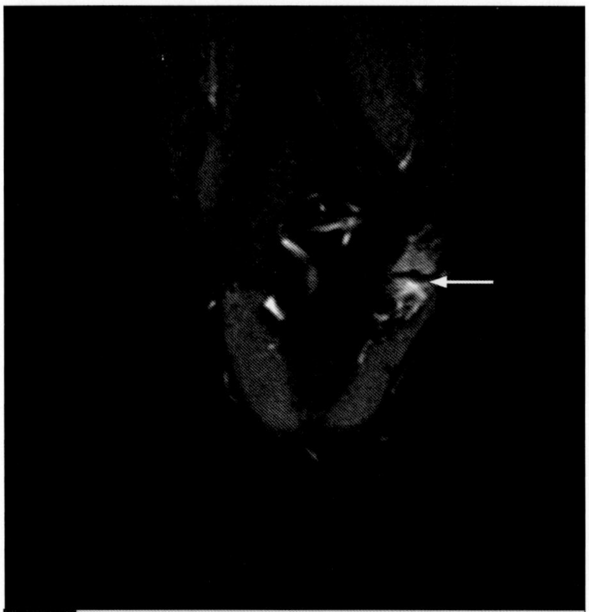

图 53-6　1 例肘关节内侧疼痛的男性患儿的肘关节 MRI 图像。冠状位压脂质子密度图像（重复时间 / 回波时间 –2210/52）显示骺板形态不规则，伴骺板增宽和周围骨水肿，提示小球员肘

肌腱扭伤或撕裂可发生于攀岩运动员，被称为登山肘（climber's elbow）。

肘关节后方最常见的疾病是肱骨后上髁炎（posterior epicondylitis），这是一种过度使用综合征，表现为肱三头肌腱病变及部分撕裂。

神经卡压的 MRI

肘关节的 3 个主要神经是尺神经、桡神经及正中神经，最常发生尺神经在肘管处的卡压。尺神经压迫是肘关节周围最常见的外周神经病变，常见于投掷运动员。MRI 可以帮助评估神经的完整性和所支配肌肉群的形态和信号强度。轴位 T1 加权成像显示尺神经的粗细和形状，而 T2 加权成像可以显示被卡压神经信号强度增高。如果出现卡压综合征，在急性期，所支配的肌肉群在压脂 T2 加权成像上信号强度异常增高。在慢性期，所支配肌肉群萎缩、体积缩小、脂肪浸润，这些变化在 T1 加权成像上最方便观察。

CT 和 CTA

CT 可以描述骨结构细节，联合关节造影可以诊断关节内病变、关节囊盂唇病变、肌腱病变和韧带损伤。现代多层 CT 扫描仪有极好的空间分辨率和对比分辨率。可以重建任何平面的影像，这有助于显示复杂的关节解剖。还可以用原始数据重建三维影像，有助于制订手术计划。

CT 的优势：比 MRI 更适于评估软组织钙化、骨化性肌炎和关节内游离体。软骨下骨受累时，骨关节炎显而易见。CT 的劣势：放射剂量。在患者需要多次检查，或者孕妇需要 CT 检查时，需要考虑放射剂量。CT 显示软组织特征的能力较差，很难发现细微的软组织损伤。骨或关节周围软组织内的金属物会造成明显的 X 线硬化伪影，这些伪影限制了周围骨和软组织的评估。

关节 CTA 需要分 2 步：关节内注射造影剂及获得 CT 图像。亚毫米各向同性多探测器计算机断层扫描（MDCT）技术的引入大大提高了 CTA

的空间分辨率和多平面重建能力，显著提高了关节CTA的诊断能力。MDCT关节造影一般用于肩关节无法进行MRI或MRI失败时，[10]具体包括关节附近有金属物（肩部术后），患者存在幽闭恐惧、肥胖等一般情况。

CTA有多个优势，包括各向同性亚毫米空间分辨率，这改善了纵向分辨率。扫描时间大大降低使运动伪影减少，也使CTA可以用于创伤和儿科患者。CTA的劣势包括有创性和射线暴露，骨髓水肿和软组织的对比分辨率较差。

有一项研究评估了肩关节MDCT关节造影的诊断精确度和指征，患者都有MRI绝对或相对禁忌证（有关节周围金属内置物），金标准是关节镜检查[11]。在42例非手术治疗的患者中，对比MDCT关节造影和关节镜检查后发现，MDCT关节造影的敏感性和特异性都在87%~100%。在28例手术治疗的患者中，MDCT关节造影的诊断敏感性为94%，而MRI仅为25%。在MDCT和MRI中，各种损伤评估的观察者间一致性近乎完美（Kappa=0.95）。用McNemar测试对比MDCT关节造影和MRI对于术后患者的评估，发现二者有显著差异（$P < 0.05$）。

肩关节

非增强CT对关节内软组织的成像不够清晰，因此使用肩关节CTA以增加关节内软组织图像的对比分辨率。适应证包括肩袖的评估、关节囊盂唇韧带复合体的评估及关节软骨的评估，尤其适用于术后有金属人造物妨碍MRI检查的患者（图53-7）。[12]

肘关节

CT被广泛用于评估肘关节周围的骨折，并显示关节内骨折和关节内小骨块。静脉含碘造影剂可以用来检查任何关节周围的血管损伤。关节内注射含碘造影剂的CTA是极好的检查关节软骨的方法。如果软骨面完整，则关节造影无法发现内部结构变化。CTA一般用于有MRI禁忌证的患者。

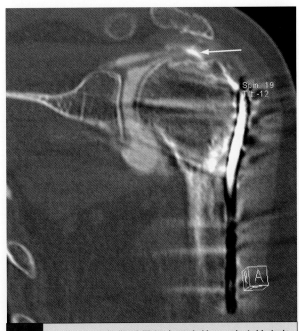

图 53-7　1例2005年做过骨折内固定的60岁女性患者的左肩关节CTA图像。患者诉上举疼痛。冠状位图像显示冈上肌下表面中度撕裂，有一个钉孔穿透了骨质全层（箭头）。图中还可以看到外侧钢板和螺钉固定的肱骨头和肱骨颈，左侧肱骨大结节骨折畸形愈合，以及与慢性起止点病相符的大结节骨囊肿和骨代谢改变

超声检查

10 MHz~18 MHz高频线性传感器的出现使肌内骨超声快速发展。与MRI相比，肌内骨超声有多个优势，包括容易获得、扫描快速、动态扫描。[13]超声检查是无创检查，没有电离辐射，操作简单、安全，可双侧对比。然而，超声检查结果非常依赖操作人员的水平，肌内骨超声的训练非常必要，因为这种技术学起来很快。超声检查无法提供肩和肘关节的复杂图像。超声检查的视野是有限的，不容易穿透骨质。超声检查可以用来检查局部的具体状况，但对于骨性异常或骨软骨病变这些深部结构的评估效果较差。

随着全景图像、视频储存、三维超声探头等技术的进步，存档的静态超声图像与MRI图像有的联系更密切了。

肩关节

超声检查可以用来评估肩袖肌腱、肱二头肌

腱，诊断滑囊炎，以及实时引导外科操作。

一项 2011 年的研究以已有临床实验为基础，探究超声诊断部分和全层肩袖撕裂的精确度。[14] 该项研究包含了 62 场研究，6007 例患者，6066 例患肩。超声诊断部分肩袖撕裂（敏感性 0.84，特异性 0.89）和全层肩袖撕裂（敏感性 0.96，特异性 0.93）的敏感性和特异性都不错。

可以使用超声从纵向和横向评估肌腱。肩袖的每根肌腱都有相应最佳的特殊检查体位。在纵向平面上，正常肩袖肌腱表现为平行走向的纤维状高回声结构；在横向平面上，正常肩袖肌腱表现为椭圆形高回声结构。超声检查可以鉴别肩袖的部分和全层撕裂，部分撕裂表现为低回声，全层撕裂表现为无回声。肩袖部分撕裂的征象包括肌腱滑囊侧或关节侧局部无回声或低回声缺损（图 53-8，53-9）。在组织谐波图像上，肌腱内部的撕裂表现为低回声线状。组织谐波图像和三维超声使得部分撕裂显像更清晰。[15]

超声诊断肩袖卡压的征象除了肩袖损伤或滑囊增厚外，还有肩外展动态扫描时发现的滑囊膨胀、滑囊内液体聚集或滑囊褶皱。许多影像科医师做肩袖卡压试验时，在超声引导下向三角肌下滑囊注射长效局部麻醉药（如丁哌卡因），通常还

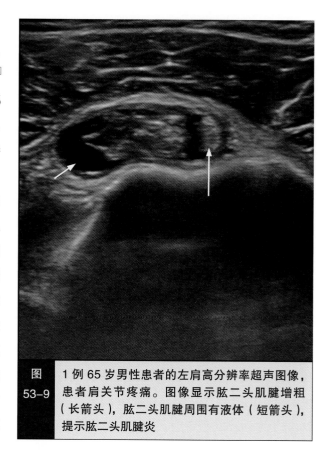

图 53-9　1 例 65 岁男性患者的左肩高分辨率超声图像，患者肩关节疼痛。图像显示肱二头肌腱增粗（长箭头），肱二头肌腱周围有液体（短箭头），提示肱二头肌腱炎

联合注射长效激素（如甲泼尼龙）作为治疗。

肘关节

超声检查常用来评估肘关节周围的软组织疾病，因为超声检查可以得到浅表结构（如韧带、肌腱和神经）的清晰图像。[16] 超声检查也可以用来探查关节积液、韧带或肌腱撕裂、尺神经异常，以及引导各种肘关节周围的介入操作。

有些疾病只有在肢体活动时才能明显表现出异常，如尺神经半脱位和肌疝，可以用动态超声评估这类疾病。超声检查可以发现 X 线或 MRI 不易发现的微小钙化或异物。超声检查可以用来引导一些外科操作，如肌腱内激素注射。多普勒超声的引导可以避免在穿刺中损伤血管。

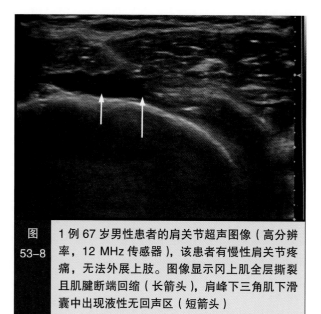

图 53-8　1 例 67 岁男性患者的肩关节超声图像（高分辨率，12 MHz 传感器），该患者有慢性肩关节疼痛，无法外展上肢。图像显示冈上肌全层撕裂且肌腱断端回缩（长箭头），肩峰下三角肌下滑囊中出现液性无回声区（短箭头）

总结

对于肩袖卡压综合征和肩袖撕裂，MRI 和超声检查都可以发现肩袖撕裂。MRA 和 CTA 都是发现盂唇撕裂的有效手段。表 53-1 总结各种影像

表 53-1

各种影像学检查对于肩关节解剖区域评估的适用性

损伤类型	MRI	MRA	CT	CTA	US
盂唇撕裂	++	+++	—	+++	—
肩袖部分撕裂（滑囊侧）	+++	++	—	++	+
肩袖部分撕裂（关节侧）	+++	+++	—	+++	+
肩袖全层撕裂	+++	+++	—	+++	+
软骨缺损	++	+++	—	+++	—
骨髓水肿	+++	+++	+	+	—

注：CTA= 计算机断层扫描关节造影；MRA= 核磁共振关节造影；US= 超声；+= 适用性弱；++= 适用性中；+++= 适用性强；—= 不适用。

学检查对不同肩关节病变评估的适用性。

对于肘关节病变，恰当序列的 MRI 更适合评估隐匿性骨性损伤和软骨异常，也更适合诊断肌腱、韧带和神经内的软组织病变。

参考文献

［1］ Bolog N, Nanz D, Weishaupt D:Muskuloskeletal MR imaging at 3.0 T:Current status and future perspectives. *Eur Radiol* 2006 ;16(6):1298-1307.

［2］ Kijowski R, Gold GE:Routine 3D magnetic resonance imaging of joints. *J Magn Reson Imaging* 2011; 33(4):758-771.

This article describes various three dimensional sequences used in musculoskeltal MRI, along with their clinical application in various joints.

［3］ Osinski T, Malfair D, Steinbach L:Magnetic resonance arthrography. *Orthop Clin North Am* 2006 ;37(3):299-319, vi.

This article describes the technique of performing MRA as well as its advantages and disadvantages over conventional MRI.

［4］ Magee T:3-T MRI of the shoulder:Is MR arthrography necessary? *AJR Am J Roentgenol* 2009 ;192(1):86-92.

The purpose of this study is to report the diagnostic sensitivity of 3-T conventional MRI versus MRA of the shoulder in the same patient population.

［5］ Shahabpour M, Kichouh M, Laridon E, Gielen JL, De Mey J:The effectiveness of diagnostic imaging methods for the assessment of soft tissue and articular disorders of the shoulder and elbow. *Eur J Radiol* 2008; 65(2):194-200.

In this article, a meta-analyisis was performed of the relevant literature, and the role of MRI of the shoulder and elbow discussed, along with a comparison of other diagnostic modalities. Level of evidence:III.

［6］ de Jesus JO, Parker L, Frangos AJ, Nazarian LN:Accuracy of MRI, MR arthrography, and ultrasound in the diagnosis of rotator cuff tears:A meta-analysis. *AJR Am J Roentgenol* 2009 ;192(6):1701-1707.

The authors of this study compared the diagnostic accuracy of MRI, MRA, and ultrasound for the diagnosis of rotator cuff tears through a meta-analysis of literature studies. Sixty-five articles met the inclusion criteria for this meta-analysis.

［7］ Shah N, Tung GA:Imaging signs of posterior glenohumeral instability. *AJR Am J Roentgenol* 2009; 192(3):730-735.

The purpose of this article is to review mechanisms of injury leading to posterior glenohumeral instability and the correlated imaging findings on CT and MRI. In patients with suspected posterior glenohumeral instability, imaging of the affected shoulder can show abnormalities of the bone, the labrum, and the joint capsule. Accurate detection and characterization of these lesions aid in both diagnosis and management.

［8］ Brunton LM, Anderson MW, Pannunzio ME, Khanna AJ, Chhabra AB:Magnetic resonance imaging of the elbow:Update on current techniques and indications. *J Hand Surg Am* 2006 ;31(6):1001-1011.

［9］ Stevens KJ, McNally EG:Magnetic resonance imaging of the elbow in athletes. *Clin Sports Med* 2010; 29(4):521-553.

This article reviews imaging of common disease conditions occurring around the elbow in athletes, with an emphasis on MRI.

［10］ Fritz J, Fishman EK, Small KM, et al:MDCT arthrography of the shoulder with datasets of isotropic resolution:Indications, technique, and applications. *AJR Am J*

Roentgenol 2012 ;198(3):635-646.

The purposes of this review were to summarize the indications MDCT arthrography of the shoulder, highlight the features of MDCT acquisition, and describe the normal and abnormal MDCT arthrographic appearances of the shoulder. MDCT arthrography is a valid alternative for shoulder imaging of patients with contraindications to MRI or after failed MRI. MDCT arthrography is accurate for assessming a variety of shoulder abnormalities and, with further validation, may become the imaging test of choice for evaluating the postoperative shoulder.

[11] De Filippo M, Bertellini A, Sverzellati N, et al:Multidetector computed tomography arthrography of the shoulder:Diagnostic accuracy and indications. *Acta Radiol* 2008 ;49(5):540-549.

In this study, diagnostic accuracy and indications of arthrography and MDCT arthrography of the shoulder with absolute and relative contraindications to MRI of the shoulder in patients with periarticular metal implants were evaluated using diagnostic arthroscopy as the gold standard. The results showed that MDCT arthrography of the shoulder is a safe technique that provides accurate diagnosis in identifying chondral, fibrocartilaginous, and intra-articular ligamentous lesions in patients who cannot be evaluated by MRI and in patients after surgery.

[12] Oh JH, Kim JY, Choi JA, Kim WS:Effectiveness of multidetector CTA for assessing shoulder pathology:Comparison with magnetic resonance imaging with arthroscopic correlation. *J Shoulder Elbow Surg* 2010; 19(1):14-20.

This study evaluated the diagnostic efficacy of CTA in the assessment of various shoulder pathologies with arthroscopic correlation. It was hypothesized that CTA would be cost-effective and comparable with MRA for assessing labral detachments and full- thickness rotator cuff tears. The sensitivity, specificity, and agreement were comparable in each imaging study for Bankart lesions, SLAP lesions, Hill-Sachs lesions, and full-thickness rotator cuff tears, but those of CTA were significantly lower than MRA for partial- thickness cuff tears. The ROC curves for CTA and MRA were not significantly different for any of the pathologies, except partial-thickness cuff tears. Level of evidence:I.

[13] Jacobson JA:Musculoskeletal ultrasound:Focused impact on MRI. *AJR Am J Roentgenol* 2009 ;193(3):619-627.

This article compares image interpretation, accuracy, observer variability, economic effect, and education with regard to musculoskeletal ultrasound and MRI because these factors will influence the growth of musculoskeletal ultrasound and the effect on MRI. The development of less expensive portable ultrasound machines has opened the market to nonradiologists, and applications for musculoskeletal ultrasound have broadened. Selective substitution of musculoskeletal ultrasound for MRI can result in significant cost saving to the healthcare system.

[14] Smith TO, Back T, Toms AP, Hing CB:Diagnostic accuracy of ultrasound for rotator cuff tears in adults:A systematic review and meta-analysis. *Clin Radiol* 2011; 66(11):1036-1048.

This study was performed to determine the diagnostic accuracy of ultrasound to detect partial- and full thickness rotator cuff tears based on all available clinical trials. Sixty-two studies assessing 6,007 patients and 6,066 shoulders were included. Ultrasonography had good sensitivity and specificity for the assessment of partial-thickness (sensitivity, 0.84 ;specificity, 0.89), and full-thickness rotator cuff tears (sensitivity, 0.96; specificity, 0.93). However, the literature poorly described population characteristics and assessor blinding and was based on limited sample sizes.

[15] Parker L, Nazarian LN, Carrino JA, et al:Musculoskeletal imaging:Medicare use, costs, and potential for cost substitution. *J Am Coll Radiol* 2008 ;5(3):182-188.

This study explores the substitution of ultrasound for MRI of musculoskeletal disorders by describing the recent use and costs of musculoskeletal imaging in the Medicare population, projecting these trends from 2006 to 2020, and estimating cost savings involved in substituting musculoskeletal ultrasound for musculoskeletal MRI, when appropriate.

[16] Lee KS, Rosas HG, Craig JG:Musculoskeletal ultrasound:Elbow imaging and procedures. *Semin Musculoskelet Radiol* 2010 ;14(4):449-460.

This article discusses the unique application of ultrasound in evaluating common elbow pathology and in advanced ultrasound-guided treatments.